# Immigrant Medicine

# Immigrant Medicine

**Patricia Frye Walker** MD, DTM&H
Medical Director
Center for International Health and
Travel Medicine Program
HealthPartners Medical Group
Assistant Professor
Department of Internal Medicine
Division of Infectious Disease
and International Medicine
University of Minnesota
St. Paul, MN
USA

**Elizabeth D. Barnett** MD
Maxwell Finland Laboratory
for Infectious Diseases
Boston Medical Center
Boston, MA
USA

**SAUNDERS**

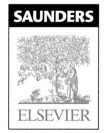

ELSEVIER

**SAUNDERS**
ELSEVIER

An imprint of Elsevier Inc.
© 2007, Elsevier Inc. All rights reserved.

First published 2007

ISBN: 978-0-323-03454-8

**British Library Cataloguing in Publication Data**
A catalogue record for this book is available from the British Library

**Library of Congress Cataloging in Publication Data**
A catalog record for this book is available from the Library of Congress

**Notice**

Medical knowledge is constantly changing. Standard safety precautions must be followed, but as new research and clinical experience broaden our knowledge, changes in treatment and drug therapy may become necessary or appropriate. Readers are advised to check the most current product information provided by the manufacturer of each drug to be administered to verify the recommended dose, the method and duration of administration, and contraindications. It is the responsibility of the practitioner, relying on experience and knowledge of the patient, to determine dosages and the best treatment for each individual patient. Neither the Publisher nor the author assume any liability for any injury and/or damage to persons or property arising from this publication.

**The Publisher**

Printed in China
Last digit is the print number:  9  8  7  6  5  4  3  2  1

Commissioning Editor: *Karen Bowler*
Development Editor Manager: *Nani Clansey*
Project Manager: *Gemma Lawson*
Design Manager: *Stewart Larking*
Illustration Manager: *Gillian Richards*
Illustrator: *Jane Fallows*
Marketing Manager(s) (UK/USA): *Clara Toombs / Kathy Neely*

# Contents

# List of Contributors

**Libby Arcel**
Associate Professor of Clinical Psychology
Institute of Psychology
University of Copenhagen
Copenhagen
Denmark

**Gregory L. Armstrong MD**
Asia/Europe Team Lead
Immigrant, Refugee & Migrant Health Branch
Division of Global Migration & Quarantine
Centers for Disease Control & Prevention
Atlanta, GA
USA

**Marilyn Augustyn MD**
Associate Professor of Pediatrics
Developmental and Behavioural Pediatrician
Department of Pediatrics
Boston University School of Medicine
Boston, MA
USA

**Linda L. Barnes PhD, MA, MTS**
Associate Professor of Family Medicine and
Pediatrics
Boston University School of Medicine
Division of General Pediatrics
Boston, MA
USA

**Elizabeth D. Barnett MD**
Maxwell Finland Laboratory for Infectious Diseases
Boston Medical Center
Boston, MA
USA

**Carol Berg RN MPH**
Community & Public Health Manager
UCare Minnesota
Minneapolis, MN
USA

**John Bernardo MD**
Professor of Medicine
Research Professor of Biochemistry
Department of Pulmonary Medicine
Boston University School of Medicine
Tuberculosis Control Officer
Massachusetts Department of Public Health
Boston, MA
USA

**Joseph R. Betancourt MD, MPH**
Director
The Disparities Solutions Center
Massachusetts General Hospital
Professor of Medicine
Harvard Medical School
The Institute for Health Policy
Boston, MA
USA

**Theresa Stichick Betancourt ScD, MA**
Assistant Professor of Child Health and Human
Rights
Department of Population and International Health
Francois-Xavier Bagnoud Center for Health and
Human Rights
Harvard School of Public Health
Boston, MA
USA

**Jeffrey M. Borkan MD, PhD**
Professor of Family Medicine
Memorial Hospital of Rhode Island
Pawtucket, RI
USA

**David R. Boulware MD, MPH, DTM&H**
Assistant Professor
Division of Infectious Disease & International
Medicine
University of Minnesota
Minneapolis, MN
USA

**Helen Bruce SCM, MTD, CNM**
Certified Nurse Midwife
Obstetrics and Gynaecology Department
HealthPartners
St Paul, MN
USA

**Nerissa Caballes MS, CRC, LPC**
Emergency Services Clinical Coordinator
Hartgrove Hospital
Chicago, IL
USA

**J. Emilio Carrillo MD, MPH**
President and Chiel Medical Officer
The New York Presbyterian Community Health
Plan
Associate Professor of Public Health
Joan and Sanford Weill Medical College of Cornell
University
New York, NY
USA

**Martin S. Cetron MD**
Director
Division of Global Migration and Quarantine
National Center for Infectious Disease
Centers for Disease Control and Prevention
Associate Professor (Adjunct) Emory University
School of Medicine and Rollins School of Public
Health
Atlanta, GA
USA

**George Clark BA, Certificate-Psychiatric Vocational Rehabilitation**
Vocational Rehabilitation Specialist
VA Boston Healthcare System
Psychology Service
Jamaica Plain, MA
USA

**Jennifer Cochran MPH**
Director
Refugee & Immigrant Health Program
Massachusetts Department of Public Health
Jamaica Plain, MA
USA

**Ellen R. Cooper MD**
Associate Professor of Pediatrics
Division of Infectious Diseases
Boston University School of Medicine
Boston Medical Center
Maxwell Finland Laboratory of Infectious Diseases
Boston, MA
USA

**Susan E. Cote RDH MS**
Program Coordinator
Program for Refugee Oral Health
Northeast Center for Research to Evaluate and
Eliminate Dental Disparities
Boston University Goldman School of Dental
Medicine
Boston, MA
USA

**Sondra S. Crosby MD**
Assistant Professor of Medicine
Section of General Internal Medicine
Department of Medicine
Boston University School of Medicine
Boston, MA
USA

**Kathleen A. Culhane-Pera MD, MA**
Community Family Physicia
East Side Family Clinic
St. Paul, MN
USA

**Allison Dubois MPH**
Vice President
Health Center Administration
Hudson River Healthcare
Peekskill, NY
USA

**David P. Eisenman MD MSHS**
Assistant Professor of Medicine
Division of General Internal Medicine and Health
Sciences Research
David Geffen School of Medicine
University of California
Los Angeles, CA
USA

**Solvig Ekblad PhD**
Associate Professor in Transcultural Psychology
Karolinska Institutet
Department of Clinical Neuroscience
Karolinska University Hospital
Stockholm
Sweden

**B. Heidi Ellis PhD**
Assistant Professor of Psychiatry and Psychology
Department of Child and Adolescent Psychiatry
Boston University Medical Center
Center for Medical and Refugee Trauma
Boston, MA
USA

**Katherine Fennelly**
Professor of Public Affairs
Hubert H. Humphrey Institute
University of Minnesota
Minneapolis, MN
USA

**Anita J. Gagnon**
Associate Professor
Department of Obstetrics and Gynaecology
MgGill, School of Nursing
Montreal, Quebec
Canada

**Roger L. Gebhard MD**
Professor of Medicine
Department of Gastroenterology
University of Minnesota
Staff Gastroenterologist
HealthPartners Medical Group
St. Paul, MN
USA

**Kristin Gebhard**
Scientist
University of Minnesota,
Department of Diagnostic and Biological Sciences
Minneapolis, MN
USA

**Paul L. Geltman MD, MPH**
Medical Director
Refugee and Immigrant Health Program
Massachusetts Department of Public Health
Associate Professor of Pediatrics
Boston University School of Medicine
Boston, MA
Staff Pediatrician
Cambridge Health Alliance
Cambridge, MA
USA

**Susan T. Goldstein MD**
Acting Associate Director for Medical Science
Division of Viral Diseases
Centers for Disease Control & Prevention
Atlanta, GA
USA

**Alexander R. Green MD, MPH**
Senior Scientist
The Disparities Solutions Center
Massachusetts General Hospital
Instructor in Medicine
Harvard Medical School
The Institute for Health Policy
Boston, MA
USA

**Peter J. Hotez MD, PhD, FAAP**
Walter G Ross Professor or Microbiology,
Immunology, and Tropical Medicine
Department of Microbiology, Immunology, and
Tropical Medicine
The George Washington University
Washington, DC
USA

**David Hunt**
President and CEO
Critical Measures, LLC
Minneapolis, MN
USA

**Randy Hurley MD**
Assistant Professor of Medicine
University of Minnesota
HealthPartners Medical Group
Regions Hospital
St. Paul, MN
USA

**James M. Jaranson MD, MA, MPH**
Consultant
Department of Psychiatry
School of Public Health
Division of Epidemiology and Community Health
University of Minnesota School of Medicine
San Diego, CA
USA

**M. Patricia Joyce MD FACP**
Medical Officer/Epidemiologist
National Center for Immunization and Respiratory
Diseases
Centers for Disease Control and Prevention
Atlanta, GA
USA

**Gregory Juckett MD, MPH**
Professor of Family Medicine
West Virginia University Health Sciences Center
Morgantown, WV
USA

**Marianne C. Kastrup MD PhD**
Head
Centre for Transcultural Psychiatry
Rigshospitalet
Copenhagen
Denmark

**Anne Kauffman Nolon MPH**
President and CEO
Hudson River HealthCare, Inc
Peekskill, NY
Visiting Professor
George Washington University
Geiger Gibson Health Policy
USA

**Jay S. Keystone MD FRCPC**
Professor of Medicine
Tropical Disease Unit
Toronto General Hospital
Toronto, Ontario
Canada

**Yae-Jean Kim MD, DTM&H**
Fellow
Department of Infectious Diseases
Fred Hutchinson Cancer Research Center
Seattle, WA
USA

**J. David Kinzie MD**
Professor of Psychiatry
Department of Psychiatry
Intercultural Psychiatric Program
Oregon Health & Science University
Portland, OR
USA

**Georgi V. Kroupin LP**
Lead Psychologist
Center for International Health
HealthPartners Medical Group
St. Paul, MN
USA

**Kevin Larsen MD**
Assistant Professor of Internal Medicine
University of Minnessota
General Internal Medicine Division
Hennepin County Medical Center
Minneapolis, MN
USA

**James H. Maguire MD, MPH**
Professor and Head, Division of International
Health
Department of Epidemiology and Preventive
Medicine
University of Maryland School of Medicine
Baltimore, MD
USA

**Susan A. Maloney MD, MHSc**
Director
International Emerging Infections Program –
Thailand
Ministry of Public Health
Muang
Thailand

**Lisa Merry N MSc(A)**
Research Coordinator
McGill School of Nursing
University Street
Montreal, Quebec
Canada

**Rajal Mody MD**
Staff Physician
Center for International Health
HealthPartners Medical Group
Saint Paul, MN
USA

**Pedro L. Moro MD, MPH**
Immunization Safety Office
Centers for Disease Control and Prevention
Atlanta, GA
USA

**Linda S. Nield MD**
Associate Professor of Pediatrics
West Virginia University School of Medicine
Robert C Byrd Health Sciences Center
Morgantown, WV
USA

**Thomas B. Nutman MD**
Head, Helminth Immunology Section
Head, Clinical Parasitology Unit
Laboratory of Parasitic Diseases
National Institutes of Health
Bethesda, MD
USA

**Ann O'Fallon RN, BSN, MA**
Minnesota Refugee Health Coordinator
Minnesota Department of Health
St. Paul, MN
USA

**Patricia J. Ohmans MPH**
Director
Health Advocates Community Health Consultants
Saint Paul, MN
USA

**Luis S. Ortega MD, MPH**
Chief
Immigrant Refugee and Migrant Health Branch
Division of Global Migration and Quarantine
Centers for Disease Control
Atlanta, GA
USA

**Elyse R. Park PhD**
Assistant Professor
Department of Psychiatry
Massachusetts General Hospital
Institute for Health Policy
Boston, MA
USA

**Patrick Pederson MD**
Medical Resident – Pediatrics
Department of Medicine
University of Minnesota
Minneapolis, MN
USA

**Nancy Piper Jenks MS, CFNP**
Director, Travel and Migrant Medicine
Hudson River HealthCare, Inc
Peekskill, NY
USA

**Linda A. Piwowarczyk MD MPH**
Assistant Professor of Psychiatry
Boston University School of Medicine
Co-Director
Boston Center for Refugee Health & Human Rights
Boston, MA
USA

**Drew L. Posey MD MPH**
Medical Epidemiologist
Immigrant, Refugee and Migrant Health Branch
Division of Global Migration and Quarantine
National Center for Infectious Diseases
Centers for Disease Control and Prevention
Atlanta, GA
USA

**Paola Ricci MD**
Assistant Professor of Medicine
University of Minnesota
Staff Hepatologist
HealthPartners -Regions Hospital
St. Paul, MN
USA

**Cathlyn Robinson RN, BScN, MSc(A)**
Clinical Nurse Specialist for Trauma
Department of Trauma
Montreal General Hospital
McGill University Health Centre
Montreal, Quebec
Canada

**Meghan Rothenberger MD**
Resident Physician,
Department of Internal Medicine
University of Minnesota
Minneapolis, MN
USA

**Peter M. Schantz VMD, PhD**
Epidemiologist & Senior Service Fellow
Division of Parasitic Diseases,
National Center for Zoonotic, Vector-Borne and
Enteric Diseases
Centers for Disease Control and Prevention,
Atlanta, GA
USA

**Jonathan Sellman MD**
Infectious Disease Consultant
HealthPartners Medical Group
Health Specialty Center
St. Paul, MN
Clinical Scholar Assistant Professor
Division of Infectious Diseases
Department of Medicine
University of Minnesota
Minneapolis, MN
USA

**Lorna Seybolt MD**
Pediatrician
Maine Medical Center
Maine Pediatric Specialty Group
Portland, ME
USA

**David R. Shlim MD**
Medical Director
Jackson Hole Travel and Tropical Medicine
Jackson Hole, WY
USA

**Harpreet Singh RDH, MS**
Clinical Instructor
Boston University School of Dental Medicine
Division of Community Health Programs
Boston, MA
USA

**John Q. Smith MD**
Associate Professor of Medicine
Johns Hopkins School of Medicine
Baltimore, MD
USA

**William M. Stauffer MD, MSPH, DTM&H**
Assistant Professor
Department of Internal Medicine
Division of Infectious Disease & International
Medicine
University of Minnesota
School of Public Health, Epidemiology
Minneapolis, MN
USA

**Andrea P. Summer MD, MSCR, DTM&H**
Assistant Professor of Pediatrics
Department of Pediatrics
Medical University of South Carolina
Charleston, SC
USA

**Sydney van Dyke MA**
Manager of Interpreter Services
Regions Hospital
St Paul, MN
USA

**Patricia F. Walker MD, DTM&H**
Medical Director
Center for International Health and
Travel Medicine Program
HealthPartners Medical Group
Assistant Professor
Department of Internal Medicine
Division of Infectious Disease and
International Medicine
University of Minnesota
St. Paul, MN
USA

**Thomas Wenzel**
Professor of Medicine
Department of Psychiatry
University Hospital
Medical University of Vienna
Vienna
Austria

**A. Clinton White, Jr. MD**
Professor
Infectious Disease Section
Department of Medicine
Baylor College of Medicine
Houston, TX
USA

**Ian T. Williams PhD**
Acting Chief, Epidemiology and Surveillance
Branch
Division of Viral Hepatitis
Centers for Disease Control and Prevention
Atlanta, GA
USA

**Mary E. Wilson MD, FACP, FIDSA**
Associate Professor of Population and International
Health
Harvard School of Public Health
Boston, MA
USA

**Linda Siti Yancey MD**
Physician
Houston Center for Infectious Diseases
Houston, TX
USA

# Acknowledgements

This book would not have been possible without those who believed in our vision to pull together the rich information about healthcare for immigrants in this volume. We thank the many authors who have contributed their valuable time and effort to this book, our colleagues who have supported us through this work, and our families who have encouraged us. We thank our patients for their courage, inspiration, wisdom and resilience. Conni Conner provided invaluable support for several authors and editors.

# Dedication

To my parents
Frederick Frye Walker and Phyllis Lane Walker
who gave me the world,

AND

to Becky Enos
who shares it with me

Patricia Frye Walker, MD, DTM&H


To my parents; and to Mustafa,
Alex, Sam and Leila.

Elizabeth D Barnett MD

# CHAPTER 1

# An Introduction to the Field of Refugee and Immigrant Healthcare

Patricia F. Walker and Elizabeth D. Barnett

Caring for immigrants has become a nearly universal experience for healthcare professionals practicing in the first decade of the twenty-first century. The inspiration for this book is our conviction that there is a rich body of international knowledge and experience in refugee and immigrant healthcare. Our overriding goal is to reduce health disparities by defining best practices in refugee and immigrant medicine and making them available to those who are working in the field. The contributors to this text have worked with immigrants and refugees in many of the domains of their lives, and they have joined us in writing about best practice models for care of immigrants and refugees.

Global migration patterns, and the speed of that migration, result in the daily recognition that there are no local diseases. As eloquently described in Thomas Friedman's book, *The Earth is Flat*, the business community was perhaps quicker than the medical community to respond competently to the fact that the global is local, and that the key to success in business is to think globally. The same is true in medicine. Every day in hospitals and clinics around the world, healthcare providers struggle with lack of adequate knowledge, skills and abilities, and attitudes to provide high-quality healthcare to new migrants. We cross many cultures in healthcare, including those related to gender, race and ethnicity, socioeconomic status, and belief systems regarding health and illness. Our personal capacity, training, and skills to reach across those cultural chasms are often inadequate to prepare us for the changing demographics of our patient populations. Physicians in training acknowledge this feeling of lack of preparation in cross-cultural healthcare.[1] In one study, healthcare providers expressed less satisfaction in clinical encounters with ethnic immigrant patients, with the greatest source of dissatisfaction being associated with patients' understanding of prevention and management of chronic disease.[2] That desire to improve outcomes is an inherent goal for most healthcare providers, and can be particularly challenging with recent immigrants. The provider in the twenty-first century must be cognizant not only of cross-cultural issues, but differences in disease prevalence by race and ethnicity, as well as country of origin. Many immigrants arrive from less-developed countries, and have a higher prevalence of infectious diseases including intestinal parasites, hepatitis B, and tuberculosis. Protocols for screening new arrivals can be complex, and management of diseases heard of only in medical school can be difficult to remember. Once the new migrant has settled, perhaps an even more difficult challenge becomes management of mental health issues (Section 5), preventive healthcare and chronic diseases (Chapter 42), as the healthy migrant advantage (Chapter 3) is lost with time and acculturation.

A complex and far-reaching group of national and international organizations including the Centers for Disease Control and Prevention, the International Organization for Migration, nongovernmental organizations, as well as many resettlement agencies, have had decades of experience in addressing health issues of refugees, the internally displaced, and migrants as they are screened for departure to new countries, as well as upon arrival. Contributing authors outline international screening protocols

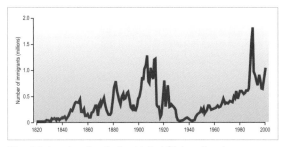

Fig. 1.1 Immigration to the United States: fiscal years 1820–2001 (millions). (From Migration Information Source. http://www.migrationinformation.org)

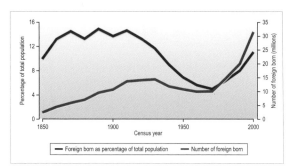

Fig. 1.2 Size of the foreign-born population and foreign born as a percentage of the total population of the United States: 1850–2000. (From Migration Information Source. http://www.migrationinformation.org)

(Chapter 10), as well as suggested best practices in screening of new arrivals to the United States (Chapter 11). Major diseases seen in refugees and immigrants are discussed in chapters on hepatitis B (Chapters 22,23), intestinal parasites (Chapter 20), and tuberculosis (Chapter 19). Many unusual diseases not seen in North America, as well as diseases with long latency periods (Chapter 17) such as leprosy (Chapter 34) and strongyloidiasis (Chapter 40), are discussed in detail. Key to the diseases and disorders section of this textbook (Section 3) are clinical pearls and common pitfalls in management of diseases seen in immigrants.

## Demographic Changes

At least 185 million people worldwide currently live outside their countries of birth, up from 80 million three decades ago.[19] The United States is currently experiencing its largest wave of immigration since the beginning of the twentieth century (Fig. 1.1).

The percentage of the entire US population represented by the foreign born was much higher in the nineteenth century, and steadily decreased until 1970. Since that time, the percentage of the foreign born in the United States has increased and, as of 2005, accounts for approximately 12% of the total population (Fig. 1.2).

International migration patterns have also had a major impact on Canada and Western as well as Eastern Europe, as shown by the percentage of foreign born in each country in 2001 (Table 1.1).

By far, most international migration takes place among countries in the southern hemisphere and goes largely unreported.[20] In the United States, the top 10 countries of origin for the foreign born are led by Mexico, at 28% (Fig. 1.3).

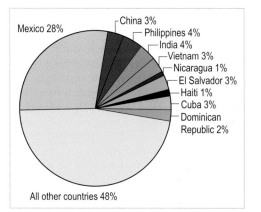

Fig. 1.3 Ten source countries with the largest populations in the United States as percentages of the total foreign-born population: 2000. (From Migration Information Source. http://www.migrationinformation.org)

**Table 1.1 Percentage of total population which is foreign born, by country, in 2001**

| | |
|---|---|
| Australia | 23.1% |
| Canada | 18.8% |
| Sweden | 11.5% |
| United States of America | 11.4% |
| Netherlands | 9.3% |
| Norway | 6.8% |
| United Kingdom | 8.3% |
| Russian Federation (1989 data) | 7.8% |

Migration Information Source, http://www.migrationinformation.org

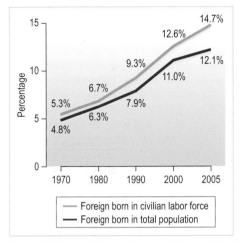

Fig. 1.4 Share of the foreign born in the total United States population and in the civilian labor force, 1970–2005. (From Migration Information Source. http://www.migrationinformation.org)

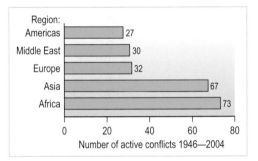

Fig. 1.5 Number of active conflicts by area, 1946–2004. (Dept of Peace and Conflict Research, Uppsala University: http://www.pcr.uu.se/)

The foreign born remain powerful contributors to the US economy, representing 12.1% of the population, and 14.7% of the civilian labor force by 2005 (Fig. 1.4).

This book focuses on refugees and recent immigrants to the West. As mobile populations created by international geopolitics, refugees and the internally displaced have always been a reality, and will continue to challenge healthcare delivery systems worldwide. Between 1946 and 2004, 229 armed conflicts occurred around the world (Fig. 1.5). Unfortunately, the number of peace agreements (Fig. 1.6) is far outnumbered by areas of ongoing strife.

As a subset of immigrants, refugees are a highly traumatized group, with long histories of difficulties in their country of origin, as well as during their escape and residence in refugee camps in countries of first asylum. Physical and mental health issues can

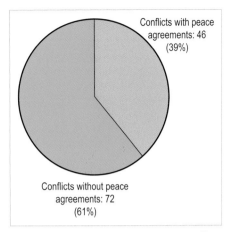

Fig. 1.6 Peace agreements in armed conflicts, 1989–2005. (Dept of Peace and Conflict Research, Uppsala University: http://www.pcr.uu.se/)

remain difficult for decades for refugees and victims of torture, and are addressed in the mental health section of this text. Refugee women and girls are a particularly vulnerable group, and are often victims of rape and sexual torture. Access to adequate contraceptives and safe prenatal care is poor, and complications of pregnancy and delivery remain a leading cause of maternal mortality worldwide. Medical problems of women refugees, and cross-cultural and clinical issues in care of women refugees, are addressed in Chapters 43 and 44.

Thirty-three million people – or nearly one in every 275 people on earth – are refugees, returned refugees, and internally displaced peoples (IDPs).[21] There are currently 12.0 million refugees and asylum seekers worldwide.[13] Afghanistan, with an estimated 2 191 100 refugees and asylum seekers, and Palestine, with 2 971 600, are by far the largest sources of refugees.[13] While the number of refugees has decreased from a high of 14.9 million in 2001, the number of internally displaced persons has continued to increase. By conservative estimate, more than 21 million people are currently displaced within the borders of their own country.[13] In a UNHCR survey of 149 countries, a record 668 000 persons submitted applications for asylum in 2005 (Table 1.2; Box 1.1).[14]

Global trafficking in people also contributes to international migration, and the International Organization for Migration estimates that criminal organizations 'traffic' four million people per year into prostitution and exploitative work in a global trade that reaps US$7 billion in profits.[18] Approximately 50 000 people, the majority of whom are women and

3

**Table 1.2 Refugees and asylum seekers worldwide (as of 31 December, 2005)[17]**

| Area | Refugees and asylum seekers |
|---|---|
| Middle East | 4 855 400 |
| Africa | 3 176 100 |
| South and Central Asia | 1 953 000 |
| East Asia and the Pacific | 1 029 400 |
| Europe | 530 200 |
| Americas and the Caribbean | 475 000 |
| **TOTAL** | **12 019 100** |

**Box 1.1**

### Refugee: 12 million[13]

The term refugee means any persons who have fled their country, are unable or unwilling to avail themselves of the protection of their country of nationality or habitual residence because of a well-founded fear of persecution on account of race, religion, nationality, membership in a particular social group or political opinion.

### Asylee: 668 000[14]

An asylee is a person who has been granted asylum, that is, granted the right to remain permanently in safety. In contrast to a refugee who underwent processing overseas, an asylee is a person who first reached another country, usually as a visitor or other non-immigrant status, and either upon or after arrival declared him/herself to be a 'refugee' based on the refugee standard described in the answer above; made a formal application for asylum; and was granted asylum by authorities of that country.

### Internally displaced: 21 million[13]

The internally displaced are people who are displaced within their own country and to whom the United Nations High Commissioner for Refugees (UNHCR) extends protection or assistance, or both, generally pursuant to a special request by a competent organ of the United Nations.

**Box 1.2**

'All European hospitals are invited to implement the Amsterdam Declaration to become migrant friendly and culturally competent organizations and develop individual, personalized services from which all patients will benefit. Investments in increased responsiveness to the needs of populations at risk will be an important step towards overall quality assurance and development.'

Migrant Friendly Hospital Group, 2004

universal application (Chapters 4, 42). In Europe, for example, the Amsterdam Declaration of December 2004 is expected to serve as the European platform for improving hospital and health services for migrants and ethnic minorities.[22] Developed by the Migrant Friendly Hospital Project Group, a group of hospitals from 12 European countries, and supported by the European Commission and the Austrian Government, the recommendations of the Amsterdam Declaration are endorsed by the European Commission, international experts, and many international and scientific organizations. The Migrant Friendly Hospital group is a European initiative to promote health and health literacy for migrants and ethnic minorities in an ethnoculturally diverse Europe (Box 1.2).

## Myths about the Cost of Caring for Immigrants

Myths abound in relationship to refugee and immigrant healthcare costs. A 2005 study by researchers from Harvard Medical School found that healthcare expenditures for US immigrants were approximately 55% less than those of US-born residents. Health expenditures for immigrant children in 1998 were 74% less than those of native-born children. Immigrants on average received US$1139 in healthcare in 1998, compared with US$2546 for native-born residents. Although immigrants accounted for 10% of the US population in 1998, they accounted for only 8% of US healthcare costs. Study coauthor Steffi Woolhandler commented, 'It's a complete myth that immigrants are a disproportionate burden. The majority have health insurance, and, even when they have insurance, they use a whole lot less.'[8] A report on the Kaiser network showed that communities with high numbers of Hispanics, immigrants, and the uninsured actually have lower usage rates for emergency departments than communities with

children, are trafficked to the United States on an annual basis for illicit purposes.[15]

While the focus of this text is on the North American migrant, many of the principles described in the text hold true for migrants worldwide. Issues of health policy, and the design of healthcare delivery systems which are effective for migrants, can have lower numbers of residents in these three groups.[9] Uninsured individuals had 16 fewer visits to the emergency department per 100 people than Medicaid beneficiaries and 20 fewer visits than seniors with Medicare. Immigrants had 17 fewer visits per 100 individuals. The study's author, Peter Cunningham, commented, 'While there are individual hospitals along the border or in some inner-city areas that may be experiencing a large increase, the larger perspective is that uninsured Hispanic immigrants generally are not heavy users of emergency departments.'[9] The uninsured often avoid medical treatment because of the expense, while illegal immigrants may be afraid of being deported.

Higher spending and availability of health insurance also does not automatically equate to more or better care. In a study comparing the health of people aged 55–64 years in the US and Britain, US residents aged 55–64 were much sicker than people in Britain in the same age group, with higher rates of diabetes, heart attack, stroke, lung disease, and cancer.[10] US patients rate their healthcare among the worst in the industrialized world, despite spending more on medical care than patients in other countries. The US ranks thirty-third in infant mortality and twenty-eighth in disease-free life expectancy, according to the World Health Organization. Meanwhile, the US spent US$6280 per capita on medical care in 2004, more than twice as much as any other industrialized nation.[11] In an Office of Management and Budget study, the cost of providing professional interpreters for limited English-speaking patient visits was estimated at 0.5% of the cost of the total visits.[23]

Currently, 49.6 million Americans (18.7% of US residents) speak a language other than English at home; 22.3 million (8.4%) have limited English proficiency, speaking English less than 'very well,' according to self ratings. Between 1990 and 2000, the number of Americans who spoke a language other than English at home grew by 15.1 million, a 47% increase, and the number with limited English proficiency grew by 7.3 million, a 53% increase (Fig. 1.7).[12] Legal and quality issues in the use of interpreters are reviewed in Chapters 5 and 6, and school readiness for immigrant children in Chapter 55.

## Redesigning the Care Delivery System: An Immigrant Perspective

Barriers of access to healthcare (Chapter 4), language and literacy (Chapter 56), and lack of adequate professional interpreters (Chapters 5, 6) are an everyday

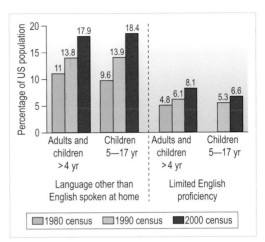

**Fig. 1.7** Percentages of Americans who speak a language other than English at home or who have limited English proficiency. (US Census Bureau)

reality. The early chapters in this text provide an eloquent testament to the importance of focusing not only on our personal preparation to care for multicultural patient populations (Chapters 7, 8, 9), but on the key importance of redesigning healthcare delivery systems, as recommended by the Institute of Medicine *Crossing the Quality Chasm Report*, to provide care which is safe, timely, effective, efficient, equitable, and patient centered for migrants.[3]

As healthcare providers and healthcare delivery systems commit to providing care based on these six principles noted above, much work remains to be done in order to achieve these goals. The quality chasm, so vast for many Americans, is arguably most gaping for those with low health literacy, limited English proficiency, and communities of color. Examples of achieving the six aims for refugees and immigrants, and the promises and system change required for care delivery systems to achieve those aims, are offered in Table 1.3.

If we commit to providing equitable care, we must first know for whom we are caring, and develop adequate demographic data sets, including not only race and ethnicity, but language and country of origin. We must then analyze quality and satisfaction data by demographic group. The National Health Plan Collaborative, a coalition of nine major health insurance companies, recently acknowledged that improving systematic data collection is crucial in helping reduce racial and ethnic discrepancies in healthcare.[4] Yet a recent survey found that only 78% of US hospitals systematically collect data on patients' race or ethnicity, and more than half relied

**Table 1.3 Achieving the 6 aims[3] to improve quality for immigrants; promises and outcomes**

| | |
|---|---|
| 'We promise your care will be safe.' | Health literacy will be assessed, and systems designed to reduce barriers related to low health literacy. All patients will receive medication instructions which are personally understood. |
| 'We promise your care will be timely.' | Same-day and walk-in care, familiar to most immigrants, will be offered in primary care settings. |
| 'We promise your care will be effective.' | Preferred spoken and written language for interacting with care delivery systems will be assessed for all patients. Professionally trained medical interpreters will be utilized for all interactions with limited English proficient patients. |
| 'We promise your care will be efficient.' | Staff demographics will reflect the communities served. Episodic care (short clinic visits) will no longer be the norm for immigrant populations. Care delivery models including community partnerships, group care, community health workers and use of modern techniques such as digital health educational materials in multiple languages, accessed from secure networks remotely, will be the norm. |
| 'We promise your care will be equitable.' | Quality and satisfaction data will be analyzed by demographic group. Care delivery systems will design and implement effective interventions to reduce disparities. Cultural competency training will be required of providers. |
| 'We promise your care will be patient centered.' | 100% of our patients will report their care is customized to their physical emotional and spiritual needs and beliefs. |

Patricia F Walker, MD, DTM&H, 2006

on registration clerks' impressions of patients' race and ethnicity rather than directly asking patients.[5] Expert panels have recommended that patients' race and ethnicity should be collected by self-report.[6] There is data presented in this textbook which suggest that, for the recent immigrant, country of origin is a better proxy for health than is race or ethnicity (Chapter 42). The heterogeneity of immigrant populations makes development of guidelines, such as new arrival screening or cancer screening protocols, more difficult. Much research is needed in this area. The ultimate goal is to understand why health disparities exist, and design care delivery models which can reduce these disparities.

The good news is that there are many national and international examples of effective care delivery models for immigrants, including hiring providers which reflect the communities served, and utilizing professional interpreters, social work/case management staff and community health workers (Chapters 4, 5, 6, 42). Physicians and other healthcare providers should be knowledgeable regarding innovative ways to reduce health disparities for migrants, and should be advocates for change in this regard.

Perhaps one of the most difficult promises to keep to immigrant patients is the provision of patient-centered care. Cross-cultural ethical dilemmas, cancer care, and end-of-life care all challenge physicians to examine their own biomedical model and healthcare belief systems, and are addressed in this text (Chapters 7, 8, 9, 42).

## Core Values in Immigrant Medicine

We believe a set of core values can and should provide the basis for all decisions related to the financing, structure and operations of healthcare delivery worldwide. Core values for providers working with refugees and immigrants include global health equity, respect, trust, cultural humility, and compassion.

### Global health equity

The tragic reality of healthcare for many migrants is the pervasive relationship of health to poverty and politics. Forty years ago, Einstein stated, 'nationalism is an infantile disease; it is the measles of mankind.' The last case of polio described in the western hemisphere, in Peru in 1991, occurred in a young boy whose clinic, from which he would have received the polio vaccine, was destroyed by the Sendero Luminoso, or Shining Path, guerrilla group. More recently, polio has spread from Nigeria to 16 other countries, after Nigerian tribal leaders, for religious and political reasons, told the populations under their control not to accept polio vaccination.[7] Cross-cultural and religious differences resulted in five cases of polio in Minnesota in a religious minority community, the Amish.[7] Dr. Bill Foege has stated, 'We must ask what is best for the world; we are dealing with closed systems.'[16] Although refugees and many immigrants clearly have improved access to quality healthcare after migration, health inequities follow them to their new countries.

## Respect

Less than 1% of the world's refugees arrive in the United States, and their journeys, when time can be taken to learn of them, are both harrowing and inspiring. For many Western clinicians, seeing a Cambodian patient brings thoughts of the killing fields of Pol Pot and the Khmer Rouge, where 1.5 million people died from genocide, disease, and starvation from 1975 through 1979. Yet to many Cambodians, their memories go back to an earlier era of the grandeur of the Angkor Empire, which culminated in building the temple complex of Angkor Wat, one of the architectural wonders of the world. Respect for the richness of our patients' personal culture, religion, and country of origin, as well as the courage and strength it takes to leave one's homeland, can create a powerful bond between clinician and patient (Box 1.3).

## Trust

Trustworthiness is a key element of successful outcomes in the care of refugees and immigrants. Care provided by bilingual, bicultural providers is one of the most effective ways to engender trust, yet many international medical graduates face daunting barriers to training and establishing practices in the United States. Having the time in the clinical encounter to address socioeconomic and cultural issues is also critical to establishing trust. The reality of financial pressures often makes such encounters difficult to attain. Providers who can effectively communicate in the patient's language or via a professional interpreter are critical to establishing trust.

> **Box 1.3**
>
> 'Heroes, all of them – at least they're my heroes, especially the immigrants, especially the refugees. Everyone makes fun of New York cabdrivers who can't speak English: they're heroes. To give up your country is the hardest thing a person can do: to leave the old familiar places and ship out over the edge of the world to America and learn everything over again different that you learned as a child, learn the language that you will never be so smart or funny in as in your true language. It takes years to start to feel semi-normal. And yet people still come – Russia, Vietnam and Cambodia and Laos, Ethiopia, Iran, Haiti, Korea, Cuba, Chile, and they come on behalf of their children, and they come for freedom. Not for our land (Russia is as beautiful), not for our culture (they have their own, thank you), not for our system of government (they don't even know about it, may not even agree with it), but for freedom. They are heroes who make an adventure on our behalf, showing by their struggle how precious beyond words freedom is, and if we knew their stories, we could not keep back the tears.'
>
> Garrison Keillor, Newsweek July 4, 1998

## Cultural humility

Cultural humility is also a positive quality for clinicians dealing with patients from other cultures. We have much to learn from our colleagues and patients worldwide. Traditional healing methods utilized for centuries including artemether-based medications derived from a plant, sweet wormwood (Chinese: 青蒿), one of the most effective antimalarials available, potato poultices for knee pain (a cheap alternative to microwave hot packs), and more recently, red yeast rice, which contains statins, for treatment of hyperlipidemia, are a few of many examples.

## Compassion

As eloquently described by Dr David Shlim (Chapter 2), compassion can be developed by clinicians, and may be one of the most powerful tools in our armamentarium to care for refugees and immigrants. It is hard to empathize with the degree of suffering many refugee and immigrant patients have experienced. Dr Steven Miles, Minnesota internist and medical bioethicist who recently published a book on Abu Graib prison and physicians, created the family tree of a young Cambodian refugee, since resettled to the United States. Color-coded to represent killings by the Khmer Rouge or Vietnamese, or death from

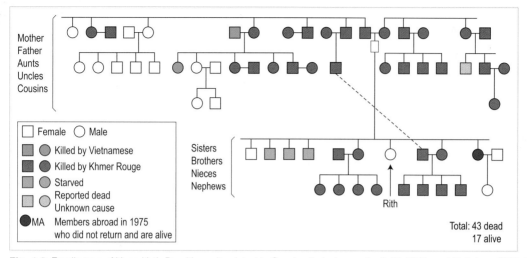

**Fig. 1.8** Family tree of Yong Yuth Banrith, as it existed in Cambodia between April 17, 1975, and October, 1979. Recorded at Khao I Dang Refugee Camp, Aranyaprathet, Thailand, October, 1979. (By personal permission, Banrith Yong Yuth and Steven Miles, M.D.)

disease and starvation, the family tree shows that Banrith Yong Yuth lost 43 members of his immediate family (Fig. 1.8).

Now married with 4 children, and owner of a successful French restaurant, Banrith Yong Yuth's story reflects the unimaginable degree of loss and suffering true for so many of our patients. Dr Shlim's chapter (Chapter 2) outlines techniques to improve the clinician's capacity for compassion, thus enhancing the clinical encounter for both immigrant patients and their care givers.

## Conclusion

Dr William Foege has stated that we must change the healthcare debate to focus on quality, equality, prevention, and outcomes, and that ultimately we should measure civilization by how people treat each other.[16] The Irish writer George Bernard Shaw reminded us, 'Do not do unto others as you would that they should do unto you – their tastes may not be the same.' We would add that their cultures, healthcare belief systems and diseases may also not be the same. The challenge of providing patient-centered care in a multicultural society means that respect for cultural differences as well as knowledge of diseases seen by race/ethnicity and country of origin should be the expectations and competencies of every healthcare provider operating in the twenty-first-century global health environment.

The motivation for publication of this book began with our recognition that healthcare disparities for refugees and immigrants are pervasive and the reasons for their existence complex. We also realized that many clinicians lacked comfort with their skills in caring for immigrants, but that this could be addressed by defining a body of knowledge for the field, and developing best-practice models of care. It also springs from the joy and privilege of interacting with patients and colleagues from around the world. Our patients teach us on a daily basis about strength, courage in the face of overwhelming adversity, respect, cultural humility, and compassion. Our patients remind us of the inadequacies of our clinical knowledge base, and challenge us to examine the biomedical model and our own cultural biases. Lessons learned from the healthy migrant can help us examine our own lifestyles and priorities, as industrialized societies struggle with epidemics of obesity, diabetes, and heart disease. Immigrants reinvent the American dream on a daily basis, focusing on family, education, and economic advancement. Our hope is that this book will help equip medical administrators, health systems experts, public health providers, and practicing clinicians, as well as the thousands of dedicated international medical graduates, promotores, social workers, and other community health workers, with some of the personal and health system tools they need to provide high-quality, culturally competent care to refugees and immigrants worldwide.

# References

1. Weissman JS, Betancourt J, Campbell EG, et al. Resident physicians' preparedness to provide cross-cultural care. JAMA 2005; 294:1058–1067.
2. Kamath CC, O'Fallon WM, Offord KP, et al. Provider satisfaction in clinical encounters with ethnic immigrant patients. Mayo Clin Proc 2003; 78:1353–1360.
3. Institute of Medicine. Crossing the quality chasm: a new health system for the 21st century/Committee on Quality Health Care in America, Institute of Medicine. Committee on Quality of Health Care in America. Washington, DC: National Academy Press; 2001.
4. HealthPartners Health Care Daily. Data collection 'crucial' for reducing gaps in care for minorities, insurers say. ACHP's Media Monitoring Report 7/10/2006.
5. Hasnain-Wynia R, Pierce D, Pittman MA. Who, what, when, where: the current state of data of collection on race and ethnicity in hospitals. New York, NY: Commonwealth Fund; 2004.
6. Bierman AS, Lurie N, Collins KS, et al. Addressing racial and ethnic barriers to effective healthcare: the need for better data. Health Aff (Millwood) 2002; 21:91–102.
7. Polio cases in Minnesota. Minnesota Department of Health. Available: http://www.health.state.mn.us Accessed 2/25/07.
8. Mohanty SA, Woolhandler S, Himmelstein DU, et al. Healthcare expenditures of immigrants in the United States: A nationally representative analysis. Am J Public Health 2005: 95;8:1431–1438.
9. Cunningham PJ. What accounts for differences in the use of hospital emergency departments across US communities? Health Affairs, Sept/Oct 2006; 25(5): w324–w336.
10. Banks J, Marmot M, Oldfield Z, et al. Disease and disadvantage in the United States and in England. JAMA 2006; 295:2037–2045.
11. Zwillich T. Survey: Americans rate US healthcare among worse in industrial world. WebMD April 4, 2006.
12. Flores G. Language barriers to healthcare in the United States. N Engl J Med 2006; 355(3):229–231.
13. US Committee for Refugees and Immigrants. Refugee Reports. 2005 Statistical issue. 2006; 27:1.
14. UNHCR (United Nations High Commission for Refugees). 2005 global refugee trends. Available: Pg 7. http://unhcr.org/statistics Accessed 2/25/07.
15. Trends in International Migration Annual Report SOPEMI 2002 Edition.
16. Foege WH. Global Public Health: Targeting Inequities. Jama 1998; 279:1931–1932.
17. US Committee for Refugee and Immigrants survey 2006.
18. International Organization for Migration 2002. Available: http://www.iom.int Accessed 2/25/07.
19. United Nations 2002
20. Migration Information: www.migrationinformation.org
21. UNHCR http://www.unhcr.org/statistics
22. Migrant Friendly Hospitals: http://www.mfh.eu.net
23. Office of Management and Budget. Report to Congress; Assessment of the Total Benefits and Costs of Implementing Executive Order No. 13166: Improving Access to Services for Persons with Limited English Proficiency. March 14, 2002.

# CHAPTER 2

# Compassion

David R. Shlim

The twelve-year-old girl's lips were blue with cold as she staggered through the thigh-deep snow. At 19 000 feet in altitude, she was buffeted by the bitter cold wind as she endured the second day of a winter blizzard. The group she was with had no warm jackets and only canvas sneakers on their feet. They couldn't turn around for two reasons: it was now harder to go back up over the pass they had just crossed than to carry on down, and if they did re-cross the pass, the army would be waiting for them.

A young man put the girl on his back. He carried her that day, and huddled with her at night, for they had no tents or sleeping bags. The next day, as he staggered through the snow with the girl on his back, he realized that she had died. He had no choice but to leave her in the snow, and try to save his own life.

The man had been so focused on carrying the young girl that he had not noticed that his feet were now frozen. He could no longer walk. His girlfriend put him on her back, and forced her way through the snow. Another day and night brought them out of the snow into a new country.

The police stopped them. These border officials were not interested in sending them back or in helping them. Their only motivation was to steal all they could from the helpless group. They took whatever valuables they could find, even extra clothing, and let them go. The ragged group carried on down a valley into the warmth of the lower altitudes.

They reached a road, and managed to get a ride for 5 hours to Kathmandu. There they found the Tibetan refugee center and a nurse. She looked at the hands and feet of the newly arrived refugees and called me to see them.

The twenty-one-year-old man who had coura-geously struggled across the highest part of the pass

with the dying girl on his back had severe frostbite. His feet had already turned completely black above his ankles and begun to shrivel. Both of his legs would need to be amputated below the knees. The others had varying degrees of frostbite: some would lose their toes, others would lose half their foot. Several people would lose parts of their fingers. They had endured this tortuous journey to achieve freedom from an oppressive occupier of their country.

If this brave group had been Americans, they would have immediately gone onto television news and talk shows, signed book contracts, and sold the film rights to their story. The fact that no one outside of a handful of people in Nepal or India was at all interested in their struggle says a lot about our view of refugees and immigrants. For a nation that prides itself on having been built by immigrants, we seem to have lost our interest in those who are still being forced to move from their native lands.

'One little girl trapped at the bottom of a Texas well had the entire nation holding its breath,' said Ted Koppel on *Nightline* in 1991. 'But millions starv-ing in Africa, as many as 25 000 drowned in Bangla-desh, over 1000 killed by cholera in Peru barely get our attention. Why?'[1]

Most readers of this textbook will have grappled with these questions already. The desire to care spe-cifically for an immigrant or refugee population sug-gests that the reader already has the ability to imagine oneself in their situation, and to want to help. We could call this desire to help compassion.

Compassion is defined in the dictionary as 'to suffer' (passio) 'with' (com). This definition is closer to sympathy and empathy than it is to the Buddhist definition of compassion which means, 'the desire to ease suffering in others.'[1] (The Tibetan word for com-passion is 'nyingje,' which literally translates as 'from the heart.') This definition resonates with a much more active feeling of wanting to help, and is actually closer to what people naturally feel when they see someone who is suffering.

All of us have compassion in relative degrees at different times. However, our ability to maintain the desire to ease suffering is often limited. It is easiest for us to care about our own families and close friends and relatives. We may also find it easier to care about people with whom we share some common heritage or beliefs. Beyond that, it becomes more difficult to demonstrate strong compassion towards those we don't know. And most of us find it almost impossible to be kind and compassionate towards those who are making it difficult for us, or have harmed us in the past. How many of us were able to feel compassion towards the September 11, 2001 hijackers along with their victims?

In addition, we may feel that we just don't have enough energy to care about what happens to people in all corners of the world. The range of suffering experienced in other parts of the world often goes so far beyond our imagination that it appears to be happening on another planet. There are very few Americans who have ever spent even a passing moment trying to imagine what it would be like to be forced from their homes by a marauding militia, fleeing on foot for days or weeks, and winding up across the Mexican border with a handful of possessions, no money, not speaking the local language, and wondering what was going to happen to them that night, much less the rest of their lives.

Those in the medical profession who take care of immigrants often do so by choice, probably because they have some sense of the suffering that many have been through, and want to try to help. An immigrant population may be needier than other patient populations. They may have language obstacles, and a lack of cultural understanding. They may have logistical, emotional, or psychological problems that make it difficult to care for them. After some time, our ability to maintain compassion may start to erode.

That situation speaks to the heart of the problem. How does one increase or stabilize compassion when one already feels that one is trying as hard as one can? Is compassion fixed like a character trait, or can it be modified through training? If our compassion can decrease – something we all unfortunately seem to experience at times – can it be increased?

Our current concept of compassion is that it is like a rechargeable battery. It can take only a finite amount of charge. Once charged, it can only run down, so we tend to use it sparingly, applying it to specific situations, and withholding it in others. When it is finally depleted, we need to get it recharged, which usually means going on a holiday. If it is a successful holiday, we will have a charged battery for a while. However, like a rechargeable battery, our ability to hold a full charge may decrease over time. Eventually, we may even declare ourselves the victims of 'professional burnout' and leave our current job.

It may be useful to look at compassion in a different way. What if there was a way to train in compassion? What if our capacity for compassion could be increased and the effort required to maintain that compassion could be decreased?

From the medical point of view, we can agree that there is a need for more compassion in our field. The focus of modern medicine began to shift in the 1920s as diseases started to replace the patient as the focus of care. We began to treat 'diabetes' rather than a person with high blood sugar. The advantages of a scientific approach to medicine seem obvious. However, this shift in emphasis has permanently affected the doctor–patient relationship, as pointed out in 1927 by Francis Peabody:

'He discerned a great irony: at the very time that medicine was improving, a decline in the physician–patient relationship was taking place. Physicians, he argued, were in danger of forsaking the patient for science.'[2]

It's not as if modern medicine is without compassion – after all, doctors and nurses work long hours, often work night shifts, or remain on call day and night. Fulfilling this schedule means making a lot of personal sacrifices to care for patients. This commitment is based on compassion. Compassion – when looked at this way – is assumed to be built into the practice of medicine: 'Of course I care for you, I'm caring for you aren't I?' This type of compassion can be called 'de facto compassion,' and it ends up feeling dissatisfying to both the patients (who aren't sure that the doctor really knows or cares about them), and the doctor (who ends up feeling unappreciated and can't understand why).

Ordinarily, when we have a problem to solve in medicine, we seek advice from experts who have studied the problem. The only experts that the author has been able to find who can describe compassion in detail and outline step-by-step ways of increasing one's own compassion appear to be the teachers of the Tibetan Buddhist tradition. The Dalai Lama is known for his profound compassion and wisdom, and there are many other teachers in the Tibetan tradition who embody these same qualities. Each of them has achieved a vast and stable form of compassion that one can appreciate if one gets to know them personally. These teachers spend their lives trying to inspire and teach others that compassion, as an inherent part of our true nature, can be expanded to an extraordinary degree through training.[3] (The Tibetan Buddhist concept of compassion stands in contrast to a less certain view of compassion in the West, as characterized by Anne Harrington: 'We understand ourselves to be emergent products of indifferent physiochemical process: and – though we have always admitted our capacity to experience and practice compassion – there is little in the stories we tell of our origins and emergence that is likely to incline us to see compassion as fundamental to our nature.')

If other experts on compassion emerge, they should be consulted as well. The idea is not to promote Buddhism, but to explore the qualities of compassion, and how these qualities can be expanded through training, and applied to the practice of Western medicine.

Medical schools have recognized a need to encourage medical students to see their patients as more than just a disease process. They encourage empathy and teach interview techniques and appropriate ways of responding in difficult situations. Students, in general, appear to benefit from these educational efforts, but as they reach the clinical wards, the need to be efficient and get one's work done trumps the desire to spend time getting to know and comfort one's patients. Indeed, the problem of the rigors of clinical training eclipsing the classroom teaching on empathy has been dubbed 'a hidden curriculum,' within medical training.[4] One doctor who studied the problem concluded that 'for many residents, fatigue cultivates anger, resentment, and bitterness, rather than kindness, compassion, or empathy.'[5]

This author is unaware of any Western models that provide the ability to directly train in increasing one's capacity and breadth of compassion. Therefore, I will outline Tibetan Buddhist concepts of training in compassion so that we can investigate for ourselves whether these insights will help us achieve the goal of being able to be compassionate towards more people more of the time. These concepts are available in much more detail in the book that I helped create entitled *Medicine and Compassion: A Tibetan Lama's Guidance for Caregivers*.[6] This book represents the teachings that Chokyi Nyima Rinpoche, a Tibetan lama with whom I have a close relationship, gave during two courses on medicine and compassion directed to medical professionals.

We need to first consider why it is difficult for us to maintain our compassion throughout our working day, let alone our careers. We can list three main reasons:

1. The compassion we have is *unstable* – it fluctuates based on our mood and the magnitude of the problems that we encounter.
2. The compassion we have is *limited* in scope – we can't automatically apply it to everyone we meet, regardless of their background or attitude.
3. When we use our compassion we are often subtly seeking an *ego reward* – we want people to recognize and thank us for our efforts. When our patients or our colleagues don't appreciate our efforts, we begin to feel discouraged.

Dealing with these three obstacles to compassion seems so normal to us that it is difficult for us to imagine their opposite: a kind of compassion that is stable, vast, and not ego-dependent. It even seems reasonable to question whether such compassion is possible.

Before we can address how to increase compassion, it's important to think about where compassion originates, and whether it is present in a form that can be modified through training. There are four major hypotheses regarding the basis of compassion:

1. It evolved through an evolutionary process of survival of the fittest.
2. It is a gift from God.
3. It is the result of how we are brought up, that is, by example and teaching.
4. It is an inherent part of our consciousness.

Those who postulate that compassion, or altruistic behavior, stems purely from evolutionary forces face a problem. Survival of the fittest implies that individuals are exclusively concerned about the propagation of their own DNA. Helping another person survive, particularly at the expense of oneself (altruistic behavior), would not appear to be the best way to accomplish this goal. Behavioral biologists explain the origin of altruism by postulating the survival value of certain forms of teamwork when compared to an individual's effort to survive.[7,8]

Those who believe that we were created by an all-knowing God would say that compassion was made part of our personalities by God, perhaps in imitation of God's own compassion for human beings.[9]

Some believe that our mind and personality are shaped to a major degree by the kinds of experiences we have as a child. In this sense, compassion could be thought of as a character trait that emerges from our formative years.

Buddhists would say that compassion is a natural part of our awareness, the part of us that is able to perceive and have experiences. The kind of vast, stable compassion that was mentioned above is said to be already present in all of us, but is currently obscured by negative thoughts and emotions. From a Buddhist point of view, the more we can clear away these obstacles to realizing our inherent nature, the more we will be able to express our natural compassion.

If we adhere to the first hypothesis, evolution, then there would appear to be little room to modify compassion through training, just as one's ability to process oxygen in endurance sports (one's $VO_2$ max) cannot be improved dramatically through training.

If we adhere to the second hypothesis, that compassion comes from God, it should be possible to increase compassion through a close connection and belief in the Creator, that is, through prayer. Traditions exist to increase compassion in this fashion through religious practices, but they are usually not widely taught to lay people.

The third hypothesis would suggest that compassion can be encouraged and modeled during formative years. In this model, compassion is a cognitive expression of a desire to help. This is the model that is most often used in medical schools.

The first three hypotheses do not suggest ways to greatly increase compassion in the individual. The fourth model postulates that a vast and stable form of compassion lies fully formed beneath our tumultuous surface of emotions. The process of training in compassion, in this model, is to allow us to recognize and stabilize our inherent compassion. As we do so, our compassion becomes more available and more effortless.

At the present time, we are often caught in a dilemma of caring. When we take care of any patient, it requires a certain amount of intellectual and psychological energy. The needier the patient, the more their suffering can pull on our emotions, draining us of the enthusiasm to keep caring for others. When we hear a story of great suffering, we often experience it as a sense of anguish in ourselves, which we eventually seek to avoid. How many of us have said that we don't want to hear any more really awful stories from patients right now because we are unable to get rid of the images and emotions? Indeed, we often feel caught between sharing their anguish – and overwhelming ourselves in the process – or

intentionally shutting out their pain, which makes us feel distant and unconcerned. At some point, this dilemma becomes a Catch 22: the only way we can care more for patients is to not care as much for an individual patient.

In order for our compassion to be stable and expansive, we would need to be able to understand the suffering of others, but not internalize it ourselves. We would need to be able to have the desire to ease that suffering, but not experience that as a burden. How can we find this middle ground?

If we look closely at ourselves, we can discover that we are most compassionate when we are most relaxed. When our minds are relaxed and undistracted by prior or future personal issues that can make us irritable, angry, or sad, we are better equipped to focus on the patient's problems. The patient experiences the relaxed, compassionate attention of the caregiver as a sure sign that the caregiver is present and willing to help.

If it's true that we are most compassionate when we are relaxed, then one way of stabilizing our compassion would be to learn how to relax. What does it actually mean to relax? If we try to relax our body, and our mind remains tense and distracted, we don't call that being relaxed. In order to be truly relaxed, we need to have a relaxed mind. Ordinarily, the only way we know how to relax our mind is to go on holiday – to get away from it all. If we have a successful holiday, we can come back relaxed, but it tends to wear off fairly quickly.

What prevents our mind from feeling relaxed? It is nothing other than our intrusive thoughts and emotions: anger, attachment, indifference, along with hope and fear. For most of us, we need to admit that our minds are just ready to feel upset. We can be feeling completely fine, and then a comment, some bad news, a new worry comes, and we can't shake the emotional reaction. If we could train to let go of these intrusive thoughts and emotions as they arise, we would be better able to maintain a sense of equilibrium, a feeling of contentment.

As long as compassion is derived from a conscious effort, it will be unstable, and ready to wear down. The more that compassion derives from a completely relaxed mind, the more stable it will be. In Buddhist philosophy, a distinction is made between these two types of compassion. Conceptual compassion refers to the type of compassion that we are familiar with, in which we become aware of someone in need, and generate the effort to help them. Nonconceptual compassion refers to a type of compassion that is already present in our mind. It doesn't need a particular stimulus to arise. It arises naturally from a mind that is free of negative emotions.

As mentioned earlier, it is easy to care about people we know and love, and who care about us. It is more difficult to care about strangers, and it is most difficult to care about people who give us trouble or cause us harm. But if we think about the people we admire for their compassion, it is all encompassing, unselective. One way to achieve this type of compassion is to train the mind in a profound form of relaxation that allows us to remain aware, but free from disturbing thoughts and emotions. The fully realized version of this type of compassion can only be achieved through personal instruction by someone who has already realized this natural state of mind. However, one can begin to achieve results through practicing specific forms of meditation.

There are, fortunately, more immediately available ways of training one's compassion. In the Buddhist tradition, someone who undertakes to improve one's compassion in a determined and courageous way is called a bodhisattva. The training of a bodhisattva is based on developing six major virtues. These virtues can be useful to apply to the practice of medicine as well.

The first virtue is generosity. When we practice medicine, it automatically implies that we will be giving of ourselves. To be more compassionate, we need to try to expand this giving quality, to be willing to do whatever is necessary to help our patients. Not just to treat them with appropriate medicine, but to be there in a way that comforts the sick person.

The second virtue is pure ethics. This refers to cultivating the willingness to do what is right without any hesitation – to be conscientious and to try to avoid being careless, lazy, or frustrated.

The third virtue is tolerance. Tolerance is necessary because patients can sometimes be challenging to deal with. Either their problems seem overwhelming, or their attitude is one of aggression or anger, or they appear incapable or unwilling to follow your recommendations. In all these situations, it is easy to lose patience and want to stop caring for such a person. We need to realize that many patients who act badly toward their caregivers are actually scared, or feeling desperate, or are in a state of panic. In this situation, you need to apply tolerance, to try to understand their situation and not take it personally. Perhaps someone else can be consulted. You need to try to maintain your caring attitude. That is the meaning of tolerance.

The fourth virtue is perseverance. This refers to the willingness to carry through. This can either be done as a sense of duty, feeling that we have no choice, or it could be accomplished with a sense of joy, a feeling of truly wanting to help the other person, to ease the suffering. The term for this kind of perseverance is *joyous diligence*. Being able to help heal someone is intrinsically good. It is a very pure way of easing suffering. Therefore, it makes sense to take joy in that activity, to gain some satisfaction from the effort one has made.

The fifth virtue is cultivating pure concentration. This means that one tries not to get distracted, to avoid making errors, as best as one can. The toil is to try to keep in mind all of the important issues in caring for someone, and not get careless.

The sixth virtue is to cultivate a specific kind of open-minded intelligence, a kind of wisdom. This type of wisdom is closely associated with cultivating a relaxed, open mind. One of the obstacles to seeing clearly, for example, might be professional pride. One may believe too much in one's own ability, and not feel comfortable consulting others when it might be appropriate to do so. One may feel jealous of others, and try to compete with them through diagnosis and treatment skills. One may feel insecure, and not want others to know that one has doubts. Wisdom means seeing through those emotions and being able to do what is best for one's patient, without worrying about what others think of oneself.

All of these virtues are achieved more easily if one cultivates a relaxed mind. However, thinking about these specific virtues can help encourage one and remind oneself of how one ultimately wants to be when taking care of others.

Since none of us, at present, has perfect compassion and wisdom, it would be foolish to act as if we did. We all get tired and frustrated. By actively training in compassion, we are trying to push back the point at which we may feel like giving up. If our motivation is to relieve suffering, we must remember that suffering is both physical and mental, and patients who are making it difficult for us may be suffering from emotional disturbances that they can't handle. When confronted with difficult patients, we need to put on what Chokyi Nyima Rinpoche calls 'our armor of patience.' Let the armor absorb the anger and fear of the patient, while we keep trying to be as compassionate as possible.

However, we must keep in mind that we all have our limits, and if we reach a point where we feel that we have tried our best and just can't do any more, it is sensible to recognize that we have reached our limit and try to step out of the situation. We want to help the other person, but we can see that it is not happening at the moment. If we have truly tried our best, we can take satisfaction in that effort. It may still be possible to arrange for someone else to step in and try to help this person. But it is important not to feel defeated or disappointed because we couldn't solve every situation. The important thing is to maintain our motivation to try, and to recognize when further pushing of ourselves will not help the patient and will only start to hurt ourselves as well.

When we begin to think about being more compassionate with patients, we need to distinguish between just acting as if we are more compassionate, and genuinely having a more compassionate attitude. Acting as if we are compassionate has been encouraged in a recent review article.[10] Although acting more compassionate is preferable to not acting compassionate at all, we need to remember that patients who are very ill are also very sensitive. They can quickly determine whether a caregiver genuinely cares about him or her, or whether they have adopted a 'bedside manner.' It is incredibly more powerful – and in the long run much easier – to cultivate a genuinely compassionate attitude.

An issue related more specifically to taking care of refugees and immigrants is trying to comprehend the suffering that so many people in the world are forced to endure. When people are uprooted, attacked, imprisoned, tortured, or forced to suffer from the horrors of war, how are we to help them deal with their trauma? Although there is much literature on how to help deal with post-traumatic stress disorder, it is also important to spend time trying to personally understand why things happen the way they do.

In the Judeo-Christian tradition it has long been a dilemma, even a challenge to one's faith, to try to understand why a compassionate and all-powerful God would allow suffering to occur. If one has faith in God, one learns to accept suffering as a test of faith, or at least a test of one's understanding, in that we may not comprehend God's plan.[11]

For those who don't have faith in God, or don't believe that God has power over everything that happens on this planet, it can be difficult to understand evil and suffering. Buddhist philosophy expresses the idea that what happens to us in the present is the result of actions committed during an endless string of past lives. This law of cause and effect is called *karma*. In the West, we express a somewhat similar belief, but we call it 'luck.' Good things

happen because a person had 'good luck.' Bad things happen because a person had 'bad luck.' But we stop short of trying to comprehend why one person had good luck and the other had bad luck. Karma is an attempt to understand the cause of good or bad luck.

In any case, it can be useful to try to understand – and accept – that bad things can happen to people, and our only recourse is to try to help relieve their suffering. If we are able to find a way to understand the causes of suffering, then each new traumatic situation that we confront will not cause us to question our own core beliefs. We will be able to absorb the suffering more skillfully, and keep our focus on the patient.

The only way that the world will see a decrease in senseless suffering and horror is when the desire to relieve suffering and promote happiness begins to outweigh the greed, anger, and revenge that spur our current conflicts. In a practical way, we can't insist that others be more compassionate than ourselves. We need to cultivate a good heart, and have confidence that the capacity of the mind is such that a good heart can have influence on others. Although at the moment the concept that one could become a completely compassionate and wise being may seem hopelessly out of reach, the sincere desire to start on a path towards this goal will have immense rewards. As with any other important endeavor, the extent to which we succeed will be proportional to the amount of effort we put into it.

# References

1. Moeller SD. Compassion fatigue: how the media sell disease, famine, war and death. New York: Routledge; 1999:22.
2. Porter R. The greatest benefit to mankind: a medical history of humanity. New York: W.W. Norton; 1997:683.
3. Harrington A. A science of compassion or a compassionate science? What do we expect from a cross-cultural dialogue with Buddhism? In: Davidson RJ, Harrington A, eds. Visions of compassion: Western scientists and Tibetan Buddhists examine human nature. Oxford: Oxford University Press; 2002:20.
4. Branch WT Jr, Kern D, Haidet P, et al. The patient–physician relationship. Teaching the human dimensions of care in clinical settings. JAMA. 2001; 286:1067–1074.
5. Green MJ. What (if anything) is wrong with residency overwork? Ann Internal Med 1995; 123:512–517.
6. Rinpoche CN, Shlim DR. Medicine and compassion: a Tibetan lama's guidance for caregivers. Boston: Wisdom; 2004:136.
7. Ruse M. A Darwinian naturalist's perspective on altruism. In: Post SG, Underwood LG, Schloss JP, et al., eds. Altruism and altruistic love: science, philosophy and religion in dialogue. Oxford: Oxford University Press; 2002:151–167.
8. Sober E. Kindness and cruelty in evolution. In: Davidson RJ, Harrington A, eds. Visions of compassion: Western

scientists and Tibetan Buddhists examine human nature. Oxford: Oxford University Press; 2002:46–65.

9. Browning DS. Science and religion on the nature of love. In: Post SG, Underwood LG, Schloss JP, et al., eds. Altruism and altruistic love: science, philosophy and religion in dialogue. Oxford: Oxford University Press; 2002:337–338.

10. Larsen EB, Yao X. Clinical empathy as emotional labor in the patient–physician relationship. JAMA 2005; 293:1100–1106.

11. Melling DJ. Suffering and sanctification in Christianity. In: Hinnells JR, Porter R, eds. Religion, health and suffering. London: Kegan Paul; 1999:48.

# CHAPTER 3

# Health and Well-being of Immigrants:
## *The Healthy Migrant Phenomenon*

Katherine Fennelly

## Introduction

A growing body of literature describes what has come to be known as the 'healthy migrant' phenomenon – the fact that, on a variety of measures, immigrants to the United States,[1-5] Canada,[6,7] Australia,[8] and Western Europe[9,10] are often healthier than native-born residents in their new countries of residence. Over time, however, the migrant health advantage diminishes dramatically.

Health status is the sum of a complex set of factors, with wide variability within and across groups. Nevertheless, researchers have noted some interesting trends in comparisons of the health status of US- and foreign-born residents. While immigrants to the United States do have higher rates of some infectious diseases than native-born residents, on measures of health risks, chronic conditions, and mortality they are generally better off. Singh and Siahpush[3] used data from the National Longitudinal Mortality Study (1979–1989) and found that immigrant men and women had significantly lower risks of mortality than their US-born counterparts. Jasso et al.[5] pooled National Health Interview Survey data between 1991 and 1996 and examined chronic conditions by year since immigration and by age of immigrants; they found that prevalence rates of chronic conditions for immigrants were much lower than those for the US-born. Similarly, Muennig and Fahs[4] compared hospital utilization and mortality rates of foreign-born and US-born residents in New York City, and concluded that immigrants were healthier and had significantly longer life

expectancies than natives. They estimated that the over-all cost of providing hospital-based care to the foreign-born residents in New York would be US$611 million less than care for an equivalent number of US-born persons in 1996. Dey and Lucas[11] calculated adjusted odds ratios of selected chronic diseases using National Health Survey data on over 196 000 respondents from 1997 to 2002, and found that foreign-born residents had lower levels of obesity, hypertension, diabetes, cardiovascular disease, and serious psychological distress than US-born residents. Other researchers have suggested that superior health may be one of the reasons for lower healthcare expenditures by immigrants, even when they are covered by health insurance.[12] Mohanty et al.[12] linked 1998 medical expenditure data to 21 241 records from the 1996–1997 National Health Interview Survey and found that the per capita health expenditures of immigrants were 55% less than those of US-born individuals, even after controlling for health insurance coverage. They note that their findings debunk the commonly held myth that immigrants consume large amounts of scarce health resources.

Kandula et al.[13] performed a comprehensive review of the literature published on the health of immigrants between 1996 and 2003, and summarized findings on the ten 'Leading Health Indicators' defined as goals for 'Healthy People 2010.' They reviewed literature on the health of foreign-born residents, and when data by place of birth were unavailable, they included studies of Latinos in the US. They caution that some comparisons of immigrants and the native-born yield contradictory or mixed results (for example, comparative studies of physical activity, sexual activity, injury, and violence), and on measures of levels of immunization and access to care, US-born residents do better. However, immigrants had superior health outcomes on measures of obesity, smoking, alcohol, and drug abuse, and each of these indicators worsened with increasing time in the US. Similarly, in a review of the national literature for which comparative data are available, Fennelly[14] found that foreign-born residents did better than the US-born residents on 12 of the 14 goals specified by the Minnesota Department of Health to eliminate health disparities. These included infant mortality, breast and cervical cancer, sexually transmitted diseases, HIV, heart disease, diabetes, teen pregnancy, unintentional injury, suicide, homicide, motor vehicle accidents, tobacco use, and alcohol use. The exception is immunization rates of foreign-born children. Children under age 3 had lower rates of Hib and hepatitis B vaccinations than US-born children. Some comparative data were not available, notably comparative rates of HIV and AIDS (according to the HIV/AIDS Bureau of the Health Research and Services Administration of the US Department of Health and Human Services);[15] and comparative data on motor vehicle accidents were not found, although it is likely that foreign-born residents have lower motor vehicle mortality rates because they are less likely to use motor vehicles. (This is the case for US Hispanics compared to non-Hispanic whites, although data are not available distinguishing US- and foreign-born Hispanics.[16])

Although not all Latinos are foreign born, studies of Latino health add to our understanding of changes in health status as individuals become more acculturated to US society. Lara et al.[17] conducted an extensive review of the literature and found that on some measures acculturation had a negative, a positive, or no effect on health, but that it exerted a positive effect on use of health services and self-perceptions of health. (This effect is likely to be attenuated in more recent studies because of the increase in numbers of undocumented Latinos who are ineligible for all but emergency services). The authors go on to conclude that 'the strongest evidence points toward a negative effect of acculturation on health behaviors overall, particularly those related to substance abuse, diet and birth outcomes (low birthweight and prematurity) – among Latinos living in the United States.' It is the focus of attention on these increasingly negative outcomes and disparities between Hispanics and non-Hispanic whites (for example) that prevents many health providers from recognizing the initial health advantage of immigrants.

One area in which immigrants may not enjoy health advantages is in the incidence of depression or other mental health conditions. Research comparing the mental health of immigrants and native-born adults leads to ambiguous conclusions. Some studies show more mental health problems among immigrants, while other suggest that they are less likely to suffer from mental health conditions. Hyman,[6] for example, cites studies demonstrating that Mexican immigrants have significantly lower rates of post-traumatic stress disorder (PTSD) and depression than US-born Mexicans. This may not be the case for other groups of immigrants. A number of researchers suggest, for example, that refugees are at high risk for mental health problems as a result of exposure to deprivation, violence, and forced migration.[18]

The healthy migrant phenomenon has also been observed in Western Europe[9,10,19] and Canada.[6] Hyman, of Health Canada, for example, conducted an extensive review of the literature on immigration and health and concluded that 'in Canada national health survey data show that recent immigrants, particularly from non-European countries, are in better health than their Canadian-born counterparts.'

The superior health of immigrants seems particularly counter-intuitive because of the poor health conditions in many of their countries of origin, and because of recent public attention to well-documented and significant health disparities between majority and minority populations in the United States. Two factors are operating to produce these contradictions. First, immigrants who leave their home countries tend to be healthier than those who remain at home.[5] Second, after migration to the US they experience a decline in health status over time, i.e. a marked deterioration in some indicators of immigrant health after settlement, and with each successive generation (see, for example Harris,[20] CAMS,[21] Hernandez,[22] LaVeist,[23] Razum et al.[9]). In what Rumbaut[24] calls the 'paradox of assimilation,' length of time in the US is positively correlated with increases in low birth weight infants,[2,25] adolescent risk behaviors,[20,26] cancer,[27] anxiety and depression,[28] and general mortality.[3,4]

Another reason for public misperceptions regarding immigrant health stems from disproportionate attention to serious, but low incidence and well-publicized conditions that affect immigrants, such as tuberculosis and other infectious diseases. Refugees represent a subgroup of immigrants who are at particularly high risk of tuberculosis (TB).[6] Although rates for immigrants are higher than for US-born individuals, tuberculosis case rates for both groups have dropped dramatically since 1992 as a result of increases in the proportion of patients who receive and complete treatment regimens.[29] The highest tuberculosis rates are found among immigrants to the US from Central and South America and the Caribbean and Western Pacific countries.[29]

## Explanations of the Healthy Migrant Effect

As mentioned earlier, Jasso et al.[5] argue that migration is selective on health, namely that individuals who migrate are a self-selected group who are much healthier than individuals in their home countries. Subsequent declines in health with time in the US can be seen as a natural 'regression to the mean.' The gradual changes from immigrant health advantages to disparities has been ascribed to 'acculturation' to an American lifestyle, raising the question of what acculturation actually means, and how it affects health. The research literature includes many different measures of acculturation, including English language proficiency, country of origin, time in the US, or scores on a variety of acculturation scales.

Noh and Kaspar[30] give a broad explanation of the loss of migrant health advantage that includes widely varying implicit definitions of acculturation:

> The more 'they' become like 'us,' immigrants and immigrant children fail to maintain their initial health advantages. The process is poorly understood, but may be the result of the adoption of our poor health behaviors and life styles, leaving behind resources (social networks, cultural practices, employment in their field of training, etc.), and ways in which the settlement process wears down hardiness and resilience.[30]

Researchers such as Hunt et al.[31] call for greater measurement precision. They point out that many studies of acculturation suffer from inadequate definitions of the construct, and – what is worse – simplistic and largely untested notions of 'traditional' culture as negative (in the literature on Hispanic health, which is their focus, this is manifested in assumptions regarding the negative effects of machismo and traditional gender roles) or positive (as in assumptions regarding the positive effects of religiosity or strong family values on health outcomes). The authors suggest that such untested assumptions may result from acceptance of cultural stereotypes:

> In reading through this body of literature one is continually struck by the juxtaposition of careful psychometric measurements, on the one hand, and such free-wheeling, meanderings about the supposed effect of unexamined cultural traits, on the other. Can the granting of such interpretive license in an otherwise rigorous genre be an indication of insidious acceptance of cultural stereotypes?[31]

## Additional explanations of the loss of the migrant health advantage

### Poverty

Vague hypotheses regarding the 'protective effects of culture' divert attention from inequalities in health access and healthcare, and the ways in which poverty leads to health risks and barriers to care among both immigrants and native-born minorities, through inadequate housing, stresses that lead to mental health problems, and adoption of unhealthy diets.

Such disparities are particularly pronounced among immigrants. Sixteen percent of foreign-born and 11% of US-born residents in the United States were living below the poverty line in 2002.[32] The percentage of immigrants in poverty varies greatly by national origin group and educational levels, but regardless of national origin, non-citizens are much more likely than citizens to be poor, even though they are equally likely to participate in the labor force.[33] Poverty levels differ for immigrants of different origins and legal statuses, and immigrants are over-represented in both high-skilled and low-skilled jobs. The largest group – Hispanic immigrants – have very high labor force participation rates, but many are relegated to low-paying jobs that offer few or no benefits. In contrast with Latinos, most Southeast Asians, Africans, Russians, and Eastern Europeans initially came to the US as refugees, or as immigrants sponsored by family members who were refugees or asylees. For these individuals the trauma of forced evacuation may make it difficult to find or maintain employment, and government bureaucratic delays in establishing eligibility for benefits may exacerbate or even cause poverty.

### Housing

One consequence of poverty is poor housing, and the lack of adequate and affordable housing has important implications for immigrant health, since over half of severely crowded households in the US are inhabited by foreign-born residents.[34] Although inadequate housing can contribute to stress and illness for all low-income residents, immigrants are especially vulnerable because of barriers of language, large family size, and their concentration in ethnic enclaves. Housing is linked to health in a variety of ways. Substandard housing can be a direct cause of accidents and physical ailments, as well as an indirect source of health problems related to barriers to receipt of services, and a barrier to stable employment and schooling. In a recent study of children in homeless shelters in New York City, McLean et al.[35] found that half of the children had symptoms consistent with asthma. They attribute this extremely high incidence to both environmental risks and to the social disruption caused when families are isolated from transportation, friends, schools, and medical services. A public health nurse in a Minnesota study described the ways in which lack of stable housing can limit access to education and health or social services.

> If children do not reside in one long-term location, going to school becomes an issue. Moving from place to place makes it more difficult to access services that may be available, such as ESL classes. Having a command of the English language is key to being able to access opportunities which may lead to a more stable life. If you don't have access to affordable housing, everything else becomes more difficult.[14]

Evans and Wells[36] have reviewed a number of studies affirming an association between housing and mental health in the general population, and Magaña and Hovey[37] have described similar links among Latino farm workers in the Midwest. In the latter study, 'rigid work demands and poor housing conditions' were associated with high levels of anxiety.

Undocumented residents and refugees have particular difficulties establishing the credit history necessary to be able to sign a lease or qualify for a mortgage. Migrant workers who travel seasonally also face special obstacles to securing affordable short-term leases. Furthermore, the fact that immigrants in general have larger families and lower incomes than do US-born adults makes it difficult for them to find suitable, affordable housing. Immigrants are also particularly susceptible to housing discrimination, either because they are unaware of their rights, or because they fear reprisals for reporting substandard housing conditions or exploitation by landlords.

## Acculturative stress

For immigrants and refugees alike, mental health problems can be caused or aggravated by the stresses of adaptation to an unfamiliar society. Depression is a common problem, especially among the elderly and the poor. Problems of job loss, unemployment and underemployment, language barriers, isolation, discrimination, and the Americanization and alienation of children are only a few of the causes of what has been termed 'acculturative stress.'

Refugees undergo health screening before being admitted to the United States, but mental health screening is often inadequate. Nationally, many refugee health programs do not perform routine mental health screening. Vergara et al.[38] surveyed nine large metropolitan refugee health programs across the US and found that only one-third performed mental status examinations, although over two-thirds offered some mental health services. A provider in Minnesota has noted that:

> The mental status exam that is used was actually developed to screen for dementia and delirium, not mental health issues. It is so culturally based as to be useless for immigrant populations. Items include counting backwards from 100 by 7s, spelling 'world' backwards, drawing a clock with hands, defining some sayings like 'A bird in hand is worth 2 in the bush,' and completing analogies such as 'eye is to seeing as ear is to ••' (Councilman R: personal communication. 2004).

The stigma of acknowledging mental health problems poses a significant barrier to help seeking on the part of some groups of immigrants. In some cultures, psychological problems – if they are recognized at all – are attributed to somatic ills.

## Nutrition

Changes in diet are frequently mentioned as behaviors that account for some of the loss of initial health advantages among immigrants who remain in the US. A prepublication report of work by Akresh[39] describes the deteriorating nutritional status of US immigrants over time. She found that 39% of a sample of 6637 foreign-born adults reported increased consumption of junk food and meat, higher body mass indices (BMI) and decreased consumption of healthy foods, such as fruits, vegetables, fish, and rice since arrival in the US.

Acculturation to an unhealthy American diet is associated with obesity, diabetes, and cancer.[40] Mazur et al.[41] discuss the ways in which time in the US increases the risk of obesity and chronic disease among Mexican-American adults because of increased consumption of fat, decreased consumption of fiber, and reduced physical activity. They describe the generally more nutritious diet of first-generation Hispanics as 'culture-based protection against adverse health effects normally associated with low income.' Similarly, Fishman et al.[42] found that Latino migrant children were less likely to eat junk food or to skip meals than their non-migrant peers, but that, over time, these differences disappeared.

## Substance abuse

Several studies have shown that rates of smoking and substance abuse among the foreign-born increase over time. For example, Gfroerer and Tan[43] analyzed data from the National Household Survey of Drug Abuse and found lower rates of tobacco, alcohol, and illicit drug use among immigrant youth, but increasing rates with greater time in the US. They speculate that 'acculturation' increases exposure to peers, adults, and mass media that could influence a youth's propensity to use substances.

## Access to care

Barriers to access to healthcare in the US have been strongly implicated as a source of increasing health disparities between immigrants and native-born residents. Riedel[44] notes that access is a problem facing all vulnerable populations in the United States, and one which health policy makers, administrators, and consumers have decried for over 30 years. The problems are particularly acute for the foreign born. In 1996, Congress passed a comprehensive welfare bill known as 'The Personal Responsibility and Work Opportunity Reconciliation Act of 1996' (PRWORA). Under the provisions of PRWORA, public assistance was denied to most legal immigrants for 5 years or until they attain citizenship. Some states enacted legislation permitting some groups of immigrants, such as refugees, time-limited access to benefits.[45] Nevertheless, as a consequence of federal and state welfare reform, there have been major reductions in legal immigrants' use of social and health benefit programs across the United States.[46] These declines coincide with increases in poverty among the children of immigrants, many of whom were born in the United States.[47] Poor citizens in the US are twice as likely as poor non-citizens to

have health insurance.[48] Recognizing this, a large number of providers have called for changes in federal and state policies regarding welfare and health benefits for immigrants.

The Kaiser Commission[33] reports that in 1999, of 9.8 million low-income non-citizens, almost 59% had no health insurance, and only 15 percent received Medicaid', (compared with 30% uninsured low-income citizens and 28% with Medicaid).

Low levels of insurance coverage for immigrants are mainly the result of two factors. First, although foreign-born residents have high rates of labor force participation, they are over-represented in jobs that do not provide health insurance. Second, federal and state legislative changes tied to Welfare Reform have resulted in severe restrictions on immigrant eligibility for Medicaid and other benefits. Restrictions are most severe for undocumented immigrants, largely Latinos.[46] Since September 11, 2001, exclusion of immigrants from access to healthcare has grown worse. In 2005, 80 bills were proposed in 20 states to cut immigrants' access to services or to require divulging their visa status to providers.[49] Although many of these proposals were not adopted, a surge of new restrictive bills has followed. As of this writing, Congress is considering legislation that would make unauthorized presence in the US or assistance to undocumented individuals a felony.

Not all of the increase in negative health outcomes among immigrants who remain in the US can be ascribed to limited access to care; there are a number of immeasurable variables in comparisons of health outcomes for immigrants, including an unknown number of individuals who enter the US and subsequently return to their home countries.[5] Furthermore, income and access to healthcare increase over time in the US, and both of these variables are important determinants of positive health.[5] In their review of the literature on acculturation and health, Lara et al.[17] found several studies showing that more-acculturated Latinos have greater access to services and higher rates of use of health services, but still demonstrate higher rates of substance abuse, poor nutrition, and worse birth outcomes than Latinos who have lived in the country for a shorter period of time. The paradoxical finding that some health indicators worsen in spite of increased access to healthcare suggests that the effects of acculturation on health cannot be explained by simple bivariate associations. Observing the same phenomenon in Canada, McDonald and Kennedy[7] speculate that with increased use of the health system recent immigrants may become more likely to be diagnosed with chronic conditions, although they note that available data do not support this hypothesis. Alternatively, it may be that immigrants' self-definitions of what constitutes 'good health' change over time in the country. Another likely explanation is that the effects of access on health interact with other characteristics of poverty and vary for particular groups. Finch et al.[50] for example, analyzed survey data from 1000 adult migrant farm workers in California and found that acculturation led to lower self-ratings of health among the most acculturated farm workers. They hypothesize that these individuals may be more vested in American society, and thus more vulnerable to the stresses of adaptation and language, or – alternatively – that the more highly acculturated individuals were demonstrating the negative health effects of longer periods of exposure to stressful and harmful conditions.

## Recommendations for Providers

What can healthcare providers do to maintain the initial advantages of first-generation immigrants and prevent the subsequent deterioration of their health? In the following section, we present a series of recommendations based upon the literature summarized in this chapter.

1. Help to dispel myths regarding the inferior health of the foreign born, and to publicly acknowledge to immigrants and US-born colleagues the positive practices that account for the healthy migrant phenomenon.

2. Effective, holistic care requires attention to the ways in which poverty reduces the health and life chances for all categories of patients. Conscientious providers need to be good listeners, and to be attentive to problems related to employment, education, child rearing, housing, and discrimination. Healthcare that does not take these external factors into account will be ineffectual.

3. Some barriers to health care and treatment can be overcome with the assistance of trained, qualified, bicultural interpreters. In addition to the obvious importance of interpreters in facilitating effective communication, these staff members can be effective 'cultural translators' for both providers and patients. Although the US Department of Health and Human Services requires agencies receiving federal funds to provide assistance to clients with limited English proficiency, such policies are unevenly implemented.[33]

4. Seek out opportunities for cross-cultural training for yourself and your colleagues. Begin by recognizing the limitations of Western medical models of health, and the educational benefits of exposure to alternate ways of conceptualizing the causes and treatment of disease. Study the backgrounds, culture, and traditions of your patients. Educate yourself regarding conditions in your patients' home countries, and the kinds of trauma to which some may have been subjected. Never underestimate the challenges of being a *consumer* of care (in the Western sense), and of seeking help in an unfamiliar environment. Recognize that many of your patients are likely to be unfamiliar with appointment systems, health insurance regulations, compliance with medical recommendations, and standard use of medications. Maintain an open mind regarding alternative health beliefs and treatments that may be more familiar to some of your patients. To the extent possible, make accommodations for different ideas of modesty and gender roles.

5. Regulations regarding eligibility for services for various categories of immigrants are extraordinarily complex and commonly misunderstood by patients and providers alike. Take steps to insure that your clients are not denied services for which they are eligible, or reluctant to come in for care because of the belief that their confidentiality and security will be violated. Take it upon yourself to educate your provider colleagues regarding the complexities of eligibility and barriers that they pose to immigrants.

6. Remember that there is more diversity within any national origin group than between any two groups of immigrants, or between immigrants and non-immigrants. Avoid making assumptions or generalizations about the beliefs, needs, or characteristics of your immigrant clients. At the same time, providers serving immigrants need to be conscious of the stresses associated with migration and acculturation to a new environment.

7. Consider what you can do to help dispel the myths about immigrants that are prevalent among many native-born citizens and elected officials. Misperceptions and xenophobia contribute to acculturative stress and also drive many of the policies that have severely curtailed access to healthcare and social benefits among immigrants in the United States.

8. Help other providers and healthcare administrators understand that working with immigrant patients requires *additional time* to follow the recommendations outlined above: careful listening, improved communication, development of trust, careful and accurate interpretation, and assistance navigating an unfamiliar healthcare system.

## Conclusion

The general public, and even many healthcare providers, share a common misperception regarding immigrant health. The marked health disparities between Hispanics and non-Hispanics, for example, obscure the fact that, on many measures, first-generation immigrants arrive in the US in better health than native-born Americans. As described in the present chapter, it is post-immigration experiences and poverty that lead to tangible stresses and risk factors that compromise health and well-being.

The notion that poverty and discrimination impede access to care and affect health status is not new. There is a substantial and growing literature demonstrating the extent to which poor Americans have reduced access to care and poor health outcomes. In addition to the recommendations for individual providers, the present research leads to a clear set of logical public policy recommendations that are, unfortunately, unlikely to be implemented. As Rank[51] has noted, the high prevalence of poverty in the United States is the result of a lack of national will to address the issue, rather than a lack of resources. His general statement that 'blaming the poor for poverty "lets us off the hook" ' is particularly relevant to the foreign born. For immigrants, the effects of poverty are compounded by discriminatory legislation mandating reductions to and denial of access even for many legal immigrants. The problems are especially acute for Latinos. Although Latino immigrants generally have very high rates of labor force participation, many of these workers are in low-wage jobs that do not offer benefits. Nationally, for example, the Hispanic uninsured rate is the highest of any racial or ethnic group.[27]

The policy implications of the healthy migrant phenomenon are significant. First, it belies the arguments of some anti-immigrant groups that immigrants pose a health threat to Americans. Second, it illustrates that the most economically sound policies would be to invest in services to maintain the good health of this important and growing segment of the population, rather than to continue to cut benefits and create barriers to preventive care. To do otherwise will prove far more costly in the long run.

## References

1. Neria J. Maternal child health risks of women from Latin America. vol. 2003: APHA The Maternal and Child Health Community Leadership Institute; 2000.
2. Fuentes-Afflick E, Hessol NA, Perez-Stable E. Testing the epidemiologic paradox of low birth weight in Latinos. Arch Pediatr Adolesc Med 1999; 153:147–153.
3. Singh GK, Siahpush M. All-cause and cause-specific mortality of immigrants and native born in the United States. Am J Public Health 2001; 91(3):392–399.
4. Muennig P, Fahs M. Health status and hospital utilization among immigrants to New York City. Prevent Med 2002; 35:225–231.
5. Jasso G, Massey DS, Rosenzweig MR, et al. Immigrant health: selectivity and acculturation. In: Anderson NB, Bulatao RA, Cohen B, eds. Critical perspectives on racial and ethnic differences in health in late life. vol Panel on Race, ethnicity, and health in later life, National Research Council: National Academy Press; 2004.
6. Hyman I. Immigration and health. Ottawa: Health Canada; 2001.
7. McDonald JT, Kennedy S. Insights into the 'healthy immigrant effect': health status and health service use of immigrants to Canada. Social Sci Med 2004; 59:1613–1627.
8. Australian Institute of Health and Welfare: Australia's Health 2000. Canberra: 2000.
9. Razum O, Zeeb H, Rohrmann. The 'healthy migrant effect' – not merely a fallacy of inaccurate denominator figures. Internat J Epidemiol 2000; 21:199–200.
10. Toma L. Immigration phenomenon and right to health in Italy. Metropolis Conference, Rotterdam, 2001.
11. Dey AN, Lucas J. Physical and mental health characteristics of USS- and foreign-born adults: United States, 1998–2003. Advance Data from Vital Health Statistics, 369.
12. Mohanty S, Woolhandler S, Himmelstein D, et al. Health care expenditures of immigrants in the United States: A nationally representative analysis. Am J Public Health 2005; 95(8):1431–1438.
13. Kandula NR, Kersey M, Lurie N. Assuring the health of immigrants: what the leading health indicators tell us. Annual Review of Public Health 25:357–376, 2004.
14. Fennelly K. Listening to the experts: provider recommendations on the health needs of immigrants and refugees. J Cultural Diversity 2006; 13(4).
15. US Department of Health and Human Services. Foreign-born populations in the US: HIV/AIDS. Reports and Statistics; September, 2003.
16. Braver E. Race, Hispanic origin, and socioeconomic status in relation to motor vehicle occupant death rates and risk factors among adults. Acc Anal Prev 2003; 35(3):295–309.
17. Lara M, Gamboa C, Kahramanian MI, et al. Acculturation and Latino health in the United States: A review of the literature and the sociopolitical context. Ann Rev Public Health 2005; 26:367–397.
18. Palinkas LA, Pickwell SM, Brandstein K, et al. The journey to wellness: stages of refugee health promotion and disease prevention. J Immigrant Health 2003; 5(1):19–28.
19. Swerdlow AJ. Mortality and cancer incidence in Vietnamese refugees in England and Wales: a follow-up study. Internat J Epidemiol 1991; 20:10–13.
20. Harris KM. The health status and risk behaviors of adolescents in immigrant families. In: Hernandez DJ, ed. Children of immigrants. Washington, DC: National Academy Press, 1999:286–315.
21. Chinese American Medical Society (CAMS). Cancers in Asian-Americans and Pacific Islanders: migrant studies. Chinese American Medical Society; 1999.

22. Hernandez DJ. Children of immigrants: health, adjustment and public finance. In: Hernandez DJ, ed. Children of immigrants. Washington, DC: National Academy Press; 1999:1–17.

23. LaVeist T. Race, Ethnicity, and health: a public health Reader. New York: Jossey-Bass; 2002.

24. Rumbaut R. Paradoxes of assimilation. Sociological Perspectives 1997; 40(3):483–511.

25. Peak C, Weeks J. Does community context influence reproductive outcomes of Mexican-origin women in San Diego, California? J Immigrant Health 2002; 4:3.

26. Hernandez DaEC. From generation to generation: the health and well-being of children in immigrant families. Washington, DC: National Academy Press; 1998.

27. Institute of Medicine BoHSPH: unequal treatment: confronting racial and ethnic disparities in health care. Washington, DC: National Academy Press; 2002.

28. Finch BK, Vega WA. Acculturation stress, social support, and self-rated health among Latinos in California. J Immigrant Health 2003; 5(3):109–117.

29. Centers for Disease Control and Prevention. Tuberculosis morbidity among US-born and foreign-born populations: United States, 2000. MMWR 2002; 51(5):101–110.

30. Noh S, Kaspar V. Diversity and immigrant health. Toronto: University of Toronto; 2003.

31. Hunt LM, Schneider S, Comer B. Should 'acculturation' be a variable in health research? A critical review of research on US Hispanics. Social Sci Med 2004; 59:973–986.

32. Martin P, Midgley E. Immigration: shaping and reshaping America. Population Bulletin 2003; 58(2).

33. Kaiser Commission on Medicaid and the Uninsured: Immigrants' Health Care Coverage and Access. Kaiser Foundation; 2003.

34. Myers D, Baer W, Choi S-Y. The changing problem of overcrowded housing. J Amer Planning Assoc 1996; 62(Winter):66–84.

35. McLean DE, Bowen S, Drezner K, et al. Asthma among homeless children. Arch Pediatr Adolesc Med 2004; 158:244–249.

36. Evans GW, Wells NM, Moch A. Housing and mental health: a review of the evidence and a methodological and conceptual critique. J Social Issues 2003; 59(3):475.

37. Magaña CG, Hovey JD. Psychosocial stressors associated with Mexican migrant farmworkers in the Midwest United States. J Immigrant Health 2003; 5(2):75–86.

38. Vergara AE, Miller JM, Martin DR, et al. A survey of refugee health assessments in the United States. J Immigrant Health 2003; 5(2):67–73.

39. Lynn A. Many new immigrants to the US change diets – and not for the better. Urbana-Champagne: News Bureau University of Illinois; 2006.

40. Li FP. Cancers in Asian Americans and Pacific Islanders: migrant studies. Asian American Pacific Island Journal of Health 1998; 6(2):123–129.

41. Mazur RE, Marquis GS, Jensen HH. Diet and food insufficiency among Hispanic youths: acculturation and socioeconomic factors in the third national health and nutrition examination survey. Am J Clin Nutrition 2003; 78(6):1120–1127.

42. Fishman A, Pearson K, Reicks K. Gathering food and nutrition information from migrant farmworker children through in-depth interviews. J Extension 1999; 33:5.

43. Gfroerer JC, Tan LL. Substance use among foreign-born youths in the United States: does the length of residence matter? Am J Public Health 2003; 93(11):1892–1895.

44. Riedel RL. Access to health care. In: Loue S, ed. Handbook of immigrant health. New York: Plenum Press; 1998: 101–124.

45. Tumlin KC, Zimmerman W, Ost J. State snapshots of public benefits for immigrants: a supplemental report to patchwork policies. Washington, DC: The Urban Institute; 1999.

46. Fix M, Passel JS. The scope and impact of welfare reform's immigrant provisions. Washington, DC: The Urban Institute; 2002.

47. Van Hook J. Poverty grows among children of immigrants in US. Migration Information Source 2003(12–1-03). On-line journal.

48. Capps R, Ku LK, Fix M, et al. How are immigrants faring after welfare reform? Washington, DC: The Urban Institute; 2002.

49. Bernstien N. Recourse grows slim for immigrants who fall ill. The New York Times, March 3, 2006.

50. Finch BK, Frank R, Vega WA. Acculturation and acculturation stress: a social-epidemiological approach to Mexican migrant farmworkers' health (1). International Migration Review 2004; 38(1):236.

51. Rank MR. One nation, underprivileged: why American poverty affects us all. New York: Oxford University Press; 2004.

# CHAPTER 4

# Action Steps to Improve the Health of New Americans

Patricia Ohmans

## Introduction

One in 10 Americans is a first-generation immigrant, according to the US Census. Since the earliest days of our nation, when European settlers joined the native population, immigrants have helped make America a more vibrant and productive place to live.

Sadly, many immigrants to the United States are poorly served by national and local health and social service programs, depending on their legal status, their education, their assets, and whether or not they have health insurance. This poor service results in health status disparities between immigrant and non-immigrant populations. The problem is manifested in a variety of ways, among them:

**Incomplete screening and treatment**: Immigrants and refugees need screening and treatment for infectious diseases, chronic conditions such as diabetes, high blood lead levels and depression. Often, they do not get them. As a result, there are higher rates of some illnesses among immigrants and refugees than among non-immigrant groups.

**Inadequate insurance coverage**: Lack of insurance and confusing payment systems discourage many immigrants from seeking the healthcare they need. Blocked from access to healthcare or insurance, many immigrants seek care only in emergency situations. Higher healthcare costs result, for what would have been preventable conditions if they had been treated earlier.

**Lack of cultural and linguistic competence**: Healthcare providers – most from very different cultures than their immigrant patients – may not be aware of significant communication barriers with the people they treat. The distinctly different clinical and social needs of immigrants are often minimized or misunderstood, resulting in lower rates of comprehension and adherence to doctors' orders by immigrant patients.

**Shortage of bilingual and bicultural providers**: Highly trained, bilingual, and capable immigrant healthcare providers are not being integrated into our current healthcare workforce. A waste of human capital occurs, as former physicians and nurses are retrained for other work.

This chapter describes eight important action steps to reduce the barriers to immigrant health described above. The chapter provides a template for broad changes within the healthcare system, with policy and program recommendations to be undertaken by healthcare providers and administrators, policy makers, academic researchers and educators, and immigrant advocates.

These recommendations were developed by the Minnesota Immigrant Health Task Force, a 2-year citizen advisory group to the Department of Health and Department of Human Services, consisting of healthcare providers, academics, policymakers, and immigrant advocates. Patricia Ohmans, MPH, served as the Task Force coordinator; Patricia Walker, MD, DTM&H, was its chairperson.

**Box 4.1**

**The Task Force on Immigrant Health recommends these eight action steps to improve immigrant health**

1. Provide equal access to care for all, regardless of immigration or insurance status.
2. Assess patients' language preference, and healthcare organizations' capacity to provide appropriate care.
3. Recognize different costs of healthcare for recent immigrants.
4. Develop clinical guidelines and best practices orders for immigrant healthcare.
5. Diversify the healthcare workforce to include more immigrant and minority providers.
6. Use trained interpreters.
7. Use bilingual and bicultural community health workers.
8. Train healthcare providers and educate immigrant patients.

The Task Force recommendations address barriers to full health for immigrants in Minnesota, but are applicable nationally, and have been amplified and annotated here to fit a national context (Box 4.1). Some of the recommendations are addressed more thoroughly in other chapters of this text. These are noted.

Sponsored by the Minnesota Department of Health and the Minnesota Department of Human Services, the Minnesota Commissioners' Task Force on Immigrant Health consisted of over 80 representatives from the state's public, private, nonprofit academic, and healthcare sectors, many of them also first-generation immigrants to the state.

The Task Force met every 2 months from July, 2002, to July, 2004, with the following mission: 'To promote quality, comprehensive and culturally competent healthcare for all recent immigrant communities, by effecting change in statewide health delivery systems.' The Task Force utilized two reports from the Institute of Medicine as the framework for its deliberations: 'Crossing the Quality Chasm: A New Health System for the 21st Century' (2001) and 'Unequal Treatment: Confronting Racial and Ethnic Disparities in Health Care' (2003), available at www/iom.edu. The complete report from the Minnesota Immigrant Health Task Force is available at www.health.state.mn.us/divs/idepc/refugee/immigrant

## Action Steps

### 1. Provide equal access to care for all, regardless of immigration or insurance status

The United States is the only developed nation in which healthcare is not universally guaranteed. Nearly 47 million Americans are uninsured and many immigrants are among them. Non-citizens are 7% of the population, but 21% of the uninsured. Their lack of access to healthcare affects us all.[1]

Access to healthcare can be crucial to achieving full health. People who lack insurance are less likely to be offered screening and treatment of many kinds. They are also less likely to benefit from medical advances, even common ones. Use of the latest treatment technology is lowest among the uninsured.[2] Differences in access to care between immigrants and non-immigrants exacerbate these and other health disparities.

Leaving people uninsured is not cost-effective. Uninsured people make greater use of emergency rooms and sometimes delay getting care until they are desperately ill.[3]

Those suffering from infectious and communicable diseases who do not receive early screening and treatment can present a threat to an entire community. Decisions to cut healthcare benefits for immigrants can have unintended and more expensive results, especially when benefits to young children are cut (Box 4.2).

### 2. Assess patients' language preference, and healthcare organizations' capacity to provide appropriate care

Improvements in care for immigrants cannot be documented without data linking immigrant status with health status. Healthcare facilities should also document their capacity to provide good care to immigrants. Healthcare organizations should collect key demographic data, including race/ethnicity, country of origin, and preferred language for interacting with healthcare providers.

Current data on the connection between immigration status and health status are inadequate.[4] The link between minority status, low income, and health disparities is increasingly clear,[5] but there is much missing in our understanding of possible links between health and immigration status or low English proficiency.

**If you are a policy maker, you can:**
Strengthen access to insurance and care for the poor. Immigrants are disproportionately poor and uninsured.

Increase funding for prevention and treatment of communicable diseases such as TB and HIV-AIDS. Screening and early treatment are cost-effective and protect the community at large from serious infectious diseases.

**If you are a healthcare administrator, you can:**
Enforce existing mandates and standards such as the standards for Culturally and Linguistically Appropriate Services (CLAS) issued by the US Department of Health and Human Services.

Allow providers to offer creative alternatives for discounted or free care.

**If you are an educator or researcher, you can:**
Document how cuts in public funding for healthcare affect health outcomes among immigrants and other minority groups.

Document health disparities between immigrants and non-immigrants and their relationship to healthcare access.

Research the impact of equitable access to health insurance and care on health outcomes.

**If you are a healthcare provider, you can:**
Become familiar with public programs that offer healthcare at free or reduced rates, and recommend these to your patients who lack insurance.

Donate a percent of your work time to volunteer or charity care for immigrant patients.

Work toward a system of universal healthcare.

**If you are an advocate for immigrants, you can:**
Lobby for a system of universal healthcare. The US is the only nation in the developed world without one.

Help immigrant patients contact legislators or policymakers to stress the importance of healthcare for all.

Information can be very revealing. Because of screening done by health authorities and researchers, we know immigrants suffer disproportionately from some health conditions, while seeming protected from others. Infectious diseases such as tuberculosis are more prevalent among the foreign born. On the other hand, birth outcomes among recent immigrant mothers are often better than those among other minority group mothers. (For a thorough discussion of the seemingly paradoxical 'healthy migrant effect' see Dr. Kathleen Fennelly's analysis in chapter 3). More data linking diseases and conditions with immigration status would help explain this paradox.

Collection and reporting of data on race, ethnicity, and primary language are legal, according to Title VI of the federal Civil Rights Act of 1964. No federal statutes prohibit this collection.[6] Further, patients agree that it is important for healthcare providers to collect and track data on race, ethnicity, and language. When they know why the information is being asked of them, they disclose it readily to healthcare providers.[7]

Healthcare organizations can do more to collect and analyze useful data.[8] Increasingly, healthcare facilities are expected to assess their capacity to serve diverse patients, including immigrants. In 2000, the US Department of Health and Human Services issued standards for culturally and linguistically appropriate services in healthcare that recommend internal audits and outcomes-based evaluations of cultural competence, as well as data collection on patients' race, ethnicity, and language preferences.[9]

The Joint Commission on Accreditation of Hospitals and the National Council on Quality Assurance both recognize the importance of data collection and assessment regarding cultural and linguistic aspects of care in the accreditation review processes.[10]

A commitment to eliminating health disparities between immigrant and non-immigrant patients should be measurable from the boardroom to the waiting room. Healthcare networks and systems should have written policies about access, language services, provider training, marketing and of course, data collection. They should also have internal quality assurance measures to track goals toward increased cultural competence.[11,12]

Data collection and assessment leads to rational funding allocations, more cost-effectiveness, better care and ultimately, better outcomes.[13] Using accurate information on the race and ethnicity of patients, providers, clinics and healthcare systems can identify health status and service disparities.[14] This vital pool of information can serve as a guide in focusing prevention and treatment efforts as well as general expenditure of health dollars (Box 4.3).

## Box 4.3
## Data and assessment: what you can do

**If you are a policy maker, you can:**
Establish mandates and expectations regarding data collection by healthcare and social service organizations.

**If you are a healthcare administrator, you can:**
Explore existing forms of data collection which provide valuable information without the need for new collection; use markers such as ER visits, increases in insured individuals, etc. to measure progress toward better care.
Routinely link organizational key quality measures to demographic data which are collected, and develop organizational responses to the results.
Develop policies and systems within your organization to support data collection at the point of the patient's first encounter with your system.

**If you are an educator or researcher, you can:**
Use existing and new data to explore the link between immigrant status and health.
Document ways that healthcare organizations are using data effectively to improve services.

**If you are a healthcare provider, you can:**
Explain the clinical importance of language and ethnicity data to patients, to overcome reluctance to provide such information.
Learn more about the relationship between immigrant status and poor health outcomes.

**If you are an advocate for immigrants, you can:**
Ensure that immigrant status is never a barrier to the provision of equitable healthcare, by monitoring collection systems and uses of data.

## 3. Recognize different costs of healthcare for recent immigrants and provide equitable payment

Because of cultural and language differences between immigrant patients and Western-trained providers, caring for such patients sometimes takes longer. This is more costly in the short run, especially given the need for interpreting, but is cost-effective in the long term.[15] We should work to eliminate financial disincentives to equitable health-

care for recent immigrants if they require an interpreter.

Current systems of payment are often inflexible, fragmented, or inadequate.[16] Payment for healthcare should reflect the varying requirements of care for all kinds of patients, including those with limited English proficiency (LEP). Having the same reimbursement system for patients who require an interpreter is unfair and leads to poor care for LEP patients. Medicaid and SCIP will reimburse healthcare providers for the cost of interpreting services, but most states have not provided mechanisms for reimbursement. Further, even though millions of Medicare patients have limited English proficiency, Medicare does not pay for interpreter services at all.[17]

More basically, immigrants who are insured through public programs may have a hard time staying covered. People who are on public assistance commonly bounce in and out of coverage because they are unfamiliar with the complex rules and regulations for retaining public benefits. Such programs should reduce the number of times a recipient must re-enroll to receive benefits[18] (Box 4.4).

## 4. Develop clinical guidelines and best practices orders for immigrant healthcare

Clinical practice and positive outcomes are enhanced through the use of evidence-based guidelines. Adherence to evidence-based best practices also ensures consistency of care.

Treatment for most health conditions must be adapted to be effective in caring for people from differing cultural backgrounds. However, guidelines reflecting the unique needs of immigrants and limited English-speaking patients are rare.

Healthcare providers should develop and follow clinical guidelines for patients who are recent immigrants (Box 4.5). Many of the chapters in this text offer such clinical guidelines. See especially chapters in Sections 2–5.

## 5. Diversify the healthcare workforce to include more immigrant and minority providers

Healthcare works best when patients and providers share backgrounds and values. Racial and ethnic similarity between patients and providers is associ-

---

**Box 4.4**

**Equitable payment: what you can do**

**If you are a policy maker, you can:**
Spread the burden of caring for the uninsured more evenly across hospitals and clinics.
Set up systems to keep patients eligible for health programs.
Reduce paperwork requirements in determining patients' eligibility for healthcare coverage.

**If you are a healthcare administrator, you can:**
Allow a longer visit time for patients who need an interpreter.
Avoid payment structures (salary and pay for performance) which are disincentives to providers to care for non-English-speaking patients.
Institute programs to hire bilingual staff whenever possible.
Emphasize billing systems based on time spent in direct patient care.

**If you are an educator or researcher, you can:**
Document the impact of financial barriers and disincentives to care for immigrants.

**If you are a healthcare provider, you can:**
Schedule more clinical time for interactions with LEP patients and other immigrants with complex needs.
Create language-specific clinics to consolidate interpreter schedules.

**If you are an advocate for immigrants, you can:**
Help immigrant patients enroll in health insurance programs.
Create health education group teaching programs for recent immigrants to familiarize them with healthcare systems.

---

**Box 4.5**

**Clinical guidelines: what you can do**

**If you are a policy maker, you can:**
Support the development of clinical guidelines for immigrant and refugee patients.

**If you are a healthcare administrator, you can:**
Train providers to recognize the importance of following clinical guidelines.
Encourage providers to use established clinical guidelines and to improve them with appropriate cultural perspectives.
Encourage the adaptation of existing standing order sets, including electronic medical record text and orders, that address linguistic and cultural aspects of care.

**If you are an educator or researcher, you can:**
Research and develop additional guidelines for treatment of conditions prevalent among immigrant patients.
Review existing guidelines and research to evaluate the impact of culturally competent care on treatment outcomes.

**If you are a healthcare provider, you can:**
Follow existing evidence-based guidelines related to appropriate care for immigrant patients, based on country of origin and race/ethnicity where available.
Develop standing orders that include appropriate cultural competence practices.
Use evidence-based guidelines and appropriately adapt them to incorporate the consideration of cultural beliefs and language differences.
Encourage the adaptation of existing standing order sets to address linguistic and cultural aspects of care.

**If you are an advocate for immigrants, you can:**
Promote the importance of research and evidence-based guidelines in improving immigrant health.

---

ated with greater patient participation, higher satisfaction, and greater adherence to treatment.[19]

The implication for immigrant healthcare providers is clear: more of them are needed in order to provide a range of cultural and linguistic perspectives on the delivery of care. But minorities and immigrants are under-represented in healthcare professions and capable foreign-trained providers are not being used to full advantage.[20]

Many foreign-trained health professionals spend years working outside their fields, because of restrictive licensing and certification systems.[21] Further, even when hired to work in US healthcare facilities, foreign-trained providers experience significant discrimination.[22]

Some states have implemented programs to incorporate foreign-trained professionals more readily. Other programs are aimed at recruitment and training of minority and immigrant students to become healthcare professionals[23] (Box 4.6).

**If you are a policy maker, you can:**
Develop funding sources and programs to encourage immigrant students to pursue healthcare careers.
Develop innovative programs to take advantage of fully trained and competent foreign-trained health providers.

**If you are a healthcare administrator, you can:**
Hire immigrant and minority physicians and nurses.
Set institutional goals for minority and immigrant recruitment.
Institute mentoring and apprentice programs to allow immigrant providers to help with patient care.

**If you are an educator or researcher, you can:**
Research ways that diversity in the healthcare workforce can be encouraged.
Recruit and support minority and immigrant students in healthcare programs.
Analyze the effect of racial, ethnic, or language concordance on health outcomes of immigrant patients.

**If you are a healthcare provider, you can:**
Encourage your professional certification or licensing body to address restrictions on immigrant providers.
Work collaboratively with foreign-trained colleagues who may need sponsorship or mentoring.
Take advantage of cultural insights offered by foreign-trained colleagues.

**If you are an advocate for immigrants, you can:**
Lobby for changes in immigration laws, certification, and licensing systems that restrict the employment of foreign-trained providers.

## 6. Use trained interpreters

A trained interpreter facilitates communication between a patient who speaks limited or no English, and the healthcare provider. Use of an interpreter with LEP patients can improve delivery of care and reduce healthcare disparities.[24,25]

Title VI of the Civil Rights Act requires healthcare facilities to offer interpreting services free of charge for those who need them. Failure to provide mean-ingful access to interpreter services can result in a loss of federal funding for hospitals and other health-care facilities.[26]

Despite existing legal mandates, many healthcare facilities are not equipped with interpreter services for LEP patients. The demand for trained medical interpreters exceeds the supply. Training is essential, since the skills required in interpreting go far beyond mere fluency in two languages.[27]

The profession is developing rapidly, with new standards for training, ethical behavior, and certification of skills (Box 4.7).[28] For a fuller description of developments in the interpreter field, see Chapter 6.

## 7. Use community health workers

Community health workers (CHWs) provide a unique service within the healthcare system. CHWs are bilingual, bicultural individuals who serve as a bridge between the healthcare system and immigrant patients.[29]

They perform a variety of functions, including informal counseling and social support, health education, enrollment in health insurance programs, advocacy, referral and follow-up services. As members of the community they serve, they can be highly effective guides to better health for immigrants.[30]

Unlike many other healthcare professions, however, there is no standardized training and credentialing program for community health workers. In the highly regulated healthcare industry, this is a barrier to employment and greater use of CHWs.[31] Additional barriers to the full use of CHWs include uncertain funding and unclear reimbursement mechanisms for CHW services, poor integration of the CHW role in the healthcare team and a need for more data on CHW effectiveness (Box 4.8).[31]

## 8. Train healthcare providers and educate immigrant patients

Patients and providers who approach each other with respect and interest can learn from one another, ensuring better health outcomes and reduced health disparities in the process.[32]

This is the essence of cultural competence, an essential aspect of healthcare for immigrants.

Healthcare providers and all those who interact with immigrant patients can be more effective if

## Box 4.7
### Trained interpreters: what you can do

**If you are a policy maker, you can:**
Enforce existing mandates and guidelines about linguistic access for patients who speak limited English.
Advocate for increased reimbursement of interpreter services in healthcare.

**If you are a healthcare administrator, you can:**
Forbid the use of patients' minor children or family members as interpreters in your healthcare organization.
Assess the languages spoken by your patient population, and plan accordingly for adequate interpreter services.
Measure the source of your interpretive services, and provide feedback to staff.

**If you are an educator or researcher, you can:**
Help deliver a training curriculum for healthcare interpreters, or train providers how to work effectively with interpreters.
Document the effect of interpreters on immigrant healthcare.

**If you are a healthcare provider, you can:**
Collaborate with interpreters to improve outreach and education of immigrant patients.
Seek training in working effectively with an interpreter as part of the healthcare team.
Schedule trained professional interpreters in all important encounters with LEP patients.

**If you are an advocate for immigrants, you can:**
Insist that immigrant patients with limited English be provided timely, free interpreting.

## Box 4.8
### Community health workers: what you can do

**If you are a policy maker, you can:**
Support the development of community health worker training and certification programs.
Advocate for reimbursement of community health worker services in healthcare.
Fund programs to reimburse healthcare organizations for the use of community health workers.

**If you are a healthcare administrator, you can:**
Hire and develop career ladder programs for community health workers in your healthcare organization.
Assess the cost-effectiveness of community health workers for your facility.

**If you are an educator or researcher, you can:**
Evaluate the effectiveness of community health worker programs in improving immigrant health and reducing health disparities.
Help develop or deliver a training curriculum for community health workers.

**If you are a healthcare provider, you can:**
Collaborate with community health workers to improve outreach and education of immigrant patients.

**If you are an advocate for immigrants, you can:**
Promote community healthcare workers' role in improving immigrant health.

they are trained to work across language and cultural differences.[33] Training in cultural awareness and sensitivity is now recognized as an essential part of healthcare education.[34]

Cross-cultural training builds the attitudes, knowledge, and skills necessary for effective clinical encounters. Medical educators strongly recommend the integration of cross-cultural education into the training of current and future health professionals.[35]

By the same token, patients who have learned about US healthcare systems adhere more readily to treatment and may have better outcomes. Patients who understand the healthcare system and how it works are more likely to be active participants in their own healthcare.[36]

Such active participation is hampered for immigrants by language and cultural barriers and sometimes by the constraints of low health literacy. Patient education, especially when delivered in a culturally appropriate fashion, can reduce such constraints and open up avenues of clear communication between patients and providers.[37]

## Box 4.9

### Training and education: what you can do

**If you are a policy maker, you can:**
Support requirements for cultural competency training for healthcare providers.
Find funds for preventive and patient education programs.

**If you are a healthcare administrator, you can:**
Require cultural competence and linguistic access training for all staff who interact with immigrant patients.
Offer incentives or recognition for providers who demonstrate cultural competence.
Institute programs to orient immigrant patients to clinical procedures.
Assess organizational needs before instituting cultural competency programs.

**If you are an educator or researcher, you can:**
Evaluate the effectiveness of provider training programs.
Help develop or deliver patient education programs for immigrant patients.
Evaluate the cost and benefits of provider training and patient education programs.

**If you are a healthcare provider, you can:**
Collaborate with community members to improve outreach and education of immigrant patients.
Seek out additional training in cultural and linguistic competence.
Assess your patients' satisfaction with their treatment.
Assume a leadership or mentoring role for colleagues who are less familiar with cultural competence.

**If you are an advocate for immigrants, you can:**
Support the development of programs to orient recent immigrants to the Western healthcare system.
Develop patient advocacy and community health worker programs.
Help develop and distribute multilingual and low-literacy patient education materials.

## References

1. Kaiser Family Foundation. How race/ethnicity, immigration status and language affect health insurance coverage, access and quality of care among the low income population. Washington, DC; 2003.
2. Institute of Medicine. Care without coverage: too little, too late. Washington DC: National Academy Press; 2002.
3. Commonwealth Fund. Staying covered: the importance of retaining health insurance coverage for low-income families. New York: Commonwealth Fund; 2002.
4. Bierman A, Lurie N, Collins K, et al. Addressing racial and ethnic barriers to effective healthcare: the need for better data. Health Affairs 2002; May/June:91–102.
5. Fiscella K, Franks P, Gold M, et al. Inequality in quality: addressing socioeconomic, racial and ethnic disparities in healthcare. JAMA 2000; 283(19):2579–2584.
6. Perot RT, Youdelman M. Racial, ethnic and primary language data collection in the healthcare system: an assessment of federal policies and practices. New York: Commonwealth Fund; 2001.
7. Baker D, Cameron K, Feinglass J, et al. Patients' attitudes toward healthcare providers collecting information about their race and ethnicity. J Gen Internal Med 2005; 20(10):895–900.
8. Regenstein M, Sickler D. Race, ethnicity and language of patients: hospital practices regarding collection of information to address disparities in healthcare. National Public Health and Hospital Institute, Washington; 2006. www.naph.org March 2006.
9. National Standards for Culturally and Linguistically Appropriate Services in Health Care Final Report. Office of Minority Health; 2001. The final standards were published in the Federal Register on December 22, 2000; 65(247):80865–80879.
10. Office of Minority Health CLAS Standards Crosswalked to 2004 Joint Commission on Accreditation of Hospitals Standards for Hospitals, Ambulatory, Behavioral Health, Long Term Care and Home Care www.jcaho.org/about+us/hlc/hlc_omh_xwalk.pdf March 3, 2006.
11. Hasnain-Wynia R, Pierce D, Pittman M. Who, when, and how: the current state of race, ethnicity, and primary language data collection in hospitals. New York: Commonwealth Fund; 2004.
12. Nerenz D, Gunter M, García M, et al. Developing a health plan report card on quality of care for minority populations. New York: Commonwealth Fund; 2002.
13. National Research Council. Eliminating health disparities: measurement and data needs. Washington, DC: National Academies Press; 2004.
14. Nerenz D. Healthcare organizations' use of race/ethnicity data to address quality disparities. Health Affairs 2005; 24(2):409–416.
15. Kravitz R. Comparing the use of physician time and healthcare resources among patients speaking English, Spanish and Russian. Med Care 2000; 38(7):728–738.
16. Institutes of Medicine. Crossing the quality chasm. Washington, DC: National Academy Press; 2001.
17. Ku L, Flores G. Pay now or pay later: providing interpreter services in healthcare. Health Affairs 2005; 24(2):435–444.
18. Commonwealth Fund. Rethinking recertification: keeping eligible individuals enrolled in New York's public health insurance programs. New York: Commonwealth Fund; 2002.
19. Cooper L, Roter D. Patient-centered communication, ratings of care and concordance of patient and physician race. Ann Internal Med 2003; 139(11):907–915.
20. Institute of Medicine. The nation's compelling interest: ensuring diversity in the healthcare workforce. Washington: National Academies Press; 2004.
21. Daviratanasilpa S, Sriaroon C, Loghmanee D, et al. Medical residency training in the US: important considerations. J Med Assoc Thailand 2003; 86(11):1073–1079.
22. Coombs A, King R. Workplace discrimination: experiences of practicing physicians. J Nat Med Assoc 2005; 97(4):467–477.
23. McDonough J, Gibbs B, Scott-Harris J, et al. A state policy agenda to eliminate racial and ethnic health disparities. New York: Commonwealth Fund; 2004.
24. Jacobs E, Lauderdale D, Meltzer D, et al. Impact of interpreter services on delivery of healthcare to limited-English-proficient patients. J Gen Intern Med 2001; 16(7):468–474.

25. Robert Wood Johnson Foundation. The right words: addressing language and culture in healthcare. New Jersey: Robert Wood Johnson Foundation; 2003.

26. The White House Executive Order 13166. Improving access to services for persons with limited English proficiency. www.usdoj.gov/crt/cor/Pubs/eolep.htm March 2006.

27. Youdelman M, Perkins J. Providing language interpretation services in healthcare settings: examples from the field. New York: Commonwealth Fund; 2002.

28. National Council on Interpreting in Health Care. 2004 and 2002 national standards of practice for interpreters in healthcare, and national code of ethics for interpreters in healthcare. http://www.ncihc.org/sop.php March 2006.

29. Annie E. Casey Foundation. The national community health advisor study. Arizona; 1998.

30. Blue Cross and Blue Shield of Minnesota Foundation. Critical links: findings and forum highlights in the use of community health workers and interpreters in Minnesota. Minnesota; 2003.

31. Brownstein J, Bone L, Dennison C, et al. Community health workers as interventionists in the prevention and control of heart disease and stroke. Am J Preventive Med 2005; 29(581):128–133.

32. Kleinman A. Patients and healers in the context of culture. Berkeley, CA: University of California Press; 1980.

33. Hudleson P. Improving patient – provider communication: insights from interpreters. Family Pract 2005; 22:311–316.

34. California Endowment. Principles and recommended standards for cultural competence education of healthcare professionals. San Francisco; 2003.

35. Weissman J, Betancourt J, Campbell E. Resident physicians' preparedness to provide cross-cultural care. JAMA 2005; 294(9):1058–1067.

36. Kamath C, O'Fallon M, Offord K, et al. Provider satisfaction in clinical encounters with ethnic immigrant patients. Mayo Clin Proc 2003; 2003(78):1353–1360.

37. Institutes of Medicine. Unequal treatment: confronting racial and ethnic disparities in healthcare. Washington, DC: National Academy of Medicine; 2002.

# CHAPTER 5

# Language Assistance for Limited English Proficient Patients:
## *Legal Issues*

David Hunt

## Introduction

An elderly male Hmong patient was recently admitted to a midwestern hospital. The patient spoke no English. No interpreter was provided to him. Instead, his attending nurse attempted to communicate with the patient via hand gestures. Each time the nurse spoke to the patient in English and gestured with her hands, the elderly gentleman would look at her, smile, and nod. After 3 days in the hospital, a Hmong interpreter was finally arranged. When the attending nurse was asked why she hadn't used an interpreter, she said that she and the patient were communicating just fine and that she didn't feel the need to call one. Under further questioning, however, the nurse acknowledged that she did not know how to access an interpreter, had received no training on how to communicate with patients via an interpreter, and had not apprised the patient of his legal right to an interpreter. Unbeknown to the nurse, the Hmong patient was blind.

This story is repeated every day in some form throughout the United States. Such stories represent an ongoing tragedy for limited English proficient (LEP) patients and their families who are denied high-quality healthcare as well as their civil rights. But they also represent a tragedy for many well-intentioned medical professionals who are unaware that their ignorance of existing laws requiring the provision of language assistance services could compromise patient care and create both legal liability

and medical malpractice exposure (see endnote EN1).

Providers' failure to ensure meaningful access to language assistance for people with limited English skills can have serious, even life or death, consequences as the following cases demonstrate:

- A hospital in South Carolina had a policy of prohibiting women with limited English skills from receiving an epidural during labor and delivery.[1]
- Hongkham Souvannarath, a 52-year-old refugee from Laos, was jailed by the Fresno California County Health Department for almost 11 months because she did not take medication for a case of tuberculosis that health officials feared could become contagious. Ms. Souvannarath stopped taking her medications, in part, because she understood a non-Laotian appointed interpreter to say that the medicine would kill her. Souvannarath was taken at gunpoint to the county jail after being told she was being taken to a hospital. There she was strip-searched and initially housed in a safety cell for 3 days because a Hmong officer misinterpreted her Laotian comment that she was 'afraid to die' as a suicide threat. While in confinement she was frequently handcuffed, shackled, and chained to her bed. Only one guard occasionally provided interpretation

services and she was unable to communicate her needs to jail personnel. A subsequent lawsuit against the county was settled for $1.2 million.[2,3]

- A young boy in Los Angeles interpreted a consent form for his father that pertained to his ailing mother. The son thought the form meant that a nurse would make daily visits to care for his mother, and the father signed the form. Instead, the mother was sent to a nursing home.[4]

This chapter is organized into two parts. In Part One, we will describe the existing framework of federal and state laws that require healthcare organizations to provide language assistance services and 'culturally appropriate care' to limited English proficient patients. In this section, we will also describe what healthcare organizations and medical professionals must do to comply with these laws. In Part Two, we will describe a variety of policy initiatives currently being discussed to promote more culturally and linguistically appropriate care and the legal issues presented by these policies. In particular, this section will discuss legal issues associated with: (1) promoting the collection of data related to race, ethnicity and primary language by health plans, hospitals and government programs; (2) providing cross-cultural medical education to doctors and nurses; and (3) implementing a comprehensive language access agenda.

## Part One: Federal and State Laws Requiring Language Assistance

The Civil Rights Act of 1964, of which Title VI is a part, created broad national powers to end discrimination in employment, places of public accommodation (such as hospitals), and programs and activities that receive federal financial assistance. The legislative history of Title VI indicates that healthcare was prominent in the minds of its authors, as passage of the 1964 Act was contemporaneous with the judicial ruling in *Simkins v. Moses H. Cone Memorial Hospital*.[5] *Simkins* was a landmark case in which the courts struck down as unconstitutional key portions of the Hill Burton Act which had authorized the use of federal funds to construct and operate segregated healthcare facilities.

Title VI of the Civil Rights Act of 1964 prevents federal money from being used to support activities and programs that discriminate on the basis of race, color, or national origin. Section 601 of Title VI states

that no person shall 'on the ground of race, color, or national origin, be excluded from participation in, be denied the benefits of, or be subjected to discrimination under any program or activity receiving Federal financial assistance.'[6] Under section 602, the Department of Health and Human Services (HHS) has issued regulations that say recipients of federal funds can not:

[U]tilize criteria or methods of administration which have the effect of subjecting individuals to discrimination because of their race, color, or national origin, or have the effect of defeating or substantially impairing accomplishment of the objectives of the program as respect to individuals of a particular race, color, or national origin.[7]

In 1974, the US Supreme Court affirmed these regulations in *Lau v. Nichols*.[8]

*Lau* involved a San Francisco, California, school district that was desegregated under court order in 1971. The desegregation process left 1800 Chinese-American students who did not speak English in schools without supplemental English language courses. The Court recognized that 'there is no equality of treatment merely by providing students with the same facilities, textbooks, teachers and curriculum, for students who do not understand English are effectively foreclosed from any meaningful education.'[9] The Court held that the school district's failure to take affirmative steps to provide language assistance constituted national origin discrimination under Title VI.[10]

Significantly, the key provisions of Title VI of the Civil Rights Act of 1964 have gradually been incorporated into virtually every major federal statute of significance to healthcare. For example, Title VI's provisions have been incorporated into Medicaid, Medicare, Medicare Plus Choice, the State Children's Health Insurance Program (SCHIP), the Hill Burton Act, the Community Health Centers Act, and the Maternal and Child Health Block Grant Programs. As a result, nearly every state and local government, health plan, hospital, and physician that receives federal monies is bound by Title VI. The requirements of Title VI apply to all recipients of federal funds, regardless of the amount of federal funds received. Further, HHS has enforced Title VI against healthcare organizations and providers that have failed to provide language assistance to LEP patients. The rationale for doing so is virtually the same as the Supreme Court's analysis in *Lau*. According to HHS, 'a recipient of Federal financial assistance that does not have the ability to communicate with LEP persons deprives such persons of an equal opportunity to participate and benefit from the federal program.' As a result:

> No persons may be subjected to discrimination on the basis of national origin in health and human services because they have a primary language other than English.[11]

## Litigating language assistance requirements under federal law

Title VI addresses two types of discrimination. The language of Title VI plainly addresses intentional discrimination. However, regulations issued pursuant to Title VI also address policies or practices that may be neutral on their face but have the *effect* of discriminating on the basis of race, color, or national origin (the 'disparate impact' theory or 'effects' test).

Until recently, immigrants and other private litigants were permitted to sue to enforce Title VI regulations prohibiting acts with discriminatory effects. However, the United States Supreme Court in the 2001 case of *Alexander v. Sandoval* ruled that there is no private right of action under the Title VI regulations.[12] *Sandoval* involved a class of non-English-speaking residents of Alabama who alleged that the state's policy of offering the driver's license exam only in English amounted to national origin discrimination under the previously mentioned 'effects' provision of the Title VI regulation. While the Court of Appeals for the Eleventh Circuit agreed, the Supreme Court ruled that private parties lacked the authority to file a lawsuit to enforce the effects provision of the Title VI regulation.

In the aftermath of *Sandoval*, immigrants and other private plaintiffs must now establish that the conduct in question amounts to intentional discrimination under Title VI (see endnote EN2).[13] Significantly, however, while *Sandoval* applies to private parties, it has no effect on the federal government's ability to pursue civil rights cases using the effects test under the Title VI regulation. The authority of agencies such as the Office for Civil Rights at the Department of Health and Human Services remains unchanged.

Immigrants can invoke the protections of Title VI in one of two ways. First, one could file a written complaint with the Office of Civil Rights (OCR). Alternatively, one could file a lawsuit under Title VI. From the standpoint of the immigrant plaintiff, there are many advantages to filing an OCR complaint. Filing an OCR complaint does not require a lawyer.

If OCR becomes involved it can investigate both allegations of intentional discrimination under Title VI and disparate impact under the Title VI regulations. If OCR investigates and makes a finding of discrimination, that can be very powerful evidence against the defendant. Moreover, the involvement of OCR frequently results in a resolution of the case, sparing both the expense and uncertainty of protracted litigation.

Once a complaint is filed, OCR will investigate its merits by reviewing the pertinent practices and policies of the hospital or provider that is the subject of the complaint, the circumstances under which the possible non-compliance occurred, and other factors relevant to a determination of whether the defendant has failed to comply with Title VI. If OCR finds non-compliance, it will first seek voluntary compliance by the provider. OCR's ultimate sanction is to terminate federal funding to the provider, either in an administrative proceeding or by referring the case to the Department of Justice for litigation.

Despite the stated advantages of filing a complaint with OCR, substantial evidence suggests that this route has severe limitations. OCR has consistently lacked the funding and the staff for conducting systematic compliance reviews (see endnote EN3). As a result, the agency has frequently been criticized as being reactive rather than proactive. Moreover, the complaint approach used by OCR has several specific problems when it comes to addressing racial and ethnic disparities in healthcare. First, immigrants generally are not prone to file complaints, whether out of fear of possible retaliation or possible deportation in the case of illegal aliens. Second, with some notable exceptions, the advocacy community has not been focused on this issue since the Supreme Court issued the *Sandoval* decision. Third, OCR's lack of technical expertise in the medical area results in few complaints being upheld. Finally, even after a complaint enters the system, OCR's investigative processes are inadequate and slow in finding violations, resulting in inordinate lengths of time for case resolution and a finding of compliance in most race-related cases. (OCR has never terminated federal funding for any provider no matter how egregious the offense.)

Although OCR's track record of effectiveness may be less than inspiring, providers dare not take it for granted. According to Thomas E. Perez, Former Director, Office for Civil Rights at the US Department of Health and Human Services, language access cases are easily OCR's most frequently encountered type of Title VI case.[14] (Ironically, as Perez notes, the large number of OCR complaints may actually understate the true extent of the problem, as many immigrants are reluctant to file complaints.)

Over the last 30 years, OCR has undertaken thousands of investigations and reviews involving language differences in healthcare. A sampling of recently settled OCR cases shows that intentional discrimination against immigrants and/or LEP patients is hardly a thing of the past:

- OCR settled a case involving Visiting Nurse Services, a home healthcare agency in western Massachusetts. Although the agency is located in an area with a significant Spanish-speaking population, complainants alleged that the agency would not provide interpreters to LEP patients and refused to accept patients for home care services if they did not speak English.
- OCR reached a settlement with the Rancho Los Amigos Rehab Hospital, a county-run hospital in Los Angeles. Complainants in the case alleged that the hospital discriminated against LEP patients by failing to provide free interpreters and by routinely requiring LEP clients to bring a family member or friend to interpret for them and routinely requiring LEP clients to pay for services.
- OCR reached a settlement with a hospital located near the US–Mexico border in McAllen, Texas, that ordered its security personnel to dress up in uniforms that closely resembled the US Border Patrol. This policy had the effect of deterring Latinos in the area from using the facility.[15]

The National Health Law Program has researched many of the formal complaints between OCR and providers. The overwhelming majority of these reviews involved hospitals. However, recently the subject matter of OCR reviews has broadened, to include investigations regarding:

- RENAL DIALYSIS: for failing to provide qualified interpreters (Cook County Hospital Renal Dialysis Center);
- MANAGED CARE: for failing to ensure that Medicaid health maintenance organizations did not engage in marketing practices which deny information or enrollment opportunities to LEP persons (Illinois Department of Public Aid);
- STATE DEPARTMENT OF HEALTH: A preliminary assessment found that the North Carolina Department of Health and Human Services has turned LEP clients away because no interpreters were available; required LEP clients to use family members and friends as interpreters; and failed to assess language needs of national origin groups, evaluate interpreter competency, have procedures to determine when written materials need translation, train staff on language access requirements, and notify LEP persons that interpreter services are available to them at no cost.

OCR representatives have indicated that the most frequently encountered language access problems are providers who: (1) directly or indirectly require patients to provide their own interpreter service, through family or friends; (2) fail to provide interpreter service, or provide untrained personnel; and (3) subject people with limited English skills to lengthy delays as a result of the lack of readily available interpreter services.[16]

Although they involve a range of providers and situations, the OCR cases share a number of common features. Specifically, they require providers to:

- Develop a written plan for providing LEP services;
- Designate a staff person to coordinate Title VI activities;
- Provide information and training to staff on these policies;
- Post translated notices that contain information on the availability of no-cost interpreters;
- Maintain effective interpreter services by emphasizing in-person interpretation and, to the extent possible, minimize telephone interpretation;
- Provide translation of important forms and documents;
- Collect and analyze data to determine if interpreter services are effective; and
- Monitor subcontractors and include a non-discrimination clause in all contracts for services.[17]

## Recent developments: Executive Order 13166 and DHHS guidance

In recent years, with immigration at record highs, there has been a spate of new federal developments with respect to the provision of language assistance services to immigrants. On August 11, 2000, President Clinton issued Executive Order 13166, entitled Improving Access to Services for Persons with Limited English Proficiency. Executive Order 13166 required every federal agency that provides federal assistance, including HHS, to publish a Title VI guidance to explain to recipients of federal funds how to provide access to LEP persons and achieve compliance with the Title VI regulations. The HHS Office of Civil Rights issued an initial guidance on this topic on August 30, 2000. Subsequently, on August 4, 2003, HHS published a revised Guidance to Federal Financial Assistance Recipients Regarding Title VI Prohibition Against National Origin Discrimination Affecting English Proficient Persons (2003 HHS LEP Policy Guidance).[18] The Guidance made clear that it did not create new obligations, but rather clarified existing Title VI responsibilities.

## What providers must do to comply with federal language access laws

The Office of Civil Rights' 2003 LEP Policy Guidance outlines the responsibilities of health and human service providers under Title VI to ensure that people with limited English skills can meaningfully access health and human services. It also provides a roadmap to assist providers in meeting their legal obligations. Providers who are subject to these obligations include hospitals, nursing homes, state Medicaid agencies, managed care organizations, home health agencies, state, county, and local health agencies, and physicians and other providers who receive federal financial assistance from HHS.

The Guidance defines a limited English proficient individual as 'individuals who do not speak English as their primary language and who have a limited ability to read, write, speak or understand English.' Significantly, LEP individuals may not only be the patient themselves but also parents and legal guardians of minors eligible for coverage.

## Four-factor test to determine language assistance obligations

The Guidance states DHHS's intent that recipients of federal funds take reasonable steps to ensure that LEP persons have '*meaningful access*' to programs and activities. 'Meaningful access' means that communications between the LEP patient and the provider are effective in promoting mutual understanding. The following four factor test will be used to evaluate whether a provider has a legal obligation to provide language assistance and, if so, whether it is providing meaningful access:

1. The number or proportion of LEP persons eligible or likely to be served by the program as determined by program-specific data along with census, school, or other community-based data from the relevant service area;
2. The frequency with which LEP individuals have or should have contact with the program;
3. The nature and importance of the program, activity, or service to people's lives; and
4. The resources available to the provider and the costs.[19]

In applying the four-factor test, providers should keep the following general principles in mind. The greater the number or proportion of LEP persons served or encountered in the eligible service population, the stronger the provider's legal obligation will be to provide language assistance services. The more frequent the contact with a particular language group, the more likely it is that enhanced language services will be needed in that language. The more important or urgent a provider's service is (e.g. a hospital emergency room), the more important language services become to help the LEP person and their families access them. Smaller providers with more limited budgets are not expected to provide the same level of language assistance as larger providers with larger budgets.

If providers have an obligation to provide language assistance, there are two major ways to discharge it:

1. ORAL LANGUAGE SERVICES: Where oral interpretation is needed, providers should develop procedures for providing competent interpreters in a timely manner. When the timeliness of services is important and delay would result in the effective denial of a benefit, service, or right, language assistance likely cannot be delayed.
2. TRANSLATION OF WRITTEN MATERIALS: An effective LEP policy ensures that vital written documents are translated into the language of each regularly encountered LEP group eligible to be served and/or likely to be affected by the recipient's program. (Technical or linguistic competence can often be assured by back translation.)[20]

## Guidelines for providing oral interpretation services to LEP patients

Where oral interpretation is needed, providers should develop procedures for providing competent interpreters in a timely manner. The DHHS Guidance describes various options for providing oral language assistance, including hiring bilingual staff or qualified staff interpreters, contracting for interpreters, using telephone interpreter lines, and using community volunteers. The Guidance makes clear that while providers may choose the means of communicating with the LEP patient, the result must be effective communication. While LEP patients may elect to use an interpreter of their own choosing, providers may not require LEP persons to use family members as interpreters.[21]

Irrespective of who is chosen to interpret, providers have a legal duty to assure that a competent interpreter is provided at no cost to the patient. According to the DHHS Guidance, competence requires more than self-identification as bilingual. Competency to interpret does not always mean formal certification, although certification is helpful. At a minimum, however, providers should insure that interpreters: demonstrate proficiency in both languages; are bound by confidentiality and impartiality; have knowledge of specialized medical terms/concepts; demonstrate the ability to convey information in both languages accurately and avoid other roles such as that of counselor or legal advisor.

The DHHS Guidance discourages the use of family members, friends, and especially children as interpreters. 'Extra caution' should be taken when the LEP person chooses to use a minor to interpret.[22] The use of family members and friends as medical interpreters is highly problematic and can compromise many aspects of patient care. While family members and friends may know more English than the patient, they may not understand medical terminology, and ad hoc interpreters are more likely than professional interpreters to commit errors of potential clinical consequences. (One case that exemplified this situation occurred in Minneapolis, Minnesota, where a 14-year-old Hmong girl tried to interpret for an older family member. The attending physician explained to the girl that further X-rays were needed, but the girl misunderstood and explained to the family that the physicians were planning to 'microwave the patient.') Using a family member or friend as an interpreter risks breaching patient privacy and confidentiality; patients may be less inclined to reveal sensitive personal or medical information when relatives or friends are present. Using minor

children to interpret also upsets the traditional family hierarchy and can subject children to information that they are not emotionally or intellectually prepared to handle.

Providers are asked to verify and monitor the competence and appropriateness of using the family member or friend to interpret, particularly in situations involving administrative hearings, child or adult protective investigations, life, health, safety or access to important benefits; or when credibility and accuracy are important to protect the individual. Moreover, if the provider determines that the family member or friend is not competent, the provider must provide competent interpreter services in place of or as a supplement to the LEP person's interpreter.

## Legal duty to provide written translated materials – safe harbors

With respect to written translation, DHHS says it will determine compliance on a case-by-case basis, taking into account the 'totality of the circumstances' in light of the four-factor test. However, the DHHS Guidance makes clear that providers have a legal obligation to translate 'vital written documents' into the languages of the most frequently encountered LEP populations eligible to receive its services. 'Vital documents' may include: consent and complaint forms; intake forms with the potential for important consequences; written notices of rights, denial, loss, or decreases in benefits or services; notices of disciplinary action; applications to receive services or benefits; and notices advising LEP persons of their right to receive free language assistance services.[23]

Significantly, DHHS also designated two 'safe harbors' that, if met, will provide 'strong evidence' of compliance with the provider's written translation obligations:

1. The [provider] provides written translations of 'vital documents' (e.g. intake forms with the potential for important consequences, consent and complaint forms, eligibility and service notices) for each eligible LEP language group that constitutes 5% or 1000, whichever is less of the population of persons eligible to be served or likely to be affected or encountered. Translation of other documents, if needed, can be provided orally; or

2. If there are fewer than 50 persons in a language group that reaches the 5% trigger above, the recipient provides written notice

in the primary language of the LEP language group of the right to receive competent oral interpretation of vital written materials, free of cost.[24]

Where providers have determined that they have a legal obligation to provide language assistance, they should develop a written LEP policy/plan. Effective plans typically have five elements:

1. Identify LEP individuals who need language assistance.
2. Provide appropriate language assistance measures.
3. Train staff on LEP policies and procedures.
4. Provide notice to LEP persons about available language assistance services at no charge.
5. Monitor and update the plan – at a minimum once every 3 years.[25]

DHHS also notes that an effective plan will set clear goals and establish management accountability for achieving them. Providers may also want to provide opportunities for community input and planning throughout the process. The August 2003 LEP Guidance notes that systems will evolve over time, and DHHS will look favorably on intermediate steps that recipients take that are consistent with the Guidance.

## Office of Minority Health cultural and linguistic access standards

Title VI is the only federal law that directly supports any aspect of cultural competency in healthcare. As currently applied, Title VI only requires language assistance for LEP patients. While the absence of language assistance is a major source of racial and ethnic disparities in healthcare, many healthcare advocates, civil rights organizations, and others have encouraged HHS' Office of Civil Rights to adopt additional recommendations including guidance on cultural competence.

In fact, HHS has already developed standards for culturally and linguistically appropriate services in healthcare. The Office of Minority Health began the process of developing national standards in 1997. On December 22, 2000, following a lengthy period of public comment and collaboration, the HHS Office of Minority Health issued National Standards on Culturally and Linguistically Appropriate Services (CLAS) in Health Care.[26] The standards 'are especially designed to address the needs of racial, ethnic, and linguistic population groups that experience

unequal access to health services . . . [and] to contribute to the elimination of racial and ethnic health disparities.'

The CLAS standards contain 14 standards, organized into three themes: culturally competent care, language access services, and organizational supports for cultural competence. The 14 standards can also be categorized by their stringency as mandates, guidelines, and recommendations.[27] Significantly, all of the mandates (Standards 4–7) deal specifically with language access. These standards are essentially restatements of existing Title VI law for purposes of recipients of federal funds and provide as follows:

- STANDARD 4: Healthcare organizations must offer and provide language assistance services, including bilingual staff and interpreter services, at no cost to each patient/consumer with limited English proficiency at all points of contact in a timely manner during all hours of operation.
- STANDARD 5: Healthcare organizations must provide to patients/consumers in their preferred language both verbal offers and written notices informing them of their right to receive language assistance services.
- STANDARD 6: Healthcare organizations must assure the competence of language assistance provided to limited English proficient patients/consumers by interpreters and bilingual staff. Family and friends should not be used to provide interpretation services (except on request by the patient/consumer).
- STANDARD 7: Healthcare organizations must make available easily understood patient-related materials and post signage in the languages of the commonly encountered groups and/or groups represented in the service area.[28]

Aside from its language assistance mandates, the CLAS Standards also include 'guidelines and recommendations.' The guidelines are activities the Office of Minority Health recommended for adoption by federal, state, and national accrediting agencies. The recommendations are suggestions the Office of Minority Health made for voluntary adoption by healthcare organizations. The guidelines and recommendations are not legally enforceable at this time, but they provide strategic direction for addressing some of the causes of racial and ethnic disparities in healthcare.

The CLAS standards are independent of DOJ and OCR guidance documents. However, because they address many of the same issues in great detail and are aimed at healthcare providers, these standards are proving helpful to providers as they devise and implement language access plans. Already, the CLAS standards are being used widely. For instance, George Washington University Center for Health Service Research and Policy has released and widely circulated model cultural competence purchasing specifications for Medicaid managed care that are based on the CLAS standards. HHS has also made cultural and linguistic competence the focus of Medicare + Choice quality improvement projects and has encouraged health plans to use CLAS standards in developing their projects. While aimed at healthcare organizations, the standards are also presented as guidelines for accreditation and credentialing agencies such as the Joint Commission on Accreditation of Healthcare Organizations, the National Committee on Quality Assurance, and peer review organizations. Finally, to the extent that the CLAS standards represent the first national standards on culturally and linguistically appropriate healthcare services, it could be argued that these standards represent a new community standard for medical malpractice purposes.

## State laws requiring language access

According to a National Health Law Program survey, 43 states have laws that address language access in healthcare settings.[29] At least 26 states and the District of Columbia have enacted legislation requiring language assistance such as interpreters and/or translated forms and other written materials for LEP patients. For example, California statutes require interpreters or bilingual staff at general acute care hospitals, county medical health programs, and intermediate care facilities.[30] Idaho requires interpreters for the purpose of obtaining consent from patients in the state's Medical Assistance Program. Massachusetts enacted the 'Emergency Room Interpreter Bill,' effective as of July 1, 2001. The law requires all public and private acute care hospitals to provide 'competent interpreter services' for all emergency room services. Rhode Island requires hospitals to provide a qualified interpreter when a bilingual clinician is unavailable for all services given to every non-English-speaking patient. This law became effective January 1, 2002.[31]

Many states have addressed linguistic access in their contracts with healthcare providers. According to George Washington University's Center for Health Services Research and Policy, the majority of Medicaid managed care contracts or requests for proposals require managed care organizations to provide materials in other languages (38 states), require services for persons whose primary language is not English (31 states), or include a cultural competency requirement (27 states).

A few states have used the law to implement broader cultural competency efforts. Recently, California has acknowledged the need for cultural competency by adding state administrative support for such efforts. A 1999 statute established an Office of Multicultural Health. The Office's duties includes performing 'an internal assessment of cultural competency, and training of healthcare professionals to ensure more linguistically and culturally competent care.' A 2000 California law established 'The Task Force on Culturally and Linguistically Competent Physicians and Dentists.' The Task Force's work has already generated additional legislation, including a bill to provide language and cross-cultural training to California physicians.[32]

Other state approaches to cultural competency vary widely. Some laws use linguistic access and cultural competency program requirements as licensing conditions. Some require managed care organizations to develop written cultural competency plans to provide effective healthcare services to members. Others establish service standards, pilot programs, research priorities, and specific programs aimed at particular racial and ethnic communities.

## Federal disabilities laws also require language assistance

Section 504 of the Rehabilitation Act of 1973 and the Americans with Disabilities Act also require federal financial recipients to provide language assistance services to handicapped and/or disabled persons. These laws merit discussion here for three key reasons. First, many immigrant and/or LEP patients are also disabled. (Recall the case of the blind Hmong patient at the start of this chapter.) Second, laws requiring healthcare organizations to provide language assistance services to the disabled pre-date more recent regulations that require the provision of such services to LEP immigrants. As a result, the courts may well look to disability law for guidance in interpreting them. Third, both sets of laws are enforced by the same administrative agency – HHS' Office of Civil Rights (OCR). Many OCR settlement agreements with providers clearly have been influenced by language assistance principles that first emerged from disability law.

Section 504 of the Rehabilitation Act of 1973 requires federal financial recipients' programs to be equally accessible to handicapped persons. DHHS regulations to Section 504 require provision of necessary auxiliary aids such as sign language interpreters to ensure equal access to federal recipients programs. In particular, they state that:

A recipient . . . that employs fifteen or more persons shall provide appropriate auxiliary aids to persons with impaired sensory, manual or speaking skills where necessary to afford such persons an equal opportunity to benefit from the service in question. . . . [A]uxiliary aids may include brailled and taped material, interpreters, and other aids for persons with impaired hearing or vision.[33]

Under Section 504 of the Rehabilitation Act of 1974, providers have a legal duty to ensure 'effective communication.' There is no distinction between inpatient and outpatient treatment with respect to this duty. However, during hospitalization, effective communication must be provided at 'critical points' during the patient's stay. Critical points would include those points during which critical medical information is communicated, such as admission, when explaining medical procedures, when an informed consent is required for treatment, and at discharge.

Title III of the Americans with Disabilities Act (ADA) prohibits discrimination against individuals with disabilities by places of public accommodation. Private healthcare providers are considered places of public accommodation under the Act. Title III of the ADA applies to all private healthcare providers regardless of the size of the office or the number of employees. It applies to providers of both physical and mental health. Hospitals, nursing homes, psychiatric and psychological services, offices of private physicians, dentists, health maintenance organizations, and health clinics are specifically included among the healthcare providers covered by the ADA.

Title III of the ADA prohibits healthcare professionals from discriminating against individuals on the basis of disability. Generally, a healthcare professional discriminates on the basis of disability if: (1) a sign language interpreter is necessary to ensure effective communication between a patient and a healthcare professional; (2) the patient has requested an interpreter, and (3) the healthcare professional refuses to provide a qualified interpreter.[34]

Under the ADA, healthcare providers have a legal duty to provide 'effective communication' to individuals who are blind, deaf, or hard of hearing. Providers can discharge that duty by using auxiliary aids and services that ensure that communication with people who have vision or hearing loss is as effective as communication with others.

To whom do providers have a duty of providing effective communication? Healthcare providers must communicate effectively with customers, clients, and other individuals with disabilities who are seeking or receiving their services.[35] Significantly, this legal duty may extend beyond the provider's patients. For example, if prenatal classes are offered as a service to both fathers and mothers, a father with a hearing loss must be given auxiliary aids or services that offer him the same opportunity to benefit from the classes as would other fathers. Similarly, a deaf parent of a hearing child may require an auxiliary aid or service to participate in the child's healthcare and to give informed consent for the child's medical treatment.

Providers may use a variety of auxiliary aids and services to discharge their legal duty to provide effective communication. Appropriate auxiliary aids and services include equipment or services a deaf or hard or hearing person needs to understand aural communication. For example, the rule includes qualified interpreters, assistive listening devices, notetakers, written materials, television decoders, and telecommunications devices for the deaf. Healthcare providers may use their discretion to determine which auxiliary aid or service is best for the patient so long as the chosen method produces effective communication.[36]

In considering what constitutes effective communication under the ADA, providers would be well advised not to rely on lip reading or written notes to communicate with deaf and hard of hearing individuals. While some deaf and hard of hearing individuals rely on lip reading for communication, very few rely on lip reading alone for exchanges of important information. Significantly, 40–60% of English sounds look alike when spoken. On the average, even the best lip readers only understand 25% of what is said to them, and many individuals understand far less. Lip reading may be particularly difficult in medical settings where complex medical terminology is used. Similarly, passing written notes to a deaf or hard of hearing individual may also not constitute effective communication depending upon the reading level of the individual. The reading level of some deaf individuals is much lower than that of hearing people. Additionally, many deaf people consider American Sign Language (ASL) to be their first language. Because the grammar and syntax of ASL differ considerably from English, writing back and forth may not provide effective communication between the deaf patient and the healthcare provider. Moreover, written communications are often slow and cumbersome in a healthcare setting and information that would otherwise be spoken may not be written. If a healthcare professional is providing less information in writing than he or she would provide when speaking to a hearing patient, writing is not an equally effective method of communication.

There are two exceptions to the ADA requirement to provide auxiliary aids and services to disabled patients.[37] First, the ADA does not require the provision of any auxiliary aid or service that would result in an 'undue burden' on the provider. An undue burden is an accommodation that would involve significant difficulty or expense to the provider. Factors to consider include the cost of the aid and/or service, the overall financial resources of the healthcare provider, the number of the provider's employees, legitimate and necessary safety requirements, the effect on the resources and operation of the provider, and the difficulty of locating or providing the aid or service. Second, the ADA does not require the provision of any auxiliary aid or service that would result in a 'fundamental alteration in the nature of the goods or services provided' by a healthcare provider. The healthcare provider still has the duty to furnish an alternative auxiliary aid or service that would not result in an undue burden or fundamental alteration.

Providers are obligated to provide a qualified interpreter when two conditions apply: (1) when an interpreter is necessary to ensure effective communication; and (2) the patient has requested one.[38] Under the ADA regulations, a qualified interpreter is defined as 'an interpreter who is able to interpret effectively, accurately, and impartially, both receptively and expressively, using any necessary specialized vocabulary.'

ADA regulations make plain that an interpreter should be present in all situations in which the information exchanged is sufficiently lengthy or complex to require an interpreter for effectively communication. Typical situations that would require an interpreter's presence would include: obtaining a patient's medical history or informed consent and permission for treatment; explaining a patient's diagnosis, prognosis, or treatment plan, communicating prior to and after major medical procedures, providing complex instructions regarding medication, explain-

ing medical costs and insurance, and explaining patient care upon discharge from a medical facility.

Providers are the ultimate decision-makers of whether an interpreter is required, not patients. The Department of Justice Technical Assistance Manual on the ADA provides that while consultation with patients is 'strongly encouraged,' the 'ultimate decision as to what measures to take to ensure effective communication rests in the hands of the physician or provider.' The power or authority to decide when an interpreter is required is balanced by the legal obligation to 'ensure that the method chosen results in effective communication.'

Healthcare providers may not charge a disabled patient for the costs of providing auxiliary aids and services either directly or through the patient's insurance carrier. Further, healthcare providers must pay for an interpreter or auxiliary aid even where the cost exceeds the provider's charge for the appointment. The somewhat surprising result can be explained as follows. A healthcare provider is expected to treat the costs of providing auxiliary aids and services as part of the annual overhead costs of operating a business. Accordingly, so long as the provision of the auxiliary aid does not impose an undue burden or fundamentally alter the provider's services, the provider must pay.

An intriguing language access issue under the ADA is whether patients can bring their own interpreter to an office visit and then bill the health professional for the cost. With respect to this situation, the Department of Justice Technical Assistance Manual states:

> The physician is not obligated to comply with the unilateral determination by the patient that an interpreter is necessary. The physician must be given an opportunity to consult with the patient and make an independent assessment of what type of auxiliary aid, if any, is necessary to ensure effective communication. If the patient believes that the physician's decision will not lead to effective communication, the patient may challenge the decision under Title III of the ADA.

## Part Two: Legal Issues Associated with Emerging Policy Initiatives

There are a variety of policy initiatives currently being discussed to promote more culturally and linguistically appropriate care. In particular, this section will discuss legal issues associated with: (1)

promoting the collection of data related to race, ethnicity, and primary language by federal, state and local governments and healthcare facilities; (2) providing cross-cultural medical education to doctors and nurses; and (3) implementing a comprehensive language access agenda.

## Racial, ethnic and language data collection

According to a report released in 2002 by the Institute of Medicines: standardized data collection is critically important in the effort to understand and eliminate racial and ethnic disparities in healthcare. Data on patient race, ethnicity, and primary language would allow for disentangling the factors that are associated with healthcare disparities, help plan monitoring performance, ensure accountability to enrolled members and payers, improve patient choice, allow for evaluation and intervention programs, and help identify discriminatory practices.[39]

It is impossible to address racial and ethnic disparities in health status without adequate data. Yet many health plans and hospitals seeking to improve care for minority populations are often hindered because they do not collect data on the race, ethnicity, or primary language status of their members and patients. Even if they had the organizational capacity to collect such data, many wonder whether they could do so legally.

The National Health Law Program (NHLP) examined this question and issued a comprehensive report detailing its findings.[40] In essence, the NHLP reached three major conclusions. First, the collection and reporting of data on race, ethnicity, and primary language are legal and authorized under Title VI of the Civil Rights Act of 1964. (No federal statutes prohibit this collection [not even HIPPA] although very few require it.) Second, federal data collection policy is not uniform at present. An increasing number of federal policies emphasize the need for obtaining racial and ethnic data. Four sets of federal health service regulations require racial and ethnic data collection and/or reporting. These health services regulations include: Medicaid, SCHIP, End-Stage Renal Disease Program, and SAMSHA. Third, no federal statutes require collection or reporting of primary language data. However, MA managed care regulations require states to inform health plans of the primary language of enrollees.[40]

State laws pertaining to the collection of race and ethnicity data vary. Many states are already collecting data on race, ethnicity, and language of preference. While no state statutes exist to bar hospitals from collecting race and ethnicity data, some states restrict health plans from doing so. For example, both California and Maryland prohibit health insurers from identifying or requesting an applicant's race, color, or national origin on an insurance application or other documents that relate to an application for insurance. New Hampshire and New Jersey have similar laws. The central concern behind such laws is that insurers would use these data to discriminate against applicants of color or substitute race and ethnicity for more legitimate underwriting criteria.

The current status of race, ethnicity, and primary language data collection activities by health plans and hospitals can be summarized as follows.

### Data collection by health plans

In 2003/04, the Robert Wood Johnson Foundation and America's Health Insurance Plans (AHIP) surveyed approximately 300 health insurance companies representing 55% of the total enrollment in managed care plans.[41] Of those surveyed, 137 plans representing 88.1 million enrollees responded. The study found that over one-half (53.5%) of enrollees are covered by plans that collect data on race and ethnicity, with most insurance companies (74.1%) accessing this information at enrollment. While most health plans are collecting some racial and ethnic information on their enrollees, wide varieties of methods are used to do so. Most plans collecting racial and ethnic information on enrollees use direct methods, such as enrollment forms or satisfaction surveys versus indirect methods to gather this information. Most Medicaid health plans (78.2%) collect racial and ethnic identifiers on enrollees as do many Medicare plans (74.3%), while only one in two commercial plans (50.9%) were found to be collecting such data.[41]

The Robert Wood Johnson Foundation/AHIP survey found that just over half of enrollees (56.4%) are covered by plans that responded to the survey and collect data on the primary language of their enrollees. Virtually 80.9% of responding plans which collect language data do so during enrollment. The most common primary languages spoken by enrollees (other than English) included: Spanish (96.7%), Chinese (76.2%), Korean (72.8%), and Vietnamese (49.1%).[41]

The most important reasons cited by health insurance plans for collecting these data were to identify enrollees with risk factors for certain conditions, reduce disparities identified in quality measures, assess variation in quality measures by racial and ethnic groups, and identify the need for translation materials. In addition, plans indicated that they use information on primary language to determine the need for interpreters and translation of materials, such as summary plan descriptions, directions, health education materials, and benefit materials.[41]

### Data collection by hospitals

In 2003, the Commonwealth Foundation contracted with the Health Research and Educational Trust to conduct a survey of hospitals' data collection practices with respect to the collection of patient race and ethnicity data.[42] A total of 272 of 1000 hospitals returned completed surveys during a 1-month time period (27% response rate). The majority of responding hospitals (78%) reported collecting race and ethnicity data. No significant relationship was found between system affiliation and the collection of data on race and ethnicity. Teaching hospitals, urban hospitals, and hospitals in states with a mandate to collect race/ethnicity data were significantly more likely to collect such data than other hospitals. With respect to collection of data on patients' primary language, the Commonwealth study found that 39% of responding hospitals collected data on patients' primary language, 52% did not, 3% of respondents did not know, and 6% did not respond to the question.[42]

Hospitals used race/ethnicity data for a variety of internal purposes including ensuring the availability of interpreter services, quality improvement or disease management programs, program/benefit design, marketing, actuarial purposes, and underwriting. Of the 78% of hospitals indicating that they collected race/ethnicity information, only 28% actually used it for quality improvement purposes.[42]

While these results are impressive, they become less so under closer scrutiny. While most hospitals reported that the primary source of information about race/ethnicity is the patient or an admitting clerk obtaining information from the patient directly, 51% of responding hospitals reported that admitting clerks determined the patient's race/ethnicity based on observation. The researchers also asked hospitals to disclose the percentage of cases where data on race or ethnicity were missing or unavailable. Responses ranged from 0 to 100 percent.[42]

In 2003, the same year as the Commonwealth study, the American Hospital Association's Annual Survey included two questions asking hospitals whether they gather information on patient race, ethnicity, and primary language.[43] The survey was sent to 6000 hospitals nationwide and had an 80% response rate. The majority of hospital respondents (78 % – exactly the same percentage as in the Commonwealth study) reported collecting race and ethnicity data about patients. A smaller percentage (59.7%) reported collecting data on patients' primary language during their hospital stay.

Most recently, a February 2006 study conducted by the National Public Health and Hospital Institute (NPHHI) found that while approximately 78.4% of US hospitals collect information on patient race, fewer than one in five hospitals used such information to improve patient care. NPHHI researchers analyzed survey data from 500 non-federal acute care hospitals on procedures for collecting information on patients' race, ethnicity, and preferred language. The study found that more than two-thirds of hospitals collect race information, 50.4% gathered ethnicity data, and 50.2% record patients' language preference. However, less than 20% of surveyed hospitals used collected information to assess and compare quality of care, utilization of health services, health outcomes, or patient satisfaction rates among various patient populations. Significantly, despite growing national attention to the issue of racial and ethnic disparities in healthcare, researchers found that more than half of non-data-collecting hospitals viewed patient information about race, ethnicity, and language as 'unimportant.'[44]

### Requiring cross-cultural medical education

A 2004 paper in the Journal of the American Medical Association (JAMA) found that among nearly 8000 graduate medical educational programs surveyed in the United States only 50.7% offered cultural competence training in 2003–2004.[45] While this figure was up from 35.7% in 2000–2001, the implication of this finding is that nearly half of today's medical students and virtually the entire complement of practicing physicians in the US have had little to no formal education on the clinical implications of cultural and linguistic differences.

Many resident physicians clearly do not feel prepared to provide cross-cultural medical care. An article in the September 7, 2005, edition of JAMA assessed residents' attitudes about cross-cultural care and preparedness to deliver quality care to diverse patient populations.[46] The authors mailed a survey to 3435 resident physicians in their final year of training at US academic health centers and obtained a 60% response rate. Substantial percentages of respondents believed that they were not prepared to provide specific aspects of cross-cultural care, including caring for patients whose health beliefs were at odds with Western medicine (25%), new immigrants (25%), and patients whose health beliefs affect treatment (20%).

A series of recent and dramatic changes, however, will assure that future physicians will receive training on cross-cultural medicine. In 2000, the CLAS Standards strongly encouraged healthcare organizations to train staff 'at all levels and across all disciplines' on 'culturally and linguistically appropriate service delivery' (see endnote EN4). In 2001, the Accreditation Council of Graduate Medical Education (ACGME) published recommended cultural competence standards.[47] Most significantly, in 2002, the prestigious Institute of Medicine (IOM) published 'Unequal Treatment', a report documenting the extensiveness of racial and ethnic disparities in the quality of medicine throughout the United States. As one important part of remedying these disparities, the IOM suggested that cross-cultural curricula be part of the training of clinicians from undergraduate to continuing medical education. Following pressure from the ACGME and the IOM, the Liaison Committee on Medical Education (LCME), in 2004, announced its cultural competence accreditation standard which requires all medical schools in the United States to integrate cultural competence into their curricula. The American Association of Medical Colleges followed up on the LCME announcement by creating a tool to assist medical schools to evaluate the effectiveness of their cultural competence training.[47]

Apart from changes in academia, significant regulatory and legislative changes have also encouraged cross-cultural medical training. In 2004, the New York State Department of Health modified its US$33 million per year Graduate Medical Education Reform Incentive Pool to reward residency programs that provide 8 hours of cultural competency training to at least 80% of residents.[48] This incentive approach worked so well that 66 of the 104 residency programs in New York State proposed new cultural competence curricula in the first year of the program. In May of 2005, New Jersey became the first state in the United States to require all physicians, as a condition of continuing licensure, to complete at least some training in cross-cultural medical care.[49] Following closely on New Jersey's heels, the California Assembly, in October of 2005, passed AB 1195, which requires that all continuing medical education courses in California include curricula on cultural and linguistic understanding. As all California physicians must take 100 hours of CME credits every 4 years, this measure insures that every practicing California physician will receive cultural competence training on an ongoing basis.[50] Several other states including Illinois, New York, and Arizona were considering similar legislation at the time that this book went to print.

## Implementing a comprehensive language access agenda

If the United States sought a comprehensive solution to the language access problem in healthcare, it would address six critical issues. First, federal and state governments should eliminate unnecessary barriers to participation in critical health programs for immigrant populations. Second, DHHS should require providers and states to collect data on race, ethnicity, and language of preference. Third, federal and state governments, health plans, and hospitals must find ways to pay for qualified interpreters for LEP patients as part of the clinical encounter. Fourth, Congress should re-establish a private right of action for disparate impact discrimination under Title VI. Fifth, federal and state civil rights enforcement agencies should receive more budgetary support to effectively enforce existing laws. Sixth, accreditation agencies such as JCAHO and NCQA should examine health plans and hospitals' language access programs as an ongoing condition of accreditation. We will discuss each of these issues in turn.

### Eliminate unnecessary barriers to participating in public programs

Identifying barriers that prevent or inhibit immigrants from seeking healthcare is key to reducing healthcare disparities among this growing segment of the American population. While the language barrier is likely the most frequently encountered challenge that immigrants face in obtaining high-quality care, several other factors are also at work. It is hard to overestimate the role that fear plays in immigrants' decisions to seek healthcare. Fear prevents many lawful American citizens and legal immigrants from applying for public aid such as Medicaid or State Children's Health Insurance Program benefits. Immigrants are fearful for at least two reasons. First, some legal immigrants fear that accessing public benefits or uncompensated care will jeopardize their pending application for citizenship. Second, immigrants fear that accessing such services may force them to disclose information about the immigration status of undocumented household members.[51]

Sometimes, immigrants' fears are unfounded. For example, any legal immigrant can access Medicaid or SCHIP benefits without jeopardizing his or her application for citizenship. But many immigrants' fears are legitimate and well founded. Many government programs and policies sometimes intentionally, sometimes not, have the effect of deterring immigrant participation. For example, a well-known Social Security Administration program kept many immigrants from accessing needed benefits as a result of one irrelevant question in the application process.[51] The Enumeration at Birth program is designed to obtain social security numbers for infants at the time of their birth. Obtaining social security numbers at birth helps babies qualify immediately for Medicaid benefits. However, the program's application form asked parents to provide their own social security numbers in order for the baby to receive one. Many immigrant parents of children born in the US do not have social security numbers. Although their children were clearly eligible to receive a social security number, this meaningless question kept many parents from applying for a social security card for their children. In turn, without a social security card, immigrant children were prevented or delayed from accessing essential health services that are vital to newborn and pediatric health. The Social Security Administration has since corrected this problem.

In other cases, however, the motives of government policy makers are not so benign. OCR initiated an investigation of the state of Georgia upon determining that Georgia's application for Medicaid benefits required all applicants to certify under penalty of perjury that all members of the household were legal residents of the United States. As former OCR Director Thomas Perez observed: '[t]he only relevant immigration question for Medicaid purposes was the immigration status of the applicant him or herself.'[51] The obvious effect of asking that question was to keep eligible applicants from applying, out of fear that the INS would discover undocumented family members. OCR's investigation revealed that Georgia's policies and practices not only deterred eligible applicants, but they violated Title VI because they had an impermissible and disproportionate impact based on applicants' national origin.[51] Georgia's application form has since been redesigned.

Based on its experience in Georgia, OCR reviewed the application forms for public benefits for all states and found many policies, practices, procedures, and questions that had the effect of deterring eligible immigrants and citizens from seeking important

benefits.[51] State officials and immigrant advocates would do well to continue to examine, challenge, and eliminate these barriers in order to maximize participation in Medicaid and SCHIP, reduce disparities, and improve immigrant health status.

## Mandate the collection of data on race, ethnicity and primary language

Despite the fact that we now live in the Information Age replete, for providers, with the advent of the electronic patient record, the sad fact is that many, if not most, healthcare organizations do not know who their patients are demographically. Without such knowledge it will continue to be impossible to eliminate racial, ethnic, and linguistic disparities in health status. While at first blush it might appear that the private sector already has this problem well in hand given the growing attention to collecting race, ethnicity, and primary language data, the reality could not be further from the truth. After an extensive examination of the hospital industry's efforts to collect just such data, researchers from the Health Research and Educational Trust concluded that there was a tremendous amount of 'both intra-organizational and inter-organizational inconsistency.'[52] While the researchers acknowledged that hospitals displayed a 'theoretical commitment to collecting race/ethnicity/primary language information and a basic understanding of its importance,' what was lacking was consistent operational policies and practices to make it happen. Given that insight, the researchers concluded that: '*the race, ethnicity, and language data that hospitals currently collect are not necessarily valid or reliable and the data collection is ineffective and inefficient*' (emphasis added).[52]

The Department of Health and Human Services already has the authority under existing Title VI regulations to require providers and states to collect data on race, ethnicity, and primary language. However, according to former OCR Director Thomas Perez, HHS does not have the legal obligation under the regulations to require the collection of data on race, ethnicity, or primary language.[53] Consequently, federal action is needed (see endnote EN5). The current data collection system within and between states is patchwork at best and shameful at worst. Congress must act to remedy this situation.

Fortunately, there appears to be growing, bipartisan support in Congress for just such legislation. In October, 2005, Senators Joseph Lieberman (D-CT) and Orrin Hatch (R-UT) introduced groundbreaking legislation that addresses two serious problems plaguing our nation's healthcare system: inconsistent healthcare quality and healthcare disparities. Their bill, called 'FairCare' would help alleviate both problems by standardizing data collection and offering new incentives for healthcare providers to raise quality standards for all patients. Specifically, FairCare would:

- Create a uniform method for collecting demographic information from patients in federally funded health programs to provide a foundation for further research on healthcare quality and disparities;
- Establish a federal grant program within the Department of Health and Human Services for data collection, quality improvement, and disparity reduction to ensure that hospitals and community health centers have the resources needed to engage in the structural adjustments necessary to expand data collection.[54]

### Find public and private means to pay for qualified interpreters

How to pay for the provision of language access services is one of the core issues at the heart of the debate over how best to end racial and ethnic disparities in healthcare. Many observers have commented that eliminating linguistic barriers to care is one of the low-hanging fruit in the disparities battle. But the issue remains fiercely divisive politically and threatens to stay that way.

In 2000, shortly before leaving the White House, President Clinton issued Executive Order 13166. Promising to continue the progress begun by the Civil Rights Act of 1964, Clinton ordered all federal agencies to issue regulations that would end discrimination against limited English proficient persons by recipients of federal funds. Applying this broad order in the healthcare context, DHHS issued standards that year requiring that providers deliver 'competent' oral interpretation and written translation services to limited English proficient patients at no cost to the patient. The standards harshly criticized the use of family members and friends as interpreters. Entirely missing from the standards was any mention of who should pay for language access.

Shortly after the election of President Bush, the Republican Congress asked the Office of Management and Budget (OMB) to conduct an analysis of the costs and benefits of implementing Executive Order 13166. To facilitate its work, OMB issued a general request for cost–benefit information from all affected constituencies. Support for EO 13166 poured in from pro-patient and pro-immigrant groups, led by the

National Health Law Program and the National Council on Interpretation in Health Care. Opposition to EO 13166 was led by the American Medical Association (AMA).

In its letter to the OMB on the subject, the AMA stated that it was 'fully committed to the importance of achieving greater access for LEP patients.' 'Nevertheless,' the AMA said:

> We are strongly opposed to allowing the burden of funding written and oral interpretation services for LEP patients to fall on physicians, as would occur under OCR's requirements. It is extremely inequitable to require physicians to fund written and oral interpretation services. The cost of hiring an interpreter, which our state survey shows can greatly vary between $30 and $400, is significantly higher than the payment for a Medicaid office visit, which in many states ranges between $30 and $50. Physicians would sustain severe economic losses if forced to cover the cost of interpretation services and thus may no longer be able to provide services to LEP patients. . . . Accordingly, the OCR requirements could reduce, not strengthen access to healthcare services for LEP patients.[55]

The OMB report was issued on March 14, 2002.[56] Making the healthcare system more accessible for LEP persons, it concluded, would produce many benefits including: 'increased patient satisfaction, decreased medical costs, improved health, sufficient patient confidentiality in medical procedures and true informed consent.' The OMB was unable to evaluate the actual costs of implementing the Executive Order due to insufficient information about the cost of providing language services. However, using data from emergency room and inpatient hospital visits and outpatient physician and dental visits, it estimated that language services would cost an extra 0.5% of the average cost per visit. (This figure was based on the total number and average cost of ER visits, inpatient hospital visits, outpatient physician visits, and dental visits.)[56]

Following the publication of the OMB report, DHHS re-issued its LEP Policy Guidance. The new Guidance adopted a much more permissive stance towards the use of family members and friends as interpreters, seeing them as a comfort issue for patients and a cost-savings device for providers.

In light of these developments, what should be done and by whom to pay the cost of language access services? As a series of first principles, it may be easiest to first indicate who should not pay for language access services. Immigrants and their families have the least ability to pay of any of the major constituent groups and should not be expected to pay for services to which they are entitled by right. Similarly, it is true that two-thirds of physician offices around the United States are small businesses. For them to assume the entire burden of language access services by themselves would clearly be onerous and likely counter-productive.[57]

There are some federal funds available for medical interpreter services. (On August 31, 2000, the Health Care Financing Administration [now the Centers for Medicare and Medicaid Services; CMS] issued a letter to all state Medicaid and SCHIP directors that clarified that federal Medicaid and SCHIP matching funds are available for state expenditures related to the provision of oral and written translation activities and services.)[58] States can obtain federal matching funds from Medicaid and SCHIP to pay for language access services if they put up their own Medicaid dollars first. At least nine states have already done so: Hawaii, Idaho, Maine, Massachusetts, Minnesota, Montana, New Hampshire, Utah, and Washington (see endnote EN6).[59] More states should follow their lead. However, with many states continuing to face severe budget deficits, this prospect may not be a realistic long-term vehicle for resolving the language access crisis.

As a result, the best-situated providers for absorbing the costs of providing language access services are health plans and hospitals. Significantly, each has ample reason and incentive to invest in language access improvements.

Health plans should invest in language access services in an attempt to keep their members healthier, thereby deterring higher medical costs. Today, with language barriers to care so imposing, many immigrants, particularly Hispanic immigrants, put off medical care until their medical needs are acute. By providing interpreters and encouraging more preventive use of the healthcare system, insurers could assist enrollees to live healthier lives and avoid the high cost of acute episodes.

There is some evidence that exactly this kind of far-reaching approach can work. Elizabeth Jacobs, MD, an emergency physician at Cook County Hospital in Chicago, has studied the impact of interpreter services on care. When Harvard Pilgrim Health Care Inc., a large insurer based in Wellesley, Massachusetts, put in place interpreter services for its Spanish- and Portuguese-speaking patients, Dr. Jacobs compared the gains in clinical and preventive services use with that of the general population.[60] Her findings showed that the use of interpreters

helped close the gap in rates of fecal occult blood testing, rectal exams, and flu immunization between English- and non-English-speaking patients, and boosted the number of prescriptions written and filled.[60] Dr. Jacobs also looked at the expense of providing interpreter services. When the cost was spread out over the entire HMO population, the plan paid only US$2.40 more per person per year. And Dr. Jacobs believes that if total patient treatment costs could be accurately measured, plans might find savings accruing in other areas.[60]

It is also in hospitals' self-interest to invest in language access services. Today, many immigrants use hospital emergency rooms inappropriately because they have not been educated on how best to use the American healthcare system. Since emergency care is the most cost-intensive form of medicine, this creates extremely high costs for hospitals and substantially increases the fiscal impact of uncompensated care because many immigrant patients have no insurance and have not applied for coverage by public programs. Investing in language access services could help immigrants learn how to use the American healthcare system more effectively and efficiently. By improving immigrants' use of primary care resources, hospitals' investment in language access services could also help to reduce the costs of uncompensated care.

Another reason why hospitals should invest in language access services is the fact that most LEP patients link their overall perceptions about quality of care with the quality of their interpreter.[61] Research has highlighted that patients with limited English proficiency have more difficulty communicating with healthcare providers and are less satisfied with the care they receive than those who are proficient in English. A recent study published in the Journal of General Internal Medicine used a survey of 2715 LEP Chinese and Vietnamese immigrant adults who received care at 11 community-based health centers across the US to highlight that those who rated their interpreters highly ('excellent' or 'very good') were more likely to rate the healthcare they received highly.[61] In sum, the perceived quality of the interpreter is strongly associated with patients' assessments of quality of care overall.

Even if more funding were provided to pay for the costs of interpreters, there is no guarantee that language access would improve. That is because physicians don't always use interpreters even when they are available and affordable. The Alameda Alliance for Health, a nonprofit health plan that primarily serves low-income people in Alameda County, California, has paid the full cost of professional medical interpreters since its inception in 1996. Yet use of interpreters was still low, according to Kelvin Quan, chief financial officer and general counsel for the plan. Quan believes that physicians have no incentives to use interpreters because physicians are largely compensated on a production basis, so spending more time with immigrant patients and their interpreters translates into lost revenue for the provider. To remedy this problem, Alameda, along with many other health plans, has set up a system where physicians receive extra compensation when dealing with LEP patients through interpreters. To Quan, the program is not intended so much as an incentive to use interpreters as it is a realistic recognition of the additional time that LEP encounters are likely to take.[62]

To improve language access, then, will take more than money. It will require a change in physician behavior. This is so because most physicians have never received any formal training on how to interact with an LEP patient through an interpreter or how to practice cross-cultural medicine. Learning these techniques can save busy clinicians time and reduce interpretation and translation costs for hospitals and health plans.

Immigrant communities should be expected to do their share as well. Many such communities have found ingenious ways to help providers and help themselves by creating community-based language banks where members of the community receive special training in medical interpreting.

### Allow immigrants to sue for disparate impact discrimination

Congress should act to restore the status quo that existed prior to the Supreme Court's decision in *Sandoval* by passing legislation to re-establish a private right of action for disparate impact discrimination under the Title VI regulation. (A number of legal commentators have advocated this reform.[63]) Passing such legislation would reinvigorate many nonprofit advocacy groups and place additional pressure on providers to comply with the law. Failing to restore individuals' pre-*Sandoval* rights will place even more pressure on an already overburdened and underfunded OCR to pursue disparate impact cases. Re-establishing this right will not open a floodgate of litigation, since providing disparate impact discrimination is extremely difficult to prove from an evidentiary point of view. Consequently, there are sound policy reasons for restoring this basic right.

### Increase budgetary support for The Office of Civil Rights

The Office for Civil Rights at HHS is the lead federal agency combating discrimination in healthcare. The first budget of HHS OCR was US$22 million in fiscal year 1980, which supported approximately 550 employees.[64] In the ensuing 20-plus years since then, OCR's budget has essentially remained stagnant. Its budget for fiscal year 2000 was also US$22 million, which supported only 215 employees. As a result, it has been difficult for OCR to carry out its mission in a fully effective manner.

Congress should increase budgetary support for the DHHS Office of Civil Rights for two critical reasons. First, despite the resource limitations on its effectiveness, OCR has established a solid body of cases that document continuing instances of discriminatory activity in violation of Title VI. There is no question that its work continues to be critically necessary. Second, budgetary support for OCR should be increased because its enforcement responsibilities have increased dramatically with the passage of new civil rights laws, such as the Americans with Disabilities Act.[64]

If additional Congressional budgetary support cannot be obtained, then DHHS should internally redirect some of the money spent for other agency purposes on civil rights enforcement. HHS spends hundreds of millions of dollars addressing racial and ethnic disparities in healthcare; OCR should have a greater share of those dollars.[64]

### Accreditation agencies should tie language access to patient safety concerns

There is ample evidence that ineffective language access systems pose compelling patient safety concerns. Both NCQA and JCAHO should place greater emphasis on the effectiveness of health plans and hospitals language access systems as a critical determinant of quality of care and patient safety. If accreditation agencies placed greater emphasis on the importance of language access systems, hospitals and health plans would also be forced to accord them a higher level of priority.

In fact, JCAHO is already in the process of taking three key initial steps towards this end. First, the Joint Commission recently approved a new requirement for the inclusion of language and communication needs in medical records (Standard IM.6.20).[65] The new requirement is one of a list of information requirements such as patient name, gender, and age. The hope is that language and communication needs will be identified in the record in a place that will allow the information to be easily shared across the continuum of care.

Second, JCAHO in partnership with the Commonwealth Fund, has commissioned a study on 'Understanding Adverse Events in Minority Patients With LEP.'[65] The purpose of the project is to learn more about the epidemiology of adverse events attributed to patient–provider communication problems due to language barriers and to identify quality improvement opportunities for inpatients with limited English proficiency. De-identified adverse event data were collected from participating hospitals through their existing incident reporting systems, stratified by English-speaking and LEP patients. These data are being examined using the Joint Commission's Patient Safety Event Taxonomy as an analytical framework, and events are deconstructed to identify causative and contributive factors related to communication and language. This project will provide important information on linguistically appropriate patient care for policy makers, researchers, and clinicians.[65]

Finally, in January 2004, JCAHO launched its 'Hospitals, Language, and Culture' program.[65] The program is a two-and-one-half-year project funded by The California Endowment that will gather data on a sample of hospitals to assess their capacity to address issues of language and culture that impact the quality and safety of patient care. According to JCAHO, the focus of this project is not to develop new standards and set new expectations for accredited organizations but instead to better understand what the current state of practice is and develop recommendations. JCAHO also hopes to explore emerging practices that can be shared with the field and replicated.[65]

## Endnotes

1. California hospitals may face possible tort liability if a limited English proficient (LEP) patient files a medical malpractice claim in an instance where a lack of communication creates a damaging barrier to adequate care, for example in the case of a lack of informed consent. The maximum amount of damages for noneconomic losses in medical malpractice actions is US$250 000. See Cal. Civil Code 3333.2. See also Harsham, P. A., 'A Misunderstood Word Worth $71 Million,' Med. Econ. 1984; June: 289–292, which reports on a successful, multimillion dollar lawsuit over a single misinterpreted word – 'intoxicado' – in a hospital emergency department. In that case, a paramedic interpreted a boy's utterance of the word 'intoxicado' as 'intoxicated,' instead of its intended meaning, which is 'nauseated.' For several days, the boy was evaluated for drug abuse. Subsequently, he was found to have damage caused by a ruptured brain aneurysm. The patient ended up a quadriplegic and was awarded US$71 million in a malpractice case.

2. Thomas Perez, the Former Director of DHHS' OCR makes an important observation on this point. Despite the Supreme Court's ruling in *Sandoval*, Perez maintains that private plaintiffs may still be able to meet the higher intent standard in language access cases. By virtue of the OCR Guidance on National Origin Discrimination Against LEP issued in 2003, Perez suggests that healthcare providers have been put on notice of their obligation under Title VI to ensure meaningful access for people with limited English skills. As a result, he says, 'a private plaintiff can argue that the failure to comply with a civil rights obligation that has been clearly communicated amounts to intentional discrimination under Title VI.' Additionally, a number of states have laws and/or regulations requiring the provision of language assistance services. Private plaintiffs can also avail themselves of these provisions even in the aftermath of *Sandoval*.

3. Numerous authors have commented on OCR's limited effectiveness. See, for example, Perez at p. 656. See also: Villazor, R. C., 'Community Lawyering: An Approach to Addressing Inequalities in Access to Health Care for Poor, Of Color and Immigrant Communities,' Legislation and Public Policy, Vol. 8, pp. 35–62, at pp. 47–48, and especially FN 85; 1 US Comm'n on Civil Rights, The Health Care Challenge: Acknowledging Disparity, Confronting Discrimination, and Ensuring Equality 1, 189–200 (1999) (reporting that OCR had failed to effectively enforce Title VI); Perkins, J., Race Discrimination in America's Health Care System, 27 Clearinghouse Rev. 371, 380 (Special Issue 1993) (questioning the efficiency of OCR complaint process.)

4. CLAS Standard number three states: 'Healthcare organizations should ensure that staff at all levels and across all disciplines receive ongoing education and training in culturally and linguistically appropriate service delivery.' The developers of the CLAS Standards have stated their belief that this standard was one of the most important of the fourteen standards. In one of the preliminary drafts of the CLAS standards it was suggested that providers receive up to 13 hours of training on the provision of culturally competent care. When healthcare industry representatives balked at the time and cost involved in implementing this recommendation, the recommendation itself was allowed to remain but all suggestions of a required amount of time spent on cultural competence training were omitted.[26]

5. It is worth noting that CLAS Standard 10 encourages the collection of race, ethnicity, and spoken and written language. However, this standard is a recommendation, not a mandate and does not have the force of law. CLAS Standard 10 states: 'Healthcare organizations should ensure that data on the individual's race, ethnicity, and spoken and written language are collected in health records, integrated into the organization's management information systems and periodically updated.'

6. The National Health Law Program surveyed the states to determine the extent to which federal funding is being used specifically to reimburse the costs associated with the provision of language services to Medicaid beneficiaries. The nine states listed reported obtaining those matching funds. States can receive reimbursement for language services as an administrative expense (equal to 50% of the costs). Idaho, Hawaii, Maine, and Utah receive reimbursement as a covered service, thus obtaining reimbursement at a higher rate. Different payment models are being used. Hawaii, Washington, and Utah contract with language interpretation agencies to which the states pay directly for services. In New Hampshire, interpreters contract with the state Medicaid agency and become participating Medicaid providers who are then reimbursed directly by the state. Idaho, Maine, and Minnesota require providers to pay interpreters and then receive reimbursement from the state.

# References

1. Perez Thomas E. The civil rights dimension of racial and ethnic disparities in health status. In: Institute of Medicine. Unequal treatment: confronting racial and ethnic disparities in healthcare. 2002:639.
2. Marcum D. Soul searching Fresno woman returns to the jail cell where she was illegally detained to claim her spirit. The Fresno Bee, April 23, 2001: A1.
3. See also: *Hongkham Souvannarath v. David Hadden et al.*, 116 Cal.Rptr.2d 7 (Cal. App.4 Dist. 2002).
4. Perez Thomas E. The civil rights dimension of racial and ethnic disparities in health status. In: Institute of Medicine. Unequal treatment: confronting racial and ethnic disparities in healthcare. 2002:641.
5. *Simkins v. Moses H. Cone Mem'l Hospital*, 323 F.2d 959 (4th Cir. 1963).
6. Pub. L. No. 88–352, Title VI, 601, 78 Stat. 241, 252 (1964) Codified as amended at 42 U.S.C. 2000d (2001).
7. 45 C.F.R. 80.3(b)(2) (2000).
8. *Lau v. Nichols*, 414 U.S. 563 (1974).
9. Id, 566.
10. Id, 568–569.
11. 45 Fed. Reg. 82,972 (Dec. 17, 1980) (Department of Health and Human Services Notice).
12. *Alexander v. Sandoval*, 121 S.Ct. 1511 (2001).
13. Perez Thomas E. The civil rights dimension of racial and ethnic disparities in health status. In: Institute of Medicine. Unequal treatment: confronting racial and ethnic disparities in healthcare. 2002:641 FN 29.
14. Perez Thomas E. The civil rights dimension of racial and ethnic disparities in health status. In: Institute of Medicine. Unequal treatment: confronting racial and ethnic disparities in healthcare. 2002:640.
15. Perez Thomas E. The civil rights dimension of racial and ethnic disparities in health status. In: Institute of Medicine. Unequal treatment: confronting racial and ethnic disparities in healthcare. 2002:639.
16. Perez Thomas E. The civil rights dimension of racial and ethnic disparities in health status. In: Institute of Medicine. Unequal treatment: confronting racial and ethnic disparities in healthcare. 2002:641.
17. Perkins J. Ensuring linguistic access in healthcare settings: an overview of current legal rights and responsibilities. National Health Law Program August 2003:13–14.
18. US Department Of Health And Human Services, Guidance To Federal Financial Assistance Recipients Regarding Title Vi Prohibition Against National Origin Discrimination Affecting Limited English Proficient Persons. Volume 68 Federal Register Number 153, Friday, August 8, 2003:47311–47323.
19. Id., 47314.
20. Id., 47315.
21. Id., 47317.
22. Id., 47318.
23. Id., 47319.
24. Id., 47318–47319.
25. Id., 47319–47320.
26. National Standards For Culturally And Linguistically Appropriate Services In Health Care. Final Report, Office Of Minority Health, U.S. Department Of Health And Human Services. March, 2001. *The final standards were published in the Federal Register on December 22, 2000 (Volume 65, Number 247, pp. 80865–80879). Complete information about the project can be found at* http://www.omhrc.gov/CLAS.
27. CLAS Standards Final Report, 3.
28. CLAS Standards Final Report, 7–13.
29. Perkins J. Ensuring linguistic access in healthcare settings: an overview of current legal rights and responsibilities. National Health Law Program August 2003:16. Updated January 2006.
30. Ikemoto L. Racial disparities in healthcare and cultural competency. 48 St. Louis Univ. Law Journal 111, 75–130. *See especially FNs 229–231, at p. 111 describing applicable California law.*
31. Id., 111–113.
32. Id.,113.
33. 45 C.F.R. 84.52(d).
34. Arizona Center for Disability Law. The duty of healthcare professionals to provide sign language interpreters: a self-advocacy guide. Revised 09/03/01 at p. 1.
35. 56 Fed. Reg. 35544 (July 26, 1991) at 35565.
36. Id., 35566–35567.
37. 28 C.F.R. 36.303(a).
38. Arizona Center for Disability Law, op. cit., p.2.
39. Institute of Medicine. Unequal treatment: confronting racial and ethnic disparities in healthcare. Washington DC: National Academy Press; 2003.
40. Perot R, Youdelman M. Racial, ethnic, and primary language data collection in the healthcare system: an assessment of federal policies and practices. New York: The National Health Law Program funding provided by the Commonwealth Fund; September 2001.
41. America's Health Insurance Plans, Collection of racial and ethnic data by health plans to address disparities: final summary report. The Robert Wood Johnson Foundation; June, 2004.
42. Health Research and Education Trust. Hasnain-Wynia R, Pierce D, Pittman M. Who, when and how: the current state of race, ethnicity, and primary language data collection in hospitals. The Commonwealth Fund: May, 2004.
43. Id. *The study by the Commonwealth Fund also summarized the results of the American Hospital Association survey of its members.*
44. National Public Health and Hospital Institute. Regenstein M, Sickler D. Race, ethnicity, and language of patients: hospital practices regarding collection of information to address disparities in healthcare. The Robert Wood Johnson Foundation; January, 2006:4–5, 8–9, 11. *According to the study, '[f]or hospitals that do not collect [race] data, the most common barrier by far was the sense that there was no need to collect the information. More than half of the hospitals that do not collect this information identified this as a barrier to collection – more than three times the rate seen among hospitals that collect this information.'*
45. Brotherton SE, Rockey PH, Etzel SI. 'US graduate medical education: 2003–2004. JAMA 2004; 292(9):1032–1037.
46. Weissman JS, Betancourt JR, et al. Resident physicians' preparedness to provide cross-cultural care. JAMA 2005; 294:1058–1067.
47. Betancourt J, Green A, Carrillo E, et al. Cultural competence and healthcare disparities: key perspectives and trends. Health Affairs 2005; April:499–505.
48. New York State Department of Health. Graduate medical education reform incentive pool. December, 2004. Available: http://www.health.state.ny.us/nysdoh/gme/main.htm 27 December 2004.
49. Adams D. Cultural competency now law in New Jersey. American Medical News, April 25, 2005. See also, New Jersey State Legislature, S144. Available: http://www.njleg.state.nj.us/2004/Bills/SO500/144_[1.htm 21 January 2005.
50. News Release. NCLR welcomes passage of cultural and linguistic competency training bill for physicians in California. October 6, 2005, National Council of La Raza. Available: http://www.nclr.org/content/news/detail/34227/
51. Perez Thomas E. The civil rights dimension of racial and ethnic disparities in health status. In: Institute of Medicine. Unequal treatment: confronting racial and ethnic disparities in healthcare. 2002:648.
52. Health Education and Research Trust, see Ref 42.
53. Perez Thomas E. The civil rights dimension of racial and ethnic disparities in health status. In: Institute of Medicine. Unequal treatment: confronting racial and ethnic disparities in healthcare. 2002:650.
54. Press Release. Summary of FairCare legislation, Office of Senator Joseph Lieberman (D-CT). October 27, 2005.

55. See Letter from Robert W. Gilmore, M.D., American Medical Association, to Brenda Aguilar, Office of Management and Budget (Dec. 21, 2001) available: http://www.ama.org
56. Office of Management and Budget, Report to Congress. Assessment of the total benefits and costs of implementing Executive Order 13166: Improving Access to Services for Persons with Limited English Proficiency (Mar. 14, 2002). Available: http://www.whitehouse.gov/omb/inforeg/lepfinal3–14.pdf.
57. Newman B. Doctor's orders can get lost in translation for immigrants. The Wall Street Journal, January 9, 2003. *This article cited the OMB's 2002 report which estimated the number of patient encounters across language barriers each year at 66 million. Were language assistance services made more widely available, that number would likely increase dramatically.*
58. CMS, Dear State Medicaid Director. Aug. 31, 2000.
59. Perkins J, op.cit., 14.
60. Hawryluk M. Lost in translation: ways to afford speaking your patients' languages. AMNews, Dec. 2, 2002.
61. Green A, Ngo-Metzger Q, et al. Interpreter services, language concordance, and healthcare quality: experiences of Asian Americans with limited English proficiency, J Gen Internal Med 2005; 20:1050.
62. Hawryluk M, op. cit. See FN 76 above for full citation.
63. Perez Thomas E. The civil rights dimension of racial and ethnic disparities in health status. In: Institute of Medicine. Unequal treatment: confronting racial and ethnic disparities in healthcare. 2002:661–662.
64. Perez Thomas E. The civil rights dimension of racial and ethnic disparities in health status. In: Institute of Medicine. Unequal treatment: confronting racial and ethnic disparities in healthcare. 2002:656.
65. See the JCAHO website at http://www.jcaho.org/about+us/hlc/home.htm In particular, consult Hospitals, Language and Culture under the drop-down menu beneath About Us. See also Resources and Standards on the About Us menu for links to useful links to pdf. files such as: a Crosswalk of Joint Commission and Culturally and Linguistically Appropriate Standards (CLAS) and Joint Commission Standards that Support the Provision of CLAS.

# CHAPTER 6

# Communicating with Limited English Proficient Patients:
*Interpreter Services*

Carol Berg and Sidney Van Dyke

The need to ensure linguistic access to healthcare for limited English proficient (LEP) patients through the use of bilingual providers or trained interpreters can be understood from four primary perspectives: regulatory, demographic, financial, and quality. The regulatory basis for the provision of interpreter services was covered in Chapter 5, so the focus here will be on the demographic, financial, and quality perspectives, all illustrated in the following patient experience.

Yee (not her real name) presented in the ER of a large urban hospital with a serious hand injury. Like large numbers of other recent immigrants to this urban center, Yee spoke fluent Hmong but almost no English. She did not bring an interpreter nor had one been arranged for her through the hospital, so her husband agreed to interpret at the physician's request. The physician asked the patient to follow up immediately at the hand clinic, but her husband interpreted the physician's request to mean that they were to follow up at their primary care clinic to have her hand seen again. It took the primary care physician two visits to realize the mistake and set up a follow-up appointment with the surgery clinic. Precious weeks were lost due to this one interpretation error and the window of opportunity to repair the nerve and ligament damage to this woman's hand had narrowed significantly. If a trained interpreter had been used for Yee's visit to the ER, the additional cost would likely not have exceeded $75. The price of saving this expense? Significant:

- The physician put his organization at risk of litigation by not offering the services of an interpreter to the patient as required by law.
- The healthcare system was burdened with the cost of two unnecessary primary care visits.
- The health outcome this patient could expect was severely compromised by her lack of understanding of follow-up instructions.

## The Demographic Perspective

According to the 2000 census,[3] more than 21 million individuals in the US have limited English proficiency or identify themselves as speaking English less than 'very well.' LEP populations grew more than 100% in fifteen states between 1990 and 2000 with significant growth occurring in rural as well as urban settings. As LEP populations have grown, so too has the need for healthcare organizations to find ways to effectively bridge the language gap between providers and their patients. A key first step in doing this is to identify the primary language groups in one's service area. The language map available through the Modern Languages Association (*www.mla.org*) is a very useful tool for accomplishing this. It allows users to search for 30 different languages by state, county, city, and zip code. Other good

LEP persons are individuals who are not able to speak, read, write, or understand the English language at a level that permits them to interact effectively with healthcare providers and social service agencies.[2]

The NCIHC defines interpreting as the process of understanding and analyzing a spoken or signed message and re-expressing that message faithfully, accurately and objectively in another language, taking the cultural and social context into account.

The following terms are helpful in understanding different means and modes of interpretation and how interpretation differs from translation:

*Ad hoc interpreter*: an untrained person who is called upon to interpret, such as a family member interpreting for parents, a bilingual staff member pulled away from other duties to interpret, or a self-declared bilingual in a hospital waiting-room who volunteers to interpret. Also called a *chance interpreter* or *lay interpreter*.

*Professional interpreter*: an individual with appropriate training and experience who is able to interpret with consistency and accuracy and who adheres to a code of professional ethics.

*Certified interpreter*: a professional interpreter who is certified as competent by a professional organization or government entity through rigorous testing based on appropriate and consistent criteria. Interpreters who have had limited training or have taken a screening test administered by an employing health, interpreter or referral agency are not considered certified.

*Consecutive interpreting*: the conversion of a speaker or signer's message into another language after the speaker or signer pauses, in a specific social context.

*Simultaneous interpreting*: converting a speaker or signer's message into another language while the speaker or signer continues to speak or sign.

*Sight translation*: translation of a written document into spoken/signed language. An interpreter reads a document written in one language and simultaneously interprets it into a second language.

*Translation*: the conversion of a written text into a corresponding written text in a different language. [Within the language professions, *translation* is distinguished from *interpreting* according to whether the message is produced *orally* (or manually) or *in writing*. In popular usage, the terms 'translator' and 'translation' are frequently used for conversion of either oral or written communications.]

sources of population estimates are community-based organizations and refugee resettlement agencies that serve new refugee and immigrant arrivals in a particular area. Collecting race/ethnicity and language preference data, covered in Chapter 7, offers an additional snapshot of the demographic trends that should shape the interpreter services developed in a particular organization.

## The Financial Perspective

Many healthcare organizations consider cost to be one of the most significant barriers to ensuring linguistic access to their LEP populations. Yet research has shown that the cost of *not* providing trained interpreters could be significantly higher than the cost of providing them. A 2002 US government report estimated that 'healthcare providers could spend up to $267.6 million on language services for approximately 66.1 million ER visits, inpatient hospital visits, outpatient physician visits, and dental visits by LEP persons. This represents about $4.04 per visit or a 0.5% premium.'[4] At the same time, there is a growing body of research documenting areas in which failure to bridge the communication gap between LEP patients and their providers is adding significant, measurable costs to the healthcare system. The most obvious of these is the increased risk of litigation due to non-compliance with federal regulations. In one high-profile malpractice case, a family was awarded $71 million when a paramedic's misinterpretation of a young boy's Spanish – taking 'intoxicado' to mean 'intoxicated' rather than 'nauseated' as was intended – led to the boy being evaluated for drug abuse over a period of several days. He was later found to have suffered a ruptured brain aneurysm. Delay in appropriate treatment left him quadriplegic.[5]

In two separate research studies, an unaddressed language barrier led to increased usage of diagnostic testing.[6,7] The Hampers and McNulty study also reported an increased rate of hospital admission in the absence of a bilingual provider or professional interpreter. The general conclusion: when faced with a language barrier, providers tend to be more cautious – and more expensive – decision-makers.

A third study, conducted to assess the impact of interpreter services on the cost and utilization of healthcare services among LEP patients, found that the provision of professional interpreter services resulted in a statistically significant increase in receipt of preventive and primary care services, which has the potential of reducing costly complications of chronic conditions such as diabetes or heart disease.[8] Similarly, research conducted at the Boston Medical Center found that the use of trained medical interpreters reduces Emergency Department (ED) services and charges. When trained interpreters were used to meet the language needs of patients in this study, there was an associated reduction in ED return rates, increased utilization of outpatient clinics, and lower 30-day charges without any concurrent increase in visit costs or length of stay.[9]

All of these studies point to the same conclusion: failure to meet the language needs of LEP individuals and their providers leads to increased financial burden on the American medical system. An appropriate response would be to view interpreter services as an investment made to avoid incurring significantly higher costs in other ways.

## The Quality Perspective

Healthcare providers should understand the critical role of language services in improving health outcomes. Language barriers and inadequate funding of language services inhibit LEP persons' access to healthcare and pose a risk to the quality of care they receive.[10,11] LEP patients are less likely to have a regular source of care,[12,13] are more likely to report overall problems with care,[14] and are more at risk of experiencing medical errors.[15]

In contrast, using trained interpreters reduces medical errors, increases patient compliance, increases patient satisfaction, and improves primary care utilization,[16] thus improving the overall quality of healthcare and health outcomes for LEP patients. A research team from the University of California, Los Angeles, analyzed data on 26 298 parents of children enrolled in the California State Children's Health Insurance Program and found that providing trained medical interpreters can substantially improve how patients experience care. Providing interpreting services to those who needed them produced a 9% improvement in the communication measure for Hispanics and a 23% improvement for Asian/Pacific Islanders.[17]

A systematic literature review was conducted in 2005 by Glen Flores on the impact of interpreter services on quality of care.[18] In his review, Flores focused on three separate categories:

1. Communication issues;
2. Patient satisfaction; and
3. Health processes, outcomes, complications, and use of health services.

The most thorough studies yielded the following conclusions:

1. Communication issues:
   - Limited English proficient patients who need an interpreter but do not have one report a poor understanding of their diagnosis and treatment and often wish their providers had 'explained things better.'
   - Untrained interpreters are more likely to make errors that have clinical consequences, have higher risk of not mentioning side effects and may ignore 'embarrassing' medical issues, particularly when children are used as interpreters.
   - Quality of psychiatric encounters is negatively impacted by use of untrained interpreters and positively impacted by bilingual providers.
2. Patient satisfaction:
   - Bilingual providers produced the highest patient satisfaction. Ad hoc interpreters showed significantly lower satisfaction. The lowest satisfaction rate was among patients who needed an interpreter but did not receive this service.
3. Health processes, outcomes, complications and use of health services:
   - Interpreter services improve preventive services utilization rates.
   - It is not clear that medical visits with interpreter services are longer than other visits.
   - Use of trained interpreter services resulted in more office visits and more prescriptions being written and filled.
   - Limited English proficient patients with no interpreter services or with ad hoc interpreters have more medical tests, higher test costs, more frequent intravenous hydration, and a higher rate of hospitalization.

Flores concludes: 'This systematic review of the literature indicates that additional studies employing rigorous methods are needed on the most effective and least costly ways to provide interpreter services to LEP patients. But available evidence suggests that optimal communication, the highest satisfaction, the best outcomes, and the fewest errors with potential clinical consequence occur when LEP patients have access to trained professional interpreters or bilingual healthcare providers.'[18]

Providing language assistance ultimately puts the patient in the forefront and in a role of control equal to any English speaker's experience, which is key to beginning to reduce the racial and ethnic disparities that exist in healthcare. Healthcare providers can be assured of accurate, reliable transmission of their communication and patients can be assured of better understanding of their diagnosis and treatment options only when professional interpreters are used to bridge the language gap.

## Ensuring linguistic access

While this chapter focuses on the appropriate use of professional interpreters to bridge the language gap, we want to acknowledge that there are a variety of ways one can effectively overcome the language barrier with LEP persons. They include the following approaches.

**Bilingual/bicultural healthcare providers** An ideal strategy is for provider and patient to speak the same language, but this requires fluency in both parties. False fluency, in which a provider believes he is more competent than he actually is, can lead to serious miscommunication. While such miscommunication can be humorous – such as during a fetal ultrasound when a provider announced to a proud mother-to-be that he saw her baby's beer (*cerveza*) instead of her baby's head (*cabeza*) – it can also have dangerous consequences. In testimony before the US Senate Committee on Health, Education, Labor and Pensions Subcommittee on Public Health, Dr. Glenn Flores told the story of a young Latino girl who, with her brother, was taken into custody by the Department of Social Services for 48 hours after a medical resident who identified himself as Spanish-speaking made a serious interpretation error. When the girl's mother was asked how the little girl had fractured her right collarbone, she responded, 'Se pegó, se pegó' or 'she fell and hit herself,' not 'she was hit' as the resident physician interpreted the response.[19]

Healthcare providers should be tested for fluency before assuming that they can satisfactorily communicate in the language of the patient. Catherine Dower, associate director of the University of California–San Francisco's Center for the Health Professions, states that a 'credentialing system' should be established to identify clinicians who are proficient in foreign languages. She also argues that they should be offered financial incentives for their bilingual skills. This would allow patients to more easily choose physicians who speak their native language.[20] Healthcare provider directories should indicate language proficiency among clinicians listed to make it easier for LEP patients to choose a physician who can provide care in their native language.

**Professional interpreters** Professional interpreters are skilled bilinguals who are trained in the skill of interpreting and the standards of practice and professional code of ethics that govern the profession. When provider and patient do not speak the same language, only trained professional interpreters should be used to bridge the communication gap. Untrained bilingual staff, family members, and friends should only be used when all sources of professional interpretation have been exhausted and it is medically imprudent to reschedule the visit. The limited fluency and weak knowledge of medical terminology in one or both languages of these individuals can seriously impair communication. Their lack of training in interpreting, coupled with little or no familiarity with professional standards of practice, often lead them to editorialize or omit key information they deem unimportant. Cultural barriers can also interfere with clear communication when family members are used to interpret. Furthermore, the use of family members, especially children, can place a serious emotional burden on the individual asked to interpret. If the patient has a poor health outcome, the family member who acted as an interpreter can blame himself or herself for it. A parent's authority can also be seriously undermined when a minor child is used as an interpreter, in effect reversing the balance of power between parent and child. Minor children should never be used as interpreters.

If a patient indicates a preference for using a family member to interpret, the provider should thank the family member for his or her support but insist that the family member would better assist the patient by being a supportive second set of ears rather than an interpreter, leaving that role to an interpreter more familiar with the complex medical vocabulary the physician may use. If a patient still insists on using a family member, the provider should document the patient's refusal to use a professional interpreter in the patient's chart and may wish to have an interpreter observe the interaction.

There are three commonly recognized methods of providing professional interpreter services to patients and providers. They are:

1. In-person interpreting, when an interpreter is physically present with the patient and provider. This service can be provided by

either staff interpreters or contracted interpreters.

2. Telephonic interpreting, which is provided by trained interpreters who work for a contracted agency or staff interpreters working a phone bank at a remote location. Phones with a speaker or dual handset work best in the exam room, while a conference call function is useful when making calls to or receiving calls from LEP patients.

3. Remote interpreting, where an audio (wireless headsets) or video (portable monitors) feed is used to access an interpreter.

In-person interpreting is the preferred method of service provision but telephonic interpreting may be the next option if an interpreter is unable to be present for an encounter. Remote interpreting options are just now being piloted in healthcare settings and, while promising, it is not yet clear how useful this technology will be in communicating with LEP patients.

**Bilingual/bicultural community health workers**
Bilingual/bicultural community health workers (CHWs) play an important role in effectively communicating health information to LEP persons. CHWs are members of the community they serve, build relationships and trust at the grassroots level, and bridge the gap between individuals, families, and communities with health and social service providers.[21] CHWs are paraprofessionals who teach community members and providers the knowledge and skills needed to understand, give and receive appropriate care and services, but they should not be used as interpreters as part of their job unless they have taken professional interpreter training.

**Employee language banks (qualified and evaluated)** If a healthcare organization chooses to have an employee language bank from which to utilize bilingual staff as interpreters on occasion, the identified staff must have professional interpreter training and should be proficiency tested prior to being added to the language bank. The employer may need to cover both training and testing if the staff does not have evidence of proper education and adequate proficiency. The staff member's interpreter role should be included as part of his or her job description and appropriate remuneration should be calculated into the salary.

**Multilingual health resources (such as written materials, audiotapes, videotapes, TV and radio programs)** Communication of health information in different languages is enhanced by using quality health resources and materials in the language of the patient. It is helpful to ask and document what the patient's preferred learning method is in order to use the most appropriate form of communication when sharing health information. There are a number of websites that offer multilingual health resources, some of which are listed under Resources at the end of this chapter.

## Financing interpreter services

The federal requirements for providers receiving federal funds to offer language assistance (identified in Ch. 3) do not provide a funding mechanism to pay for these services. The 2002 Office of Management and Budget report mentioned earlier determined that it would cost the nation $268 million a year to provide interpreting services for inpatient hospital, outpatient physician, ED and dental visits.[4] The OMB's estimate did not discount the costs of interpreter services already being provided or discount for reductions in other health costs that might occur if there were better patient–provider communication. The net additional costs of expanding interpreter services would be expected to be lower.

Ku and Flores[22] suggest several payment models for language services:

• Secure insurance reimbursement for professional interpreters, paid hourly or per visit. Currently, legislation regarding reimbursement is inconsistent from state to state and differs significantly depending on whether an individual carries publicly or privately funded insurance.
• Allow providers to seek reimbursement from insurers for services provided by telephone interpretation firms, contracted through these insurers. Reimbursement for telephonic interpreting is not standard across insurers and payers.
• Fund community organizations to create 'language banks' that recruit, train, and organize medical interpreters for healthcare facilities.
• Modify standard healthcare reimbursements for medical appointment of LEP patients. One example is to modify a physician's relative value scale payment when serving an LEP patient, raising reimbursement by X dollars or Y percent because of the added

services needed for these patients. Healthcare institutions would then be able to use the additional funds they generate to increase the number of bilingual healthcare providers they employ or fund contract or staff interpreters.

Further exploration is needed to identify ways in which the many sectors of society dependent on the availability of high-quality interpreter services can partner to share the financial responsibility for providing these services.

## Assuring interpreting competency

Underlying all these various reimbursement models is a need to assure the competency of interpreters. Many groups are working across the country to increase the number of interpreters who have completed professional training, but training programs are not yet available in some areas and no national certification process currently exists for healthcare interpreters. Until adequate training is more widely available in educational institutions and a certification process is in place, medical organizations and interpreter agencies must work independently or in partnership with each other to ensure that they have a competent pool of medical interpreters on their staff or roster.

The National Council on Interpreting in Health Care (NCIHC) has identified four steps needed at the national level to further professionalize the field of healthcare interpreting and standardize the quality expectations healthcare professionals and patients should have of interpreters:

1. Develop a single *code of ethics*. A national code of ethics was issued by NCIHC in 2004 (Box 6.2).
2. Develop a unified set of *standards of practice* defining best practices in healthcare interpreting. NCIHC published a national set of standards in 2005.[24] The full set of 32 standards is available at *www.ncihc.org* The standards are grouped under 9 headings that show the relationship between each standard and a corresponding ethical principal from the NCIHC Code of Ethics. These headings are: accuracy, confidentiality, impartiality, respect, cultural awareness, role boundaries, professionalism, professional development, and advocacy.
3. Develop standards for healthcare interpreter training programs.

---

> **Box 6.2**
>
> **NCIHC National Code of Ethics for Interpreters in Health Care[23]**
>
> - The interpreter treats as confidential, within the treating team, all information learned in the performance of professional duties, while observing relevant requirements regarding disclosure.
> - The interpreter strives to render the message accurately, conveying the content and spirit of the original message, taking into consideration its cultural context.
> - The interpreter strives to maintain impartiality and refrains from counseling, advising or projecting personal biases or beliefs.
> - The interpreter maintains the boundaries of the professional role, refraining from personal involvement.
> - The interpreter continuously strives to develop awareness of his/her own and other (including biomedical) cultures encountered in the performance of professional duties.
> - The interpreter treats all parties with respect.
> - When the patient's health, well-being, or dignity is at risk, the interpreter may be justified in acting as an advocate. Advocacy is understood as an action taken on behalf of an individual that goes beyond facilitating communication, with the intention of supporting good health outcomes. Advocacy must only be undertaken after careful and thoughtful analysis of the situation and if other less intrusive actions have not resolved the problem.
> - The interpreter strives to continually further his/her knowledge and skills.
> - The interpreter must at all times act in a professional and ethical manner.

4. Create a national certification process that will set a standard for qualifications as a professional healthcare interpreter.

In the meantime, efforts are being made in many states to assure that persons providing interpreter services are screened for language proficiency, demonstrate understanding of the professional code of ethics and standards of practice, and provide evidence of their interpreting.

Both medical organizations hiring staff interpreters and agencies recruiting interpreters on contract should thoroughly assess each candidate's qualifications and capacity to work as a medical interpreter. The assessment process recommended by the NCIHC includes a thorough review of credentials, an employment interview, and an assessment of interpreter skills using such methods as language competency testing, an ethical case study, and a medical terminology test.[25]

While healthcare organizations and interpreter agencies have traditionally had to develop their own competency assessments, resulting in wasted resources and a serious lack of standardization, there have been advances in evaluating the skills of bilingual persons who wish to act as interpreters. For instance, Language Line University (www.languageline.com) offers a number of testing services aimed at evaluating language and interpreting skills and can tailor testing requests to specific disciplines, including healthcare. Another option is Language Testing International, or LTI (www.languagetesting.com), which serves as the testing branch of the American Council on the Teaching of Foreign Languages. LTI testing is not specific for healthcare settings and does not offer a test of interpreting skills but can test for general language proficiency in 48 different languages.

Others have pooled their resources to create assessment tools and/or do joint assessments of bilingual persons interested in serving as interpreters in their common service area. For example, a group of eight hospitals and healthcare institutions in Dane County, Wisconsin, created the Dane County Health Care Providers Interpreter Services Group in 1994, which partners to standardize interpreter policies and testing and offers training opportunities to bilingual applicants. This allows them to maintain a pool of qualified interpreters on a roster published for all participating institutions. Interpreters must successfully pass the screening process, agree to abide by the National Code of Ethics for Interpreters in Health Care and complete the policy requirements of the participating institutions (i.e. background checks, safety and infection control training). The collaborative has also developed a medical interpreter assessment for Spanish interpreter candidates. All freelance Spanish interpreters wishing to be added to the roster must take and pass this assessment. Partner organizations share the administrative costs for this collaboration, which amount to $3,000–$4,000 per year.

Interpreter agencies that contract with healthcare organizations to provide interpreter services are generally expected to assess and assure the competency of the interpreters they provide. However, assessment and practice standards vary widely from agency to agency, so healthcare organizations wishing to contract with an interpreter agency should make every effort to understand the ways in which the agencies assure the competency of their interpreters. The document entitled *How to Choose and Use a Language Agency* provides useful guidance. It is available through the California Endowment at www.calendow.org

## What Healthcare Providers Can Do?

Healthcare providers can play a key role in improving language access in the following concrete ways:

1. Ensure compliance with linguistic access laws in your own practice. The Department of Justice suggests taking these five steps:[26]
   • Identify patients who need language assistance.
   • Offer information on ways in which language assistance will be provided.
   • Develop a written policy regarding language access that will ensure meaningful communication.
   • Train staff members so they understand the policy and are capable of implementing it.
   • Monitor to ensure that LEP patients have meaningful access to healthcare and update the policy as needed.

One key method for understanding access in your setting is to measure *how* services are being provided, as illustrated in Figure 6.1.

A helpful resource for implementing all five of these steps is 'Addressing Language Access Issues in Your Practice: A Toolkit for Physicians and Their Staff Members,' available from the California Academy of Family Physicians.

2. Learn about reimbursement available for interpreter services in your state. As of 2005, 11 states allow reimbursement for interpreter services provided for Medicaid and State Children's Health Insurance (SCHIP) enrollees. These states are Hawaii, Idaho, Kansas, Maine, Massachusetts, Minnesota, Montana, New Hampshire, Utah, Vermont, and Washington.[27] You may contact the state agency that administers the Medicaid program in your state for more information. Medicaid agency contact information by state is available at www.nasmd.org

3. Receive training in techniques of working with interpreters (Box 6.3). Many

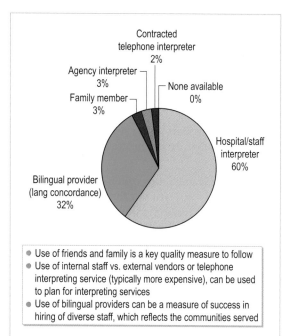

Contracted
telephone interpreter
2%

Agency interpreter
3%

None available
0%

Family member
3%

Hospital/staff
interpreter
60%

Bilingual provider
(lang concordance)
32%

- Use of friends and family is a key quality measure to follow
- Use of internal staff vs. external vendors or telephone interpreting service (typically more expensive), can be used to plan for interpreting services
- Use of bilingual providers can be a measure of success in hiring of diverse staff, which reflects the communities served

**Figure 6.1** Meeting the needs of the LEP patient. Quality measurement tool utilized by the Center for International Health, St Paul, MN (P. Walker MD, DTM&H, personal communication, 2006).

**Box 6.3**

## Guidelines for working with interpreters[28]

To facilitate good communication when speaking through an interpreter it is helpful to follow these guidelines:

- Use qualified interpreters to interpret.
- Don't depend on children or other relatives and friends to interpret.
- Have a brief pre-interview meeting with the interpreter.
- Establish a good working relationship with the interpreter.
- Plan to allow enough time for the interpreted session.
- Address yourself to the interviewee, not the interpreter.
- Don't say anything that you don't want the other party to hear.
- Use words, not just gestures, to convey your meaning.
- Speak in a normal voice, clearly, and not too fast.
- Avoid jargon and technical terms.
- Keep your utterances short, pausing to permit the interpretation.
- Ask only one question at a time.
- Expect the interpreter to interrupt when necessary for clarification.
- Expect the interpreter to take notes if things get complicated.
- Be prepared to repeat yourself in different words if your message is not understood.
- Have a brief post-interview meeting with the interpreter.
- Make sure the interpreter understands his or her role before you begin.
- Use the simplest vocabulary that will express your meaning.
- Speak in short and simple sentences.
- Check to see if the message is understood.

organizations and agencies offer training to healthcare providers in the techniques of working effectively with interpreters.

4. Articulate support for appropriate language services through your professional association. Many organizations, including the American College of Physicians and the American Hospital Association, have endorsed a formal statement of principles on language access in healthcare (Appendix A). These principles were developed in 2005 by a collaborative group which included representation from numerous healthcare, language and accrediting organizations, among others. Interested organizations may sign on to the Principles by contacting the National Health Law Program (see Resource section below).

5. Identify and work with those who may be collaborating in your area to improve interpreter training and interpreter service delivery. For instance, you can contact the professional interpreter association that serves your area to see what resources are available and what interpreter issues are being addressed locally. A list of healthcare

interpreting associations in the US is available through the National Council on Interpreting in Health Care's website (www.ncihc.org).

6. Advocate for public policy for language access and interpreter services. One example of a group working to improve public policy in this area is the Medical Leadership Council on Language Access, which was founded in 2002 by the California Endowment and convened by the California Academy of Family Physicians. The 28

organizations of the Council developed a set of organizing principles focused on provider education, workforce issues, organization and access, written resources, quality assessment, and payment. They also developed policy recommendations for Medicaid/Medicare and managed care organizations.

## Resources for Interpreting Services

If you would like to know more about interpreter services in your state, you may go to the website of the National Council on Interpreting in Health Care (www.ncihc.org) that lists the professional interpreter associations by state and region. Many of these groups are involved in working with healthcare providers in their area to address interpreter service concerns and improve service delivery.

Other helpful resources for interpreting issues include the following:

- The LEP.gov (www.lep.gov) website offers guidance for assuring language access to federal programs and federally assisted programs. It is a clearinghouse that provides information, tools, and technical assistance regarding limited English proficiency and language services for federal agencies, recipients of federal funds, users of federal programs and federally assisted programs, and other interested parties.
- The National Health Law Program is a national public interest law firm that aims to improve healthcare for America's working and unemployed poor, minorities, the elderly, and persons with disabilities. On their website, www.healthlaw.org, click on 'Language Access' for language services news and resources including the Language Access in Health Care Statement of Principles and the Language Services Action Kit: Interpreter Services in Health Care Settings for People with Limited English Proficiency.
- The California Academy of Family Physicians website (www.familydocs.org) includes two key resources mentioned earlier in this chapter: (1) Addressing Language Access Issues in Your Practice: A Toolkit for Physicians and Their Staff Members, and (2) Public Policy Principles for Language Access and Interpreter Services in California.

- The American Translators Association (ATA) (www.atanet.org) is a professional association founded to advance the translation and interpreter professions and foster the professional development of individual translators and interpreters. Their Interpreters Division website (http://www.ata-divisions.org/ID/) contains a wealth of information pertaining specifically to medical interpreting.
- The Massachusetts Department of Public Health website (http://www.mass.gov/dph/) is home to Best Practice Recommendations for Hospital-Based Interpreter Services.
- The Modern Language Association (www.mla.org) Language Map is an excellent resource to determine primary languages other than English spoken in specific US geographic locations, down to individual zip codes.
- The National Guideline Clearinghouse has posted an evidence-based protocol for interpreter facilitation for persons with limited English proficiency on their website (http://www.guideline.gov/).

Examples of websites for multilingual health resources to use in patient education include:

- CultureMed (www.sunyit.edu/library/html/culturemed): This website (based at the Peter J. Cayan Library, SUNY Institute of Technology in Utica, NY) provides access to materials that promote culturally competent healthcare for refugees and immigrants.
- Ethnomed (www.ethnomed.org): Offers patient education materials in a variety of languages as well as cultural information resources for immigrant populations. It is a joint project of University of Washington Health Sciences Library and the Harborview Medical Center's Community House Calls Program.
- LA Health Plan: This health maintenance organization received funding from the California Endowment to provide health-related material in the 10 languages most commonly found in Los Angeles County (http://www.lacare.org/opencms/opencms/en/providers/document_search/index.html).
- Multilingual Health Resource Exchange (www.health-exchange.net): Over a dozen healthcare organizations in Minnesota share

the responsibility and cost of creating and distributing health education materials for LEP patients. Providers working with the participating partners are able to download multilingual health resources on the site. Guests to the website are able to learn more about health education for LEP audiences and view the materials list.

## APPENDIX A    Language Access in Health Care Statement of Principles

- Effective communication between healthcare providers and patients is essential to facilitating access to care, reducing health disparities and medical errors, and assuring a patient's ability to adhere to treatment plans.
- Competent healthcare language services are essential elements of an effective public health and healthcare delivery system in a pluralistic society.
- The responsibility to fund language services for LEP individuals in healthcare settings is a societal one that cannot fairly be visited upon any one segment of the public health or health-care community.
- Federal, state, and local governments, and healthcare insurers should establish and fund mechanisms through which appropriate language services are available where and when they are needed.
- Because it is important for providing all patients with the environment most conducive to positive health outcomes, linguistic diversity in the healthcare workforce should be encouraged, especially for individuals in direct patient contact positions.
- All members of the healthcare community should continue to educate their staff and constituents about LEP issues and help them identify resources to improve access to quality care for LEP patients.
- Access to English as a Second Language instruction is an additional mechanism for eliminating the language barriers that impede access to healthcare and should be made available on a timely basis to meet the needs of LEP individuals, including LEP healthcare workers.
- Quality improvement processes should assess the adequacy of language services provided when evaluating the care of LEP patients, particularly with respect to outcome disparities and medical errors.
- Mechanisms should be developed to establish the competency of those providing language services, including interpreters, translators, and bilingual staff/clinicians.
- Continued efforts to improve primary language data collection are essential to enhance both services for, and research identifying the needs of, the LEP population.
- Language services in healthcare settings must be available as a matter of course, and all stakeholders, including government agencies that fund, administer or oversee healthcare programs, must be accountable for providing or facilitating the provision of those services. (Source: National Health Law Program, 2005.)

## References

1. Standards, Training and Certification Committee, National Council on Interpreting in Health Care. The Terminology of Health Care Interpreting: A Glossary of Terms, NCIHC Working Paper Series; 2001:3–8. Available: http://www.ncihc.org
2. Minnesota Department of Human Services Glossary; 2006. Available: http://www.dhs.state.mn.us/main/groups/agencywide/documents/pub/dhs_id_016420.hcsp
3. US Bureau of the Census, Ability to Speak English; 2000 (Table QT-P17). Available: http://factfinder.census.gov
4. Office of Management and Budget. Report to Congress: Assessment of the Total Benefits and Costs of Implementing Executive Order No. 13166: Improving Access for Persons with Limited English Proficiency. Washington, DC: Office of Management and Budget; 2002:56. Available: http://www.whitehouse.gov/omb/inforeg/lepfinal13–14.pdf
5. Harsham P. A misinterpreted word worth $71 million. Med Econ 1984; June:289–292.
6. Hampers LC, Cha S, Gutglass DJ, et al. Language barriers and resource utilization in a pediatric emergency department. Pediatrics 1999; 103:1253–1256.
7. Hampers LC, McNulty JE. Professional interpreters and bilingual physicians in a pediatric emergency department: effect on resource utilization. Arch Pediatr Adolescent Med 2002; 156:1108–1113.
8. Jacobs EA, Shepard DS, Suaya JA, et al. Overcoming language barriers in healthcare: costs and benefits of interpreter services. Am J Public Health 2004; 94:866–869.
9. Bernstein J, Bernstein E, Dave A, et al. Trained medical interpreters in the emergency department: effects on services, subsequent charges and follow-up. J Immigrant Health 2002; 4:171–176.
10. Kaiser Commission on Medicaid and the Uninsured, Caring for Immigrants. Health Care Safety Nets in Los Angeles, NY, Miami and Houston. Kaiser Permanente; 2001:ii–iii. Available: http://www.kff.org/uninsured/2227-index.cfm

11. Smedley B, Stith A, Nelson A. Unequal treatment: confronting racial and ethnic disparities in healthcare. Washington, DC: Institute of Medicine; 2002:71–72.

12. Kirkman-Liff B, Mondragon D. Language of interview: relevance for research of Southwest Hispanics. Am J Public Health 1991; 81:1399–1404.

13. Weinick R, Krauss N. Racial/ethnic differences in children's access to care. Am J Public Health 2000; 90:1771–1774.

14. Carrasquillo O, Orav EJ, Brennan TA, et al. Impact of language barriers on patient satisfaction in an emergency department. J General Med 1999; 14:82–87.

15. Gandhi TK, Burstin HR, Cook EF, et al. Drug complications in outpatients. J General Internal Med 2000; 15:149–154.

16. Like R. Cross-cultural communication in healthcare: building organizational capacity. US Department of Health and Human Services, Health Resources and Services Administration satellite broadcast, June 4, 2003.

17. Morales, LS. The impact of interpreters on parents' experiences with ambulatory care for their children, Med Care Res Rev 2006; 63:110–128.

18. Flores G. The impact of medical interpreter services on the quality of healthcare: a systematic review. Med Care Res Rev 2005; 62:255–299.

19. Testimony by Glenn Flores, MD, FAAP Chair, Latino Consortium, American Academy of Pediatrics Center for Child Health Research and Associate Professor of Pediatrics, Epidemiology & Health Policy Director, Community Outcomes Associate Director, Center for the Advancement of Urban Children Department of Pediatrics, Medical College of Wisconsin Before the United States Senate Committee on Health, Education, Labor and Pensions Subcommittee on Public Health Hearing on Hispanic Health: Problems with Coverage, Access, and Health Disparities September 23, 2002. Available: http://www.mcw.edu/display/displayFile.asp?docid=10229&filename=/User/akrimmer/CAUC/Senate_Testimony.doc

20. Dower C. As quoted in Hochman M. Interpreters needed even after doctors study languages. Boston Globe, Sept 5, 2005. Available: http://www.boston.com/news/globe/health_science/articles/2005/09/05/interpreters_needed_even_after_doctors_study_languages/

21. Dower C, Knox M, Lindler V, O'Neil E. Advancing Community Health Worker Practice and Utilization: The Focus on Financing. San Francisco, CA: National Fund For Medical Education, 2006.

22. Ku L, Flores G. Pay now or pay later: providing interpreter services in healthcare. Health Affairs 2005; 24:435–444.

23. National Council on Interpreting in Health Care. A National Code of Ethics for Interpreters in Health Care. July, 2004.

24. Standards, Training and Certification Committee, National Council on Interpreting in Health Care. National Standards of Practice for Interpreters in Health Care. September, 2005.

25. Standards, Training and Certification Committee, National Council on Interpreting in Health Care. Guide to Initial Assessment of Interpreter Qualifications. April, 2001.

26. US Department of Justice. Guidance to Federal Financial Assistance Recipients Regarding Title VI Prohibition Against National Origin Discrimination Affecting Limited English Proficient Persons, Federal Register, June 18, 2002. Vol 67, No 117:41455–41472.

27. National Health Law Program. Medicaid/SCHIP Reimbursement Models for Language Services 2005 Update. December, 2005.

28. Downing B. Guidelines for working with interpreters. Program in Translation and Interpreting, University of Minnesota, 2000.

# CHAPTER 7

# Multicultural Medicine

Kathleen A. Culhane-Pera and Jeffrey M. Borkan

Refugees and immigrants enter this country with knowledge, values, and behaviors about health, illness, and treatment that may be drastically different than those which underlie Western bio-medicine and the American healthcare delivery system. Healthcare professionals must take on the potentially complicated tasks of diagnosing and treating these newcomers in manners that are appropriate and effective, overcoming barriers of language, concepts, and expectations. Though not all refugees or immigrants experience difficulties with the American medical system, the potential pitfalls for patients and providers are numerous.

Part A of this chapter describes seven general concepts about healing systems that are pertinent for healthcare professionals who strive to provide culturally competent medical care to refugees and immigrants. Part B provides six recommended fundamental principles for applying the information in clinical settings to help professionals provide quality healthcare and promote therapeutic alliances. Though these concepts and frameworks illuminate multicultural care for immigrants, it is important to emphasize that they are relevant to all healthcare encounters.

## Part A: General Concepts about Healing Systems

Cultures around the world and through time have created healing systems to respond to sickness and life-cycle changes such as pregnancy, birth, puberty, aging, and death. All healing systems have beliefs about what constitutes health, how the body functions normally, what happens to make it function abnormally, and what people can do to restore health.[1-4]

According to Sharma, there are three minimum requirements for a healing system: it must claim to be curative, have a systematized body of knowledge or theory, and a specified technical intervention that can be applied by an expert practitioner.[5] These features are applicable to the healing systems in all cultures, irrespective of their origin or content, or whether they are primarily folk, traditional, or professional in nature. They apply to ancient systems, such as the Chinese traditional medicine, or modern, such as biomedicine. And they apply to healing systems with hundreds of millions of adherents, such as the Indian Ayurvedic system, or small healing systems whose devotees are counted in the hundreds, such as those in remote areas of Africa and South America.

It is important for healthcare professionals to have at least a basic understanding of the various cultural healing systems to which their patient populations adhere. Immigrants and refugees bring elements of their healthcare systems with them, often adapting and modifying them to their new homes, adding to the healing cacophony. To help impart some order, we provide information on seven general concepts of healing systems.

## Concepts of bodily functions, health, and disease

All healing systems have beliefs about what constitutes health and disease, and a coherent system of knowledge about how bodies function normally and abnormally.[1-4] Understanding these may be a first step in gaining insights into health behaviors and forming therapeutic partnerships. For example, the traditional Indian system of Ayurvedic medicine is built on the ancient knowledge in the Atharvaveda text about the three humors – *Vita*, *Pitta*, and *Kapha*.[6] Each person's prescribed lifestyle of diet, exercise, and meditation is designed to maintain his or her specific balance between the three humors. Ayurvedic medicine has influenced other Asian systems, such as the Thai. The traditional Han Chinese system conceives of humans as being part of the universe that is modulated by the opposing *yin* and *yang* forces (male/female, hot/cold, wet/dry, dark/light), which are always changing.[7,8] Health is maintained by balancing *yin* and *yang* forces and diseases are treated by restoring the balance. The Chinese traditional concepts of health and disease permeated other Asian healing systems, such as Vietnamese traditional healing, including the *am/duong* (or *yin/yang*) forces, and in turn had probably been influenced by them.[9] Traditional Mexican beliefs of health include the importance of balancing hot/cold and wet/dry, concepts that probably were swayed by traditional concepts of the native peoples, such as the Mayan and Aztec, and by concepts brought to the New World by Spaniards whose practices had originated with Hippocrates' theory of disease and the four humors.[10,11]

Every healing system has ideas about how natural, social, and supernatural aspects of life are related to health, illness, and healing.[2] The *natural realm* describes the connections between people and the earth, such as dirt, water, air, plants, animals, etc. The *social realm* describes the connections between people of different ages, genders, lineages, and ethnic groups. And the *supernatural realm* describes the connections between the spiritual world and the human world and includes religious beliefs about birth, death, and the afterlife.

Healing systems are indivisible from the cultures in which they are present and are interwoven with other sociocultural elements ranging from familial relations to concepts of the universe.[1–4] No connections or influences on health systems may be stronger than those of religion and spiritual beliefs.[12] For example, Chinese medicine is interwoven with and influenced by Taoism, Ayurvedic medicine by Hinduism, and Tibetan medicine by Buddhism. Santeria healing rituals comes from Santeria, the syncretic religion formed from Yoruba gods and Catholicism, when Yoruba slaves in the West Indies were forbidden to practice their traditional religion but discovered their gods in Catholic saints. Similarly, people's religious beliefs are intertwined with their interpretations and experiences of health and disease. The Islamic faith, for instance, teaches that all life events come from God or *Allah*, and that illness may be sent as a punishment, or an opportunity to atone

for sins.[13,14] Some Muslims believe that Allah has predetermined life events, and all statements about the future include the phrase *Insha Allah*, 'If *Allah* wills,' to acknowledge and accept God's authority. Muslims try to endure their illnesses, and accept their experiences without losing faith or patience with God.

## Theories of disease causation

Every healing system has explanations about etiologies. Determining causation has several functions: it guides therapy prospectively, confirms treatments retrospectively, and provides solace and meaning to human suffering. Helman organizes causations into four categories – individual, natural, social, and supernatural causes – with overlap between the categories.[2] Some healing systems focus more on the individual and natural areas (such as biomedicine), while other systems know that all illnesses are ultimately caused by supernatural forces (such as the Azande). Still other systems examine the intertwined natural and supernatural reasons (such as Aztec, Haitian, Hmong, Mayan, and Yoruba). In the latter situations, people may identify a single cause for some illnesses, such as change in weather or a germ; for other illnesses, people may recognize an underlying supernatural cause, such as soul fright, which subsequently renders the person more vulnerable to a natural cause, such as a germ; while for other illnesses, particularly chronic life-threatening illnesses, people may suspect and address multiple causations over time.

Another method of categorizing disease causation distinguishes between 'internal' and 'external' etiologies.[15] Internal etiologies refer to pathophysiological mechanisms in the body and identify proximate causes, i.e. what specifically caused the internal disorder or disease. Models for understanding proximate causation vary greatly from culture to culture. In Chinese traditional medicine, etiologies invariably involve alterations in the flow of energy or *qi*. In Western biomedical models, disease is usually the result of alterations or disorders of internal physiological homeostatic systems (e.g. electrolyte abnormalities or cancers) or the passage of external pathogens or mechanisms of disease and injury into the physical body (e.g. infectious agents, toxins, or bullets). Note that in the Western system, there is no disease state until such harmful items are 'internalized,' where they can disrupt homeostasis.

In contrast, external etiologies refer to mechanisms outside the body and identify the ultimate causes, i.e. what is the external root of the internal disorder or disease. These tend to focus on spiritual, religious, and philosophical reasons, such as ancestral spirits, divine providence, or fatalism. They may be the primary focus of concern, or may be an adjunct to help consider questions such as 'why me?' or 'why now?' In contrast, Western biomedicine has tended to ignore such topics. In some cultures, for example among the Azande in Africa, ultimate causation is often the dominant issue. As E. E. Evans-Pritchard discovered in the 1920s, if Azande people were cut while running down a path, the wounds were only part of their concern; they would hope to discover which spirit they had offended or who had bewitched them.[16] Their focus was not on the specific and proximate mechanism of injury, but rather on the spiritual, or ultimate cause.

## Classification of diseases

Each medical system classifies illnesses into discrete entities, similar to the manner in which biomedical professionals categorize diseases.[2] Some systems have been carefully mapped out and written down, such as the Chinese and Ayurvedic systems. Others come from oral traditions, and have only recently been written, such as the Hmong in Laos, and Badaga in India. While all people may recognize abnormal bodily symptoms, such as diarrhea or fever, various healing systems classify them differently. For example, the Maya in Chiapas, Mexico, have eight types of diarrhea while an ethnic group in Mozambique has seven types of diarrhea.[17] The Pakistani folk classification system describes several types of diarrhea, such that Pakistani mothers are more willing to use oral rehydration solution for some types of diarrhea than for others.[18] In another example, Hmong have a disease classification system about childhood fevers with rashes (ua qoob) that differs from Western classification, which has caused conflicts between parents and providers about conducting septic evaluations of fever and about obtaining measles vaccinations in a measles outbreak.[19]

Different systems ascribe different names and different meanings to a disease, such that there may be no direct translations and no similar interpretations between systems. For Amharic people from Ethiopia, their traditional word for illnesses with jaundice such as hepatitis is yewof bashiyta, which means 'bat disease,' because jaundice was understood to be transmitted by bat urine when bats flew through the air in Ethiopia. To avoid this connotation, interpreters at Harborview Medical Center in Seattle, WA, use the word gubbät or 'liver disease' when discussing hepatitis.[20]

Unique entities that are recognized by one healing system but not by others, particularly biomedicine, have been called folk-illnesses or culture-bound syndromes.[2,21] Culture-bound syndromes have a specific cluster of symptoms, signs, or behavioral changes recognized by members of the cultural group, and responded to in a standardized way. They usually have a range of symbolic meanings – moral, social, or psychological – for both the victims and others around them. Culture-bound illnesses often link individual cases of illness with wider concerns, including victims' relationships with the community, supernatural forces, antisocial emotions, and social conflicts, in a culturally patterned way. Ideally, the response to the illness can lead to the expression and resolution of these wider concerns.

The psychiatric Diagnostic and Statistical Manual of Mental Disorders, version IV, includes categories for culture-bound syndromes, including Latino susto, Malaysian amok, and Laotian latah.[22] However, folk illnesses can also pertain to physical conditions and not just to psychiatric conditions, including Latino empacho (abdominal pain attributed to intestinal blockage by food), ataques de nervios (attacks of nerves, caused by social anxieties), and caida de la mollera (fallen fontanelle caused by handling a baby roughly or pulling the breast out of an infant's mouth quickly).[23] Western societies are not immune to the attribution of culture-bound syndromes. Examples from the USA include high blood, colds, and chills, while the French may suffer from a particular type of liver pain (crise de foie).[2] Like the other culture-bound syndromes that may seem more exotic to biomedical providers, each is identified as a unique disorder, mainly recognized and meaningful to individuals from particular cultures. Biomedical physicians may make psychiatric or medical diagnoses, such as psychosis, upper respiratory infection, appendicitis, heart attacks, or dehydration.

As folk illnesses are studied, it is apparent that some are not limited to one cultural group, but are shared by many cultures. For example, koro or genital shrinking is found among a wide range of Asian cultures; nervios is found in various Latino American and Mediterranean cultures; and evil eye has similar features between Latin Americans' mal de ojo and the Arab's evil eye.[21] Similarly, neck pain and headache are routine among white collar employees and back pain among blue collar workers in many cultures around the world. While these may have pathophysiological ramifications, they also provide expression for personal, familial, communal, and social issues and forces. Other illnesses that start as folk illnesses, such as chronic fatigue syndrome and premenstrual syndrome, have become part of the biomedical lexicon, which entitles them to be designated as 'true' diseases worthy of medical treatment.

For Western medical practitioners treating immigrants and refugees, accurately diagnosing diseases and not overdiagnosing or underdiagnosing is a challenge. Health professionals must avoid providing too many and too few cultural diagnoses when they are not appropriate. For example, diagnosing *ataques de nervios* when a seizure disorder is present is an injustice. Similarly, diagnosing psychosis in immigrants or refugees who speak with their ancestors when they are from cultures where people communicate with spirits and ghosts is a disservice. Difficult dilemmas arise in some situations such as spousal abuse or child brides or female circumcision when cultural norms allow those behaviors. In these cases, the norms and laws of the new land generally prevail, but sensitive interventions are required.

## Interpretations of signs and symptoms

The question of how people know they are sick is far from simple. People's interpretations of their bodily signs and symptoms are influenced by their healing system's general concepts of normal and abnormal bodily functions, disease causation, and treatment options.[2] People must first decide if a sign or symptom is normal or abnormal. For example, refugees and immigrants who are accustomed to seeing pus draining from children's ears may not interpret draining ears as abnormal. Similarly, refugees and immigrants who are usually malnourished do not interpret obesity as a health problem, and those who are asymptomatic with hypertension or diabetes may not recognize they have a disease. If people decide their sign or symptom is abnormal, they must determine the meaning of the abnormality, and decide whether it's trivial enough to ignore or important enough to label as a sickness.

People's interpretations are based in individuals' lived experiences and in their group's cultural healing system. Kleinman[24-26] calls people's ideas about an illness their explanatory model (EM). Explanatory models have five aspects: timing and mode of onset of symptoms, pathophysiological processes, the etiology of the condition, natural history and severity of illness, and appropriate treatments. The sick person, family members, social network, and providers have their own explanatory models about the sickness event, which may be complemen-

tary or contradictory. Kleinman conceives that the more agreement between the patient, family, and provider's explanatory models, the smoother their interactions are, while the more disagreement between the concepts, the more conflicts there are.

## Treatment options – sectors of care

Treatments are closely linked to a healing system's concepts of bodily functions, causation, and classification of diseases.[2] For example, in Western biomedicine, specialists use medicines and operations to tackle physical diseases caused by proximate natural processes that work internally to disrupt bodily systems. In Chinese traditional medicine, therapies such as acupuncture and herbal medicines aim to rebalance energy flow that was disrupted by external natural or metaphysical forces.[7,8] In Azande traditional systems, a spiritual healer divines the ultimate supernatural cause and sets about to eliminate that cause, such as by appeasing displeased spirits.[16]

Every society has a multiplicity of options for the treatment of diseases and illnesses as part of its healthcare system. This is true whether we speak about a village in the Kalahari Desert or the downtown area of any US city. Every healing system has medicines. Plants, animals, or earth materials are eaten, inhaled, worn, burned, or applied as poultices in order to soothe physical symptoms, restore metaphysical balance, ward away offending spirits, or bring inner peace and strength.[27] Most systems also have physical therapies, such as Mexican abdominal massage to relieve *empacho*;[28] Southeast Asian cupping, coining, and moxibustion to relieve built-up wind and bad blood;[9] Chinese *tai chi* movements and acupressure to manipulate *qi*;[7,8] and allopathic surgical interventions. Spiritual healing approaches are unique to each healing system's connection with the spiritual world. Prayer, incantations, rituals, burning of incense, and sacrifice of animals are performed with different meanings and different interpretations in different religious traditions.[27]

With the abundance of therapeutic options, both patients and providers need to define and categorize therapies. Kleinman describes three sectors of healers that are overlapping and interconnected: the lay or popular sector, the folk sector, and the professional sector (Table 7.1).[25] In the lay sector, treatments are provided by family members or by the sick person, and may include medicines, massage, coining, cupping, burning, incantations, or wound dressings. The folk sector is comprised of healers that emanate from the secular or sacred ethnic or

**Table 7.1 Sectors of care**

| Sector | Basis of authority | Providers | Payment |
|---|---|---|---|
| Popular/lay | Individual and family based. Culturally integrated and congruent. | Family members and nonspecialist community members. | Often nonmonetary, such as gratitude, appreciation, or exchange. |
| Folk | Training. Social nexus and community based. Culturally integrated and congruent. | Traditional healers or religious leaders such as bonesetters, herbalists, priests, or shamans. | Gifts, rather than fees. These many be monetary, material items, or involve exchange. |
| Professional: conventional | Formal education and licensure in allopathic or osteopathic Western biomedicine. | Physicians, nurses, dentists, pharmacists. | Third-party insurance or cash payments. |
| Professional: complementary alternative medicine | Formal education, apprenticeship, or other pathways. | Acupuncturists, homeopaths, Ayurvedic, Chinese medicine specialists, etc. | Third-party insurance or cash payments. |

religious traditions (such as priests, shamans, or herbalists) and treatments generally require some sort of payment, whether money or gift. Many societies have professional medical personnel, including conventional allopathic and complementary/alternative medicine healers, where formal education and licensing are required and monetary payment is standard.

Healers from these three sectors may refer to each other, ignore each other, or compete with each other. In many societies, multiple folk healers exist side by side, providing generalized or specialized services. For example, among Arab Bedouin tribes in the Middle East, wise men or women with knowledge of traditional herbs may deal with simple ailments; amulet-makers tend to illnesses requiring more intensive or spiritual care; and dervishes are the ultimate authorities, reserved for more severe or recalcitrant cases.[29]

When refugees and immigrants arrive in this country, they bring along their traditional healers and healing methods. There may be barriers to the availability, accessibility, and affordability of these healing methods, from legal laws to financial barriers to structural constraints. But in every American community where immigrants and refugees settle, there are traditional herbalists, acupuncturists, masseuses, injectionists, ministers, midwives, magicians, or spiritual healers who are providing services to their ethnic group and to other populations as well. Mexican-American communities have access to traditional healers, such as *curanderos* who diagnose

and treat natural illnesses with massage and herbal medicines that they grow or import from Latin America; *yerberos* who specialize in herbal medicines to prevent and treat illnesses; *sobadors* who treat bodily pain with massage; and *brujos or brujas*, sorcerers and witches, who treat supernatural illnesses with incantations and curses. In addition, there are *botanicas*, or shops that sell religious and spiritual products for healing.[28,30]

One might ask whether all these healing systems and options for care in the various sectors actual 'work,' i.e. demonstrate efficacy in terms of health and healing. The simple answer is 'yes,' but the reasons are complex.[31] All cultural groups have had a vested interest in discovering the healing effects of their actions, and in passing along their knowledge to subsequent generations of healers. Generally, humans have discovered efficacious therapies over time, by objective and subjective evaluation, trial and error, and systematic observation, whether or not the tests were done by scientific principles. Indeed, the efficacy of some traditional therapeutics has been confirmed by modern scientific methods, such as aspirin from willow bark used by people from Assyria, Egypt, Greece, North America, and Sumer; quinine from bark of South American cinchona trees used by Native Americans; and acupuncture, acupressure, and *tai chi* from Chinese traditional medicine. In addition, all cultures have passed along their knowledge to new healers, whether or not their wisdom was written down or passed along orally.

Several other reasons are also relevant. One, most illnesses are self-limited and people either get better or die. Two, the placebo effect means that people's desires to be healed and their beliefs in their system promote healing. Three, people tend to remember their successes rather than their failures. Four, failures support the system; patients are blamed for not following the treatment adequately or not seeking help soon enough; practitioners are blamed for not diagnosing the disease correctly or not administering the treatment accurately; the disease is blamed for being too strong; and spirits or fate or the impermanent nature of life are blamed for deaths.

## Medical decision-making

The decision-making process is complex, and includes cultural beliefs and social factors.[2,25,27] Once the sick individual or the therapeutic management group (such as the extended family) decides the sick person needs healing assistance, they have to decide whom to consult in the lay, folk, and professional sectors. The vast majority of illnesses are treated in the popular sector, as self-therapy and home-therapy are the first approaches to many ailments. When lay therapies are inadequate responses to the sickness, people may seek help from folk healers or professionals. This search for cures is referred to as the hierarchy of resort. Patients may utilize various healers from any of the sectors in a variety of patterns, ranging from sequential use of healers and treatments to simultaneous use of healers and treatments, to a mixture (Table 7.2).

Cultural beliefs such as the explanatory model influence people's decision about which healers to consult and which methods to use, as well as influence people's evaluation of the treatment's effectiveness. A study of Southeast Asians 10 years after their arrival found that ethnic Lao were most likely and Hmong were least likely to seek biomedicine, while Vietnamese started with traditional therapies before seeking biomedical care, and Cambodians didn't

seem to have a preference for either system, easily using both.[32]

Social factors influence whether healers or professionals are available, accessible, and affordable, such as location, hours of operation, direct costs, indirect costs, insurance, language, socioeconomic class, and ethnic identity. Also, who decides is influenced by social structure. In many social systems, the family rather than the individual sick person makes medical decisions, such as among Arabs,[14] Hmong,[33] and Latinos.[28,30]

Studies around the world have found that people's cultural beliefs about tuberculosis (TB) play an important role in people's interpreting their symptoms, seeking healthcare, and taking medications for TB.[34] But social factors – including access to treatment centers, direct cost of buying medications and indirect costs of losing work, fear of social stigma and rejection by family and community members, language concordance between patients and providers, feeling disrespected and lacking trust with providers – are also important, and may be more important in medication adherence. In a fruitful combination of medical anthropology and public health, Paul Farmer's Partners in Health TB treatment program has illustrated how creating solutions to healthcare that are aimed at community social and economic realities, rather than aimed at community health beliefs, can be successful.[35] Healthcare providers and administrators need to integrate community beliefs about disease as well as community social and economic factors into creating successful healthcare system programs.

While immigrant and refugee ethnic identity is initially strong and plays a considerable role in medical decision-making, acculturation changes ethnic identify over time. Acculturation is not a predictable process that changes people from aligning with their traditional healing system to people who accept the mainstream healing system. Rather, acculturation is an irregular, dynamic, bidirectional process that results in considerable variation for individuals, families, and communities.[36] Change is not always away from traditional healing practices. One study found that highly educated Korean-Americans were more likely to see traditional herbalists than noneducated Korean-Americans.[37] Other studies document how people move away from traditional practices, such as fewer Hmong seeking shaman as they become Christians and fewer Somali girls having female circumcision operations due to legal sanctions and change in people's assessment of the procedure. However, this movement along the Western acculturation continuum is often

---

**Table 7.2  Hierarchy of resort**

***Temporal sequence of treatments***
1. Sequential:
   Popular → Folk → Professional (conventional or CAM)
   Popular → Professional → Folk
2. Simultaneous resort
3. Mixed resort: utilization of sequential and simultaneous resort

individual and nonlinear, and may revert back in times of crises, such as illness events.

## Healer–sick person relations

Every healing system has expectations about the relationship between the sick person, family, and healer. The domains of this relationship – communication styles, expected and inappropriate topics, the power dynamics – are culturally and socially influenced. The cultural and social rules of engagement in the United States may seem strange, rude, or unacceptable to immigrants and refugees. For example, refugee and immigrant patients from many backgrounds (i.e. Amharic, Arabs, Chinese, Oromo, Koreans, and others) may not be comfortable talking about sexuality, may not expect to have physical examinations, and may be offended by genital exams.[8,14,20]

Styles of interacting vary between cultural groups. For example, many Latino patients prefer an interaction based on *personalismo*, which means that trusting relationships are developed through personal, warm, and friendly relationships that include connections with personal and family life beyond the strictly medical context.[28,30] Muslim patients may prefer that husbands speak for their sick wives, and may expect providers to interact with family members as well as the sick person, including telling family members rather than telling the sick person about serious life-threatening diagnoses.[13,14] Hmong patients may expect providers to tell bad news in indirect expressions, such as 'If you don't have this operation, then you may not get better, and the sky will get blacker and blacker,' rather than directly, 'If you don't have this operation, then you will die,' as words have power and can cause events to happen.[33]

The power differential between patients, families, and providers can be both helpful and harmful to patients.[2,38,39] Immigrants and refugees are most vulnerable to the adverse effects of the power differential, given differences in language, socioeconomic class, and expectations of the healer–sick person relationship. For example, during interactions between Hmong parents and physicians about septic work-ups for febrile children, parents are more likely to agree with physicians' evaluations and consent if the parents feel respected, than if they feel disrespected and 'treated like dogs.'[19]

## Part B: Multicultural Care in Clinical Settings

This section provides a framework for applying some of the general concepts of traditional and bio-medical healing systems presented in Part A. The goal is to assist healthcare professionals in applying cultural information to the clinical encounter with a specific patient and family in order to provide quality healthcare. There are six recommended fundamentals for providing multicultural care: healthcare providers must know themselves as cultural beings; know their patients as cultural beings; have attitudes that express respect and engender trust; develop communication skills that facilitate mutual understanding; apply the LEARN model and similar models in clinical encounters; and develop multicultural negotiation skills that build therapeutic relationships. These six elements are common to many advocated approaches to culturally competent care.[4,33,40-44] The goal is to provide healthcare interactions that are medically, linguistically, and culturally appropriate, irrespective of the background of the patient and provider, in order to provide excellent healthcare with optimal healthcare outcomes.

## Know yourself as a cultural being

'Culture' is not just something the patient possesses; it is something that *all* humans possess. Being aware of one's own cultural beliefs, values, and assumptions is extremely important in providing quality care that addresses cultural components.[33,40,43,45,46] All healthcare professionals are socialized into cultural systems, as children in homes and in communities, as students in healthcare professions, and as adults in a complex world filled with multiple cultural, ethnic, and religious perspectives. These cultural processes affect healthcare professionals' interpretations of disease, preferred treatments, healthcare-seeking behaviors, and expectations of patient–provider relationships. Without self-awareness, biases and unchallenged assumptions can adversely affect healthcare delivery, particularly when interacting with people who have different cultural beliefs, values, and ethics.

Multicultural care requires self-assessment and identification of one's awarenesses, 'sensitivities,' reactions, biases, and 'centrisms' (e.g. ethnocentrism). Techniques to become aware of such barriers or facilitators are common in intercultural work, such as the Peace Corps but less common in healthcare.[47] Knowing oneself and working to recognize and overcome biases is a first step towards cultural competence. The Institute of Medicine report *Unequal Treatment* explored research that studied disparities in healthcare delivery and found that patients from nonmainstream ethnic and racial groups received worse medical care than mainstream patients because of providers' unacknowledged biases, assumptions, and stereotypes that surface in the face of busy schedules and uncertainties.[46]

## Know others as cultural beings

In order to serve refugees and immigrants, healthcare professionals should strive to become familiar with the group's cultural background.[2,4,33,40,43,45] This includes being familiar with traditional lifestyles, religions, social structures, histories (particularly historical events that led to migration or refugee flight), and prior experiences with healthcare, ranging from lay and traditional healing systems to Western biomedicine. This knowledge has utilitarian value in everything from understanding patients' health-related behaviors to forming therapeutic alliances. There are many ways to learn: reading books, articles and websites; listening to patients, interpreters, and community leaders; attending community events and classes; and doing ethnographic fieldwork in the country of origin and in the US.

It may be particularly helpful for professionals to identify similarities and differences between the immigrant's traditional system and biomedicine's perspective, which are pertinent to healthcare delivery. What are the similarities and differences in nonverbal communication styles, in concepts of time and personal space, in ideas of disease causation and preferred treatment, and in approaches to decision-making? Finding common ground and identifying points of divergence can be key to creating best practices and delivering excellent healthcare.

Similarly, providers can identify potential areas of congruence and incongruence in the culture's general expectations of patient–provider relationships.[48] How is trust established? What behaviors demonstrate respect? What are patients', providers', and institutions' roles and responsibilities? How is healthcare information shared? How are patients' best interests determined? What constitutes good healthcare decision-making? If the immigrant or refugee group has orientations that are vastly different from biomedical care's orientations to these questions, healthcare professionals will face more challenging situations than when their expectations are similar. In the latter case, providers may need to change their behaviors, their recommendations, and their approaches to families and patients.

## Have attitudes that express respect and engender trust

Immigrants and refugees may respond best to professionals who can express respect and engender trust across cultural gaps, and providers need to engage in behaviors that patients, families, and communities interpret as respectful. Indeed, attitudes of respect, interest, patience, and empathy may be even more important in delivering quality care than specific cognitive knowledge about cultural differences.[2,4,33,40,43,45] One challenge to professionals is that respect is a cross-cultural concept. People from different cultural groups demonstrate and experience respect in different ways. For example, professionals may mean to express friendliness with an open mouth and toothy grin but patients may interpret it as being silly and childish. Similarly, professionals may want their firm handshake to be engaging, but patients may find it aggressive or the contact may be taboo if it is between men and women.

Cultural humility is an exemplary attitude as well as an overall ethical approach to providing multicultural healthcare. 'Cultural humility incorporates a lifelong commitment to self-evaluation and self-critique, to redressing the power imbalances in the patient–physician dynamic, and to developing mutually beneficial and nonpaternalistic clinical and advocacy partnerships with communities on behalf of individuals and defined populations.'[49]

## Develop nonverbal and verbal communication skills that facilitate mutual understanding

Communication skills are paramount in healthcare for all patients, but perhaps even more important when patients and providers come from dissimilar origins.[2,4,33,43,45,50] A phrase, a word, or gesture may have vastly different meanings depending on people's cultural milieu. It is highly recommended that healthcare professionals be familiar with differences in nonverbal and verbal communication for the immigrant and refugee groups they serve.

Nonverbal communication is replete with multiple meanings, so that cross-cultural miscommunication can easily occur. Providers should understand the group's general nonverbal communication patterns, such as eye contact (Is direct eye contact experienced as engaging or belligerent?), personal space (Is being close experienced as reassuring or invasive?), gestures (Is using the left hand experienced as neutral or offensive?), greetings (Is shaking hands experienced as welcoming or odd?), touching (Is a gentle touch on the shoulder experienced as reassuring or seductive?), and body parts (Is touching the head permissible or offensive?).

Verbal communication differences must also be addressed. Ideally, healthcare professionals can become fluent in the languages of the people they serve. If this is not possible, it is highly recommended to learn basic greetings and medical words. However, irrespective of one's level of fluency, it is essential for healthcare providers at all levels to become proficient in working with interpreters. There is a vast range of interpreters and interpretive services available, from telephone consultations to professional interpreters who are appropriately matched to patients. Guidelines generally encourage working with trained interpreters, rather than adult family members, children, or untrained individuals who happen to know the language. It is important to choose interpreters who are acceptable to patients and family members in terms of their ethnic group and gender, and who can translate directly in first-person singular style, 'word for word,' rather than summarizing. It may also be helpful if they can act as a cultural broker in addition to providing linguistic interpretation. (For more information on interpreters, see Ch. 6.)

## Apply patient-centered multicultural communication models in clinical encounters

There are several approaches to applying knowledge, attitudes, and skills to clinical encounters in order to provide excellent healthcare to immigrants. One approach is articulated in patient-centered medicine.[51] The patient-centered medicine model encourages clinicians to explore both the patient's disease perspective and illness experience; understand the whole person in the context of individual development, the family life cycle, and the larger socioeconomic and cultural context of people's lives; find common ground in the clinical encounter with good patient communication skills that lead to mutual decisions; incorporate prevention and health promotion; and enhance the patient–clinician relationship, while being realistic about the realities of clinical medicine.

Another model is the LEARN model, or Listen-Explore-Acknowledge-Recommend and Negotiate.[52] This model flows well with the typical clinical encounter, and supports clinicians eliciting, and

**Table 7.3 Kleinman's modified questions**

1. What do you (or other people) think is wrong? What do you call it?
2. What do you (or other people) think has caused the problem?
3. How has this problem affected your life (and other people's lives)?
4. What are you (or other people) afraid of?
5. What healing methods have you (or other people) tried?
6. What do you (or other people) think will help?
7. Who usually helps you make (or makes) decisions about your healthcare?
8. What concerns do you (or other people) have about seeking US healthcare services for this problem?

responding to patients' and families' specific social and cultural needs.

**L = Listen** Healthcare professionals must listen to patients' illness stories, including their beliefs, fears, values, and desires for care in the healthcare system. This information facilitates the diagnostic work for disease identification and treatment planning as well as the development of a therapeutic relationship.

Exploring patients' and families' cognitive explanatory models and knowing one's own explanatory models can aid professionals as they meet patients' and families' healthcare needs.[24–26] The areas of congruence and conflict between patients', families', and providers' explanatory models can influence the interaction between patients, families, and healthcare professionals, both positively and negatively. Also, eliciting and hearing patients' narratives is a rich and easily accessible portal to their culture, experiences, and world view and can be gathered with simple questions about their life and healthcare prior to immigration, their story of passage between lands, and their encounters in their new home.

Kleinman has eight questions designed to elicit patients' explanatory models (Table 7.3).[25] Seaburn et al. have an expanded list of questions to elicit the patient's story as well as the family's story (Table 7.4).[53] In addition, Carrillo et al. have created the 'social context review of systems,' encouraging providers to ask about (1) changes in community context, (2) social stressors and support network, (3) material resources and healthcare access issues, and (4) literacy and language.[54] And Smith recommends using open-ended interviewing techniques and following

**Table 7.4 Seaburn et al.'s questions: eliciting the patient's and family's story**

*History of the illness/problem*
1. How long have you had this problem?
2. How did you first notice it?
3. How did the family and friends react to changes you were going through?
4. Who first suggested that you seek medical help?
5. How many physicians and other healthcare providers have been involved in your care? How have they been helpful? Not helpful?
6. What tests or procedures were needed to diagnose this problem? Have you been hospitalized? What medications are you taking?
7. What is your understanding of the current status of your health?

*Impact of the illness on the individual*
1. How has your daily functioning changed?
2. What do you miss most from before you were ill?
3. What have you learned from this illness that has been useful to you?
4. What do you think will happen with the illness in the future?
5. How has your view of the future changed?
6. What do you hope for?

*Impact of illness on the family*
1. What changes have occurred in the family since the illness began?
2. How are family members coping with this difficulty?
3. Do you talk about the illness as a family?
4. Who has been most affected? Least affected?
5. Who has the greatest responsibility for caring for the ill family member? How does the primary caregiver get support?
6. In general, how do you support one another? How do you express emotions?
7. Does this experience remind you or your family of other difficulties the family has faced?
8. How well do you feel the family is coping? Is there anything the family wishes they could do differently?

*Meaning of the illness, and family resources*
1. Why do you think this illness has occurred?
2. How long do you think it will last?
3. Are there times when the illness seems stronger than you or the family? Are there times when you or the family seems stronger than the illness?
4. Do you or your family have religious or spiritual beliefs about this illness? If so, what are they?
5. What are the strengths of your family? What keeps you going?

Modified by David Hatem, MD, Workshop, International Conference on Communication in Health Care, Chicago, Illinois, October 2005.

patients' leads in interviews to place their illnesses into the broader context of their lives.[55]

Once some information is collected – whether gathered briefly or in-depth, whether gathered in one encounter or over many encounters – that information can be built upon in the remainder of the clinical interaction, such as in the LEARN model.

**E = Explain** Healthcare professionals always need to explain their medical perspective, including desired diagnostic tests, recommended treatments, and diagnoses and prognosis, in words and concepts that patients can understand. This may be a challenge with any patient, but more so when treating immigrants or refugees whose medical concepts may be unfamiliar, where translation into other languages may be required, and where levels of health literacy may be difficult to assess. Nonetheless, providers working with multicultural patient populations should work to tailor their explanations to take into account their patients' language abilities, literacy levels, and cultural concepts.

**A = Acknowledge** Once healthcare professionals know their patients' models, perspectives, and fears, and have explained their medical perspective in a linguistically and culturally appropriate manner, they can then acknowledge the similarities and differences between the two perspectives. Statements that may be helpful include, 'You said you're worried about cancer, and I hear you. I want you to be reassured that I don't find any evidence of cancer,' or 'We both agree that this could be serious, but we have different ideas about what disease you may have.'

R = **Recommend** Healthcare professionals can make recommendations, such as about diagnostic tests, medications, operations, or other therapeutic approaches. Recommending care and then obtaining patients' responses as to whether they agree with this approach is more respectful of patients' cultural orientations than ordering care and expecting patients to comply.

N = **Negotiate** Ultimately, healthcare professionals must be ready to negotiate about their diagnostic and therapeutic recommendations. If patients do not agree with the recommended medical approach, then it is best for providers to know about patients' and families' reactions, discuss their desires, pursue options, and negotiate alternative approaches. If differences are due to cultural beliefs, values, and ethical formulations, they can be elicited and responded to.

### Develop multicultural negotiation skills

Difficulties delivering healthcare in multicultural settings that require negotiation may arise from different patient and provider health beliefs, expectations of life-cycle events, desires for treatment, moral values, or ethical principles. If professionals have objections to patient or family requests for care or refusals of care, they have to decide if they are objecting based on challenges to their personal preferences (i.e. objecting to patients wearing amulets to ward off evil spirits during an operation), personal moral beliefs (i.e. objecting to animal sacrifice in healing rituals), or professional integrity (i.e. families asking to withdraw a ventilator when the patient is not terminally ill).[48] In the first two situations, providers need to discuss alternatives with the patient, family, and perhaps community members and try to negotiate other actions. If negotiation is unsuccessful, the provider must either accommodate the patient or transfer care to another provider. In the third situation, challenges to professional integrity may also be resolved via negotiating with the patient, but if not, they may need assistance from an ethics committee that has community input.

During negotiation, providers have to be aware of the power differentials that exist between themselves, patients, and families.[38,39] Most often, physicians have more power than patients and family members because they have more biomedical knowledge, institutional support, and language skills. Inadvertently, this power can operate to put patients at a disadvantage. Studies illustrate how providers' unrecognized biases and prejudices can result in poor healthcare services. To avoid harmful consequences of unintentional biases, physicians must (1) be aware that disparities in healthcare exist, (2) be aware of their own unchallenged assumptions and preferences, and (3) take actions so that their biases do not impair care.[46]

## Conclusion

Immigrants and refugees arrive in this country with traditional healing systems, whether intact or impaired by the deprivations that led to migration or refugee flight. It is imperative that healthcare professionals learn about the immigrant and ethnic groups that they serve, including their traditional and changing healing system, medical decision-making processes, acculturation influences, social factors that influence availability, accessibility, and affordability of traditional healers, and social factors that influence power dynamics and expectations of biomedical providers. This knowledge is invaluable to provide efficient, effective, patient-centered, quality care. Quality multicultural care requires that providers understand themselves and their patients as cultural beings, have attitudes that express respect and engender trust, develop communication skills that facilitate mutual understanding, apply these knowledge, attitudes, and skills in clinical encounters, and develop multicultural negotiation skills.

### Websites

Asian and Pacific Islander American Health Forum http://www.apiahf.org
Association for Asian Pacific Community Health Organizations http://www.aapcho.org
Center for Cross-cultural Health http://www.crosshealth.com
Country Studies, Library of Congress http://lcweb2.loc.gov/frd/cs
Cross Cultural Health Care Program http://www.xculture.org
Cultural Profiles, Center for Applied Linguistics http://www.culturalorientation.net/fact.html
Ethnomed http://www.ethnomed.org Profiles on immigrants and refugees in Seattle WA, including Amharic, Cambodia, Chinese, Eritrean, Hispanic, Oromo, Somali, Tigrean, Vietnamese, and others, prepared by University of Washington Harborview Medical Center.
Hablamos Juntos Resource Center http://www.hablamosjuntos.org/resourcecenter/default.asp

Hmong Health http://www.hmonghealth.org

Islamic Health and Human Services http://hammoude.com/Ihhs.html

National Alliance for Hispanic Health http://www.hispanichealth.org

National Center for Cultural Competence http://www.cultural@georgetown.edu

National Council on Interpretation in Health Care http://www.diversityrx.org

National Health Law Program http://www.healthlaw.org

National Hispanic Medical Association http://www.nhmamd.org/

Provider's Guide to Quality and Culture http://erc.msh.org
  Profiles on African-Americans, Arab-Americans, Asian-Americans, Central Asians, Hispanics/Latinos, Muslims, Native Americans, Pacific Islanders, and South Asians.

Resources for Cross-cultural Health http://www.diversityrx.org

Vietnamese Community Health Promotion Project http://www.suckhoelavang.org/

World Education; Culture, Health and Literacy http://www.worlded.org/us/health/docs/culture/about.html

# References

1. Ember CR, Ember E eds. Encyclopedia of medical anthropology: health and illness in the world's cultures. New York: Kuwer Academic/Plenum Publishers; 2004.
2. Helman CG. Culture, Health and illness: an introduction for health professionals. 4th edn. Woburn: Butterworth-Heinemann; 2000.
3. Bigby JA, ed. Cross-cultural medicine. Philadelphia: American College of Physicians; 2003.
4. Purnell LD, Paulanka BJ, eds. Transcultural healthcare: a culturally competent approach. 2nd edn. Philadelphia: FA Davis; 2003.
5. Sharma U. Complementary medicine today: practitioners and patients. London: Tavistock, Routledge; 1992.
6. Khanna SK. JAT. In: Ember CR, Ember E, eds. Encyclopedia of medical anthropology: health and illness in the world's cultures. New York: Kuwer Academic/Plenum Publishers; 2004:777–782.
7. Liu X. Han. In: Ember CR, Ember E, eds. Encyclopedia of medical anthropology: health and illness in the world's cultures. New York: Kuwer Academic/Plenum Publishers; 2004:703–717.
8. Wang Y. People of Chinese heritage. In: Purnell LD, Paulanka BJ, eds. Transcultural healthcare: a culturally competent approach. 2nd edn. Philadelphia: FA Davis; 2003:106–121.
9. Nowak TT. People of Vietnamese heritage. In Purnell LD, Paulanka BJ, eds. Transcultural healthcare: a culturally competent approach. 2nd edn. Philadelphia: FA Davis; 2003:327–343.
10. Berlin E, Berlin B, Stepp JR. Maya of highland Mexico. In: Ember CR, Ember E, eds. Encyclopedia of medical anthropology: health and illness in the world's cultures. New York: Kuwer Academic/Plenum Publishers; 2004:838–849.
11. Huber BR. Nahua. In: Ember CR, Ember E, eds. Encyclopedia of medical anthropology: health and illness in the world's cultures. New York: Kuwer Academic/Plenum Publishers; 2004:863–872.
12. Barnes L. Spirituality and religion in healthcare. In: Bigby JA, ed. Cross-cultural medicine. Philadelphia: American College of Physicians; 2003:161–194.
13. Hammoud MM, Siblani MK. Care of Arab Americans and American Muslims. In: Bigby JA, ed. Cross-cultural medicine. Philadelphia: American College of Physicians; 2003:161–194.
14. Kulwicki AD. People of Arab heritage. In: Purnell LD, Paulanka BJ, eds. Transcultural healthcare: a culturally competent approach. 2nd edn. Philadelphia: FA Davis; 2003:90–105.
15. Stoeckle JD, Barsky AJ. Attributions: uses of social science knowledge in the 'doctoring' of primary care. In: Eisenberg L, Kleinman AD, eds. The relevance of social science for medicine. Dordrecht: Reidel; 1981:223–240.
16. Evans-Pritchard EE. Witchcraft, oracles, and magic among the Azande. Oxford: Oxford University Press; 1976.
17. Berlin E. Diarrhea. In: Ember CR, Ember E, eds. Encyclopedia of medical anthropology: health and illness in the world's cultures. New York: Kuwer Academic/Plenum Publishers; 2004:353–359.
18. Mull JD, Mull DS. Mothers' concept of childhood diarrhoea in rural Pakistan: what ORT program planners should know. Social Sci Med 1988; 27:53–67.
19. Culhane-Pera KA, Thao V. Hmong health beliefs and practices concerning childhood fevers. In: Culhane-Pera KA, Vawter DE, Xiong P, et al., eds. Healing by heart: clinical and ethical case studies of Hmong families and western providers. Nashville: Vanderbilt University Press; 2003:120–128.
20. Ethnomed. Harborview Medical Center, Seattle, Washington. http://www.ethnomed.org November 20, 2005.
21. Rebhun LA. Culture-bound syndromes. In: Ember CR, Ember E, eds. Encyclopedia of medical anthropology: health and illness in the world's cultures. New York: Kuwer Academic/Plenum Publishers; 2004:319–327.
22. Diagnostic and Statistical Manual of Mental Disorders, IV. Text Revision, 4th edn. Washington, DC: American Psychiatric Association; 2000.
23. Guarnaccia PJ, Rogler LH. Research on culture-bound syndromes: new directions. Am J Psychiatr 1999; 156(9):1322–1327.
24. Kleinman A. Concepts and a model for the comparison of medical systems as cultural systems. Soc Sci Med 1978; 12(2B):85–94.
25. Kleinman A. Patients and healers in the context of culture: an exploration of the borderland between anthropology, medicine, and psychiatry. Berkeley: University of California Press; 1980.
26. Kleinman A, Eisenberg L, Good B. Culture, illness and care: clinical lessons from anthropologic and cross-cultural research. Ann Intern Med 1978; 88:251–258.
27. O'Connor BB. Healing practices. In: Loue S, eds. Handbook of immigrant health. New York: Plenum Press; 1998: 145–162.
28. Morales S. Care of Latinos. In: Bigby JA, ed. Cross-cultural medicine. Philadelphia: American College of Physicians; 2003:61–94.
29. Borkan JM, Morad M, Schvarts S. Universal healthcare? The views of Negev Bedouin Arabs on health services. Health Policy Plan 2000; 15(2):207–216.
30. Zoucha R, Purnell LD. People of Mexican heritage. In: Purnell LD, Paulanka BJ, eds. Transcultural healthcare: a culturally competent approach. 2nd edn. Philadelphia: FA Davis; 2003:264–278.
31. Borkan J. Why therapies work. Presentation, Brown University, Providence, RI.
32. Brainard J, Zaharlick A. Changing health beliefs and behaviors of resettled Laotian refugees: ethnic variation in adaptation. Soc Sci Med 1989; 29(7):845–852.
33. Culhane-Pera KA, Vawter DE, Xiong P, et al., eds. Healing by heart: clinical and ethical case studies of Hmong families and western providers. Nashville: Vanderbilt University Press; 2003.
34. Shrestha-Kuwahara R, Wilce M, Joseph HA, et al. Tuberculosis research and control. In: Ember CR, Ember E, eds. Encyclopedia of medical anthropology: health and illness in the world's cultures. New York: Kuwer Academic/Plenum Publishers; 2004:528–542.
35. Farmer P. Pathologies of power: health, human rights, and the new war on the poor. Berkeley: University of California Press; 2003.

36. Lara M, Gamboa C, Kahramanian MI, et al. Acculturation and Latino health in the United States: a review of the literature and its sociopolitical context. Ann Rev Public Health 2005; 26:367–397.

37. Miller JK. Use of traditional Korean healthcare by Korean immigrants to the United States. Sociol Social Res 1990; 75(1):38–48.

38. Brody H. The healers' power. New Haven: Yale University Press; 1992.

39. Candib L. Medicine and the family: a feminist perspective. New York: Basic Books; 1995.

40. Campinha-Bacote J. The process of cultural competence in the delivery of healthcare services: a culturally competent model of care. 3rd ed. Cincinnati: Transcultural C.A.R.E. Associates; 1998.

41. Betancourt JR, Green AR, Carrillo JE. Ananeh-Firempong. Defining cultural competence: a practical framework for addressing racial/ethnic disparities in health and healthcare. Public Health Reports 2003; 118(4):293–302.

42. Immigrant Health Task Force. Immigrant Health: A Call to Action: Recommendations from the Minnesota Immigrant Health Task Force. MN Department of Health and MN Department of Human Services. January, 2005. Available: http://www.health.state.mn.us/divs/idepc/refugee/immigrant/immhealthrpt.pdf November 21, 2005.

43. Leininger M, McFarland MR. Transcultural nursing: concepts, theories, research, and practice. 3rd ed. New York: McGraw-Hill; 1995.

44. US Department of Health and Human Services. National Standards on Culturally and Linguistically Appropriate Services (CLAS) in Health Care. 2000. Available: http://www.omhrc.gov/clas/November 21, 2005.

45. Epstein R. Mindful practice. JAMA 1999; 282(9):833–839.

46. Smedley BD, Stith AY, Nelson AR, eds. Unequal treatment: confronting racial and ethnic disparities in healthcare. Institute of Medicine, Washington, DC: National Academies Press; 2002.

47. Borkan JM, Neher JO. A developmental model of ethnosensitivity in family practice training. Fam Med 1991; 23(3):212–217.

48. Vawter DE, Culhane-Pera KA, Babbitt B, et al. The healing by heart model of culturally responsive care. In: Culhane-Pera KA, Vawter DE, Xiong P, et al., eds. Healing by heart: clinical and ethical case studies of Hmong families and western providers. Nashville: Vanderbilt University Press; 2003:297–356.

49. Tervalon M, Murray-Garcia J. Cultural humility versus cultural competence: a critical distinction in defining physician training outcomes in multicultural education. J Health Care Poor Underserved 1998; 9(2):117.

50. Salimbene S. What language does your patient hurt in?: A practical guide to culturally competent patient care. Amherst: Amherst Educational Publishing; 2001.

51. Stewart M, Brown JB, Weston WW, et al. Patient-centered medicine transforming the clinical method. Thousand Oaks: Sage Publications;1995.

52. Berlin EA, Fowkes WS. A teaching framework for cross-cultural healthcare. West J Med 1983; (139):934.

53. Seaburn DB, Lorenz AD, Gunn WB, et al. Models of collaboration: a guide for mental health professionals working with healthcare professionals. New York: Basic Books; 1996.

54. Carrillo JE, Green AR, Betancourt J. Cross-cultural primary care: A patient based approach. Ann Intern Med 1999; 130:829–834.

55. Smith RC. The patient's story: integrated patient doctor interviewing. Boston: Little-Brown; 1996.

# CHAPTER 8

# Cultural Competence:
## *A Patient-Based Approach to Caring for Immigrants*

Alexander R. Green and Joseph R. Betancourt

## Background

It has long been said that America is a nation of immigrants. With 28.4 million foreign-born residents in this country (according to a 2000 US Census report),[1] this is as true today as ever. But clinicians often care for patients – sometimes for years – without knowing much about where they came from, why they came, and how they have been affected by the change to life in this country. While some people are able to make a fluid transition to the new way of life, others have greater difficulty. On a very practical level, patients may have difficulty negotiating the unfamiliar new customs and environment, particularly those of the American medical system. At times, patients may seem 'difficult' when they are accustomed to a very different healthcare system.

In Long Island City, New York, just over the 59th Street Bridge connecting Manhattan to the borough of Queens, there is a community health center that provides primary care to immigrants from over 40 countries who speak more than 25 different languages. This center also provides care to their sons and daughters and grandchildren, many born in this country, among other patients whose American, Italian, Greek, Jewish, and African ancestry dates back decades or centuries. The physicians, nurses, and other clinical staff are keenly aware that practicing medicine in this setting is unique in many ways. Some thrive on the challenges this incredible diver-

sity poses and learn ways to deal with the unique situations that arise. Others are easily frustrated – even angered. They wish their patients would be 'easier' to deal with, rather than learning how to adapt their own paradigms and expectations to meet their patients' needs.

While this community health center presents a striking example of diversity in healthcare, many community health centers, public hospitals, and even private medical practices today provide care for a growing and incredibly diverse immigrant population. But what exactly can we do to address the challenges that providing healthcare to new immigrants poses? Isn't it enough to just be thoughtful, kind, and caring? These questions have led us to develop a curriculum for health professionals entitled *The Patient-based Approach to Cross-cultural Care*. Our goal was to identify the key issues that practicing physicians and other healthcare professionals face when caring for patients of diverse sociocultural backgrounds and to come up with some practical advice on how to manage these issues when they present themselves. This chapter provides a summary of how these principles of cross-cultural care apply to immigrant medicine. First, we will cover the basic concepts of cross-cultural care; next, we will present our framework which consists of first assessing core cross-cultural issues; second, exploring the meaning of the illness; third, determining the social context; and fourth, engaging in negotiation.

## Context

Cultural competence is the ability to provide high-quality healthcare to patients from diverse socio-cultural backgrounds. Concern about cultural competence in healthcare has increased in recent years as providers and policy makers aim to close the quality of care gap between people of different racial, ethnic, and sociocultural backgrounds.[2] The greater attention given to the issue of racial/ethnic disparities in healthcare, and the potential role cultural competence can play in their elimination, has further raised the expectations for this field. It is undeniable that healthcare providers today face the challenge of caring for patients from diverse cultural backgrounds who may have limited English proficiency, different levels of acculturation, limited socioeconomic means, and unique ways of understanding illness and healthcare. The 2000 US Census reported that there are 28.4 million foreign-born residents living in the United States, and about 47 million residents (18% of the total population) who speak a language other than English at home.[3] In some states, such as California, the figure is as high as 40% of the population who speak a language other than English at home. Nearly half of these individuals have difficulty speaking and understanding English. Patient satisfaction and adherence to medical recommendations are closely related to the effectiveness of communication and the doctor–patient relationship.[4] However, immigrants face additional challenges to communication that are not just related to their potential limited English proficiency. Sociocultural differences between doctor and patient can include those related to health and treatment be-liefs, values, styles of communication and decision-making, immigration experiences and related fears, and trust, which among others can lead to major communication and relationship barriers that extend beyond language. Health professionals are now challenged to learn a new set of skills and a knowledge base necessary to overcome these barriers.

This chapter is designed to provide practical guidelines and suggestions on how to manage cross-cultural issues in the delivery of healthcare to immigrants.

## The Categorical Approach to Cross-Cultural Healthcare

Culture is a learned system of beliefs, values, rules, and customs that is shared by a group and used to interpret experiences and to direct patterns of behavior.[5,6] While it is increasingly common that multiple social and cultural influences blur the distinguishing lines between cultural or ethnic groups, many immigrants to the United States may identify strongly with a nationality or ethnic group – Hmong, Afghani, or Haitian for example. It would then make sense to understand some of the characteristics that help to define these groups in order to better understand them. Many Hmong, for instance, have strong spiritual beliefs about health and healing and may have a certain degree of mistrust towards Western medicine. The problem is, there are hundreds of distinct ethnicities, nationalities, and cultural groups in the US, each with its own complex set of beliefs, values, and health behaviors. It would be nearly impossible to learn meaningful and clinically relevant information about all of these groups, and equally difficult to fit it into one book chapter.

One way that some have dealt with this issue is by lumping many smaller groups together into larger categories such as Asian and Hispanic/Latino, but this raises different problems. Latinos may have some commonalities (the Spanish language, for example) but they represent many different countries, ethnicities, and cultures, each with very different characteristics. There are Mexicans of Mayan descent, Argentineans with Italian roots, and Cubans of African ancestry, for example. Even within these subgroups there is a tremendous diversity based on social status, acculturation, age, local environment, and individuality, among other factors. The complex cultural and personal characteristics that make human beings as diverse as they are also makes any standardized guide to dealing with them cumbersome, stereotypic, and fairly useless. As such, we will not provide a 'manual' of how to care for patients from different racial, ethnic, or cultural groups. Instead, we will teach a practical framework to allow one to ascertain from the individual patient what social and cultural factors influence the patient's health values, beliefs, and behaviors, and thus their interaction with the health professional.

## The Patient-Based Approach

The patient-based approach to cross-cultural healthcare[7] involves principles of both patient-centered care and cultural competence. Rather than learning about individual cultures and their characteristics – which is impractical, impossible, and can lead to stereotyping and assumptions – this approach focuses on the issues that arise most commonly due to cultural differences, and how they may impact interaction with any patient.

Referring back to the Hmong patient example, we mentioned the issue of mistrust of Western medicine and the use of traditional or spiritual forms of healing. This is not specific to Hmong patients. This may also be an issue with Afghanis and Haitians, and is in fact common in cross-cultural encounters with many different groups. Rather than learn all about characteristics of the Hmong people, we can learn how to explore traditional healing practices with any patient whose culture is different than our own, along with ways to approach this issue. We can also learn how to identify mistrust, think about its causes, and learn trust-building strategies that are effective with all patients. Integrating these skills into routine medical practice can lead to more effective care, and can even save time by avoiding miscommunication and getting to the root of challenging interpersonal issues. Cross-cultural questions can be used selectively, similar to a review of systems.

Of course, it is still very helpful to explore the beliefs, values, and customs, as well as the demographic and historical experiences of the cultural groups that one sees most frequently following the principles of community-oriented care. This may be especially true with new immigrant groups, who may reside in the same neighborhood, share the immigration experience (which can be positive or negative), and have common beliefs about disease and illness, as well as specific expectations about healthcare. Working with a specific population or community for years imparts a level of cultural competence with that particular group that is hard to come by any other way. Those who gain this level of understanding often do so by taking the time to learn from their patients directly, and do not follow any manual but instead balance the knowledge they have with a patient-centered approach that prevents them from falling prey to stereotypes. Balancing learning about the individual while learning about groups is one of the key tightropes of cross-cultural healthcare, and one that must be understood clearly. Ultimately, it is important to realize that the patient before one is absolutely the best source of information regarding how social and cultural factors impact their health beliefs and behaviors.

## Culture in the Clinical Encounter

When seeing a patient, it is important to understand that it isn't just the patient's culture that is at play, but one's own culture, as well as the culture of medi-

cine. All three of these cultures interact in ways we need to be sensitive to and aware of, as they influence the outcome of the encounter. To understand patients who are culturally different from ourselves, it is first necessary to recognize our own cultural beliefs, values, and behaviors as well as how our life experiences influence the way we think about healthcare, and how it shapes the way we make clinical decisions. Reflecting on what our parents did for us when we were sick, did we go to the doctor right away? Did we wait it out? Were doctors respected and trusted? Throughout this chapter, as culturally based issues are discussed, we must think about our own perspectives and anticipate how they impact our clinical behavior.

There is also a very powerful culture of medicine, which has its own particular beliefs, values, and customs – for example, the idea of patient autonomy and the value placed on scientific evidence. Looking at these cultural norms and how patients may differ, we can predict some of the cross-cultural conflicts and difficulties that may arise. For instance, patients may have a different view of the cause of illness based not on science but on folk beliefs, religious ideas, or their own common-sense explanations. They may appear skeptical about the efficacy of pharmaceutical medication or feel that surgery is too invasive. They may make decisions as a family unit rather than individually, and the hurried manner of health professionals may make them seem mistrustful. Their style of communicating may not be directly in line with the standard patient history format, and sometimes they may just not seem to 'get it.' They may be mistrustful of the organization we represent. The culture of medicine, as well as our own culture, must always be considered in our cross-cultural encounters.

## The Triad of Empathy, Curiosity, and Respect

At the heart of any meaningful and successful medical encounter (especially one across cultures) are three core values: empathy, curiosity, and respect. As the old metaphor goes, they are like three legs of a stool. When one is missing, the stool collapses. The stool represents our connectedness with our patients, and our ability to understand who they are, and what makes them unique. This is more than just fluff. Patients who feel their doctors listen to them, understand them, and care about them are less likely to file malpractice suits, and this type of connection can lead to better health outcomes.[8] And yet, we tend not to connect with people that are different from us.

The death of thousands in an earthquake in Turkey affects most of us much less than the death of a member of our own community, even if we don't know that person. It is normal for us to care more about people who are like us, and we tend to like people who are similar to us. But imagine being a patient and feeling that your doctor doesn't connect with you or care about you so much because you are somehow different. As physicians and healthcare providers, we are morally obligated to try to overcome these tendencies, and to care about all of our patients as equally as possible. We need to develop our ability to empathize with, be curious about, and respectful of all people, both for the sake of our patients and for our own personal growth.

*Empathy* is perhaps the most crucial of the three values to put into practice. It can be defined as an active process of learning about an individual, and perceiving and responding to his or her thoughts and feelings. The central techniques for this are actually quite straightforward. They involve: (1) identifying a thought or emotion that a patient is experiencing, (2) identifying the source of the thought or emotion, and (3) responding in a way that shows you have made the connection between the first two steps.[9,10] Maintaining an attitude of *curiosity* towards our patients is of particular importance when dealing with people who are more likely to think and act in ways that are unfamiliar. People are fascinating when you make a small effort to learn about them. We have an entire world of cultural influences and perspectives right in our own hospital beds and waiting rooms. And as healthcare providers we have a privileged window into the lives of people with whom we may have otherwise had only the most superficial contact, if any. *Respect* in cross-cultural interactions means that regardless of differences, people should be treated with dignity and their perspectives should be taken into account. We are used to reserving our respect for people whom we feel deserve it. We tend to have less respect for those who do not fit our expectations of how people 'should be,' and those expectations differ according to cultural norms. We have to be careful as providers of healthcare to apply a basic level of respect to all individuals regardless of differences in values and behavior.

The triad of empathy, curiosity, and respect represents core values that are fundamental to the practice of medicine in a diverse society. They may have a tendency to wane under the burden of long hours, heavy caseloads, time pressures, and less-than-perfect role models. By holding on to them and inte-grating them into your daily practice our patients will benefit – as will we. Nowhere is this triad more important than in the care of immigrants, with whom we may have little baseline connection due to cultural and linguistic barriers and lack of personal experience.

## The Framework for Cross-Cultural Care

### Assess core cross-cultural issues

Interactions between immigrant patients and healthcare professionals often lead to misunderstandings that reflect inherent differences in cultural values and expectations. These misunderstandings can originate from healthcare providers being inattentive to 'hot-button' issues which can lead to outcomes ranging from mild discomfort, to noncooperation, to a major lack of trust that disintegrates the therapeutic relationship. As previously discussed, the vast number of cultural and ethnic groups in the US and their heterogeneity makes it impractical if not impossible to learn specific aspects of each that could influence the medical encounter. Fortunately, certain core cross-cultural issues tend to recur across cultures. For example, one study found a lower level of patient autonomy, and an emphasis on the role of the family in medical decision-making among both Korean and Hispanic patients compared to African-Americans and European-Americans.[11]

Rather than attempt to learn an encyclopedia of culture-specific issues, a more practical approach is to explore the various types of problems that are likely to occur in cross-cultural medical encounters, and to learn to identify and manage these as they arise. Box 8.1 lists five core cross-cultural issues that should be taken into account with immigrant patients in order to avoid cross-cultural misunderstanding. Once a potential core issue is recognized, it can be explored further by inquiring about the patient's own belief or preference, which may be quite different from the 'cultural norm.' Box 8.2 describes three case vignettes which we will refer to in this chapter to highlight some of these core cross-cultural issues.

### Styles of communication

Differences in styles of communication between patient and provider can lead to discomfort and potential miscommunication. This includes culturally based customs around both verbal communica-

## Core cross-cultural issues

Styles of communication
Mistrust and prejudice
Decision-making and family dynamics
Traditions, customs, and spirituality
Sexual and gender issues

## Three case vignettes

An 8-year-old boy whose family emigrated from Vietnam several years ago is brought into an urgent care center with an asthma exacerbation. While talking to the family, the physician pats the boy on the head and notices that this seems to make his parents very uncomfortable. During the examination, the physician notices several red streaks on the boy's chest, which appear to be caused by trauma. Worried about the possibility of abuse, he discusses the case with a colleague who is familiar with the custom of coining. She states that among some Southeast Asians, to treat certain maladies, a coin is rubbed briskly over the skin in several places, raising linear, red lesions, a technique known as coining.

A 33-year-old Haitian woman presented for routine care to a family medicine practice along with her 2-year-old son. She was employed but had a low enough income to qualify for the Women, Infants, and Children program, a federally sponsored program designed to provide enhanced nutrition for low-income mothers and their young children. The physician strongly encouraged her to sign up for the program and provided paperwork and a brief explanation. When she returned the next time, she had not enrolled, so the physician referred her to a social worker. The woman became upset, refusing to fill out any forms against her will.

A 45-year-old, healthy Egyptian woman presents as a new visit to a male physician, accompanied by her husband. Her husband is somewhat overbearing, answering all of the medical history questions himself. When the conversation is shifted back to the patient, he states that she does not speak English very well. During the physical examination, the husband is respectfully asked to leave the room, and it becomes clear that the patient is quite proficient in English. A history of menstrual irregularity is elicited which had been denied or minimized previously. While the patient remains comfortable during the examination, she becomes very anxious and refuses a breast examination.

tion and nonverbal communication such as eye contact, touch, and personal space. The first case vignette illustrates how some cultures may be offended by what is perceived to be inappropriate physical contact, in this case touching a patient's head. Direct eye contact may also be avoided in some cultures while in others it is a sign of respect. Providers should be aware of their own behaviors and be sensitive to the preferences of their patients. Other aspects of communication include level of assertiveness, which may range from very deferent to very aggressive (often influenced substantially by culture). It is helpful not to assume that a patient agrees with the plan outlined by the provider (a mistake made in the second vignette). A deferent patient may simply be hesitant to voice a conflicting view, making it crucial to ask for the patient's input and encourage verbalization of any disagreement.

More complex communication issues include preferences regarding relating 'bad news' to a patient. Providers often assume that patients should be told just as they themselves would want to hear it. Yet personal and/or cultural preferences for a direct or indirect approach may vary, and should be elicited from patients, ideally before ordering an important test. This technique is often used in HIV pretest counseling, and an abbreviated version can be adapted prior to a colonoscopy or CT scan, for example.

### Adapting to different communication styles and customs

- Get a sense for the patient's general communication style and adapt your style of communicating to fit best with it.
- Try to draw out indirect or reserved patients by making them feel comfortable, asking open-ended questions, and making it acceptable to voice their opinion. Do not assume that lack of resistance means agreement with your plan or recommendations.
- Determine how the patient prefers to receive bad news (e.g. test results), for example:
  'I am going to check the report of your sonogram tomorrow and would like to let you know the results. Some of my patients want to be told directly, no matter what the test shows, even over the phone. While I don't suspect that there will be anything serious, I would like to know how you prefer to hear the results.'

- Get a sense for whether the patient is more stoic or expressive of pain and symptoms. Avoid judging patients based on one's own cultural perspective.
- Pay attention to cultural differences in personal space, eye contact, body language. Try to be flexible without being misled by differences in meaning.

## Mistrust and trust-building

Trust is a crucial element in the therapeutic alliance between patient and healthcare provider. It facilitates open communication and is directly related to patient satisfaction and adherence to provider recommendations.[12] Yet research highlights that public trust in healthcare has dropped to an all-time low from 1966 to 2002.[13] While trust in one's own personal physician has stayed somewhat higher in general, many minority patients have less inherent trust in the healthcare system due to historical mistreatment and fear of discrimination.[14] While much of the literature in this area focuses on African-American patients, a recent survey by the Kaiser Family Foundation showed that Latinos and Asians also are much more likely than whites to worry that they will be treated unfairly by the healthcare system due to their race/ethnicity.[13] Previous bad experiences, poor communication, disrespectful treatment, and the general loss of control that patients experience when ill can compromise trust by patients across all cultural, ethnic, racial, and socioeconomic backgrounds, but may be a particularly sensitive issue for immigrants.

In the second case vignette, the origins of the patient's anger and mistrust were multifactorial. She felt that the physician was being condescending to her by assuming that she wasn't able to provide for herself and her son. Also, she was afraid that filling out government forms could lead to her deportation. It is wise for providers not to blindly assume that patients will trust them fully. Being aware of cues that may be signs of some degree of mistrust is particularly helpful. Patients may express concerns about whether a particular test is necessary, or they may mention some bad experience in the past, for example. These should be taken seriously and should lead to direct efforts at reassurance and trust-building. This includes developing good rapport, communicating effectively, allowing patients a decision-making role in their own care, and respecting patients' needs, fears, and concerns. Here is a list of helpful suggestions for building trust with patients, especially across cultures.

### Suggestions for trust-building across cultures

- Discuss mistrust openly. If the patient seems open to it, discuss why the patient might feel mistrustful of doctors or medical care. Reassure them of your intentions to help.

  'You've mentioned that you don't really like coming to doctors. Was there anything in particular that led you to feel that way? (Any bad experiences or concerns?)

- Understand the patient's perspective and what's important for the patient, especially when different than one's own.

  'What are your thoughts about having this operation?'

  'What were you hoping that I could do for you today?'

- Provide focused reassurance. After determining the patient's perspective and what causes the greatest concern, focus the reassurance on those concerns.

  'You've told me that the pain is what you're really worried about so I'm going to make absolutely sure that you'll have enough pain medication after the operation.'

- Build a partnership with patients. Many mistrustful patients respond well to being given options and some control over their healthcare decisions.
- Communicate clearly and effectively. Listen carefully, avoid medical jargon, and check regularly for feedback from the patient.

## Decision-making and family dynamics

Making decisions about healthcare can be stressful for patients. As clinicians, we try to give patients as much information as possible and then help guide them to make a decision that is right for them while fully valuing their 'autonomy.' However, in some cultures, autonomy is not the norm and family members or others tend to be very involved in the decision-making process. In some cases, families may even wish to exclude the patient from these decisions in order to avoid what they perceive could cause them undue stress.[11] The family may look to a specific authority figure as the decision maker, and this role may be determined by gender, position in the family, or level of acculturation. Many immigrant families have to rely on their children to help negotiate medical situations because of their limited English proficiency (though this should be avoided through the use of interpreters).

The third case vignette in Box 8.2 shows how attitudes toward authority in the family may give rise to a challenging situation. In this case, the patient's husband acts as the authority figure in the encounter, answering questions and making decisions regarding his wife's medical care. Another common issue in medical decision-making occurs when a family asks the healthcare team to withhold a terminal diagnosis from a patient. In this situation, the family is acting together as a unit and trying to do what they feel is best for the individual patient. However, this conflicts with the mainstream medical system, which places great value on patient autonomy and the 'right to know.' A compromise might be reached in these situations if the patient agrees to allow the family to make medical decisions on the patient's behalf.

### Understanding cultural differences in decision-making and family dynamics

*   Introduce yourself respectfully to the patient and others in the room and determine their relation to the patient, keeping in mind that in some cultures it is appropriate to speak only to certain individuals.
*   Find out if the patient is an autonomous decision maker or would prefer the family, or someone else in particular, to be involved.
    'How much do you want your family to be involved in making decisions regarding your healthcare (such as tests or medications)?'
*   Find out if there is an authority figure in the family, or a community or religious leader to consult, and involve that person in important decisions when appropriate.
    'Is there anyone in particular who we should talk to about your healthcare besides you – someone who makes decisions in your family (or community)?'
*   Consider allowing a patient to waive the right to know (legal documents can be signed in this case) when the family wants to withhold information.

*   When a dominant family member is not allowing direct communication with the patient, explain the situation tactfully. If this fails, try ways to obtain information directly from the patient without offending the relative.
    'I appreciate what you're saying Mr. –; your input is very important. From a medical standpoint, though, it's also very important for me to hear a description of the problem from the patient, so I can make a more accurate diagnosis.'
*   Realize that in many cultures it is typical (and important) for family members to stay with the patient in the hospital at all times, sometimes even five or ten of them. If this leads to difficulty for the staff, it should be negotiated openly.

### Traditions, customs, and spirituality

Of the myriad traditions and customs that help to shape a person's cultural environment, some may have a significant relationship to health and illness. For example, issues relating to dietary practices, folk remedies, and certain religious customs, among others, may impact directly on the medical encounter. While it is impossible to describe even a fraction of these medically relevant traditions and customs, it is important to have an awareness of their importance, as well as the openness and skills to explore them further. For example, a physician discussing diabetes with a recent immigrant from Bangladesh inquires about the patient's typical diet. After getting the appropriate information, the physician mentions the importance of regularity of diet in controlling diabetes. The physician then learns that the patient is a Muslim and is about to start a fast for Ramadan, raising concern for potential hypoglycemic episodes.

The first case in Box 8.2 deals with a traditional folk remedy. In this case, familiarity with the custom of coining, or at least openness to the possibility, helps to prevent inappropriate suspicion and involvement of child protective services. While it is impractical to memorize an encyclopedia of medically relevant traditions and customs, it is worth the effort to learn about some of the more important ones among one's patient population. Again, it is crucial to explore these with the individual rather than attempting to predict a patient's thoughts or behavior based on the patient's culture.

Many of these health-based traditions and customs are directly related to the patient's world-view, religion, or spiritual beliefs. Illness and death are among the most powerful and mysterious phenomena in our existence and people often seek meaning in these experiences through some form of spirituality. Several recent studies have shown that physicians undervalue the importance of addressing spiritual concerns with patients in the primary care setting.[15,16] Patient expressions of spirituality should be discussed when appropriate and relevant to the clinical interaction.[17]

## Questions for clinicians about customs, religion, and spirituality

- 'Can you tell me anything about your customs that might affect your healthcare? What about your diet?'
- 'How important is religion (or spirituality) in your life?'
- 'Some patients have spiritual or religious beliefs that prevent them from having certain tests or treatments, such as blood transfusions. Do you?'
- 'How important are these beliefs to you, and do they influence how you care for yourself or what type of care you might receive?'

## Sexual and gender issues

In many parts of the Middle East, Africa, and South Asia, and among other regions and cultures, gender roles are strictly defined and enforced. The male role is commonly seen as that of protector and spokesperson for the family, especially for the women who may play a more domestic role. Cultural differences in attitudes towards sexuality and gender roles can be 'hot-button' issues and should be negotiated with tact and respect to maintain the therapeutic relationship. Difficult situations may arise due to patient and provider being of different (or the same) gender, discomfort with genital, breast, or rectal exams, or shame in discussing sexual issues, among others. Referring back to the third case in Box 8.2 reveals substantial overlap between this issue and the issue of authority/autonomy. The husband's domineering role may clash dramatically with the attitude of the provider, potentially compromising care. It is important for providers to recognize and temporarily set aside their own values in potentially volatile situations such as this. It is also important to try to elicit the patient's personal perspective and desires for how he or she may interact with the Western care delivery system. The goal is to provide quality medical care, which requires a trusting and empathic provider–patient relationship.

Another aspect of this same case vignette is the female patient's discomfort with the male physician performing a breast examination. Some Muslim patients may refuse to have a male physician altogether. Others may have no problem with this. Some Hassidic Jewish men are prohibited from touching a woman of childbearing age to whom they are not married. Many American women prefer a female gynecologist. Healthcare providers should keep these sexual and gender issues in mind when dealing with patients of all cultures, but especially when the patient appears to be traditional or conservative.

## Sexual and gender issues, customs, and taboos

- Be aware of the different ways that patients and families view gender roles and try to accommodate them when feasible.
  'Unfortunately, we have no female obstetricians in clinic today, but if you are willing to reschedule your appointment, I can make sure that your wife will see a female doctor next week.'
- Keep in mind that a judgmental attitude toward patients will doubtfully change their behaviors and values, but may compromise both the physician–patient relationship and the physician's ability to provide good healthcare.
- Ask patients/family what is acceptable to them rather than making assumptions based on limited information (name, clothing, etc.).
  'I perform breast examinations on all of my female patients to look for signs of breast cancer or other problems. Is this OK with you?'
- Be particularly sensitive to the patient's views on discussing sexual issues openly. State that you will be asking about some personal issues and explain why, especially in interactions where you are unfamiliar with the patient's cultural background.
  'I generally ask all patients about some very personal matters at this point, which are important for doctors to know about. Are you comfortable talking about these things with me?'
- Recognize that patients' views and language regarding sexuality and sexual orientation may differ. Ask whether patients have had sexual partners who are men or women rather than whether they are gay, bisexual, etc.

## Explore the meaning of the illness

When patients seek care for a medical issue, they generally come with certain beliefs about the cause of their symptoms, concerns about their illness, and expectations about potential treatment. The overall conceptualization of the illness experience has been called the patient's explanatory model.[18] In essence, the explanatory model represents the 'meaning of the illness' for the patient, or how the patient understands and explains the condition. This concept may seem abstract but it is actually very basic. For example, many people believe that the common cold is caused by going out into a cold, damp climate without proper clothing, or even from air conditioning. This is despite evidence that shows that upper respiratory tract infections are more common in cold climates because people tend to be in closed spaces where the transmission of viruses that lead to these conditions is facilitated. Nevertheless, 'catching a cold' is a popular explanatory model commonly expressed among mainstream Americans. Many people also believe that colds should be treated with antibiotics to prevent bronchitis or pneumonia – a constant source of frustration for primary care providers trying to limit overuse of antibiotics. Patients' explanatory models can range from the mundane to what would be considered by the medical profession to be strange and exotic, and they may be more complex than is initially apparent. Exploring and understanding these can be extremely useful with all patients, but particularly for immigrant patients whose cultural backgrounds and perspectives on health and illness may differ significantly from the Western model of biomedicine. The case in Box 8.3 illustrates this.

Common sense and lay health beliefs are probably the most typical type of explanatory model that clinicians will encounter. Because they seem to make sense and have often been learned and reinforced over years, patients may strongly adhere to them. Limited education, low health literacy, lack of information, or mistrust of medicine may lead people to develop their own ideas about the causes, consequences, and appropriate treatment of their illness. The patient's understanding of his foot pain, in case study 1, may have been partly his own conceptualization, and partly a belief shared by other fishermen who suffered similar symptoms. Sometimes beliefs are simply misunderstandings about medical information, as with the idea that diabetes can be controlled by simply avoiding sugar. There is obviously individual variation in how tightly people adhere to their beliefs. Some will be happy to learn 'the truth'

---

**Box 8.3**

**Case study 1**

An affable but somewhat stubborn 62-year-old fisherman from the Azore Islands of Portugal came in to see his new physician for the second time. He had some allergic rhinitis and benign prostate enlargement, but his main problem was his diabetes. He had been on oral medications for a couple of years but his HgbA1c had stayed high and his fingerstick glucose levels (on the rare occasions when he checked them) were always very high. Over the past year or so, he had been complaining a lot about numbness and pain in his feet – probably diabetic neuropathy. When he was eventually switched to insulin injections he was not happy with the idea. His previous physician had tried to convince him of the seriousness of his condition and need for insulin, but had not realized that the patient had an entirely different understanding about diabetes and his foot pain. He knew that diabetes was a disease of sugar, and was convinced that if he avoided sweets (which he did determinedly) he should have no problem. He did not believe that the diabetes was causing his foot pain. He attributed this to years of net fishing, which he would do barefoot, exposing his feet to rocks, shells, and thousands of bites from a certain type of small fish.

---

from a physician. Others will ignore whatever they are told if it doesn't take into account their own particular perspective and respect their common sense.

Box 8.4 summarizes a set of questions helpful for exploring patients' explanatory models.[18] While patients may be initially hesitant to reveal their beliefs and fears, this can often be overcome through further respectful questioning and reassurance. Focusing on what others may believe, or on hypothetical situations, may take some of the pressure off the patient. The questions can also be adapted for use in various contexts besides illness. For example, they may be used to explore the meaning of a particular procedure or treatment for a patient, such as a breast biopsy or chemotherapy.

The use of traditional remedies, healing practices, or other forms of alternative therapy deserves specific mention here, as they may have particular relevance to the care of immigrant patients. The recent Institute of Medicine Report on Complementary and Alternative Medicine found that over one-third of

---

**Box 8.4**

**Questions for exploring the patient's explanatory models**

**1. What do you think has caused the problem?**
This question gets at the patient's beliefs about the cause of illness, probably the most fundamental and important aspect of the explanatory model. There are many ways to ask about this, and different clinicians have developed their own styling and phrasing, modified to suit the particular situation.

**2. What do you call the problem?**
This question is especially helpful when you suspect the patient believes a particular folk illness to be causing the symptoms. Another way to phrase this would be, 'Do you have a name for this sickness (in your language)?'

**3. Why do you think it started when it did?**
This can link the illness to certain events in the patient's life that may be important elements of the explanatory model. A related question is, 'What was going on in your life at the time that this illness started?'

**4. What do you know about the illness and how it works?**
This gets at the patient's deeper understanding of the illness and how it affects him or her. Many patients may not be able to describe how the illness works at this level, just as patients who believe that viruses cause colds cannot necessarily describe how this works.

**5. How severe is the illness? How worried are you about it?**
Patients may be very worried about an illness while the physician is not: for example, when there are symptoms that do not suggest any concerning disease but are very upsetting to the patient. The opposite may be true, when the patient feels the illness to be minor and does not believe the physician's diagnosis. This is important to discuss as openly as possible.

**6. What kind of treatment do you think you should receive? What are the most important results you hope to get from this treatment?**
Part of the patient's understanding of the illness has to do with beliefs about its treatment. Traditional and alternative healers and remedies play a large role in many a patient's perspective on health and illness. The patient may also have opinions on Western medical therapy as well, and these should be taken into consideration.

**7. What are the chief problems the sickness has caused?**
This is a good way to discuss the effect that the illness has had on the patient's life and daily routine. Understanding this allows better insight into the patient's unique illness experience. Other ways to phrase this include, 'How has this illness affected your life?' or 'What has changed in your life since this illness started?'

**8. What do you fear most about the sickness?**
This is a crucial question because it allows the physician to tailor the explanation of the illness and its treatment to the patient's concerns. This can be extremely helpful for a patient's perspective on a particular medication or procedure.

---

Americans rely on unconventional practices either in conjunction with medications or in place of them.[19] The case in Box 8.5 illustrates this.

The following can be helpful for exploring patients' use of complementary/alternative medicine.

- Ask patients in a nonjudgmental, open-minded way about nonmedical, alternative practices (can be asked after 'medications' in the medical history).

  'A lot of my patients use other forms of treatment, such as home remedies, herbs, or acupuncture that can be helpful.

  Besides the medications that you mentioned, have you used any other types of therapy?'

- Check to see whether alternative therapies are safe and look for any interactions with medications.

- Negotiate the use of alternative therapies along with standard medicine when safe and important to the patient, and discuss reasons to discontinue any dangerous ones.

---

**Box 8.5**

**Case study 2**

A 42-year-old Chinese-American man presented with moderate asthma. He had always been extremely skeptical of medications, instead relying on Chinese herbs for his asthma, which he felt had helped somewhat. He began having episodes of dizziness and on several occasions nearly passed out. He decided to see a physician who noted a heart murmur and sent him for an echocardiogram, which showed hypertrophic obstructive cardiomyopathy (a serious heart condition). On a follow-up visit, he recommended starting verapamil to improve the symptoms, but the patient refused. He continued to refuse medication on subsequent visits, but began to get more concerned about his health. Rather than continuing to push him to take the medicine, the physician began expressing interest in the herbal medications and how he felt about them, looking them up to make sure they were safe. On the next visit he asked if it would be alright to speak to the herbalist, for whom the patient had great respect. The herbalist was very happy that the physician had called. He had not realized that the patient had a heart condition or that he was refusing Western medication in favor of the herbs. He agreed to discuss this with the patient and to let him know that for his condition it was advisable to take Western medications in addition to herbs. On his return visit, the patient agreed to a trial of the verapamil.

## Determine the social context

The manifestations of a person's illness are inextricably linked to those factors that make up the individual's social environment.[20,21] This social context is not limited to socioeconomic status, but also encompasses migration history, social networks, literacy, and other factors. There is a vast literature defining the relationship of these social factors to health status[22-25] and elucidating the effects of social class barriers between patient and doctor.[26] The social context can be broken down into three specific areas with particular relevance to the clinical encounter: (1) change in environment (such as migration); (2) literacy and language; and (3) life control, social stressors and supports.

### Environment change

Environment change refers to any migration, whether from a different country, city, town, or even neighborhood, that requires adaptation to new physical and social surrounding. While some individuals may be able to make a fluid transition to the new way of life, others have greater difficulty. On a very practical level, there may be difficulty negotiating the unfamiliar new customs and physical environment, particularly those of the American medical system. More complex issues arise when patients are accustomed to a very different health system. For example, a recent Russian immigrant presented with a headache and was very insistent that he receive a CT scan. He was used to a health system where expensive tests are tightly rationed, and only offered to those with very convincing arguments. Similarly, a woman from rural Ecuador described a long list of complaints. In her previous healthcare experience, visits to the doctor were few and far between, and she was raised to believe that it was her responsibility to inform the doctor of any symptom she had experienced in the interim. Understanding these may improve negotiation and management of patients who may be perceived as 'difficult.'

On another level, the adaptation to an entirely new way of life presents an enormous source of stress to the individual. The reasons for the migration, ranging from fleeing political persecution and torture to attending an American university, may be crucial in understanding past and present stresses. A resulting change in status (e.g. from physician to lab technician) may also be relevant. Mental illness and psychosomatization are potential consequences of stress and should be recognized and managed with sensitivity and awareness of the social context. The questions in Box 8.6 are examples of how to begin exploring a patient's change in environment.

Understanding the patient's unique migration experience can help the healthcare provider to build rapport and trust, allay certain concerns (such as fear of deportation), acknowledge a source of distress which may be causing psychological or psychosomatic problems, and focus on interventions which facilitate the patient's transition.

### Language and literacy

According to the 2000 Census, 47 million United States residents speak languages other than English at home.[3] This represents 18% of the total population (up from 14% in 1990), and in some states, such as California, the figure is as high as 40%. Nearly half of these individuals have difficulty speaking and understanding English. This is clearly an issue posing challenges for immigrants trying to obtain

**Environment change**

- Where are you from originally? When did you come here?
- What made you decide to come to this country (city, town)?
- How have you found life here compared to life in your country (city, town)?
- What was medical care like there compared to here?

**Life control, social stressors, and supports**

- What is causing the most stress in your life? How do you deal with this?
- Do you have friends or relatives that you can call on for help? Do they live with you or close by?
- Are you involved in a religious or social group?
- Do you feel that God (or a higher power) provides a strong source of support in your life?
- Do you ever feel that you are not able to afford food, medications, medical expenses, etc.?
- How do you keep track of appointments/medications?
- Are you more concerned about how your health affects you right now, or how it might affect you in the future?
- Do you feel that you have the ability to affect your own health (or particular medical condition) or is it out of your control?
- Do you ever feel that you are treated unfairly by the healthcare system for any reason (e.g. socioeconomic status, insurance status, race/ethnicity, language, etc)?

**Language and literacy**

- Do you have trouble reading your medication bottles, instructions, or other patient information?
- Do you have trouble reading in general?

healthcare. Language barriers present a major threat to quality of care in several ways. Compared to English speaking patients, patients with limited English proficiency have been shown to be: less likely to have a regular source of healthcare and to receive timely eye, dental, and physical examinations;[27] less likely to receive preventive services such as cervical screening, mammography, and breast examination;[28] more likely to report medication complications;[29] and less satisfied with both provider communication[30] and with their healthcare overall.[31] As a result, assessing a patient's language proficiency and assuring that there are appropriate interpreter

services available (either trained interpreter or telephone interpreter service) are essential components of delivering care to immigrant populations.

Along these lines, research has shown that more than 30% of the US population is functionally illiterate and innumerate. This refers to just general literacy and numeracy, not the more complicated issue of health literacy or the ability to understand health information. Many studies have documented that approximately 45% of patients have low health literacy.[32] Assessing a patient's general literacy and numeracy, as well as health literacy, is essential and probably more important for immigrant patients who may be illiterate in both English and their native language. The key for both of these issues is that although we may not be able to solve them, we need to identify them and use or refer immigrant patients to the appropriate resources.

### Life control, social stressors and support

As it relates to health and healthcare, a patient's lack of control over the environment can have a clear effect on the health seeking behavior and symptom threshold. Some patients will present at the earliest stages of their disease. Others will tolerate a great deal of symptomatic distress before feeling sick enough to present to the medical system, or before finding the time needed to do so. While part of this may be cultural or a matter of individual character, there is undeniably a socioeconomic component to this issue. Knowing this helps the healthcare provider develop a plan that is sensitive to the patient's concerns, which might include accessing available financial supports and social services. Similarly, patients' illness experience can be very much related to the social stressors and supports they have. Two patients may have the exact same medical condition, but they may manifest their condition in drastically different ways, one much more severely if they are socially isolated, and one much less severely if they have a broad set of social supports. For immigrants who may have limited means of small networks of social support, assessing these factors takes on additional importance.

Box 8.6 lists several interview questions designed to elicit this information. These should serve as a social context 'review of systems.' Like the traditional review of systems, they are used selectively, in a focused, problem-oriented fashion. They are guidelines that may be modified to fit the clinical scenario.

# Engage in negotiation

Clinicians and patients rarely see things in exactly the same way. Cross-cultural interactions add additional layers of complexity to this situation which may be especially pronounced when caring for immigrant patients. For example, in many cultures, questioning an authority figure (such as a healthcare professional) is considered inappropriate or impolite. Culture also affects patients' perspectives on illness and treatment, and their trust in clinicians' recommendations. Much of the emphasis of cross-cultural communication has to do with exploring patients' perspectives. But when their views differ significantly from our views and recommendations, what are we to do? While there is no simple answer to this question, we can often turn to the process of cross-cultural negotiation for some guidelines.

Social and cultural factors determine differences in expectations, agendas, concerns, meanings, and values between patients and physicians.[33] The healthcare provider serves as the expert on disease, while the patient experiences and expresses a unique illness. Thus, even when sociocultural backgrounds are similar, substantial differences may exist because of these separate perspectives.

The knowledge and skills presented previously provide insights that facilitate the process of cross-cultural negotiation. Negotiating a mutually acceptable agreement between patient and provider is described in six phases: relationship building, agenda setting, assessment, problem clarification, management, and closure.[34]

The six phases are integrated with the strategies of Katon and Kleinman to provide a framework for cross-cultural negotiation.[35] Skills developed can be utilized both to negotiate explanatory models and to negotiate management options (Box 8.7).

Negotiation of explanatory models involves an acknowledgement of differences in belief systems between patient and provider. A compromise of explanatory models is reached by explaining that although blood pressure does go up when the patient is stressed, the arteries are under stress all the time, which the patient may not feel. Taking the medication regularly helps to relieve this stress; however, it cannot take away the stresses of life. For this, the patient may need measures such as counseling and relaxation techniques. Patients whose beliefs are less ingrained may be quick to accept the biomedical model; others may require more creative negotiation.

## Box 8.7
## A framework for cross-cultural negotiation

### Step 1. Explore the patient's perspective
This may involve asking open-ended questions about the patient's understanding and concerns about the illness and its treatment.

### Step 2. Explain your own perspective
This requires providing the patient with an explanation in terms that are understandable and familiar, including explaining why you think your perspective is in the patient's best interest.

### Step 3. Acknowledge the difference in opinion
Do this in a way that is nonjudgmental and accepting of difference.

### Step 4. Create common ground
This may mean offering a compromise or asking the patient what he or she is willing to do, and often requires some back and forth discussion in an environment where the patient feels free to be open with you.

### Step 5. Settle on a mutually acceptable plan
Once a plan is developed, check with the patient again to make sure that it is acceptable. Look for any sign of hesitation on the patient's part and discuss this openly.

Cultural differences cannot be solved by arguing that the physician's perspective is right and the patient's perspective is simply wrong. These are values and perspectives, not black and white facts, and all people generally feel strongly about their personal values. Only through negotiation can a mutually acceptable agreement be reached. This is not in conflict with one's duties as a clinician in most cases; in fact, it is one's duty as a clinician.

Negotiation is not about trying to convince patients who are refusing medical treatment that they should accept what we say. It is about getting beyond the notion that whatever we think as physicians and medical professionals is automatically right for everyone. It is also about teaching people what we know in a way that they can understand and that also values their system of beliefs. This can be done in an efficient, effective way by considering the steps presented in Box 8.7.

## Conclusion

Communicating effectively across cultures is a critical component of providing quality healthcare to diverse populations, and even more crucial in the care of immigrants. Given what we know about immigration patterns, we need to be prepared to care for patients from anywhere in the world. It is obviously impossible to learn everything about every culture, and we should not be expected to do so. Instead, we should learn about the immigrant communities we care for, but more importantly have a framework to care for any immigrant patient – or any patient in general – regardless of race, ethnicity, or cultural background.

The patient-based approach to cross-cultural care described here enables healthcare providers to cut through perceptual barriers and lift veils of social and cultural misunderstanding. This approach can facilitate all medical encounters, but is particularly important in the setting of cultural and social differences. These tools are based on the key tenets of listening, asking the right questions, and meeting the patients where they are. Our goal has been to identify the key issues that practicing physicians and other healthcare professionals face when caring for patients of diverse sociocultural backgrounds, and to come up with some practical advice on how to manage these issues when they present themselves. The model of assessing core cross-cultural issues, exploring the meaning of the illness, determining the social context, and engaging in negotiation should help us to do a better job in the care of immigrant patients.

## References

1. US Census 2000. Available: http://www.census.gov March 7, 2003.
2. Unequal treatment: confronting racial and ethnic disparities in healthcare. Washington, DC: Institute of Medicine; 2003.
3. Language use and English-speaking ability: 2000. Available: http://www.census.gov March 7, 2003.
4. Betancourt JR, Carrillo JE, Green AR. Hypertension in multicultural and minority populations: linking communication to compliance. Curr Hypertens Rep 1999; 1(6):482–488.
5. Robins LS, Fantone JC, Hermann J, et al. Improving cultural awareness and sensitivity training in medical school. Acad Med 1998; 73(10 Suppl):S31–S34.
6. Donini-Lenhoff FG, Hedrick HL. Increasing awareness and implementation of cultural competence principles in health professions education. J Allied Health 2000; 29(4):241–245.
7. Carrillo JE, Green AR, Betancourt JR. Cross-cultural primary care: a patient-based approach. Ann Intern Med 1999; 130(10):829–834.
8. Levinson W, Roter DL, Mullooly JP, et al. Physician–patient communication. The relationship with malpractice claims among primary care physicians and surgeons. JAMA 1997; 277(7):553–559.
9. Stepien KA, Baernstein A. Educating for empathy. a review. J Gen Internal Med 2006; 21(5):524–530.
10. Puchalski C. The role of spirituality in healthcare. Baylor University Medical Center Proceedings 2001; 14(4):352–357.
11. Blackhall LJ, Murphy ST, Frank G, et al. Ethnicity and attitudes toward patient autonomy. JAMA 1995; 274(10):820–825.
12. Doescher M, Saver B, Franks P, et al. Racial and ethnic disparities in perceptions of physician style and trust. Arch Fam Med 2000; 9(10):1156–1163.
13. Race, ethnicity and medical care, a survey of public perceptions and experiences. Kaiser Family Foundation; 2005.
14. Thom D, Campbell B. Patient–physician trust: an exploratory study. J Fam Pract 1997; 44(2):169–176.
15. Ehman J, Ott B, Short T, et al. Do patients want physicians to inquire about their spiritual or religious beliefs if they become gravely ill? Arch Intern Med 1999; 159(15):1803–1806.
16. Maugans T, Wadland W. Religion and family medicine: a survey of physicians and patients. J Fam Pract 1991; 32(2):210–213.
17. Post S, Puchalski C, Larson D. Physicians and patient spirituality: professional boundaries, competency, and ethics. Ann Intern Med 2000; 132(7):578–583.
18. Kleinman A, Eisenberg L, Good B. Culture, illness, and care: clinical lessons from anthropologic and cross-cultural research. Ann Intern Med 1978; 88(2):251–258.
19. Complementary and alternative medicine in the United States. Washington, DC: Institute of Medicine; 2005.
20. De La Cancela V, Guarnaccia P, Carrillo JE. Psychosocial distress among Latinos: a critical analysis of ataques de nervios. Humanity Society 1986; 10:431–447.
21. Helman C. Culture, health and illness: an introduction for health professionals. 3rd edn. Boston: Butterworth-Heinemann; 1994.
22. Sorlie P, Backlund E, Keller J. US mortality by economic, demographic, and social characteristics: the National Longitudinal Mortality Study. Am J Public Health 1995; 85:949–956.
23. Kaplan G, Keil J. Socioeconomic factors and cardiovascular disease: a review of the literature. Circulation. 1993; 88(4):1973–1978.
24. Feinstein J. The relationship between socioeconomic status and health: a review of the literature. Milbank Q 1993; 71:279–322.
25. Carrillo JE. A rationale for effective smoking prevention and cessation interventions in minority communities. Discussion Paper Series, Institute for the Study of Smoking Behavior and Policy. Cambridge, MA. Harvard University, John F. Kennedy School of Government; 1987:1–40.
26. Quill T. Barriers to effective communication. In: Lipkin MJ, Putnam S, Lazare A, eds. The medical interview: clinical care, education, and research. New York: Springer-Verlag; 1995:110–121.
27. Hu D, Covell R. Healthcare usage by Hispanic outpatients as function of primary language. West J Med 1986; 144:490–493.
28. Woloshin S, Schwartz LM, Katz SJ, et al. Is language a barrier to the use of preventive services? J Gen Intern Med.1997; 12(8):472–477.
29. Gandhi JK, Burstin HR, Cook EF, et al. Drug complications in outpatients. J Gen Internal Med 1998; 15:149–154.
30. Morales LS, Cunningham WE, Brown JA, et al. Are Latinos less satisfied with communication by healthcare providers? J Gen Intern Med 1999; 14(7):409–417.
31. Carrasquillo O, Orav EJ, Brennan TA, et al. Impact of language barriers on patient satisfaction in an emergency department. J Gen Intern Med. 1999; 14(2):82–87.

32. Health literacy: a prescription to end confusion. Washington, DC: Institute of Medicine; 2004.

33. Kleinman A. Patients and healers in the context of culture: an exploration of the borderland between anthropology, medicine, and psychiatry. Berkeley: Univ. of California Press; 1980.

34. Botelho RJ. A negotiation model for the doctor–patient relationship. Fam Pract 1992; 9(2):210–218.

35. Katon W, Kleinman A. Doctor–patient negotiation and other social science strategies in patient care. In: Eisenberg L, Kleinman A, eds. The relevance of social science for medicine. Higham, Mass: D. Reidel Publishing; 1980.

# CHAPTER 9

# Cultural Competence:
## Healthcare Disparities and Political Issues

Joseph R. Betancourt and Alexander R. Green

## Background

*Cultural competence* has recently gained increasing attention from healthcare policy makers, providers, insurers, and educators as a strategy to improve quality of care and eliminate racial/ethnic disparities in healthcare. Cultural competence is grounded in two basic principles:[1] first, it is important to explore and understand the sociocultural factors that influence a patient's values, beliefs, and behaviors related to health and healthcare; and second, it is critical to develop multilevel strategies in the design and delivery of healthcare in an effort to bridge the gaps in quality that result from sociocultural and linguistic barriers. Ultimately, the goal of cultural competence is to create a healthcare system and workforce that are capable of delivering the highest quality of care to every patient, regardless of race, ethnicity, culture, or language proficiency. Such a system would be equitable, of high quality, and free of disparities based on individual patient characteristics. Bringing this to fruition requires action by various sectors of healthcare, yet each may have different motivations, approaches, and leverage points for advancing cultural competence.

The purpose of this chapter is to present the perspectives on cultural competence as expressed by experts in the field within government, academia, managed care, and community healthcare. Through key informant interviews we were able to identify how individuals in these different sectors view cultural competence – including their motivation, vision, and experience in making it 'actionable' – as well as how efforts in this area link to quality improvement and the elimination of racial and ethnic disparities in healthcare.

## Cultural Competence Emerges

Cultural competence has emerged as an important healthcare issue for three very practical reasons. First, as the US becomes more diverse, clinicians will increasingly see patients with a broad range of thoughts regarding health and well-being, oftentimes influenced by their social or cultural background. Culture can be seen as an integrated pattern of learned beliefs and behaviors that can be shared among groups and includes thoughts, styles of communicating, ways of interacting, views on roles and relationships, values, practices and customs. Culture is shaped by multiple influences, including race, ethnicity, nationality, language, and gender, but also extending to socioeconomic status, physical and mental ability, sexual orientation, and occupation, among others. For instance, patients may present their symptoms quite differently from the way healthcare providers have read about them in their medical textbooks; they may have limited English proficiency, thus limiting their ability to communicate; they may have different thresholds for seeking care, or expectations about the care they receive; and they may hold beliefs that influence whether or not they adhere to our recommendations.[2]

Second, research has shown that effective provider–patient communication is directly linked to improved patient satisfaction, adherence and, subsequently, health outcomes.[3] Thus, patient dissatisfaction, nonadherence, and poorer health outcomes may result when sociocultural differences between the patient and the provider are not effectively addressed in the clinical encounter.[4] This is further complicated by situations in which the patient has limited English proficiency or low health literacy. Ultimately, these barriers do not just apply to minority groups (African-Americans, Hispanics, Asian, Pacific Islanders, and Native Americans/ Alaska Natives: taken from US Office of Management and Budget definition [OMB-15 Directive]), but may just be more pronounced in these cases.

Finally, two recent Institute of Medicine Reports – Crossing the Quality Chasm[5] and Unequal Treatment[6] – both highlighted the importance of patient-centered care, evidence-based guidelines, and cultural competence as a means of improving quality, achieving equity, and eliminating the significant racial/ethnic disparities in healthcare that persist today. These recommendations are based on the premise that improving health systems and provider–patient communication are important components of addressing racial and ethnic disparities in healthcare that occur even when variations in such factors as insurance status, income, age, comorbid conditions, stage of presentation, and symptom expression are taken into account.

In our previous research[1,7] we have described three main levels of cultural competence in healthcare:

- *Organizational cultural competence* focuses on increasing the diversity of the healthcare workforce and leadership as a means of improving quality of care.
- *Systemic cultural competence* focuses on strategies that address structural processes of care, including implementing racial/ ethnic and language preference data collection (as a way of monitoring quality of care); developing specific culturally competent quality improvement projects to address disparities; ensuring interpreter services and culturally and linguistically appropriate health education materials and signage; and creating mechanisms for community assessment and input.
- *Clinical cultural competence* focuses on educational and training strategies that highlight the importance of sociocultural factors on patients' health values, beliefs, and behaviors, and equip providers with the tools and skills to effectively address these in the clinical encounter.

It is felt that this practical framework for cultural competence has the potential to broaden access, improve quality, and eliminate racial/ethnic disparities in healthcare.

## Perspectives from the Field

The authors conducted interviews with national experts in cultural competence from academia (residency programs, medical schools, and professional organizations) community health centers, managed care, and the government (including representatives from agencies of the Department of Health and Human Services and state and county Departments of Health). Key informants were asked to define cultural competence in their domain of healthcare, identify key actionable components of cultural competence, describe leverage points for action and implementation, and identify links to quality and the elimination of racial/ethnic disparities in healthcare. Key informants were selected from lists of:

1. Nationally recognized experts in cultural competence who had presented at one of a series of national meetings on the topic. (National Conference Quality Health Care to Culturally Diverse Populations. The New York Academy of Medicine, October 1998; Providing care to diverse Populations: State Strategies for Promoting Cultural Competency in Health System. AHRQ ULP Program, June 1999; Difference Matters: Multiculturalism in Medical Education. Harvard Medical School, June 1999; Kaiser Family Foundation's Conference 'Race, Ethnicity, and Medical Care: Improving Access in a Diverse Society,' October 1999.)
2. Members of national expert cultural competence advisory panels. (HCFA QISMC Cultural Competence Quality Measure Review Panel; Association of American Medical Colleges Diversity Project Team; Office of Minority Health CLAS Project Advisory Group; New York Academy of Medicine Working Group on Racial/Ethnics Disparities.)
3. Snowball sampling using sequential recommendations from initial key informants.

A total of 37 interviews were completed in the Spring and Summer of 2002 (individuals and affiliations listed in Appendix). Interviews were taped, transcribed, and qualitatively coded by three independent coders according to a coding structure that disseminated major themes according to frequency and relevance. The coding scheme was designed and overseen by a qualitative methods expert, and the final themes were reviewed for content appropriateness by an expert in cultural competence. Below, we describe the major issues that arose among the different stakeholder groups.

## Government

### Increasing access to quality healthcare for the most vulnerable

Given the roles and responsibilities of federal, state, and local government in developing and managing healthcare delivery and financing systems for some of America's most vulnerable populations (including children, the elderly, and socioeconomically disadvantaged groups), the overarching motivation for cultural competence was couched in terms of 'increasing access to quality care for all patient populations'.

'. . . to increase accessibility to our services through working to have our staff and providers really understand the cultural attitudes and beliefs patients have towards health.'

The implied assertion was that many groups, including minorities who experience sociocultural barriers, have difficulty getting appropriate, timely, high-quality care due to several issues such as having a different cultural perspective about health and healthcare, having different expectations about diagnosis and treatment, or experiencing language barriers in the clinical encounter. As such, 'cultural competence' aims to move what many consider on the whole to be a 'one size fits all' healthcare system to be more responsive to the needs of an increasingly diverse nation and patient population.

'. . . it's being able to communicate with people with different social mores, different languages, different views, different religions, any kind of differences. It's a means of overcoming the barriers that have been created in the systems and messages we're presenting.'

### Key capacities of cultural competence

Key informants in government highlighted three essential components underlying the delivery of culturally competent care:

1. Organizational capacities, including diversity among staff and providers, and strategies for diversity in hiring practices and recruitment. Across the board, it was seen as critical to have the diversity of the communities being served also represented among the providers and staff who are providing healthcare.

'We're not keeping up with our demographic changes, and we're going to continue to have disparities if we don't start increasing diversity in the health professions.'

2. Systemic capacities, including data collection methods to both assess the needs of the patient populations that are served (not only quantitatively, but qualitatively through the development of community linkages and mechanisms for community advising) and track progress in improving health outcomes (with ties to accountability); improving the capacity to care for limited English proficient patients through the development of effective interpreter services; and exploring the use of emerging technologies (evidence-based computer aides, voice recognition) to help us meet the challenges of caring for diverse populations.

'. . . the issue of language is probably the one that has been studied the most and that we have the best data for making the case for cultural competence and what happens when you don't have the appropriate translation.'

3. Training capacities, including cultural competence education for senior management, healthcare providers, and staff. This training should focus on knowledge and skills, and should equip providers with tools and skills to deliver quality care to all patients (with an acknowledgement that systems need to be in place to facilitate this goal).

'. . . if we can develop cross-cultural education curricula for the various health professions I think we can at least start making an impact on the attitudes, knowledge and skills of practitioners when they start serving more diverse populations.'

## Purchasing power as leverage to advance cultural competence

Various strategies and approaches were delineated to facilitate the evolution and development of cultural competence in healthcare. Among them, the influence of government as the largest healthcare purchaser, and the use of contractual requirements (federal and state), emerged as the strongest leverage points. Experts agreed that healthcare purchasers – both government based, as through Medicare, and private, through large purchasing coalitions seen in industry – could help stimulate change if they understood the impact of healthcare delivery that was not culturally competent.

> 'The trick of course is getting the purchaser to be interested and educated enough about [cultural competence] to be able to develop the right policy . . . and so that makes the purchaser–advocate partnership really critical.'

The role of the Centers for Medicare and Medicaid Services, the Joint Commission on Accreditation of Healthcare Organizations, and state healthcare provider licensure and medical school accreditation organizations were also named specifically, as well as the need to make the 'business model' for these interventions.

> '. . . we're not going to convince purchasers or business people unless we make the business model.'

## Cultural competence as one step toward eliminating disparities

Informants developed a clear link between cultural competence and eliminating racial/ethnic disparities in healthcare. However, there was agreement that disparities are multifactorial (due to socioeconomic disparities, educational disparities, etc.) and that cultural competence alone could not address this problem. There was a sense, however, that cultural competence was crucial to systems and quality improvement, especially given disparities in our longstanding populations, and the emergence of new populations. It was also stated that, in fact, these cultural competence 'adjustments' in healthcare delivery are synergistic with the larger movement of quality improvement, and should occur at the level of systems, and at the level of the clinical encounter.

> 'That's what we're talking about in terms of cultural competency . . . providing quality care to individuals who in the past have not received

it . . . and when I think of quality care, that's what we're looking for all Americans, not only for diverse populations.'

The Culturally and Linguistically Appropriate Services (CLAS) Standards project was often referred to as an effective blueprint for improving the cultural competence of our healthcare system. (This project was developed by the Office of Minority Health and can be found at http://www.omhrc.gov/clas)

## Academia

### Training the future healthcare workforce to care for diverse populations

Key informants in academic medicine were motivated to advance cultural competence as an educational strategy to prepare the future healthcare workforce to care for diverse patient populations. This group tended to view cultural competence primarily from the standpoint of the provider–patient interaction, with a focus on communication. They stressed the importance of providers having an awareness and understanding of culture (one's own and that of others), knowledge of the relationship between cultural beliefs and behaviors, and the ability for introspection. Many described cultural competence as a level of self-awareness or self-reflection and knowledge, but equally referred to the development of skills needed to improve quality of care.

> '. . . the ability of medical practitioners to identify cultural indicators in the history taking, diagnosis, and treatment of any patients.'

Despite this, some expressed concern that there is still too much focus on stereotyping strategies or 'cookbook practices' (i.e. treat 'Hispanics' this way and 'African-Americans' another way), and little focus on the factors that impact the individual patient. They mentioned additional components that needed to be integrated into training such as the importance of empathy, the impact of socioeconomic class on patients' ability to obtain quality care, the development of communication skills, and the importance of addressing racism and bias in the clinical encounter.

> 'I think too often we want to leap to the knowledge and skill base rather than going to the mental assumptions and biases that are brought to the medical interaction . . . and

understanding issues of context and culture and language.'

## Cultural competence education gaining momentum

When discussing the practical aspects of operationalizing cultural competence, key informants referred to the implementation of programs on cross-cultural education in the health professions. Many cited regulatory/accreditation pressures (including those from the Accreditation Council of Graduate Medical Education for residency training and the Liaison Council on Medical Education for medical schools), societal pressures, and the growing diversity of patients, students, and faculty as leverage for moving agendas forward. Funding opportunities that have developed, especially through professional societies, foundations, and government, also provide an important incentive.

'I think the funding issue is particularly relevant for medical education . . . Very often just getting things started is enough to allow for things to happen. But you have to make that initial commitment. And with the best of intentions sometimes it actually takes the resources and the resources are usually dollars.'

Many agreed that there is currently a greater awareness of cultural competence being an important part of training in medical schools and residency, particularly those that serve diverse communities. Reasons for this increased included changing patient demographics, an increased awareness of health disparities, a climate of healthcare consumerism, and managed care.

'It is certainly beginning to increase again in interest, partly due to the increasing diversity of the populations we are serving.'

A few participants stated that although the climate is better than before, there was still a long way to go. Several concerns were expressed about the present climate being fragile and misappropriated, and about the great attention the field is currently receiving at the risk of being transient.

'But in the faddish sense, in academic medicine, people are coming to it now because if there is grant money, you have to say something about cultural competence . . . if you are going to get a grant from the NIH, you have to mention that word.'

## A need for better standardization and quality of educational programs

The field of cultural competence training (or cross-cultural education) has suffered from a lack of a uniform approach or set of standards. This is typical in an area that is young and can be defined so broadly. Although there was a perception that cross-cultural training efforts were well intentioned and helpful overall, informants often described them as 'piecemeal' and not coming out of a unified conceptual framework. Many cited great variability as to whether cultural competence education is being offered, the quality of training, and the lack of faculty development in the area at medical schools and residency training programs. Educating faculty, not just students, was seen as crucial since they play such an important role in the 'informal curriculum' and the role modeling of behavior in the clinical setting. A major challenge is that faculty currently may not have the awareness and skills to teach (or even role model) culturally competent care.

'The basic problem is that the faculty does not understand it very well and it is hard to teach about it then.'

## Education a necessary vehicle to address disparities

Racial/ethnic disparities in health were seen as major factors leading to increased awareness of the need for cultural competence in healthcare. Several participants cited disparities initiatives set forth by Former President Clinton and Surgeon General Satcher as being particularly important while others mentioned the recent increase in literature on healthcare disparities. However, studies on outcomes of cultural competence training interventions have been sparse and variable. Nevertheless, most informants felt that cultural competence training could help reduce disparities, and some called for a formal regulatory body to report on the growing body of evidence for this link as it develops.

'It would be very nice to see something created analogous to the US Preventive Services Taskforce which could be called the US Health Disparities and Cultural Competence Taskforce that could periodically examine and report on the evidence base that supports this link whether in education, research, legislation or policy efforts.'

## Managed care

### Cultural competence a business and quality imperative

Key informants in managed care viewed the evolution of cultural competence within this area as being driven by both business and quality imperatives. Time and time again, they highlighted cultural competence as a mechanism of being responsive to a diverse membership, not only from the standpoint of those already enrolled, but from the standpoint of attracting new patients and increasing market share.

> 'It's a business strategy . . . I get people that drive 60 miles to get their healthcare here because they come to see a physician who looks like them and is able to speak the same language or whose family may have come from the same village.'

As a precursor to this, the issue of assessment was stressed heavily. It was felt to be extremely important to understand not only who is in one's catchment area and currently part of one's membership, but what are their needs, and how can one help meet them. Only through this thorough assessment could one be certain to have the appropriate systems and staff in place to maximize health outcomes and control costs.

### Leadership, systems, and education are key

Key informants highlighted the 'multilevel' nature of cultural competence with the understanding that interventions should occur at several tiers of the healthcare delivery continuum ('from the organization right down to the clinical encounter').

1. Organizational capacities, including diversity in leadership of healthcare delivery systems, and in the healthcare workforce (most especially the healthcare provider network). The need for diverse leadership was particularly pronounced, as lack of diversity on Board of Trustees and Senior Management was mentioned as a persistent problem.

   > '. . . I see it all the time when I talk to Trustee Groups . . . we don't see representation from some of our vulnerable populations . . . we don't see people of color at the table . . . I will look into a group of 250 and not see one person of color. If we don't have people of color

and the diverse populations we serve at the table, you can be sure that policy making and program design is also going to be exclusionary as well.'

2. Systemic capacities, including mechanisms for conducting effective needs assessments (on catchment area and population served), data collection, cross-cultural marketing, services to deal with patients with limited English proficiency, flexible patient scheduling strategies, language-appropriate telephone systems, and quality and outcomes measurement (including patient satisfaction). It was stressed that cultural competence should be addressed systematically.

   > 'We need to have the right systems in place, the right technology, the right environment, and the right people.'

3. Training capacities, including cultural competence training for healthcare providers and staff. One issue that was raised was the need for 'cultural competence training' not to be taught in categories (African-Americans behave this way, Hispanics behave that way) as this would lead to stereotyping and is not in the spirit of true cross-cultural training and provision of skills. This group felt that training, however, should be standardized and evidence-based as much as possible, with appropriate monitoring for completion as part of being in a provider network as a 'process' issue (perhaps as a way of distinguishing health plans).

   > 'On the process side, you can get into things such as training. Does the plan offer cultural competence training programs? You can count them, you can count the hours invested in them, you can count the number of people who attend them.'

### Cultural competence clearly links to quality improvement and addressing disparities

Key informants felt that managed care can play a key role in advancing cultural competence, and that quality improvement was one of the strongest levers. There was unanimous sentiment that, in theory, purchasers can be instrumental in moving this issue forward. However, they expressed skepticism about the current state of affairs, given the multiple competing interests (including rising healthcare costs and premiums, drug costs, etc.) purchasers face, and their lack of knowledge about the issue.

'I am impressed by the influence of purchasers over managed care organizations. They care about quality, cost . . . but in my direct experience the issue of disparities and then cultural and linguistic competence as a vehicle for reducing disparities isn't front and center right now.'

Two methods were discussed to facilitate this process. First, the incorporation of culturally competent, or health disparity quality measures as part of HEDIS, which would allow employers and purchasers to respond to evidence-based outcomes (including data showing clinical impact of interventions such as reducing hospitalization, increasing satisfaction, and improving market share and member loyalty, etc.); and second, by informing employees about disparities and cultural competence and empowering them to request more culturally appropriate services from the managed care provider their employee has contracted with. Regulatory methods, aside from the Joint Commission on Accreditation of Healthcare Organizations, were mentioned much less frequently. In general, information, research, and activism were the suggested combination of actions to facilitate cultural competence in managed care.

All informants made a link between cultural competence and eliminating racial/ethnic disparities in healthcare. However, they were measured in terms of its impact in achieving that goal. They acknowledged that there are many causes for disparities, and felt that cultural competence efforts at multiple levels were an important component of efforts to address this problem.

'I'm very convinced that specific cultural competence techniques can help reduce disparities, though in no way do I think it's the whole solution. There is no single bullet that is going to eliminate disparities.'

## Community healthcare

### Fulfilling the mission and responding to the needs of the community

Key informants in this area spoke about a longstanding motivation for culturally competent care, rooted in the mission and evolution of community health centers. Overall, there was a general feeling that cultural competence is something that has been going on for a long time in the community health setting starting from a grass-roots level, often with few resources, and becoming a part of the fabric of the organization.

'. . . cultural competence and cultural, racial, and ethnic diversity is a part of the makeup of who we are as an organization and who our patients are so it's not like a new issue.'

Another important issue that arose was the importance of community evaluation and developing an understanding of the target community being cared for. This stemmed from the idea that issues of cultural competence may vary from place to place, although there was agreement that there are some unifying concepts that should be known by all who provide care in these settings.

'It's the ability to understand and respond effectively to the needs of the community . . . people from all backgrounds.'

Key informants cited an understanding of health beliefs and behaviors of certain populations and the need to consider the social, political, and economic environment as important aspects of cultural competence. They also mentioned educating and training patients to understand the medical system and to be better healthcare consumers.

'For example, with immunizations there is a lot of misunderstanding about side effects and a lot of myths with the Latino community about disease, and the health education messages need to include the cultural beliefs and values of the community.'

### Involving community to advance cultural competence

Informants discussed the value of systemically involving community members in the process of developing culturally competent practices.

'Well, I think that being culturally competent means that you are going to do better outreach.'

They suggested formally including culturally diverse community health advocates or mentors, gathering input on community affairs, empowering consumers, and recruiting staff from different communities. Others mentioned linkages with organizations, particular community-based organizations, but also environmental and immigration agencies, as an important way for community health centers to help push forward the cultural competence agenda. Some of the recommendation included:

1. Building trust with communities, includes working on other social needs besides health, and providing language and other services important to patients in the community.
2. Orientating and training the community, educating consumers in the community to understand the healthcare industry and how it pertains to them.
3. Orienting and training of providers to increase communication and sensitivity, to use interpreters, to deliver appropriate health education materials, and to deal with issues of bias.
4. Investing in programs to improve interpreter services, hire bilingual staff, and provide educational materials in several languages.

### Using benchmarks to advance cultural competence and address disparities

The link between cultural competence, quality, and disparities was clearly made. Experts described the need to use tools and benchmarks to evaluate outcomes – 'creating a standard of care for evaluation of care' – and the need to translate cultural competence into quality indicators or outcomes that can be measured, monitored, evaluated, or mandated. Doing this, in and of itself, was seen as a tool to eliminate barriers and disparities.

> '[Cultural competence] is being talked about a lot and it is a beautiful goal but we need to translate this into quality indicators or outcomes that can be measured, monitored, evaluated, or mandated.'

Important outcomes included early identification of disease through better screening, better compliance in treatment programs, decreasing barriers to healthcare (social, cultural, and linguistic), and following the CLAS standards as a blueprint.

## Current Trends in Cultural Competence

Recent trends in several healthcare sectors bear out the key informants' perspectives on cultural competence. For example, health insurers, such as Aetna,[8] Blue Cross–Blue Shield of Florida,[9] and Kaiser Permanente[10] among others, have developed initiatives in cultural competence from both the quality and educational sides as a means of addressing disparities. Large healthcare purchasing coalitions, such as

the Washington Business Group on Health,[11] have been active in informing their membership about the issues of cultural competence and racial/ethnic disparities in healthcare, as well as exploring contracting language to move this issue forward. Accreditation agencies, including the National Committee on Quality Assurance,[12] and the Joint Commission on Accreditation of Healthcare Organizations,[13] are also exploring opportunities to include measures that track disparities and cultural competence.

From the standpoint of medical education, the Accreditation Council on Graduate Medical Education (as part of its 'Outcomes Project'),[14] as well as the Liaison Council on Medical Education,[15] have developed accreditation standards for cultural competence education. Taking this a step further, the New York State Department of Health is providing incentives (by way of bonus funds through the graduate medical education reform incentive pool) for those residency programs that provide a set amount of cultural competence training and are involved in minority recruitment.[16] The state of New Jersey has legislation passed that would require cultural competence continuing education as part of the mandatory licensure process of healthcare professionals.[17] Even professional societies, such as the American Medical Association[18] and the American Nursing Association[19] have statements in support of, and are pursuing active agendas in, cultural competence education.

The federal government has also been advancing this agenda in various ways. For instance, the Health Resources and Services Administration in partnership with the Institute for Healthcare Improvement has developed a 'Disparities Collaborative' focused on eliminating disparities by working with community health centers.[20] Part of this work focuses on developing culturally competent systems of care. In addition, the National Institutes of Health (through the National Center for Minority Health and Health Disparities)[21] and the Agency for Healthcare Research and Quality,[22] have funded research and education in cultural competence over the last few years.

## Conclusion

Key informants from government, academia, managed care, and community health presented various perspectives about the issue of cultural competence in healthcare. In general, there was a strong sense that the field is emerging, and that organizational, systemic, and clinical facets are central to the advancement of cultural competence. Additionally, all saw a clear link between cultural competence, improving quality of care, and eliminating racial and ethnic disparities in healthcare. National trends seem to confirm this viewpoint, as many major healthcare stakeholders have responded to the need to improve quality and address racial and ethnic disparities in healthcare by supporting efforts in cultural competence. Yet the motivations for advancing the issue of cultural competence – and the approaches different stakeholders are taking to make cultural competence actionable – vary depending on each group's mission, goals, and sphere of influence. Despite these differences, there are many synergies that should allow for the continuing development of cultural competence in healthcare. In summary, cultural competence seems to be evolving from a marginal to a mainstream healthcare policy issue, and as a strategy to improve quality and address disparities.

## APPENDIX

Dennis Andrulis, Ph.D.
Department of Medicine
State University of
New York-Downstate,
New York, NY

Lisa Cooper-Patrick,
M.D., M.P.H.
Assistant Professor of
Medicine and Health
Policy
Johns Hopkins
University
Baltimore, MD

Sherlyn Dahl, R.N.,
M.P.H.
Executive Director
Family Health Care
Center
Fargo, ND

Maria Fernandez
South L.A. Health
Projects
Los Angeles, CA
Luis F. Guevara, Psy.D.
Manager of Cross
Cultural Training
White Memorial
Medical Center
Los Angeles, CA

Michael Katz
Centers for Medicare
and Medicaid
Services,
Baltimore, MD

Charles Aswad, M.D.
Council on Graduate
Medical Education
New York State,
Albany, NY

Denice Cora-
Bramble, M.D.
Former Director
Quality Center
Bureau of Primary
Health Care
Bethesda, MD

Deborah Danoff, M.D.
Vice President,
Division of Medical
Education
Association of
American Medical
Colleges
Washington, DC

Iris Garcia, Ph.D.
Former Health Policy
Analyst,
Massachusetts
Division of Medical
Assistance, Office of
Clinical Affairs
Boston, MA

Melba Hinojosa,
M.A., R.N.
Health Plan Advisor,
MediCal Managed
Care California
Department of Health
Los Angeles, CA

Ed Christian, M.D.
Thomas Jefferson
Medical School
Director, Office of
Minority Affairs
Philadelphia, PA

Kathleen Culhane-
Pera, M.D., M.A.
Department of Family
Practice
University of
Minnesota

Tom Delbanco, M.D.
Professor of Medicine
Harvard Medical
School
Beth Israel Deaconess
Hospital
Boston, MA

Ron Garcia, Ph.D.
Asst. Dean of
Minority Affairs
Stanford Medical
School
Palo Alto, CA

Miya Iwataki
Director
Diversity Programs
Los Angeles County
Department of Health,
Los Angeles, CA

Kathryn Linde, M.P.H.
Blue-Cross/Blue-
Shield of Minnesota

Karan Cole, Sc.D.
Assistant Professor of
Medicine
Johns Hopkins
Baltimore, MD

Merle Cunningham,
M.D., M.P.H.
Medical Director
Lutheran Medical
Center,
Brooklyn, NY

Len Epstein
Senior Advisor on
Quality and Culture,
The Quality Center
Bureau of Primary
Health Care
Health Services
Resource
Administration,
Rockville, MD

Tawara Goode
Associate Director
Community Planning,
Center for Child and
Human Development
Georgetown
University
Washington, DC

Bonnie Jacques,
M.S.W.
Chief
Office of
Administrative
Resources
Washington State

David Nerenz, Ph.D.
Director,
Institute for Health
Care Studies,
Michigan State
University

Tom Perez, J.D.
Former Director
Office of Civil Rights
Washington, DC

Christy Swanson
Washington Free
Clinic
Washington, D.C.

Valerie Welsh
Project Officer
Office of Minority
Health
Washington, DC

Robert Like, M.D., M.S.
Associate Professor of
Family Medicine
Robert Wood Johnson
Medical School
Newark, NJ

Ana Nunez, M.D.
Director
Women's Health
Education Program
MCP-Hahnemann
Philadelphia, PA

Julia Puebla-Fortier
Director
Resources for Cross
Cultural Health Care
Silver Springs, MD

Gayle Tang, R.N.,
M.S.N.
Director,
National Linguistic
and Cultural
Programs
Kaiser Permanente,
San Francisco, CA

John O'Brien, M.B.A.
Former CEO,
Cambridge Health
Alliance,
Cambridge, MA

Robert Putsch, M.D.
Professor of Medicine
University of
Washington Cross
Cultural Health Care
Program
Seattle, WA

Melanie Tervalon, MD
Co-Chair, Culture and
Behavior in the
Curriculum
University of
California, San
Francisco

Department of Social
and Health Services
Olympia, WA

Molly McNees, M.A.
Medical
Anthropologist
Lutheran Medical
Center
Brooklyn, NY

Guadelupe Pacheco
Project Officer
Office of Minority
Health
Washington, DC

Beau Stubblefield-Tave,
M.B.A.
Health Policy
Consultant

Melissa Welch, M.D., M.P.H.
Formerly at the
Division of General
Internal Medicine
University of
California, San
Francisco

## References

1. Betancourt JR, Green AR, Carrillo JE. Cultural competence in healthcare: emerging frameworks and practical approaches. The Commonwealth Fund Field Report; 2002.
2. Berger JT. Culture and ethnicity in clinical care. Arch Int Med 1998; 158:2085–2090.
3. Stewart M, Brown JB, Boon H, et al. Evidence on patient–doctor communication. Cancer Prevent Control 1999; 3:25–30.
4. Williams DR, Rucker TD. Understanding and addressing racial disparities in healthcare. healthcare financing review (Health Care Financing Administration). 2000; 21:75–90.
5. Institute of Medicine. Crossing the quality chasm: a new health system for the 21st century. Washington, DC: National Academy Press; 2001.
6. Institute of Medicine. Unequal treatment: confronting racial and ethnic disparities in healthcare. Washington, DC: National Academy Press; 2002.
7. Betancourt JR, Green AR, Carrillo JE, et al. Defining cultural competence: a practical framework for addressing racial/ethnic disparities in health and healthcare. Public Health Rep 2003; 118:293–302.
8. 'Aetna supports efforts to reduce disparities in healthcare.' Press release. Available: http://www.aetna.com/news/2003/pr_20031222.htm 15 August 2004.
9. Blue Cross–Blue Shield of Florida Diversity Program. Available: http://www.bcbsfl.com/index.cfm?section=&fuseaction=Careers.diversityProgram 15 August 2004.
10. Kaiser Permanente Diversity and Inclusion Program. Available: http://www.kaiserpermanentejobs.org/workinghere/diversity.asp 15 August 2004.
11. Washington Business Group on Health. 'Health Disparities Solution Series: Cultural Competency in Health Care.' Available:http://www.wbgh.com/pdfs/913_agenda.pdf15 August 2004.
12. National Committee on Quality Assurance received grant to examine measures that would allow identification of health disparities. Personal Communication, Ignatius Bau, Program Officer, The California Endowment. March 2004.
13. Joint Commission on the Accreditation of Healthcare Organizations. Hospitals, language, and culture. Available: http://www.jcaho.org/about+us/hlc/home.htm15 August 2004.
14. Accreditation Council on Graduate Medical Education. ACGME Outcome Project. Available: http://www.acgme.org/outcome/comp/compMin.asp 15 August 2004.
15. Liaison Committee on Medical Education. Accreditation Standards. Available: www.lcme.org/standard.htm 15 August 2004.
16. New York State Department of Health Graduate Medical Education Reform Incentive Pool. Available: http://www.health.state.ny.us/nysdoh/gme/main.htm15 August 2004.
17. New Jersey State Legislation. Available: Bill S144 http://www.njleg.state.nj.us/15 August 2004.
18. American Medical Association. 'Ethics and Health Disparities Program.' Available: http://www.ama-assn.org/ama/pub/category/9421.html 15 August 2004.

19. American Nursing Association. 'Many Faces of Diversity Program.' Available: http://www.nursingworld.org/ojin/topic20/tpc20lnx.htm 15 August 2004.
20. Institute for Healthcare Improvement. 'Health Disparities Collaboratives.' Available: http://www.ihi.org/IHI/Topics/Improvement/SpreadingChanges/Literature/HealthDisparitiesCollaboratives.htm 15 August 2004.
21. National Center on Minority Health and Health Disparities. Available: http://ncmhd.nih.gov. 15 August 2004.
22. Agency for Healthcare Research and Quality. Cultural competence guides now available to aid managed care plans. Available: http://www.ahrq.gov/research/nov02/1102ra14.htm15 August 2004.

# Overseas Medical Screening for Immigrants and Refugees

Susan A. Maloney, Luis S. Ortega, and Martin S. Cetron

## Introduction

Migration is a major human and global phenomenon, with many complex linkages to economic, trade, social, security, and health policies. In the dynamic relationship between migration and health, immigration has long been recognized to have a large impact on disease epidemiology and the use of health services in migrant receiving nations.[1] For example, the impact of immigration on disease epidemiology is demonstrated by the global epidemiology of tuberculosis (TB). Tuberculosis is a leading global cause of infectious disease morbidity and mortality; however, rates of TB in most regions of the developing world are many times higher than those in the developed world (i.e. the TB prevalence gap), and decreasing at a much slower rate.[2] Many migration receiving countries in the developed world have had stable or increased migration of persons from regions with high TB prevalence, while at the same time have successfully decreased TB incidence in their native-born population, further exacerbating this prevalence gap. Consequently, the majority of TB cases in migration receiving countries such as the US and Canada are now being diagnosed in foreign-born populations from high-prevalence source countries.[3,4]

Many immigration receiving countries have pre-arrival medical examination requirements and protocols for entering migrants, which vary both by the types of populations screened, and the diseases for which examination is required. As an example, the US currently does not require a sputum culture for TB diagnosis, while it is required by some other receiving countries. The health conditions tested through the medical examination procedures required by countries such as Australia, Canada, New Zealand, the United Kingdom, and the United States of America are determined on the basis of the risk or danger that these conditions can represent to public health and safety and the additional costs that may be incurred by national public services expenditures.[5-9] In general, these medical examination procedures include a review of the past medical history, a physical examination, and tests that include a chest X-ray and laboratory analyses. The diseases most frequently tested for to determine visa eligibility or the admissibility of a migrant are infectious diseases such as tuberculosis, sexually transmitted diseases, and mental or behavioral conditions. Immigration regulations in some of these countries do allow for the consideration of medical waivers to inadmissible health conditions. Although many immigration receiving countries in Europe either do not require pre-arrival health evaluations or have fewer requirements and only limited grounds for refusal of admission based on health grounds, most have provisions for notification and inspection if a communicable or serious health condition is recognized or suspected.[10,11]

## US Migration and Health Screening Policies

The number of foreign-born persons living in the US, approximately 28 million, is greater than ever before in the nation's history.[12] In 2004, the foreign-born proportion of the total US population reached approximately 12%, a proportion comparable to the peak reached during the great immigration wave at the turn of the twentieth century. In contrast to the previous twentieth-century US immigration wave, which was dominated by Eastern Europeans who were driven from their countries of origin by factors such as persecution and poverty (so called 'push factors'), the twenty-first-century immigration wave, which began in the 1970s, is characterized predominantly by Hispanic migrants followed by Asian migrants who are attracted to the US for economic opportunities (or 'pull factors'). In both waves of migration, migrants have brought with them not only skills and cultural traditions that enriched US economic and social fabrics, but also diseases and disease exposures which were different from those existing in US receiving communities. In addition, twenty-first-century migrants are more mobile and remain connected to their countries of birth, typically making several back and forth journeys to visit friends and relatives (VFR). New immigrants and refugees who cross disease prevalence gaps and their frequent VFR travel patterns constitute potentially high-risk populations for translocating communicable diseases of public health significance.

The Department of Homeland Security has reported that approximately 60 000 000 migrants enter the United States annually (Table 10.1).[13] These migrants include immigrants, refugees, migrants adjusting their visa status, persons with non-immigrant visas, persons in short-term transit status, and other groups of migrants who entered the United States without inspection, including undocumented migrants. The majority of these migrants are not required to undergo medical screening prior to US entry. Given the immense numbers of persons crossing US borders and finite resources for evaluation and surveillance, US migrant health screening policy focuses on migrants planning to establish permanent US residence, as this group has the largest potential long-term impact both on disease epidemiology and healthcare resources utilization. Currently, the Immigration and Nationality Act (INA) requires that medical screening examinations be performed overseas for all US-bound immigrants and refugees, and in the United States for migrants applying to adjust their visa status to permanent residence (i.e. 'green cards').[8,9,14,15] In 2003, approximately 700 000 immigrants, refugees, and migrants seeking visa status adjustment underwent medical screening examinations. The remainder of this chapter will discuss US overseas medical screening issues for US-bound immigrants and refugees. The two following chapters will address screening programs and individual health assessments for new immigrants on arrival in the US.

## Required Overseas Medical Screening Examinations for US-Bound Immigrants and Refugees

On average, approximately 400 000 documented immigrants and refugees arrive in the US annually; immigrants comprise approximately 90% of arrivals, and refugees close to 10%.[13] Trends in the number

**Table 10.1** Categories and number of migrants entering the United States by medical screening requirements, 2003

| Category | Annual number | Medical screening | Screening site | Screening location |
|---|---|---|---|---|
| Immigrants | 358 411 | Yes | Panel physicians | Overseas |
| Refugees | 28 306 | Yes | Panel physicians | Overseas |
| Status adjusters | 347 416 | Yes | Civil surgeons | US |
| Non-immigrants | 27 849 443 | No | | |
| Short-term transit | ≈30 000 000 | No | | |
| Others* | ≈1 500 000 | No | | |
| TOTAL | ≈60 000 000 | | | |

Source: US Department of Homeland Security.
* Others include migrants who entered the United States without inspection, including those who entered with and without proper documentation.

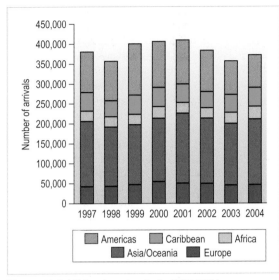

**Figure 10.1** US immigrant arrivals 1997–2004.

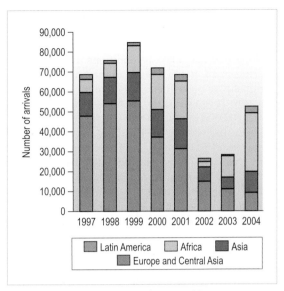

**Figure 10.2** US refugee arrivals 1997–2004.

and regions of origin for US-arriving immigrants and refugees are presented in Figures 10.1 and 10.2. From 1997 to 2004, over 3 million immigrants arrived in the US; the number of arrivals and regions of origin remained relatively stable over the 8 years examined. Between 357 000 and 410 000 immigrants arrived annually; 43% from Asia/Oceania, 26% from the Americas (with the majority of these arrivals [roughly 60%] from Mexico), 13% from the Caribbean, 12% from Europe, and 7% from Africa. From 1997 to 2004, close to 560 000 refugees arrived in the US; in contrast to immigrants, the number of arrivals and regions of origin have changed markedly over the 8 years examined. From 1997 to 2001, the number of refugees entering the US remained stable at approximately 70 000 per year. However, after the September 11 terrorist attacks, increased security requirements delayed some refugee processing, and therefore the number of refugees arriving in 2002 and 2003 decreased to 30 000 or less. It is reported that almost 53 000 refugees arrived in the US by the end of 2004. The number and proportions of arriving refugees from different regions of the world also changed over the 8 years examined. In 1997, the majority (70%) of arriving refugees were from Europe and Central Asia, with only 9% of arriving refugees from Africa. In contrast, in 2004, almost 55% (approximately 29 000 refugees) arrived from Africa. These trends have important implications for medical evaluation and treatment of refugees, both overseas and stateside, as refugees from Africa have relatively high rates of certain diseases, including human

immunodeficiency (HIV), TB, malaria, intestinal helminth infections, and other tropical diseases (e.g. schistosomiasis), and likely lack routine vaccinations.

All immigrants and refugees migrating to the United States are required to have a medical screening examination overseas, which is performed by local physicians (panel physicians) appointed by the local US embassy.[8,9] The mandated medical examination focuses primarily on detecting diseases determined to be inadmissible conditions for the purposes of visa eligibility. These diseases include certain serious infectious diseases such as infectious tuberculosis, human immunodeficiency virus infection, syphilis, and other sexually transmitted infections, and infectious Hansen's disease. Other diseases (noninfectious) designated as inadmissible conditions include mental disorders associated with harmful behavior, and substance abuse. For the purposes of determining the inadmissibility of an applicant, medical conditions are categorized as class A or B. Class A conditions are defined as those conditions which preclude an immigrant or refugee from entering the US. Class A conditions require approved waivers for United States entry and immediate medical follow-up upon arrival. These conditions include communicable diseases of public health significance, a physical or mental disorder associated with violent or harmful behavior, and drug abuse or addiction. Class B conditions are defined as significant health problems: physical or mental abnormalities, diseases, or disabilities serious in degree or permanent in nature amounting to a substantial departure from normal well-being. Follow-up evaluation soon after US arrival is recommended for migrants with class B conditions. If immigrants or refugees are found to have an inadmissible condition that may make them ineligible for a visa, a visa may still be issued after the illness has been adequately treated or after a waiver of the visa eligibility has been approved by US Customs and Immigration Services.

In 1996, a new subsection was added to the Immigration and Nationality Act requiring that persons seeking immigrant visas for permanent residency show proof of receipt of at least the first dose of all vaccination series recommended by the Advisory Committee for Immunization Practices (ACIP), if these vaccines are available in the originating country. Although these regulations apply to all adult immigrants, and most immigrant children, internationally adopted children who are younger than 10 years of age have been exempted from the immunization requirements as a consequence of strong objections posed by advocacy groups who cited safety concerns over immunization practices in several origin countries. Refugees are not required to meet the INA immunization requirements at the time of initial entry into the United States but must show proof of vaccination at the time they apply for permanent US residence, typically within 3 years of US arrival.

The Centers for Disease Control and Prevention (CDC), Division of Global Migration and Quarantine (DGMQ), is responsible for providing technical guidance to the panel physicians in performing the overseas medical screening examination.[14] The testing modalities recommended for the medical examination are outlined in Table 10.2, and the algorithm for the required overseas medical screening examination is presented in Figure 10.3. The CDC, DGMQ, is also responsible for monitoring the quality of the overseas medical examination process at over 650 panel physician sites (healthcare staff, radiology facilities, vaccination protocols, and laboratories) worldwide, through its Quality Assurance Program (QAP). Due to limited resources, not all panel physician sites can be visited and assessed annually. Sites are prioritized for monitoring, based upon the number of immigrant and refugee visas processed and country-specific prevalence of such diseases as tuberculosis and human immunodeficiency virus. In addition, DGMQ performs remediation visits when medical screening examination deficiencies have been identified. In an effort to share experiences regarding the optimization of immigration

**Table 10.2 Testing for required overseas medical screening examination**

| Health condition | Testing |
| --- | --- |
| Tuberculosis | Chest radiograph; AFB smear if CXR+ |
| HIV | Serology |
| Syphilis | Serology |
| Other sexually transmitted diseases | Physical examination |
| Hansen's disease | Physical examination |
| Mental disorders with associated harmful behavior | History |
| Drug abuse or addiction | History, physical exam |
| Vaccinations | History, vaccination records, serology |

Source: CDC, DGMQ.

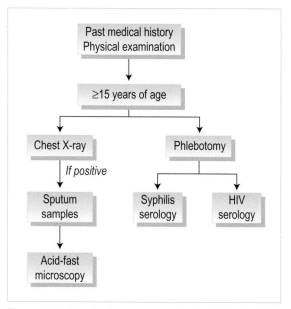

**Figure 10.3** Required overseas medical screening examination.

medical processes, technical aspects of the medical screening, the performance evaluation of panel physicians, and review policies, regulations, and practices of the various resettlement nations, DGMQ has met with sister agencies from other countries to discuss possible approaches to common challenges such as health information systems, privacy, confidentiality, and resource utilization and constraints.

The CDC, DGMQ, is also responsible for notifying state and local health departments of all arriving refugees and those immigrants with class A or B health conditions who are resettling in their jurisdiction and need follow-up evaluation and possible treatment in the US.[8,9] Under the current system, US Department of State forms summarizing the results of the overseas medical examination, including classification of health conditions, are manually collected at US ports of entry. This information is transmitted to state and local health departments through the US mail. State and local health departments are asked to report to DGMQ the results of these US follow-up evaluations, and any significant public health conditions occurring among recently arrived immigrants and refugees, as a way to better understand epidemiological patterns of disease in recently arrived migrants and to monitor the quality of overseas medical examination. Public health models for accomplishing these goals are discussed in Chapter 11.

## Health Conditions Identified Through Required US Overseas Medical Screening Examinations

The number and types of health conditions identified through required overseas medical screening examinations among the approximately 2 million immigrants and 280 000 refugees who arrived in the US from 2000 to 2004 are summarized in Table 10.3. For both refugees and immigrants, the most frequent conditions identified were suspect active and inactive tuberculosis.

The underlying objective of the overseas tuberculosis screening process is to limit the entry of persons seeking long-term US residence who have infectious (defined as acid-fast bacilli (AFB) smear-positive) active TB, and therefore pose an immediate public health risk, and to refer others with suspect active and inactive TB for further evaluation and treatment in the US, where diagnostic facilities and mycobacterial culture capability are generally more readily available and treatment can more easily be monitored and supervised. Suspect active tuberculosis (e.g. class A and B1) was identified in 0.96% of immigrants and 0.77% of refugees examined overseas from 1999 through 2003. A recently published study assessing the performance of US overseas TB screening has demonstrated that the ability of the current overseas TB screening algorithm (based on chest radiographs and AFB smear microscopy) to detect pulmonary tuberculosis disease is low. The sensitivity, specificity, and positive and negative predictive values for serial AFB smears (compared to the gold standard of mycobacterial culture) were 34.4%, 98.1%, 76.8%, and 89.1%, respectively, and nearly two-thirds of immigrants with positive cultures were not identified overseas using the current algorithm.[16] These data, in conjunction with a recent outbreak of TB and MDR TB among Hmong refugees in Thailand, underscore the need for improved diagnostic methods and enhanced screening measures to enrich identification and control of TB among migrants.[17] CDC is currently working on revising the recommendations for overseas TB screening to improve and enhance TB diagnosis and treatment and to prevent disease importation.

**Table 10.3 Number of health conditions identified through overseas medical screening examination among immigrants and refugees, 2000–2004**

| Health conditions (2000–2004) | Immigrants | Refugees | Total |
|---|---|---|---|
| Infectious (AFB +) active TB: class A | 20 | 5 | 25 |
| Not infectious (AFB −) active TB: class B1 | 20 196 | 2378 | 22 574 |
| Not active TB: class B2 | 16 318 | 7057 | 23 375 |
| HIV | 134 | 1165 | 1299 |
| Syphilis | 221 | 199 | 420 |
| Hansen's disease | 13 | 4 | 17 |
| Mental disorder associated with harmful behavior | 36 | 10 | 46 |
| Drug abuse or addiction | 6 | 1 | 7 |
| TOTAL | 36 944 | 10 819 | 47 763 |

Data from Division of Global Migration and Quarantine, Centers for Disease Control and Prevention.

Previous studies have reported that during US follow-up, pulmonary TB disease was diagnosed in 3.3–14.0% of immigrants and refugees classified overseas as having suspect active TB.[18-24] If these estimates are used to calculate expected rates of active TB among newly arrived US immigrants and refugees with suspect active TB, the expected rates of pulmonary TB disease for immigrants would be between 29 and 134 per 100 000 persons and for refugees between 23 and 208 per 100 000 persons. These rates are as high and likely higher than the reported TB rate among all foreign-born persons in the US in 2002 (23.6 per 100 000).[3] Further, compared to the US native-born TB rates (2.8 per 100 000), these expected rates are higher by several orders of magnitude.

The high rates of TB in newly arrived immigrants and refugees underscore the importance of both enhancing overseas TB screening procedures and assuring timely and appropriate US follow-up evaluation of immigrants and refugees with suspect active TB, as the yield for TB case finding is high. Although rates of follow-up for immigrants and refugees identified overseas as class B1 or class B2 are relatively high (63–99%),[18] problems exist with late or lost arrival notifications in up to 30% of notifications (CDC, unpublished data). These deficiencies in the current manual notification process can delay the evaluation and treatment of TB cases among immigrants and refugees after arrival in the US, and can potentially contribute to increased TB morbidity and mortality and disease transmission. A CDC initiative to develop an electronic disease notification system for arriving refugees and immigrants is already underway to address these deficiencies, and will be discussed in a later section of this chapter.

The number of HIV infections identified during the overseas medical screening examination is relatively small. Early identification of HIV infections among immigrants and refugees is important to assure appropriate notification and linkages to medical services in resettlement communities. Current regulations require that syphilis infections be treated before departure to the US. During the time period examined, a total of approximately 400 immigrants and refugees infected with syphilis were identified overseas. In reference to other inadmissible conditions listed in Table 10.3, fewer than 20 cases of Hansen's disease, fewer than 50 cases of mental disorder associated with harmful behavior, and only 7 cases of drug abuse or addiction were identified among US-bound immigrants and refugees.

## Program Initiatives to Address Challenges and Improve Immigrant and Refugee Health

### Electronic disease notification system

The Division of Global Migration and Quarantine is currently embarked upon a long-term, multiyear initiative to develop a comprehensive electronic disease notification system to communicate with both national and international partners about diseases and disease outbreaks occurring among mobile populations entering the United States. Such mobile populations include immigrants, refugees, migrants, and international travelers (including temporary visitors). The system, called the Electronic Disease Notification (EDN) system, will integrate data from multiple sources and surveillance systems and will include modules dedicated to specific populations and disease entities of public health importance, such as tuberculosis. The EDN-Tuberculosis (EDN-TB) module was prioritized for implementation due to the crucial role it can play in enhancing tuberculosis control and prevention efforts among arriving immigrants and refugees, and is currently being piloted in several US states. The objectives of the EDN-TB module are to: (1) use the CDC secure data network to electronically notify health departments of newly arriving immigrants and refugees with class A and class B tuberculosis, (2) provide an electronic system for health departments to inform other health departments of secondary migration of immigrants and refugees with TB conditions within the US, (3) provide health departments with an electronic system to record and evaluate the outcome of domestic follow-up examinations, (4) provide federal and state public health officials with data to evaluate the effectiveness of follow-up of immigrants and refugees with suspect tuberculosis, and (5) allow comparison of overseas health assessments with domestic follow-up outcomes as part of a comprehensive quality assessment program for overseas TB screening examinations. This module has initially been deployed to a limited number of states for real-time operation. Monitoring the system performance will identify improvements needed and guide the implementation and deployment of the system to additional states.

### Enhanced refugee health assessment programs

It has long been recognized that immigrants and refugees may carry significant disease burdens which are determined by geographic origin, ethnicity, and living and health conditions in countries of origin or departure.[25] These migrants can suffer from a multitude of health conditions, including infectious diseases (such as tuberculosis and many tropical and parasitic diseases), malnutrition, reproductive health needs, and mental health disorders, often caused by tenuous circumstances in their countries of origin or departure.[25-31] Such disease burdens can seriously hamper migrants' ability to successfully integrate and optimally contribute to their resettlement communities, and may cause strain on health and social services systems in the US.[28] Most of these health conditions are not addressed during the required overseas medical examination process.

Refugees do receive stateside evaluation and treatment, usually conducted at state or local health departments, within 3 months of US arrival, but currently there is no standardized nationwide protocol for post-arrival health assessment, and therefore the content of post-arrival refugee health evaluations varies from state to state, and funding sources are often noted to be inadequate to provide comprehensive services. Further, both refugees and immigrants often have other daily demands to achieve integration into their new living environment which may compete with their need for health evaluations and treatment. Optimizing migrant health prior to resettlement, and addressing migrant health needs early in the migration process can therefore be cost-effective and can prevent larger expenditures later.[23,32-34] Realization of this fact has led to the development of the Enhanced Refugee Health Programs (ERHPs), pilot programs aimed at achieving an integration of the health needs of migrant populations and host and receiving countries. The US CDC has developed these programs in collaboration with the US Bureau of Population and Migration (PRM), the International Organization for Migration (IOM), and often with US state and local health departments, to begin to address the healthcare needs of US-destined refugees while they are still overseas, and to facilitate and promote appropriate stateside evaluation and treatment. These programs focus on refugees for a number of reasons: (1) refugees comprise vulnerable populations, exposed to a variety of harsh environmental conditions and diverse disease exposures with limited access to healthcare; (2) a unique opportunity exists to address refugee health concerns during required overseas health assessments; (3) the language and charge of the US Refugee Act provide more latitude to address conditions of public health concern among refugees (in addition to

inadmissible conditions); and (4) lessons learned from a focus on the smaller number of refugees may be potentially applicable to the larger numbers of immigrants, or other migrant groups.

The ERHP strategy is to utilize the required overseas medical examination process as a unique opportunity to assess and improve the health status of refugees overseas, and to incorporate both required screening components for inadmissible conditions and additional expanded components, which are tailored to specific refugee population needs and targeted to diseases of public health importance. The program first ensures quality staffing and infrastructure in the field by evaluating, training, and lending resources to support the capacity currently in place, when necessary. Extending health services in the country of origin or transit allows patients to be served by health providers who are closer geographically and often culturally to the patients' circumstances and health needs. Further, through the development of enhanced and electronic data exchange systems, ERHPs also promote more timely transmission of population-based health and medical examination data acquired overseas to US health departments in resettlement communities, facilitating appropriate follow-up and treatment of refugees after arrival in the US. In the future, programs will strive to support and standardize follow-up evaluation and treatment of refugees after US arrival by state and local health departments and other community health providers.

Since 1997, the US CDC has undertaken enhanced refugee health programs for at least eight large-scale, emergent movements of refugee populations, and one US-based intervention among the Lost Boys and Girls of Sudan. These programs have included components to provide presumptive pre-departure treatment for malaria, intestinal parasites, and other tropical diseases, expanded tuberculosis diagnosis and treatment, HIV services, appropriate immunizations, dental and mental health assessments, chronic disease evaluations, and post-arrival treatment for schistosomiasis and Strongyloides infection (Table 10.4). These programs have successfully prevented thousands of cases of intestinal parasitosis, malaria, and vaccine-preventable diseases, and hundreds of cases of tuberculosis and other communicable diseases among US-bound refugees.[35-39] Other integral components of the ERHP initiative have been efforts to provide linkages to US programs in host countries, such as Global AIDS Program (GAP), which can provide diagnostic treatment and prevention services to refugees awaiting US resettlement. Such efforts are aimed to assure that refugees have access

**Table 10.4 US CDC Enhanced Refugee Health Programs, by population group and program components, 1997–2005**

| Program components | Population group, year, (n) | | | | | | | | |
|---|---|---|---|---|---|---|---|---|---|
| | Somali Barawans, 1997 (4000) | Kosovars, 1999 (10 000) | Burmese, 2001 (1000) | Vietnamese Montagnards, 2002 (1000) | Somali Bantu, 2003 (15 000) | Liberians, 2003 (8000) | Lost Boys of Sudan, 2004 (5000) | Laotian Hmong, 2004/2005 (15 000) | Burmese, 2004/2005 (3000) |
| **Overseas** | | | | | | | | | |
| ***Pre-departure treatment:*** | | | | | | | | | |
| Malaria | X | | | | X | X | | X | X |
| Intestinal parasites | X | | | | X | X | | | |
| ***Screening/targeted treatment:*** | | | | | | | | | |
| Malaria | X | | X | X | X | X | | X | X |
| Schistosomiasis | X | | | | | | | X | X |
| Immunizations (emergent) | X | | | X | | | | X | X |
| Immunizations (routine) | | | | | | | | X | |
| Expanded tuberculosis diagnosis and treatment | | X | X | X | | X | | X | X |
| Expanded HIV services | | X | | | | X | | X | X |
| Emergent disease surveillance | | | | | X | X | | X | X |
| Outbreak response | | | | | X | X | | X | |
| Enhanced notification and data transmission | | | | | | | | | |
| Electronic notification and data transmission | X | X | X | X | X | X | | X | X |
| **US/stateside** | | | | | | | | | |
| ***Post-arrival treatment for:*** | | | | | | | | | |
| Malaria | | X | | X | | | | | |
| Schistosomiasis | | | | | | | X | | |
| Strongyloides | | | | | | | X | | |
| Scabies | | | | | | | | | |
| Acute and primary care | | X | | | | | | | |
| Chronic disease evaluation | | X | | | | | | | |
| Mental health | | X | | | | | | | |
| Dental health | | X | | | | | | | |
| Immunizations (routine) | | X | | X | | | | | |
| Expanded TB evaluation | | X | | X | | X | X | X | X |
| Hepatitis screening | | | | X | | | | | |
| Outbreak response | | | | | | | | X | |

Source: CDC, DGMQ.

118

to needed healthcare services in a prompt manner even while still in asylum countries prior to US resettlement, and to reduce the burden placed on host country resources, as overseas interventions can decrease refugee health utilization once in the US, reduce treatment costs, and avoid overburdening the domestic health system.

Vaccine-preventable diseases are a source of significant morbidity and mortality in developing countries, and refugees are known to be under-vaccinated due to collapsing public health infra-structures in countries of origin or departure and lack of access to healthcare. In addition, outbreaks of measles, rubella, and varicella among US-bound Liberian refugees in Côte d'Ivoire, varicella among the Somali Barawans in Kenya in 1997 and Somali Bantu refugees in Kenya in 2003 and 2004, and hepatitis A among Hmong refugees in Thailand in 2004 were identified and controlled during ERHP programs.[40(and CDC unpublished data)] As a result of these and other disease outbreaks, the movement of refugees has frequently been significantly delayed and necessitated substantial additional per capita investments in the resettlement process (e.g. last-minute cancellation of nonrefundable commercial airline tickets and the need for dedicated refugee charter flights), not to mention the obvious risks to refugee health and threat of importation and spread of disease in receiving communities. To prevent morbidity, mortality, and the threats of disease importation along with the avoidance of costly delays in refugee resettlement, CDC, DGMQ recommends that refugees also receive age-appropriate immunizations listed in the *Technical Instructions to Panel Physicians for Vaccination Requirements* (for immigrants) if the vaccines are available in-country or easily obtained. CDC recognizes that some vaccines may not be available in all host countries and therefore vaccination with some vaccines may not be feasible. However, common vaccines that can be routinely obtained overseas for use in many originating countries include DPT, Td, OPV, MMR, hepatitis B, and varicella; an initial dose of vaccines in these series should be administered as early as possible before migration, to maximize utility and protection. The following vaccinations may not be easily obtained in host countries: *Haemophilus influenzae* type b (Hib), pneumococcal, and influenza. If vaccines are not available in host countries, they should be administered as soon as possible after resettlement in the United States.

Although ERHPs have clearly proven to be successful for targeted groups of refugees and specific conditions, such as malaria and intestinal parasites,

more substantial investment is needed to optimize overseas health assessment and intervention for more refugees. In the last 2 years, the CDC and the US government have responded to 11 international and domestic outbreaks of infectious diseases among US-bound refugees, including measles, rubella, vari-cella, cholera, hepatitis A, O'nyong-nyong fever, and multidrug-resistant tuberculosis. These outbreaks, which were associated with importation of infectious diseases in the US and secondary domestic transmission, including multidrug-resistant tuberculosis and congenital rubella syndrome, have taxed the resources of state and local health departments and represent an obstacle to the US plans for elimination of tuberculosis and vaccine-preventable diseases, including measles and rubella. In addition to the public health resources for outbreak response, these outbreaks halted resettlement and cost hundreds of thousands of dollars in flight cancellations and other expenses. These outbreaks highlight the need to enhance overseas health screening and treatment for US-bound refugees and other migrants. Investment in and enhancement of overseas capacity for disease diagnosis and treatment for US-bound refugees is a cost-effective strategy for reducing US imported cases, decreasing the healthcare burden on US health providers, and improving overall US health security.[41,42] Current challenges to effective overseas refugee health screening and treatment include inadequate healthcare funding resources; insufficient authorizations and appropriations; inadequate overseas investment in screening, diagnosis, treatment, and prevention; and limited domestic public health resources.

## Directions for the Future

Future directions for achieving more integrated and comprehensive overseas immigrant and refugee health screening programs and policies include:

1. Identifying sustainable funding to support overseas migration health programs, in both receiving and host countries.
2. Continuing efforts to tailor migration health policies to incorporate the unique needs of migrant populations and to provide flexibility to address emerging global health issues.
3. Expanding the role of migration health assessments in enhancing the health of migrants and protecting the public health of

receiving and host country populations.
Priority areas should include:

- Support for delivery of essential
  preventive and treatment interventions,
  such as vaccinations, treatment for
  malaria and other parasitic diseases,
  tuberculosis, HIV, and waterborne
  diseases;
- Creation of effective surveillance systems
  for emerging infectious diseases;
- Development of emergency response
  capacity; and
- Inclusion of components to address
  emerging infectious diseases,
  reproductive and mental health needs,
  and other diseases of public health
  importance.

4. Applying new information technology to
   secure electronic information exchange
   among numerous international and
   interagency partners and assuring real-time
   communication of health data along the
   migration pathway.

5. Promoting public–private partnerships to
   address migrant health issues.

6. Developing international and interagency
   partnerships to facilitate harmonization of
   policies and the integration of global
   migration and health issues.

Ultimately, health and migration are intimately
linked and interdependent. Early investment in
addressing and integrating the health needs of
refugees and immigrants in both host and receiving
communities will facilitate the migration process,
improve migrant health, and decrease associated
morbidity and mortality, avoid long-term health
resource and social costs, and protect global public
health.

## References

1. Gushalak BD, MacPherson DW. Globalization of infectious
   diseases: the impact of migration. Clin Infect Dis 2004;
   38:1742–1748.
2. Corbett EL, Watt CJ, Walker N, et al. The growing
   burden of tuberculosis: global trends and interactions
   with the HIV epidemic. Arch Intern Med 2003;
   163(9):1009–1021.
3. Centers for Disease Control and Prevention. Reported
   tuberculosis in the United States, 2002. Atlanta, Georgia: US
   Department of Health and Human Services, CDC;
   September 2003.
4. Health Canada. Tuberculosis Statistics 2002. Health Canada
   2003; no. H49–108/2002.
5. Citizenship and Immigration Canada. http://www.cic.
   gc.ca/manuals-guides/english/op/index.html Accessed
   2/1/07.

6. Department of Immigration and Multicultural and
   Indigenous Affairs, Australian Government. http://www.
   immi.gov.au/media/fact-sheets/22health.htm Accessed
   2/1/07.
7. New Zealand Immigration Service. http://www.
   immigration.govt.nz/migrant Accessed 2/1/07.
8. Immigration and Nationality Act. US Department of
   Homeland Security. http://www.uscis.gov/portal/site/uscis
   Accessed 2/1/07.
9. 42 Code of Federal Regulations (CFR) Part 34.3. Scope of the
   Examination. http://www.access.gpo.gov/nara/cfr/
   waisidx_03/42cfr34_03.html Accessed 2/1/07.
10. United Nations High Commission for Refugees. http://
    www.unhcr.org/cgi-bin/texis/vtx/home March 16, 2006.
11. European Economic Area Nationals. Annex E – General
    Guidance. http://www.ind.homeoffice.gov.uk/documents/
    ecis/ Accessed 2/1/07.
12. Center for Immigration Studies (CIS). http://www.cis.org
    Accessed 2/1/07.
13. The Office of Immigration Statistics (OIS), Office of
    Management, Department of Homeland Security (DHS):
    Yearbook of Immigration Statistics. http://www.dhs.gov/
    ximgtn/statistics/ Accessed 2/1/07.
14. Centers for Disease Control and Prevention. Division of
    Global Migration and Quarantine. Technical Instructions
    for Panel Physicians. http://www.cdc.gov/ncidod/dq/panel.
    htm Accessed 2/1/07.
15. Centers for Disease Control and Prevention. Division of
    Global Migration and Quarantine. Technical Instructions
    for Civil Surgeons. Available: http://www.cdc.gov/ncidod/
    dq/civil.htm Accessed 2/1/07.
16. Maloney SA, Fielding KL, Laserson KL, et al. Assessing the
    performance of overseas tuberculosis screening programs: a
    study among US-bound immigrants in Vietnam. Arch
    Intern Med 2006; 166:234–240.
17. Centers for Disease Control and Prevention. Multidrug-
    Resistant Tuberculosis in Hmong Refugees Resettling From
    Thailand into the United States, 2004–2005. MMWR 2005;
    54(30):741–744.
18. Binkin NJ, Zuber PLF, Wells CD, et al. Overseas screening
    of tuberculosis in immigrants and refugees to the United
    States: current status. Clin Infect Dis 1996; 26;1226–1232.
19. Zuber PLF, Knowles LS, Binkin NJ, et al. Tuberculosis
    among foreign-born persons in Los Angeles County, 1992–
    1994. Tuberc Lung Dis 1996; 77:524–530.
20. Centers for Disease Control and Prevention. Tuberculosis
    among foreign-born persons who have recently arrived in
    the United States–Hawaii, 1992–1993, and Los Angeles
    County, 1993. MMWR 1995; 44:703–707.
21. Zuber PLF, Binkin NJ, Ignacio AC, et al. Tuberculosis
    screening for immigrants and refugees. Diagnostic
    outcomes in the state of Hawaii. Am J Respir Crit Care Med
    1996; 154:151–155.
22. Wells CD, Zuber PLF, Nolan CM, et al. Tuberculosis
    prevention among foreign-born person in Seattle–King
    County, Washington. Am J Respir Crit Care Med 1997;
    156:573–577.
23. Sciortino S, Mohle-Boetani J, Royce SE, et al. B notifications
    and the detection of tuberculosis among foreign-born recent
    arrivals in California. Int J Tuberc Lung Dis 1999; 3:778–785.
24. Granich RM, Moore M, Binkin NJ, et al. Drug-resistant
    tuberculosis in foreign-born persons from Mexico, the
    Philippines, and Vietnam–United States, 1993–1997. Int J
    Tuberc Lung Dis 2001; 5(1):53–58.
25. Stauffer WM, Kamat D, Walker PF. Screening of
    international immigrants, refugees, and adoptees. Prim
    Care Clin Office Pract 2002; 29:879–905.
26. Barnett ED. Infectious disease screening for refugees
    resettled in the United States. Clin Infect Dis J 2004;
    39:833–841.
27. Catanzaro A, Moser RJ. Health status of refugees from
    Vietnam, Laos and Cambodia. JAMA 1982; 247(9):1303–1308.
28. Paxton LA, Slutsker L, Schultz LJ, et al. Imported malaria in
    Montagnard refugees settling in North Carolina:

implications for prevention and control. Am J Trop Med Hyg 1996; 54(1):54–57.

29. Sachs WJ, Adair R, Kirchner V. Enteric parasites in East African immigrants. Minnesota Med 2000; 83:25–28.

30. Peterson MH, Konczyk MR, Amrosino K, et al. Parasitic screening of a refugee population in Illinois. Diagnost Microbiol Infect Dis 2001; 40:75–76.

31. Vergara AE, Miller JM, Martin DR, et al. A survey of refugee health assessments in the United States. J Immigr Health 2003; 5(2):67–73.

32. Thomas RE, Gushulak B. Screening and treatment of immigrants and refugees to Canada for tuberculosis: implications of the experience of Canada and other industrialized countries. Can J Infect Dis 1995; 6(5):246–255.

33. Anderson JP, Moser RJ. Parasite screening and treatment among Indochinese refugees, cost-benefit/utility and the general health policy model. JAMA 1985; 253(15):2229–2235.

34. Muennig P, Pallin D, Sell RL, et al. The cost-effectiveness of strategies for the treatment of intestinal parasites in immigrants. N Engl J Med 1999; 340:773–779.

35. Centers for Disease Control and Prevention. Enhanced medical assessment strategy for Barawan Somali refugees–Kenya, 1997. MMWR 1998; 46:1250–1254

36. Miller JM, Boyd HA, Ostrowski SH, et al. Malaria, intestinal parasites, and schistosomiasis among Barawan Somali refugees resetting to the United States: A strategy to reduce morbidity and decrease risk of imported infections. Am J Trop Med Hyg 2000; 62(1):115–121.

37. Geltman PL, Cochran J, Hedgecock C. Intestinal parasites among African refugees resettled in Massachusetts and the impact of an overseas pre-departure treatment program. Am J Trop Med Hyg 2003; 69(6):657–662.

38. SA Maloney. Migration health policies: shifting the paradigm from exclusion to inclusion. Immigrant and Refugee Health: Focus on North America. Pre-Meeting Course for 53rd Annual Meeting of the American Society of Tropical Medicine and Hygiene, Miami, Florida, November 6–7, 2004.

39. Posey DL, O'Rourke TO, Weinberg M, et al. Urgent resettlement of Liberian refugees to the United States, 2003: an enhanced refugee health response. Fourth European Conference on Travel Medicine: Travel and Safety. Rome, Italy, March 29–31, 2004.

40. Posey D, Guerra M, Weinberg M, et al. Varicella outbreak among Liberian refugees in Côte d'Ivoire: clinical epidemiology and impact of mass varicella vaccination. 42nd Annual Meeting of the Infectious Diseases Society of America, Boston, Massachusetts, September 30–October 3, 2004.

41. Schwartzman K, Oxlade O, Barr RG, et al. Domestic returns from investment in control of tuberculosis in other countries. N Engl J Med 2005; 353:1008–1020.

42. Bloom BR, Salomon JA. Enlightened self-interest and the control of tuberculosis. N Engl J Med 2005; 353:1057–1059.

# CHAPTER 11

# US Medical Screening for Immigrants and Refugees
## *Public Health Issues*

Jennifer Cochran, Ann O'Fallon, and Paul L. Geltman

## Introduction

This chapter will present an overview of the refugee health screening process within the larger context of refugee resettlement. Included will be summaries of refugee health needs as justification for health screening, the legal and regulatory basis for refugee health screening, the historical perspective of health screening of migrants to the US, and the overseas screening process as it relates to the domestic counterpart. Details of overseas screening and the clinical content of domestic health screening are described in other chapters. The process of refugee health screening will be described through discussion of its relationship with other resettlement services provided to refugees, funding mechanisms and public health infrastructure, different models used by states for implementing health screening programs, and the role of public health agencies in data collection and disease surveillance, monitoring, and reporting. Lastly, the chapter will conclude with a discussion of the cultural, linguistic, and demographic challenges for the future of refugee health screening. While the focus of this chapter is refugee screening, the guidance offered is appropriate for many foreign-born persons, regardless of immigration status.

In this chapter, the term 'refugee' refers to individuals eligible for federal refugee benefits and services, including immigrants holding a refugee visa from the US government. To receive refugee status, an individual must meet international standards of having suffered persecution or have a fear of persecution on account of race, religion, nationality, membership in a particular social group, or political opinion. Often, the persecution is conducted or tolerated by the government. As defined by international laws, the refugee has fled his or her country of origin, and is unable or unwilling to return to that country because of this persecution or fear. The term, as used here, also includes other immigration classifications such as Cuban and Haitian entrants, certain Amerasians, asylees and victims of a severe form of trafficking.

## The Health Needs of Refugees Justify Prompt Health Screening in the United States

The health needs of refugees resettled in the United States have been well documented. Although this is particularly so for refugees from Southeast Asia and the former Soviet Union, more recent reviews have incorporated findings from African refugee populations.[1-8] These studies highlight the increased health morbidity of refugees, both adults and children. Refugees of many backgrounds now enter the country with a wide array of unmet health needs, including nutritional deficiencies, anemia, hepatitis B infection, tuberculosis infection, parasitosis, and other acute and chronic physical illnesses. While war and civil unrest have worsened the already poor health status of developing nations that are the sources of many refugees, developed countries such as those of the former Soviet Union and Yugoslavia have seen marked deterioration in national health status attributable to the turmoil in those regions.[9,10]

In addition to these physical health concerns is the vast burden of potentially long-term mental illness and emotional distress.[11-13] Mental health concerns (including alcohol and drug abuse[14]) increasingly are garnering greater attention among the refugee resettlement and health communities. This is due both to the recognition of the violence directed at civilian populations in recent civil conflicts such as those of Bosnia, Rwanda, Somalia, and Sudan and an understanding of the impact of such violence on human beings.[15-17] Alternatively, economic deterioration in the formerly socialist countries of Eastern Europe (such as the USSR) is believed to have contributed greatly to the declining quality of life and concurrent rise in alcohol and drug abuse there.[10] Lastly, increased use of government-sponsored torture and child soldiers has exacerbated mental health issues for adults and children. Amnesty International has estimated that over 150 countries around the world practice government-sponsored torture against their citizens.[18] Refugee populations have historically included high proportions of survivors of torture who have serious physical and mental health concerns related to their torture experiences.[19]

These health concerns may confer significant functional limitations on refugees of all ages. Functional limitations may then limit a refugee's ability to integrate successfully into US society through completion of many of the tasks necessary for resettlement, such as job placement and English language training for adults and school attendance and performance for children. Health screening of newly arrived refugees in the US will allow follow-up of health conditions identified overseas and new identification of other health conditions that may negatively affect their functional health status.

## The Legal and Regulatory Basis of Refugee Resettlement and Health Screening

The Refugee Act of 1980[20] amended the Immigration and Nationality Act to establish a domestic refugee resettlement program. This legislation marked the inauguration of the modern resettlement era as it currently exists. The Refugee Act delineated the philosophical approach and the role of government in facilitating refugee resettlement, stating the objectives 'to provide a permanent and systematic procedure for the admission to this country of refugees of special humanitarian concern to the United States, and provide comprehensive and uniform provisions for the effective resettlement and absorption of those

refugees who are admitted.'[21] The Act defined the term *refugee*, outlined the process for the annual admission of refugees, and established the Office of Refugee Resettlement (ORR) in the Department of Health and Human Services, through which resources for domestic resettlement would be made available.

The Refugee Act codified the US definition of a refugee, similar to that noted earlier. Allowance is made for the President to include in this definition individuals who are within their country of nationality; that is, individuals who have not crossed an international border prior to seeking consideration for refugee status from the US. Such in-country processing has been conducted in Vietnam, Cuba, and countries of the former Soviet Union.

In accordance with the Refugee Act, and as part of a consultative process on refugee admissions, the President annually provides Congress with information on refugee admissions priorities.[22] Proposed admission numbers are ceilings and not goals. In addition to refugees from overseas, other individuals are eligible for refugee benefits and services, including the domestic health assessment. Recipients of political asylum must meet the same 'well-founded fear of persecution' test as a refugee, but they make their claims from within the US rather than another country. Asylees may then petition for visas for family members who arrive from overseas and are also eligible. Cuban and Haitian entrants have special immigration statuses that confer eligibility for refugee program participation. Finally, the Trafficking Victims Protection Act of 2001 granted certified victims of a severe form of trafficking eligibility for refugee benefits and services.

Public health activities delineated in the Refugee Act include notification to state or local health officials of each refugee's arrival and monitoring of refugees to insure that they receive appropriate and timely treatment for health conditions of public health significance that are identified overseas.[23] Furthermore, the 'Director [of the Office of Refugee Resettlement] is authorized to make grants to, and enter into contracts with, State and local health agencies for payments to meet their costs of providing medical screening and initial medical treatment to refugees.'[24]

The implementing regulations of the Refugee Act further delineate the opportunity for states to provide domestic health assessment services with federal refugee funding support.[25] To qualify, state health assessments need to be in accordance with ORR requirements, be approved in writing by the ORR director, and, if done within the first 90 days after a refugee's entry into the US, can be provided to all individuals eligible for the federal refugee program.

## Historical Perspective of the Health Screening of Refugees and Immigrants

Medical and public health screening of refugees and immigrants has a long tradition, which began with centuries-old attempts to control the spread of leprosy. This tradition eventually expanded to include screening and quarantine programs. In recent times, the goal of health screening of refugees and immigrants has been to control the spread of infectious diseases and other health conditions and diseases of public health importance. To meet US admission requirements, refugees and immigrants complete an overseas screening, which is valid for a maximum of 1 year. Then, after arriving in the US, refugees generally complete a voluntary domestic screening as well.

Since refugees often have high health morbidity and come from situations of poor hygienic conditions, most US states have a refugee health assessment program which goes beyond the exclusionary focus of overseas screening and emphasis on screening out individuals with communicable diseases. The 1-year validity of the overseas evaluation allows the possibility of refugees acquiring new diseases or conditions before resettlement; thus, domestic health assessments are encouraged by US Office of Refugee Resettlement regulations to take place within 90 days after the refugee's arrival in the US.

The International Organization of Migration (IOM) conducts overseas screening of most refugee migrants to the US. IOM is an intergovernmental agency based in Switzerland that manages refugee movements for third-country resettlement. While destination countries such as the US, Canada, and Australia have different medical examination requirements and exclusionary criteria, IOM officials state the overarching goals of medical screening of migrants in four points: (1) to identify individuals with communicable diseases and thus to protect the public health in the receiving nation; (2) to prevent entry of individuals with health problems because they may constitute a financial burden or impose excessive demand on public health and medical services; (3) to ensure that as future residents the migrants will be healthy and productive (fit to work); and (4) to identify individuals in need of medical care in order to prepare the host country's healthcare system to meet their needs.[26,27]

Countries such as the US that receive large numbers of immigrants and refugees have seen dramatic declines over time in domestic rates of some infectious diseases such as tuberculosis[28] and vaccine-preventable diseases such as measles.[29] In the face of an increasingly mobile global population, some infectious diseases such as these in the US are becoming concentrated among recently migrated immigrant populations.[22,23] Consequently, US and IOM public health officials have recognized the need to rethink strategies for the overseas screening of immigrants and refugees.

## Recent Trends in Overseas Screening and Implications for Refugee Health Programs in the US

After a refugee's application for US resettlement has been approved by US immigration authorities, refugees undergo a health screening that is overseen by the CDC and implemented by the Migration Health Services of the IOM or local panel physicians under contract with US consular staff. The overseas screening is intended to identify conditions that will exclude the refugee from entering the US ('class A conditions') or warrant follow-up in the US ('class B conditions'). The screening is limited in its scope and focused mainly on detection of infectious disease of public health significance (tuberculosis, HIV, and syphilis) and mental health or other problems that may result in harmful behavior towards himself/herself or others. The content is fully described in the *Technical Instructions for Medical Examination of Aliens* (Atlanta, GA: Centers for Disease Control and Prevention; June 1991: http://www.cdc.gov/ncidod/dq/technica.htm) and summarized in the preceding chapter.

Following the historic infection control tradition of refugee health assessment, class A conditions are generally infectious diseases. Other class A conditions include mental illness that is associated with violent or harmful behavior and substance abuse. While class A conditions are grounds for exclusion from the US, refugees may complete treatment to render the condition noninfectious or apply for a waiver to permit entry. The most notable of class A conditions are active infectious tuberculosis and HIV infection. Because of the humanitarian nature of their resettlement, unlike other immigrants, refugees with HIV infection may use a simplified waiver process to enter the US that releases them from the requirement of not being a public charge risk. Class

B conditions are physical defects, diseases, or disabilities significant enough to cause functional impairment or require follow-up.

In the past decade, overseas screening of refugees has been the focus of applying modern epidemiologic and screening techniques.[20] Recent attention has been placed on identifying health needs of specific refugee populations that are to resettle in third countries such as the US in order to improve health among that community and reduce transmission of disease among the future resettlement community.[20,30,31] Thus, interest in the control and prevention of certain diseases among refugees has been rejuvenated by efforts to control infectious diseases at different levels: the whole population through mass empiric treatment and the individual migrant through targeted screening for and treatment of specific conditions.[20,22]

Once in the US, the question of how to address the health needs of refugees broadens beyond infectious disease screening. Domestic refugee health programs must consider the impact of changing overseas screening and empiric treatment on their clinical protocols and health needs of refugees while seeing them for screening. Similarly, as more empiric treatment is implemented overseas, chronic disease and mental health become more prominent as public health issues in the US at the state and local level. As such, one refugee health assessment program has implemented an innovative mental health screening program.[32] Providing access to mental health services in appropriate languages and with cultural sensitivity is also an added burden on local health resources in resettlement communities. Refugees experience inequities in access to and quality of primary care in many Western countries that resettle refugees, as described in a paper from Great Britain.[33] Inequities arise from the cumulative effects of local clinicians inexperienced with refugee health needs, deleterious mental health problems, extra time and expense required to overcome language and cultural barriers in primary care, and the need for comprehensive national strategies. These issues are all strikingly familiar to those faced by refugees and clinicians in the US.

## Health Screening within the Process of Refugee Resettlement in the US

Unlike immigrants, most of whom are required to be self-reliant or supported by family on arrival in the US, newly arrived refugees are provided services by a network of agencies receiving federal funds. The Department of State has cooperative agreements with nine private, nonprofit national voluntary agencies (VOLAGs) and the State of Iowa to provide initial reception and placement (R&P) services through their networks of local affiliate offices (Table 11.1).

The R&P period is generally considered to be the first 30 days after arrival in the US. R&P services address immediate and essential needs of housing, clothing, and food as well as referral for health assessment and support to complete Social Security card applications, benefits applications (Medicaid, Transitional Assistance, and Food Stamps), and school enrollment for children. Orientation to life in the US and referral to services that will facilitate employment are also vital activities.

**Table 11.1 Agencies that have cooperative agreements with the US Department of State to resettle refugees**

| National VOLAG | Website |
|---|---|
| Church World Service | www.churchworldservice.org/Immigration/ |
| Episcopal Migration Ministries | www.episcopalchurch.org/emm.htm |
| Ethiopian Community Development Council | www.ecdcinternational.org/ |
| Hebrew Immigrant Aid Society | www.hias.org/ |
| US Committee for Refugees and Immigrants | www.refugees.org/ |
| International Rescue Committee | www.theirc.org/ |
| Lutheran Immigrant and Refugee Services | www.lirs.org/ |
| United States Conference of Catholic Bishops | www.usccb.org/mrs/ |
| World Relief Corporation | www.wr.org/ |
| State of Iowa, Bureau of Refugee Services | www.dhs.state.ia.us/refugee/resettlement/ |

Resettlement benefits and services funded by ORR are designed to extend beyond R&P, with the objective of facilitating refugee self-sufficiency. Benefits include time-limited cash and medical assistance (currently 8 months from date of entry). Services focus on employment preparation and job placement, skills training, English language training, and social adjustment. While the primary focus is on recently arrived refugees, social service funds can be used for refugees who are within 5 years of US entry.

The network of refugee service providers delivering ORR-funded services is far broader than the VOLAGs funded through R&P agreements. Mutual Assistance Associations (MAAs), as described by ORR, are 'agencies organized and directed by refugees to address community building, facilitate cultural adjustment and integration of refugees, and deliver mutually supportive functions such as information exchange, civic participation, resource enhancement, orientation and support to newly arriving refugees and public education to the larger community on the background, needs and potential of refugees.'[34] Because MAAs, by definition, depend upon refugee community involvement for their organization and vitality, they are more typically found in areas where there are significant resettled ethnic populations. As a result, all communities do not have MAAs. Other private and public agencies that form part of the refugee service network include English language training providers, employment service agencies, community health agencies, and numerous public agencies such as departments of education, health, employment, and welfare.

The domestic health assessment occurs within the first 90 days after arrival in the US, at a time when refugees are concurrently engaged in other immediate tasks and activities noted above. Further, refugees are learning about activities of daily living and managing finances, having children attend school, and establishing new routines in a new home and country. In this context, health and healthcare are often a lower priority for refugees, particularly if there are no acute health problems. Yet, neglected health problems, for example chronic diseases such as hypertension in adults or developmental delay and undernutrition in children, have the potential to impair successful resettlement, especially if defined by the current focus on job placement and retention (and similarly school achievement for children).

Accomplishing the domestic health screening within the first 3 months of arrival is ideal for the purposes of identifying and treating infectious dis-

eases. However, challenges that range from health education and orientation to utilizing the American healthcare system to the management of chronic or long-neglected health conditions cannot be well served during a time when the refugee is preoccupied with the urgent demands of adjusting to life in the US.

## Funding and Public Health Infrastructure for Refugee Health Screening in the US

The domestic health assessment differs significantly in scope and purpose from the overseas assessment. The domestic assessment is designed to eliminate health-related barriers to successful resettlement while also protecting the health of the US population. The refugee health assessment is usually considered to be very important for successful resettlement; however, the domestic assessment is a voluntary program for refugees.

State refugee health programs, most often run by departments of health or public health, are responsible for the design and implementation of the assessment. ORR provides guidance in its 'Medical Screening Protocol for Newly Arriving Refugees' (ORR State Letter #95–37, Nov. 11, 1995). As defined in this document, the purpose of domestic screening is to:

1. Ensure follow-up of class A and B conditions identified overseas;
2. Identify persons with communicable diseases of public health importance; and
3. Identify personal health conditions that adversely impact on effective resettlement (e.g. job placement or attending school).

Health screening for refugees is elective for both states and refugees. As a result, the range of what constitutes a health screening varies among states. Some states screen refugees only for TB; other states add screening for conditions of particular concern to their own public health authorities. At the other end of the spectrum of state health screenings for refugees are states that see this initial contact with refugees as an opportunity to orient them to the local healthcare system, educate them on age, sex, or risk-specific issues (such as contraceptive use, cancer self-exams, and substance abuse), and connect these new client–patients with sensitive and capable providers for follow-up. In between these two extremes of what makes up a 'refugee health screening' are various combinations of testing for diseases (e.g.

serologic testing for hepatitis B virus), screening for abnormalities (e.g. vision, hearing, oral health, or mental health), referrals for ancillary services (e.g. for WIC enrollment), education/orientation (e.g. HIV/AIDS risk factors, exercise, or prevention measures), and medical referrals (both for primary care follow-up and sub-specialty care as indicated). Further discussion of the clinical aspects of domestic refugee health screening is addressed in the following chapter.

One of the factors that influence what each state includes in its refugee health screening is the organization and payment of services. Funding for health screening may come from a number of sources: federal Refugee Medical Assistance (RMA) administered by ORR, state-administered Medicaid funds, discretionary preventive health grants funded by ORR and, at times, state and local governments.

ORR regulations allow states to use RMA funds to reimburse directly for refugee health assessment services without determining eligibility for Medicaid provided that the state has an approved health assessment protocol and service plan approved by ORR. Those states that do not have an approved, RMA-funded health assessment program rely on a combination of funding from Medicaid (for those refugees categorically eligible for Medicaid) and RMA (for those refugees not eligible for Medicaid) to reimburse for services through the state's Medicaid program. In cases such as this, the scope of services is dependent on the state's Medicaid plan and entry to care is dependent on receipt of Medicaid coverage. Regardless of the funding stream, all refugees entering the US are eligible for some package of screening services provided by the states.

The actual clinical settings for health screenings vary from state to state as well. Many states use networks of county and local public health clinics to screen and treat refugees. Other states use the competitive bidding process to identify private (generally not-for-profit) clinics to provide these services in areas where refugees are most concentrated. Still other states rely on physicians and clinical practices that accept Medicaid to perform screenings as they see fit, without guidance or standard requirements by the state.

To enter the US, refugees must pass through one of a limited number of ports of entry that have staffed quarantine stations. Members of the US Public Health Service operate these stations. The quarantine officers review refugees' medical documents and perform a limited inspection to look for obvious signs of illness. The officers notify state or county public health authorities in the refugee's point of destination of the arrival as well as the overseas medical documentation. These state and county authorities, in turn, coordinate the domestic refugee health assessments for refugees arriving in their jurisdictions.

The domestic health assessment, while restricted in scope, serves as a refugee's first encounter with the US healthcare system. Given these limitations, the general approach taken by refugee health assessment programs is one that incorporates consideration of epidemiology, screening, and follow-up resources, refugee experiences, and the role of health assessment as an entrée to primary care.

Most refugee health assessment programs at a minimum include follow-up of class A and B conditions identified during the overseas medical examination and evaluation for tuberculosis. In many larger areas, the assessment also includes medical history and physical examination; evaluation for TB, hepatitis B, anemia, pregnancy, parasitic infections; lead poisoning; immunizations; and screening of vision, hearing, and dentition.[35] As stated earlier in this chapter, additional services and programs may complement the health screening. The extent of how these components are implemented, like the screening content, will vary considerably among states.

## Public Health Models for Refugee Health Assessment Programs

The variation among health assessment program models found in the US partly reflects the organization of public health and healthcare services at the state and local level. Many refugees resettle in larger metropolitan areas, but significant numbers also resettle in rural communities or small cities that host industries or businesses that are attractive as employers to refugee populations. Therefore, while it is recommended to use a consistent statewide screening protocol, different models of screening may work better in different jurisdictions within a state. Three models are highlighted in this chapter: (1) an ORR-approved public–private model funded solely through RMA; (2) the public health clinic model; and (3) a private provider model funded through Medicaid and/or RMA.

Certain elements of the screening process are consistent throughout different models and states. Collaboration with VOLAGs and their case managers is critical. Once the resettlement agency knows the date of arrival for a given refugee or refugee family, the case manager usually contacts the clinic where the health assessment will take place to provide contact information and initiate the scheduling process.

## The RMA funded, public–private model

Massachusetts is among a handful of states, primarily in New England, that do not have county health departments. Rather, each of the 351 cities and towns has a municipal health department that is responsible for public health activities required by Massachusetts general laws and state and local regulations. Most do not provide direct clinical services. As a result, when organized refugee resettlement began in Massachusetts, health departments were not an option for screening refugees.

By 1994, efforts by the Massachusetts Department of Public Health to facilitate health screening for newly arrived refugees through the Medicaid system had failed to raise the very low assessment rates. As such, the screening process was ineffectual for infection control and prevention efforts. Private medical providers or clinics usually did the health assessments prior to that time and were under no obligation to follow state refugee health screening guidelines that were issued in 1987. The reliance on Medicaid to reimburse providers directly for screening services also contributed to low rates of initiation and limited laboratory and other testing. This occurred because the time lag between arrival in the US and the receipt of Medicaid benefits effectively left refugees uninsured for the first months after arrival. Consequently, Massachusetts requested and received ORR approval for a RMA-funded refugee health assessment plan. The Massachusetts Department of Public Health implemented the plan in 1995 as the Refugee Health Assessment Program.

Essential elements of the Refugee Health Assessment Program are: (1) a defined protocol with core elements and targeted testing options to provide consistent and uniform care while affording flexibility for clinicians to address individual health needs of refugee patients; (2) creation of a network of qualified private sector providers (usually community health centers that serve the geographic areas that are home to refugee populations) under contract with the Department of Public Health – essentially a 'preferred provider network;' and (3) linkages with other public health programs at the local and state level. The philosophical approach recognizes the importance of a service delivery model that provides linguistically and culturally appropriate services in a manner that responds to the unique experiences of refugees.

By contracting with a limited number of clinics, the clinicians and staff at the sites become more knowledgeable about and responsive to the health needs of refugees, many of whom continue at the site as primary care patients. Shaped by the preexisting infrastructure of the public health system in Massachusetts, the consolidation of the health screening at these clinics significantly improved access, quality, and timeliness of health assessments in Massachusetts.[36] Prior to the creation of the Refugee Health Assessment Program, only 35% of eligible refugee arrivals completed health screening. Within 3 years of its implementation, over 90% completed screening, including 95% of those with class A or B conditions.

## The public health clinic model

In many states, public health clinics exist at the county level and incorporate refugee health assessments into their operations. This is the case in the three largest counties in Minnesota, where public health clinics are staffed to complete the refugee screenings. Bilingual, bicultural staff members often act as interpreters and cultural brokers for refugees. Staffing at public clinics is fairly stable and provides an environment for continuous sharing of knowledge among all cultures represented. The screening, which includes a comprehensive examination, is completed over the course of three separate visits. The clinics maintain pharmacy stocks of commonly prescribed medications. Since these public health clinics do not offer primary care, all conditions needing follow-up must be referred; each has a close working relationship with the respective county tuberculosis clinic.

In the late 1970s, Minnesota began receiving large numbers of Southeast Asian arrivals and health screening efforts were initiated, but not funded. It was difficult for the Minnesota Department of Health (MDH) to do more than send out notice of arrival and a blank screening form to appropriate Local Public Health (LPH) agencies. With the passage of the Refugee Act in 1980, federal funding became available and MDH generated subcontracts with LPH agencies in the counties most heavily impacted by arrivals. A standardized screening form was generated for each refugee and, upon notification, the forms were sent to counties to initiate screening. The LPH agencies were charged with accomplishing the screening, as described above, or making arrangements to have the screening completed elsewhere, and returning the completed screening forms to MDH. The state had no authority in this matter and the quality and completeness of screenings varied.

A combination of Medicaid and RMA pays for the screenings in Minnesota. Public and private clinics alike bill the state Medicaid office directly for the services they have provided. For those refugees who do not qualify for Medicaid, the MDH Refugee Health Program (RHP) uses RMA funds to reimburse providers at a flat fee.

In 1993, MDH hired the first Refugee Health Coordinator who began to develop a more comprehensive refugee health program. With this move MDH provided leadership and more clearly defined expectations for screening newly arrived refugees. Strong efforts were put in place to increase collaboration among all agencies working with refugees and the Metro Refugee Health Task Force was born. This Task Force includes concerned community and health professionals who continue to meet monthly to discuss topics of general interest.

This model of accomplishing refugee screening continues in Minnesota today, though both the state and local programs have grown much stronger over time. Local public health agencies now expect to organize screenings for refugees, are invested in their screening rates, and know how to contact the RHP when they have a concern.

Even though visibility and expectations were much clearer, in 1999 the overall screening rate in Minnesota was still only 74%. The MDH RHP initiated a series of efforts to improve the screening rates and experienced a rise to 85% in 2000 and 97% in 2004. These efforts included meeting with community colleagues one-on-one, asking how MDH could collaborate to improve screening quality and outcomes. For LPH agencies, MDH offered an in-service for their staff, highlighting their arrival numbers and screening rates followed by a discussion about what could be done to make things better. In areas where adversarial working relationships had developed, MDH met with VOLAGs and LPH agencies and helped them achieve a better appreciation for their differing, but complementary, missions. For private clinics, MDH offered a lunch or evening presentation on refugee health (sometimes paired with a tuberculosis update) emphasizing the importance of screening for communicable diseases within their communities as well as local demographics and screening results. These efforts were combined with others described in the following section of this chapter.

## The private provider model

Another health assessment model is similar to the system that was in place in Massachusetts before implementation of the RMA-funded system of publicly contracted private providers. It is frequently used in rural areas of Minnesota without county health clinics. In this system, county agencies typically have an identified refugee health contact, usually a public health nurse. This public health nurse works with private clinics in the community to achieve the refugee screening. The volume of refugee arrivals to counties can vary greatly, as do the resources available. Public health nurses and providers may be unfamiliar with working with non-English-speaking persons and need guidance through the process of completing the refugee health assessment. Finding an interpreter and transportation in rural areas is often a challenge. The centralized RHP at the state level makes an extra effort to support rural public health personnel as they accomplish the health assessment.

Expectations for the public health nurse are critical to success. These start with contacting the refugee and the community clinic to arrange for the health screening examination. The nurse must determine the new arrival's health insurance coverage and provide assistance with facilitation of transportation and interpretation if needed. The nurse may offer immunization and tuberculosis screening if the county agency has this capacity. The nurse must also ensure the refugee has copies of all pertinent medical forms to take to the clinic, i.e. any record of immunizations or class A or B tuberculosis information. If the state has refugee health screening protocols or guidelines, the nurse will also assess the clinic's experience with these protocols and educate clinic staff regarding their content, as needed. The nurse will also ask the healthcare provider to return a completed reporting form to the public health agency, review the returned form for completion, and determine if any follow-up is needed on the part of the local public health agency (e.g. TB treatment, follow-up on pending lab results, immunizations, etc.). Finally, the nurse will send completed assessment forms to the centralized state office.

## Data Collection and Reporting, Monitoring and Disease Surveillance, and Quality Assurance and Program Oversight

Public health departments are responsible for administrative oversight and quality assurance of statewide screening programs. In addition, they may have regulatory obligations related to monitoring and epidemiological surveillance of health conditions of public health significance. As such, public health departments usually request that health assessment providers report individual refugee health assessment findings. State-specific health assessment forms provide the framework for this reporting. In many areas, payment for services is contingent upon reporting, essentially guaranteeing high rates of return.

Quality assurance in refugee health assessment includes monitoring to determine timeliness of services, adherence to protocols, and appropriate linkage with follow-up services in the public or private sector. For those conditions that are followed in the public health sector – particularly infectious disease conditions such as tuberculosis, hepatitis B, and STDs – standard reporting mechanisms complement the health assessment form. As required by public health regulations, reporting of positive laboratory findings generates case investigations. In areas where the public health system utilizes bilingual, bicultural community outreach educators to extend public health services to refugees, health assessment providers often report findings to the health department to facilitate linkage with follow-up services, such as for evaluation of positive tuberculin skin tests.

Data from health assessments also may form the basis for an improved understanding of population-specific refugee health status that is more comprehensive than can be learned from the overseas medical examination. Such knowledge enables the improvement of services that are provided to refugees. By evaluating health screening data from state or county programs with large enough populations, findings are more generalizable than those reported from smaller clinic-based evaluations, and analyses of subsets (such as gender or nationality) are possible. As newer refugee populations become smaller and more diverse, however, states may even need to pool their data to allow for meaningful, generalizable conclusions. Efforts of this nature have been initiated.

At the level of the state health assessment program, analysis of screening data by national origin or ethnicity can yield findings that provide benefit to that community at large. Such data offer public and private healthcare professionals an estimate of the prevalence of certain common conditions in newly arrived refugees. The information can be used to prioritize and strategize health education and interventions for specific communities. Individual clinicians benefit by having a heightened index of suspicion for common diseases, or prompting the inclusion of appropriate conditions in a differential diagnosis.

Health assessment data can also be reviewed in light of the quality and scope of the overseas medical examination. Positive consequences of CDC's pre-departure empiric albendazole treatment program for African refugees were observed in health assessment data from Massachusetts: on a population basis, rates of parasitic infections were significantly lower after this program was implemented.[6] Although rare, conditions of public health significance that should have been identified prior to US entry are diagnosed during the health assessment. By providing feedback to the CDC, an evaluation of physician practice and laboratory quality at an overseas site can be initiated, if warranted. In 2005, cases of active TB, including some with multidrug-resistant organisms, in Hmong refugees arriving from Thailand were diagnosed soon after arrival in the US. Reports from state health departments generated an investigation by CDC that resulted in a revised algorithm for screening and treatment of refugees in Thailand.[37]

As noted above, through centralized coordination at the state level, domestic health screening can produce data that inform health screening of both refugees and immigrants. For example, the documentation of elevated blood lead levels among refugees in Massachusetts[5] and a subsequent CDC investigation of lead poisoning in New Hampshire[38] led to the issuance by the ORR[39] and CDC[40] of guidelines on screening for and follow-up of lead poisoning among refugee children. Minnesota has piloted the guidelines at one clinic while Massachusetts has fostered collaboration with its state childhood lead poisoning prevention program to direct prevention activities and follow-up for refugee children. Following reports from state and local refugee health programs of positive syphilis tests among refugee children from areas with endemic yaws,[41] the CDC issued guidelines on screening for yaws that have been piloted by the Minnesota program. Similarly, coordinated domestic screening facilitates rapid response to data that suggest revision or expansion of screening protocols to meet newly identified health needs. When the CDC identified high rates of strongyloidiasis among Sudanese at a mass screening it conducted, states such as Massachusetts and Minnesota were quickly able to implement screening guidelines for their RHA clinics. After chart reviews of West African refugee children in Minnesota revealed high rates of subclinical malaria, Massachusetts implemented a new protocol for screening African refugees for malaria. Like the issue of lead poisoning, such a malaria screening policy is also relevant to the healthcare of the broader population of African immigrants such as Nigerians who may also be at high risk for *Plasmodia* spp. parasitemia.

Also important in quality assurance is determining which refugees fail to complete a health assessment and possible reasons why. Many programs survey health assessment providers, requesting explanation for why an examination was not completed. Common reasons include being unable to locate the refugee or the refugee having moved to another jurisdiction. Programs prioritize tracking refugees within their first 90 days so that, even if there is a jurisdictional change, the health assessment can be completed. Programs can use utilization data to recruit new providers if, for example, refugees resettle distant from existing sites and poor access to care is due to clinic location. Generally speaking, screening rates have increased with the maturity of the program.

## Challenges Facing Public Health Screening Programs for Refugees

In recent years, there has been a dramatic shift away from resettlement of large refugee populations over an extended period of years (e.g. Vietnamese, former Soviet Union refugees) to smaller populations representing increased national, ethnic, and cultural diversity and a range of refugee experiences. Priority populations have been identified, processed overseas for US resettlement, and resettled as a group, all over a relatively short span of 1–2 years. Recent examples include the approximately 15 000 Hmong resettled from Thailand in fiscal year 2005 (FY05), 8000 at-risk Liberians resettled from Côte d'Ivoire in FY05, and 10 000 Somali Bantu resettled from Kenya in FY04–05. In contrast, resettlement of thousands of religious minorities from the former Soviet Union has been ongoing for two decades.

This increasing diversity, particularly among African refugees who now comprise approximately half of refugee arrivals, creates significant logistical difficulties in providing healthcare. Among refugees are a multitude of cultures, languages, experiences, and histories. Literacy levels reflect educational opportunities; low literacy rates are common. Providers offering refugee screening must be continuously cognizant of how recently these refugees have arrived in the US, what life experiences brought

them here, and how culturally based beliefs affect health behaviors.

Health systems, clinics, and providers must begin with knowing what communities they are likely to serve in refugee screening. Providers will benefit from awareness that disease prevalence rates vary among refugee populations. Similarly, differences may be manifest in the history and culture of new refugee groups, their knowledge of and names for different health conditions and their treatments, and past experiences with healthcare systems in their homelands and refugee camps. Clinics may be well versed in and capable of addressing the health needs of existing refugee or immigrant communities, but their competency may be strained by new arrivals with different cultural and linguistic needs as well as educational and literacy levels.

A significant challenge to public health is the limited pool of migrants who are eligible for domestic health assessment. In contrast to refugees who have access to government-funded health assessment services immediately upon entry in the US, the vast majority of migrants to the US, including many coming from similar situations and areas where infectious diseases are prevalent, do not receive any kind of organized health screening after arrival in the US. In the absence of a formal public health program, medical screening of migrants remains irregular, limited in scope, and dependent on health insurance coverage. Physicians and other medical professionals who care for these populations may, however, apply lessons learned from refugee health screening. The screening results of various ethnic groups can efficiently guide providers seeing non-refugee foreign-born patients toward appropriate screening tests. Many refugee health programs have developed educational materials useful for a broad range of patients. For example, the Refugee Health Assessment Pocket Guide (Fig. 11.1) would be useful in structuring a first clinic visit for all newly arrived foreign-born individuals. Many other health education resources and screening results can be found online at state health department sites such as those for Minnesota and Massachusetts:

- www.health.state.mn.us/refugee
- www.mass.gov/dph/cdc/rhip/wwwrihp.htm

## Conclusion

Improved collaboration between all levels of public health and the US private medical community is

# REFUGEE HEALTH ASSESSMENT POCKET GUIDE

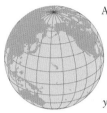

All refugees should have a comprehensive health screening within 90 days of arrival in the U.S. After the exam, complete the MDH Initial Refugee Health Assessment Form and *return it to your county health department.*

## THIS SCREENING SHOULD INCLUDE:

### HEALTH HISTORY, PHYSICAL EXAM INCLUDING VISION/HEARING/DENTAL ASSESSMENT

### IMMUNIZATION REVIEW AND UPDATE

- Record previous vaccines, lab evidence of immunity or history of disease; doses are valid if given according to Minnesota child or adult schedules.
- Do not restart a vaccine series.
- Update immunizations as indicated.
- If no documentation, assume patient is unvaccinated. Give age-appropriate vaccinations per the MN child or adult schedule.

### TUBERCULOSIS SCREENING

- Apply Mantoux tuberculin skin test for patients >6 months of age, regardless of BCG history.
- Read Mantoux within 48-72 hours (measure mm of induration, not erythema).
- Chest x-ray MUST be done if:
  - Mantoux is positive (>10mm induration) OR
  - Refugee has a Class A or B TB condition (per overseas exam) OR
  - Patient is symptomatic, regardless of Mantoux results.
- Record whether treatment was prescribed and date started.

### TUBERCULOSIS (TB) IN MINNESOTA

- 30-50% of MN refugees have latent TB infection.
- More than 80% of TB cases in MN are foreign-born.
- Foreign-born persons are more than twice as likely to have drug-resistant TB.
- MDH provides free TB medications.

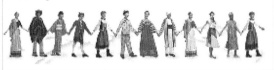

### HEPATITIS B SCREENING

- Screen all new arrivals for HBsAg and anti-HBs.
- Vaccinate all susceptibles (i.e., negative for both HBsAg and anti-HBs).
- Patients testing positive for anti-HBs are immune, no hep B vaccine needed.
- Refer all carriers (HBsAg positive) for additional medical evaluation. All susceptible household and sexual contacts of carriers should be screened and vaccinated.

### SEXUALLY TRANSMITTED INFECTIONS (STI)

- Screen for syphilis with VDRL or RPR; confirm all positives.
- At provider's discretion, screen sexually active patients for other STIs.
- Use urine testing for GC/chlamydia, if possible.

### PARASITE SCREENING

- Collect 3 stool specimens more than 24 hours apart. Eosinophilia requires further evaluation for pathogenic parasites, even with 3 negative stools.

### MALARIA SCREENING

- Screen if symptomatic or if from an endemic area and suspicious history. Obtain 3 thick and thin smears to screen.

### LEAD SCREENING

- Screen if child is ≤5 years
- Refer to Public Health and medical follow-up if BLL ≥10mg/DL

### RECOMMENDED LAB TESTS FOR FIRST VISIT

- Varicella titer if no report of disease history or vaccination
- Hepatitis B screening (anti-HBs, HBsAg, and per provider discretion, anti-HBc)
- VDRL or RPR, urine GC/chlamydia if indicated
- Hemoglobin/hematocrit
- Pregnancy test, if indicated
- UA/UC, if indicated
- Blood lead level if ≤5 years
- Stools for ova and parasites; send home containers and instruct patient on collection
- CBC with differential
- Malaria screening if history or symptoms are suspicious of malaria
- Other labs, as appropriate, for follow up

### REFUGEE HEALTH RESOURCES

- **MDH Refugee Health Program, Tuberculosis Prevention and Control Program**
  **612-676-5414**
  **www.health.state.mn.us/refugee**
  **www.health.state.mn.us/tb**
- **Minnesota Immunization Hotline**
  **1-800-657-3970**
  **www.health.state.mn.us/immunize**

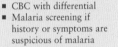

IC# 141-0569

2004

**Fig. 11.1** Refugee health assessment pocket guide.

increasingly sought as attention to global health issues has increased. This collaboration is especially relevant in refugee health assessment where overseas protocols can affect domestic screening in a most immediate manner and state screening programs can identify and address conditions of public health concern. Each state will benefit from establishing a model of refugee health screening that plays to the strengths of their public and private

health infrastructure. Centralized planning and two-way communications from the state are critical to the success of a comprehensive program with high screening rates.

It is critical for providers to remember that the domestic health assessment is the refugee's first interaction with US medicine and as such is a great learning opportunity for both the refugee and provider. This assessment will make a strong impression upon the refugee about what it is like to seek and receive healthcare in the US. While the opportunities for cultural and linguistic miscommunications are high, incorporating trained medical interpreters and bilingual, bicultural staff in delivery models together with clinicians well versed in refugee health, will promote mutual understanding. Refugee health assessment can start the process of refugees building healthy lives in the US.

# References

1. Ackerman LK. Health problems of refugees. J Am Board Fam Pract 1997; 10:337–348.
2. Hayes EB, Talbot SB, Matheson ES, et al. Health status of pediatric refugees in Portland, ME. Arch Pediatr Adolesc Med 1998; 152:564–568.
3. Lifson AR, Thai D, O'Fallon A, et al. Prevalence of tuberculosis, hepatitis B virus, and intestinal parasitic infections among refugees to Minnesota. Public Health Reports 2002; 117:69–77.
4. Geltman PL, Radin M, Zhang Z, et al. Growth status and related medical conditions among refugee children in Massachusetts, 1995–1998. Am J Public Health 2001; 91:1800–1805.
5. Geltman PL, Brown MJ, Cochran J. Lead poisoning among refugee children resettled in Massachusetts, 1995–1999. Pediatrics 2001; 108:158–162.
6. Geltman PL, Cochran J, Hedgecock C. Intestinal parasites among African refugees resettled in Massachusetts and the impact of an overseas pre-departure treatment program. Am J Tropical Med Hygiene 2003; 69:657–662.
7. Cote S, Geltman PL, Nunn M, et al. Dental caries of refugee children compared to US children. Pediatrics 2004; 114: e733–e740.
8. Garg PK, Perry S, Dorn M, et al. Risk of intestinal helminth and protozoan infection in a refugee population. Am J Trop Med Hyg 2005; 73(2):386–391.
9. Centers for Disease Control and Prevention. Status of public health – Bosnia and Herzegovina, August – September 1993. MMWR 1993; 42:973, 979–982.
10. Notzon FC, Komarov YM, Ermakov SP, et al. Causes of declining life expectancy in Russia. JAMA 1998; 279:793–800.
11. Marshall GN, Schell TL, Elliott MC, et al. Mental health of Cambodian refugees 2 decades after resettlement in the United States. JAMA 2005; 294:571–579.
12. Lopes Cardozo B, Vergara A, Agani F, et al. Mental health, social functioning, and attitudes of Kosovar Albanians following the war in Kosovo. JAMA 2000; 284:569–577.
13. Sabin M, Cardozo BL, Nackerud L, et al. Factors associated with poor mental health among Guatemalan refugees living in Mexico 20 years after civil conflict. JAMA 2003; 290:635–642.
14. Nelson KR, Bui H, Samet JH. Screening in special populations: a 'case study' of recent Vietnamese immigrants. Am J Med 1997; 102:435–440.
15. Basoglu M, Livanou M, Crnobaric C, et al. Psychiatric and cognitive effects of war in former Yugoslavia. JAMA 2005; 294:580–590.
16. Toole MJ, Waldman RJ. The public health aspects of complex emergencies and refugee situations. Annu Rev Public Health 1997; 18:283–312.
17. Gellert GA. Humanitarian responses to mass violence perpetrated against vulnerable populations. Br Med J 1995; 311:995–1001.
18. Amnesty International. Amnesty International Annual Report. London: Amnesty International Secretariat, 1997.
19. Jaranson JM, Butcher J, Halcon L, et al. Somali and Oromo refugees: correlates of torture and trauma history. Am J Pub Health 2004; 94:591–598.
20. Public Law 96–212.
21. Refugee Act of 1980. PL 96–212. Section 101(b).
22. See www.state.gov/g/prm
23. Refugee Act of 1980. PL 96–212. Section 412 (b)(4)(C-D).
24. Refugee Act of 1980. PL 96–212. Section 412 (b)(5).
25. 45 CFR Chapter IV Part 400.017.
26. Gushulak B, ed. Immigration medical screening: a move towards public health risk management. Migration and Health Newsletter 1998; 2:1–3.
27. Weekers J, Siem H. Overseas screening of migrants: justifiable? Public Health Reports 1997; 112:397–402.
28. Centers for Disease Control and Prevention. Trends in Tuberculosis – United States, 2005. MMWR 2006; 55: 305–308.
29. Centers for Disease Control and Prevention. Measles – United States, 2005. MMWR 2006; 55:1348–1351.
30. Miller JM, Boyd HA, Ostrowski SR, et al. Malaria, intestinal parasites, and schistosomiasis among Barawan Somali refugees resettling to the United States: a strategy to reduce morbidity and decrease the risk of imported infections. Am J Trop Med Hyg 2000; 62:115–121.
31. Centers for Disease Control and Prevention. Enhanced medical assessment strategy for Barawan Somali refugees – Kenya, 1997. MMWR 1998; 46:1520–1524.
32. Savin D, Seymour DJ, Littleford LN, et al. Findings from mental health screening of newly arrived refugees in Colorado. Public Health Reports 2005; 120:224–229.
33. Jones D, Gill PS. Refugees and primary care: tackling the inequalities. Br Med J 1998; 317:1444–1446.
34. Office of Refugee Resettlement. Federal Register. 2004; 69:22291.
35. Vergara AE, Miller JM, Martin DR, et al. A survey of refugee health assessments in the United States. J Immig Health 2003; 5:67–73.
36. Geltman PL, Cochran J. A private-sector preferred provider network model for public health screening of newly resettled refugees. Am J Public Health 2005; 95:196–199.
37. Centers for Disease Control and Prevention. Multidrug-resistant tuberculosis in Hmong refugees resettling from Thailand into the United States, 2004–2005. MMWR 2005; 54:741–744.
38. Centers for Disease Control and Prevention. Elevated blood lead levels in refugee children – New Hampshire, 2003–2004. MMWR 2005; 54:42–46.
39. Office of Refugee Resettlement. State Letter 05–01. 2005. Available: www.acf.hhs.gov/programs/orr/policy/sl05–01. htm Accessed 2/17/07.
40. Centers for Disease Control and Prevention. CDC recommendations for lead poisoning prevention in newly arrived refugee children. 2005. Available: www.cdc.gov/nceh/lead/Refugee%20Recommendations.pdf Accessed 2/17/07.
41. Centers for Disease Control and Prevention. Notice to readers: recommendation regarding screening of refugee children for treponemal infection. MMWR 2005; 54:933–934.

# CHAPTER 12

# US Medical Screening for Immigrants and Refugees:
## *Clinical Issues*

Lorna Seybolt, Elizabeth D. Barnett, and William Stauffer

## Background

Millions of people become refugees, seek political asylum, are adopted, or immigrate for another reason each year. Many of these people originate from the developing world and thus infectious diseases are a common focus of medical assessment. In addition, this population is at high risk for other medical conditions such as lead poisoning, dental caries, certain cancers, and mental health problems. Therefore, domestic health assessment must address issues of both infectious and noninfectious illnesses.

People immigrate for multiple and varied reasons. They may be resettled as refugees due to political or environmental issues or they may seek asylum from persecution. They may move to attend school or to seek work. In addition, it is becoming increasingly common to adopt children from other countries. These diverse reasons for immigration bring a wide variety of people to the United States, all of whom have their own unique exposures to communicable diseases and environmental hazards. Thus, immigrants have different risks than the native population and those risks vary by the category of immigrant and the individual experiences prior to immigration. Understanding these differences helps to ensure adequate and appropriate healthcare during the assessment process and subsequent follow-up.

Depending on their immigration status, immigrants may undergo medical assessment prior to departure from their country of origin or first asylum. The main purpose of this process is to prevent the importation of communicable diseases

of public health significance. This overseas assessment process is detailed in a separate chapter in this text. It may be difficult in the clinical setting to know whether this assessment has taken place, especially with patients who are reluctant to discuss their immigration status. In general, those seeking permanent resident status from outside the US, refugees, and internationally adopted children are most likely to have undergone screening before arrival. In the US, the Federal Refugee Act requires domestic medical screening of refugees to be provided at the state level. Several excellent articles have been published recently which review the screening process for immigrants of all ages and discuss both infectious and noninfectious issues.[1-4] This chapter will review the purposes and components of domestic health assessment. Detailed information on screening rationale and strategies for testing for specific diseases found in immigrant populations will be provided. Some information on initial management of positive tests will be presented here; detailed management of these diseases can be found in chapters addressing each condition.

## Purpose of Domestic Health Assessment

The goals of domestic health assessment are twofold: to protect the health of the population by identifying and treating communicable diseases, and to ensure the health of the individual immigrant. To accomplish both goals, a complete health assessment that goes beyond screening to focus on the individual needs of the patient is desirable. An approach that combines the use of universal screening with targeted screening for specific groups is optimal. The two groups of immigrants for which there are the most data to inform such a process are refugees and internationally adopted children. Several surveys of specific immigrant groups are also available. For other immigrant groups, such as migrant workers, undocumented immigrants, and short-term visitors, less is known about specific disease risks and susceptibilities. For this reason, this chapter will build the case for evidence-based universal plus targeted screening based on the groups for which the most data are available.

Health screening for refugees entering the US is encouraged after arrival by federal regulations and funds that are available for these programs. The Office of Refugee Resettlement developed a protocol to assist states in the development of health assessment programs[5] and has issued guidelines for the use of Refugee Medical Assistance funds for these screening programs.[6] Refugee Medical Assistance funds may be available to cover the costs of screening and prevention not covered by existing Medicaid or other state or local health programs. These funds do not extend to immigrants who have nonrefugee status. Experts in the field of international adoption have developed recommendations for assessment of internationally adopted children upon arrival in the US. The requirement for health insurance as a condition for eligibility to adopt internationally makes it easier to provide comprehensive health assessments for these children. For many immigrant groups, however, there are no defined protocols for screening, and financial constraints limit significantly what screening can be done.

There are currently no recognized universal guidelines for screening or assessing the health status of new immigrants. Recommended empiric treatment and screening tests vary widely by state, local clinic, and the immigration status of the individual. There is, however, general agreement in the literature regarding basic elements of the health assessment. These generally accepted elements include a complete history and physical examination, basic screening laboratory evaluation, testing for tuberculosis, immunizations as needed, dental evaluation, hearing and vision screening, and mental health screening (Table 12.1). Other testing and evaluation can be done based on the results of the initial general screening. Healthcare providers caring for immigrants should be familiar with any existing state guidelines and availability of specific screening tests in their area. Each state makes

| Table 12.1 Recommended components of domestic health assessment |
| --- |
| Review all available records, chest radiograph |
| Complete history and physical examination |
| Vision and hearing screening |
| Dental evaluation |
| Mental health assessment |
| Tuberculin skin testing |
| Laboratory testing |
|    CBC with differential |
|    Serum chemistries |
|    Hepatitis B serology |
|    Malaria smear/PCR (see text) |
|    Urinalysis |
|    Stool O&P |
|    Lead level (children) |
| Immunizations as needed |

arrangements for screening while some states utilize state or county public health clinics for screening; others contract with private providers.[7] Detailed information about public health models for assessing health status on new immigrants can be found in Chapter 11.

The goals of a comprehensive screening program for refugees in Colorado illustrate a thoughtful and thorough approach to screening.[8] Seven goals were set out: establish a multidisciplinary team effective in providing health screening and care, establish a comprehensive system for screening, enhance services to provide a full assessment of all refugees, create a system for data collection, enhance provider cultural competency, establish systems for referral and follow-up, and ensure competent interpreter services.

Screening of immigrants should also be tailored to known epidemiologic risk factors. Much is known about geographic risk factors for certain infectious diseases but good evidence on which to base screening programs may be lacking. An overview of medical screening is presented but it should be recognized that these recommendations will vary with time, population shifts, and resources available.

## Components of Domestic Health Assessment

### History

As with all patient encounters, a thorough history is the foundation on which further evaluation is based (Table 12.2). Though details of the past medical

**Table 12.2 Recommended components of domestic health assessment history**

Current symptoms
Recent concerns
Past medical history
    Hospitalizations
    Surgeries
    Blood transfusions
    Episode(s) of jaundice
    Immunizations
    Malaria
Medications
    Current and past
    Traditional medicines
    Herbal remedies
Allergies
Review of systems
    Fever
    Night sweats
    Weight loss
    Pruritus
    Skin lesions
    Cough
    Diarrhea
    Rash
    Jaundice
Family history
Social history
    Family structure
    Occupational history
    Tobacco, alcohol, other substances
Travel history
    Country of birth
    Residence in other areas
    Residence in refugee camp
Mental health screen

history are desirable, initial questions should focus on the immediate health concerns of the patient, and these should be addressed during the visit, even if it means delaying some components of the health assessment.

The medical history should include questions about prior surgical procedures, transfusions, history of varicella infection, episodes of jaundice, and hospitalizations. Review of systems should include questions relevant to possible exposures during the course of migration to the US: hematuria (exposure to schistosomiasis), pruritis or limb swelling (filarial disease), skin lesions (leprosy, leishmaniasis), etc. (see Ch. 14, Differential Diagnosis of Ill Immigrants by Organ System). Questions regarding current or past medications should include traditional and herbal remedies and any known allergies. Family

history should be elicited if possible, though patients may not have knowledge of specific illnesses of interest such as diabetes, heart disease, or cancer. A complete travel history should be elucidated as many immigrants will have lived in several countries or regions prior to arrival and some will have spent extensive periods of time outside their country of origin. Knowledge about different geographic exposures as well as residence in specific refugee camps can be helpful in focusing the screening process. The social history should include questions about use of tobacco, including smokeless tobacco, alcohol, or other substances as well as questions about current and past family structure. Previous occupational history as well as current occupation, if already employed, may be useful to determine exposures to chemical and environmental risks. For children, school attendance and grade is helpful; for both children and adults assessment of literacy level is helpful. A mental health screen is an important aspect of the history, though may be difficult to elicit before a trusting relationship is developed between the patient and health professional. Psychological stressors can be identified for most new immigrants (separation from family members, moving to a new and unfamiliar place, language barriers) but the presence of stressors alone does not necessarily mean the patient has a mental health problem. Identifying and acknowledging patients' strengths and coping strategies is often as important as identifying specific stressors. Mental health screening is discussed in detail in Chapter 48.

The history will, in many cases, be obtained via an interpreter. Some centers have interpreter services available to provide a trained interpreter who will be in the room with the patient. Other centers use telephone interpreters. In either case providers should be comfortable working with interpreters and understand that these visits will require extra time and that some concepts of disease may be difficult to translate. In small communities, patients may prefer the use of anonymous telephone interpreters rather than discuss health issues with an interpreter who may be known to them, or is a member of their community. Working with interpreters is discussed in Chapter 6.

## Physical examination

A complete physical examination should be performed on all immigrants (Table 12.3). Some individuals may request same-gender providers; eliciting patient preferences for a same-gender provider is

## Table 12.3 Recommended components of domestic health assessment physical examination

General appearance
Vital signs
Weight, height
Head circumference for those younger than 3 years
Vision and hearing
Dental examination
  Caries
  Missing teeth
  Gingivitis
Cardiovascular
  Heart murmurs
Lymphadenopathy
Abdomen
  Hepatosplenomegaly
Genitourinary
  Female circumcision
Skin
  Pallor
  Rash
  Ritual scarification
Evidence of traditional health practices

appropriate when this is possible. Providers should be sensitive to the fact that this may be the first complete examination for some patients. Examination should include height and weight and, for children less than 36 months, head circumference. Growth parameters should be plotted on the appropriate growth charts for all children and sexual maturity rating should be determined. Note should be made of discrepancies of age based on examination compared with information provided on immigration paperwork. This discrepancy of growth may reflect a true physical state (i.e. secondary to nutritional deficiency) or may be due to mistakes/inaccuracies in documentation. Pulse and blood pressure should be measured. Attention should be paid to the dental and skin examination. Note should be made of scarification and evidence of traditional health practices including female circumcision. Attention should also be paid to the cardiovascular examination for previously undiagnosed murmurs and the abdominal examination for hepatosplenomegaly. Vision and hearing should be assessed during the initial evaluation if possible or persons should be referred to appropriate sites for screening. Pelvic examination is almost never appropriate in the first health assessment visit, unless there is a specific medical indication and the ability to explain in an appropriate setting the reason for the examination and the procedures to be done.

## Review of immunization status and provision of needed immunizations

Immunization records, if available, should be reviewed at the first screening visit. Individuals with refugee status and international adoptees are not required to receive immunizations prior to arrival but many will have received some vaccines and some may have documentation. Those persons with immigrant visa status have been required to show proof of immunization prior to immigration but records should be reviewed on arrival as not all recommended vaccines are available in other countries. Vaccination schedules for routine and catch-up childhood immunizations as well as recommendations for adults are available from several sources. Recommendations are updated periodically and the most current information can be found on the internet from the Centers for Disease Control and Prevention or from national authorities in other countries.[9-11]

Vaccines may be accepted as valid if they conform to local standards for age at initiation and interval between doses. History of or examination findings consistent with varicella are considered acceptable but history of other vaccine-preventable diseases is not considered proof of immunity. Serologic screening may be considered prior to immunization as discussed in Chapter 13.

Immunization catch-up should begin at the first screening visit. Immunizations should be completed at subsequent visits or immigrants should be referred to appropriate sites to complete vaccines. All immigrants should receive an immunization document on which all doses given are documented. This record will be needed for school enrollment, employment, and on application for permanent resident status.

## Assessment of dental health

Dental problems are commonly encountered in the immigrant population. Dental caries were the most common finding on examination in pediatric refugees resettled in Portland, Maine, with a prevalence of 16.7% (22/132).[12] In Buffalo, New York, 42% of 107 pediatric refugees required referral for dental care.[13] Of 1825 refugee children screened in Massachusetts, 62% had dental caries.[14] The physical examination should include an oral examination to evaluate for caries, missing teeth, and gingivitis.

Dental care for immigrants is problematic in many areas due to insurance inequities and lack of public assistance dental programs. A detailed discussion of dental health issues in immigrant populations is provided in Chapter 45.

## Mental health assessment

Refugees and immigrants have frequently experienced war, trauma, and torture. Post-traumatic stress disorder and depression are the most common psychiatric disorders encountered in these populations. Despite cultural differences, symptoms of post-traumatic stress disorder may be remarkably similar across populations with hyperarousal, avoidance, and difficulties with concentration and memory being common.[4] It may be difficult to initiate discussion of such exposures during the initial screening visits but a detailed history and a mental status examination should be performed as part of a complete evaluation. Attention should also be paid to symptoms suggestive of psychiatric problems with consideration of ethnic and cultural differences of immigrants. A detailed discussion of mental health issues affecting immigrants can be found in a separate section of this text.

## Laboratory screening tests

There is some agreement that testing for tuberculosis and hepatitis B and obtaining a complete blood count are appropriate screening tests for all immigrants. Medical screening tests should meet minimum accepted criteria for population-based screening tests: the condition sought should be an important health problem, there should be a latent or asymptomatic disease state, there should be a suitable test (acceptable sensitivity, specificity, negative and positive predictive values), the test should be acceptable to the population, there should be an acceptable treatment and an agreed upon strategy of whom and how to treat, and the diagnosis and treatment should be cost-effective. Laboratory screening tests currently thought to be beneficial in most groups include tuberculin skin testing, complete blood count with differential, serum chemistries including renal function tests, and hepatitis B serologies. Tests most appropriately done in specific groups of immigrants include blood lead testing, serologic tests for parasitic diseases, examination of blood smears (or serum PCR) for malaria, hepatitis C testing, HIV, and testing for syphilis. Tests that are not currently recommended for universal screening, and for which insufficient information is available to direct targeted screening, include testing for CMV, hepatitis A, and *Helicobacter pylori*. Table 12.4 indicates strength of evidence to support universal testing, and specific groups of immigrants for whom testing may be indicated. The following sections discuss the different screening tests and the evidence to support universal or targeted screening.

## Tuberculin skin testing

Tuberculin skin testing should be performed in all new immigrants over the age of 6 weeks. As rates of

**Table 12.4 Strength of evidence to support universal versus targeted screening**

| Test | Strength of evidence to support universal screening | Specific groups for which targeted screening is appropriate |
|---|---|---|
| Tuberculin skin test | Strong | |
| Hepatitis B surface antigen | Strong | |
| Anemia | Strong | |
| Intestinal parasites | Good | |
| Hepatitis C | Poor | Standard risk factors; immigrants from Egypt; Children adopted from China, Southeast Asia, Russia, and Eastern Europe |
| Lead | Poor | Children |
| Hepatitis A | Poor | Those with hepatitis B or C |
| Malaria | Poor | Fever, splenomegaly, thrombocytopenia in those from endemic areas |
| *Helicobacter pylori* | Fair-poor | Signs or symptoms of disease associated with *H pylori* infection |

tuberculosis among US-born persons decline, an increasing proportion of cases in the US are among immigrants. The proportion of cases in foreign-born individuals in the US rose from 27% in 1992 to 50% in 2002 and continues to rise.[15] The highest risk of developing active disease is within the first 2 years after exposure. Treatment of latent tuberculosis infection can prevent progression to active disease in most persons. A study of tuberculosis among persons in Manhattan demonstrated that among foreign-born persons most disease is due to reactivation of latent infection, whereas most cases in US-born persons result from recent transmission.[16]

The World Health Organization estimates that one in three persons is infected with *Mycobacterium tuberculosis* worldwide. Based on this estimate, the US Centers for Disease Control and Prevention estimate at least 7 million foreign-born persons in the US are infected.[17] Treatment of active and latent tuberculosis in this population is complicated by the rising incidence of multidrug resistant tuberculosis in the developing world. Providers should have knowledge of resistance trends in the countries of origin of their patients as well as any other regions of long-term residence prior to immigration.

A positive tuberculin skin test is one of the most common findings on screening of immigrants. Of over 92 000 refugees screened throughout the US in 1993–1995, 43.2% had positive tuberculin skin tests.[4] Rates ranged from 10.1% to 70% in different groups of immigrants tested (Table 12.5). In Buffalo, New York, 17 of 83 (20%) screened refugee children had positive skin tests.[13] In Portland, Maine, 35.2% (45/128) of refugee children were positive.[12] A larger study in Minnesota of refugees of all ages found an overall prevalence of positive skin tests of 49% (1145/2355).[25] Males, those over age 18 years, and persons from Southeast Asia and sub-Saharan Africa were more likely to test positive.

Screening has been found to be effective in finding patients earlier and reducing the period during which they are infectious in a study of over 800 immigrants in the Netherlands.[26] Patients found by screening were less likely to have smear-positive sputum, had fewer hospitalizations, were symptomatic for shorter periods, and had shorter periods of infectiousness compared with patients who were detected passively.

Some immigrants will have been screened for tuberculosis before arrival in the US. Pre-departure chest radiographs are required of refugees over 14 years of age (≥2 years for Southeast Asia). This is done to identify and exclude persons with active tuberculosis until they are treated and no longer infectious. Because chest radiographs do not diagnose latent tuberculosis infection (LTBI) nor can they identify extrapulmonary tuberculosis, tuberculin skin testing (TST) should be done on all newly arrived immigrants over 6 weeks of age. A trained healthcare provider should read the test 48–72 hours after placement. Interpretation should be done without regard to Bacille Calmette-Guerin (BCG) vaccine status. BCG does not affect the sensitivity of the TST which is 99% in immunocompetent individuals.[27] The effect on the specificity of the TST varies with the age at receipt of last BCG. For those whose only BCG was during infancy, the TST specificity is 95% and declines to 75% for those who received BCG after age 5 years. In areas of high prevalence, the positive predictive value (PPV) of the TST remains high despite use of BCG. In regions where the prevalence of tuberculosis is low and BCG is used, the PPV will be lower and interpretation of the TST becomes more problematic. A newer blood-based assay (detection of release of interferon gamma in response to tuberculosis antigens) was recently recommended for use interchangeably with the TST by the Centers for Disease Control and Prevention.[28] A study is currently underway in Minnesota to assess the utility in screening refugees.

In most cases, positive TST is defined as 10 or more millimeters of induration. For those with a known tuberculosis contact, signs or symptoms of tuberculosis, an abnormal chest radiograph, or who are immunocompromised, a cutoff of 5 millimeters should be used.[29] Persons with a positive skin test should have a chest radiograph to evaluate for pulmonary tuberculosis. A chest radiograph should also be performed in any person with symptoms of pulmonary tuberculosis such as cough, weight loss, fevers, or night sweats. Symptomatic patients should have a chest radiograph regardless of the results of tuberculin skin testing. Extrapulmonary tuberculosis may account for up to half of the tuberculosis in this population and persons with chronic constitutional symptoms should be evaluated thoroughly with a high index of suspicion for tuberculosis.

LTBI (positive TST, negative chest radiograph, no symptoms) should be treated with 9 months of daily isoniazid. Resistance to isoniazid is increasing around the world but current guidelines still recommend its use as first-line therapy in most cases. Treatment of active tuberculosis consists of a multidrug regimen and should be undertaken under the supervision of a specialist knowledgeable about resistance patterns (see Ch. 19).

**Table 12.5 Screening test results for selected immigrant and refugee groups**

| Population | Positive TST | HBsAg positive | Anemia | Eosinophilia | Pathogenic intestinal parasites | Hepatitis C | Elevated blood lead | Dental caries |
|---|---|---|---|---|---|---|---|---|
| Refugees, US, 1993–1995[4] | 43.2% (n = 92 838) | 6.1% (n = 44 299) | | | 29.9% (n = 57 761) | | | |
| Refugees, Minnesota, 1993–1995 (n = 19,115)[4] | 10.1% (Cuba) – 53.2% (Somalia) | 0.5% (Cuba) –16% (Ethiopia) | | | 18.8% (Cuba) – 62.6 (Somalia) | | | |
| African immigrants, Minneapolis, 1997[18] | 52% (n = 91) | 14% (n = 73) | | | | 3% (n = 59) | | |
| Latino immigrants, San Francisco, 1978–1983[19] | 53% (n = 1232) | | | | | | | |
| Refugee children, Massachusetts, 1995–1998[14] | 25% (n = 1737) | | 12% <2 years of age: 28% (n = 1247) | | 21% (n = 1642) | | | |
| Refugees, Minnesota, 1997[4] | 34.9% (n = 979) | 5.3% (n = 885) | | | 39.5% (n = 792) | | | |
| Refugees, Minnesota, 1999[25] | 49% (n = 2355) | 7% (n = 2353) | | | 22% (n = 2129) | | | |
| Vietnamese immigrants, Boston, 1994–1995[20] | 70% (n = 94) | 14% (n = 96) | | | 32.5% (n = 80) | | | |
| Refugee children, Maine, 1994–1995[12] | 35.2% (n = 128) | 4% (n = 124) | 19.7% (n = 127) | | 43.7% (n = 87) | | 16.7% (<6 years) (n = 30) | |

**Table 12.5 Screening test results for selected immigrant and refugee groups—cont'd**

| Population | Positive TST | HBsAg positive | Anemia | Eosinophilia | Pathogenic intestinal parasites | Hepatitis C | Elevated blood lead | Dental caries |
|---|---|---|---|---|---|---|---|---|
| Southeast Asian immigrants, ages 1–24, Los Angeles, 1981[21] | 22.9% (n = 606) | | 13.3% (n = 623) | | 58.7% (n = 574) | | | |
| Refugee children, Buffalo NY, 1991–1993[13] | 20% (n = 83) | 7% (n = 81) | 6.5% (n = 107) | | 21.8% (n = 87) | | | 42% (n = 107) |
| Central American immigrant children, 1981–1982[22] | | | | | 65% (n = 96) | | | |
| Latin American immigrant children, 1984–1989[23] | | | | | 35% (n = 124) | | | |
| Immigrant women, 1984–1985[24] | | 5.9% (n = 288) | | | | | | |
| Jewish refugees from the former Soviet Union, 1990–1993[31] | | 0.4% (n = 496) | | | | | | |
| Liberian, 2004. MN. (unpublished) | 43% (n = 103) | 15% (n = 103) | 24% (n = 103) | 28% (n = 103) | 13% (n = 103) | | | |
| Highland Lao (Hmong), 2004. MN. (unpublished) | 14% (n = 217) | 7.3% (n = 218) | 20% (n = 218) | 17% (n = 218) | 75% (n = 190) | 1.5% (n = 81) | 1.5% (n = 61) | |

**Table 12.6 Hepatitis B serology interpretation**

| HBsAg | Anti-HBsAg | Anti-HBc IgM | Anti-HBc IgG | HBeAg | Anti-HBeAg | HBV DNA | Interpretation |
|---|---|---|---|---|---|---|---|
| + | − | + | − | + | − | + | Acute infection |
| − | + | − | + | − | + | − | Resolved infection |
| − | + | − | − | − | − | − | Immunization |
| + | − | − | + | + | − | + | Chronic infection Active carrier |
| + | − | − | + | − | + | − | Chronic infection Inactive carrier |

## Hepatitis B

Hepatitis B infection is common among immigrants, especially those from East and Southeast Asia and sub-Saharan Africa. Testing for surface antigen to hepatitis B (HBsAg) yielded positive results in 0.4–16% of those tested at various screening sites (see Table 12.5). HBsAg was found in 7% of children in Buffalo, New York, 4% of children in Portland, Maine, and 7% of all refugees tested in Minnesota.[12,13,25] Of particular concern is the finding of HBsAg in almost 6% of foreign-born women screened at a prenatal clinic in New York. Almost one-third of these women also tested positive for e antigen, a marker for infectivity. Infants born to these mothers have a nearly 90% chance of chronic hepatitis B infection with persistent positive HBsAg if not given preventative Rx at birth.[30] In Minnesota, higher prevalence was seen in those over 18 years of age but it is clear from these three studies that children are potentially infected as well. Jewish refugees from the former Soviet Union and immigrants from Cuba had much lower rates (0.4% and 0.5%, respectively) of hepatitis B surface antigen than immigrants from Asia and Africa.[4,31]

Hepatitis B screening is recommended for all immigrants because there is an intervention for those who are susceptible and because there are significant consequences, including chronic hepatitis and hepatocellular carcinoma, of hepatitis B infection. Hepatitis B is transmissible to intimate partners and household contacts; screening has the potential for reduction of disease in contacts by education about transmission and by immunizing those contacts.[32] The availability of treatment options also makes it important to identify and monitor those who are infected with this virus. Although Hurie et al.[31] make the case that a prevalence rate of HBsAg of 0.4 % in the refugees they tested might suggest

that testing is not of value, the fact that an additional 22% had evidence of past infection with hepatitis B, and therefore would not be candidates for vaccine, suggests that screening for hepatitis B would still be important in this population in terms of cost savings and reduction of visits to healthcare professionals to receive the three-dose vaccine series.

Optimal screening for hepatitis B consists of testing for hepatitis B surface antigen, antibody to hepatitis B core antigen (anti-HBc), and hepatitis B surface antibody (anti-HBsAg). Interpretation of hepatitis B serology can be challenging (Table 12.6). HBsAg is present in those recently infected and chronically infected. Those who recover from acute infection will develop antibody to the surface antigen and the surface antigen will disappear from the blood. Antibody to the core antigen can be used to distinguish those persons vaccinated (will not have core antibody) from those who have recovered from the illness. Those persons who do not clear surface antigen are chronically infected. Two general states of chronic infection exist. Inactive carriers will have surface antigen and core antibody but will have low or undetectable levels of hepatitis B DNA. These persons do not have evidence of ongoing inflammation and damage. Active carriers or those experiencing a flare of the disease will have high levels of DNA as well as evidence of inflammation (elevated liver enzymes). Those persons with high levels of DNA as well as the presence of e antigen are more infectious. Consultation with a gastroenterologist or infectious diseases specialist with expertise in this area may be helpful (see Ch. 22).

Those found to be susceptible to hepatitis B should receive a three-dose series of hepatitis B vaccine. Those found to be infected should be counseled about how to prevent transmission and referred for ongoing follow-up, either by their primary care provider or a hepatologist, and their household and sexual contacts should be tested and vaccinated if susceptible. Individuals with chronic hepatitis B should also have periodic (every 6–12 months) screening for hepatocellular carcinoma with serum alpha fetoprotein and liver ultrasound because hepatocellular carcinoma can develop in the absence of cirrhosis. Inactive carriers should have periodic screening with liver function tests to detect flaring disease. Those with hepatitis B infection should also be tested for hepatitis A and C; those found to be hepatitis A nonimmune should receive vaccine. Those with hepatitis C should be counseled about the implications of this coinfection and informed of strategies to reduce their risk of further liver damage (avoidance of alcohol, caution in using certain medications, etc.) (see Ch. 22 on Hepatitis B and Ch. 31 on Hepatitis C).

Identification of carriers who are women of childbearing age is particularly important to prevent perinatal transmission. Perinatal infection is much more likely to result in chronic infection than infection later in life and such children are at increased risk of developing chronic liver disease and/or hepatocellular carcinoma.

## Complete blood count

A complete blood count with white cell differential and red cell indices can identify anemia, thrombocytopenia, and eosinophilia, and may provide clues to the presence of other hematologic or infectious conditions. Anemia is seen commonly in immigrants and may be due to one or a combination of factors. Common reasons for anemia include iron deficiency, thalassemia, other hemoglobinopathies, infection with hookworm, and malaria. Lymphopenia may be seen with HIV infection. Thrombocytopenia may be seen with malaria although persons with asymptomatic malaria usually have normal hemoglobin and platelet levels. Eosinophilia (absolute eosinophil count >450 cells/microliter) may be due to parasitic infection and warrants further investigation as described below.

## Screening for parasitic diseases

**Intestinal parasites** Gastrointestinal parasites are commonly found on screening stool examinations of immigrants and refugees. Frequently encountered nonpathogens are *Endolimax nana*, *Entamoeba coli*, *Entamoeba hartmanni*, *Iodamoeba butschlii*, *Chilomastix mesnili*, and *Blastocystis hominis*. With the possible exception of *Blastocystis hominis*, these organisms are considered nonpathogenic and should not be treated.

| Table 12.7 Gastrointestinal parasites | |
| --- | --- |
| **Pathogens** | **Nonpathogens** |
| *Giardia lamblia* | *Endolimax nana* |
| *Entamoeba histolytica* | *Entamoeba coli* |
| *Trichuris trichiura* | *Entamoeba dispar* |
| *Ascaris lumbricoides* | *Entamoeba hartmanni* |
| *Hymenolepis nana* | *Iodamoeba butschlii* |
| Hookworm | *Chilomastix mesnili* |
| *Strongyloides stercoralis* | *Blastocystis hominis* (?) |
| *Schistosoma* species | |
| *Dientamoeba fragilis* | |

Common organisms considered pathogens include *Giardia lamblia*, *Entamoeba histolytica*, *Trichuris trichiura*, *Hymenolepis nana*, *Ascaris lumbricoides*, hookworm, *Strongyloides stercoralis*, *Schistosoma* species, and *Dientamoeba fragilis* (Table 12.7). Other, more unusual, parasitic infections are occasionally identified, such as the fluke infections (i.e. *Ophisthorchis* spp.).

Prevalence of parasites in refugee children in Buffalo, New York, was 21.8% (19/87),[13] similar to that seen in refugees of all ages in Minnesota (22%, 462/2129).[25] A higher percentage was found in refugee children in Portland, Maine, 43.7% (38/87).[12] About a third (31.1%, 75/241) of refugee children in Miami–Dade County, Florida, had pathogens found on stool O&P.[33]

Empiric overseas pre-departure treatment of refugees in sub-Saharan Africa with albendazole has been ongoing since 1999 (excluding pregnant women and those <2 years of age). Reductions in detection of intestinal parasites were seen in a before-and-after study of refugees arriving in Massachusetts.[34] Significant reductions in both helminths and protozoa including hookworm, *Trichuris*, *Ascaris*, and *Entamoeba histolytica* were observed. It should be noted that in this population eosinophilia is frequently residual from a parasitic infection prior to departure. In fact, eosinophilia in this pretreated group has only a 12% positive predictive value for the subsequent detection of a potentially pathogenic parasite in the stool. Newer comprehensive treatment regimen recommendations aimed at empiric treatment of *Strongyloides stercoralis* and *Schistosoma* spp. may broaden the overseas treatment and will empirically treat most cestode, nematode, and trematode parasites.

Routine examination of stool for ova and parasites (stool O&P) is currently recommended for individuals arriving from the developing world or who resided in refugee camps or areas where sanitation services were disrupted due to natural disasters or political conditions. Any person with symptoms suggesting a gastrointestinal parasite regardless of their prior living conditions should also be tested. Eosinophilia is also strongly suggestive of infection with parasites. The specificity of eosinophilia in a nontreated refugee (absolute eosinophil count above 400–500/microliter) has been shown to be greater than 95%.[35] While multiple stool specimens increase the likelihood of finding a pathogen, the optimal number is not clear.[36-38] One to three specimens should be adequate in most cases. *Strongyloides* is present in many parts of the world and is difficult to detect on stool O&P: even three properly collected stool examinations only identify half of those infected. Autoinfection can result in infection lasting decades. This is of concern due to the risk of disseminated infection and death when patients become immunosuppressed from human immunodeficiency virus (HIV) infection, malignancy, or medications (steroids, chemotherapy). Most infected individuals will have eosinophilia. This parasite should be considered when a patient has eosinophilia with no source identified in the stool. In this case, serologic evaluation may identify the infection and lead to appropriate treatment.

*Entamoeba dispar* cysts cannot be distinguished from *E. histolytica* by microscopy. An asymptomatic refugee who has *E. histolytica/dispar* complex identified should have serologic evaluation and/or stool antigen testing and undergo treatment only if the diagnosis of *E. histolytica* is confirmed. In many settings, these tests may not be available, and some experts choose to treat these patients with a 7-day course of paromomycin to assure eradication of potentially harmful cysts.

Collection of stool will be done in the home, and specimen containers contain toxic preservative material. Clear instructions should be given to patients in their own language via an interpreter if necessary to avoid receipt of unusable specimens and inadvertent exposure to the preservative.

Recently, the Centers for Disease Control and Prevention established recommendations for presumptive treatment of strongyloidiasis and schistosomiasis for Sudanese refugees.[39] These recommendations were based on findings of a serosurvey showing that almost 70% of the Lost Boys and Girls of Sudan tested positive for schistosomiasis or strongyloidiasis and over 20% tested positive for both. Current recommendations are presumptive treatment for all Sudanese refugees who are not pregnant or lactating and do not have evidence of neurocysticercosis. For those not tested for Loa loa, recommended treatment is a 7-day course of albendazole (400 mg twice a day) for those over 1 year of age and two doses of praziquantel (20 mg/kg 6–8 hours apart) for those 4 years of age and over. For those who have tested negative for Loa loa and weigh more than 15 kg, ivermectin (200 mcg/kg, one dose) was recommended for treatment of strongyloidiasis. Those persons over 1 year of age were also recommended to receive one dose of albendazole (600 mg) for treatment of other intestinal parasites and the above noted dose of praziquantel for schistosomiasis. Testing for schistosomiasis and strongyloidiasis is available at the Centers for Disease Control and Prevention for persons who meet the exclusion criteria for presumptive treatment. It is unclear at this time whether these recommendations are being followed by those seeing refugees and immigrants from Sudan, or whether these recommendations can be generalized to include other immigrant groups. Many experts who screen refugees prefer to make specific diagnoses and generate targeted treatment plans, while monitoring the course of eosinophilia over time. The most important finding to come of these studies may be to prompt clinicians to consider screening high-risk asymptomatic individuals, even those without eosinophilia, for parasitic diseases, especially strongyloidiasis.

**Screening for parasites in immigrants with eosinophilia** Eosinophilia (absolute eosinophil count >450 cells/microliter) is a common finding on screening blood count. The most common cause of eosinophilia worldwide is infection with helminthic parasites.[35] It is most often associated with asymptomatic infection but some may have signs and symptoms suggestive of specific parasites. For instance, hematuria suggests *Schistosoma hematobium* while skin complaints suggest filarial infection or cutaneous larva migrans. Some parasites will be identified on stool O&P. If after three such examinations an etiology is not identified, additional testing is warranted. This testing will be focused by signs and symptoms if present and by potential exposures if asymptomatic. A thorough travel history is important in this evaluation to determine risks for specific infections. Infections to consider include strongyloidiasis, schistosomiasis, filariasis, and toxocariasis. In a study of Southeast Asian refugees with persistent eosinophilia and no diagnosis after a comprehensive screening evaluation, a significant number were subsequently found to have infection with hookworm and *Strongyloides stercoralis*.[40]

In a study of newly arrived refugees, eosinophilia (absolute eosinophil count >450 cells/microliter) was present in 12% (266/2224). Of those with eosinophilia, 29% had stool pathogens. Serologic evidence of parasitic infection with *Strongyloides*, *Schistosoma* and/or filaria was seen at all levels of eosinophilia and in patients with and without stool pathogens. An approach agreed upon by many experts for evaluation for parasites in asymptomatic persons with eosinophilia from endemic areas includes stool O&P examination, *Strongyloides* serology for all patients, and *Schistosoma* and filaria serology when geographically appropriate.[41] In refugees with no pathogenic infections identified, an eosinophil count should be repeated in 3–6 months.

A detailed description of the evaluation of eosinophilia is presented in Chapter 21.

**Screening for malaria** Individuals arriving from malaria endemic areas may be asymptomatic but harbor malaria parasites. A study in Minnesota of newly arrived Liberian refugee children found the prevalence of malaria to be 60% (34/57).[42] Fever, splenomegaly, and thrombocytopenia were predictive of malaria but 29% of children were asymptomatic. In Spain, 44% (56/125) of children from sub-Saharan Africa were found to have malaria and of these, 12.5% (7/56) were asymptomatic.[43] A study of immigrants presenting to a tropical medicine hospital in Madrid showed a prevalence of malaria of 15.1% (149/988). The prevalence was higher in short-term (<3 months since arrival in Spain) immigrants (26.7%) than long-term (>18 months) immigrants (7.1%).[44] Refugees from selected areas now receive pre-departure treatment, generally with pyrimethamine-sulfadoxine, if they are 2 years of age or older and not pregnant. This treatment is not universal and would not apply to those arriving with nonrefugee status. Even with this intervention, a study of 103 asymptomatic Liberian refugees who received screening by smears, rapid antigen testing kits, and PCR found 8.7% were still infected with *P. falciparum* malaria 1 month after arrival. Although some experts have recommend screening all refugees from endemic areas based on increasing reports of symptomatic illness developing in persons after resettlement,[45] this former study found both thick and thin blood smear to be very insensitive (20%). Currently, PCR is not widely available. Given these and other restrictions on diagnosis, some experts recommend empiric treatment of all refugees from highly endemic areas (all sub-Saharan Africa except Nairobi and South Africa) if they did not receive pre-departure empirical treatment. The CDC is currently revising recommendations to implement more effective pre-departure regimens (see Ch. 37).

## Urinalysis

Urinalysis is used to screen for a variety of problems including undiagnosed sexually transmitted infections (sterile pyuria), *Schistosoma hematobium* (hematuria), and renal disease (proteinuria). Glucose identified in the urine indicates that further evaluation for diabetes is necessary.

## Targeted screening tests appropriate for specific immigrant groups

**Lead** Refugees are at risk for elevated blood lead levels upon arrival and remain at risk after resettlement. Risk factors include traditional medicines and pottery, environmental lead pollution, and parental occupational exposures both overseas and after resettlement. Some refugee health programs include lead screening for children as part of routine testing but the American Academy of Pediatrics and the Centers for Disease Control and Prevention do not include foreign birth as a risk factor.

In Massachusetts, refugee children were found to have greater than twice the prevalence of elevated lead levels compared with US-born children and newly elevated levels were found more than 6 months after resettlement in some children.[46] These children were younger than 7 years of age and had venous blood lead level testing done within 90 days of arrival as part of routine health assessment. Six hundred and ninety-three children were tested and 11% had elevated levels (>10 micrograms/dL). Country of birth was found to be the strongest predictor of elevated lead level, with those children from Central America and the Caribbean having the highest prevalence at 40% and those from Northern Eurasia having levels comparable to US-born children. Levels did not vary by age or gender.

Lead testing guidelines were developed in New Hampshire after the death of a Sudanese refugee child in 2000. Screening consists of capillary blood testing within 90 days of arrival for children 6 months to 15 years of age followed by venous testing 3–6 months after initial testing for children younger than 6 years old. Preliminary data indicate that 14% (13/92) had elevated lead levels at both time points.[47] High rates of elevated blood lead levels have also been reported in refugee children in Maine[12] and Miami–Dade County, Florida.[33] The appropriate age cutoff for lead testing has not been determined.

The Centers for Disease Control and Prevention is working to ensure lead testing for all refugee children.[44] The recommendation is for testing children younger than 6 years with blood lead level and hemoglobin as well as a nutritional assessment within 3 months of arrival. Lead testing should be repeated 3–6 months after resettlement. Multivitamins with iron should be provided to children younger than 59 months of age and screening should be considered in older children with risk factors. Individual states may choose other approaches: in Massachusetts, the Refugee Health Assessment Program recommends lead testing for all individuals 16 years of age and younger.

**Hepatitis C** Routine screening for hepatitis C is not recommended at this time. Rates of hepatitis C vary widely among immigrant groups and prevalence of hepatitis C is higher in many countries from which immigrants arrive than it is in the US. Estimates of hepatitis C prevalence rates in adults are 5% in Africa, 3% in China, and 2.5% in Southeast Asia.[48] Perinatal transmission occurs at much lower rates than for hepatitis B. Especially high rates of infection are seen in all ages in Egypt[49] and persons emigrating from there should be screened. The American Academy of Pediatrics recommends screening of internationally adopted children from China, Southeast Asia, Russia, and Eastern Europe.[50] Screening of more than 700 refugees resettled in Massachusetts identified a very low number of infected individuals.[51] Immigrants may, however, have some of the standard risk factors for hepatitis C infection, such as blood transfusion, use of potentially contaminated needles, or organ transplant. If these are identified, testing for hepatitis C is appropriate. No data are available on the cost-effectiveness of screening immigrants for hepatitis C.

Those found to be infected with hepatitis C should be counseled regarding transmission prevention and should receive hepatitis B and hepatitis A vaccines if not already immunized or immune. Treatment options for hepatitis C are evolving rapidly. The decision to treat is based on a number of factors including the genotype of the virus, the extent of liver damage based on biopsy, the age of the patient, and medical and psychiatric comorbidities. Persons with chronic hepatitis C should be referred to a specialist for management and consideration of treatment (see Ch. 31).

**Sexually transmitted infections** Testing for syphilis is done for refugees and some other categories of immigrants before arrival in the US for individuals 15 years of age and older. Testing for syphilis should be considered strongly for individuals who arrive

without test results, especially when risk factors or signs or symptoms of disease are present. Rapid Plasma Reagin (RPR) or Venereal Disease Research Laboratory (VDRL) tests are both acceptable. Younger persons who are sexually active or who report a history of rape or sexual abuse should also be tested; these situations may not be disclosed at the initial visit. Other sexually transmitted infections are not screened for routinely. Those patients with a history or examination suggestive of a sexually transmitted infection should have targeted testing performed. The availability of urinary antigen testing has facilitated testing for sexually transmitted diseases in a noninvasive way.

Recent recommendations from the Centers for Disease Control and Prevention call for screening of all children arriving from areas where treponemes are endemic with RPR or VDRL.[52] This recommendation was prompted by reports of positive tests among refugee children from Liberia and Somalia. Those who test positive on screening non-treponemal testing should have confirmatory treponemal testing performed. No data are available on the prevalence of positive tests or the cost-effectiveness of this strategy, and the use of this strategy by those screening immigrants has not been assessed.

**Human immunodeficiency virus** Human immunodeficiency virus (HIV) testing is performed on all immigrants ≥15 years prior to departure from the country of origin (or first asylum). Some younger children may have been tested under certain circumstances such as known HIV infection in the mother. HIV is an excludable condition in the US but infected persons can receive a waiver. Testing with a method that detects both HIV-1 and HIV-2 is preferred. Testing should be considered in those persons with risk factors such as receipt of a blood transfusion, receipt of immunizations with non-sterile needles, or multiple sexual partners. Those who have been diagnosed with another sexually transmitted infection should also be considered for testing. Any person with signs or symptoms suggestive of an immunodeficiency should be tested. In the US, consent must be obtained before testing for antibody to HIV. Immigrants should be afforded the same pre- and post-test counseling offered to non-immigrants. Management of those who test positive should be in consultation with specialists with expertise in the field.

**Hepatitis A** Universal screening for hepatitis A is not recommended, but those who are identified as infected with hepatitis B or C, who plan to travel to areas with a high risk of hepatitis A exposure, or who have other risk factors for hepatitis A disease, may be candidates for serotesting. Hepatitis A is an acute, self-limited disease in most cases; occasionally, fulminant hepatic disease develops but there is no chronic form of this infection. Immunization against hepatitis A is now part of the routine immunization schedule in the US. Many immigrants come from areas of high hepatitis A incidence and are immune; because the disease is generally mild in young children, a negative history does not rule out the possibility of prior exposure and immunity.[53]

**Helicobacter pylori** Universal screening for *Helicobacter pylori* is not recommended at this time. *H. pylori* is one of the most common bacterial infections in humans.[54] It has a wide geographic distribution and is found in all ages. Those in developing countries are infected at earlier ages and the prevalence in these areas is greater than in the developed world.[54] Most children in developing countries are infected before age 10 years and the prevalence in adults is greater than 80%. Overcrowding and lack of access to potable water are risk factors for early acquisition of this infection. The importance of *H. pylori* is its association with gastric cancer. About 40% of these cancers are attributable to this organism, resulting in as many as 350 000 cases of gastric cancer worldwide. Gastric lymphoma is also associated with *H. pylori*. The association with colon cancer remains controversial.

Noninvasive testing for *H. pylori* can be done by serology to detect IgG and IgA antibodies, stool antigen assays, and urea breath tests. All tests have acceptable sensitivity and specificity in adults but the breath test and serology are unreliable in children under 6 years of age. In older individuals, serologic tests may be of variable specificity due to geographic variability of strains of *H. pylori* requiring local validation of the tests used.[55] Endoscopy is the most accurate method of diagnosis and is appropriate in the setting of gastric ulcer, concern about lymphoma, those with alarming symptoms (anemia, GI bleeding, weight loss), and those over age 50. Because of the high prevalence of *H. pylori* in many countries, testing may be appropriate in individuals with compatible symptoms and those taking acid-suppressive medications for acid reflux disease. The association of *H. pylori* and dyspepsia remains controversial; for individuals from endemic areas with dyspepsia and positive serology or positive breath test, a trial of therapy seems appropriate.

Cost-effectiveness data for screening asymptomatic persons in the immigrant population are not available. At this time, when there is no universally accepted screening test, universal screening of asymptomatic immigrants cannot be supported. It may be reasonable to test adults with compatible clinical signs or symptoms arriving from the developing world where prevalence rates are high. Testing of internationally adopted children has been reviewed recently.[56] A high index of suspicion for disease was recommended, but universal screening was not felt to be appropriate until suitable screening tests become available.

**Cancer screening** Rates of specific types of cancer vary with geography and ethnic group, reflecting variation in risk factors related to environmental exposures, infectious diseases, and behaviors. For instance, stomach, liver, esophagus, and uterine cervix cancer are all more common in the developing world.[57] Routine screening recommended for the local population should be afforded to all immigrants. This may not be achieved during the initial health assessment visits but should be included in routine follow-up. Screening mammography, colonoscopy, and Pap smears should be provided to all persons regardless of their immigration status. As noted above, those with chronic hepatitis B infection require screening for hepatocellular carcinoma with serum alpha fetoprotein and liver ultrasound every 6 months. Those with hepatitis C and cirrhosis should have the same screening. Because these procedures are more invasive than most of the screening tests described above, and require detailed explanations of the purpose of the test, the process of testing, and, in some cases, of the preparation that needs to be done before the test, none of these tests is suitably done as part of the initial health assessment. Arrangements for these tests to be done should be made at appropriate times within the primary care setting, preferably allowing sufficient time to explain the testing in detail.

## Conclusion

Refugees, immigrants, and international adoptees arrive with multiple potential health problems that may be identified on initial history, examination, or laboratory evaluation. Some of these are of public health concern and some may pose barriers to the successful resettlement of individuals. Initial assessment should include a thorough review of all records available, including immunization records. A complete history and physical examination with attention to any areas identified in old records or current symptoms of the patient should be performed. Screening laboratory tests should include a complete blood count with white blood cell differential and red cell indices, serology for hepatitis B, lead level in children, urinalysis, and stool for ova and parasites. Tuberculin skin testing should be performed and immunizations should be updated as needed, based on current vaccine recommendations. All immigrants deserve access to healthcare consistent with the norms of the country of resettlement.

## References

1. Barnett ED. Infectious disease screening for refugees resettled in the United States. Clin Infect Dis 2004; 39:833–841.
2. Stauffer WM, Maroushek S, Kamat D. Medical screening of immigrant children. Clin Pediatr 2003; 42:763–773.
3. Stauffer WM, Kamat D, Walker PF. Screening of international immigrants, refugees, and adoptees. Prim Care Clin Office Pract 2002; 29:879–905.
4. Walker PF, Jaranson J. Refugee and immigrant healthcare. Med Clin North Am 1999; 83:1103–1120.
5. Department of Health and Human Services, Office of Refugee Resettlement. Medical screening protocol for newly arriving refugees. ORR state letter #95-37. Washington, DC: Department of Health and Human Services; 1995:1–8.
6. Department of Health and Human Services, Office of Refugee Resettlement. Guidelines regarding the use of RMA health screening programs. ORR state letter #04-10. Washington, DC: Department of Health and Human Services; 2004:1–2.
7. Geltman PL, Cochran J. A private-sector preferred provider network model for public health screening of newly resettled refugees. Am J Public Health 2005; 95:196–199.
8. Kennedy J, Seymour DJ, Hummel BJ. A comprehensive refugee health screening program. Public Health Rep 1999; 114:469–477.
9. Centers for Disease Control and Prevention. Recommended adult immunization schedule by vaccine and age group, United States October 2006–September 2007. http://www.cdc.gov/nip/recs/adult-schedule.pdf Accessed 2/16/07.
10. Centers for Disease Control and Prevention. Recommended immunization schedules for persons aged 0–18 years, United States 2007. http://www.cdc.gov/mmwr/preview/mmwrhtml/mm5551a7.htm?s_cid=mm5551a7_e Accessed 2/16/07.
11. Centers for Disease Control and Prevention. Catch-up immunization schedule for persons aged 4 months–18 years who start late or who are more than one month behind, United States 2007. http://www.cdc.gov/mmwr/preview/mmwrhtml/mm5551a7.htm?s_cid=mm5551a7_e Accessed 2/16/07.
12. Hayes EB, Talbot SB, Matheson ES, et al. Health status of pediatric refugees in Portland, Maine. Arch Pediatr Adolesc Med 1998; 152:564–568.
13. Meropol SB. Health status of pediatric refugees in Buffalo, New York. Arch Pediatr Adolesc Med 1995; 149:887–892.
14. Geltman PL, Radin M, Zhang Z, et al. Growth status and related medical conditions among refugee children in Massachusetts, 1995–1998. Am J Public Health 2001; 91:1800–1805.
15. Bloom BR. Tuberculosis – the global view. New Engl J Med 2002; 346:1434–1435.
16. Geng E, Kreiswirth B, Driver C, et al. Changes in the transmission of tuberculosis in New York City from 1990 to 1999. New Engl J Med 2002; 346:1453–1458.
17. Centers for Disease Control and Prevention. Recommendations for prevention and control of tuberculosis among foreign-born persons. MMWR 1998; 47(RR-16):1–35.
18. Adair R, Nwaneri MO. Communicable disease in African immigrants in Minneapolis. Arch Int Med 1999; 159:83–85.
19. Perez-Stable EJ, Slutkin G, Paz EA, et al. Tuberculin reactivity in United States and foreign-born Latinos: results of a community-based screening program. Am J Public Health 1986; 76:643–646.
20. Nelson KR, Bui H, Samet JH. Screening in special populations: a 'case study' of recent Vietnamese immigrants. Am J Med 1997; 102:435–440.
21. Goldenring JM, Davis J, McChesney M. Pediatric screening of Southeast Asian immigrants. Clinical Pediatrics 1982; 21:613–616.
22. Sarfaty M, Rosenberg Z, Siegel J, et al. Intestinal parasites in immigrant children from Central America. Western J Med 1983; 139:329–331.
23. Bass JL, Mehta KA, Eppes B. Parasitology screening of Latin American children in a primary care clinic. Pediatrics 1992; 89:279–283.
24. Friedman SM, DeSilva LP, Fox HE, et al. Hepatitis B screening in a New York City obstetrics service. Am J Public Health 1988; 78:308–310.
25. Lifson AR, Thai D, O'Fallon A, et al. Prevalence of tuberculosis, hepatitis B virus, and intestinal parasitic infections among refugees to Minnesota. Public Health Reports 2002; 117:69–77.
26. Verver S, Bwire R, Borgdorff. Screening for pulmonary tuberculosis among immigrants: estimated effect on severity of disease and duration of infectiousness. Int J Tuberc Lung Dis 2001; 5(5):419–425.
27. Centers for Disease Control and Prevention. Targeted tuberculin testing and treatment of latent tuberculosis infection. MMWR 2000; 49(RR-6):1–51.
28. Centers for Disease Control and Prevention. Guidelines for using the QuantiFERON®-TB Gold Test for detecting *Mycobacterium tuberculosis* infection, United States. MMWR 2005; 54(RR-15):49–55.
29. American Academy of Pediatrics. Tuberculosis. In: Pickering LK, ed. American Academy of Pediatrics. Red Book: 2006 Report of the Committee on Infectious Diseases. 27th edn. Elk Grove Village, IL: American Academy of Pediatrics; 2006:678–698.
30. American Academy of Pediatrics. Hepatitis B. In: Pickering LK, ed. American Academy of Pediatrics. Red Book: 2006 Report of the Committee on Infectious Diseases. 27th edn. Elk Grove Village, IL: American Academy of Pediatrics; 2006:335–355.
31. Hurie MB, Gennis MA, Hernandez LV, et al. Prevalence of hepatitis B markers and measles, mumps, and rubella antibodies among Jewish refugees from the former Soviet Union. JAMA 1995; 273:954–956.
32. Hurie MB, Mast EE, Davis JP. Horizontal transmission of hepatitis B virus infection to United States-born children of Hmong refugees. Pediatrics 1992; 89:269–273.
33. Entzel PP, Fleming LE, Trepka MJ, et al. The health status of newly arrived refugee children in Miami-Dade County, Florida. Am J Public Health 2003; 92(2):286–288.
34. Geltman PL, Cochran J, Hedgecock C. Intestinal parasites among African refugees resettled in Massachusetts and the impact of an overseas pre-departure treatment program. Am J Trop Med Hyg 2003; 69:657–662.
35. Rothenberg ME. Eosinophilia. N Engl J Med 1998; 338:1592–1600.
36. Gyorkos TW, MacLean JD, Law CG. Absence of significant differences in intestinal parasite prevalence estimates after exam of either one or two stool specimens. Am J Epidemiol 1989; 130:976–980.

37. Marti H, Koella JC. Multiple stool exams for ova and parasites and rate of false-negative results. J Clin Microbiol 1993; 31:3044–3045.

38. Muennig P, Pallin D, Sell RL, et al. The cost-effectiveness of strategies for the treatment of intestinal parasites in immigrants. N Engl J Med 1999; 340:773–779.

39. Centers for Disease Control and Prevention. Recommendations for the presumptive treatment of schistosomiasis and strongyloidiasis among the Lost Boys and Girls of Sudan and other Sudanese refugees. Available: http://www.cdc.gov/ncidod/dq/lostboysandgirlssudan/presumptive_tx_recc.htm March 25, 2006.

40. Nutman TB, Ottesen EA, Ieng S, et al. Eosinophilia in Southeast Asian refugees: evaluation at a referral center. J Infect Dis 1987; 155:309–313.

41. Seybolt LM, Christiansen D, Barnett ED. Diagnostic evaluation of newly arrived asymptomatic refugees with eosinophilia. Clin Infect Dis 2006; 42:363–367.

42. Maroushek SR, Aguilar EF, Stauffer W, et al. Malaria among refugee children at arrival in the United States. Pediatr Infect Dis J 2005; 24:450–452.

43. Huerga H, Lopez-Velez R. Infectious diseases in sub-Saharan African immigrant children in Madrid, Spain. Pediatr Infect Dis J 2002; 21:830–834.

44. Lopez-Velez R, Huerga H, Turrientes MC. Infectious diseases in immigrants from the perspective of a tropical medicine referral unit. Am J Trop Med Hyg 2003; 69:115–121.

45. Seys SA, Bender JA. The changing epidemiology of malaria in Minnesota. Emerg Infect Dis 2001; 7:993–995.

46. Geltman PL, Brown MJ, Cochran J. Lead poisoning among refugee children resettled in Massachusetts, 1995 to 1999. Pediatrics 2001; 108:158–162.

47. Centers for Disease Control and Prevention. Elevated blood lead levels in refugee children – New Hampshire, 2003–2004. MMWR 2005; 54:42–46.

48. Debonne JM, Nicand E, Boutin JP, et al. Hepatitis C in tropical areas. Med Trop 1999; 59(4 Pt 2):508–516.

49. Walsey A, Alter MJ. Epidemiology of hepatitis C: geographic differences and temporal trends. Semin Liver Dis 2000; 20:1–16.

50. American Academy of Pediatrics. Medical evaluation of internationally adopted children for infectious diseases. In: Pickering LK, ed. American Academy of Pediatrics. Red Book: 2006 Report of the Committee on Infectious Diseases. 27th edn. Elk Grove Village, IL: American Academy of Pediatrics; 2006:182–188.

51. Quinn K, Christiansen D, Barnett E, et al. Prevalence of hepatitis C virus infection in refugee children. Presented at the 7th Conference of the International Society of Travel Medicine, Innsbruck, Austria, May 2001. Program Volume 1, page 186.

52. Centers for Disease Control and Prevention. Recommendations regarding screening of refugee children for treponemal infection. MMWR 2005; 54(37):933–934.

53. American Academy of Pediatrics. Hepatitis A. In: Pickering LK, ed. American Academy of Pediatrics. Red Book: 2006 Report of the Committee on Infectious Diseases. 27th ed. Elk Grove Village, IL: American Academy of Pediatrics; 2006:326–335.

54. Pounder RE, Ng D. The prevalence of *Helicobacter pylori* infection in different countries. Ailment Pharmacol Ther 1995; 9(Suppl 2):33–39.

55. Suerbaum S, Michetti P. *Helicobacter pylori* infection. N Engl J Med 2002; 347(15):1175–1186.

56. Miller LC. *Helicobacter pylori*. In: Miller LC, editor. The handbook of international adoption. New York: Oxford University Press; 2005:286–291.

57. Parkin DM, Bray F, Ferlay J, et al. Global cancer statistics, 2002. CA Cancer J Clin 2005; 55:74–108.

# CHAPTER 13

# Immunizations for Immigrants

Elizabeth D. Barnett

## Introduction

Immigrants arrive in the US with a range of needs for immunizations. Some arrive with records indicating up-to-date immunizations; others have no records but have received multiple vaccines; still others enter the country with no recollection of having received vaccines. Many forces act to encourage and promote immunizations in the US: requirements for child care and school entry, occupational health requirements, provision of immunizations during health assessments for refugees, US immigration law requiring that internationally adopted children begin immunizations within 30 days of arrival in the US, and the requirement that review of the immunization record be part of the process of changing immigration status (obtaining a 'green card') in the US. Still, many immigrants without access to these systems may miss out on needed immunizations, and others, because of population mobility, lack of permanent or portable immunization documents, and lack of recognition of prior immunity, may be immunized for the same disease many times. Strategies to provide immunizations for immigrants ideally should be based on reliable data about prior immunizations and presence of antibody, risk of vaccine-preventable diseases, and should address existing health disparities.

Healthcare professionals must be prepared to evaluate foreign immunization documents and provide immigrant families with information about US immunization recommendations, including requirements for enrolling in childcare programs, school entry, and immigration. Knowledge of the relative merits of testing for antibody to vaccine-preventable diseases versus immediate immunization is also helpful in reducing the number of needless vaccines and appointments. In this chapter we describe the existing health disparities in immunizations relevant to immigrants, the process of reviewing overseas records, immunization recommendations for children and adults, screening for antibody versus immediate immunization, and future strategies for improving immunization rates in immigrants.

## Health Disparities and Risk of Vaccine-Preventable Diseases in Immigrants

Health disparities in immunizations can be assessed by comparing rates of vaccine-preventable diseases (VPDs), immunization coverage, or seroprevalence of antibody to vaccine-preventable diseases in selected populations to these rates in a reference population. Identifying where there is increased susceptibility to vaccine-preventable diseases is the first step in identifying priorities for immunization in the immigrant population.

Risk of disease is greater outside the US for many vaccine-preventable diseases. Endemic measles, rubella, and polio no longer occur in the US, and disease due to diphtheria and *Haemophilus influenzae* type b has been eliminated almost completely.[1-5] The fact that tetanus occurs only rarely in the US is a result of high vaccine coverage.[6] Varicella and pneumococcal disease in young children have been reduced by routine infant immunization.[7,8] Pertussis has been decreased significantly by infant immunization, though outbreaks continue to occur, especially in adolescents and adults.[9]

A number of vaccines given in the US are not administered routinely in other countries. Lack of widespread availability of *Haemophilus influenzae* type b (Hib) and hepatitis B vaccines was reflected in significant differences in vaccination coverage levels between foreign-born and US-born 19–35-month-old children in 1999–2000. For Hib, coverage rates were 87.2% in foreign-born children compared with 95% in the US-born; for > 3 doses of hepatitis B vaccine, rates were 73.6% for foreign-born and 89.4% for US-born children.[10] For adults, gaps exist in pneumococcal immunization rates among ethnic populations compared to the US general population. A survey of Cambodian and Vietnamese adults revealed rates of pneumococcal immunization below those of the US general population: 18% for the Cambodian group, 40% for the Vietnamese group, and 62% for the US general population.[11] Other vaccines given in the US that are not available routinely in some other countries include varicella, hepatitis A, and meningococcal vaccines. In early 2006, a vaccine against rotavirus was licensed in the United States for use in infants; a second vaccine is licensed in some other countries.[12,13] Immigrants are likely to have been exposed repeatedly to rotavirus in their countries of origin, as are most children and adults in the US. Current CDC recommendations call for immunizing all females at age 11–12 with human papillomavirus vaccine (http://www.cdc.gov/mmwr/preview/mmwrhtml/rr5602a1.htm?s_cid=rr5602a1_e).

Immigrants who have easy access to the US health system, children who attend public schools and therefore must meet immunization requirements to attend, and those who require immunizations to meet occupational requirements are likely to be offered catch-up immunization and may not differ from local populations in risk for vaccine-preventable diseases. Unfortunately, not all immigrants have easy access to healthcare. Undocumented status, language barriers, prohibitive costs, competing priorities, and lack of understanding of need for preventive health measures all may serve as barriers to adequate immunization. It is helpful to identify, where possible, the groups of immigrants that remain susceptible to VPDs, so that interventions can focus on decreasing meaningful disparities in immunization. Measuring disparities in vaccine coverage is the critical first step to informing public health policy around targeting specific groups for interventions. As discussed by Barker et al., statistically significant differences may not, however, be meaningful from a public health standpoint.[14] When public health programs are not practical or available to address health disparities in immunizations, the burden falls on the individual health professional. Individual practices may need to make special efforts to identify and immunize the young Hispanic woman against rubella, the elderly Cambodian gentleman against pneumococcal disease, and school-aged Somali children against hepatitis B. The following sections address differences in susceptibility to vaccine preventable-diseases in immigrants compared to US-born populations, and identify populations or groups at greatest risk of disease. These points are summarized in Table 13.1.

## Measles

There is at this time no endemic measles virus circulating in the United States and vaccine coverage appears to be sufficient to prevent sustained transmission of measles within the US. The gap in coverage with measles vaccine between white and nonwhite children was reduced from 18% in 1970 to 2% in the 1990s.[15] Measles cases that were imported or import-related accounted for 80% of the 216 measles cases reported in 2001–2003 in the United States.[16] The largest number of imported cases was from China or Japan and included cases in international visitors as well as US residents traveling abroad.[16] Internationally adopted children from China have been associated with outbreaks of measles that have resulted in documented transmission within the US.[17,18]

Most immigrants to the US will have received measles-containing vaccine or will have had natural infection with measles. In fact, foreign-born children from 19–35 months of age were significantly more likely to have received measles-containing vaccine than US-born children in one study.[10] High prevalence of measles antibody in immigrant groups has been documented in several studies, and is similar to the calculated population immunity of 93% in the US general population and the 91% prevalence of antibody in a study of 508 young blood donors (Table 13.2).[19-25] Older children and adults who arrive in the US without immunization records are unlikely to be susceptible to measles, but efforts to limit needless immunization suffer from inability to determine quickly and easily who has immunity to measles. Immigrants at highest risk of developing measles in the US are infants or other individuals who did not yet receive measles-containing vaccine, and who were exposed before departure for the US.

## Mumps

A dramatic reduction in cases of mumps in the US occurred, beginning in the early 1990s. Fewer than

### Table 13.1 Immunization issues for immigrants by disease

| Disease | Risk of contracting disease in the US compared to US-born population | Special considerations for immigrants and their contacts |
| --- | --- | --- |
| Measles | Same or decreased | Infants may be at increased risk of importing disease; assure protection of US-born who will have contact with immigrant infants |
| Mumps | Unknown | |
| Rubella | Increased in some groups | Assure protection of Hispanic individuals, especially those in the child-bearing years |
| Varicella | Increased in some groups | Serotesting cost-effective in most cases (especially older children and adults) before immunizing |
| Tetanus | Same or increased | Increased risk in some groups, such as Mexican-born and island populations |
| Diphtheria | Same or increased | Increased risk in some groups, such as Mexican-born |
| Hepatitis B | Increased | Immunize new arrivals after testing for disease; immunize household contacts of new arrivals |
| Polio | Unknown | Immigrants recently immunized with OPV may shed vaccine strain virus for some time after arrival in the US |
| Hepatitis A | Decreased in older individuals; may be increased in young children | Immunize household contacts of new arrivals |
| Pertussis | Unknown | |

### Table 13.2 Prevalence of antibody to measles, mumps, rubella, and varicella in selected immigrant groups and US reference populations

| | Reference number | Measles (%) | Mumps (%) | Rubella (%) | Varicella (%) |
| --- | --- | --- | --- | --- | --- |
| US reference population | 17,18 (measles) 24 (mumps) 29 (rubella) 39 (varicella) | 91–93% | 87.7 | 92 (6–11 yrs) 83 (12–19) 85 (20–29) ≥93 (≥40) | 86 (6–11 yrs) ≥99 (>40 yrs) |
| 669 refugees ages 0–20 | 19 | 82 | | 82 | 64 |
| Pregnant immigrant women in Ireland | 28 | | | 80.3 | 94.4 |
| 772 immigrants in Hawaii | 20 | Asian: 99 PI: 70 | | Asian: 97 PI: 73 | Asian: 84 PI: 82 |
| 70 internationally adopted children (Boston) | 21 | 90 | 66 | 79 | |
| 1392 adult immigrants in Montreal | 22 | 94 | 74 | 83 | 82 |
| 496 Jewish refugees from the former Soviet Union | 23 | 93 | 95 | 95 | |

PI, Pacific Islander.

300 cases of mumps were reported in the US each year until December 2005, when an outbreak of mumps began in the state of Iowa, spreading to involve more than 5000 individuals in 45 states as of October 2006.[26,26a] There are no data to suggest that a disproportionate number of cases occurred in immigrants. Mumps vaccine is not included in routine immunizations in many countries, though many individuals may be protected after natural disease. A serosurvey in US Navy and Marine Corps recruits measured an antibody prevalence of 87.7%.[27] Seroprevalence studies of several immigrant groups documented antibody to mumps in 66% of internationally adopted children, 74% of new immigrants to Canada, and 95% of Jewish refugees from the former Soviet Union.[23-25]

## Rubella

Elimination of endemic transmission of rubella in the United States was confirmed by an independent panel of experts convened in October 2004.[6] Since 1998, the majority of cases of rubella in the United States occurred in individuals born outside the country, mostly in the Western hemisphere. In 1998–1999, more than half of reported cases occurred in foreign-born individuals; for the 432 individuals for whom country of origin was known, 75% were born outside the US. Most cases occurred in individuals of Hispanic ethnicity.[28] In addition, almost all infants with congenital rubella syndrome (96% of 23 infants) in 1998–2000, and another affected infant born in 2005, were born to non-US-born women.[29,30] Rubella vaccine is not routine in many countries but many individuals are protected by immunity from disease. Seroprevalence data available from immigrants from several countries suggest that most individuals are protected (see Table 13.1).[21-25,31] For comparison, seroprevalence rates in the US have been reported as 92% in those ages 6–11, 83% in those 12–19, 85% in those 20–29 years, 89% in those 30–39 years, and > 93% in those > 40 years.[32] The imperative to prevent congenital rubella syndrome makes it important to assure the ability to identify and immunize susceptible immigrants, especially women in their child-bearing years.

## Tetanus and diphtheria

Fewer than 50 cases of tetanus are reported in the US each year. Since 1984, only three cases of neonatal tetanus have been reported; two in children of women born outside the US who had not received immunization with tetanus toxoid.[33] There was an average of 43 cases of tetanus reported each year in the US in 1998–2000; although incidence was higher in persons of Hispanic ethnicity, countries of origin of those infected were not reported.[34] Tetanus can be prevented only by immunization; immigrants who are not immunized by the time of arrival will not be protected by high immunization rates in the US.

Diphtheria is rare in the US with 53 cases reported from 1980 to 2001.[35] Risk of contracting diphtheria is likely higher for most immigrants in their country of origin than in the US. The National Immunization Survey of 1999–2000 reported that foreign-born children 19–35 months of age were less likely to have received four or more doses of tetanus- and diphtheria-containing vaccine.[10]

In a population-based serosurvey of tetanus immunity in the US as of 1988–1991, 69.7% of Americans > 6 years of age had protective levels of tetanus antibodies (>0.15 IU/mL), though Mexican-Americans had a significantly lower rate of immunity (57.9%) compared to non-Hispanic whites (72.7%) or non-Hispanic blacks (68.1%).[36] A small study of tetanus antibodies in adults > 65 years of age showed that 45% of those born outside the US had adequate antibody levels (>0.17 IU/mL) compared with 53% of those born in the US.[37] Subsequent serosurveys of tetanus and diphtheria antibodies from 1988 to 1994 continued to show that Mexican-American adults were less likely compared with the non-Hispanic white reference population to have protection against tetanus (66% versus 74%) and diphtheria (55% versus 60%).[38] A serosurvey of blood donors in Toronto showed that foreign-born individuals were more likely to be susceptible to diphtheria (27% versus 18%) and tetanus (27% versus 12%) than those born in Canada (Table 13.3).[39]

Limited seroprevalence data from refugees and internationally adopted children document a range of antibody levels.[23,40,41] Differences in testing methods and cutoff values chosen for various studies and lack of agreement on standardized cutoffs make comparison of results from different groups challenging. In the absence of simple and cost-effective ways to determine immunity to tetanus and diphtheria, healthcare professionals must be prepared to provide a complete three-dose primary series of tetanus toxoid to all, and to plan for boosters every 10 years throughout life. In the spring of 2005, two tetanus, diphtheria, and acellular pertussis (Tdap) vaccine products were licensed for use in adolescents and, for one product, adults.[42] For individuals age 11 and over who do not have a documented series of tetanus and diphtheria vaccine, it is recommended that one dose, preferably the first, of

**Table 13.3 Prevalence of antibody to polio, tetanus, and diphtheria in selected immigrant groups and US reference populations**

| | Reference number | Polio-1 | Polio-2 | Polio-3 | Tetanus | Diphtheria |
|---|---|---|---|---|---|---|
| US reference population | 96 (polio)<br>36 (tetanus)<br>38 (tetanus, diphtheria) | ≥95.0 | ≥95 | ≥92 | 69.7–72.3 | 60.5 (≥0.1 IU/mL) |
| 415 Kosovar refugee children ages 0–10 | 40 | 95.2 | 95.5 | 93 | | 68 (>0.1 IU/mL)<br>81 (>0.01 IU/mL) |
| 145 immigrant workers in Israel | 51 | 99.3 | 98.6 | 99.3 | | |
| Refugees in southern Italy (Kosovar and Kurds) | 41 | | | | | 45.2 ('full')<br>69.9 ('basic') |
| 70 internationally adopted children (Boston) | 23 | 58 | 65 | 62 | 61 | 88 |

the series be Tdap. For those who have completed a primary series, it is recommended that the adolescent booster dose be Tdap, as long as at least 2 years have passed since the most recent dose of DTaP, DTP, or Td.[42] Adults may be given a dose of Tdap to replace one of their usual Td boosters.[42a]

## Varicella

Before introduction of varicella vaccine in the US, a large (21 288 participants) serosurvey of varicella antibody found that 86% of children 6–11 years of age and > 99% of those 40 years of age or older were seropositive. Non-Hispanic black children were 40% less likely to be seropositive compared with white children.[43] Varicella transmission has decreased in the US since initiation of routine childhood immunization.[7] Outbreaks continue to occur, and risk to immigrants will be related directly to whether they are immune to varicella when they arrive in the country. Seroprevalence studies indicate that although the majority of immigrants show evidence of antibody to varicella, some groups, especially those from the hottest parts of the tropics, or living in isolated communities before emigration, may be more likely to lack sufficient antibody.[21,24,44] A study in military recruits found that those enlisting from outside the continental US, especially those from island territories, were less likely to have antibody to varicella.[27] Seroprevalence data for selected immigrant groups are listed in Table 13.3.

Because some immigrants may be at increased risk of varicella, especially those from isolated rural areas or from tropical areas with high ambient temperatures, healthcare providers will need to assure varicella immunity, by vaccination or serotesting, in all new arrivals.

## Hepatitis B

Rates of infection with hepatitis B are well known to be higher in many countries outside the United States (see Ch. 22; Hepatitis B). Immigrants who live in the US may be at greater risk of acquiring hepatitis B due to increased exposure to infected relatives or household members from countries with higher rates of hepatitis B infection, and because they may be less likely to have received hepatitis B vaccine. The greater problem, though, is the number of immigrants who arrive in the US already infected with hepatitis B (Table 13.4). Almost half (8/19) of acute hepatitis B cases in children and adolescents ages 0–19 reported in 2001–2002 were born outside the US; six cases were in internationally adopted children.[45] Hepatitis B infection occurs overall in about 5–7% of internationally adopted children, though higher rates have been reported, especially in adoptees from Romania.[46] Risk also may be greater in older adoptees and those adopted from countries in Asia and sub-Saharan Africa, especially where hepatitis B vaccine is not administered. Immigrant groups at increased risk of hepatitis B include those

**Table 13.4 Hepatitis B status of selected immigrant groups**

| | Reference number | HBsAg positive (%) | HBsAb or HbcoreAb (%) |
|---|---|---|---|
| 310 immigrant women in Sicily | 100 | 4.2 | 24.5 |
| 132 refugee children in Maine | 99 | 4 | 21 |
| 107 refugee children in Buffalo, New York | 98 | 7 | 43 |
| 2545 refugees, Minnesota | 97 | 7 | 37 – HBsAb*<br>36 – HbcAb* |
| 96 adult Vietnamese immigrants | 101 | 13 | 83 |
| 496 Jewish refugees from the former Soviet Union | 25 | 0.4 | 22 |

* Percentages of those who were HBsAg negative.

**Table 13.5 Screening for hepatitis B, interpretation of results, and suggested immunization action**

| Hepatitis B tests | Results | Interpretation | Action |
|---|---|---|---|
| Surface antibody<br>Core antibody<br>Surface antigen | Negative<br>Negative<br>Negative | Susceptible | Offer vaccine |
| Surface antibody<br>Core antibody<br>Surface antigen | Positive<br>Negative<br>Negative | Immune (from vaccine or disease)<br>OR<br>maternal antibody | No vaccine needed<br><br>Retest to assess loss of maternal antibody |
| Surface antibody<br>Core antibody<br>Surface antigen | Positive<br>Positive<br>Negative | Immune (from vaccine or disease)<br>OR<br>maternal antibody | No vaccine needed<br><br>Retest to assess loss of maternal antibody |
| Surface antibody<br>Core antibody<br>Surface antigen | Negative<br>Negative<br>Positive | Chronic infection or carrier | No vaccine needed<br>Immunize household and other contacts |
| Surface antibody<br>Core antibody<br>Surface antigen | Negative<br>Positive<br>Positive | Acute or chronic infection | No vaccine needed<br>Immunize household and other contacts |
| Surface antibody<br>Core antibody<br>Surface antigen | Negative<br>Positive<br>Negative | Recovering from acute infection*<br>OR<br><br>Immune; surface antibody BDL*<br>OR<br>False positive core antibody: susceptible*<br>OR<br>Chronic infection; undetectable HBsAg*<br>OR<br>Maternal antibody* | No vaccine needed<br><br><br>No vaccine needed<br><br>Vaccine needed<br><br>No vaccine needed |

* Five possible interpretations for these findings; repeat testing may help clarify the situation.
BDL, below detectable limits; HBsAg, hepatitis B surface antigen.

from Asia and sub-Saharan Africa. For this reason, it is important to screen individuals from such groups for hepatitis B infection before immunizing (Table 13.5).

Protection against hepatitis B is especially important in immigrant communities with increased rates of hepatitis B infection. In addition, identification of those who are infected is important because it may identify those eligible for treatment or monitoring for chronic liver disease and liver cancer, as well as identify opportunities for prevention of transmission. Strategies to improve immunization coverage in these groups must address the context in which the disease is perceived, and must be undertaken with attention to factors that may serve as barriers to acceptance of vaccine.[47-49] Cost is also cited as a common barrier to completion of the hepatitis B vaccine series. In some states, such as Massachusetts, state funds are available to pay for hepatitis B vaccine provided to high-risk contacts.

## Polio

Endemic transmission of polio no longer occurs in the US, though a recent outbreak in an unimmunized community emphasizes the importance of maintaining high vaccine coverage.[50] Because oral polio vaccines remain in use in many parts of the world, vaccine strains of virus will continue to enter the US because of shedding of virus for a period of time following oral administration of vaccine. There is also the possibility of importation of wild-type strains of poliovirus by those arriving from areas that continue to have endemic wild-type disease. Outside the international adoption literature, there are few serosurveys of immigrant protection against polio in US immigrants, though serosurveys have been done of Kosovar children resettling in Italy and immigrant workers in Israel (see Table 13.1).[23,40,51] Many countries, however, participate in polio eradication campaigns, and immigrants are likely to have received immunization against polio. Foreign-born children between 19 and 35 months of age were as likely as US-born children to have received three or more doses of poliovirus vaccine.[10] All immigrants should receive a primary series of three doses of vaccine, with a booster in adulthood if traveling to an area of endemic polio.

## Hepatitis A

Immigrants may be candidates for hepatitis A vaccine either because they resettle in an area where this vaccine is recommended, they have another health problem such as hepatitis B infection for which hepatitis A vaccine is recommended, or they meet other criteria for which hepatitis A vaccine is recommended. In the prevaccine-era in the US (before 1995), serologic evidence of hepatitis A varied by age and ethnicity: prevalence was 9% in those 6–11 years, 19% for those 20–29 years, 33% for those 40–49 years, and 75% in those > 70 years of age. Prevalence was highest among Mexican-Americans (70%) compared with non-Hispanic blacks (39%) and non-Hispanic whites (23%).[52] Since

the late 1990s, hepatitis A rates have declined more rapidly in children than adults, and have become similar in all age groups. Racial/ethnic differences in rates have narrowed, but rates remain higher in Hispanics than non-Hispanics.[52a] Immigrants, especially those born and raised in developing countries, are likely to have been infected in childhood and are more likely to be immune to hepatitis A than US-born individuals. Seroprevalence studies of immunity to hepatitis A show that many immigrants are immune to hepatitis A: 87% of 1392 recently arrived adult immigrants to Canada had evidence of hepatitis A antibody.[24] Two studies of hepatitis immunity in adult patients seen for pre-travel consultation documented presence of antibody in 95% (Boston) and 80% (Honolulu) of those tested.[53,54] Cost-effectiveness studies show consistently that testing for hepatitis A antibody before initiating the two-dose vaccine series is cost-effective when prevalence of antibody to hepatitis A exceeds about 30%, a value exceeded in many immigrant groups.[54-56]

In 1999, the Immunization Practices Advisory Committee (ACIP) expanded recommendations for hepatitis A vaccination in the US to include routine immunization of children in states, counties, and communities with rates of infection > 20 cases per 100 000 population, and considering immunization in areas where rates were between 10 and 20 cases per 100 000 population.[52] In 2005, the ACIP voted to recommend universal immunization of children 12–23 months of age with hepatitis A vaccine.[57] All hepatitis A vaccines now available in the US are licensed for use beginning at 1 year of age.

Most immigrants, therefore, are likely to be at lower risk of hepatitis A in the US than they were in their country of origin, with the exception of those arriving from countries with lower rates of hepatitis A than the US. Special attention, however, needs to be paid to a few categories of immigrants, or of those who have close contact with immigrants, in order to provide optimal protection. First, children of migrant workers, especially those living along the US–Mexico border who travel frequently to their parents' country of origin, are at increased risk of hepatitis A.[58] A position paper prepared by the Migrant Clinician's Network outlines recommended strategies for addressing risk of hepatitis A in migrant health workers and their families.[59] Second, families who adopt children from overseas may be at increased risk of hepatitis A. Hepatitis A has been transmitted from an internationally adopted child to a family member.[60] Clinicians caring for internationally adopted children and their families may want to offer protection against hepatitis A as well as other

**Table 13.6  Resources about immunizations of special value for immigrant health**

| Information | URL |
| --- | --- |
| Childhood immunization schedule | http://www.cdc.gov/nip/recs/child-schedule.htm#Printable |
| Adult immunization schedule | http://www.cdc.gov/nip/ress/adult-schedule.htm |
| Catch-up immunization schedule | http://www.cdc.gov/nip/recs/child-schedule.htm#catchup. |
| Vaccine requirements for immigrant applicants | http://www.cdc.gov/ncidod/dq/pdf/TI.pdf. |
| Vaccination requirements for internationally adopted children | http://travel.state.gov/pdf/DS-1981.pdf. |
| Vaccine requirements for change of immigration status | http://www.cdc.gov/ncidod/dq/pdf/ti-03/appdx-a_693vacc.pdf |
| Translation of vaccine terms from English into other languages | http://www.immunize.org/izpractices/p5122.pdf |
| Translation of vaccine terms from other languages into English | http://www.immunize.org/izpractices/p5121.pdf |
| Vaccine names used worldwide | http://www.immunize.org/izpractices/p5120.pdf<br>http://www.immunization-sd.org/docs/iz78.pdf |
| General immunization information | http://www.immunize.org<br>http://www.cdc.gov/nip |

vaccine-preventable diseases before the adoption.[61,62] Lastly, the youngest immigrants as well as children of immigrants who have never visited their parents' countries of origin may be at increased risk of hepatitis A when they return to visit relatives and friends.[63] Clinicians caring for immigrant families may want to maintain awareness of travel plans and be prepared to offer appropriate vaccines at this time (see Ch. 58; Visiting Friends and Relatives).

## Sources of Information on Vaccine Requirements

Immunization schedules for children are updated regularly by the Immunization Practices Advisory Committee (ACIP) and publicized widely (Table 13.6). The most current schedule can be accessed at http://www.cdc.gov/nip/recs/child-schedule.htm#Printable. Adult immunization has received increased attention lately as a means to prevent both acute disease (influenza, for example) and diseases that have long-term sequelae (hepatitis B). Adult immunization schedules are also updated as needed, and the most recent version is available at http://www.cdc.gov/nip/recs/adult-schedule.pdf

Immigrants may have needs related to immunization that go beyond those experienced by the native-born population. Immigrants may arrive without having received vaccines in the routine US immunization schedules, such as varicella, *Haemophilus influenzae* type b, and meningococcal vaccines. It is helpful for professionals caring for immigrant patients to have access to the catch-up schedules published by CDC and available at: http://www.cdc.gov/nip/recs/child-schedule.htm#catchup

Documentation of immunizations and providing a durable and permanent record of vaccines to the recipient is critical. The first step is to transcribe all vaccines given overseas onto the US record (see below: Evaluation of Overseas Immunization Documents). Only written documentation of vaccines received should be accepted. The requirements for immunizations by category of immigrant are complex, and it is important to recognize that not all categories of immigrants are required to receive immunizations before arriving in the US. Those applying outside the US for immigrant visas are required to be up to date for the immunizations available in the country from which they are applying. Refugees are not required to have any vaccines before resettlement, and parents of internationally adopted children sign a waiver agreeing to initiate immunizations within 30 days of arrival in the US. For those who would like to review the recommendations in detail, the following links may be helpful: http://www.cdc.gov/ncidod/dq/pdf/TI.pdf (for immigrant visas), and http://travel.state.gov/pdf/DS-1981.pdf (for internationally adopted children). Finally, immigrants requesting immunizations for change in immigration status ('green card' application) will need to have an immunization document completed by a Civil Surgeon. Immunization requirements for change of immigration status are based on ACIP recommendations; the form is available at http://www.cdc.gov/ncidod/dq/pdf/ti-03/appdx-a_693vacc.pdf.

## Evaluation of Overseas Immunization Documents

Immigrants may arrive in the US with vaccine records though the records may need to be trans-lated or may contain names of vaccines unfamiliar in the US. Translations of records should be done by those familiar with medical terminology; care should be taken to avoid transposing month and day when transcribing records from many countries outside the US. Resources available for evaluating these records include a list of translations of vaccine-preventable disease terms into other languages (http://www.immunize.org/izpractices/p5122.pdf) and a table that can aid in translating foreign records into English (http://www.immunize.org/izpractices/p5121.pdf). Because trade names of vaccines differ in other countries, components of combination vaccines should be checked carefully. The Immuniza-tion Action Coalition and several state and local health departments have developed lists of vaccine names available worldwide for reference. These resources are available at: http://www.immunize.org/izpractices/p5120.pdf and http://www.immunization-sd.org/docs/iz78.pdf. Entering the name of the unfamiliar vaccine into an internet search engine often yields helpful information as well.

It is almost always possible to accept as valid immunization doses given at appropriate ages and intervals and documented in an apparently valid written record.[64] Care should be taken to note any vaccines documented in the record that do not meet the ACIP requirements. The most common example is measles or measles-containing vaccine given before 1 year of age; a child now residing in the US will still require two doses of vaccine given after 1 year of age, or documentation of presence of measles antibody.

Concerns about falsification of vaccine records and other discrepancies between vaccine records and immunity to vaccine-preventable diseases have been raised with regard to records of internationally adopted children.[65,66] Schulte and colleagues evaluated acceptability and completeness of overseas records for 504 internationally adopted children, of whom 35% had written immunization records. Ninety-four percent of records were valid (had dates of administration and no doses recorded before the child's date of birth) and recorded vaccine doses that were acceptable and up to date by current immunization schedules. Three records (<1%) had one or more doses given before the date of birth.[67] Although in most cases it will be appropriate to accept records for internationally adopted children, healthcare practitioners may at times have to use their best judgment, or call upon the expertise of those familiar with the international adoption process, to assess these records.

## Relationship between immunization documents and prevalence of antibody

The most detailed work to date examining the relationship between documented vaccines and presence of antibody has been done in the community of internationally adopted children.[65] Concern about protection of internationally adopted children against diseases for which they had documentation of immunization was raised in 1998 when data on 26 adoptees from China, Russia, and Eastern Europe were presented. Investigators compared children adopted from orphanages with children adopted from noninstitutional settings, primarily family-based foster care. Protective titers to diphtheria and tetanus were found in only 12% of children living in orphanages who had received three or more doses of DPT vaccine; 78% of the nine children living in foster homes had protection against the two diseases. The authors speculated on a number of reasons for their results: falsification of records, decreased potency of vaccine distributed to orphanages, and poor immune response due to prolonged institutionalization.[68] Based on these findings, the American Academy of Pediatrics (AAP) supported repeating previously documented immunizations if validity of vaccine records was in question.[69]

Protection against disease in relation to receipt of vaccine in internationally adopted children has been discussed in subsequent papers. A 1999 report documented suboptimal protection against polio vaccine in four children adopted from Lithuania, Russia, and China.[70] Subsequent work by the same investigator explored the possible relationship between nutritional status and vaccine response and differences in response to vaccines administered in orphanages compared with those given to children living in the community. Although lack of antibody ranged from 3% for tetanus and diphtheria to 50% for pertussis, no relation was found between presence of antibody and nutritional status (as measured by Z-scores for height, weight, and head circumference), residence in an orphanage, or medical problems of the child, including presence of parasitic infections, anemia, rickets, or positive tuberculin skin test. The authors proposed measuring antibody to vaccine-preventable diseases as a method of guiding decisions about immunization of international adoptees.[71] Subsequent studies of the correlation between vaccine records and presence of protective antibody in internationally adopted children have yielded conflicting results. Different cutoff values and methods used to detect antibody add to the challenge of comparing results from different studies. A study from the Netherlands documented antibody levels to tetanus and diphtheria similar to those from Dutch children in adoptees from all countries except China, and suboptimal levels of antibody to diphtheria, tetanus, and polio in 98 children adopted from China. The authors recommended testing for antibody in children adopted from China, but could not recommend repeating vaccines without testing because of unknown long-term consequences of repeated immunizations.[72] Most internationally adopted children from 11 countries evaluated in Cincinnati who had documentation of two or more doses of DTP and hepatitis B vaccines were found to be protected adequately against diphtheria, tetanus, and hepatitis B. The authors identified measurement of antibody as a useful method of assuring proper immunization and avoiding excess doses of vaccine.[73]

Few comparable data exist comparing documented immunizations and prevalence of antibody in other immigrant populations. A comparison of antibody prevalence in refugees with documented immunization showed that 96% of 51 individuals immunized against measles had antibody as measured by commercial ELISA; corresponding figures for rubella and varicella were 90% of 51 and 70% of 27, respectively (Michael Sylvia, personal communication, 2005). A seroprevalence study of 772 Asian and Pacific Islander immigrants to Hawaii documented antibody to measles in 89% of those with documented receipt of vaccine; antibody to rubella and varicella was 95% and 66%, respectively, in those who were immunized against rubella and varicella.[22]

## Risk of vaccine-preventable diseases in US-born family members and contacts of recent immigrants

The potential for transmission of vaccine preventable diseases from immigrants to those residing in the US is of public health concern. In general, this is a rare occurrence, but certain individuals who have close contact with immigrants may be at increased risk. Horizontal transmission of hepatitis B has been described in Southeast Asian refugees after resettlement in the US.[74] Family members of internationally adopted children are at risk of contracting vaccine-preventable diseases from these children. Measles, hepatitis A, and hepatitis B have been transmitted to caretakers of internationally adopted children.[17,18,60,75-78] In most cases, transmission occurred because of either failure to provide appropriate immunizations to US-based family members and close contacts of the new arrivals, or failure of healthcare professionals to screen or to treat those with infectious diseases upon arrival in the US. The potential for spread of imported diseases is a reminder to healthcare providers to be vigilant about immunization coverage for all adult and pediatric patients. Screening and treating immigrants for transmissible infectious diseases, especially those such as hepatitis B that may not be evident clinically, at their initial health assessment will decrease risk of disease transmission after arrival (see Ch. 11).

## Risks due to excess immunization

Repeating immunizations is generally safe, though it is recommended that children receive no more than six doses each of tetanus and diphtheria toxoids before age 7 years because of the potential for local and systemic adverse events.[79,80] Similarly, administration of more than two doses of pneumococcal polysaccharide vaccine is not recommended due to insufficient data on rates of adverse events following three or more vaccine doses.[81] The major deterrents to repeating immunizations may be the extra costs and healthcare visits required as well as the pain associated with injections.[82] Finally, in an era of unpredictable vaccine supply and periodic vaccine shortages, judicious use of vaccine resources is the most prudent approach.

## Acceptability of multiple vaccines at a single visit

Concern about potential harm due to multiple simultaneously administered vaccines is not new. One study reported that physicians had more concerns than parents about administration of multiple vaccines. The primary concern of both parents and pediatricians was pain.[83] Another study reported that parents overwhelmingly agreed for their child to receive multiple immunizations when recommended by their child's doctor.[84] Recent data indicate that deferral of vaccine doses may be associated with delayed immunization by age 2.[85] These findings emphasize the importance of pain management during vaccine administration along with the importance of providing all needed vaccines at the time they are due.

## Cost-Effectiveness of Screening Versus Immunization

Cost-effectiveness studies are helpful in informing providers whether testing or repeating immunizations is the most appropriate strategy for specific vaccines in specific populations. One study examining screening refugees for varicella antibody demonstrated cost-effectiveness of screening children 5 years of age and older before immunizing.[86] A recent study examined the least costly strategy among vaccination versus screening then vaccination for hepatitis A and B, varicella, measles, and tetanus vaccines in adults and adolescents in Catalonia. Only for varicella and for hepatitis A in adults > 24 years of age was screening then vaccination less costly.[55] The model proposed in this study is particularly applicable to immigrant populations when seroprevalence of antibody is known. It is worth noting that the seroprevalence at which serotesting for hepatitis B becomes cost-effective for adults is 27% in this study; a rate that is exceeded by some immigrant groups. It should be kept in mind, however, that hepatitis B represents a special case in which immunizing without testing is not recommended for immigrants, especially those from countries with high rates of hepatitis B, due to the importance of identifying those who are already infected. Finally, an economic analysis of testing versus presumptively immunizing internationally adopted and immigrant infants determined that serotesting for polio increased cost per patient and decreased the proportion of infants protected against polio, while serotesting for diphtheria and tetanus increased the cost per patient and also increased the proportion of patients protected against both diseases.[87] Cost-effectiveness studies are unavailable for other scenarios involving internationally adopted children and immigrants and for other vaccines.

## Recommendations for immunization of immigrants

Current approaches to immunizing immigrants include the following options: (1) repeating or administering all doses of vaccines when immunization records are unavailable or cannot be relied upon; (2) accepting as valid immunizations for which there is documentation of doses of vaccines administered according to current US vaccine schedules and administering or repeating all others; and (3) judicious use of serotesting to assess presence of antibody to selected vaccine-preventable diseases and making decisions about what vaccines to administer based on these results.[88] Primary care providers determining the best approach to completing a patient's immunizations will need to consider the number of doses of vaccines needed if all doses are given or repeated, number of visits required to administer these doses, availability of serologic tests, costs of testing, and barriers to childcare, school, or job initiation while awaiting test results. The risk of contracting a vaccine-preventable disease while completing immunizations may also be a factor, though few data exist that allow quantification of risk of disease while awaiting serologic results and subsequent immunization of those who are not protected.

Table 13.7 lists options for immunization and serologic testing for specific antibodies by vaccine. These options can be discussed with the patient or parent and the best option chosen for the individual. Schedules for catch-up immunization are listed in Table 13.8.

## Relationship between response to vaccine and stress/nutritional status

The relationship between stress, nutritional status, and response to immunization is receiving international attention. Psychological status and recent stress were related to immune response to vaccination in a study of healthy young women.[89] In malnourished children, secretory IgA antibody was delayed in appearance and did not achieve levels

**Table 13.7 Recommended and alternative approaches to immunizations for immigrants by vaccine**

| Vaccine | | Recommended (R) and alternative (A) approaches | | Supporting information and reference number(s) | Comments |
|---|---|---|---|---|---|
| Hepatitis B | R | Test for HBsAg, HBsAb, and HBcoreAb before immunizing. If HBsAg positive, no vaccine needed. If HBsAb positive, complete series; no additional vaccine if three doses. If HBcoreAb positive, may have acute, resolved, or chronic infection | R | Consensus regarding screening for hepatitis B[88]. Testing before immunizing may be cost-effective in populations where there is a high prevalence of infection and immunity to hepatitis B[55] | Individuals with HBsAg require additional evaluation to assess status of infection[102]. Those with < three documented doses who are screened and have positive results for HBsAb still must complete the series for long-term protection. Provide immunization for families of internationally adopted children |
| | A | Begin vaccine series at the same time as sending above tests; continue or stop vaccine accordingly | | | |
| DTP, DTaP, Td, Tdap | R | Continue age-appropriate immunizations; test for antibody to tetanus and diphtheria toxoids if severe local reaction | R | Severe local reactions may be related to high antibody concentrations at the time of immunization[79] | Serologic tests may not be available in all areas. Assessment of pertussis immunity not available[103]. Single antigen pertussis vaccine not available; must give DTaP to protect against pertussis in children <7 years of age. Children adopted from China may be at increased risk for lack of protective antibody against tetanus and diphtheria[72]. Single dose of Tdap can be given to those ≥11 years[42,42a] |
| | A₁ | Test for antibody to tetanus and diphtheria toxoids before immunizing | R | Most individuals with ≥ three doses documented will have protection against diphtheria and tetanus[71–73] | |
| | A₂ | Administer single dose, then test in one month; if non-immune, continue vaccine per schedule; if immune, provide booster doses per current recommendations | | | |
| | A₃ | Repeat all doses without screening when serologic testing is not available and receipt of immunologic vaccine cannot be assured | | | |

| | | | | |
|---|---|---|---|---|
| Polio | R | Accept documented doses of vaccine and complete immunization with IPV per recommended schedule | | Serologic tests may not be available in all areas<br>Cost of testing may be prohibitive<br>No consensus about number of additional doses needed if antibody lacking for ≤ three serotypes |
| | A | For children with ≥ three doses, measure antibody to polioviruses types 1, 2, and 3<br>OR<br>Give single dose IPV and then measure antibody to poliovirus types 1,2, and 3.<br>If antibody present to all three serotypes, complete immunization with IPV per recommended schedule. If antibody absent consider repeating the series. | | |
| MMR | R | Age-appropriate immunization with MMR | A | Serotesting unlikely to be cost-effective[55] Two doses of MMR are recommended by the AAP[105] | Special outreach for Hispanic women in childbearing years is appropriate to assure protection against rubella[28]<br>Provide documentation of immunity in durable, permanent immunization record; otherwise patient may face barriers to childcare and school entry if fewer than the required number of MMR doses are documented |
| | A | Test for all three antibodies and immunize accordingly | | |
| Varicella | R | Serologic testing followed by age-appropriate immunization if antibody negative | R | Cost-effectiveness of serotesting documented for specific groups (refugees 5 years of age and older; groups with high antibody prevalence)[55,86] | Provide documentation of immunity or presence of varicella scars in durable, permanent immunization record; otherwise patient may face barriers to childcare and school entry or bureaucratic documents if fewer than the required number of doses are documented |
| | R | Age-appropriate immunization | R | History of varicella may be less reliable in immigrants[106] | |
| | R | If scarring due to previous varicella infection present no vaccine needed | | |
| *Haemophilus influenzae* type b | R | Age-appropriate immunization | | | Foreign-born children less likely to have age-appropriate immunization[10] |
| Pneumococcus | R | Age-appropriate immunization | | | |
| Hepatitis A | R | Age-appropriate immunization for infants and young children | R | Cost-effective to test before immunizing in older individuals from high-prevalence areas[54-56] | Protect household members and close contacts of internationally adopted children, migrant workers, and other newly arriving immigrants[58-60] |
| | R | Serotesting before immunization for older individuals from high-prevalence countries | | |

**Table 13.8 Catch-up immunization schedule for persons aged 4 months–18 years who start late or who are ≥1 month behind – United States, 2007**

The table below provides catch-up schedules and minimum intervals between doses for children whose vaccinations have been delayed. A vaccine series does not need to be restarted, regardless of the time that has elapsed between doses. Use the section appropriate for the child's age.

| Vaccine | Minimum age for Dose 1 | Catch-up schedule for persons aged 4 months–6 years | | | |
|---|---|---|---|---|---|
| | | Minimum interval between doses | | | |
| | | Dose 1 to dose 2 | Dose 2 to dose 3 | Dose 3 to dose 4 | Dose 4 to dose 5 |
| Hepatitis B[1] | Birth | 4 weeks | 8 weeks (and 16 weeks after first dose) | | |
| Rotavirus[2] | 6 weeks | 4 weeks | 4 weeks | | |
| Diphtheria, tetanus, Pertussis[3] | 6 weeks | 4 weeks | 4 weeks | 6 months | 6 months[3] |
| Haemophilus influenzae type b[4] | 6 weeks | 4 weeks If first dose administered at age <12 months 8 weeks (as final dose) If first dose administered at age 12–14 months No further doses needed If first dose administered at age ≤15 months | 4 weeks[4] If current age <12 months 8 weeks (as final dose)[4] If current age ≤12 months and second dose administered at age <15 months No further doses needed If precious dose administered at age ≤15 months | 8 weeks (as final dose) This dose only necessary for children aged 12 months–5 years who received 3 doses below age 12 months | |
| Pneumococcal[5] | 6 weeks | 4 weeks If first dose administered at age <12 months and current age <24 months 8 weeks (as final dose) If first dose administered at age ≤12 months or current age 24–59 months No further doses needed for healthy children if first dose administered at age ≤24 months | 4 weeks If current age <12 months 8 weeks (as final dose) If current age ≤12 months No further doses needed for healthy children if previous dose administered at age ≤24 months | 8 weeks (as final dose) This dose only necessary for children aged 12 months–5 years who received 3 doses below age 12 months | |
| Inactivated Poliovirus[6] | 6 weeks | 4 weeks | 4 weeks | 4 weeks[6] | |
| Measles, Mumps, Rubella[7] | 12 months | 4 weeks | | | |
| Varicella[8] | 12 months | 3 months | | | |
| Hepatitis A[9] | 12 months | 6 months | | | |

## Catch-up schedule for persons aged 7–18 years

| Vaccine | Minimum age for Dose 1 | Minimum interval between doses | | | |
|---|---|---|---|---|---|
| | | Dose 1 to dose 2 | Dose 2 to dose 3 | Dose 3 to dose 4 | Dose 4 to dose 5 |
| Tetanus, diphtheria Tetanus, Diphtheria, | 7 years[10] | 4 weeks | 8 weeks If first administered at age <12 months | 6 months If first dose administered at age <12 months | |
| Pertussis[10] | | | 6 months If first dose administered at age ≤12 months | | |
| Human Papillomavirus[11] | 9 years | 4 weeks | 12 weeks | | |
| Hepatitis A[1] | 12 months | 6 months | | | |
| Hepatitis B[1] | Birth | 4 weeks | 8 weeks (and 16 weeks after first dose) | | |
| Inactivated Poliovirus[6] | 6 weeks | 4 weeks | 4 weeks | 4 weeks[6] | |
| Measles, Mumps, Rubella[7] | 12 months | 4 weeks | | | |
| Varicella[8] | 12 months | 4 weeks If first dose administered at age ≤13 years 3 months If first dose administered at age <13 years | | | |

[1] **Hepatitis B vaccine (MepB).** *(Minimum age: Birth)*
- Administer the 3-dose series to those who were not previously vaccinated.
- A 2-dose series of Recombivax HB® is licensed for children age 11–15 years.

[2] **Rotavirus vaccine (Rota).** *(Minimum age: 6 weeks)*
- Do not start the series later than age 12 weeks.
- Administer the final dose in the series by age 32 weeks. Do not administer a dose later that age 32 weeks.
- Data on safety and efficacy outside of these age ranges are insufficient.

[3] **Diphtheria and tetanus toxoids and acellular pertussis vaccine (DTaP).** *(Minimum age: 6 weeks)*
- The fifth dose is not necessary if the fourth dose was administered at age ≤4 years.
- DTaP is not indicated for persons aged ≤7 years.

[4] **Haemophilus influenzae type b conjugate vaccine (Hib).** *(Minimum age: 6 weeks)*
- Vaccine is not generally recommended for children aged ≤5 years.
- If current age <12 months and the first 2 doses were PRP-OMP (PedvaxHIB® or Comvax® [Merck], the third (and final) dose should be administered at age 12–15 months and at least 8 weeks after the second dose.
- If first dose was administered at age 7–11 months. administer 2 doses separated by 4 weeks plus a booster at age 12–15 months.

[5] **Pneumococcal conjugate vaccine (PCV).** *(Minimum age: 6 weeks)*
- Vaccine is not generally recommended for children aged ≤5 years.

[6] **Inactivated poliovirus vaccine (IPV).** *(Minimum age: 6 weeks)*
- For Children who received an all-IPV or all-oral poliovirus (OPV) series, a fourth dose is not necessary if third dose was administered at age ≤4 years.
- If both OPC and IPV were administered as part of a series, a total of 4 doses should be administered, regardless of the child's current age.

[7] **Measles, mumps, and rubella vaccine (MMR).** *(Minimum age: 12 months)*
- The second dose of MMR is recommended routinely at age 4–6 years but may be administered earlier if desired.
- If not previously vaccinated, administer 2 doses of MMR during any visit with ≤4 weeks between the doses.

[8] **Varicella vaccine.** *(Minimum age: 12 months)*
- The second dose of varicella vaccine is recommended routinely at age 4–6 years but may be administered earlier if desired.
- Do not repeat the second dose in persons aged <13 years if administered ≤28 days after the first dose.

[9] **Hepatitis A vaccine (HepA).** *(Minimum age: 12 months)*
- HepA is recommended for certain groups of children, including in areas where vaccination programs target older children. see MMWR 2006;55(No. RR-7):1–23.

[10] **Tetanus and diphtheria toxoids vaccine (Td) and tetanus and diphtheria toxoids and acellular pertussis vaccine (Tdap).** *(Minimum age: 7 years for Td, 10 years for BOOSTRIX®, and 11 years for ADAOEL™)*
- Tdap should be substituted for a single dose of Td in the primary catch-up series or as a booster if age appropriate; use Td for other doses.
- A 5-year interval from the last Td dose is encouraged when Tdap is used as a booster dose. A booster (fourth) dose is needed if any of the previous doses were administered at age <12 months. Refer to ACIP recommendations for further information. See MMWR 2005;55(No. RR-3).

[11] **Human papillomavirus vaccine (HPV).** *(Minimum age: 9 years)*
- Administer the HPV vaccine series to females at age 13–18 years if not previously vaccinated.

Information about reporting reactions after immunization is available online at http://www.vares.hhs.gov or by telephone via the 24-hour national toll-free information line 800-822-7967. Suspected cases of vaccine-preventable diseases should be reported to the cases or local health department, including precautions and contra indications for immunization. Is available from the National Center for Immunization and Respiratory Diseases at http://www.cdc.gownip.default.htm or telephone. 800-CDC-INFO (800-232-4638)

From Centers for Disease Control and Prevention, http://www.cdc.gov/mmwr/preview/mmwrhtml/mm5551a7.htm?s_cid=mm5551a7_e.

comparable to those observed in healthy controls following immunization with oral polio and live attenuated measles vaccines.[90] Coadministration of vitamin A to Indian infants at the time of immunization with oral polio vaccine enhanced response to poliovirus type 1.[91] The WHO recommends that infants in vitamin A deficient countries received vitamin A at the time of measles vaccination.[82] In contrast, response to hepatitis B vaccine was not impaired in 31 infants with protein calorie malnutrition.[93] Detailed investigations of specific markers of immune response and relation to specific and non-specific nutritional deficiencies are lacking, but data demonstrating delayed progression of HIV disease following vitamin administration suggest that this is an area of potential investigation.[94]

## Future Directions for Research

Future directions for research could include continued development of combination vaccines to permit reduction in the number of immunizations, standardized and more widely available testing for antibody to vaccine-preventable diseases, and cost-effectiveness studies to inform decisions about screening versus immediate immunization. A recent abstract highlighted a rapid diagnostic test for identification of antibody to vaccine-preventable diseases that has the potential to be used in a clinical setting for on-site decisions about immunizations.[95] Although it is important to protect immigrants from vaccine-preventable diseases soon after arrival to the US, the interaction between repletion of nutritional status and response to vaccine is not well understood and it may be important for malnourished individuals to achieve better nutrition to optimize vaccine response.

Primary care providers will be called upon to determine appropriate immunization schedules for new immigrants. Repeating every vaccine dose is the most conservative approach to assure immunity, but may be impractical due to financial or logistical constraints. Combining selected serotesting with immediate immunization may optimize resources and increase patient and provider satisfaction. Building a body of knowledge about quality of immunization records, cost-effectiveness of various immunization and serotesting strategies, vaccine response and nutritional status, and acceptability of various strategies by patients will inform future vaccine recommendations for immigrants.

## References

1. Centers for Disease Control and Prevention. Measles – United States, 2000. MMWR 2002; 51:120–123.
2. Centers for Disease Control and Prevention. Elimination of rubella and congenital rubella syndrome – United States, 1969–2004. MMWR 2005; 54:279–282.
3. Centers for Disease Control and Prevention. Certification of poliomyelitis elimination – the Americas, 1994. MMWR 1994; 43:720–722.
4. Bisgard KM, Hardy IRB, Popovic T, et al. Respiratory diphtheria in the United States, 1980–1995. Am J Public Health 1998; 88:787–791.
5. Adams WG, Deaver KA, Cochi SL, et al. Decline of childhood *Haemophilus influenzae* type b (Hib) disease in the Hib vaccine era. JAMA 1993; 269:221–226.
6. Centers for Disease Control and Prevention. Notifiable diseases and deaths. MMWR 2005; 54:1108–1118.
7. Zhou F, Harpaz R, Jumaan AO, et al. Impact of varicella vaccination on healthcare utilization. JAMA 2005; 294:797–802.
8. Centers for Disease Control and Prevention. Direct and indirect effects of routine vaccination of children with 7-valent pneumococcal conjugate vaccine on incidence of invasive pneumococcal diseases – United States, 1998–2003. MMWR 2005; 54:893–897.
9. Centers for Disease Control and Prevention. Pertussis – United States, 1997–2000. MMWR 2002; 51:73–76.
10. Strine TW, Barker LE, Mokdad AH, et al. Vaccination coverage of foreign-born children 19 to 35 months of age: Findings from the National Immunization Survey, 1999–2000. Pediatrics 2002; 110:e15.
11. Centers for Disease Control and Prevention. Health status of Cambodians and Vietnamese – Selected communities, United States, 2001–2002. MMWR 2004; 53:760–767.
12. Vesikari T, Matson DO, Dennehy P, et al. Safety and efficacy of a pentavalent human-bovine (WC3) reassortant rotavirus vaccine. N Engl J Med 2006; 354:23–33.
13. Ruiz-Palacios GM, Perez-Schael I, Velazquez FR, et al. Safety and efficacy of an attenuated vaccine against severe rotavirus gastroenteritis. N Engl J Med 2006; 354:11–22.
14. Barker LE, Luman ET, McCauley MM, et al. Assessing equivalence: an alternative to the use of difference tests for measuring disparities in vaccination coverage. Am J Epidemiol 2002; 156:1056–1061.
15. Hutchins SS, Jiles R, Bernier R. Elimination of measles and of disparities in measles childhood vaccine coverage among racial and ethnic minority populations in the United States. J Infect Dis 2004; 189(Suppl 1):S146–S152.
16. Centers for Disease Control and Prevention. Epidemiology of Measles – United States 2001–2003. MMWR. 2004; 53:713–716.
17. Centers for Disease Control and Prevention. Measles outbreak among internationally adopted children arriving in the United States, February–March 2001. MMWR 2002; 51:1115–1116.
18. Centers for Disease Control and Prevention. Multistate investigation of measles among adoptees from China – April 2004. MMWR 2004; 53:309–310. Available: http://www.cdc.gov/mmwr/preview/mmwrhtml/mm53d409a1.htm (Accessed 1/31/07)
19. Hutchins SS, Bellini WJ, Coronado V, et al. Population immunity to measles in the United States, 1999. J Infect Dis 2004; 189(Suppl 1):S91-97.
20. Ehresmann KR, Crouch N, Henry PM, et al. An outbreak of measles among unvaccinated young adults and measles seroprevalence study: implications for measles outbreak control in adult populations. J Infect Dis 2004; 189(Suppl 1): S104–S107.
21. Barnett ED, Christiansen D, Figueira M. Seroprevalence of measles, rubella, and varicella in refugees. Clin Infect Dis 2002; 35:403–408.

22. Lasher L, Yin C, Park SY, et al. Seroprevalence of antibodies to measles, rubella, and varicella in Asian and Pacific Islander immigrants. Presented at the 43rd annual meeting of the Infectious Disease Society of America, October 6–9, 2005, San Francisco.

23. Miller LC, Comfort K, Kelly N. Immunization status of internationally adopted children (letter). Pediatrics 2001; 108:1050–1051.

24. Greenaway C, Boivin JF, Dongier P, et al. Susceptibility to vaccine-preventable diseases in newly arrived immigrants and refugees in Montreal, Canada. Presented at the 44th Interscience Conference on Antimicrobial Agents and Chemotherapy, Oct 30–Nov 2, 2004, Washington DC.

25. Hurie MB, Gennis MA, Hernandez, LV, et al. Prevalence of hepatitis B markers and measles, mumps, and rubella antibodies among Jewish refugees from the former Soviet Union. JAMA 1995; 273:954–956.

26. Centers for Disease Control and Prevention. Update: Multistate outbreak of mumps – United States, January 1–May 2, 2006. MMWR 2006; 55(Dispatch):1–5.

26a. Centers for Disease Control and Prevention. Update: Mumps activity – United States, January 1–October 7, 2006. MMWR 2006; 55:1152–1153.

27. Struewing JP, Hyams KC, Yueller JE, et al. The risk of measles, mumps, and varicella among young adults: a serosurvey of US Navy and Marine Corps recruits. Am J Public Health 1993; 83:1717–1720.

28. Reef SE, Frey TK, Theall K, et al. The changing epidemiology of rubella in the 1990s: on the verge of elimination and new challenges for control and prevention. JAMA 2002; 287:464–472.

29. Centers for Disease Control and Prevention. Elimination of rubella and congenital rubella – United States, 1969–2004. MMWR 2005; 54:279–281.

30. Centers for Disease Control and Prevention. Brief report: imported case of congenital rubella syndrome – New Hampshire, 2005. MMWR 2005; 54:1160–1161.

31. Knowles SJ, Grundy K, Cahill I, et al. Susceptibility to infectious rash illness in pregnant women from diverse geographical regions. Communicable Dis Pub Health 2004; 7:344–348.

32. Dykewicz CA, Kruzson-Moran D, McQuillan GM, et al. Rubella seropositivity in the United States, 1988–1994. Clin Infect Dis 2001; 33:1279–1286.

33. Craig AS, Reed GW, Mohon RT, et al. Neonatal tetanus in the United States: a sentinel event in the foreign-born. Pediatr Infect Dis J 1997; 16:955–959.

34. Pascal FB, McGinely EL, Zanardi LR, et al. Tetanus surveillance – United States, 1998–2000. In: Surveillance Summaries, June 20, 2003. MMWR 2003; 52(No. SS-3): 1–8.

35. Centers for Disease Control and Prevention. Summary of Notifiable Diseases – United States, 2001. MMWR 2001; 50(No. 53):90–96.

36. Gergen PJ, McQuillan GM, Kiely M, et al. A population-based serologic survey of immunity to tetanus in the United States. New Engl J Med 1995; 332:761–767.

37. Alagappan K, Rennie W, Kwiatkowski T, et al. Seroprevalence of tetanus antibodies among adults older than 65 years. Ann Emerg Med 1996; 28:18–21.

38. McQuillan GM, Kruszon-Moran D, Deforest A, et al. Serologic immunity to diphtheria and tetanus in the United States. Ann Intern Med 2002; 136:660–666.

39. Yuan L, Lau W, Thipphawong J, et al. Diphtheria and tetanus immunity among blood donors in Toronto. Can Med Assoc J 1997; 156:985–990.

40. Germinario C, Chironna M, Quarto M, et al. Immunosurveillance on Kosovar children refugees in southern Italy. Vaccine 2000; 18:2073–2074.

41. Chironna M, Germinario C, Lopalca PL, et al. Immunity to diphtheria among refugees in southern Italy. Vaccine 2003; 21:3157–3161.

42. Broder KR, Cortese MM, Iskander JK, et al. Preventing tetanus, diphtheria, and pertussis among adolescents: use of tetanus toxoid, reduced diphtheria toxoid and acellular pertussis vaccines. MMWR 2006; 55 (No.RR-3):1–34. Available: http://www.cdc.gov/mmwr/preview/mmwrhtml/rr55e223a1.htm Accessed 1/31/07.

42a. Centers for Disease Control and Prevention. Preventing tetanus, diphtheria, and pertussis among adults: use of tetanus toxoid, reduced diphtheria toxoid and acellular pertussis vaccine. MMWR 2006; 55(RR17):1–33. Available at: http://www.cdc.gov/mmwr/preview/mmwrhtml/rr5517a1.htm?s_cid=rr5517a1_e Accessed 1/24/07.

43. Kilgore PE, Kruszon-Moran D, Seward JF, et al. Varicella in Americans from NHANES III: implications for control through routine immunization. J Med Virol 2003; 70(Suppl 1):S111–S118.

44. Mandal BK, Mukherjee PP, Murphy C, et al. Adult susceptibility to varicella in the tropics is a rural phenomenon due to the lack of previous exposure. J Infect Dis 1998; 178(Suppl 1):S52–S54.

45. Centers for Disease Control and Prevention. Acute hepatitis B among children and adolescents – United States, 1990–2002. MMWR 2004; 53:1015–1018.

46. Johnson DE, Miller LC, Iverson S, et al. The health of children adopted from Romania. JAMA 1992; 268: 3446–3451.

47. Au L, Tso A, Chin K. Asian-American adolescent immigrants: the New York City schools experience. J School Health 1997; 67:277–279.

48. Burke NJ, Jackson JC, Thai HC, et al. 'Honoring tradition, accepting new ways': development of a hepatitis B control intervention for Vietnamese immigrants. Ethnicity and Health 2004; 9:153–169.

49. Taylor VM, Yasui Y, Burke N, et al. Hepatitis B testing among Vietnamese American men. Cancer Detect Prevent 2004; 28:170–177.

50. Centers for Disease Control and Prevention. Poliovirus infections in four unvaccinated children – Minnesota, August–October 2005. MMWR 2005; 54:1053–1055.

51. Calderon-Margalit R, Sofer D, Gefen D, et al. Immune status to poliovirus among immigrant workers in Israel. Preventive Med 2005; 40:685–689.

52. Centers for Disease Control and Prevention. Prevention of hepatitis A through active or passive immunization: recommendations of the Immune Practices Advisory Committee (ACIP). MMWR 1999; 48(RR12):1–37. Available: http://www.cdc.gov/mmwr/preview/mmwrhtml/rr4812a1.htm Accessed 1/31/07.

52a. Centers for Disease Control and Prevention. Prevention of hepatitis A through active or passive immunization: Recommendations of the Advisory Committee on Immunization Practices (ACIP). MMWR 2006; 55(RR07): 1–23. Available at: http://www.cdc.gov/mmwr/preview/mmwrhtml/rr5507a1.htm Accessed 1/31/07.

53. Barnett ED, Holmes AH, Harrison TS, et al. Immunity to hepatitis A in people born and raised in endemic areas. J Travel Med 2003; 10:11–14.

54. Fishbain JT, Eckart RE, Harner KC, et al. Empiric immunization versus serologic screening: developing a cost-effective strategy for the use of hepatitis A immunization in travelers. J Travel Med 2002; 9:71–75.

55. Plans-Rubio P. Critical prevalence of antibodies minimizing vaccination costs for hepatitis A, hepatitis B, varicella, measles and tetanus in adults and adolescents in Catalonia, Spain. Vaccine 2004; 22:4002–4013.

56. Schwartz E, Raveh D. The prevalence of hepatitis A antibodies among Israeli travelers and the economic feasibility of screening before vaccination. Int J Epidemiol 1998; 27:118–120.

57. Centers for Disease Control and Prevention: Provisional Recommendations for Hepatitis A Vaccination of Children. Available at: http://www.cdc.gov/nip/recs/provisional_recs/hepA_child.pdf Accessed 1/31/07.

58. Weinberg M, Hopkins J, Farrington L, et al. Hepatitis A in Hispanic children who live along the United States–Mexico border: the role of international travel and food-borne exposures. Pediatrics 2004; 114:e68–e73. Available: http://pediatrics.aappublications.org/cgi/content/abstract/114/1/e68 Accessed 1/31/07.

59. Migrant Clinicians Network, Inc. Hepatitis screening, immunization and testing for mobile populations and immigrants from Mexico, Central and South America, and the Caribbean. 2005. Available: http://www.migrantclinician.org/_resources/Hep_MCN_Position_Paper.pdf Accessed 1/31/07.

60. Wilson ME, Kimble J. Posttravel hepatitis A: probable acquisition from an asymptomatic adopted child. Clin Infect Dis 2001; 33:1083–1085.

61. Chen LH, Barnett ED, Wilson ME. Preventing infectious diseases before and after international adoption. Ann Intern Med 2003; 139:371–378.

62. Barnett ED, Chen LH. Prevention of travel-related infectious diseases in families of internationally adopted children. Pediatr Clin N Am 2005; 52:1271–1286.

63. Bacaner N, Stauffer B, Boulware DR, et al. Travel medicine considerations for North American immigrants visiting friends and relatives. JAMA 2004; 291:2856–2864.

64. Centers for Disease Control and Prevention. General Recommendations on Immunization. MMWR 2006; 55(RR15):1–48. Available: http://www.cdc.gov/mmwr/preview/mmwrhtml/rr5515a1.htm Accessed 1/31/07.

65. Barnett ED. Immunizations and infectious disease screening for internationally adopted children. Pediatr Clin N Am 2005; 52:1287–1309.

66. Miller LC. Immunizations and vaccine-preventable diseases. In: Miller LC. Handbook of international adoption. New York: Oxford University Press; 2005: 292–299.

67. Schulte JM, Maloney S, Aronson J, et al. Evaluating acceptability and completeness of overseas immunization records of internationally adopted children. Pediatrics 2002; 109:e22. Available: http://pediatrics.aappublications.org/cgi/content/full/109/2/e22 Accessed 1/31/07.

68. Hostetter MK, Johnson DJ. Immunization status of adoptees from China, Russia, and Eastern Europe (abstract). Pediatr Res 1998; 43:147A.

69. American Academy of Pediatrics. Medical evaluation of internationally adopted children for infectious diseases. In: Pickering LK, ed. 2000 Red Book: Report of the Committee on Infectious Diseases. 25th edn. Elk Grove Village, IL: American Academy of Pediatrics; 2000:148–152.

70. Miller LC. Internationally adopted children – immigration status (letter). Pediatrics 1999; 103:1078.

71. Miller LC, Comfort K, Kelly N. Immunization status of internationally adopted children. Pediatrics 2001; 108:1050–1051.

72. Schulpen TWJ, van Seventer AHJ, et al. Immunisation status of children adopted from China. Lancet 2001; 358:2131–2132.

73. Staat MA, Daniels D. Immunization verification in internationally adopted children (abstract). Pediatr Res 2001; 49:468A.

74. Hurie MB, Mast EE, Davis JP. Horizontal transmission of hepatitis B virus infection to United States-born children of Hmong refugees. Pediatrics 1992; 89:269–273.

75. Friede A, Harris JR, Kobayashi JM, et al. Transmission of hepatitis B virus from adopted Asian children to their American families. Am J Public Health 1988; 78:26–29.

76. Hershow RC, Hadler SC, Kane MA. Adoption of children from countries with endemic hepatitis B: transmission risks and medical issues. Pediatr Infect Dis J 1987; 6:431–437.

77. Sokal EM, Van Collie O, Buts JP. Horizontal transmission of hepatitis B from children to adoptive parents (letter). Arch Dis Child 1995; 72:191.

78. Vernon TM, Wright RA, Kohler PF, et al. Hepatitis A and B in the family unit: nonparenteral transmission by asymptomatic children. JAMA 1976; 235:2829–2831.

79. Rennels MB, Deloria MA, Pichichero ME, et al. Extensive swelling after booster doses of acellular pertussis-tetanus-diphtheria vaccines. Pediatrics 2000; 105:e12.

80. Edsall G, Elliott MW, Peebles TC, et al. Excessive use of tetanus toxoid boosters. JAMA 1967; 202:17–19.

81. Centers for Disease Control and Prevention. Prevention of pneumococcal disease: recommendations of the Advisory Committee on Immunization Practices (ACIP). MMWR 1997; 46(No. RR-8):1–24.

82. Feikema SM, Klevens RM, Washington ML, et al. Extraimmunization among US children. JAMA 2000; 283:1311–1317.

83. Woodin KA, Rodewald LE, Humiston SG, et al. Physician and parent opinions: are children becoming pincushions from immunizations? Arch Pediatr Adolesc Med 1995; 149:845–849.

84. Melman ST, Nguyen TT, Ehrlich E, et al. Parental compliance with multiple immunization injections. Arch Pediatr Adolesc Med 1999; 153:1289–1291.

85. Meyerhoff AS, Jacobs RJ. Do too many shots due lead to missed vaccination opportunities? Does it matter? Preventive Med 2005; 41:540–544.

86. Figueira M, Christiansen D, Barnett ED. Cost-effectiveness of serotesting compared with universal immunization for varicella in refugee children from 6 geographic regions. J Travel Med 2003; 10:203–207.

87. Cohen AL, Veenstra D. Economic analysis of prevaccination serotesting compared with presumptive immunization for polio, diphtheria, and tetanus in internationally adopted and immigrant infants. Pediatrics 2006; 117:1650–1655.

88. American Academy of Pediatrics. Medical evaluation of internationally adopted children for infectious diseases. In: Pickering LK, ed. Red Book: 2006 Report of the Committee on Infectious Diseases. 27th edn. Elk Grove Village, IL: American Academy of Pediatrics; 2006:182–188.

89. Snyder BK, Roghmann KJ, Sigal LH. Effect of stress and other biopsychosocial factors on primary antibody response. J Adol Health Care 1990; 11:472–479.

90. Chandra RK. Reduced secretory antibody response to live attenuated measles and poliovirus vaccines in malnourished children. Br Med J 1975; 2(5971): 583–585.

91. Bahl R, Bhandari N, Kant S, et al. Effect of vitamin A administered at Expanded Program on Immunization contacts on antibody response to oral polio vaccine. Eur J Clin Nutrition 2002; 56:321–325.

92. Ross DA, Cutts FT. Vindication of policy of vitamin A with measles vaccination. Lancet 1997; 350:81–82.

93. el-Gamal Y, Aly RH, Hossny E, et al. Response of Egyptian infants with protein calorie malnutrition to hepatitis B vaccination. J Trop Pediatr 1996; 42:144–145.

94. Fawzi WW, Msamanga GI, Spiegelman D, et al. A randomized trial of multivitamin supplements and HIV disease progression and mortality. N Engl J Med 2004; 351:23–32.

95. Sylvia MJ, Barnett ED, Maloney SA, et al. Comparison of a new rapid ImmunoDot method vs. standard ELISA testing for antibody to varicella, measles, rubella, tetanus and diphtheria in refugees (abstract #1059) Presented at the 42nd Annual Meeting of the Infectious Diseases Society of America, Boston, September, 2004.

96. Prevots DR, Pascual FB, Angellili ML, et al. Population immunity to polioviruses among preschool children from four urban underserved low income communities, United States, 1997–2001. Pediatr Infect Dis J 2004; 23:1130–1136.

97. Lifson AR, Thai D, O'Fallon A, et al. Prevalence of tuberculosis, hepatitis B virus, and intestinal parasitic infections among refugees to Minnesota. Public Health Reports 2002; 117:69–76.

98. Meropol SB. Health status of pediatric refugees in Buffalo, New York. Arch Pediatr Adolesc Med 1995; 149:887–892.

99. Hayes EB, Talbot SB, Matheson ES, et al. Health status of pediatric refugees in Portland, Maine. Arch Pediatr Adolesc Med 1998; 152:564–568.

100. Bonura F, Sorgi M, Perna AM, et al. Pregnant women as a sentinel population to target and implement hepatitis B virus (HBV) vaccine coverage: A three-year survey in Palermo, Sicily. Vaccine 2005; 23:3243–3246.

101. Nelson KR, Bui H, Samet JH. Screening in special populations: a 'case study' of recent Vietnamese immigrants. Am J Med 1997; 102:435–440.

102. American Academy of Pediatrics. Hepatitis B. In: Pickering L, ed. 2006 Red Book: Report of the Committee on Infectious Diseases 27th ed. Elk Grove Village, IL: American Academy of Pediatrics; 2006:335–355.

103. American Academy of Pediatrics. Pertussis. In: Pickering L, ed. 2006 Red Book: Report of the Committee on Infectious Diseases 27th ed. Elk Grove Village, IL: American Academy of Pediatrics; 2006:498–520.

104. American Academy of Pediatrics. Mumps. In: Pickering L, ed. 2006 Red Book: Report of the Committee on Infectious Diseases 27th ed. Elk Grove Village, IL: American Academy of Pediatrics; 2006:464–468.

105. American Academy of Pediatrics. Rubella. In: Pickering L, ed. 2006 Red Book: Report of the Committee on Infectious Diseases 27th ed. Elk Grove Village, IL: American Academy of Pediatrics; 2006:574–579.

106. Christiansen D, Barnett ED. Comparison of varicella history with presence of varicella antibody in refugees. Vaccine 2004; 22:4233–4237.

# CHAPTER 14

# Differential Diagnoses of Ill Immigrants by Organ System

Linda S. Nield and Meghan Rothenberger

## Introduction

Every year thousands of individuals leave their countries of birth to settle in the United States (US). In fact, nearly 12% of the people residing in the US are foreign born.[1] Although certain regions have a higher percentage of this population, all 50 states are home to immigrants from a wide range of geographical regions. Therefore, American healthcare providers will likely be involved in the care of an immigrant patient at some point in time, regardless of their practice location or medical specialty. Unfortunately, US-trained clinicians are often unaccustomed to diagnosing and treating many of the illnesses that disproportionately burden immigrants, such as tuberculosis (TB), malaria, intestinal parasites, and rheumatic heart disease. This chapter, organized by organ system, is intended to provide healthcare providers with an overview of many of the diseases commonly encountered in immigrant patients. By taking into account the predominantly affected organ system, presenting symptoms, patient's homeland, timing of immigration, and exposure history, an appropriate differential diagnosis may be generated. Determining this differential diagnosis facilitates timely diagnostic testing and aids in the development of appropriate management strategies.

## Nervous System

In an immigrant population, a number of both infectious and non-infectious diseases, can present with neurological symptoms (Box 14.1). Several of the most commonly encountered symptoms include headache, focal deficits, weakness, sensory changes, seizures, and psychological complaints.

## Headache

A sudden, severe headache is concerning for subarachnoid hemorrhage. Although this may be due to rupture of a congenital aneurysm, rupture of a mycotic aneurysm secondary to infective endocarditis should also be considered in an immigrant patient. Cerebral gnathostomiasis, most common in immigrants from Thailand and Laos, may also present with acute intracranial bleed.

A progressively worsening headache may be due to increased intracranial pressure caused by space-occupying lesions such as neoplasm or localized infection. Cysticercosis, the most common parasitic brain infection worldwide, is endemic in Mexico, Central and South America, sub-Saharan Africa, and Asia.[2] It often presents with chronic headache or afebrile seizures. Intracranial tuberculomas due to infection with *Mycobacterium tuberculosis* can also cause headache without evidence of extracranial disease. Other infections associated with space-occupying lesions include toxoplasmosis, trichinosis, echinococcosis, schistosomiasis, amoebiasis, and paragonimiasis.

Headache associated with fever, confusion, or nuchal rigidity may indicate meningitis or encephalitis. Bacterial meningitis due to *Neisseria meningitis* is of particular concern in individuals who have lived in or traveled through the 'meningitis belt' of

171

---

**Box 14.1**

**Differential diagnosis of common neurological disorders**

Headache
**Stroke/intracranial hemorrhage**
Cerebral gnathostomiasis
Chagas' disease
Endocarditis with septic emboli
Hypertension
Moya Moya
Rheumatic heart disease
Sickle cell disease
Syphilis
Takayasu's arteritis

**Space occupying lesions**
Amoebiasis
Cysticercosis
Echinococcus
*E. histolytica*
Malignancy (primary or metastatic lesions)
*Paragonimus* spp.
Schistosomiasis
Toxoplasmosis
Trichinosis
Tuberculoma

**Meningitis/encephalitis**
Babesiosis
Dengue fever
*Hemophilus influenza* type b
Herpes
Human immunodeficiency virus
Japanese encephalitis
Listeria
Lyme Disease
Malaria
Measles
Mumps
*Neisseria meningitidis*
Rabies

*Streptococcus pneumoniae*
Syphilis
Trypanosomiasis
Tuberculosis
West Nile virus

**Focal motor deficits, weakness and/or sensory loss**
**Infectious**
Gnathostomiasis
HIV
Leprosy
Paralytic rabies
Polio
Schistosomiasis
Spinal tuberculosis
Syphilis
Tropical spastic paralysis (HTLV related)

**Noninfectious**
Diabetes mellitus
Guillain-Barré
Nutritional deficiencies
Space occupying lesions (see above)
Stroke (see above)
Toxic exposures
Tropical ataxic neuropathy

**Cognitive deficits/behavioral disturbances**
Anxiety disorder
Depression
Metabolic disorders
Nutritional deficiencies
Post-traumatic stress disorder
Somatoform disorders
Substance abuse
Toxic exposures/heavy metals
Traumatic brain injury

---

sub-Saharan Africa.[3] Those who have taken part in the annual Muslim Hajj pilgrimage are also at increased risk.[4] Infection caused by *Streptococcus pneumoniae* and *Haemophilus influenza* type b may occur at a higher rate in newly relocated immigrant children due to lack of routine immunization in most developing areas. Other bacterial pathogens that cause meningitis and encephalitis include *L. monocytogenes*, *Treponema pallidum*, and *M. tuberculosis*. Viral etiologies include members of the flaviviridae family (dengue fever, Japanese encephalitis, West Nile virus), arboviruses, enteroviruses, human immunodeficiency virus (HIV), *herpes simplex* virus (HSV), measles, and mumps. Tick-borne illnesses such as Lyme disease and babesiosis, as well as other insect-borne infections such as malaria and trypanosomiasis must also be considered in the differential diagnosis of immigrants with headache and fever.

## Focal motor deficits

Although many of the diseases mentioned above can present with focal neurological signs, cerebrovascular accident (CVA) must always be considered in any patient presenting with new focal findings. Worldwide, cerebrovascular disease accounts for over four million deaths yearly; nearly 70% of these deaths occur in less affluent countries.[5] While the common risk factors for cerebrovascular disease, such as hypertension, diabetes, hyperlipidemia, and smoking, are important in immigrant populations, other unique causes of stroke must be considered in this population as well. In young patients presenting with stroke, rheumatic heart disease, Chagas' disease, sickle cell disease, and tertiary syphilis are possible underlying etiologies. Moya Moya disease, a vascular condition most common in Asians, can present with stroke. Asians, particularly young women, may present with stroke related to Takayasu's arteritis.

## Weakness

Weakness may be the result of brain, spinal cord, peripheral nerve, or muscle pathology. Cerebral vascular accident and space-occupying lesions are important central causes. Spinal cord disease can be secondary to TB, metastatic malignancies, HIV, schistosomiasis, gnathostomiasis, or syphilis. Human T-lymphotropic virus (HTLV), a retrovirus endemic to most of the tropical developing world, has been shown to play a causative role in HTLV-associated myelopathy/tropical spastic paresis (HTLV/TSP).[6] This condition presents with slow-onset spastic paresis associated with bladder dysfunction and variable degrees of sensory deficits and must be differentiated from Guillain-Barré syndrome. Both polio and rabies can present with paralysis. Given that the incubation period of rabies can be months, immigrants may present with new infection after being in the US for an extended period of time; it is therefore very important to ask about any history of animal contact, even remote, in patients presenting with weakness.[7]

## Sensory deficits

Sensory changes may be associated with several of the infectious agents that cause weakness including polio, HTLV-1 (tropical spastic paresis), HIV, and rabies. A progressive symmetrical peripheral neuropathy in individuals from the tropics may be due to lepromatous leprosy. Noninfectious causes of sensory changes are also common. Guillain-Barré syndrome, a disease thought to be autoimmune in etiology, can present with sensory deficits and

weakness. Immigrants may present with a slowly progressive sensorimotor neuropathy associated with ataxia; this condition, known as tropical ataxic neuropathy, is associated with heavy consumption of cassava, a root commonly consumed in regions of Africa, Asia, and Latin America.[8] With the increasing worldwide incidence of diabetes mellitus, diabetic peripheral neuropathy is commonly seen as well.

Nutrient deficiency is another important cause of sensory dysfunction. Thiamine deficiency (beriberi), a particular problem in refugee populations that subsist on rice-based foods, is associated with ataxia and peripheral neuropathy.[9] Deficiencies of vitamins $B_6$, $B_{12}$, and niacin (pellagra) can also cause peripheral neuropathy.

## Various neurologic abnormalities

In addition to causing peripheral nerve symptoms, nutrient deficiencies and malnutrition can cause numerous other neurological symptoms. Iodine deficiency can lead to mental retardation. Irritability, apathy, and lethargy may result from kwashiorkor, marasmus, pellagra, and iron deficiency. In advanced cases of pellagra, dementia and eventual death can occur.

Varied neurologic signs and symptoms, including cognitive deficits, may be due to exposure to toxins such as lead, mercury, and arsenic. Lead poisoning is particularly prevalent in refugee children.[10] Even after resettlement in the US, continued exposure may occur through imported ceramics, traditional medications, cosmetics, and paint in older homes. Many immigrants are not aware of the dangers of lead exposure.[11] Malnutrition and iron deficiency, both prevalent in the refugee populations, increase the likelihood of lead toxicity.[11] Chronic lead exposure is associated with hyperactivity, developmental delay, irritability, behavioral problems, peripheral neuropathy, and hearing loss. These symptoms can easily be confused with attention deficit disorder.

As with lead toxicity, exposure to methyl mercury results in numerous neurological symptoms. Toxicity generally presents with irritability, paresthesias of the limbs and perioral area, ataxia, muscle weakness, dysarthria, paralysis, difficulty with swallowing, and seizures. The degree to which mercury poisoning causes neurologic abnormalities in resettled populations is unknown. However, historically, there have been several large outbreaks of methyl mercury toxicity. In Iraq, thousands of people were affected after consuming bread made from mercury-contaminated grain.[12] Release of methyl mercury into the Minamata Bay in Japan led to hundreds of cases of toxicity via consumption of contaminated fish.[12] In other parts of the world, such as the Amazon, high mercury levels are thought to be due to gold mining and agricultural practices.[13] Arsenic toxicity, most common in immigrants from Bangladesh and India, can cause peripheral neuropathy and skin changes.[14] It should also be kept in mind that traditional medications may contain neurotoxic materials such as strychnine and arsenic, so it is always important to ask patients specifically about the use of traditional remedies.[15]

## Psychological complaints

Although organic disorders can produce mood and sleep disturbances, anxiety, irritability, sexual dysfunction, hallucinations, panic attacks, and cognitive deficits, these symptoms may be seen in an immigrant suffering from a mental illness. An estimated two-thirds of refugees experience some form of anxiety or depression.[16] Exposure to violence, trauma, and upheaval prior to immigration as well as poverty, unemployment, social isolation, and language difficulties following immigration likely contribute to the increased rate of psychiatric complaints.[16,17] The most common psychiatric disorder amongst this population is post-traumatic stress disorder (PTSD); refugees are nearly 10 times more likely to develop PTSD than age-matched native-born controls.[16,18] Compared to native-born populations, somatoform disorders occur with increased frequency in resettled populations.[19,20] These disorders are particularly challenging for clinicians, as it is often very difficult to determine if symptoms have an organic basis. It is vitally important for healthcare providers to address these mental health conditions, especially given the risk of suicide with untreated disease.[18] Screening for alcohol and substance abuse is also important; although immigrants do not appear to be at greater risk for abuse than US-born individuals, abuse is still very prevalent and has significant health and social consequences.[21]

## Eye

According to the World Health Organization (WHO), there are 37 million people worldwide with bilateral blindness (3/60 visual acuity or less); an additional 161 million individuals have severe impairment in both eyes (visual acuity less than 6/18 but better than 3/60).[22] It has been estimated that 90% of cases

---

**Box 14.2**

**Differential diagnosis of ophthalmologic conditions**

**Acute infections**
Chagas' disease
Dengue fever
Gonorrhea
Leprosy
Leptospirosis
Measles
Typhoid fever
Viral hemorrhagic fevers

**Chronic infections**
Cysticercosis
Chagas' disease (decreased night vision)
Filariasis
Leprosy
Toxocariasis
Trachoma
Trichinosis
Trypanosomiasis
Syphilis
Toxoplasmosis (chorioretinitis)

**Noninfectious**
Cataracts (congenital and acquired)
Diabetic retinopathy
Exposure to traditional medications
Trauma
Vitamin A deficiency

---

of blindness occur in developing regions.[23] Congenital defects, defects secondary to aging, infections, and nutritional deficiency can all affect the eye adversely (Box 14.2). Given the scope of this problem and the high likelihood of caring for an immigrant with ophthalmologic complaints, it is important for clinicians to have a basic understanding of several of the most common ophthalmologic conditions encountered in this population.

The most common cause of blindness worldwide is cataracts, both congenital and age-related.[22,23] The high prevalence of cataracts in developing regions is largely due to poor access to surgical correction.[24] Diabetic retinopathy is another common cause of visual impairment. In immigrants, disease may be quite advanced at time of presentation due to lack of routine screening and poor diabetic control prior to immigration.

Trachoma, caused by *Chlamydia trachomatis*, is yet another important cause of visual impairment; an estimated 84 million people worldwide are currently infected.[25] Trachoma causes progressive visual loss through scarring and revascularization of the cornea. Since treatment with antibiotics and surgery (in more advanced cases) can halt the progression to blindness, it is very important to recognize this condition.[25]

A number of other infections cause ophthalmologic symptoms. Amongst protozoan infections, filariasis (*Loa loa* in tropical Africa and *Onchocerca volvulus* in Africa, South America, and the Middle East) and toxocariasis can cause an array of complications including conjunctivitis, photophobia, keratitis, uveitis, optic atrophy, and blindness. Congenital toxoplasmosis frequently leads to visual impairment; interestingly, loss of visual acuity and new eye lesions may occur as late as the third or fourth decades of life.[26] Systemic diseases such as leptospirosis, dengue fever, and measles are often associated with characteristic ophthalmologic symptoms. For example, conjunctival suffusion is a classic sign of leptospirosis, and retro-orbital pain is typical of dengue fever. Chagas' disease may mimic periorbital cellulitis (Romaña's sign). Although less common than in past generations, leprosy still exists and can also cause visual damage.

Ophthalmologic problems in immigrant children may be due to vitamin A deficiency. This condition, known as xerophthalmia, is the most common cause of childhood blindness worldwide, affecting over 1.5 million children.[24] The symptoms and signs associated with xerophthalmia include night blindness, Bitot's spots (irregular gray or white conjunctival patches), corneal xerosis, ulceration, scarring, and eventual blindness.[9] Treatment can reverse many of these complications, so timely and proper diagnosis is imperative.

Immigrants, particularly those from regions of unrest, may present with trauma-related eye complaints. These traumatic injuries are often due to land mines.[24] Corneal ulcerations may also result from use of traditional ophthalmologic medications; questions regarding the use of these medications should be included in the evaluation of immigrant patients presenting with ophthalmologic complaints.

## Cardiovascular System

Cardiovascular diseases most commonly seen in immigrant populations can be separated into the broad categories of congenital anomalies, valvular disorders, vascular abnormalities, pericardial disease, myocarditis, and cardiomyopathies (Box 14.3). Despite

---

**Box 14.3**

**Differential diagnosis of cardiovascular conditions**

**Congenital heart defects**
Patent foramen ovale
Atrial septal defect
Ventricular septal defect
Patent ductus arteriosus
Pulmonary stenosis
Tetralogy of Fallot
Aortic stenosis
Aortic coarctation

**Valvular disorders**
Rheumatic heart disease
Infective endocarditis
Congenital defects (i.e. bicuspid aortic valve)

**Vascular disorders**
Coronary artery disease
Aortitis secondary to syphilis
Sickle cell disease

**Pericarditis/myocarditis**

**Infectious causes**
Viral (echoviruses, adenoviruses, coxsackieviruses, HSV, HIV)
Bacterial (*Staphylococcus*, *Pneumococcus*, tuberculosis, brucellosis, rickettsial organisms)
Protozoal (Chagas' disease, toxoplasmosis, malaria, leishmaniasis)
Helminthic (trichinosis, echinococcosis, schistosomiasis, filariasis)

**Noninfectious causes**
Connective tissue disorders
Renal failure
Hypothyroidism
Medications
Neoplasm

**Congestive heart failure**
May result from many of the disease processes listed above
May also be due to:

    Alcohol abuse
    Postpartum cardiomyopathy
    Toxin exposure
    High output states (anemia, hyperthyroidism, beriberi)

the differences in underlying pathology, it is important to remember that many of these conditions will present similarly.

Congenital heart anomalies may be diagnosed because of an asymptomatic murmur; however, they may also present with heart failure, cyanosis, dyspnea, polycythemia, or digital clubbing. Although congenital heart diseases occur with similar frequencies in developed and developing regions, far more children in developing nations remain undiagnosed and untreated.[27] It is therefore important for clinicians to perform thorough cardiac examinations on all immigrant patients, not only children, keeping in mind the possibility of congenital abnormalities. The most commonly encountered congenital heart diseases include ventricular and atrial septal defects, patent ductus arteriosis, and pulmonary stenosis. However, a clinician may also discover unexpected conditions such as tetralogy of Fallot or aortic coarctation, even in adolescent patients.

An estimated twelve million individuals worldwide have rheumatic heart disease; the prevalence is particularly high in Africa and the Pacific Islands.[28] As with congenital heart disease, rheumatic valve disease may present as an asymptomatic murmur but may also cause heart failure or stroke. Valvular disease in an immigrant may also be caused by infective endocarditis; it is particularly important to consider this if systemic symptoms are present, although long-term valvular defects can result from previous episodes of endocarditis. Aortitis secondary to syphilis can cause aortic valve dysfunction as well.

Chest pain in an immigrant may be due to coronary artery disease. As the prevalence of cardiac risk factors such as diabetes mellitus, hypertension, obesity, and smoking are increasing in developing regions, coronary artery disease is becoming increasingly common in individuals from these areas. In fact, according to the WHO, 60% of the global burden of coronary artery disease is in the developing world.[29] Furthermore, once immigrants move to the US and adopt often unhealthy Western habits, their risk likely increases further. Acute chest crisis secondary to sickle cell disease should also be considered when an immigrant (particularly if the patient is of African heritage) presents with chest pain.

Chest pain may also be the presenting symptom of pericarditis and myocarditis. Most common viral causes of pericarditis include the echoviruses, adenoviruses, and coxsackieviruses. Bacterial causes include both Gram-positive and Gram-negative organisms as well as TB. Parasitic etiologies include *Entamoeba*, *Echinococcus*, and *Toxoplasma*.

Noninfectious causes include connective tissue diseases, renal failure, hypothyroidism, neoplasms, and medications.

Like pericarditis, myocarditis also has many diverse causes. Infectious etiologies include viruses such as coxsackieviruses, *herpes simplex* virus, Epstein-Barr virus (EBV), and HIV; rickettsial diseases such as scrub typhus; bacterial infections including brucellosis, TB, and leptospirosis; protozoal infections such as toxoplasmosis, malaria, and leishmaniasis; and helminth infections such as trichinosis, echinococcosis, schistosomiasis, and filariasis.[30-32] In immigrants from Central and South America, Chagas' disease, caused by the protozoa *Trypanasoma cruzi*, is a common cause of myocarditis and cardiomyopathy.[33]

Noninfectious etiologies of cardiomyopathy (CM) include alcohol abuse, malnutrition, postpartum CM, and toxin exposure. High-output states such as beriberi, uncontrolled hyperthyroidism, and severe anemia can also result in heart failure.

## Respiratory Tract

Respiratory complaints such as dyspnea or cough in immigrants may be due to infections, chronic noninfectious lung diseases, vascular pathology, or malignancy (Box 14.4).

Acute lower respiratory tract infections are the leading cause of infection-related mortality worldwide.[34] Overcrowding and inadequate sanitation often found in refugee camps facilitate person-to-person spread of respiratory pathogens. Many of the viruses and bacteria that cause acute lung infections in refugees and recent immigrants are the same pathogens responsible for disease in the US (such as pneumococcus and influenza). Given that one-third of the world's population is infected with TB and that nearly 55% of cases in the US are in foreign-born individuals, it is extremely important to consider this infection in any patient with pulmonary complaints.[35] All immigrants and refugees must be screened for TB, and the diagnosis should be strongly suspected in any individual with chronic cough, chest pain, hemoptysis, or weight loss. However, it should be remembered that over 40% of TB cases in immigrants are extrapulmonary at time of diagnosis, so classic pulmonary symptoms may not be seen.[36-39] Pulmonary anthrax is of great public concern with its high mortality rate, but it is quite rare and generally limited to endemic areas.

Given the high rate of parasitic disease in immigrants, these infections must be considered in

## Box 14.4

### Differential diagnosis of respiratory tract conditions

#### Acute symptoms
#### Infectious causes
Bacterial (*Staphylococcus*, *Pneumococcus*, *Chlamydia pneumoniae*, *Mycoplasma pneumoniae*, melioidosis)
Viral (influenza, adenovirus, parainfluenza, respiratory syncytial virus, measles, SARS)
Protozoal (malaria, *amoebiasis*)
Migratory phase of helminth infections (*Ascaris*, *Strongyloides*, hookworm)
Tuberculosis

#### Noninfectious causes
Acute chest crisis in patient with sickle cell disease
Toxic exposure
Asthma exacerbation
Pneumothorax

#### Chronic symptoms
#### Infectious causes
Bacterial (tuberculosis, atypical mycobacterium, melioidosis)
Fungal infections
Migratory phase of helminth infections (*Strongyloides*, filariasis)
Parasitic infections (paragonimiasis)

#### Noninfectious causes
Chronic obstructive pulmonary syndrome
Asthma
Malignancy
Occupational exposures
Pulmonary hypertension
Cystic fibrosis
Sarcoidosis

patients presenting with respiratory complaints. The migratory phase of parasitic infections such as *Ascaris lumbricoides*, *Strongyloides stercoralis*, toxocariasis, and hookworm can cause coughing and wheezing. It is particularly important to evaluate patients from endemic regions for *Strongyloides* infection prior to any steroid or immunosuppressive treatment, as hyperinfection syndrome may be precipitated by these treatments. This syndrome is associated with respiratory failure and/or Gram-negative sepsis and carries a 30–70% mortality rate.[40] Other parasitic infections that can cause pulmonary symptoms include malaria, amoebiasis, filariasis, and paragonimiasis. Pulmonary hypertension,

which can be caused by schistosomiasis, can also present with dyspnea.[41] In immigrants from Southeast and Northern Asia with pulmonary symptoms, melioidosis (caused by infection with the bacteria *Burkholderia pseudomallei*) should be considered. This infection can be dormant for years; in fact, there have been cases of active disease developing up to 29 years after exposure.[42]

Pulmonary complaints, both acute and chronic, may also be due to noninfectious etiologies. Acute chest syndrome in a patient with sickle cell anemia can present with severe chest pain, dyspnea, cough, and infiltrates on chest radiograph. Chronic pulmonary complaints may be due to asthma or chronic obstructive pulmonary disease. Although often regarded as diseases of the developed world, environmental exposures and cigarette use have contributed to increasing rates of chronic lung conditions in developing regions. In Costa Rica for example, an estimated 13% of the population suffers from asthma.[43]

Lung cancer should be considered in immigrants with chronic pulmonary complaints and no evidence for infectious cause. Over two million men in developing nations are estimated to die each year from smoking-related diseases, the most common of these being lung cancer.[5] Pollution and occupational exposures may also increase immigrants' risks of developing malignancy.

## Gastrointestinal Tract

Gastrointestinal (GI) symptoms in a sick refugee or immigrant may include diarrhea, nausea, vomiting, abdominal pain or distension, jaundice, anorexia, and organomegaly. Although infectious etiologies account for many gastrointestinal problems, there are also several very important noninfectious causes that must be considered (Box 14.5).

### Diarrhea

Diarrhea is a major cause of morbidity and mortality among displaced populations; its high prevalence is often due to inadequate water supplies and sanitation facilities. In determining the most likely etiology of diarrhea, it is useful first to consider whether the diarrhea is acute (less than 2 weeks' duration) or chronic (over 2 weeks). Any of the viral or bacterial pathogens (such as rotavirus, *Escherichia coli*, *Shigella*, and *Salmonella*) commonly encountered in the US may also be the cause of acute diarrhea in an immigrant. Serious systemic infections such as

**Box 14.5**

**Differential diagnosis of gastrointestinal complaints**

**Diarrhea**

**Acute (less than 2 weeks' duration)**
Adenovirus
*Campylobacter* spp.
*E. coli*
Norovirus
Rotavirus
*Salmonella* spp.
*Shigella* spp.
Systemic infections (malaria, measles, Legionella, the
    hemorrhagic fevers)
*Vibrio cholerae*

**Chronic (more than 4 weeks)**
Chagas' disease with pseudo-obstruction
*E. histolytica*
Inflammatory bowel disease
Malabsorption
    Chronic pancreatitis
    Cryptosporidium
    Giardia and other parasites
    Lactose intolerance
    Strongyloides
Tropical sprue
Metabolic disorders

**Abdominal pain**
Gastroesophageal reflux
Helminth infection
Lead toxicity
Malignancy
Pancreatitis
Peptic ulcer disease (*Helicobacter pylori* infection)
Reproductive tract disorders
Sickle cell disease with abdominal crisis
Tuberculosis related strictures
Appendicitis

**Jaundice**
Hepatocellular damage
    Acute infection (EBV, adenovirus, CMV,
      leptospirosis)
    Alcohol abuse
    Bantu siderosis
    Hepatitis B
    Hepatitis D in patient with hepatitis B

Hepatitis C
Hepatocellular carcinoma
Indian childhood cirrhosis
Other infectious hepatitides
Schistosomiasis
Toxic ingestions
Yellow fever
Portal vein disease
    Schistosomiasis
    Veno-occlusive disease
Biliary disease
    *Ascaris* infection
    *Clonorchiasis* spp.
    *Echinococcus* spp.
*Opisthorchis* spp.
Hemolysis

**Abdominal distension**

**Ascites**
Heart failure
Intra-abdominal tuberculosis
Liver failure
Pulmonary hypertension

**Masses**
Megacolon due to Chagas' disease
Ovarian neoplasms
Primary GI malignancies
Amoebiasis

**Splenomegaly**
Brucellosis
Cytomegalovirus
Epstein Barr virus
Fungal infections
Heart failure
Hemoglobinopathies
Hyper-reactive malarial splenomegaly
Liver cirrhosis
Malignancies (especially lymphoproliferative disorders)
Salmonella
Schistosomiasis
Sequestration
Tuberculosis
Visceral leishmaniasis

malaria, measles, *Legionella*, relapsing fever, melioidosis, the hemorrhagic fevers, and anthrax may be associated with acute diarrhea. Although outbreaks of cholera have occurred in several refugee camps, there have been few cases imported into the US.[9,44]

The differential diagnosis of chronic diarrhea in an immigrant is broader than that of acute diarrhea. If the patient reports blood in stools, malignancy, inflammatory bowel disease, an infection with *E. histolytica* should be considered. If the patient reports no blood in stools but has signs of malnutrition, malabsorption syndromes are likely. Both primary GI disease and systemic diseases can cause malabsorption.

Tropical enteropathy is a form of primary malabsorption associated with intestinal mucosal morphological abnormalities.[45] Parasitic infections such as *Giardia* and *Cryptosporidium* can cause severe secondary malnutrition.[46] Deficiency of digestive enzymes as seen in chronic pancreatitis, liver failure, or biliary disease is another possible etiology. Chagas' disease can lead to malabsorption and diarrhea by causing pseudo-obstruction.[47] Endocrine/metabolic diseases such as hyperthyroidism can also cause chronic diarrhea. Lactose intolerance is yet another cause of nonresolving diarrhea; this may become evident as immigrants adopt a Western diet and consume increased amounts of dairy products.

## Abdominal pain

Epigastric abdominal pain may be secondary to gastritis, gastroesophageal reflux, or peptic ulcer disease. *Helicobacter pylori* infection is particularly prevalent in the developing world. In some regions, up to 70% of children are infected by the age of 10 years compared to only 10% of children in the US.[48]

Colicky abdominal pain is suggestive of helminth infection; *Ascaris lumbricoides* is estimated to infect a quarter of the world's population.[49] Infection with *Strongyloides stercoralis* is a common etiology of abdominal complaints in immigrants although a variety of other cestodes, nematodes, and trematodes may also cause abdominal problems. However, it is important to note that most intestinal helminth infections cause no signs or symptoms. Colicky abdominal pain may also be the presenting symptom of TB-induced intestinal strictures or lead poisoning, particularly in children. Other causes of abdominal pain to consider include pancreatitis (which can be caused by migrating nematodes), malignancy, hepatosplenomegaly, or vaso-occlusive abdominal crisis in a sickle cell patient. In women with lower abdominal pain, pelvic inflammatory disease and ectopic pregnancy must be considered.

## Jaundice

There are many possible infectious and noninfectious diseases that can cause jaundice in immigrant populations. Jaundice may be the result of intrinsic hepatocellular disease, biliary disease, or hemolysis. Acute hepatitis may be secondary to viral infection; although the majority of patients with acute hepatitis

C infection are generally asymptomatic, patients with acute hepatitis B, hepatitis E, or hepatitis D (in patients with chronic hepatitis B) may present with jaundice and acute liver failure.[50–52] Many immigrants are from regions where hepatitis A is endemic; therefore, adults are less likely to present with severe liver dysfunction related to this infection. Other causes of acute hepatitis include yellow fever and other viral hemorrhagic diseases, brucellosis, and leptospirosis. These causes are especially important in newly arrived immigrants.

Chronic hepatocellular disease, which can present with progressive jaundice, ascites, encephalopathy, coagulopathy, and GI hemorrhage, may be related to chronic hepatitis B or C infection. Symptoms may not become evident for years after infection. Chronic hepatitis B and C infections are associated with an increased risk of developing hepatocellular carcinoma (HCC). The risk of HCC is particularly high in patients with hepatitis B and cirrhosis; among this group, an estimated 1.5% per year will develop HCC.[53] In Africa and Asia, 60% of cases of HCC are attributed to hepatitis B; in US-born citizens, only 20% of cases are attributed to this infection.[54] In addition to high rates of exposure to hepatitis B, immigrants are at increased risk of developing HCC because of aflatoxin exposure. Given these risk factors, the rate of HCC in immigrants is significantly higher than in native-born individuals. In fact, in some areas, immigrants are over 30 times more likely to die of HCC than native controls.[54]

Chronic liver disease is also associated with schistosomiasis, which has been estimated to affect over 200 million people in 75 countries.[55] Infection can cause portal fibrosis resulting in hepatomegaly, portal hypertension, and eventually ascites, varices, and splenomegaly. Interestingly, there appears to be little associated hepatocellular damage. Isolated portal hypertension may also be related to veno-occlusive disease, a form of hepatic outflow tract obstruction associated with ingestion of alkaloids found in herbal teas and contaminated grains.[56] This disorder has been found in populations from numerous tropical areas including the Middle East, Caribbean, India, and southern Africa.

Miscellaneous causes of end-stage liver disease are plentiful. Alcohol-related liver failure should be included in the differential of an immigrant with cirrhosis. Iron overload is yet another possible cause; Bantu siderosis, a form of iron overload thought to be due to the combination of increased iron intake and an inherited genetic mutation, can be found in up to 10% of the population in certain rural communities in Africa.[57] Young children from India, Malaysia, Burma, and Sri Lanka may present with a form of idiopathic liver failure known as Indian childhood cirrhosis. As with Wilson's disease, this is associated with high serum copper levels.

Biliary disease can be caused by *Ascaris* infection. These nematodes are found worldwide, from Asia (including India) to Africa to Latin America. Although infected individuals are often asymptomatic, organisms may migrate through the biliary system, producing biliary colic or cholangitis.[58] *Echinococcus granulosis*, endemic worldwide, can form hydatids that communicate with the biliary tree. When hydatids rupture, obstructive jaundice, cholangitis, and cholecystitis can result.[59]

Liver fluke infections occur in Japan, Korea, China, Vietnam, Laos, Thailand, Europe, and former Soviet Union. Certain species migrate through the biliary system producing biliary colic, cholelithiasis, and occasionally cholangitis.[60] Other species (Opisthorciasis) may enter the liver parenchyma and may not become evident until years after immigration.[61] Chronic infection with liver flukes is also associated with the development of cholangiocarcinoma, which is usually rapidly fatal.

### Abdominal distension

As with the other GI signs and symptoms presented thus far, the differential diagnosis of an immigrant presenting with abdominal distension is very broad. Ascites may result from liver disease, heart failure, or severe pulmonary hypertension. Megacolon caused by Chagas' disease can cause significant distension.

Intra-abdominal TB or malignancies are other possible etiologies to consider.

### Splenomegaly

Splenomegaly in an immigrant may be due to both infectious and noninfectious causes. Hyper-reactive malaria syndrome (also known as tropical splenomegaly syndrome or hyper-reactive malarial splenomegaly syndrome) should be considered in an immigrant from a region with endemic malaria. Although malarial parasitemia may not be demonstrated in these patients, it is thought that exposure to malaria triggers an exaggerated stimulation of polyclonal B lymphocytes leading to immune dysregulation and eventual splenomegaly.[62] Other infectious causes of splenomegaly include TB, schistosomiasis, visceral leishmaniasis, brucellosis,

cytomegalovirus (CMV), *Salmonella*, fungal diseases, and acute EBV infection. In addition to these infectious causes, malignancies, particularly B-cell lymphoproliferative disorders, should be considered in immigrants found to have splenomegaly.

## Genitourinary Tract

Many diseases of the genitourinary system that affect immigrants are similar to those seen in the native US population (Box 14.6). However, many of these conditions will present at more advanced stages in immigrants due to poor access to healthcare prior to immigration. Some disorders, such as schistosomiasis and TB-related renal disease, will be more common in certain immigrant populations.

### Chronic renal disease

Several of the most common causes of chronic kidney disease in international populations are glomerulonephritis, chronic interstitial nephritis, diabetes mellitus, and hypertension.[63-65] The most common causes of glomerular disease in developing regions include poststreptococcus glomerulonephritis, malaria, hepatitis B and C, IgA nephropathy, and HIV.[66] Interstitial nephritis, most common in immigrants from India and Pakistan, may result from TB, visceral leishmaniasis, or industrial and environmental toxins.[65,66] The global prevalence of diabetes mellitus is staggering; an estimated 171 million people are diabetic.[67] Rates are increasing alarmingly, particularly in developing nations. Immigrants may have had diabetes for a prolonged period of time, but were never appropriately managed, making the likelihood of developing diabetic nephropathy higher than in the domestic population. Hypertension also affects millions of individuals worldwide and is an important cause of renal disease.[64]

### Hematuria

In an immigrant presenting with hematuria, infection with *Schistosoma hematobium* must be considered. Urinary schistosomiasis is endemic in sub-Saharan Africa and often presents with gross, painless hematuria. If left untreated, schistosomal infections can progress to renal failure secondary to obstructive uropathy. These infections are also associated with the development of squamous cell bladder

**Differential diagnosis of genitourinary disorders**

**Chronic renal disease**

Glomerulonephritis
   Poststreptococcal
   IgA nephropathy
   HIV
   Hepatitis B or C
   Malaria
   Schistosomiasis
Nephritis
   Tuberculosis
   Toxins/medications
   Visceral leishmaniasis
Diabetic nephropathy
Hypertensive nephropathy

**Hematuria**

Schistosomiasis
Sickle cell disease with renal infarctions
Bladder malignancy
Bladder/kidney stones
Poststreptococcal glomerulonephritis

**Milky/tan urine**

Bancroftian filariasis

**Genital lesions**

Sexually transmitted disease
   Gonorrhea
   Syphilis
   HSV
   *Haemophilus ducreyi*
   *Lymphogranuloma venereum*
Other infections
   Genital schistosomiasis
Malignancy
   Penile carcinoma
   Cervical cancer
   Vulvar cancer
Trauma
Female genital manipulation/excision

with rupture or fistula formation into the urinary tract.[70]

## Genital lesions

Genital lesions, especially when associated with dysuria or penile/vaginal discharge raise the possibility of sexually transmitted infections (STIs). Millions of individuals are infected yearly with syphilis, gonorrhea, chlamydia, HSV, and trichomoniasis. The majority of these infections occur in developing regions, where testing and treatment options are often more limited than in the US. It is therefore vital to screen for STIs in any immigrant with symptoms or suggestive history. The importance of screening for HIV, particularly in patients with other STIs, cannot be overemphasized given the high prevalence of this infection in many regions of the world. In addition to more common STIs, infections uncommon in the US such as *lymphogranuloma venereum* and chancroid (due to *Haemophilus ducreyi*) may be seen in immigrants. Nonsexually transmitted infections such as schistosomiasis and amoebiasis can also cause genital lesions; these lesions can easily be mistaken for those caused by STIs.

Genital lesions may also be due to noninfectious causes. Penile lesions may be secondary to carcinoma; although rare in the US, penile carcinoma accounts for nearly 10% of all malignancies in some regions of Africa and South America.[71] In Uganda, it is the most commonly diagnosed cancer.[71]

Cervical cancer is also important to include on the differential diagnosis of a female immigrant with constitutional, abdominal, or genital complaints. It is estimated that over 80% of cases of cervical cancer occur in developing regions; this disproportionately high burden of disease is likely due to lack of screening.[72] Given the high rates of sexual violence in regions of upheaval, genital lesions in refugees should also alert the clinician to the possibility of inflicted trauma. Rape, torture, or sexual assault may present with unusual vulvar lesions, ecchymoses, and lacerations.

Clinicians caring for female immigrants and refugees will likely encounter cases of female genital manipulation (also referred to as female genital excision, female genital mutilation, female circumcision). This is a relatively common practice in many parts of the world; an estimated 120 million girls and women have undergone some form of genital manipulation.[73] Although most common in Africa, this is also practiced in areas of Southeast Asia, the Middle East, and Central and South America.

carcinoma.[68] Other causes of hematuria include renal infarcts due to sickle cell disease, bladder cancer (which may be related to industrial or environmental toxins as well as schistosomiasis), and bladder or kidney stones. Interestingly, studies have shown that Hmong immigrants are more likely to develop uric acid stones than the general population.[69] Milky-tan colored urine in an immigrant may be due to chronic bancroftian filariasis, which causes lymphatic obstruction leading to duct engorgement

Long-term complications of these procedures include localized pain, significant discomfort with menstruation, dyspareunia, and recurrent urinary tract infections.[19]

## Hematologic System

### Anemia

Immigrants may present with a variety of hematologic disorders (Box 14.7). Anemia is the most common blood disorder worldwide; it is estimated that two billion people – over 30% of the global population – have anemia.[74] For the purpose of establishing a differential diagnosis of the cause of anemia, it is helpful to separate this disorder into the broad categories of microcytic, macrocytic, normocytic, and hemolytic.

The most common cause of microcytic anemia in the world is iron deficiency.[75] Based on WHO estimates, nearly five billion people in the world are iron deficient; four out of five of these people are from developing regions.[74] The causes of iron deficiency include poor nutrition, malabsorption, and blood loss. An estimated 750 million people worldwide are infected with hookworm, a common infection in immigrants.[76] Given that an estimated 0.25 mL of blood per worm is lost per day, heavy infections can account for up to 100 mL blood loss per day.[77] It is therefore important to consider evaluation for hookworm in any immigrant with iron deficiency anemia who is from an endemic region.

The thalassemias are another potential cause of microcytic anemia in an immigrant population. This group of hemoglobin disorders is one of the most common genetic conditions in the world, affecting almost 5% of the world's population.[78] Both alpha and beta thalassemia are found across a large geographic range stretching from the equatorial region of Africa through the Mediterranean, Middle East, India, and Southeast Asia. Beta thalassemia is particularly prevalent in Thailand, Cambodia, and southeast China.

Macrocytic anemias are most commonly associated with vitamin $B_{12}$ and folate deficiencies. $B_{12}$ deficiency is often due to malabsorption syndromes such as tropical sprue. Pure nutritional deficiencies are rare except in alcoholics, strict vegans, or those who have been in nutritionally deprived refugee situations. Folate deficiency is most common in pregnant women, those with chronic hemolytic anemia, and in individuals who cook their food for prolonged

---

**Box 14.7**

**Differential diagnosis of common hematologic disorders**

**Anemia**
**Microcytic**
Iron deficiency
    Blood loss (hookworm infection, hemolysis, urinary losses)
    Inadequate intake
    Malabsorption
Spherocytosis and other hemoglobinopathies
Thalassemias

**Macrocytic**
$B_{12}$ deficiency
Folate deficiency
Liver failure
Thyroid disease

**Normocytic**
Acute blood loss
Acute infections
Chronic disease
Early iron deficiency
G6PD deficiency
Malaria
Mixed anemia (i.e. combined iron and folate deficiency)
Sickle cell disease
Celiac disease

**Hemolytic**
G6PD deficiency
Malaria
Sickle cell disease

**Thrombocytopenia**
Many acute infections (malaria, typhoid, dengue fever)
Splenic sequestration

**Eosinophilia**
Parasitic infections (especially helminth infections)
Allergies
Collagen vascular disease
Drug reactions
Fungal infections
Malignancy
HIV infection

---

periods of time. Children who subsist on goat milk products to the exclusion of cow milk products are also at increased risk for folate deficiency. Thyroid dysfunction and liver disease are other potential causes of macrocytic anemia.

Normocytic anemia may result from acute blood loss, early iron deficiency, chronic disease, mixed anemias (i.e. iron deficiency with folate deficiency), or sickle cell disease. The differential diagnosis of hemolytic anemia is broad, but in an immigrant population, sickle cell disease, G6PD deficiency, malaria, and other acute infections should be considered.

## Thrombocytopenia

Thrombocytopenia, often associated with disorders of other cell lines, may be related to acute infectious etiologies such as malaria, typhoid, or dengue fever. Chronic thrombocytopenia may be related to splenic sequestration due to various underlying diseases, but malaria, leishmaniasis, and schistosomiasis must be given high consideration in immigrants from endemic areas.

The combination of anemia, thrombocytopenia, and coagulopathy is suggestive of disseminated intravascular coagulation, which can result from a number of causes including severe infection or sepsis. Unusual etiologies of bleeding and petechiae endemic in regions of Asia, Africa, and Eastern Europe include Lassa fever, Crimean-Congo hemorrhagic fever, dengue hemorrhagic fever, and Ebola and Marburg viral infections. Although rarely imported into the US, these entities deserve special mention because they are life threatening, often highly contagious, and could potentially threaten public health if not quickly recognized and contained with appropriate precautions.

## Eosinophilia

Eosinophilia is a very common finding in immigrants, particularly those from tropical regions. An eosinophil count over 450 cells per cubic millimeter is most commonly due to tissue-invasive parasitic helminths, including cestodes such as *Hymenolepis nana*, nematodes such as *loa loa, Strongyloides, Ascaris*, and *Trichinella*, and trematodes such as *Schistosoma*. Non-helminth causes of eosinophilia include allergies, drug reactions, collagen vascular diseases such as polyarteritis nodosa (which should especially be considered in patients with hepatitis B), malignancies, rarely fungal infections, and HIV.[79,80]

## Musculoskeletal System

Musculoskeletal conditions, both acute and chronic, are extremely prevalent worldwide. Several large

---

**Box 14.8**

**Differential diagnosis of musculoskeletal complaints**

**Arthralgias/arthritis**

**Infectious/postinfectious**
Alphaviruses (such as Chikungunya virus and Ross River virus)
Bartonellosis
Brucellosis
Chlamydia
Cytomegalovirus
Epstein Barr virus
Gram-negative enteric pathogens
HIV
Leptospirosis
Lyme disease
Parvovirus
Psittacosis
Q fever
Rheumatic fever
Rubella

**Noninfectious**
Connective tissue disorders
Familial Mediterranean fever
Osteoarthritis

**Myalgias/myositis**
Lyme disease
Coxsackieviruses
Echoviruses
HIV
HTLV
Influenza
Tropical pyomyositis
Various parasites and protozoans

**Skeletal deformities**
Congenital syphilis
Genetic syndromes
Rickets
Trauma
Scoliosis
Congenital hip dysplasia

---

studies conducted in developing regions have found that up to one-third of the population has at least one musculoskeletal complaint.[81] Although a clinician may see infection-related musculoskeletal conditions more frequently in an immigrant population compared to the general population, noninfectious etiologies will also be encountered (Box 14.8).

## Arthralgias/arthritis

An immigrant patient may complain of arthralgias, myalgias, or display frank arthritis. The sudden onset of arthralgias, especially when associated with systemic symptoms, is most likely due to infection. Bacterial infections such as bartonellosis, brucellosis, leptospirosis, psittacosis, and Q fever can all produce joint symptoms. Monoarticular joint findings are particularly concerning for septic arthritis. Migratory arthritis may be due to rheumatic fever. Infectious causes of arthritis that can be both acute and chronic in nature include parvovirus, EBV, CMV, Lyme disease, and the alphaviruses, particularly Ross River virus in individuals from the Pacific Islands, and Chikungunya virus in those from Africa and Asia.[82] Reactive arthritis may develop after infection with *Chlamydia* or enteric Gram-negative bacteria such as *Salmonella, Shigella, Yersinia,* or *Campylobacter*;[83] it is therefore important to inquire about recent illness in any patient presenting with new arthritis. HIV infection has been associated with a number of joint conditions including reactive arthritis, psoriatic arthritis, and undifferentiated spondyloarthropathies.[84] Recurrent arthritis can be seen in patients with familial Mediterranean fever; this should be considered in immigrants from the appropriate geographical area.

Immigrants may also have arthritis secondary to connective tissue disorders; studies have shown that the prevalence of rheumatologic diseases is roughly equivalent in developed and developing regions.[85] Chronic arthritis that is not associated with systemic symptoms may be due to osteoarthritis, one of the most common causes of musculoskeletal complaints in the world.[81] Lower back and knee pain are particularly common in women and men who have a history of carrying large, heavy burdens on their back or head for many years.

## Myalgias/myositis

Myositis, which generally presents with severe myalgias, generalized weakness, and fever, can be caused by a number of organisms including HIV, HTLV, influenza, coxsackieviruses, echoviruses, and *Borrelia burgdorferi.* Tropical pyomyositis, associated with deep cutaneous infections with *Staphylococcus aureus,* can be life threatening if not promptly recognized.[86] Myalgias and myositis may occur secondary to protozoan or parasitic infections including cysticercosis, malaria, trichinosis, and trypanosomiasis.

Parasites are the more likely etiology when the patient is afebrile.

## Skeletal deformities

Skeletal deformities in an immigrant, particularly in a child, may be due to rickets, or in certain populations, fluorosis. Although initially thought to be due only to vitamin D deficiency, calcium deficiency is now also recognized as a cause of rickets.[87] Young children will most often present with vitamin D-related rickets, while adolescents and occasionally adults, particularly those from South Africa, Nigeria, and Bangladesh, will present with calcium-related rickets.[87] Skeletal deformities in children may also be due to genetic syndromes, untreated scoliosis, congenital syphilis, or unrecognized congenital hip dysplasia. Given the high prevalence of accidents worldwide, trauma is yet another common cause of skeletal deformities in immigrants.

## Skin

A myriad of dermatologic signs and symptoms due to an array of conditions are possible in a patient who has immigrated to the US (Box 14.9). It is especially important for the clinician to recognize the skin manifestations of several severe systemic infections, as these infections can be life threatening and can pose significant public health risks.

## Petechiae/purpura

Any patient presenting with petechiae and purpura must be evaluated promptly, as these skin lesions often accompany severe, potentially lethal systemic infections such as meningococcosis, leptospirosis, rickettsial infections, severe malaria, and viral hemorrhagic fevers (such as dengue fever, yellow fever, and Lassa fever). Other severe systemic infections with skin manifestations that should not be missed include measles, acute HIV, disseminated gonococcus, and syphilis.

## Migratory lesions

Migratory lesions are likely due to parasitic infections; these infections are often associated with eosinophilia. One of the most common migratory rashes is cutaneous larva migrans (CLM). Symptoms result when the larvae of hookworms (usually

### Differential diagnosis of dermatologic conditions

**Petechiae/purpura**
Acute HIV
Disseminated gonococcus
Leptospirosis
Malaria
Measles
Meningococcus
Rickettsial diseases
Syphilis
Viral hemorrhagic fevers (yellow fever, Lassa fever, dengue fever)

**Migratory lesions**
Cutaneous larva migrans
Gnathostomiasis
*Loa loa*
Paragonimiasis
*Strongyloides stercoralis*

**Nodules**
Cysticercosis
Echinococcus
Kaposi's sarcoma (HIV and non-HIV associated)
Leprosy
Onchocerciasis
Schistosomiasis
Skin cancer
Sporotrichosis
Sparganosis

**Ulcers**
**Infectious**
Anthrax (often with eschar)
Cutaneous leishmaniasis
Granuloma inguinale
*H. ducreyi*
Leprosy
*M. ulcerans*
Rickettsial infections
Syphilis
Yaws

**Noninfectious**
Chronic arsenic exposure
Nutritional deficiencies

**Various skin lesions**
Autoimmune disorders (vitiligo, pemphigus)
Traditional healing practices (cupping, coining, scarification)
Trauma
Skin cancer

*Ancylostoma braziliense*) penetrate the skin and migrate through superficial tissues. Larvae can migrate for weeks to months if not treated.[88] *Strongyloides* can also cause transient serpiginous lesions, most commonly on the buttocks, groin, and trunk as opposed to the usual foot involvement of CLM. Gnathostomiasis, most common in Asia, can present with intermittent creeping eruptions due to migration of the immature adult. As with scabies, this is often associated with severe pruritis and may uniquely cause bruising. Loiasis, caused by the *Loa loa* worm, is endemic in much of Africa. This infection causes pruritus and intermittent swelling of subcutaneous tissues (known as Calabar swellings). Individual worms can also occasionally be seen migrating across the conjunctiva.

## Nodules

Skin nodules frequently have infectious etiologies. Infection with the filarial nematode *Onchocerca volvulus*, most common in Africa but also found in Mexico, Central America, and South America, causes not only diffuse dermatitis, but also nodular subcutaneous lesions. Nodules are often found on bony prominences, upper back, and head. The incubation period of this infection can be years; therefore, new symptoms may occur in an immigrant that has been in the US for an extended period of time.[89] Nodular lesions are also seen with Kaposi's sarcoma. Although many of these cases are associated with HIV infection (atypical Kaposi's), there is also a form of Kaposi's that is endemic in Africa; this form is not associated with HIV infection and generally affects individuals at a younger age.[90] Other important infectious causes of nodular lesions include sporotrichosis, leprosy, *Echinococcus*, cysticercosis, sparganosis, and schistosomiasis.

## Ulcers

Ulcers, like nodular lesions, have many possible causes. Painless ulcers may result from cutaneous leishmaniasis, primary syphilis, or granuloma inguinale. Ulcers associated with eschars may be due to anthrax or rickettsial infections. Leprosy may result in numerous neuropathic ulcers, and mycobacterial infections, particularly *M. ulcerans*, can cause severe ulcerations. Yaws, a re-emerging spirochete infection found in Africa, Asia, Oceana, and South America, is characterized by numerous papillomas; with time, these lesions may ulcerate.

## Various skin lesions

Noninfectious etiologies must also be included in the differential diagnosis of the immigrant with a dermatologic complaint. Protein malnutrition leads to depigmentation, desquamation, edema, hair color changes (black hair becomes red and brown hair becomes blond), and nail thinning. Pellagra is characterized by dermatitis, usually over sun-exposed areas. Chronic arsenic exposure can cause hyperpigmentation, hyperkeratosis of the palms and soles, and characteristic nail findings.[14]

Skin cancers are far less common in dark skinned individuals than in those with fair coloring; however, melanoma, basal cell carcinoma, and squamous cell carcinoma (which may develop at sites of chronic ulceration) should be considered in any patient with skin lesions. Autoimmune disorders, such as vitiligo and pemphigus, can also be seen in immigrant populations. Various forms of pemphigus are endemic to well-defined regions of South and Central America and Africa.[91] Fungal skin infections are very common in the tropics and are seen frequently in newly arrived immigrants and refugees. Linear or circular lesions may be due to cupping or coining, two traditional healing practices frequently seen in Asian immigrants. Bruising or scarring may indicate recent or past trauma.

## Conclusion

Given the increasing number of immigrants in the US, it is vitally important for clinicians to have an understanding of the healthcare issues affecting this group. When caring for an immigrant, timely diagnosis and treatment is crucial, not only for the well-being of the individual, but also for the health of the general population. As outlined in this chapter, symptoms, examination findings, and personal history must all be taken into account when caring for an ill immigrant. Meticulous attention to these details enables the clinician to generate and narrow a list of potential diagnoses. An appropriate differential diagnosis can then be used to develop a focused and rational diagnostic strategy, a critical step on the pathway to prompt diagnosis and treatment.

## References

1. Camarota SA, Center for Immigration Studies (Washington DC). Economy slowed, but immigration didn't: the foreign-born population, 2000–2004. Washington, DC: Center for Immigration Studies; 2004.
2. Montano SM, Villaran MV, Ylquimiche L. Neurocysticercosis: association between seizures, serology, and brain CT in rural Peru. Neurology 2005; 65:229–233.
3. Robbins JB, Schneerson R, Gotschlich EC, et al. Meningococcal meningitis in sub-Saharan Africa: the case for mass and routine vaccination with available polysaccharide vaccines. Bull World Health Organ 2003; 81:745–750; discussion 751–755.
4. Nicolas P, Ait M'barek N, Al-Awaidy S, et al. Pharyngeal carriage of serogroup W135 Neisseria meningitidis in Hajjees and their family contacts in Morocco, Oman and Sudan. APMIS 2005; 113:182–186.
5. Murray CJ, Lopez AD. Mortality by cause for eight regions of the world: Global Burden of Disease Study. Lancet 1997; 349(9061):1269–1276.
6. Proietti FA, Carneiro-Proietti AB, Catalan-Soares BC, et al. Global epidemiology of HTLV-1 infection and associated diseases. Oncogene 2005; 24:6058–6068.
7. Hemachudha T, Wacharapluesadee S, Mitrabhakdi E, et al. Pathophysiology of human paralytic rabies. J Neurovirol 2005; 11(1):93–100.
8. Kumar A. Movement disorders in the tropics. Parkinsonism Relat Disord 2002; 9:69–75.
9. Centers for Disease Control and Prevention. Famine-affected, refugee, and displaced populations: recommendations for public health issues. MMWR Recomm Rep 1992; 41(RR-13):1–76.
10. Geltman PL, Brown MJ, Cochran J. Lead poisoning among refugee children resettled in Massachusetts, 1995 to 1999. Pediatrics 2001; 108:158–162.
11. Centers for Disease Control and Prevention. Elevated blood lead levels in refugee children – New Hampshire, 2003–2004. MMWR 2005; 54:42–46.
12. Clarkson TW, Magos L, Myers GJ. The toxicology of mercury – current exposures and clinical manifestations. N Engl J Med 2003; 349:1731–1737.
13. Boudou A, Maury-Brachet R, Coquery M, et al. Synergic effect of gold mining and damming on mercury contamination in fish. Environ Sci Technol 2005; 39:2448–2454.
14. Sengupta MK, Mukherjee A, Hossain MA, et al. Groundwater arsenic contamination in the Ganga-Padma-Meghna-Brahmaputra plain of India and Bangladesh. Arch Environ Health 2003; 58:701–702.
15. Ernst E. Toxic heavy metals and undeclared drugs in Asian herbal medicines. Trends Pharmacol Sci 2002; 23:136–139.
16. Fazel M, Wheeler J, Danesh J. Prevalence of serious mental disorder in 7000 refugees resettled in Western countries: a systematic review. Lancet 2005; 365(9467):1309–1314.
17. Marshall GN, Schell TL, Elliott MN, et al. Mental health of Cambodian refugees 2 decades after resettlement in the United States. JAMA 2005; 294:571–579.
18. Carta MG, Bernal M, Hardoy MC, et al. Migration and mental health in Europe (the state of the mental health in Europe working group: appendix 1). Clin Pract Epidemol Ment Health 2005; 1:13.
19. Adams KM, Gardiner LD, Assefi N. Healthcare challenges from the developing world: post-immigration refugee medicine. Br Med J 2004; 328(7455):1548–1552.
20. Ritsner M, Ponizovsky A, Kurs R, et al. Somatization in an immigrant population in Israel: a community survey of prevalence, risk factors, and help-seeking behavior. Am J Psychiatry 2000; 157:385–392.
21. Brown JM, Penne CC, Groerer JC. Immigrants and substance use: findings from the 1999–2001 National Surveys on Drug Use and Health. 2005, Department of Health and Human Services Substance Abuse and Mental Health Services Administration, Office of Applied Studies: Rockville, MD. Publication No. SMA 04 3909, Analytic Series A-23.
22. Resnikoff S, Pascolini D, Etya'ale D, et al. Global data on visual impairment in the year 2002. Bull World Health Organ 2004; 82:844–851.

23. Taylor H. Towards the global elimination of trachoma. Nat Med 1999; 5:492–493.

24. Whitcher JP, Srinivasan M, Upadhyay MP. Corneal blindness: a global perspective. Bull World Health Organ 2001; 79:214–221.

25. Kumaresan J. Can blinding trachoma be eliminated by 20/20? Eye 2005; 19:1067–1073.

26. Jones J, Lopez A, Wilson M. Congenital toxoplasmosis. Am Fam Physician 2003; 67:2131–2138.

27. Giamberti A, Mele M, Di Terlizzi M, et al. Association of children with heart disease in the world: 10-year experience. Pediatr Cardiol 2004; 25:492–494.

28. Rheumatic fever and rheumatic heart disease. World Health Organ Tech Rep Ser, 2004. 923:1–122, back cover.

29. Mackay J, Mensah G, eds. Atlas of heart disease and stroke. Lyon: World Health Organization; 2004:46.

30. Kirchhoff LV, Weiss LM, Wittner M, et al. Parasitic diseases of the heart. Front Biosci 2004; 9:706–723.

31. Shah SS, McGowan JP. Rickettsial, ehrlichial and *Bartonella* infections of the myocardium and pericardium. Front Biosci 2003; 8:e197–e201.

32. Fairley CK, Ryan M, Wall PG, et al. The organisms reported to cause infective myocarditis and pericarditis in England and Wales. J Infect 1996; 32:223–225.

33. Higuchi ML, De Morais CF, Pereira Barreto AC, et al. The role of active myocarditis in the development of heart failure in chronic Chagas' disease: a study based on endomyocardial biopsies. Clin Cardiol 1987; 10:665–670.

34. Church DL. Major factors affecting the emergence and reemergence of infectious diseases. Clin Lab Med 2004; 24:559–586, v.

35. Centers for Disease Control and Prevention. Reported tuberculosis in the United States, 2004. Atlanta, GA: US Department of Health and Human Services; 2005.

36. Chemtob D, Weiler-Ravell D, Leventhal A, et al. Epidemiologic characteristics of pediatric active tuberculosis among immigrants from high to low tuberculosis-endemic countries: the Israeli experience. Isr Med Assoc J 2006; 8:21–26.

37. Cowie RL, Sharpe JW. Tuberculosis among immigrants: interval from arrival in Canada to diagnosis. A 5-year study in southern Alberta. Can Med Assoc J 1998; 158:599–602.

38. Farah MG, Meyer HE, Selmer R, et al. Long-term risk of tuberculosis among immigrants in Norway. Int J Epidemiol 2005; 34:1005–1011.

39. Kempainen R, Nelson K, Williams DN, et al. *Mycobacterium tuberculosis* disease in Somali immigrants in Minnesota. Chest 2001; 119:176–180.

40. Newberry AM, Williams DN, Stauffer WM, et al. Strongyloides hyperinfection presenting as acute respiratory failure and Gram-negative sepsis. Chest 2005; 128:3681–3684.

41. Morris W, Knauer CM. Cardiopulmonary manifestations of schistosomiasis. Semin Respir Infect, 1997; 12:159–170.

42. Cheng AC, Currie BJ. Melioidosis: epidemiology, pathophysiology, and management. Clin Microbiol Rev 2005; 18:383–416.

43. Bousquet J, Bosquet PJ, Godard P, et al. The public health implications of asthma. Bull World Health Organ 2005; 83:548–554.

44. Weber JT, Levine WC, Hopkins DP, et al. Cholera in the United States, 1965–1991. Risks at home and abroad. Arch Intern Med 1994; 154:551–556.

45. Nath SK. Tropical sprue. Curr Gastroenterol Rep 2005; 7:343–349.

46. Bai JC. Malabsorption syndromes. Digestion 1998; 59:530–546.

47. Hirano I, Pandolfino J. Chronic intestinal pseudo-obstruction. Dig Dis 2000; 18:83–92.

48. Czinn SJ. *Helicobacter pylori* infection: detection, investigation, and management. J Pediatr 2005; 146(3 Suppl): S21–S26.

49. Hall A, Holland C. Geographical variation in *Ascaris lumbricoides* fecundity and its implications for helminth control. Parasitol Today 2000; 16:540–544.

50. Lin KW, Kirchner JT. Hepatitis B. Am Fam Physician 2004; 69:75–82.

51. Mondelli MU, Cerino A, Cividini A. Acute hepatitis C: diagnosis and management. J Hepatol 2005; 42(Supp)l: S108–S114.

52. Wang L, Zhuang H. Hepatitis E: an overview and recent advances in vaccine research. World J Gastroenterol 2004; 10:2157–2162.

53. Hayashi PH, Di Bisceglie AM. The progression of hepatitis B- and C-infections to chronic liver disease and hepatocellular carcinoma: epidemiology and pathogenesis. Med Clin North Am 2005; 89:371–389.

54. Bosch FX, Ribes J, Cleries R, et al. Epidemiology of hepatocellular carcinoma. Clin Liver Dis 2005;9:191–211, v.

55. Vennervald BJ, Dunne DW. Morbidity in schistosomiasis: an update. Curr Opin Infect Dis 2004; 17:439–447.

56. DeLeve LD. Vascular liver diseases. Curr Gastroenterol Rep 2003; 5:63–70.

57. Gangaidzo IT, Moyo VM, Saungweme T, et al. Iron overload in urban Africans in the 1990s. Gut 1999; 45:278–283.

58. Carpenter HA. Bacterial and parasitic cholangitis. Mayo Clin Proc 1998; 73:473–478.

59. Sezgin O, Altintas E, Saritas U, et al. Hepatic alveolar echinococcosis: clinical and radiologic features and endoscopic management. J Clin Gastroenterol 2005; 39:160–167.

60. Liu LX, Harinasuta KT. Liver and intestinal flukes. Gastroenterol Clin North Am 1996; 25:627–636.

61. Stauffer WM, Sellman JS, Walker PF. Biliary liver flukes (opisthorchiasis and clonorchiasis) in immigrants in the United States: often subtle and diagnosed years after arrival. J Travel Med 2004; 11:157–159.

62. Crane GG. Hyperreactive malarious splenomegaly (tropical splenomegaly syndrome). Parasitol Today 1986; 2:4–9.

63. Alebiosu CO, Ayodele OE. The global burden of chronic kidney disease and the way forward. Ethn Dis 2005; 15:418–423.

64. Naicker S. End-stage renal disease in sub-Saharan and South Africa. Kidney Int Suppl 2003; 83:S119–122.

65. Barsoum RS. Chronic kidney disease in the developing world. N Engl J Med 2006; 354:997–999.

66. Barsoum RS. Overview: end-stage renal disease in the developing world. Artif Organs 2002; 26:737–746.

67. Wild S, Roglic G, Green A, et al. Global prevalence of diabetes: estimates for the year 2000 and projections for 2030. Diabetes Care 2004; 27:1047–1053.

68. Patton SE, Hall MC, Ozen H. Bladder cancer. Curr Opin Oncol 2002; 14:265–272.

69. Portis AJ, Hermans K, Culhane-Pera KA, et al. Stone disease in the Hmong of Minnesota: initial description of a high-risk population. J Endourol 2004; 18:853–857.

70. Dreyer G, Noroes J, Figueredo-Silva J, et al. Pathogenesis of lymphatic disease in bancroftian filariasis: a clinical perspective. Parasitol Today 2000; 16:544–548.

71. Misra S, Chaturvedi A, Misra NC. Penile carcinoma: a challenge for the developing world. Lancet Oncol 2004; 5:240–247.

72. Mandelblatt JS, Lawrence WF, Gaffikin L, et al. Costs and benefits of different strategies to screen for cervical cancer in less-developed countries. J Natl Cancer Inst 2002; 94:1469–1483.

73. Weir E, Female genital mutilation. Can Med Assoc J 2000; 162:1344.

74. Iron deficiency anaemia: assessment, prevention, and control. WHO/UNICEF/UNU. Geneva: World Health Organization; 2001.

75. Massey AC. Microcytic anemia. Differential diagnosis and management of iron deficiency anemia. Med Clin North Am 1992; 76:549–566.

76. de Silva NR, Brooker S, Hotez PJ, et al. Soil-transmitted helminth infections: updating the global picture. Trends Parasitol 2003;19:547–551.

77. Kucik CJ, Martin GL, Sortor BV. Common intestinal parasites. Am Fam Physician 2004; 69:1161–1168.

78. Rund D, Rachmilewitz E. Beta-thalassemia. N Engl J Med 2005; 353:1135–1146.

79. Moore TA, Nutman TB. Eosinophilia in the returning traveler. Infect Dis Clin North Am 1998; 12:503–521.

80. Rothenberg ME. Eosinophilia. N Engl J Med 1998; 338:1592–1600.

81. Brooks PM. Impact of osteoarthritis on individuals and society: how much disability? Social consequences and health economic implications. Curr Opin Rheumatol 2002; 14:573–577.

82. Suhrbier A, La Linn M. Clinical and pathologic aspects of arthritis due to Ross River virus and other alphaviruses. Curr Opin Rheumatol 2004; 16:374–379.

83. Leirisalo-Repo M. Early arthritis and infection. Curr Opin Rheumatol 2005; 17:433–439.

84. Tehranzadeh J, Ter-Oganesyan RR, Steinbach LS. Musculoskeletal disorders associated with HIV infection and AIDS. Part I: infectious musculoskeletal conditions. Skeletal Radiol 2004; 33:249–259.

85. World Health Organization. Global burden of musculoskeletal disease revealed in new WHO report. Bull World Health Organ 2003; 81:853–854.

86. Chauhan S, Jain S, Varma S, et al. Tropical pyomyositis (myositis tropicans): current perspective. Postgrad Med J 2004; 80:267–270.

87. Pettifor JM. Rickets and vitamin D deficiency in children and adolescents. Endocrinol Metab Clin North Am 2005; 34:537–553, vii.

88. Richey TK, Gentry RH, Fitzpatrick JE, et al. Persistent cutaneous larva migrans due to Ancylostoma species. South Med J 1996; 89:609–611.

89. Brattig NW. Pathogenesis and host responses in human onchocerciasis: impact of Onchocerca filariae and Wolbachia endobacteria. Microbes Infect 2004; 6:113–128.

90. Ablashi DV, Chatlynne LG, Whitman JE Jr, et al. Spectrum of Kaposi's sarcoma-associated herpesvirus, or human herpesvirus 8, diseases. Clin Microbiol Rev 2002; 15:439–464.

91. Abreu-Velez AM, Hashimoto T, Bollag WB, et al. A unique form of endemic pemphigus in northern Colombia. J Am Acad Dermatol 2003; 49:599–608.

# CHAPTER 15

# Diseases by Country of Origin

Mary E. Wilson

## Introduction

Infectious disease risks vary by geographic region and can change over time. Because many infections can persist in an individual for years and sometimes for a lifetime, the geographic regions of previous residence, and, to a lesser extent, travel, are relevant in the evaluation of immigrants, whether or not they have symptoms. Because many immigrants have families and relatives in their country of origin, they and their children may visit, placing them at risk for infections that may be absent or rare in the United States. Previous exposures, infections, and healthcare may place them at lower or higher risk for specific infections. For example, most people who grew up in developing countries are immune to hepatitis A because of infection in childhood (which may have been mild or inapparent and unrecognized), though as sanitation facilities improve in many countries, levels of immunity to hepatitis A are decreasing.[1,2] On the other hand, people who reside in tropical and subtropical areas are much less likely to be immune to varicella (chickenpox) than are residents of temperate areas, where most people (in the pre-vaccine era) became infected in childhood. Varicella infections occur in adult immigrants and are more likely to be severe than cases acquired in childhood.[3] In the US between 1985 and 1994 about 20% of all adult varicella deaths were in foreign-born adults.[4] Immigrants may be susceptible to other infections because vaccinations were not given or were ineffective, for example, because of poor vaccine quality, inadequate dose or number of doses, or poor immune response because of age, nutritional status, coincidental infections, or other factors. Older immigrants who have been in the US for a long time may lack immunity to tetanus because they have never received a primary series of tetanus toxoid (and a booster dose after an injury will not provide adequate protection).[5,6]

Clinicians caring for immigrants and their families need to know what persisting infections or sequelae of past infections in immigrants may be clinically or epidemiologically relevant today and in the future.[7-9] This chapter provides a series of tables that describe infectious diseases by geographic region of the world.[10,11] The geographic areas chosen are those that have been the origin of the largest number of immigrants to the United States, especially in recent years.[12-16] Specific countries are listed within some regions. Although space does not permit listing of all countries of the world, other countries in a given region may share similarities in infectious disease risk. The majority of immigrants to the US before 1950 came from Europe and Canada, areas where many infectious disease risks are similar to those in the US. Thus, infectious disease risks in those areas are not listed separately.

The infections chosen for the tables are those that may be associated with morbidity weeks to decades after a person has left a country of origin.[9] Where data are available and relevant, some description of the distribution and incidence is provided. The estimated incidence of tuberculosis is given by country and, when available, the percentage of cases with multidrug resistance is included. The incidence for many infections has decreased over time in many regions (HIV is a notable exception). Current incidence of infection may not accurately reflect the risk of acquiring infection when the immigrant lived in a country 10 or 20 years earlier. This is especially true for chronic infections, such as syphilis, tuberculosis, onchocerciasis, lymphatic filariasis, leprosy, and schistosomiasis. For example, global prevalence of leprosy has fallen by almost 90% in the last 20 years. The epidemiological situation in earlier years may be more relevant than the current prevalence or current rates of transmission for persons who resided in another country many years earlier.

The tables also detail the means of transmission, in part to help the clinician assess risk factors that might have led to infection and also to review whether infection might pose any risk to family and close contacts, including sexual partners, and whether any specific precautions might be needed.[17-19] Some of the infections can be transmitted from mother to child (including via breastfeeding) and by blood transfusion or organ or tissue transplantation. Additional comments provide other points that may be useful clinically (e.g. clinical findings, drug resistance patterns, time of appearance, and others).

Many of the infections listed can persist for prolonged periods, some for the lifetime of the host. A broad framework that can be used in thinking about consequences of past infections includes: active infection (primary, persistent, or reactivation), latent infection, immunity to infection, and other sequelae of infection.[20] In contrast to most viral infections, in which infection is followed by immunity that protects against subsequent infections with that pathogen, infection with one dengue serotype can increase the probability that infection with a different serotype can be associated with severe or complicated infection. This is relevant for immigrants from dengue-endemic areas who visit areas with dengue outbreaks. Patients with hepatitis B may be chronic carriers with or without symptoms; patients infected with tuberculosis may have latent infection, which can reactivate. Infection with HIV is persistent, typically with progression, if no interventions are applied. Other consequences of infection include malignancies related to infections (e.g. hepatitis B and C and liver cancer; papillomaviruses and cervical cancer).[21,22] Scarring and mechanical effects related to active or past infection can obstruct a ureter (e.g. tuberculosis), biliary tree (e.g. fascioliasis or echinococcal cyst), or be associated with liver fibrosis and portal hypertension (e.g. schistosomiasis). Allergic or hypersensitivity reactions may follow the release of antigen-rich material, e.g. leaking echinococcal cyst. Focal lesions and masses can lead to seizures (e.g. neurocysticercosis) and focal neurologic deficits. In many instances, the infection may have been clinically silent for years

and the patient may have no knowledge of it. The clinical presentation may not lead the clinician on initial evaluation to think that the process was the result of infectious disease, and certainly not one acquired long ago. Many of these late consequences of infection are not associated with fever.

Immigrants bring with them microbiologic and parasitic baggage related to past residences. Return trips to visit friends and family put them at risk for acquiring new infections that may be unfamiliar to many clinicians in the US. Those whose purpose of travel is visiting friends and relatives (VFRs) are at increased risk for a number of infections, including malaria, enteric fever (typhoid and paratyphoid), and hepatitis A.[23,24] Immigrants who have previously lived in malaria-endemic areas and are familiar with the infection may not realize that the immunity from previous infections that gave partial protection against severe malaria wanes over time. Many fail to take chemoprophylaxis and develop malaria.[25] In Europe during the period 1991–2001, non-nationals accounted for 43% of malaria cases registered at major centers. Children who visit high tuberculosis incidence countries are more likely to be tuberculin positive. A study in California found that US-born children who traveled to or had a visitor from a country with a high prevalence of tuberculosis were, respectively, 4.7 and 2.4 times more likely to have a positive tuberculin skin test than control children.[18]

A section follows each of the tables and lists additional infections, primarily short-incubation infections that pose a risk to persons visiting that country. Children with immigrant parents may be an especially vulnerable group because they lack the immunity their parents have to some infections and may not receive adequate pre-travel preparation, including vaccines and chemoprophylaxis.

During residence in the United States, immigrant populations and their families may have exposures related to visits from relatives as well as from travel to their country of origin. Tuberculosis is an infection that can be transmitted by household visitors, as noted above. Human infections due to *Mycobacterium bovis* have recently increased in the US after having been almost eliminated by control of infection in dairy herds and routine pasteurization of milk. At least 35 cases (and at least one death) were identified in New York City from 2001 to 2004.[26] *M. bovis* accounted for 34% of the culture-confirmed cases of TB in children aged less than 15 years in San Diego, California, during 1980–1997. About 90% of these children were born in the US to Hispanic families. Fresh cheese brought from Mexico was thought to be the source of many of these infections.

It has been estimated that about 20% of cow's milk in Mexico that is used to make fresh cheeses is not pasteurized. A study published in 2000 found that 17% of cows sampled at a meat processing plant in Mexico were infected with *M. bovis*. *M. bovis* is characterized by resistance to pyrazinamide, a marker that may help to distinguish it from *Mycobacterium tuberculosis*.

Brucellosis, another infection associated with consumption of contaminated milk products,[27] has been diagnosed after travel to endemic areas, including Mexico, but also in immigrants in the US after consumption of unpasteurized goat milk or cheese brought from Mexico.

With some parasitic infections, such as filariasis and schistosomiasis, individuals repeatedly exposed or infected at a young age may manifest clinical findings that differ from those in persons from nonendemic areas who are first exposed at an older age.[28,29]

The number of legal immigrants reflects only a part of the pool of foreign-born in the US. For example, although the estimated number of legal immigrants from Mexico entering the US per year was 175 000 (2002 statistics), the number of undocumented migrants was 961 600 and temporary visitors from Mexico was 633 078.[30]

## Limitations

The tables (Table 15.1 to Table 15.11) are based on the best information available, including materials from the World Health Organization, Pan American Health Organization, (PAHO), Centers for Disease Control and Prevention (CDC), and other regional or country-based institutions.[31,32] For many infections, data are absent or incomplete and reflect the best estimate of infection based on published reports of cases, outbreaks, seroepidemiological surveys, or other studies. In some instances, immigrants come predominately or exclusively from one part of a country, whereas the only incidence data are from the country as a whole. Many of the infections are not reportable, so information by geographic region is incomplete, outdated, and may be incorrect.

**Table 15.1 Africa**

| Diseases | Distribution/incidence | Transmission | Comment |
|---|---|---|---|
| Amoebiasis/amoebic liver abscess | Widespread in areas of poor sanitation | Fecal contamination of food/water; sexually (oral/anal) | Will most commonly manifest within weeks to months of exposure |
| Echinococcosis | Widespread in cattle-raising areas; especially northern and eastern Africa | Ingestion of eggs; transfer from fingers or from contaminated food, water, or soil | May first become apparent decades after exposure. Cystic lesions most often found in liver, lung |
| Filariasis, lymphatic | Widespread in tropical/subtropical Africa. Almost 500 million people inhabit at-risk areas. | Bite of infective mosquito | Lymphangitis, lymphedema, elephantiasis; eosinophilia; parasites can survive 10 years or longer |
| Hepatitis A | High prevalence of immunity to hepatitis A by age 5–10 years in most areas | Fecal contamination of food/water; sexually (oral/anal) | In areas with good sanitation, children and young adults may be susceptible |
| Hepatitis B | Chronic infection rates as high as 7–24%; seroprevalence of hepatitis B surface antigen >8% in most areas | Percutaneous/permucosal contact with blood, body fluids; perinatal; sexually; unsafe injections; transfusions | Chronic infection associated with increased risk of liver cancer |
| Hepatitis C | Seroprevalence 2–9% in many countries | Unsafe injections; unscreened transfused blood; rare perinatal and sexually | Chronic infection associated with increased risk of liver cancer |

**Table 15.1 Africa—cont'd**

| Diseases | Distribution/incidence | Transmission | Comment |
|---|---|---|---|
| HIV/AIDS | Seroprevalence in adults ranges from 1% to 39%. Countries with seroprevalence >20% include: Botswana, Namibia, South Africa, Swaziland, Zimbabwe | Sexual exposures; perinatal; breastfeeding; unsafe injections; transfusion of blood/blood products | High rates of co-infection with tuberculosis |
| HTLV-I/II | Endemic in parts of western and central Africa; seropositivity 5–14% in some areas | Mother to child (transplacental and via breastfeeding); sexually; blood transfusion and contaminated needles | Chronic, indolent infection. Dermatitis, adult T-cell leukaemia/lymphoma; myelopathy |
| Intestinal parasites | Most common are *Ascaris*, *Dientamoeba fragilis*, *Giardia*, hookworm, *Strongyloides*, *stercoralis*, *Trichuris trichiura*. *Hymenolepis nana* found, especially in children | Penetration of skin by larvae in soil (*Strongyloides stercoralis*, hookworm); ingestion of infective ova (*Ascaris*, *Trichuris*, *Hymenolepis nana*) or cysts (*Giardia*). Person-to-person transmission can occur with hymenolepiasis | Co-infection with multiple parasites common. *Strongyloides stercoralis* and *Hymenolepis nana* can persist indefinitely via autoinfective cycle. *Strongyloides stercoralis* can disseminate in immunocompromised |
| Leishmaniasis, cutaneous (CL), visceral (VL) | CL: especially savannah, Sudan, and highland areas VL: especially Ethiopia, Kenya, Sudan, Uganda, and savannah areas | Bite of infective phlebotomine (sandfly) | VL may manifest years after initial infection; HIV infection, other immunosuppressing conditions may lead to reactivation |
| Leprosy | Present in all countries. Highest prevalences in Madagascar, Mozambique (>30/100 000) | Probably from secretions from nasal mucosa of infected person to respiratory tract and skin of another | Indolent; may persist for decades |
| Liver flukes (fascioliasis) | Found in sheep and cattle-raising areas. Most common in northern Africa, especially Egypt | Ingestion of metacercariae (usually with raw or undercooked food, often water plants) | Adult worm in biliary tree can survive for years |
| Lung flukes (*Paragonimus africanus* and *P. uterobilateralis*) | Endemic; especially common in SW Cameroon and eastern Nigeria | Ingestion of metacercariae (infective larvae), usually in shellfish | Can persist a decade or longer; lung infection can resemble tuberculosis |
| Loiasis (African eye worm; Calabar swellings) | Central and western Africa | Bite of infective fly (*Chrysops*) | Adult worms can survive >10 years |
| Malaria | Widespread; hyperendemic in many areas | Mosquito-borne; rare transfusion, congenital, needlestick transmission | Predominantly *P. falciparum*; infections with *P. malariae* may manifest decades after initial infection; immigrants may be reinfected during visits to country of origin |
| Neurocysticercosis | Widespread except in strictly Muslim areas | Ingestion of eggs shed in feces of human tapeworm carrier | Often manifests with seizures |

**Table 15.1 Africa—cont'd**

| Diseases | Distribution/incidence | Transmission | Comment |
|---|---|---|---|
| Onchocerciasis (river blindness) | Western and central equatorial Africa | Bite of infective female blackfly, genus *Simulium* | Adult worm can survive 10–15 years |
| Papillomaviruses, human (HPV) | Widespread; estimated 68 000 cases of cervical cancer yearly in Africa | Direct contact, usually through sexual contact | Cervical cancer, caused by oncogenic HPV, is most common cancer in women in sub-Saharan Africa |
| Schistosomiasis, primarily *Schistosoma mansoni* and *S. haematobium* | Widespread in freshwater lakes and streams in Africa | Penetration of intact skin or mucosa by live cercariae in fresh water | Adult worm may survive >10 years; chronic sequelae may develop long after initial infection |
| Syphilis and endemic treponematoses | Widespread; common infection. Disease caused by endemic *Treponema pallidum* subspecies *pertenue* (yaws) has been reported from many countries in Africa | Direct contact with spirochete, usually via sexual contact; can be transmitted transplacentally and via transfusion or transplantation of infected tissue | Protean manifestations; infected person can transmit infection years after acquisition; syphilis serology positive in endemic treponematoses |
| Trypanosomiasis, African | Est. prevalence 300 000 to 500 000. *T. brucei gambiense* is more common than *T. b. rhodesiense*. Recent expansion of geographic areas and cases | Bite of infective tsetse fly | Infection with *T. brucei gambiense* (West Africa) can be chronic (months to years) |
| Tuberculosis | High rates of infection; estimated incidence/100 000 population (2003): DR Congo 369; Ethiopia 356; Kenya 610; South Africa 536; Uganda 411; Zimbabwe 659 | Inhalation of airborne droplet nuclei from infected person | Co-infection with HIV common in some populations. Multidrug resistance estimated in 1–2.3% of new cases |
| Typhoid and paratyphoid fevers (enteric fever) | Widespread; risk highest in areas with poor sanitation. Incidence in South Africa 850/100 000 in 1980s | Ingestion of bacteria in fecally contaminated food or beverages; direct fecal oral spread | 1–5% of patients with typhoid fever become chronic biliary carriers; food handlers can contaminate food; chronic urinary carriage can occur in patients with urinary tract schistosomiasis |
| Varicella | Young adults from tropical areas may be susceptible to varicella | Person-to-person; droplet or airborne spread; via freshly soiled articles; transplacental and blood transfusion (rare) | Serologic testing is advised for adults without history of varicella. Vaccine can be offered to nonimmunes |

Immigrants visiting friends and relatives in this region are also at risk for shorter incubation infections, such as acute viral infections (e.g. dengue, chikungunya, hemorrhagic fevers (some*) including yellow fever, others), brucellosis, diarrhea-causing infections (including cholera)*, hepatitis E, meningococcal infections, leptospirosis, rabies, rickettsial infections, vaccine-preventable infections (such as measles, rubella, varicella and polio)*.
*Transmissible by close contact.

**Table 15.2 Caribbean: Haiti, Dominican Republic, Jamaica**

| Diseases | Distribution/incidence | Transmission | Comment |
|---|---|---|---|
| Amoebiasis/amoebic liver abscess | Highest risk in areas with poor sanitation | Fecal contamination of food/water; sexually (oral/anal) | Will most commonly manifest within weeks to months of exposure |
| Endemic mycoses | Outbreaks of histoplasmosis have occurred in the Caribbean | Inhalation of airborne conidia from soil | Viable organisms can persist for decades; can reactivate; increased risk in immunocompromised |
| Filariasis, lymphatic | High prevalence in parts of Haiti. Endemic in 9 of 13 municipalities in DR | Bite of infective mosquito | Lymphangitis, lymphedema, elephantiasis; eosinophilia; parasites can survive 10 years or longer |
| Hepatitis A | Area of high endemicity (seroprevalence of antibodies 80% in children 6–10 yrs in DR[7]) | Fecal contamination of food/water; sexually (oral/anal) | In areas with good sanitation, children and young adults may be susceptible |
| Hepatitis B | Seroprevalence of hepatitis B surface antigen 2–7% | Percutaneous/permucosal contact with blood, body fluids; perinatal; sexually; unsafe injections; transfusions | Chronic infection associated with increased risk of liver cancer |
| Hepatitis C | Seroprevalence estimated to be <2% | Unsafe injections; unscreened transfused blood; rare perinatal and sexually | Chronic infection associated with increased risk of liver cancer |
| HIV/AIDS | Haiti: 4.5%; DR: 2.5%. Seroprevalence among pregnant women 1.8–7% in Haiti; >2% in DR; 1.4% in Jamaica | Sexual exposures; perinatal; breastfeeding; unsafe injections; transfusion of blood/blood products | High rates of co-infection with tuberculosis, especially in Haiti |
| HTLV-I/II | Seroprevalence as high as 5–14% reported in the Caribbean | Mother to child (transplacental and via breastfeeding); sexually; blood transfusion and contaminated needles | Chronic, indolent infection. Dermatitis, adult T-cell leukemia/lymphoma; myelopathy |
| Intestinal parasites | Most common are *Ascaris*, *Dientamoeba fragilis*, *Giardia*, hookworm, *Strongyloides stercoralis*, *Trichuris trichiura*. *Hymenolepis nana* found, especially in children | Penetration of skin by larvae in soil (*Strongyloides stercoralis*, hookworm); ingestion of infective ova (*Ascaris*, *Trichuris*, *Hymenolepis nana*) or cysts (*Giardia*). Person-to-person transmission can occur with hymenolepiasis | Co-infection with multiple parasites common. *Strongyloides stercoralis* and *Hymenolepis nana* can persist indefinitely via autoinfective cycle. *Strongyloides stercoralis* can disseminate in immunocompromised |
| Leishmaniasis, cutaneous | Reported from the Dominican Republic | Bite of infective phlebotomine (sandfly) | Chronic, indolent infection |
| Leprosy | Prevalence 3/100 000 in DR, 2004 | Probably from secretions from nasal mucosa of infected person to respiratory tract and skin of another | Indolent; may persist for decades |

**Table 15.2 Caribbean: Haiti, Dominican Republic, Jamaica—cont'd**

| Diseases | Distribution/incidence | Transmission | Comment |
|---|---|---|---|
| Liver flukes (fascioliasis) | Sporadic cases reported | Ingestion of metacercariae (usually with raw or undercooked food, often water plants) | Adult worm in biliary tree can survive for years |
| Malaria | Widespread in Haiti; focal in Dominican Republic | Mosquito-borne; rare transfusion, congenital, needlestick transmission | Predominantly falciparum malaria. |
| Neurocysticercosis | Cases reported from Haiti and DR | Ingestion of eggs shed in feces of human tapeworm carrier | May manifest as focal CNS lesion, seizure |
| Papillomaviruses, human (HPV) | High incidence of cervical cancer (87/100 000 in Haiti)[39] | Direct contact, usually through sexual contact | Cervical cancer, caused by oncogenic HPV, is a leading cause of cancer in women |
| Schistosomiasis due to *S. mansoni* | In DR main foci of infection have been in eastern part of country. An estimated 3000 were infected in the 1980s. | Penetration of intact skin or mucosa by live cercariae in fresh water | Adult worm may survive >10 years; chronic sequelae may develop long after initial infection |
| Syphilis and endemic treponematoses | Common. Disease caused by endemic *Treponema pallidum* subspecies has been reported from Haiti | Direct contact with spirochete, usually via sexual contact; can be transmitted transplacentally and via transfusion or transplantation of infected tissue | Protean findings; infected person can transmit infection years after acquisition; syphilis serology positive in endemic treponematoses |
| Tuberculosis | Estimated incidence (2003) per 100 000: Haiti 323; DR 96 New smear-positive cases per 100 000 (2001) Haiti 138; DR 59 | Inhalation of airborne droplet nuclei from infected person | Primary drug resistance to INH 16%; rifampin 2.5%. Prevalence of latent tuberculosis among 30-year-old immigrants: Haiti: 51%; DR 24% |
| Typhoid and paratyphoid (enteric fever) | Widespread; risk highest in areas with poor sanitation | Ingestion of bacteria in fecally contaminated food or beverages; direct fecal oral spread | 1–5% of patients with typhoid fever become chronic biliary carriers; food handlers can contaminate food |
| Varicella | Adults who have always lived in tropical areas are more likely to be susceptible than residents of temperate areas | Person-to-person; droplet or airborne spread; via freshly soiled articles; transplacental and blood transfusion (rare) | Serologic testing advised for adults without history of varicella. Vaccine can be offered to nonimmunes |

Immigrants visiting friends and relatives in this region are also at risk for shorter-incubation infections, such as acute viral infections (e.g. dengue, others), diarrhea-causing infections, leptospirosis, rabies, rickettsial infections, and vaccine-preventable infections (such as measles, rubella, and varicella). *Angiostrongylus cantonensis* caused an outbreak of eosinophilic meningitis in visitors to Jamaica in 2000.

**Table 15.3 Mexico**

| Diseases | Distribution/incidence | Transmission | Comment |
|---|---|---|---|
| Amoebiasis/amoebic liver abscess | Widespread; highest risk in areas with poor sanitation; incidence of intestinal amoebiasis/100 000 population in 2004 was 792 | Fecal contamination of food/water; sexually (oral/anal) | Will most commonly manifest within weeks to months of exposure |
| Echinococcosis | Endemic in areas where animals graze | Ingestion of eggs; transfer from fingers or from contaminated food, water, or soil | May first become apparent decades after exposure. Cystic lesions most often found in liver, lung |
| Endemic mycoses (coccidioidomycosis, histoplasmosis, paracoccidioidomycosis) | Cocci: large endemic area; histo: widely endemic and outbreaks, including related to exposures in gold and silver mines. Paracocci: also present | Inhalation of airborne conidia from soil | Infections can be acute or chronic and can reactivate; more severe infection in immunocompromised |
| Hepatitis A | Area of high endemicity (seroprevalence of antibodies almost 70% in children 6–10 yrs old[7]) | Fecal contamination of food/water; sexually (oral/anal) | In areas with good sanitation, children and young adults may be susceptible |
| Hepatitis B | Seroprevalence of hepatitis B surface antigen <1% | Percutaneous/permucosal contact with blood, body fluids; perinatal; sexually; unsafe injections; transfusions | Chronic infection associated with increased risk of liver cancer |
| Hepatitis C | Seroprevalence estimated to be 1–1.9% | Unsafe injections; unscreened transfused blood; rare perinatal and sexually | Chronic infection associated with increased risk of liver cancer |
| HIV/AIDS | Overall seroprevalence in adults < 1% (estimated 0.3% in 2003) | Sexual exposures; perinatal; breastfeeding; unsafe injections; transfusion of blood/blood products | Most infections are in men who have sex with men |
| Intestinal parasites | Especially in rural areas. Most common are *Ascaris*, *Dientamoeba fragilis*, *Giardia*, hookworm, *Strongyloides stercoralis*, *Trichuris trichiura*. *Hymenolepis nana* found, especially in children | Penetration of skin by larvae in soil (*Strongyloides stercoralis*, hookworm); ingestion of infective ova (*Ascaris*, *Trichuris*, *Hymenolepis nana*) or cysts (*Giardia*). Person-to-person transmission can occur with hymenolepiasis | Co-infection with multiple parasites common. *Strongyloides stercoralis* and *Hymenolepis nana* can persist indefinitely via autoinfective cycle. *Strongyloides stercoralis* can disseminate in immunocompromised |
| Leishmaniasis, cutaneous (CL), mucocutaneous (ML); visceral (VL) | Endemic in parts of Mexico, especially Yucatan; primarily CL, though ML and VL also reported | Bite of infective phlebotomine (sandfly) | ML and VL may manifest years after initial infection; HIV infection, other immunosuppressing conditions may lead to reactivation |

**Table 15.3 Mexico—cont'd**

| Diseases | Distribution/incidence | Transmission | Comment |
|---|---|---|---|
| Leprosy | Decreasing prevalence 1/100 000 (2004); prevalence 21/100 000 in 1990 | Probably from secretions from nasal mucosa of infected person to respiratory tract and skin of another | Indolent; may persist for decades |
| Liver flukes (fascioliasis) | Sporadic infection in humans | Ingestion of metacercariae (usually with raw or undercooked food, often water plants) | Adult worm in biliary tree can survive for years. |
| Lung flukes (*Paragonimus mexicanus*) | Cases have been reported | Ingestion of metacercariae (infective larvae), usually in shellfish | Can persist a decade or longer; lung infection can resemble tuberculosis |
| Malaria | Continued transmission in some rural areas | Mosquito-borne; rare transfusion, congenital, needlestick transmission | Vivax malaria predominates. No reported resistance to chloroquine |
| Neurocysticercosis | Seroprevalence 5% to >10% in some communities; 1000–2000 new cases/yr diagnosed in US, majority in Hispanic immigrants | Ingestion of eggs shed in feces of human tapeworm carrier | Common cause of focal CNS lesions and seizures; occasional acquisition in the US from tapeworm carrier |
| Onchocerciasis | Three endemic foci exist (Oaxaca, Northern Chiapas, Southern Chiapas) | Bite of infective female blackfly, genus *Simulium* | Ivermectin has been used since 1989 to help control infection. The size of the at-risk population was earlier estimated at 280 000 |
| Papillomaviruses, human (HPV) | Incidence of cervical cancer up to 33/100 000 | Direct contact, usually through sexual contact | Cervical cancer, caused by oncogenic HPV, is a leading cancer in women |
| Syphilis and endemic treponematoses | Disease caused by endemic *Treponema pallidum* subspecies has been reported from Mexico in the past | Direct contact with spirochete, usually via sexual contact; can be transmitted transplacentally and via transfusion or transplantation of infected tissue | Protean manifestations; infected person can transmit infection years after acquisition; syphilis serology positive in endemic treponematoses |
| Trypanosomiasis, American (Chagas') | An estimated 15 million are at risk of infection. Seroprevalence in blood banks was 0.8% in 1995. Estimated >50 000 infected Latin American immigrants reside in the US | Primarily via direct contact between broken skin (or mucosal surface) and infective feces from triatomine bug; also transplacental and via transfusion, organ transplantation; food-borne outbreak reported in 2005 in Brazil | Sequelae of chronic infection may occur 10 years or longer after onset of infection; reactivation in AIDS patients may be associated with CNS findings, including meningoencephalitis |

**Table 15.3 Mexico—cont'd**

| Diseases | Distribution/incidence | Transmission | Comment |
|---|---|---|---|
| Tuberculosis | Estimated incidence 33/100 000 (2003) | Inhalation of airborne droplet nuclei from infected person | Prevalence of MDR[†] resistance in three states 2.4% (1997). *Mycobacterium bovis* remains endemic in Mexican cattle |
| Typhoid and paratyphoid (enteric fever) | Remains endemic. Annual incidence was 20/100 000 in 1980s and 0.6% of the population were chronic carriers | Ingestion of bacteria in fecally contaminated food or beverages; direct fecal-oral spread | Chronic carriage is most common in older persons with biliary disease. |
| Varicella | National serosurvey 1987–1988 found 8.4% aged 20–24 years and 5.0% of those 25–29 years still susceptible to varicella | Person-to-person; droplet or airborne spread; via freshly soiled articles; transplacental and blood transfusion (rare) | Serologic testing advised for adults without history of varicella. Vaccine can be offered to nonimmunes |

Immigrants visiting friends and relatives in this region are also at risk for shorter-incubation infections, such as acute viral infections (e.g. dengue, others), diarrhea-causing infections (including amoebiasis), brucellosis, leptospirosis, rabies, and rickettsial infections. Hepatitis E caused a large waterborne outbreak in the past. Outbreaks of histoplasmosis have occurred in short-term travelers. Vaccine coverage for measles is high, and country has been certified polio free. Scorpion bites are a problem (especially in infants and young children) in 16 states, where >100 000 cases were recorded in 1996.
[†]multiple drug resistance.

**Table 15.4 Central America: El Salvador and Guatemala**

| Diseases | Distribution/incidence | Transmission | Comment |
|---|---|---|---|
| Amoebiasis/amoebic liver abscess | Widespread; highest risk in areas with poor sanitation | Fecal contamination of food/water; sexually (oral/anal) | Will most commonly manifest within weeks to months of exposure |
| Echinococcosis | Endemic in cattle-grazing areas | Ingestion of eggs; transfer from fingers or from contaminated food, water, or soil | May first become apparent decades after exposure. Cystic lesions most often found in liver, lung |
| Endemic mycoses (coccidioidomycosis, histoplasmosis, paracoccidioidomycosis) | Histo and cocci are endemic in focal areas of Central America. Paracocci is less common | Inhalation of airborne conidia from soil | Infections can be acute or chronic and can reactivate; more severe infection in immunocompromised |
| Hepatitis A | High prevalence of immunity to hepatitis A by age 5–10 years in most areas | Fecal contamination of food/water; sexually (oral/anal) | In areas with good sanitation, children and young adults may be susceptible |
| Hepatitis B | Seroprevalence of hepatitis B surface antigen 2–7% in most areas | Percutaneous/permucosal contact with blood, body fluids; perinatal; sexually; unsafe injections; transfusions | Chronic infection associated with increased risk of liver cancer |
| Hepatitis C | Seroprevalence estimated to be <1% to 1.9% | Unsafe injections; unscreened transfused blood; rare perinatal and sexually | Chronic infection associated with increased risk of liver cancer |

**Table 15.4 Central America: El Salvador and Guatemala—cont'd**

| Diseases | Distribution/incidence | Transmission | Comment |
|---|---|---|---|
| HIV/AIDS | Adult seroprevalence >1% in Guatemala; in El Salvador prevalence was 16% among street-based sex workers | Sexual exposures; perinatal; breastfeeding; unsafe injections; transfusion of blood/blood products | Co-infection with tuberculosis may be present |
| Intestinal parasites | Most common are *Ascaris*, *Dientamoeba fragilis*, *Giardia*, hookworm, *Strongyloides stercoralis*, *Trichuris trichiura*. *Hymenolepis nana* found, especially in children | Penetration of skin by larvae in soil (*Strongyloides stercoralis*, hookworm); ingestion of infective ova (*Ascaris*, *Trichuris*, *Hymenolepis nana*) or cysts (*Giardia*). Person-to-person transmission can occur with hymenolepiasis | Co-infection with multiple parasites common. *Strongyloides stercoralis* and *Hymenolepis nana* can persist indefinitely via autoinfective cycle. *Strongyloides stercoralis* can disseminate in immunocompromised |
| Leishmaniasis, cutaneous (CL), mucocutaneous (ML) | Reported from all countries in Central America; primarily cutaneous | Bite of infective phlebotomine (sandfly) | ML may manifest many years after initial infection |
| Leprosy | Low prevalence | Probably from secretions from nasal mucosa of infected person to respiratory tract and skin of another | Indolent; may persist for decades |
| Liver flukes (fascioliasis) | Sporadic human infections reported from Central America | Ingestion of metacercariae (usually with raw or undercooked food, often water plants) | Adult worm in biliary tree can survive for years |
| Lung flukes (*Paragonimus mexicanus*) | Cases have been reported from Central America | Ingestion of metacercariae (infective larvae), usually in shellfish | Can persist a decade or longer; lung infection can resemble tuberculosis |
| Malaria | Present in focal rural areas | Mosquito-borne; rare transfusion, congenital, needlestick transmission | Vivax malaria predominates |
| Neurocysticercosis | Widespread | Ingestion of eggs shed in feces of human tapeworm carrier | Common cause of focal CNS lesion, new-onset seizures in adults |
| Onchocerciasis | Endemic | Bite of infective female blackfly, genus *Simulium* | Residents in 3 endemic foci in Guatemala are being treated with ivermectin |
| Papillomaviruses | High incidence of cervical cancer in Central America | Direct contact, usually through sexual contact | Cervical cancer, caused by oncogenic HPV, is a leading cancer in women |
| Syphilis and endemic treponematoses | Syphilis present. Disease caused by endemic *Treponema pallidum* subspecies has been reported from region in the past | Direct contact with spirochete, usually via sexual contact; can be transmitted transplacentally and via transfusion or transplantation of infected tissue | Protean manifestations; infected person can transmit infection years after acquisition; syphilis serology positive in endemic treponematoses |

**Table 15.4 Central America: El Salvador and Guatemala—cont'd**

| Diseases | Distribution/incidence | Transmission | Comment |
|---|---|---|---|
| Trypanosomiasis, American (Chagas') | Highly endemic in some areas. Transmission most common in rural areas with poor housing. Estimated >50 000 infected Latin American immigrants reside in the US | Primarily via direct contact between broken skin (or mucosal surface) and infective feces from triatomine bug; also transplacental and via transfusion, organ transplantation; food-borne outbreak reported in 2005 | Sequelae of chronic infection may occur 10 years or longer after onset of infection; reactivation in AIDS patients may be associated with CNS findings, including meningoencephalitis |
| Tuberculosis | Estimated incidence (2003): El Salvador 57/100 000; Guatemala 74/100 000 | Inhalation of airborne droplet nuclei from infected person | Estimated incidence in both countries in 1990 was about 100/100 000 |
| Typhoid and paratyphoid (enteric fever) | Widespread; risk highest in areas with poor sanitation | Ingestion of bacteria in fecally contaminated food or beverages; direct fecal-oral spread | 1–5% of patients with typhoid fever become chronic biliary carriers; food handlers can contaminate food |
| Varicella | Young adults from tropical areas may be susceptible to varicella | Person-to-person; droplet or airborne spread; via freshly soiled articles; transplacental and blood transfusion (rare) | Serologic testing advised for adults without history of varicella. Vaccine can be offered to nonimmunes |

Immigrants visiting friends and relatives in this region are also at risk for shorter-incubation infections, such as acute viral infections (e.g. dengue, others), diarrhea-causing infections (including amoebiasis), hepatitis E, leptospirosis, rabies, rickettsial infections, and vaccine-preventable infections (such as measles, rubella, and varicella).

**Table 15.5 South America: Focus on Ecuador (with comments about some diseases in other South American countries)**

| Diseases | Distribution/incidence | Transmission | Comment |
|---|---|---|---|
| Amoebiasis/amoebic liver abscess | Widespread; highest risk in areas with poor sanitation | Fecal contamination of food/water; sexually (oral/anal) | Will most commonly manifest within weeks to months of exposure |
| Echinococcosis | Endemic in cattle-grazing areas of Ecuador and other countries | Ingestion of eggs; transfer from fingers or from contaminated food, water, or soil | May first become apparent decades after exposure. Cystic lesions most often found in liver, lung |
| Endemic mycoses (coccidioidomycosis, histoplasmosis, paracoccidioidomycosis) | Cocci and histo: focal distribution in tropical and subtropical S. America. Paracocci: endemic in tropical and subtropical S. America | Inhalation of airborne conidia from soil | Infections can be acute or chronic and can reactivate; more severe infection in immunocompromised |
| Filariasis, lymphatic | Not endemic in Ecuador; endemic in Brazil, northeastern S. America | Bite of infective mosquito | Lymphangitis, lymphedema, elephantiasis; eosinophilia; parasites can survive 10 years or longer |

**Table 15.5 South America: Focus on Ecuador (with comments about some diseases in other South American countries)—cont'd**

| Diseases | Distribution/incidence | Transmission | Comment |
|---|---|---|---|
| Hepatitis A | High prevalence of immunity to hepatitis A by age 5–10 years in most areas | Fecal contamination of food/water; sexually (oral/anal) | In areas with good sanitation, children and young adults may be susceptible |
| Hepatitis B | Seroprevalence of hepatitis B surface antigen <2% in Ecuador; seroprevalence >8% in some parts of S. America | Percutaneous/permucosal contact with blood, body fluids; perinatal; sexually; unsafe injections; transfusions | Chronic infection associated with increased risk of liver cancer |
| Hepatitis C | Seroprevalence estimated to be < 1% in Ecuador; up to 1.9% in parts of S. America | Unsafe injections; unscreened transfused blood; rare perinatal and sexually | Chronic infection associated with increased risk of liver cancer |
| HIV/AIDS | Estimated overall HIV prevalence in adults 0.3% (2003), but 12–21% in men who have sex with men (urban areas) | Sexual exposures; perinatal; breastfeeding; unsafe injections; transfusion of blood/blood products | High rates of co-infection with tuberculosis |
| HTLV-I/II | Foci of high endemicity in S. America, including in Argentina, Brazil, Colombia, Venezuela, Chile | Mother to child (transplacental and via breastfeeding); sexually; blood transfusion and contaminated needles | Chronic, indolent infection. Dermatitis, adult T-cell leukemia/lymphoma; myelopathy |
| Intestinal parasites | Most common are *Ascaris*, *Dientamoeba fragilis*, *Giardia*, hookworm, *Strongyloides stercoralis*, *Trichuris trichiura*. *Hymenolepis nana* found, especially in children | Penetration of skin by larvae in soil (*Strongyloides stercoralis*, hookworm); ingestion of infective ova (*Ascaris*, *Trichuris*, *Hymenolepis nana*) or cysts (*Giardia*). Person-to-person transmission can occur with hymenolepiasis | Co-infection with multiple parasites common. *Strongyloides stercoralis* and *Hymenolepis nana* can persist indefinitely via autoinfective cycle. *Strongyloides stercoralis* can disseminate in immunocompromised |
| Leishmaniasis, cutaneous (CL), mucocutaneous (ML), visceral (VL) | Found in all countries of S. America except Chile and Uruguay; especially common in Peru and Brazil | Bite of infective phlebotomine (sandfly) | VL and ML may manifest years after initial infection; HIV infection, other immunosuppressing conditions may lead to reactivation |
| Leprosy | Prevalence per 100 000 <10 in most countries; 46/100 000 in Brazil (2004) | Probably from secretions from nasal mucosa of infected person to respiratory tract and skin of another | Indolent; may persist for decades |
| Liver flukes (fascioliasis) | High prevalence of infection with *Fasciola hepatica* in parts of Peru, Ecuador, Bolivia | Ingestion of metacercariae contaminating plants or water | Adult worm in biliary tree can survive for years |
| Lung flukes (*Paragonimus mexicanus*) | Endemic in Ecuador (estimated 500 000 cases) and Peru | Ingestion of metacercariae (infective larvae), usually in shellfish | Can persist a decade or longer; lung infection can resemble tuberculosis |

**Table 15.5 South America: Focus on Ecuador (with comments about some diseases in other South American countries)—cont'd**

| Diseases | Distribution/incidence | Transmission | Comment |
|---|---|---|---|
| Malaria | Present in areas at altitudes <1500 meters | Mosquito-borne; rare transfusion, congenital, needlestick transmission | Vivax malaria predominates |
| Neurocysticercosis | Endemic in Ecuador; also important in Peru, Brazil, Bolivia | Ingestion of eggs shed in feces of human tapeworm carrier | Found in 50% or more of adult-onset seizures |
| Onchocerciasis | Endemic focus in Esmeraldas Province; also present in Brazil, Colombia, Venezuela | Bite of infective female blackfly, genus *Simulium* | Chronic indolent infection. Adult worms can survive >10 yrs |
| Papillomaviruses, human (HPV) | Incidence of cervical cancer is up to 87/100 000 in Ecuador and adjacent countries | Direct contact, usually through sexual contact | Cervical cancer, caused by oncogenic HPV, is a leading cancer in women |
| Schistosomiasis due to *S. mansoni* | Not found in Ecuador but present in parts of Brazil, Surinam, Venezuela | Penetration of intact skin or mucosa by live cercariae in fresh water | Adult worm may survive >10 years; chronic sequelae may develop long after initial infection |
| Syphilis and endemic treponematoses | Widespread in region; Disease caused by endemic *Treponema pallidum* subspecies has been reported from Ecuador, Colombia, Venezuela, Surinam | Direct contact with spirochete, usually via sexual contact; can be transmitted transplacentally and via transfusion or transplantation of infected tissue | Protean manifestations; infected person can transmit infection years after acquisition; syphilis serology positive in endemic treponematoses |
| Trypanosomiasis, American (Chagas') | Endemic. Rates of transmission are highest in coastal region. Estimated >50 000 infected immigrants (from Latin America) reside in the US | Primarily via direct contact between broken skin (or mucosal surface) and infective feces from triatomine bug; also transplacental and via transfusion, organ transplantation; food-borne outbreak reported in 2005 | Sequelae of chronic infection may occur 10 years or longer after onset of infection; reactivation in AIDS patients may be associated with CNS findings, including meningoencephalitis |
| Tuberculosis | Estimated incidence 138/100 000 (2003) in Ecuador (202 for Peru) | Inhalation of airborne droplet nuclei from infected person | Estimated incidence in 1990 was 202/100 000 in Ecuador |
| Typhoid and paratyphoid (enteric fever) | Widespread; risk highest in areas with poor sanitation | Ingestion of bacteria in fecally contaminated food or beverages; direct fecal-oral spread | 1–5% of patients with typhoid fever become chronic biliary carriers; food handlers can contaminate food |
| Varicella | Young adults from tropical areas may be susceptible to varicella | Person-to-person; droplet or airborne spread; via freshly soiled articles; transplacental and blood transfusion (rare) | Serologic testing advised for adults without history of varicella. Vaccine can be offered to nonimmunes |

Immigrants visiting friends and relatives in this region are also at risk for shorter-incubation infections, such as acute viral infections (e.g. dengue, yellow fever, others), diarrhea-causing infections, leptospirosis, rabies, rickettsial infections, and vaccine-preventable infections (such as measles, rubella, and varicella).

**Table 15.6 Southeast Asia with focus on Cambodia, Laos, and Vietnam**

| Diseases | Distribution/incidence | Transmission | Comment |
|---|---|---|---|
| Amoebiasis/amoebic liver abscess | Present; highest risk in areas with poor sanitation | Fecal contamination of food/water; sexually (oral/anal) | Will most commonly manifest within weeks to months of exposure |
| Echinococcosis | Not common. Sporadic cases reported | Ingestion of eggs; transfer from fingers or from contaminated food, water, or soil | May first become apparent decades after exposure. Cystic lesions most often found in liver, lung |
| Endemic mycoses (*Penicillium marneffei*) | Penicilliosis is endemic in Southeast Asia | Inhalation or ingestion of spores | Can reactivate; increased risk of dissemination in HIV, immunocompromised |
| Filariasis, lymphatic | Endemic in region. Vietnam started mass drug administration in 2004 | Bite of infective mosquito | Lymphangitis, lymphedema, elephantiasis; eosinophilia; parasites can survive 10 years or longer |
| Hepatitis A | High prevalence of immunity to hepatitis A by age 5–10 years in most areas | Fecal contamination of food/water; sexually (oral/anal) | In areas with good sanitation, children and young adults may be susceptible |
| Hepatitis B | Seroprevalence of hepatitis B surface antigen >8% in most countries of region | Percutaneous/permucosal contact with blood, body fluids; perinatal; sexually; unsafe injections; transfusions | Chronic infection associated with increased risk of liver cancer |
| Hepatitis C | Seroprevalence estimated to be 2–2.9% | Unsafe injections; unscreened transfused blood; rare perinatal and sexually | Chronic infection associated with increased risk of liver cancer |
| HIV/AIDS | Cambodia: adult HIV prevalence rate estimated 2.6% (2003); Vietnam: <1% overall but high rates in injecting drug users | Sexual exposures; perinatal; breastfeeding; unsafe injections; transfusion of blood/blood products | High rates of co-infection with tuberculosis |
| HTLV I/II | HTLV-II found in Vietnam | Mother to child (transplacental and via breastfeeding); sexually; blood transfusion and contaminated needles | Chronic, indolent infection. Dermatitis, adult T-cell leukemia/lymphoma; myelopathy |
| Intestinal parasites | Most common are *Ascaris, Dientamoeba fragilis, Giardia*, hookworm, *Strongyloides stercoralis, Trichuris trichiura. Hymenolepis nana* found especially in children | Penetration of skin by larvae in soil (*Strongyloides stercoralis*, hookworm); ingestion of infective ova (*Ascaris, Trichuris, Hymenolepis nana*) or cysts (*Giardia*). Person-to-person transmission can occur with hymenolepiasis | Co-infection with multiple parasites common. *Strongyloides stercoralis* and *Hymenolepis nana* can persist indefinitely via autoinfective cycle. *Strongyloides stercoralis* can disseminate in immunocompromised |

**Table 15.6 Southeast Asia with focus on Cambodia, Laos, and Vietnam—cont'd**

| Diseases | Distribution/incidence | Transmission | Comment |
|---|---|---|---|
| Leprosy | Prevalence per 100 000 in 2004: Cambodia 3.6; Laos 2.5; Vietnam 1.5 | Probably from secretions from nasal mucosa of infected person to respiratory tract and skin of another | Indolent; may persist for decades |
| Liver flukes (clonorchiasis, opisthorchiasis, fascioliasis) | Clonorchiasis: Vietnam and other areas; opisthorchiasis found throughout area, especially in Thailand; fascioliasis; sporadic cases | Ingestion of raw or undercooked fish (clonorchiasis, opisthorchiasis) or water or plants (fascioliasis) containing metacercariae | Adult worms of clonorchiasis and opisthorchiasis in biliary tree can persist >20 years; associated with cholangiocarcinoma |
| Lung flukes (*Paragonimus westermani*) | Endemic in Southeast Asia | Ingestion of metacercariae, usually in shellfish | Can persist a decade or longer; lung infection can resemble tuberculosis |
| Malaria | Present in much of region, especially rural areas | Mosquito-borne; rare transfusion, congenital, needlestick transmission | Chloroquine and mefloquine resistance is present in parts of area |
| Neurocysticercosis | Cases reported from the area | Ingestion of eggs shed in feces of human tapeworm carrier | Can cause focal CNS lesion and seizures |
| Papillomaviruses, human (HPV) | Incidence of cervical cancer in Cambodia up to 87/100 000 | Direct contact, usually through sexual contact | Cervical cancer, caused by oncogenic HPV, is a leading cancer in women |
| Schistosomiasis due to *S. mekongi* | At-risk population estimated at 140 000 in Cambodia and Laos | Penetration of intact skin or mucosa by live cercariae in fresh water | Adult worm may survive >10 years; chronic sequelae may develop long after initial infection |
| Syphilis and endemic treponematoses | Widespread in region. High prevalence found in Cambodia (4%). Disease caused by endemic *Treponema pallidum* subspecies has been reported from Cambodia | Direct contact with spirochete, usually via sexual contact; can be transmitted transplacentally and via transfusion or transplantation of infected tissue | Protean manifestations; infected person can transmit infection years after acquisition; syphilis serology positive in endemic treponematoses |
| Tuberculosis | Estimated incidence per 100 000 (2003): 549 for Cambodia, 157 for Laos, 178 for Vietnam | Inhalation of airborne droplet nuclei from infected person | In Cambodia, estimated 4.2% of new cases have multidrug resistance |
| Typhoid and paratyphoid (enteric fever) | Widespread; risk highest in areas with poor sanitation. Incidence in Vietnam 414/100 000 young children (2–4 years) | Ingestion of bacteria in fecally contaminated food or beverages; direct fecal-oral spread | 1–5% of patients with typhoid fever become chronic biliary carriers; food handlers can contaminate food |
| Varicella | Serosurvey in Thailand found 24% young adults (20–29 years) seronegative[62] | Person-to-person; droplet or airborne spread; via freshly soiled articles; transplacental and blood transfusion (rare) | Serologic testing advised for adults without history of varicella. Vaccine can be offered to nonimmunes |

Immigrants visiting friends and relatives in this region are also at risk for shorter-incubation infections, such as acute viral infections (e.g. dengue, Japanese encephalitis, others), diarrhea-causing infections, hepatitis E, leptospirosis, rabies, rickettsial infections, and vaccine-preventable infections (such as measles, rubella, and varicella).

**Table 15.7 Asia: China and Taiwan**

| Diseases | Distribution/incidence | Transmission | Comment |
|---|---|---|---|
| Amoebiasis/amoebic liver abscess | Present; highest risk in areas with poor sanitation | Fecal contamination of food/water; sexually (oral/anal) | Will most commonly manifest within weeks to months of exposure |
| Echinococcosis | Endemic in northern and western areas, especially where sheep are raised; grazing areas of mainland China | Ingestion of eggs; transfer from fingers or from contaminated food, water, or soil | May first become apparent decades after exposure. Cystic lesions most often found in liver, lung |
| Endemic mycoses (*Penicillium marneffei*) | Penicilliosis is endemic in China. | Inhalation or ingestion of spores | Can reactivate; increased risk of dissemination in HIV, immunocompromised |
| Filariasis, lymphatic | Endemic in large areas in the past. Participated in elimination program | Bite of infective mosquito | Lymphangitis, lymphedema, elephantiasis; eosinophilia; parasites can survive 10 years or longer |
| Hepatitis A | High prevalence of immunity to hepatitis A by age 5–10 years in many areas | Fecal contamination of food/water; sexually (oral/anal) | In areas with good sanitation, increasing percentage of children and young adults are susceptible |
| Hepatitis B | Seroprevalence of hepatitis B surface antigen >8% | Percutaneous/permucosal contact with blood, body fluids; perinatal; sexually; unsafe injections; transfusions | Chronic infection associated with increased risk of liver cancer |
| Hepatitis C | Seroprevalence estimated to be 2–2.9% | Unsafe injections; unscreened transfused blood; rare perinatal and sexually | Chronic infection associated with increased risk of liver cancer |
| HIV/AIDS | Now present in all regions of China; rapid spread in some areas because of injecting drug use and paid sex | Sexual exposures; perinatal; breastfeeding; unsafe injections; transfusion of blood/blood products | May be co-infected with TB |
| HTLV-I/II | Serosurvey of blood donors in southern China found 0.15% positive | Mother to child (transplacental and via breastfeeding); sexually; blood transfusion and contaminated needles | Chronic, indolent infection. Dermatitis, adult T-cell leukemia/lymphoma; myelopathy |
| Intestinal parasites | Most common are *Ascaris*, *Dientamoeba fragilis*, *Giardia*, hookworm, *Strongyloides stercoralis*, *Trichuris trichiura*. *Hymenolepis nana* found especially in children | Penetration of skin by larvae in soil (*Strongyloides stercoralis*, hookworm); ingestion of infective ova (*Ascaris*, *Trichuris*, *Hymenolepis nana*) or cysts (*Giardia*). Person-to-person transmission can occur with hymenolepiasis | Co-infection with multiple parasites common. *Strongyloides stercoralis* and *Hymenolepis nana* can persist indefinitely via autoinfective cycle. *Strongyloides stercoralis* can disseminate in immunocompromised |
| Leishmaniasis cutaneous (CL), visceral (VL) | VL: NE, NW China; CL: northwest | Bite of infective phlebotomine (sandfly) | VL may manifest years after initial infection; HIV infection, other immunosuppressing conditions may lead to reactivation |

**Table 15.7 Asia: China and Taiwan—cont'd**

| Diseases | Distribution/incidence | Transmission | Comment |
|---|---|---|---|
| Leprosy | Prevalence per 100 000 population (2004): China 0.3; Hong Kong 0.5 | Probably from secretions from nasal mucosa of infected person to respiratory tract and skin of another | Indolent; may persist for decades |
| Liver flukes (clonorchiasis, fascioliasis) | Clonorchiasis is endemic in China (estimated 15 million infected in 2004), Taiwan, Hong Kong; fascioliasis also found in China | Ingestion of metacercariae in raw or undercooked fish (clonorchiasis) or contaminating water or water plants (fascioliasis) | Adult worms of clonorchiasis in biliary tree can persist >20 years; associated with cholangiocarcinoma |
| Lung flukes (*Paragonimus westermani* and other species) | Endemic in China and Taiwan. Estimated 20 million are infected in China | Ingestion of metacercariae (infective larvae), usually in shellfish | Can persist a decade or longer; lung infection can resemble tuberculosis |
| Malaria | Present in focal rural areas | Mosquito-borne; rare transfusion, congenital, needlestick transmission | Chloroquine resistance present in some areas |
| Neurocysticercosis | Cases have been reported from area | Ingestion of eggs shed in feces of human tapeworm carrier | Many manifest years or more than a decade after initial exposure; CNS focal lesions and seizures |
| Papillomaviruses, human (HPV) | Annual incidence of cervical cancer <10/100 000 population in China | Direct contact, usually through sexual contact. | Screening and treatment can reduce risk of cervical cancer |
| Schistosomiasis, *S. japonicum* | At risk population estimated to number 60 million | Penetration of intact skin or mucosa by live cercariae in fresh water | Occupational risk especially for farmers and fishers |
| Syphilis and endemic treponematoses | Increases in rates of syphilis (including congenital) were reported in China in 1990s. Disease caused by endemic *Treponema pallidum* subspecies has been reported in the past | Direct contact with spirochete, usually via sexual contact; can be transmitted transplacentally and via transfusion or transplantation of infected tissue | Protean manifestations; infected person can transmit infection years after acquisition; syphilis serology positive in endemic treponematoses |
| Tuberculosis | Estimated incidence per 100 000 (2003): China 102; Hong Kong 77 | Inhalation of airborne droplet nuclei from infected person | Multidrug resistance in mainland China in 1996–1999 ranged from 2.8–10.8% |
| Typhoid and paratyphoid (enteric fever) | Risk highest in areas with poor sanitation | Ingestion of bacteria in fecally contaminated food or beverages; direct fecal oral spread | Infection caused by *S. paratyphi* more common than *S. typhi* in some areas |
| Varicella | Young adults who have resided in tropical areas may lack immunity to varicella | Person-to-person; droplet or airborne spread; via freshly soiled articles; transplacental and blood transfusion (rare) | Serologic testing advised for adults without history of varicella. Vaccine can be offered to nonimmunes |

Immigrants visiting friends and relatives in this region are also at risk for shorter-incubation infections, such as acute viral infections (e.g. dengue, hemorrhagic fever with renal syndrome, Japanese encephalitis, others), diarrhea-causing infections, hepatitis E, leptospirosis, polio, rabies, rickettsial infections, and vaccine-preventable infections (such as measles, rubella, and varicella).

**Table 15.8 Asia: India (and selected comments on Pakistan)**

| Diseases | Distribution/incidence | Transmission | Comment |
|---|---|---|---|
| Amoebiasis/amoebic liver abscess | Widespread; highest risk in areas with poor sanitation | Fecal contamination of food/water; sexually (oral/anal) | Will most commonly manifest within weeks to months of exposure |
| Echinococcosis | Endemic in cattle-grazing areas | Ingestion of eggs; transfer from fingers or from contaminated food, water, or soil | May first become apparent >decade after exposure. Cystic lesions most often found in liver, lung |
| Filariasis, lymphatic | Widespread. 454 million live in at-risk areas in India | Bite of infective mosquito | Lymphangitis, lymphedema, elephantiasis; eosinophilia; parasites can survive 10 years or longer |
| Hepatitis A | High prevalence of immunity to hepatitis A by age 5–10 years in many areas | Fecal contamination of food/water; sexually (oral/anal) | In areas with good sanitation, increasing percentage of children and young adults are susceptible |
| Hepatitis B | Seroprevalence of hepatitis B surface antigen 2–7% | Percutaneous/permucosal contact with blood, body fluids; perinatal; sexually; unsafe injections; transfusions | Chronic infection associated with increased risk of liver cancer |
| Hepatitis C | Seroprevalence estimated to be 1–1.9% in India; >2.9% in Pakistan | Unsafe injections; unscreened transfused blood; rare perinatal and sexually | Chronic infection associated with increased risk of liver cancer |
| HIV/AIDS | Estimated 5.1 million infected in India (2003); HIV prevalence >5% in some antenatal clinics | Sexual exposures; perinatal; breastfeeding; unsafe injections; transfusion of blood/blood products | High rates of co-infection with tuberculosis |
| HTLV-I/II | 1–9% high-risk patients were seropositive in India in one study[14] | Mother to child (transplacental and via breastfeeding); sexually; blood transfusion and contaminated needles | Chronic, indolent infection. Dermatitis, adult T-cell leukemia/lymphoma; myelopathy |
| Intestinal parasites | Most common are *Ascaris*, *Dientamoeba fragilis*, *Giardia*, hookworm, *Strongyloides stercoralis*, *Trichuris trichiura*. *Hymenolepis nana* found especially in children | Penetration of skin by larvae in soil (*Strongyloides stercoralis*, hookworm); ingestion of infective ova (*Ascaris*, *Trichuris*, *Hymenolepis nana*) or cysts (*Giardia*). Person-to-person transmission can occur with hymenolepiasis | Co-infection with multiple parasites common. *Hymenolepis nana* can persist indefinitely via autoinfective cycle. *Strongyloides stercoralis* can disseminate in immunocompromised |
| Leishmaniasis, cutaneous (CL), visceral (VL) | Major epidemics (VL) in eastern India (especially Assam and Bihar states); endemic in Pakistan; CL: Pakistan and NW India | Bite of infective phlebotomine (sandfly) | VL may manifest years after initial infection; HIV infection, other immunosuppressing conditions may lead to reactivation |
| Leprosy | Prevalence 26/100 000 in India, 2004 | Probably from secretions from nasal mucosa of infected person to respiratory tract and skin of another | Indolent; may persist for decades |

**Table 15.8 Asia: India (and selected comments on Pakistan)—cont'd**

| Diseases | Distribution/incidence | Transmission | Comment |
|---|---|---|---|
| Liver flukes (fascioliasis) | Sporadic cases reported | Ingestion of water or plants contaminated with metacercariae | Adult worm in biliary tree can survive for years |
| Lung flukes (*Paragonimus westermani*) | Endemic in Manipur Province, India | Ingestion of metacercariae (infective larvae), usually in shellfish | Can persist a decade or longer; lung infection can resemble tuberculosis |
| Malaria | Widespread at altitudes <2000 meters | Mosquito-borne; rare transfusion, congenital, needlestick transmission | Chloroquine-resistant falciparum malaria documented |
| Neurocysticercosis | Endemic in area | Ingestion of eggs shed in feces of human tapeworm carrier | Many manifest years to more than decade after exposure; focal CNS lesion; seizures |
| Papillomaviruses, human (HPV) | Incidence of cervical cancer up to 33/100 000 in India | Direct contact, usually through sexual contact | Cervical cancer, caused by oncogenic HPV, is a leading cancer in women |
| Schistosomiasis due to *S. haematobium* | Ill-defined focus in west | Penetration of intact skin or mucosa by live cercariae in fresh water | Adult worm may survive >10 years; chronic sequelae may develop long after initial infection |
| Syphilis and endemic tryponematoses | Widespread. Disease caused by endemic *Treponema pallidum* subspecies has been reported from India and Pakistan | Direct contact with spirochete, usually via sexual contact; can be transmitted transplacentally and via transfusion or transplantation of infected tissue | Protean findings; infected person can transmit infection years after acquisition; syphilis serology positive in endemic treponematoses |
| Trypanosomiasis | One case reported (2004) of infection with *Trypanosoma evansi*, an animal trypanosome; district of Chandrapur | | Unclear whether this was isolated event |
| Tuberculosis | Estimated incidence per 100 000 (2003): 163 India, 181 Pakistan (WHO, 2003).[†] Average annual risk of TB infection in India estimated at 1.5% in study 2000–2003[51] | Inhalation of airborne droplet nuclei from infected person | New TB cases in India with MDR estimated at 3.4%; MDR in previously treated cases has varied from 8% to >50%; in Pakistan estimated 9.6% new TB cases are MDR |
| Typhoid and paratyphoid (enteric fever) | Highly endemic in Indian subcontinent. Incidence in India 980/100 000. | Ingestion of bacteria in fecally contaminated food or beverages; direct fecal oral spread | Multidrug resistance increasingly common |
| Varicella | 31% rural adults seronegative at age 25 years;[63] 9% negative at 31–40 years[61] | Person-to-person; droplet or airborne spread; via freshly soiled articles; transplacental and blood transfusion (rare) | Serologic testing advised for adults without history of varicella. Vaccine can be offered to nonimmunes |

Immigrants visiting friends and relatives in this region are also at risk for shorter-incubation infections, such as acute viral infections (e.g. dengue, Japanese encephalitis, others), diarrhea-causing infections (including cholera), hepatitis E, leptospirosis, rabies, rickettsial infections, and vaccine-preventable infections (such as measles, rubella, varicella, and polio).
[†]multidrug resistance.

**Table 15.9 Asia: South Korea (Republic of Korea)**

| Diseases | Distribution/incidence | Transmission | Comment |
|---|---|---|---|
| Amoebiasis/amoebic liver abscess | Present; highest risk in areas with poor sanitation | Fecal contamination of food/water; sexually (oral/anal) | Will most commonly manifest within weeks to months of exposure |
| Filariasis, lymphatic | Endemic in parts of country | Bite of infective mosquito | Lymphangitis, lymphedema, elephantiasis; eosinophilia; parasites can survive 10 years or longer |
| Hepatitis A | High prevalence of immunity to hepatitis A among adults | Fecal contamination of food/water; sexually (oral/anal) | In areas with good sanitation, increasing percentage of children and young adults are susceptible |
| Hepatitis B | Seroprevalence of hepatitis B surface antigen >8% | Percutaneous/permucosal contact with blood, body fluids; perinatal; sexually; unsafe injections; transfusions | Chronic infection associated with increased risk of liver cancer |
| Hepatitis C | Seroprevalence estimated to be 2–2.9% | Unsafe injections; unscreened transfused blood; rare perinatal and sexually | Chronic infection associated with increased risk of liver cancer |
| HIV/AIDS | Prevalence in adults estimated <0.1% in 2003 | Sexual exposures; perinatal; breastfeeding; unsafe injections; transfusion of blood/blood products | High rates of co-infection with tuberculosis |
| HTLV-I/II | Seroprevalence was 0.76% (Cheju Island) and 0.13% (blood donors) | Mother to child (transplacental and via breastfeeding); sexually; blood transfusion and contaminated needles | Chronic, indolent infection. Dermatitis, adult T-cell leukemia/lymphoma; myelopathy |
| Intestinal parasites (low rates of infection in recent years) | Most common are *Ascaris*, *Dientamoeba fragilis*, *Giardia*, hookworm, *Strongyloides stercoralis*, *Trichuris trichiura*. *Hymenolepis nana* found especially in children | Penetration of skin by larvae in soil (*Strongyloides stercoralis*, hookworm); ingestion of infective ova (*Ascaris*, *Trichuris*, *Hymenolepis nana*) or cysts (*Giardia*). Person-to-person transmission can occur with hymenolepiasis | Co-infection with multiple parasites common. *Strongyloides stercoralis* and *Hymenolepis nana* can persist indefinitely via autoinfective cycle. *Strongyloides stercoralis* can disseminate in immunocompromised |
| Leprosy | Prevalence 1.1/100 000 in Korea, 2004 | Probably from secretions from nasal mucosa of infected person to respiratory tract and skin of another | Indolent; may persist for decades |
| Liver flukes (clonorchiasis) | Endemic area for clonorchiasis | Ingestion of raw or undercooked fish containing metacercariae | Adult worms of clonorchiasis in biliary tree can persist >20 years; associated with cholangiocarcinoma |

**Table 15.9 Asia: South Korea (Republic of Korea)—cont'd**

| Diseases | Distribution/incidence | Transmission | Comment |
|---|---|---|---|
| Lung fluke (*Paragonimus westermani*) | Endemic area | Ingestion of metacercariae (infective larvae), usually in shellfish | Can persist a decade or longer; lung infection can resemble tuberculosis |
| Malaria | Vivax malaria re-emerged 1993. >4000 cases reported in 2000 | Mosquito-borne; rare transfusion, congenital, needlestick transmission | Most cases have been in military personnel. No chloroquine resistance |
| Neurocysticercosis | Cases reported | Ingestion of eggs shed in feces of human tapeworm carrier | Focal CNS lesions and seizures |
| Papillomaviruses, human (HPV) | Incidence of cervical cancer up to 16.8/100 000 | Direct contact, usually through sexual contact | Screening combined with treatment can reduce risk of cervical cancer |
| Syphilis and endemic treponematoses | Syphilis is present in the region. | Direct contact with spirochete, usually via sexual contact; can be transmitted transplacentally and via transfusion or transplantation of infected tissue | Protean manifestations; infected person can transmit infection years after acquisition; syphilis serology positive in endemic treponematoses |
| Tuberculosis | Estimated incidence per 100 000 (2003): 87 | Inhalation of airborne droplet nuclei from infected person | Studies in 1999 showed MDR in new TB cases 2.2% |
| Typhoid and paratyphoid (enteric fever) | Present, especially in areas with poor sanitation | Ingestion of bacteria in fecally contaminated food or beverages; direct fecal oral spread | 1–5% of patients with typhoid fever become chronic biliary carriers; food handlers can contaminate food |

Immigrants visiting friends and relatives in this region are also at risk for shorter-incubation infections, such as acute viral infections (e.g. hemorrhagic fever with renal syndrome, Japanese encephalitis, others), diarrhea-causing infections, hepatitis E, leptospirosis, rabies, rickettsial infections, and vaccine-preventable infections (such as measles, rubella, and varicella).

**Table 15.10 Asia: Philippines**

| Diseases | Distribution/incidence | Transmission | Comment |
|---|---|---|---|
| Amoebiasis/amoebic liver abscess | Present; highest risk in areas with poor sanitation | Fecal contamination of food/water; sexually (oral/anal) | Will most commonly manifest within weeks to months of exposure |
| Filariasis, lymphatic | Endemic in many areas. Began mass drug administration in 2004 | Bite of infective mosquito | Lymphangitis, lymphedema, elephantiasis; eosinophilia; parasites can survive 10 years or longer |
| Hepatitis A | High prevalence of immunity to hepatitis A by age 5–10 years in many areas | Fecal contamination of food/water; sexually (oral/anal) | In areas with good sanitation, increasing percentage of children and young adults are susceptible |

**Table 15.10 Asia: Philippines—cont'd**

| Diseases | Distribution/incidence | Transmission | Comment |
|---|---|---|---|
| Hepatitis B | Seroprevalence of hepatitis B surface antigen >8% | Percutaneous/permucosal contact with blood, body fluids; perinatal; sexually; unsafe injections; transfusions | Chronic infection associated with increased risk of liver cancer |
| Hepatitis C | Seroprevalence estimated to be 2–2.9% | Unsafe injections; unscreened transfused blood; rare perinatal and sexually | Chronic infection associated with increased risk of liver cancer |
| HIV/AIDS | Estimated overall HIV prevalence in adults <0.1% (2003) | Sexual exposures; perinatal; breastfeeding; unsafe injections; transfusion of blood/blood products | 33% of reported cases (2004) were in overseas Filipino workers |
| Intestinal parasites | Most common are *Ascaris*, *Dientamoeba fragilis*, *Giardia*, hookworm, *Strongyloides stercoralis*, *Trichuris trichiura*. *Hymenolepis nana* found especially in children | Penetration of skin by larvae in soil (*Strongyloides stercoralis*, hookworm); ingestion of infective ova (*Ascaris*, *Trichuris*, *Hymenolepis nana*) or cysts (*Giardia*). Person-to-person transmission can occur with hymenolepiasis | Co-infection with multiple parasites common. *Strongyloides stercoralis* and *Hymenolepis nana* can persist indefinitely via autoinfective cycle. *Strongyloides stercoralis* can disseminate in immunocompromised |
| Leprosy | Prevalence 4.2/100 000 in 2004 | Probably from secretions from nasal mucosa of infected person to respiratory tract and skin of another | Indolent; may persist for decades |
| Liver flukes (fascioliasis) | Sporadic cases reported. | Ingestion of raw or undercooked fish containing metacercariae | Adult worm in biliary tree can survive for years |
| Lung flukes (*Paragonimus westermani*) | Endemic area for paragonimiasis | Ingestion of metacercariae (infective larvae), usually in shellfish | Can persist a decade or longer; lung infection can resemble tuberculosis |
| Malaria | Focal areas of risk below 600 meters in some rural areas | Mosquito-borne; rare transfusion, congenital, needlestick transmission | Chloroquine resistance confirmed |
| Neurocysticercosis | Cases have been reported from area | Ingestion of eggs shed in feces of human tapeworm carrier | Focal CNS lesions and seizures |
| Papillomaviruses, human (HPV) | Incidence of cervical cancer up to 25.8/100 000 | Direct contact, usually through sexual contact. | Cervical cancer, caused by oncogenic HPV, is a leading cancer in women |
| Schistosomiasis due to *S. japonicum* | At risk population estimated at 6 million (dogs and pigs are reservoir) | Penetration of intact skin or mucosa by live cercariae in fresh water | Adult worm may survive >10 years; chronic sequelae may develop long after initial infection |

**Table 15.10 Asia: Philippines—cont'd**

| Diseases | Distribution/incidence | Transmission | Comment |
|---|---|---|---|
| Syphilis and endemic treponematoses | Syphilis is widespread in region | Direct contact with spirochete, usually via sexual contact; can be transmitted transplacentally and via transfusion or transplantation of infected tissue | Protean manifestations; infected person can transmit infection years after acquisition; syphilis serology positive in endemic treponematoses |
| Tuberculosis | Estimated incidence per 100 000 (2003): 296 | Inhalation of airborne droplet nuclei from infected person | Estimated incidence per 100 000 in 1990: 336 |
| Typhoid and paratyphoid (enteric fever) | Widespread | Ingestion of bacteria in fecally contaminated food or beverages; direct fecal oral spread | 1–5% of patients with typhoid fever become chronic biliary carriers; food handlers can contaminate food |
| Varicella | 28% Filipino nurses age 20–25 years seronegative[59] | Person-to-person; droplet or airborne spread; via freshly soiled articles; transplacental and blood transfusion (rare) | Serologic testing advised for adults without history of varicella. Vaccine can be offered to nonimmunes |

Immigrants visiting friends and relatives in this region are also at risk for shorter-incubation infections, such as acute viral infections (e.g., dengue Japanese encephalitis, others), diarrhea-causing infections (including cholera), hepatitis E, leptospirosis, rabies, rickettsial infections, and vaccine-preventable infections (such as measles, rubella, and varicella).

**Table 15.11 Eastern Europe: Poland, former USSR, Yugoslavia**

| Diseases | Distribution/incidence | Transmission | Comment |
|---|---|---|---|
| Amoebiasis/amoebic liver abscess | Present; highest risk in areas with poor sanitation | Fecal contamination of food/water; sexually (oral/anal) | Will most commonly manifest within weeks to months of exposure |
| Echinococcosis | Endemic, including infection caused by *E. multilocularis* | Ingestion of eggs; transfer from fingers or from contaminated food, water, or soil | May first become apparent decades after exposure. Cystic lesions most often found in liver, lung |
| Hepatitis A | High prevalence of immunity to hepatitis A among adults | Fecal contamination of food/water; sexually (oral/anal) | In areas with good sanitation, increasing percentage of children and young adults are susceptible |
| Hepatitis B | Seroprevalence of hepatitis B surface antigen 2–7% in most areas; >8% in some areas | Percutaneous/permucosal contact with blood, body fluids; perinatal; sexually; unsafe injections; transfusions | Chronic infection associated with increased risk of liver cancer |
| Hepatitis C | Seroprevalence 2–2.9% in most of region | Unsafe injections; unscreened transfused blood; rare perinatal and sexually | Chronic infection associated with increased risk of liver cancer |

**Table 15.11 Eastern Europe: Poland, former USSR, Yugoslavia—cont'd**

| Diseases | Distribution/incidence | Transmission | Comment |
|---|---|---|---|
| HIV/AIDS | Adult HIV prevalence estimated <1.1% (2003), but increasing rapidly in parts of Russian Federation; prevalence in prison population 2–4% | Sexual exposures; perinatal; breastfeeding; unsafe injections; transfusion of blood/blood products | Most transmission is through sex and injecting drug use |
| Intestinal parasites (low rates of infection in recent years) | Most common are *Ascaris*, *Dientamoeba fragilis*, *Giardia*, hookworm, *Strongyloides stercoralis*, *Trichuris trichiura*. *Hymenolepis nana* found especially in children | Penetration of skin by larvae in soil (*Strongyloides stercoralis*, hookworm); ingestion of infective ova (*Ascaris*, *Trichuris*, *Hymenolepis nana*) or cysts (*Giardia*). Person-to-person transmission can occur with hymenolepiasis | Co-infection with multiple parasites common. *Strongyloides stercoralis* and *Hymenolepis nana* can persist indefinitely via autoinfective cycle. *Strongyloides stercoralis* can disseminate in immunocompromised |
| Leishmaniasis | Mediterranean littoral and southern regions of former Soviet Union | Bite of infective phlebotomine (sandfly) | May first manifest many decades after infected |
| Liver flukes (*Opisthorchis felineus*) | Population of 12.5 million estimated to be at risk for opisthorchiasis in Kazakhstan, Russian Federation, Siberia, Ukraine | Ingestion of raw or undercooked fish containing metacercariae | Adult worms of opisthorchiasis in biliary tree can persist >20 years; associated with cholangiocarcinoma |
| Malaria | Malaria present in focal areas in Azerbaijan, Georgia, Turkmenistan, Uzbekistan | Mosquito-borne; rare transfusion, congenital, needlestick transmission | No chloroquine resistance reported |
| Neurocysticercosis | Cases reported from Eastern Europe | Ingestion of eggs shed in feces of human tapeworm carrier | Focal CNS lesions and seizures |
| Papillomaviruses, human (HPV) | Incidence of cervical cancer varies | Direct contact, usually through sexual contact. | Screening combined with treatment can reduce risk of cervical cancer |
| Syphilis and endemic treponematoses | Syphilis is widespread. Major epidemics of syphilis occurred in newly independent states in 1990s. Rates remain high (including congenital syphilis) | Direct contact with spirochete, usually via sexual contact; can be transmitted transplacentally and via transfusion or transplantation of infected tissue | Protean manifestations; infected person can transmit infection years after acquisition; syphilis serology positive in endemic treponematoses |
| Tuberculosis | Estimated incidence per 100 000 (2003): Russia 126 | Inhalation of airborne droplet nuclei from infected person | In studies in 1998–1999 MDR[†] in new TB cases was 6.5 and 9% |
| Typhoid and paratyphoid (enteric fever) | Focal outbreaks continue to occur | Ingestion of bacteria in fecally contaminated food or beverages; direct fecal oral spread | 1–5% of patients with typhoid fever become chronic biliary carriers; food handlers can contaminate food |

Immigrants visiting friends and relatives in this region are also at risk for shorter-incubation infections, such as acute viral infections (e.g. hemorrhagic fever with renal syndrome, tick-borne encephalitis, others), diarrhea-causing infections, leptospirosis, rabies, rickettsial infections, and vaccine-preventable infections (such as measles, rubella, and varicella).
[†] multidrug resistance.

## References, General

1. Jacobsen KH, Koopman JS. Declining hepatitis A seroprevalence: a global review and analysis. Epidemiol Infect 2004; 132:1005–1022.
2. Nelson KE. Global changes in the epidemiology of hepatitis A virus infection. Clin Infect Dis 2006; 42:1151–1152.
3. Nicholas R, Pugh H, Omar RI, et al. Varicella infection and pneumonia among adults. Int J Infect Dis 1998; 2(4):205–210.
4. Meyer PA, Seward JF, Jumaan AO, et al. Varicella mortality: trends before vaccine licensure in the United States, 1970–1994. J Infect Dis 2000; 182:383–390.
5. Alagappan K, Donohue B, Guzik H, et al. Seroprevalence of tetanus antibodies among immigrants over age 50: a comparison to an aged-matched US-born population. Ann Intern Med 2004; 44(4):S126–S127.
6. Talan DA, Abrahamian FM, Moral GJ, et al. Tetanus immunity and physician compliance with tetanus prophylaxis practices among emergency department patients presenting with wounds. Ann Emerg Med 2004; 43:305–314.
7. Lopez-Velez R, Huerga H, Turrientes MC. Infectious diseases in immigrants from the perspective of a tropical medicine referral unit. Am J Trop Med Hyg 2003; 69(1):115–121.
8. Pockros PJ, Capozza TA. Helminthic infections of the liver. Current Infect Dis Reports 2005; 7(1):61–70.
9. Wilson ME. A world guide to infections: diseases, distribution, diagnosis. New York: Oxford University Press; 1991.
10. Adair R, Mwaneri MO. Communicable disease in African immigrants in Minneapolis. Arch Intern Med 1999; 159:83–85.
11. Oldfield EC, Rodier GR, Gray GC. The endemic infectious diseases of Somalia. Clin Infect Dis 1993; 16(suppl3): S132–S157.
12. Office of Immigration Statistics. 2002 Yearbook of immigration statistics – October 2003. Washington, DC: Department of Homeland Security; 2003.
13. Lifson AR, Thai D, O'Fallon A, et al. Prevalence of tuberculosis, hepatitis B virus, and intestinal parasitic infections among refugees to Minnesota. Public Health Rep 2002; 117:69–77.
14. Nelson KR, Bui H, Samet JH. Screening in special populations: a 'case study' of recent Vietnamese immigrants. Am J Med 1997; 102:435–440.
15. White AC, Atmar RL. Infections in Hispanic immigrants. Clin Infect Dis 2002; 34:1627–1632.
16. Worm HC, van der Poel WHM, Brandstatter G. Hepatitis E: an overview. Micro Infect 2002; 4:657–666.
17. Hurie MB, Mast EE, Davis JP. Horizontal transmission of hepatitis B virus infection to United States-born children of Hmong refugees. Pediatrics 1992; 89:269–273.
18. Lobato MN, Hopewell PC. *Mycobacterium tuberculosis* infection after travel to or contact with visitors from countries with a high prevalence of tuberculosis. Am J Respir Crit Care Med 1998; 158:1871–1875.
19. Milas J, Ropac D, Mulie R, et al. Hepatitis B in the family. Eur J Epidemiol 2000; 16:203–208.
20. Wilson ME, Pearson RD. Fever and systemic symptoms. In: Guerrant RL, Walker DH, Weller PF, eds. Tropical infectious diseases: principles, pathogens and practice. 2nd edn. Philadelphia: Elsevier; 2006:1459–1477.
21. El-Serag H, Mason AC. Rising incidence of hepatocellular carcinoma in the United States. N Engl J Med 2005; 340(10):745–750.
22. Parkin DM, Pisani P, Ferlay J. Estimates of the worldwide incidence of 25 major cancers in 1990. Int J Cancer 1999; 80:827–841.
23. Bacaner N, Stauffer B, Boulware DR, et al. Travel medicine considerations for North American immigrants visiting friends and relatives. JAMA 2004; 291:2856–2864.
24. Behrens RH. Visiting friends and relatives. In: Keystone JS, Kozarsky PE, Freedman DO, et al., eds. Travel medicine. London: Mosby; 2004:281–285.
25. Schlagenhauf P, Steffen R, Loutan L. Migrants as a major risk group for imported malaria in European countries. J Travel Med 2003; 10:106–107.
26. Centers for Disease Control and Prevention. Human tuberculosis caused by *Mycobacterium bovis* – New York City, 2001–2004. MMWR 2005; 54(24):605–608.
27. Pappas G, Papadimitriou P, Akritdis N, et al. The new global map of human brucellosis. Lancet Infect Dis 2006; 6:91–99.
28. Klion AD, Massougbodji M, Sadeler B-C, et al. Loiasis in endemic and non-endemic populations: immunologically mediated differences in clinical presentation. J Infect Dis 1991; 163:1318–1325.
29. McCarthy JS, Ottesen EA, Nutman TB. Onchocerciasis in endemic and nonendemic populations: differences in clinical presentation and immunologic findings. J Infect Dis 1994; 17:736–741.
30. Schwartzman K, Oxlade O, Barr RG, et al. Domestic returns from investment in the control of tuberculosis in other countries. N Engl J Med 2005; 353(10):1008–1020.
31. Centers for Disease Control and Prevention. Health Information for International Travel 2005–2006. Atlanta: US Department of Health and Human Services, Public Health Service; 2005.
32. Wilson ME. Geographic distribution of potential health hazards for travelers, In: Centers for Disease Control and Prevention. Health Information for International Travel 2005–2006. Atlanta: US Department of Health and Human Services, Public Health Service; 2005:47–93.

## References, Specific to Infections Included in Table 15.1 and Cited in other Tables

### Amoebiasis

1. Haque R, Huston CD, Hughes M, et al. Current concepts: amoebiasis. New Engl J Med 2003; 348:1565–1573.

### Echinococcosis

2. Schantz PM, Kern P, Brunetti E. Echinococcosis. In: Guerrant RL, Walker DH, Weller PF, eds. Tropical infectious diseases: principles, pathogens, and practice, 2nd edn. Philadelphia: Elsevier; 2006:1304–1326.

### Filariasis, lymphatic

3. Boggild AK, Keystone JS, Kain KC. Tropical pulmonary eosinophilia: a case series in a setting of nonendemicity. Clin Infect Dis 2004; 39:1123–1128.
4. Erlanger TE, Keiser J, Castro MCD, et al. Effect of water resource development and management on lymphatic filariasis, and estimates of populations at risk. Am J Trop Med Hyg 2005; 73(3):523–533.
5. World Health Organization. Global programme to eliminate lymphatic filariasis. Weekly Epidemiol Rec 2005; 23:202–212.

### Hepatitis A

6. Barnett ED, Holmes AH, Geltman P, et al. Immunity to hepatitis A in people born and raised in endemic areas. J Travel Med 2003; 10:11–14.
7. Tanaka J. Hepatitis A shifting epidemiology in Latin America. Vaccine 2000; 18:S57–S60.

8. Weinberg M, Hopkins J, Farrington L, et al. Hepatitis A in Hispanic children who live along the United States–Mexico border: the role of international travel and food-borne exposures. Pediatrics 2004; 114:e68–e73.

## Hepatitis B

9. Andre F. Hepatitis B epidemiology in Asia, the Middle East and Africa. Vaccine 2000; 18(Suppl):20–22.
10. Taylor VM, Yasui Y, Burke N, et al. Hepatitis B testing among Vietnamese-American men. Cancer Detect Prevent 2004; 28:170–177.

## Hepatitis C

11. Kim WR. Global epidemiology and burden of hepatitis C. Microb Infect 2002; 4:1219–1225.
12. Shepard CW, Finelli L, Alter MJ. Global epidemiology of hepatitis C virus infection. Lancet Infect Dis 2005; 5:558–567.

## HIV/AIDS

13. UNAIDS. Report on the global HIV/AIDS epidemic, Geneva: Joint United Nations Programme on HIV/AIDS (UNAIDS); 2004 June. Report No.: UNAIDS/04.16E. http://www.unaids.org/en/geographical = area/by = country/

## HTLV-I/II

14. Ramalingam S, Kannangai R, Prakash KJ, et al. A pilot study of HTLV-I infection in high-risk individuals and their family members from India. Indian J Med Res 2001; 113:201–209.
15. Vrielink H, Reesink HW. HTLV-I/II prevalence in different geographic locations. Transfusion Med Rev 2004; 18(1):46–57.

## Intestinal parasites

16. Ekdahl K, Andersson Y. Imported giardiasis: impact of international travel, immigration, and adoption. Am J Trop Med Hyg 2005; 72(6):825–830.
17. Garg PK, Perry S, Dorn M, et al. Risk of intestinal helminth and protozoan infection in a refugee population. Am J Trop Med Hyg 2005; 73(2):386–391.
18. Geltman PL, Cochran J, Hedgecock C. Intestinal parasites among African refugees resettled in Massachusetts and the impact of an overseas pre-departure treatment program. Am J Trop Med Hyg 2003; 69(6):657–662.
19. Loutfy MR, Wilson M, Keystone JS, et al. Serology and eosinophil count in the diagnosis and management of strongyloidiasis in a non-endemic area. Am J Trop Med Hyg 2002; 66:749–752.
20. Maggi P, Brandonisio O, Carito V, et al. Hymenolepis nana parasites in adopted children. Clin Infect Dis 2005; 41(15 Aug):571–572.
21. Muennig P, Pallin D, Sell RL, et al. The cost effectiveness of strategies for the treatment of intestinal parasites in immigrants. N Engl J Med 1999; 349:773–779.
22. Rice JE, Skull SA, Pearce C, et al. Screening for intestinal parasites in recently arrived children from East Africa. J Paediatr Child Health 2003; 39:456–459.

## Leishmaniasis, cutaneous and visceral

23. Jeronimo SMB, Sousa ADQ, Pearson RD. Leishmaniasis, In: Guerrant RL, Walker DH, Weller PF, eds. Tropical infectious diseases: principles, pathogens, and practice. 2nd edn. Philadelphia: Elsevier; 2006:1095–1113.

## Leprosy

24. World Health Organization. Global leprosy situation, 2004. Weekly Epidemiol Rec 2004; 13:118–124.
25. World Health Organization. Global leprosy situation, 2005. Weekly Epidemiol Rec 2005; 80(34):289–295.

## Liver flukes (fascioliasis)

26. Graham CS, Brodie SB, Weller PF. Imported Fasciola hepatica infection in the United States and treatment with triclabendazole. Clin Infect Dis 2001; 33:1–5.
27. Lun Z-R, Gasser RB, Lai D-H, et al. Clonorchiasis: a key foodborne zoonosis in China. Lancet Infect Dis 2005; 31:31–41.
28. Mas-Coma MS, Esteban JG, Bargues MD. Epidemiology of human fascioliasis: a review and proposed new classification. Bull WHO 1999; 77(4):340–346.
29. Stauffer WM, Sellman JS, Walker PF. Biliary liver flukes (Opisthorchiasis and Clonorchiasis) in immigrants in the United States: often subtle and diagnosed years after arrival. J Travel Med 2004; 11:157–160.

## Lung flukes

30. Keiser J, Utzinger J. Emerging foodborne trematodiasis. Emerg Infect Dis 2005; 11(10):1507–1514.

## Loiasis

31. Klion AD, Nutman TB. Loiasis and Mansonella infections. In: Guerrant RL, Walker DH, Weller PF, eds. Tropical infectious diseases: principles, pathogens, and practice. 2nd edn. Philadelphia: Elsevier; 2006:1163–1175.

## Malaria

32. Centers for Disease Control and Prevention. Yellow fever vaccine requirements and information on malaria risk, by country. In: Health Information for International Travel, 2005–2006. Atlanta: US Department of Health and Human Services, Public Health Service; 2005:325–372.

## Neurocysticercosis

33. Del La Garza Y, Graviss EA, Daver NG, et al. Epidemiology of neurocysticercosis in Houston, Texas. Am J Trop Med Hyg 2005; 73(4):766–770.
34. Schantz PM, Wilkins PP, Tsang FCW. Immigrants, imaging, and immunoblots: the emergence of neurocysticercosis as a significant public health problem. In: Scheld WM, Craig WA, Hughes JM, eds. Emerging infections 2. Washington DC: ASM Press; 1998:213–242.
35. White AC Jr. Neurocysticercosis: updates on epidemiology, pathogenesis, diagnosis, and management. Ann Rev Med 2000; 51:187–206.
36. Yancey LS, Diaz-Marchan PJ, White AC. Cysticercosis: recent advances in diagnosis and management of neurocysticercosis. Current Infect Dis Reports 2005; 7(1):39–47.

## Onchocerciasis

37. World Health Organization. Onchocerciasis (river blindness). Report from the fourteenth InterAmerican conference on onchocerciasis, Atlanta, Georgia, United States. Weekly Epidemiol Rec 2005; 80:257–260.

## Papillomaviruses

38. Bosch FX, Manos MM, Munoz N, et al. Prevalence of human papillomavirus in cervical cancer: a worldwide perspective. J Natl Cancer Inst 1995; 87:796–802.

39. Schiffman M, Castle PE. The promise of global cervical cancer prevention. N Engl J Med 2005; 353:2101–2104.

## Schistosomiasis

40. Grobusch MP, Muhlberger N, Jelinek T, et al. Imported schistosomiasis in Europe: sentinel surveillance data from TropNetEurop. J Travel Med 2003; 10(3):164–169.
41. Whitty DJM, Mabey DC, Armstrong M, et al. Presentation and outcome of 1107 cases of schistosomiasis from Africa diagnosed in a non-endemic country. Trans R Soc Trop Med Hyg 2000; 94:531–534.

## Syphilis and endemic treponematoses

42. Antal GM, Lukehart SA, Meheus AZ. The endemic treponematoses. Microb Infect 2002; 4:83–94.
43. Centers for Disease Control and Prevention. Recommendation regarding screening of refugee children for treponemal infection. Morb Mort Weekly Report 2005; 54(37):933–934.
44. Goh BT. Syphilis in adults. Sex Transm Infect 2005; 81:448–452.
45. Miller LC. Syphilis. In: The handbook of international adoption medicine. New York: Oxford University Press; 2005:276–285.
46. Tikhonova L, Salakhov E, Southwick K, et al. Congenital syphilis in the Russian Federation: magnitude, determinants, and consequences. Sex Transm Infect 2003; 79:106–110.
47. World Health Organization. Estimated new cases of syphilis among adults, 1999. http://www.who.int/tdr/dw/syphilis2004.htm May 7, 2006.

## Trypanosomiasis, African

48. Chritien J-P, Smoak BL. African trypanosomiasis: changing epidemiology and consequences. Current Infect Dis Reports 2005; 7:54–60.
49. World Health Organization. African trypanosomiasis. In: WHO report on global surveillance of epidemic-prone infectious diseases. Geneva, Switzerland: World Health Organization; 2005.

## Trypanosomiasis, American

50. Kirchhoff LV. American trypanosomiasis (Chagas' disease). In: Guerrant RL, Walker DH, Weller PF, eds. Tropical infectious diseases: principles, pathogens, and practice. 2nd edn. Philadelphia: Elsevier; 2006:1082–1094.

## Tuberculosis

51. Chadha VK. Tuberculosis epidemiology in India: a review. Int J Tuberc Lung Dis 2005; 9(10):1072–1082.
52. Granich RM, Balandrano S, Santaella AJ, et al. Survey of drug resistance of *Mycobacterium tuberculosis* in 3 Mexican states, 1997. Arch Intern Med 2000; 160:639–644.
53. Khan K, Muennig P, Behta M, et al. Global drug-resistance patterns and the management of latent tuberculosis infections in immigrants to the United States. N Engl J Med 2002; 347(23):1850–1859.
54. Smith B, Ryan MAK, Gray GC, et al. Tuberculosis infection among young adults enlisting in the United States Navy. Int J Epidemiol 2002; 31:934–939.
55. World Health Organization. Global tuberculosis control: surveillance, planning, financing. WHO report 2005. Geneva, Switzerland: World Health Organization; 2005.
56. Young J, O'Connor ME. Risk factors associated with latent tuberculosis infection in Mexican American children. Pediatrics 2005; 115:e647–e653.

## Typhoid and paratyphoid fever

57. Bhan MK, Bahl R, Bhatnagar S. Typhoid and paratyphoid fever. Lancet 2005; 366:749–762.

## Varicella

58. Alvarez y Munoz MT, Otrres J, Damasio-Santana L, et al. Susceptibility to varicella-zoster infection in individuals 1 to 29 years of age in Mexico. Arch Med Res 1999; 30(1):60–63.
59. Lee BW. Review of varicella-zoster seroepidemiology in India and Southeast Asia. Trop Med Internat Health 1998; 3(11):886–890.
60. Leikin E, Figueroa R, Bertkau A, et al. Seronegativity to varicella-zoster virus in a tertiary care obstetric population. Ob Gynecol 1997; 90:511–513.
61. Lokeshwar MR, Agrawal A, Subbarao SD, et al. Age-related seroprevalence of antibodies in varicella in India. Indian Pediatr 2000; 37(7):714–719.
62. Lolekha S, Tanthiphabha W, Sornchai P, et al. Effect of climatic factors and population density on varicella-zoster virus epidemiology within a tropical country. Am J Trop Med Hyg 2001; 64(3):131–136.
63. Mandel BK, Mukherjee PP, Murphy C, et al. Adult susceptibility to varicella in the tropics is a rural phenomenon due to the lack of previous exposure. J Infect Dis 1998; 178(Suppl 1):S52–S54.

# CHAPTER 16

# Diseases by Race/Ethnicity

Andrea P. Summer and William Stauffer

## Summary Points

- Diseases vary by population. Genetic determinants of disease will become increasingly clear with the explosion of genetic mapping expression studies and techniques.
- Immigrants and refugees have many conditions related to their race and ethnicity which impact their health after migration.
- Providers must be aware of unique or prevalent diseases affecting the populations they serve.

## Introduction

Any discussion of diseases by race/ethnicity must be prefaced by a discussion of the present debate over use of these terms. The terms 'race' and 'ethnicity' do not have universally accepted definitions, which alludes to the complexity of the connotations. Francis Collins, director of the National Human Genome Research Institute, stated in a recent article:[1]

' "Race"and "ethnicity" are poorly defined terms that serve as flawed surrogates for multiple environmental and genetic factors in disease causation.'

It will become apparent throughout the course of this chapter that racial and ethnic differences in diseases are influenced as much by socioeconomic and environmental factors as they are by cultural and genetic factors. Leading causes of death have varying evidence for genetic influence (Fig. 16.1). This chapter will focus on evidence as it relates to cardiovascular diseases, diabetes, obesity, cancer, and hemoglobinopathies.

## Cardiovascular Disease

Cardiovascular disease is the most common cause of death in the Western world and is emerging as one of the most common causes of death in the developing world (Figs 16.2–16.5). Migrants to developed countries have variable risks of morbidity and mortality from heart disease that may be associated with their race or ethnic background, as well as multiple environmental and personal risk factors. Cardiovascular disease is known to have a multifactorial etiology including genetic determinants, environmental exposures, and lifestyle factors. Urbanization in Africa and rapid economic development in Asia have resulted in an increased burden of chronic vascular diseases in developing countries and exposed important ethnic differences regarding causation. Studies in the United Kingdom have compared variations in cardiovascular risk for people of South Asian and African descent.[2,3] South Asians have been observed to have an elevated risk of ischemic heart disease when compared to Europeans and African-Caribbeans. More recent investigations have demonstrated that these differences in risk are primarily related to metabolic abnormalities that include insulin resistance, hyperglycemia, and dyslipidemia which have been shown to be more common in South Asians.[4] A genetic basis for these differences has been postulated but not yet identified.

In the early part of the twentieth century, African-Americans in the United States had a similar risk of ischemic heart disease as had recently been described in African-Caribbeans in the UK. However, with

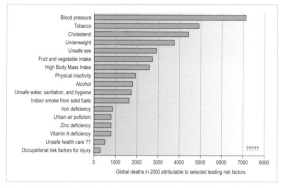

**Fig. 16.1** Global deaths in 2000 attributable to selected leading risk factors.

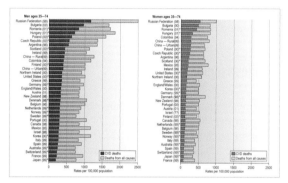

**Fig. 16.2** Death rates for total cardiovascular disease, coronary heart disease, and stroke, and total deaths in selected countries. http://www.ehponline.org/members/2004/112–15/cvdratesbg.jpg

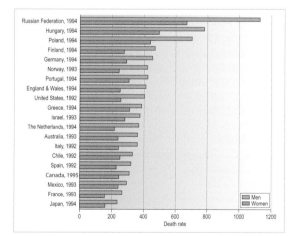

**Fig. 16.3** Age standardized rates of death from cardiovascular disease in several countries in the mid-1990s. (Source: 1995 World health statistics annual, World Health Organization. In: Disease and stroke in Canada. Ottawa: Heart and Stroke Foundation of Canada; 1997:8.) http://epe.lac-bac.gc.ca/100/201/300cdn_medical_association/cmaj/vol-157/issue-12/images/1659fig1.gif

acculturation, these discrepancies have disappeared, with African-Americans now demonstrating a higher incidence of ischemic heart disease than US whites.[5] These recent findings imply that in persons originally of African descent, socioeconomic and environmental factors may be more powerful determinants of ischemic heart disease than genetic causes. In contrast to the lower prevalence of coronary heart disease, Africans have consistently been shown to have increased rates of hypertension and stroke even prior to urbanization.[6] In addition to the increased risks of hypertension, migration to urban areas in Africa has also been shown to lead to a higher prevalence of atherosclerosis and coronary artery disease, presumably heavily influenced by change in lifestyle and environmental modifications.[7] This evidence would suggest that although genetic factors play an important role, migration and the corresponding change in environmental and social factors greatly influence cardiovascular disease rates in African immigrants and refugees.

The burden of cardiovascular disease in Hispanics who have immigrated to the US is thought to be similar to that of non-Hispanic whites. Studies in the early 1990s suggested that Hispanics often have higher traditional risk factors but lower rates of ischemic heart disease, implying a component of genetic protection.[8] More recently, however, the risk of cardiovascular disease in Hispanics living in the US has been shown to parallel that of non-Hispanic whites.[9,10]

In Eastern Europe, the prevalence of cardiovascular disease has increased rapidly since the collapse of the Soviet Union in 1991. Mortality from cardiovascular disease in Russia has been shown to be significantly higher than that of Western Europe and the US and resulted in an estimated 800 deaths per 100 000 in 2000.[11] Interestingly, the sharp rise in cardiovascular mortality in Russia appears to be only partially related to classic risk factors for cardiovascular disease such as cigarette smoking, blood pressure and serum cholesterol. It has also been driven by excessive alcohol consumption which is pervasive within certain segments of this population.[12,13]

In summary, rates of cardiovascular disease and its related morbidity and mortality are overwhelmingly influenced by lifestyle and socioeconomic factors, and generally increase after immigration from less developed to developed countries, across all ethnic groups. Any genetic difference in cardiovascular disease noted among a particular race or ethnic group appears to be significantly minimized after immigration and acculturation.

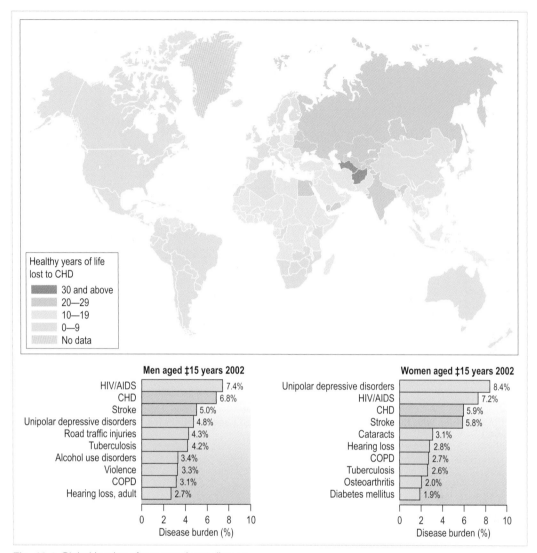

**Fig. 16.4** Global burden of coronary heart disease.

## Metabolic Syndrome, Obesity, and Diabetes

The prevalence of obesity, diabetes, and the metabolic syndrome is increasing globally and has reached epidemic proportions in many areas (Tables 16.1, 16.2; Fig. 16.6). The incidence of obesity in all age and racial groups continues to rise worldwide (Fig. 16.7). In children, the risk of being overweight and obese in affluent countries is greater for those from lower-income families, whereas the opposite occurs in low-income countries.[14] In the US, ethnic minority children are disproportionately overweight

and are thus at risk of obesity in adulthood. Ironically, although overweight and obese, these children are at risk of nutritional deficiencies due to the poor nutritional value of the calorie-rich foods frequently available to low-income populations in developed countries. In both males and females in the US, the prevalence of obesity is higher in African-Americans and Mexican-Americans compared with Caucasians. Duration of residence in the US influences rates of obesity. Goel et al. found that immigrants who had resided in the US for less than 1 year had a rate of obesity of approximately 8% that rose to a rate of 19%, approaching the rate of 22% for US-born

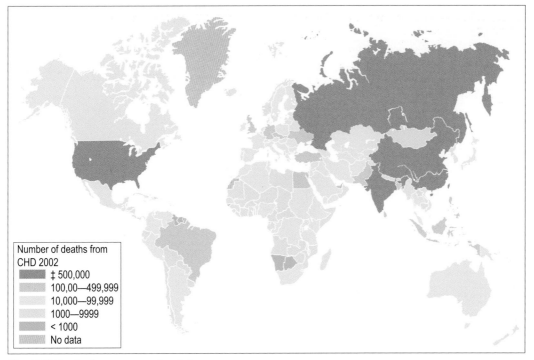

**Fig. 16.5** Deaths from coronary heart disease.

**Table 16.1 List of countries with the highest numbers of estimated cases of diabetes for 2000 and predicted for 2030**

| | 2000 | | 2030 | |
|---|---|---|---|---|
| Ranking | Country | People with diabetes (millions) | Country | People with diabetes (millions) |
| 1 | India | 31.7 | India | 79.4 |
| 2 | China | 20.8 | China | 42.3 |
| 3 | US | 17.7 | US | 30.3 |
| 4 | Indonesia | 8.4 | Indonesia | 21.3 |
| 5 | Japan | 6.8 | Pakistan | 13.9 |
| 6 | Pakistan | 5.2 | Brazil | 11.3 |
| 7 | Russian Federation | 4.6 | Bangladesh | 11.1 |
| 8 | Brazil | 4.6 | Japan | 8.9 |
| 9 | Italy | 4.3 | Philippines | 7.8 |
| 10 | Bangladesh | 3.2 | Egypt | 6.7 |

individuals, after 15 years of residence. They were also able to show that this change in obesity rates was associated with assimilation of dietary and physical activity patterns.[15] Furthermore, racial differences in the distribution of adiposity have been observed. Caucasians generally have excess fat in the upper body regions including the abdominal viscera compared to African-Americans and Mexicans. Asian Indians also appear to have a greater amount of intra-abdominal fat as well as an overall higher

**Table 16.2 Estimated numbers of people with diabetes by region for 2000 and 2030 and summary of population changes**

| 2000 Percentage of change in urban population | Number of people with DM | 2030 Number of people with DM | Percentage of change in number of people with DM | 2000–2030 Percentage of change in total population* | Percentage of change in population >65 years of age* |
|---|---|---|---|---|---|
| **Established market economies** N/A | 44 268 | 68 156 | 54 | 9 | 80 |
| **Former socialist economies** N/A | 11 665 | 13 960 | 20 | −14 | 42 |
| **India** 101 | 31 705 | 79 441 | 151 | 40 | 168 |
| **China** 115 | 20 757 | 42 321 | 104 | 16 | 168 |
| **Other Asia & South Pacific Islands** 91 | 22 328 | 58 109 | 148 | 42 | 198 |
| **Sub-Saharan Africa** 192 | 7 146 | 18 645 | 161 | 97 | 147 |
| **Latin America and the Caribbean** 56 | 13 307 | 32 959 | 148 | 40 | 194 |
| **Middle Eastern crescent** 94 | 20 051 | 52 794 | 163 | 67 | 194 |
| **World** 61 | 171 228 | 366 212 | 114 | 37 | 134 |

DM, diabetes mellitus.
* A positive value indicates an increase, a negative value indicates a decrease.

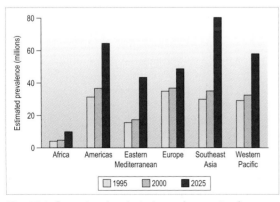

Fig. 16.6 Current and projected prevalence rates for diabetes worldwide.

percentage of body fat relative to body mass index, placing them at increased risk for insulin resistance and dyslipidemia, which is commonly referred to as the metabolic syndrome.[4,16]

The concept of the metabolic syndrome was established several decades ago. The term denotes a constellation of risk factors that are defined as any three of the following:

- Abdominal obesity (waist circumference >102 cm in men and >88 cm in women);
- Elevated blood pressure (>130/85);
- Elevated triglycerides (>150 mg/dL);
- Low HDL cholesterol (40 mg/dL in men and < 50 mg/dL in women);
- Fasting glucose > 110 mg/dL.

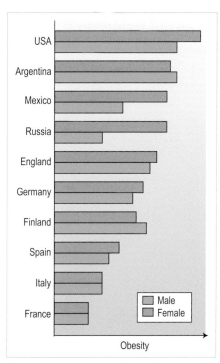

USA
Argentina
Mexico
Russia
England
Germany
Finland
Spain
Italy
France

Male
Female

Obesity

**Fig. 16.7** Proportion of obesity in selected countries. http://www.foodmuseum.com/images/ obesworldobesityflags.jpg

Metabolic syndrome is associated with undesirable health outcomes including diabetes and coronary heart disease. The syndrome is age dependent, with the prevalence rising substantially in individuals over 60 years of age. Prevalence has also been demonstrated to vary by race/ethnicity within the US, with Mexican-American women having the highest prevalence followed by Mexican-American men and finally African-American women.[17,18] Studies that have examined insulin resistance and obesity in migrant populations within the UK have found Asian Indians to have a significantly higher prevalence of the metabolic syndrome compared with individuals from other ethnic backgrounds. Recent investigations exploring the role of underlying genetic or early-life adverse events in the pathogenesis of the metabolic syndrome have revealed that the proteins adiponectin and resistin may contribute to insulin resistance; however, the mechanism is unclear.[16] As with cardiovascular disease, lifestyle and environmental factors are important determinants in the development of the metabolic syndrome.

One undesirable consequence of the metabolic syndrome is the development of type 2 diabetes. The global increase of type 2 diabetes was noted in adults many years ago and recently has been shown to be occurring among children and adolescents as well (Figs 16.3, 16.4).[19] In the US, adolescent and adult immigrants have been found to be disproportionately affected by type 2 diabetes. Specifically, African-Americans, Hispanic-Americans, Asian-Americans and Pacific Islanders are at increased risk.[20] The etiology of the observed ethnic disparity in the prevalence and incidence of type 2 diabetes is thought to be multifactorial, involving both genetic and environmental factors. Studies have demonstrated higher degrees of insulin resistance among West African descendants, including native Ghanaians, African-Americans and Hispanics compared to whites.[21,22] Interestingly, a study with a cohort of approximately 3000 individuals with impaired glucose tolerance found that the risk of progression to diabetes did not vary across race or ethnic groups.[23] This finding implies that genetic or ethnic components predisposing to diabetes must wield the greatest impact during the transition from normal metabolism to impaired glucose tolerance.

## Cancer

Global patterns of cancer incidence and mortality reveal striking diversity among geographic regions, suggesting environmental and lifestyle factors comprise a significant component of risk (Table 16.3; Figs 16.8, 16.9). Cancer has begun to emerge as the leading cause of death in the world (Fig. 16.10). Lung cancer is the most common cancer in the world and because it is highly lethal it is also responsible for the most cancer deaths. Since exposure to tobacco remains the major risk factor, regions with a high prevalence of tobacco smoking have a high incidence rate of lung cancer. Tobacco smoking has risen sharply in many low- and middle-income countries in recent years and resulted in a significant increase in lung cancer and all-cause mortality in these areas (Fig. 16.11). Many immigrants from developing countries may have a history of tobacco use, particularly women (Fig. 16.12). Unfortunately, a number of studies have revealed delayed presentation of lung cancer and more advanced stage of disease for ethnic minorities in the US,[24,25] stressing disparities in care for these populations. This discrepancy serves to remind the clinician of the importance of identifying individuals who may be at risk so that appropriate education and interventions may be offered.

Breast cancer is the second most common cancer worldwide and the most common cause of cancer

**Table 16.3 Global incidence of the five most common cancers***

| Rank | Developing nations | | Developed nations | |
| --- | --- | --- | --- | --- |
| | Males | Females | Males | Females |
| 1 | Lung | Breast | Lung | Breast |
| 2 | Stomach | Cervical | Prostate | Colorectal |
| 3 | Liver | Colorectal | Colorectal | Lung |
| 4 | Esophagus | Stomach | Stomach | Stomach |
| 5 | Colorectal | Lung | Bladder | Ovary |

* Data from Parkin DM, Pisani P, Ferley J. Global Cancer Statistics. CA Cancer J Clin 1999; 49:33–64.

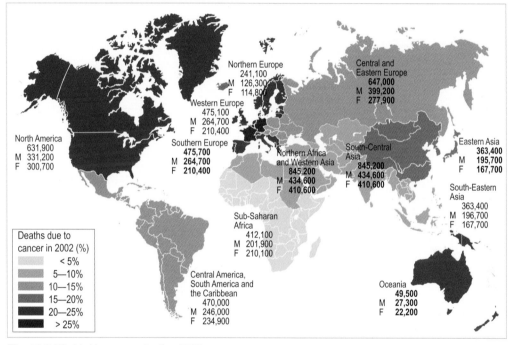

**Fig. 16.8** Worldwide cancer deaths, 2002.

mortality in women (Fig. 16.13). More than half of cases are in the developed world, especially North America and Europe, but data show that incidence rates are increasing in most countries around the world (Fig. 16.14).[26] At the cellular level, ethnic and racial differences in tumor biology and estrogen metabolism have been observed. For the individual, diet, exercise, reproductive history, level of stress, and exogenous hormone use are all important factors related to breast cancer risk.[27] Immigrants from low-risk countries typically experience an increased risk when they migrate to more industrialized nations, lending further support to the importance of environmental and cultural factors in the development of breast cancer.[28] As an example, Asian women have some of the lowest rates of breast cancer in the world but after migration to the US begin to experience some of the highest rates.[29] Women of color have lower rates of mammographic screening for breast cancer. It has been shown that active, culturally

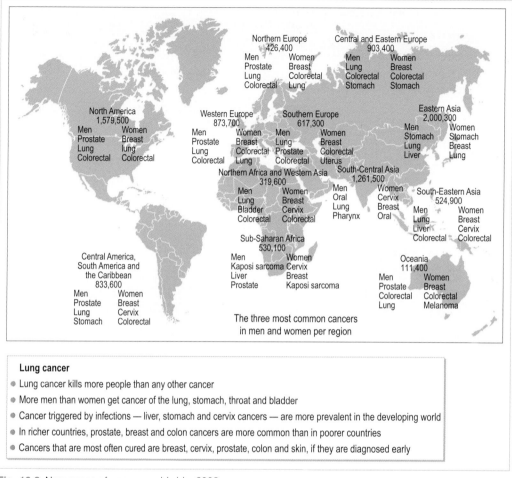

**Northern Europe**
426,400

| Men | Women |
|---|---|
| Prostate | Breast |
| Lung | Colorectal |
| Colorectal | Lung |

**Central and Eastern Europe**
903,400

| Men | Women |
|---|---|
| Lung | Breast |
| Colorectal | Colorectal |
| Stomach | Stomach |

**North America**
1,579,500

| Men | Women |
|---|---|
| Prostate | Breast |
| Lung | lung |
| Colorectal | Colorectal |

**Western Europe**
873,700

| Men | Women |
|---|---|
| Prostate | Breast |
| Lung | Colorectal |
| Colorectal | Lung |

**Southern Europe**
617,300

| Men | Women |
|---|---|
| Lung | Breast |
| Prostate | Colorectal |
| Colorectal | Uterus |

**Eastern Asia**
2,000,300

| Men | Women |
|---|---|
| Stomach | Stomach |
| Lung | Breast |
| Liver | Lung |

**Northern Africa and Western Asia**
319,600

| Men | Women |
|---|---|
| Lung | Breast |
| Bladder | Cervix |
| Colorectal | Colorectal |

**South-Central Asia**
1,261,500

| Men | Women |
|---|---|
| Oral | Cervix |
| Lung | Breast |
| Pharynx | Oral |

**South-Eastern Asia**
524,900

| Men | Women |
|---|---|
| Lung | Breast |
| Liver | Cervix |
| Colorectal | Colorectal |

**Central America,
South America and
the Caribbean**
833,600

| Men | Women |
|---|---|
| Prostate | Breast |
| Lung | Cervix |
| Stomach | Colorectal |

**Sub-Saharan Africa**
530,100

| Men | Women |
|---|---|
| Kaposi sarcoma | Cervix |
| Liver | Breast |
| Prostate | Kaposi sarcoma |

**Oceania**
111,400

| Men | Women |
|---|---|
| Prostate | Breast |
| Colorectal | Colorectal |
| Lung | Melanoma |

The three most common cancers
in men and women per region

**Lung cancer**

- Lung cancer kills more people than any other cancer
- More men than women get cancer of the lung, stomach, throat and bladder
- Cancer triggered by infections — liver, stomach and cervix cancers — are more prevalent in the developing world
- In richer countries, prostate, breast and colon cancers are more common than in poorer countries
- Cancers that are most often cured are breast, cervix, prostate, colon and skin, if they are diagnosed early

**Fig. 16.9** New cases of cancer worldwide, 2002.

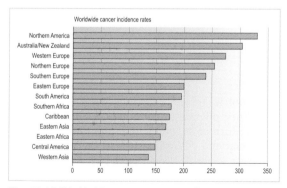

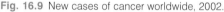

**Fig. 16.10** Worldwide cancer rates. http://www.healthextension.net/archives/2005/04/

tailored, intervention strategies may substantially increase screening rates in these migrant populations.[29]

Cancers of the colon and rectum now rank third in overall incidence. The overall highest prevalence occurs in many industrialized countries, with rates remaining low in Africa and Asia, and intermediate in southern regions of South America (Figs 16.15. 16.16). The notable geographic differences are presumably related to dietary factors, primarily consumption patterns of meat, fat, and fiber, which have been demonstrated to significantly impact the risk of cancers of the large bowel. Similar to observations made with regard to previously mentioned cancers, when individuals migrate from low-risk to high-risk areas, the incidence of colorectal cancer rises sharply

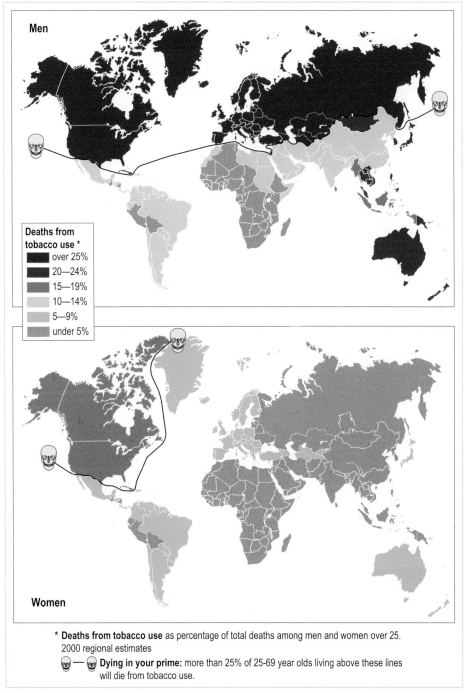

Fig. 16.11 Worldwide burden of tobacco abuse, and health consequences.

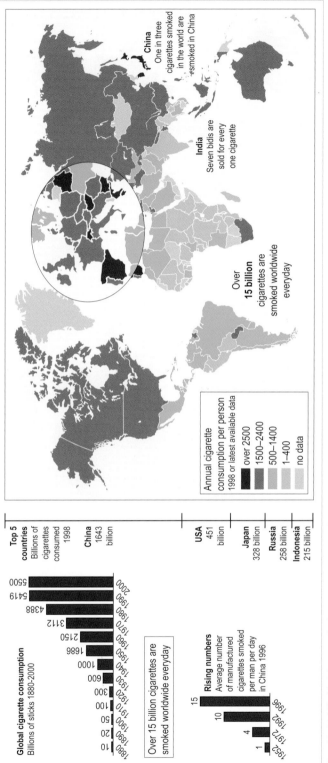

**Fig. 16.12** Worldwide use of tobacco products by females, and consequences.

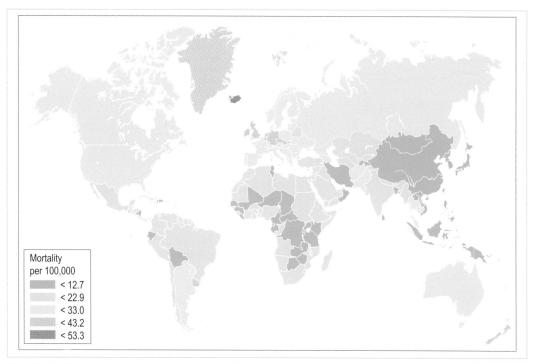

**Fig. 16.13** Global breast cancer mortality rates. http://www.proteinbiotechnologies.com/images/maps/ Breast-Mortality-Map.jpg

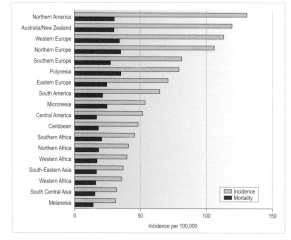

**Fig. 16.14** Global breast cancer incidence. http://www. proteinbiotechnologies.com/images/maps/ Breast-1%26M-BarChart.jpg

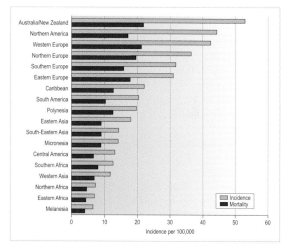

**Fig. 16.15** Global incidence and mortality rates among females of colorectal cancer. Global breast cancer incidence.

within the first generation, irrespective of racial or ethnic background.[30]

Stomach cancer was previously the second most common cancer but now ranks fourth in frequency. However, because it is an aggressive malignancy, it continues to rank second in mortality. The etiology of the worldwide decline in the incidence of gastric cancer is unknown but may reflect dietary modifications and a decreasing prevalence of *Helicobacter pylori* infection.[31] The majority of cases continue to

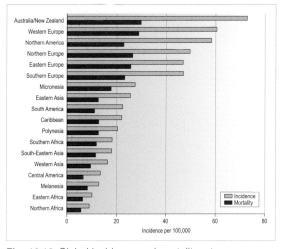

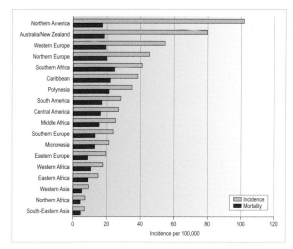

**Fig. 16.16** Global incidence and mortality rates among males of colorectal cancer.

**Fig. 16.17** Global incidence and mortality rates of prostate cancer.

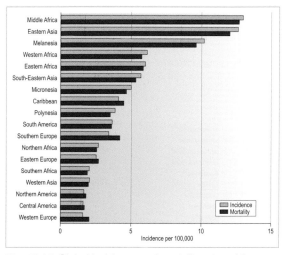

**Fig. 16.18** Global incidence and mortality rates of liver cancer among women.

occur in developing countries where *H. pylori* infection is extremely common and tends to occur at a young age. The only exception is sub-Saharan Africa where *H. pylori* infection is ubiquitous, yet in general the region has a low prevalence of gastric cancer, which implies the presence of a host protective/inhibitory factor in these populations.[32] East Asia has the highest percentage of cases, particularly China with recent estimates as high as 40% of total cancers being gastric in origin. A strong environmental component has been proposed, and earlier studies suggest that exposure to *H. pylori* during childhood is crucial.[33,34] Migrants from high- to low-risk areas do show a significant decline in risk gradually over time, particularly if migration occurs at an early age.[35]

Prostate cancer is the fifth most common cancer overall and second most common in men (Fig. 16.17). Ethnic variation in risk has been observed within countries, including the US where African-Americans have the highest risk followed by whites. Asians have been shown to have a considerably lower risk of prostate cancer. Migrants from low-risk (e.g. Japan and China) to high-risk (e.g. US, Australia) areas demonstrate a sharp increase in risk for reasons that are not completely understood but that are presumably at least partially related to environmental changes such as an increase in the consumption of dietary fat.[36–38] In addition, certain types of soy proteins that are commonly found in the Asian diet have been shown to be protective against prostate cancer.[38]

Cancer of the liver ranks sixth with regards to numbers of new cases, but because of its poor prog-

nosis, it is the third most common cause of cancer deaths (Figs 16.18, 16.19). The majority of cases and deaths occur in developing countries, where the primary risk factors for liver cancer are infection with hepatitis B and C and exposure to aflatoxins (Figs 16.20, 16.21). In the US, ethnic variations in the prevalence of hepatocellular cancer are related to ethnic differences in the prevalence of major risk factors, particularly chronic viral hepatitis rates. Recent immigrants from areas with a high prevalence of hepatitis B infection such as countries in sub-Saharan Africa and China retain rates of liver cancer that are similar to those for their native countries.[39,40] Risk of cancer for immigrants from high-risk areas has been shown to diminish gradually over subsequent generations, presumably related to the routine use of hepatitis B immunization throughout the industrialized world. Approximately 10–25% of liver cancers are cholangiocarcinoma, a tumor of the epithelium of the intrahepatic bile ducts, which appears to be increasing worldwide. Overall, there is minimal international variation; however, in areas where infections with liver flukes are common, such as northeast Thailand, China, and Laos, a high incidence of cholangiocarcinoma is typically found.[41] First-generation immigrants from these high-risk areas have also been observed to have increased risk of this cancer. In addition, migrants from areas highly endemic for liver flukes, such as Southeast Asia, have been shown to harbor these parasites for years after migration, likely predisposing them to cholangiocarcinoma.[42]

## Hemoglobinopathies

Hemoglobin disorders have a global impact due to the rise in migration of individuals from endemic areas in the Mediterranean, Asia, and Africa.[43] For many of the genetic-based hematologic disorders, a theory of selective advantage for survival during malarial infections has been proposed, which correlates with the geographic distribution of these disorders. The region with the highest number of carriers of hemoglobin disorders is Southeast Asia

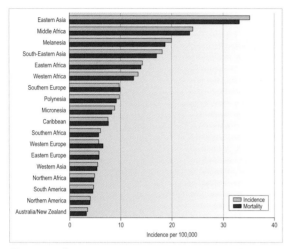

**Fig. 16.19** Global incidence and mortality rates of liver cancer among men.

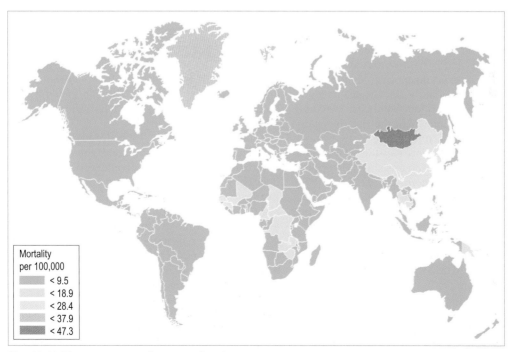

**Fig. 16.20** Liver cancer mortality among females.

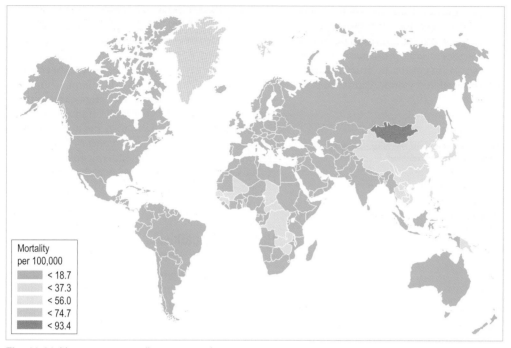

**Fig. 16.21** Liver cancer mortality among males.

where thalassemias are very common. In addition, glucose-6-phosphate dehydrogenase (G6PD) deficiency and RBC membrane defects are also prevalent in persons of Southeast Asian descent.[44] The thalassemia syndromes are inherited in an autosomal recessive pattern and result in heterogeneous clinical diseases. Both α- and β-thalassemias are characterized by ineffective erythropoiesis that results from mutations in the globin gene. Groups at high risk for thalassemias include Southeast Asians, South Asians, and Africans. With the rise in Asian migration over the past several years, many hemoglobin genotypes that were once considered uncommon in North America are now increasingly detected, particularly in California where approximately 10% of births are Asians.[45,46] Routine screening with hemoglobin electrophoresis should be performed in at-risk newborn infants and in any immigrant or refugee with an unexplained anemia.

Sickle cell disease is thought to have originated in India and Africa. In Africa, the prevalence of sickle cell has been estimated at 5–40%, with the majority of cases occurring in persons in western and central regions. Evidence suggests that those with sickle cell trait receive protection against clinically significant malaria, particularly during early childhood when they are most vulnerable to severe disease. However,

because of limited resources, the treatment of patients with sickle cell disease in Africa is generally poor.[47] In India, distribution of the sickle gene is most concentrated among Dravidians, and pre-Dravidians, who originally inhabited regions endemic for falciparum malaria in southern India. Prevalence varies dramatically among different groups with higher estimates found in the central and western parts of India. Patients in India with homozygous disease generally have milder manifestations than those in Africa.[48]

Glucose-6-phosphate dehydrogenase (G6PD) deficiency is an X-linked condition that affects approximately 400 million people worldwide. G6PD deficiency is most common among individuals who live in Africa, the Middle East, and Southeast Asia. See Chapter 46 for more details regarding hematologic issues in immigrants. Over 400 G6PD variant alleles have been described that differ in degree of enzyme deficiency. Different populations tend to have different types of mutations which lead to variations in clinical manifestations. However, due to the X-linked inheritance pattern, males tend to be more severely affected regardless of the mutation type. As with the other hemoglobin disorders, G6PD deficient RBCs provide a barrier to malaria parasites. Immigrants from malaria endemic areas in Africa,

Asia, and the Middle East are at higher risk. Immigrants from these regions may be more likely to be prescribed medications which can cause hemolysis in patients with G6PD deficiency, such as sulfas and primaquine, and should be screened for G6PD deficiency prior to use of such medications.

Other hemoglobin variants that are often observed, particularly in immigrants from Asia, include hemoglobin E. This hemoglobin disorder results from a single amino acid substitution in the β-globin gene. Heterozygous states are generally clinically silent; however, when hemoglobin E occurs with a β-thalassemia deletion, a significant hemolytic anemia may result.[44] Patients who present with a microcytic anemia should be screened with a hemoglobin electrophoresis, as well as for iron deficiency.

## Conclusion

Ethnicity and race play an important role in the risk of disease acquisition. For many diseases it is difficult to separate the role of ethnicity and race from environmental, geographic, and other factors affecting disease. By studying global migration, and thereby determining the influence of geography and environment, as well as by using evolving genetic techniques, researchers and clinicians will increasingly be able to define the various factors which determine disease in specific populations.

## References

1. Collins FS. What we do and don't know about 'race', 'ethnicity', genetics and health at the dawn of the genome era. Nat Genet 2004; 36(11 Suppl):S13–S15.
2. Chaturvedi N. Ethnic differences in cardiovascular disease. Heart 2003; 89(6):681–686.
3. Cappuccio FP. Ethnicity and cardiovascular risk: variations in people of African ancestry and South Asian origin. J Hum Hypertens 1997; 11(9):571–576.
4. Tillin T, Forouhi N, Johnston DG, et al. Metabolic syndrome and coronary heart disease in South Asians, African-Caribbeans and white Europeans: a UK population-based cross-sectional study. Diabetologia 2005; 48(4):649–656.
5. Clark LT. Issues in minority health: atherosclerosis and coronary heart disease in African Americans. Med Clin North Am 2005; 89(5):977–1001.
6. Muna WF. Cardiovascular disorders in Africa. World Health Stat Q 1993; 46(2):125–133.
7. Vorster HH. The emergence of cardiovascular disease during urbanisation of Africans. Public Health Nutr 2002; 5(1A):239–243.
8. Sorlie PD, Backlund E, Johnson NJ, et al. Mortality by Hispanic status in the United States. JAMA 1993; 270(20):2464–2468.
9. Pandey DK, Labarthe DR, Goff DC, et al. Community-wide coronary heart disease mortality in Mexican Americans equals or exceeds that in non-Hispanic whites: the Corpus Christi Heart Project. Am J Med 2001; 110(2):81–87.
10. Lerman-Garber I, Villa AR, Caballero E. Diabetes and cardiovascular disease. Is there a true Hispanic paradox? Rev Invest Clin 2004; 56(3):282–296.
11. Levintova M. Cardiovascular disease prevention in Russia: Challenges and opportunities. Public Health 2006; 120(7):664–670.
12. Tunstall-Pedoe H, Vanuzzo D, Hobbs M, et al. Estimation of contribution of changes in coronary care to improving survival, event rates, and coronary heart disease mortality across the WHO MONICA Project populations. Lancet 2000; 355(9205):688–700.
13. Averina M, Nilssen O, Brenn T, et al. Factors behind the increase in cardiovascular mortality in Russia: apolipoprotein AI and B distribution in the Arkhangelsk study 2000. Clin Chem 2004; 50(2):346–354.
14. Wang Y. Cross-national comparison of childhood obesity: the epidemic and the relationship between obesity and socioeconomic status. Int J Epidemiol 2001; 30(5):1129–1136.
15. Goel MS, McCarthy EP, Phillips RS, et al. Obesity among US immigrant subgroups by duration of residence. JAMA 2004; 292(23):2860–2867.
16. Misra A, Vikram NK. Insulin resistance syndrome (metabolic syndrome) and obesity in Asian Indians: evidence and implications. Nutrition 2004; 20(5):482–491.
17. Ford ES, Giles WH, Dietz WH. Prevalence of the metabolic syndrome among US adults: findings from the third National Health and Nutrition Examination Survey. JAMA 2002; 287(3):356–359.
18. Cossrow N, Falkner B. Race/ethnic issues in obesity and obesity-related comorbidities. J Clin Endocrinol Metab 2004; 89(6):2590–2594.
19. Pinhas-Hamiel O, Zeitler P. The global spread of type 2 diabetes mellitus in children and adolescents. J Pediatr 2005; 146(5):693–700.
20. Egede LE, Dagogo-Jack S. Epidemiology of type 2 diabetes: focus on ethnic minorities. Med Clin North Am 2005; 89(5):949–975, viii.
21. Osei K, Gaillard T, Schuster DP. Pathogenetic mechanisms of impaired glucose tolerance and type II diabetes in African-Americans. The significance of insulin secretion, insulin sensitivity, and glucose effectiveness. Diabetes Care 1997; 20(3):396–404.
22. Osei K, Schuster DP, Owusu SK, et al. Race and ethnicity determine serum insulin and C-peptide concentrations and hepatic insulin extraction and insulin clearance: comparative studies of three populations of West African ancestry and white Americans. Metabolism 1997; 46(1):53–58.
23. Knowler WC, Barrett-Connor E, Fowler SE, et al. Reduction in the incidence of type 2 diabetes with lifestyle intervention or metformin. N Engl J Med 2002; 346(6):393–403.
24. Finlay GA, Joseph B, Rodrigues CR, et al. Advanced presentation of lung cancer in Asian immigrants: a case-control study. Chest 2002; 122(6):1938–1943.
25. Bach PB, Cramer LD, Warren JL, et al. Racial differences in the treatment of early-stage lung cancer. N Engl J Med 1999; 341(16):1198–1205.
26. Parkin DM, Bray FI, Devesa SS. Cancer burden in the year 2000. The global picture. Eur J Cancer 2001; 37(Suppl 8): S4–S66.
27. Masi CM, Olopade OI. Racial and ethnic disparities in breast cancer: a multilevel perspective. Med Clin North Am 2005; 89(4):753–770.
28. Hortobagyi GN, de la Garza SJ, Pritchard K, et al. The global breast cancer burden: variations in epidemiology and survival. Clin Breast Cancer 2005; 6(5):391–401.
29. Kelly AW, Fores CM, Wollan PC, et al. A program to increase breast and cervical cancer screening for Cambodian women in a midwestern community. Mayo Clin Proc 1996; 71(5):437–444.
30. Parkin DM, Bray F, Ferlay J, et al. Global cancer statistics, 2002. CA Cancer J Clin 2005; 55(2):74–108.

31. Plummer M, Franceschi S, Munoz N. Epidemiology of gastric cancer. IARC Sci Publ 2004; (157):311–326.

32. Segal I, Ally R, Mitchell H. Gastric cancer in sub-Saharan Africa. Eur J Cancer Prev 2001; 10(6):479–482.

33. Coggon D, Osmond C, Barker DJ. Stomach cancer and migration within England and Wales. Br J Cancer 1990; 61(4):573–574.

34. Ma JL, You WC, Gail MH, et al. *Helicobacter pylori* infection and mode of transmission in a population at high risk of stomach cancer. Int J Epidemiol 1998; 27(4):570–573.

35. McMichael AJ, McCall MG, Hartshorne JM, et al. Patterns of gastro-intestinal cancer in European migrants to Australia: the role of dietary change. Int J Cancer 1980; 25(4):431–437.

36. Brawley OW, Knopf K, Thompson I. The epidemiology of prostate cancer, part II: the risk factors. Semin Urol Oncol 1998; 16(4):193–201.

37. Shimizu H, Ross RK, Bernstein L, et al. Cancers of the prostate and breast among Japanese and white immigrants in Los Angeles County. Br J Cancer 1991; 63(6):963–966.

38. Sonn GA, Aronson W, Litwin MS. Impact of diet on prostate cancer: a review. Prostate Cancer Prostatic Dis 2005; 8(4):304–310.

39. El Serag HB. Epidemiology of hepatocellular carcinoma. Clin Liver Dis 2001; 5(1):87–107, vi.

40. Kulkarni K, Barcak E, El Serag H, et al. The impact of immigration on the increasing incidence of hepatocellular carcinoma in the United States. Aliment Pharmacol Ther 2004; 20(4):445–450.

41. Khurana S, Dubey ML, Malla N. Association of parasitic infections and cancers. Indian J Med Microbiol 2005; 23(2):74–79.

42. Stauffer WM, Sellman JS, Walker PF. Biliary liver flukes (opisthorchiasis and clonorchiasis) in immigrants in the United States: often subtle and diagnosed years after arrival. J Travel Med 2004; 11(3):157–159.

43. Angastiniotis M, Modell B. Global epidemiology of hemoglobin disorders. Ann NY Acad Sci 1998; 850:251–269.

44. Jeng MR, Vichinsky E. Hematologic problems in immigrants from Southeast Asia. Hematol Oncol Clin North Am 2004; 18(6):1405–1422, x.

45. Vichinsky EP, MacKlin EA, Waye JS, et al. Changes in the epidemiology of thalassemia in North America: a new minority disease. Pediatrics 2005; 116(6):e818–e825.

46. Lorey F, Cunningham G. Impact of Asian immigration on thalassemia in California. Ann NY Acad Sci 1998; 850:442–445.

47. Diallo D, Tchernia G. Sickle cell disease in Africa. Curr Opin Hematol 2002; 9(2):111–116.

48. Mohanty D, Mukherjee MB. Sickle cell disease in India. Curr Opin Hematol 2002; 9(2):117–122.

# CHAPTER 17

# Diseases with Long Latency Periods

David R. Boulware

- Initial immigrant screening is aimed at communicable diseases and routine health conditions but may miss latent infections.
- Latent infections may be detected at screening, by incidental laboratory testing, at reactivation, or with the development of end-stage disease or malignancy.
- Eosinophilia is always abnormal. More than 75% of immigrants will have a parasite with an absolute count > 450 cells/μL. Strategies are:
  1. Three stool examinations for ova and parasites (stool O&P);
  2. Serology for long-lifespan parasites: *Strongyloides* and *Schistosoma*;
  3. Empiric treatment with ivermectin 200 mcg/kg for 2 days or albendazole 400 mg for 3 days and verifying eosinophilia resolution in 3–6 months.
- Cancer can occur with chronic infection and inflammation caused by: biliary flukes, hepatitis B and C, Helicobacter pylori, HPV, and schistosomiasis.
- Chagas' disease may be present in asymptomatic immigrants from rural Latin America presenting with later gastrointestinal and cardiac complications.

## Introduction

There are a wide variety of diseases which can present months or years after immigration. Latent infections may be cryptic, with non-specific symptoms, or asymptomatic until chronic end-stage disease develops. Even end-stage disease of conditions common in the developing world may be difficult to recognize years removed from immigration to industrialized countries. This chapter focuses on the wide spectrum of infectious diseases that may manifest remotely from emigration.

## Initial Screening

Diseases with long latency periods may be recognized upon initial immigration screening. Recognition and treatment per national guidelines is appropriate. New-arrival screening is not comprehensive and is targeted primarily at communicable diseases. Many noncommunicable diseases may not be detected. Further, although it is recommended that all immigrants receive new-arrival screening, this is rarely performed outside specific groups such as those arriving under refugee status.

The general, North American approach to refugee screening is to verify internationally obtained testing and perform additional testing as recommended. Abnormal international medical records should be interpreted per a physician's judgment as to their accuracy, with repeat diagnostic verification or treatment as appropriate. In the United States, 'class A' conditions, such as active tuberculosis (TB), syphilis, and HIV, typically are excludable conditions warranting prohibition of immigration into the US unless treated or a specific waiver is given.

## Tuberculosis

Latent tuberculosis infection (LTBI) is commonly identified. Current World Health Organization (WHO) estimates indicate that one-third of the world's population is infected with tuberculosis, with the incidence increasing by 1% every year; the incidence is 44% in Southeast Asia, 35% in Africa and the Western Pacific, 29% in the Eastern Mediterranean, 18% in the Americas, and 15% in Europe.[1] An individual with a positive tuberculin skin test (TST), i.e. PPD, should always have chest radiographs performed to exclude abnormalities suspicious for active pulmonary TB. In persons with LTBI, the standard recommendation is 9 months of isoniazid therapy. One large caveat exists. Should immunosuppression with corticosteroids or anti-TNF-alpha medications be anticipated in the near future, a more aggressive LTBI treatment regimen may be appropriate.[2] Anti-TNF-alpha antagonists, such as infliximab and etanercept, are associated with a 15- and 50-fold higher incidence of active TB, respectively.[3-5] Time of onset of an opportunistic infection varies by TNF antagonist, but 50% of TB cases will appear within 90 days of initiation of infliximab and within 1 year for etanercept.[5] Ideally, LTBI therapy should be started for 2 months prior to immunosuppression.

## Syphilis

Another common occurrence is a positive VDRL or RPR syphilis screen in asymptomatic immigrants. In one study of 750 Ethiopian immigrants, 12% of adults had positive treponemal tests without clinical disease or neurologic deficit.[6] In rural Gambia, 17% of asymptomatic persons were VDRL seropositive.[7] It is unclear whether such scenarios represent an unusual natural history of infection, cross-reaction to yaws or with other treponemal diseases, partial treatment, or false positives. Indiscriminate antibiotic usage could cause syphilis or yaws to remain subclinical yet not eradicated.[7] Yaws can relapse with ulcerative skin lesions as long as 5–10 years after initial infection or with tertiary manifestations with bone, joint, or soft tissue deformities occurring. Neurologic abnormalities do not occur with yaws. Examination of cerebrospinal fluid (CSF) among VDRL-positive Ethiopian and Thai immigrants has been shown to be of low yield.[6,8] Thus, among HIV-negative individuals, an individual with a positive low-titer VDRL and who has no neurologic symptoms can be treated for possible latent infection safely without CSF examination. Treatment consists of a series of 3-weekly penicillin G benzathine intramuscular injections of 2.4 million units or alternatively, in patients who are penicillin allergic and not pregnant, doxycycline 100 mg orally twice daily for 28 days.[6] Tetracyclines cannot be used to treat neurosyphilis. A confirmatory treponemal-specific test, such as TP-PA, FTA-AS, should be performed. Follow-up VDRL or RPR at 6 months should demonstrate a fourfold decline in the titer; specific treponemal tests remain positive for life.

## Hepatitis B

Hepatitis B testing is routinely recommended at initial screening with determination of the hepatitis B surface antibody (anti-HBs) and surface antigen (HBsAg). One is classified as immune if anti-HBs positive, and as a chronic carrier if the HBsAg is positive. If both antibody and antigen are negative, one is susceptible and should be vaccinated. Chronic carriers are at long-term risk for cirrhosis and hepatocellular carcinoma. As the consequences of hepatitis A superinfection can be devastating in persons with underlying liver damage from chronic hepatitis B infection, chronic hepatitis B carriers should have hepatitis A antibody status determined. If hepatitis A susceptible (antibody negative), patients should be offered hepatitis A vaccination.

## Schistosomiasis

Hepatosplenomegaly may indicate many diseases but the most likely infections with a long latency include schistosomiasis, visceral leishmaniasis, or chronic malaria (tropical splenomegaly). Chronic intestinal schistosomiasis, S. mansoni or S. japonicum species, may cause liver cirrhosis with subsequent portal hypertension and splenomegaly.

Chronic urinary schistosomiasis (5.hematobium) has been associated with squamous cell carcinoma of the bladder, obstruction of the ureters, and renal failure. In additions, ova swept into the verous system can go to virtually any organ in the body, with a predilection for the CNS.

## Visceral leishmaniasis

Visceral leishmaniasis (VL) may have a chronic, insidious course with fever, malaise, night sweats, and weight loss with the eventual development of hepatosplenomegaly, pancytopenia, and elevated total IgG. Approximately 500 000 visceral infections occur annually, with 90% in the five countries of Sudan, Bangladesh, Brazil, India, and Nepal.[9] Hepatosplenomegaly and emigration from a high-prevalence country should prompt diagnostic evaluation. Although splenic aspirate is the gold standard and classic technique for diagnosis in the developing world, other diagnostic evaluation is available to the clinician in the developed world. All patients with VL will have a positive IgG serology. If negative, the diagnosis of VL can be eliminated from the differential. Bone marrow biopsy should be performed on those with a clinical presentation and positive serology. A reference laboratory familiar with VL should be contacted prior to biopsy to secure appropriate culture media and assure collection of adequate samples.

## Malaria

Another frequent cause of splenomegaly is hyperreactive malarial splenomegaly that results from an aberrant immunological response to malaria with high antimalarial antibodies and high serum IgM content. In non-malaria regions, diagnosis can be made by elimination of other diagnosis (i.e. visceral leishmaniasis and schistosomiasis) demonstrating elevated malaria antibodies and elevated immunoglobulins, particularly malaria specific IgM. Treatment results in decrease of the malaria specific antibody. Splenomegaly may remain.[10] This is perhaps one of few occasions when malaria serology may be helpful. A geographic context is important as in regions also with leishmaniasis, malaria serologies may be equivocal for diagnostic purposes.[11,12] Splenomegaly may be present, coupled with chronic malaria infection years after immigration.[13]

## Incidental Laboratory Testing

Immigrants receive primary health examinations from a variety of healthcare professionals, where a

**Table 17.2 Incidental laboratory abnormalities**

| Laboratory abnormality | Clues to diagnosis |
| --- | --- |
| Eosinophilia >450 cells/mm$^3$ | Parasitic infection in >75% immigrants<br>Length of residency in nonendemic area<br>Long lifespan: *Strongyloides*, *Schistosoma*, *Opisthorchis*, *Fasciola*<br>Filarial infections in persons from West, Central Africa |
| Alkaline phosphatase, bilirubin elevation | Biliary flukes (*Clonorochis*, *Opisthorchis*) 50–75%<br>Biliary cryptosporidium >90%<br>*Fasciola hepatica* 50% |
| Anemia, microcytic | Hookworm (3–5 year max lifespan)<br>Malaria<br>Anemia of chronic disease (due to chronic infections)<br>Multiple noninfectious etiologies |
| Anemia, megaloblastic | *Diphyllobothrium latum* (fish tape worm) 2%<br>Chronic diarrhea, malabsorption, and/or small bowel bacterial overgrowth. |
| AST, ALT elevation | Chronic hepatitis B, C<br>Chronic schistosomiasis<br>Chronic fascioliasis<br>Visceral leishmaniasis |

spectrum of knowledge of latent infections may be encountered. One of the most commonly encountered incidental findings (Table 17.2) is eosinophilia. Frequently, when concern arises regarding the possibility of latent parasitic infections, three stool ova and parasite examinations are repeated if geohelminths are considered. While repeat stool O&P testing may discover a difficult-to-diagnosis helminth, such as *Strongyloides*, typically blind testing is low yield, unless a specific clue is present. Often, laboratory clues may be inadvertent or incidental in nature and testing will need to go beyond just stool O&Ps.

General knowledge of US physicians in training about helminths, and appreciation of the level of eosinophilia considered abnormal is poor compared to international trainees.[14] Eosinophilia is considered to be an absolute count >450 cells/mm$^3$ An absolute differential count is more specific than using a relative 5% of the differential.[14] Although there may be other etiologies for an asymptomatic eosinophilia such as ectopic disease, eosinophilia in this population overwhelmingly marks an undiagnosed parasitic infection. In a study of Australian immigrants, the presence of eosinophilia had a positive predictive value of > 75% for an intestinal parasite even years after immigration.[15] Depending on the region of immigration, common parasites with a *very long* lifespan include *Strongyloides* and *Schistosoma*, with which eosinophilia is present in ≈85% and ≈60%, respectively.[14,16] Chronic filarial infections typically also will be accompanied by eosinophilia. With eosinophilia, three stool O&Ps are warranted although these are frequently negative with parasitic diseases with long latency periods; therefore, serologic testing and other diagnostic maneuvers are frequently necessary (see eosinophilia in Ch. 21).

Rarer trematodes, such as *Fasciola hepatica* (sheep liver fluke) can develop relatively asymptomatic, chronic infections which may be accompanied by eosinophilia (46–92%) and mild elevations in alkaline phosphatase (46%) and gamma glutamyl transpeptidase (GGT) with normal transaminases (ALT and AST).[17-19] These chronic *Fasciola* infections, as well as the biliary liver flukes *Opisthorchis* and *Clonorchis*, may present later with obstructive biliary fascioliasis, accompanied by acute onset of jaundice that may clinically be confused with cholelithiasis, cholangitis, or pancreatitis.[20,21,22] *Fasciola hepatica* is endemic worldwide in regions where sheep, cattle, or goats are raised and is associated with consumption of uncooked watercress or alfalfa juice.[23] Heavy burdens of infection may cause a normocytic normochromic anemia in children.[24]

Cestodes, such as *Diphyllobothrium latum*, the fish tapeworm, are known to be associated with megaloblastic anemia. Their overall incidence is quite rare, as is anemia (<2%), but 40% may have a low vitamin $B_{12}$ level due to competition for $B_{12}$ by the tapeworm.[25] Generally, this parasite is either detected in the stool O&P examination or when the patient asymptomatically passes the parasite which may be many feet in length. Chronic diarrhea, malabsorption, and small bowel overgrowth are more common causes of vitamin $B_{12}$ deficiency.[26]

Amoebiasis continues to be diagnosed in the United States, primarily among Hispanic and Asian male immigrants who typically present with fever and right-upper quadrant pain.[27] Amoebic liver abscess may be incidentally diagnosed by an abdominal ultrasound in the evaluation of suspected cholangitis. The diagnosis is confirmed by a characteristic liver abscess by ultrasound accompanied by positive IgG serology. *Entamoeba histolytica* IgG serology will be positive in 95% when performed *after* 7 days of symptoms.[28] There is no available IgM serology. The latency period is relatively short, with amoebic liver abscesses typically presenting within 3 months and all within 6 months of immigration or returning travel.[29]

## Reactivation of Latent Infections

### Tuberculosis

In immigrants with latent TB infection, the lifetime risk of reactivation is highest within the first year, with approximately half the cases in this population occurring within 2 years of relocation.[30] However, the risk of pulmonary tuberculosis remains elevated for at least the first 10 years after immigration.[31] Approximately half the TB in the immigrant population presents as extrapulmonary TB. It is unclear whether this increased risk is due to intrinsic reactivation influenced by stress, dietary changes/deficiencies (e.g. vitamin D deficiency) or due to transmission within immigrant communities post-immigration. Genotypic relationship data of TB cases from Norway suggest the majority of pulmonary TB is due to reactivation.[32] However, national screening and treatment policies for LTBI may influence the relative amount of transmission within immigrant communities. In the US, LTBI therapy is recommended for all individuals unless there is a specific contraindication. Age is no longer considered a contraindication.

*Mycobacterium bovis* is an infection classically of cattle occurring in developing countries. *M. bovis* is part of the *M. tuberculosis* complex and can be mistaken for pyrazinamide-resistant TB in laboratory testing. *Mycobacterium bovis* should be suspected when there is isolated pyrazinamide resistance and further speciation should be performed. Exposure occurs either by consumption of unpasteurized dairy products or close contact with livestock due to occupation.[33,34,37] In the US, *M. bovis* predominantly occurs among Mexican immigrants (80%) due to immigration patterns, but livestock worldwide can be infected with *M. bovis*.[35] In a study of Mexican meat-processing plants, 17% of cattle sampled were infected with *M. bovis* and a recent outbreak occurred in New York from imported, unpasteurized Mexican cheese.[36] Of *M. bovis* infections 50–60% are extrapulmonary, and infection may occur in the US-born children of immigrants.[33,35,37]

## Melioidosis

Another latent infection that may reactivate is melioidosis caused by *Burkholderia pseudomallei* with sporadic occurrence in the tropics worldwide. The highest incidence of melioidosis occurs in northeastern Thailand where seroepidemiological surveys showed that infection, mostly latent, occurred in 80% of children by 4 years of age.[38] The lung is the organ most commonly affected; however, it may also cause liver and splenic abscesses, osteomyelitis, and sepsis. Pulmonary melioidosis may present either as an acute fulminant pneumonia or as an indolent cavitary disease mimicking tuberculosis. In nonendemic regions, patients with melioidosis more typically present with reactivation disease occurring months to years after initial exposure.[39] Immunosuppression, diabetes, alcoholism, and chronic renal disease are risk factors for reactivation.[40] *B. psuedomallei* is a Gram-negative bacterium that is not difficult to grow but may be misidentified as an aminoglycoside-resistant *Pseudomonas* species by microbiology laboratories in nonendemic areas.[38,39]

## Cancer and Latent Infections

Unfortunately, many immigrants may present with a malignancy due to a chronic, unrecognized infection. Several malignancies are linked to chronic infection (Table 17.3). In the developing world, some exposures are near universal, such as *H. pylori* and human herpes virus-8 (HHV-8) acquisition during childhood.[41] *H. pylori* is clearly associated with mucosa associated lymphoid tissue (MALT) lymphoma. It is worth noting that once MALT lymphoma develops therapy against *H. pylori* can prompt a remission in up to 90%.[42] While Kaposi's sarcoma's (KS) association with HHV-8 and HIV is well known, in some areas in Africa half of KS occurs in persons without HIV.[43]

## Hepatitis B

Hepatitis B occurs worldwide and is considered endemic to Southeast Asia, with nearly 10% chronically infected, and past exposure among approximately 50% of Laotian and Cambodian immigrants.[44] Hepatocellular carcinoma occurs at a 15-fold higher rate among those with chronic infection at a rate of up to 2.5% per patient per year, and hepatitis

**Table 17.3 Malignancies associated with chronic infections**

| Infection | Cancer |
| --- | --- |
| Clonorchiasis and *Opisthorchis* spp. | Cholangiocarcinoma |
| *Fasciola hepatica* | May mimic cholangiocarcinoma[22] or gall stones |
| Epstein-Barr virus | Burkitt and Hodgkin lymphoma |
| *Helicobacter pylori* | Gastric, MALT lymphomas |
| Hepatitis B virus | Hepatocellular carcinoma |
| HHV-8 (Kaposi's herpes virus) | Kaposi's sarcoma, lymphoma |
| Human papillomavirus | Cervical cancer |
| HTLV-1 (human T-cell lymphotrophic virus) | Adult T-cell leukemia[48] |
| Schistosomiasis (*S. haematobium*) | Bladder cancer |

B is one of the leading known causes of cancer worldwide.[45-47] Screening for hepatocellular carcinoma should occur, and is covered extensively in Chapter 12.

## Human papillomavirus

Human papillomavirus (HPV) infection also occurs worldwide, but cervical cancer screening is not routine in developing countries, and a complete pelvic examination is not required as part of a US immigration physical examination. However, in most developing countries, cervical cancer still remains the number-one cancer in women. In Thailand, 26 per 100 000 women developed invasive cervical cancer per year.[47] Among Southeast Asian Hmong immigrants to California, the incidence of invasive cervical cancer is similar to Thailand at 37.5 per 100 000 women annually.[49] Risk factors are well established, including HPV infection, early age of first coitus, smoking, and number of lifetime sexual partners per couple. In countries where commercial sex workers (CSWs) operate openly, the number of visits to CSWs by husbands also correlates with risk for cervical cancer.[47] Sexual violence among female refugees is unfortunately higher, increasing these risks. In the US, the greatest risk factor for cervical cancer death is lack of preventative screening.

Pelvic examinations are particularly difficult among previously traumatized women, among women with certain cultural or religious backgrounds, and when interpreters are not available. Gynecologic care is a vital screening tool, particularly among young women. Cross-cultural competency and female providers may maximize patient acceptance. In women older than 65 years of age, cervical cancer is low risk and deferment is practical and consistent with national guidelines.[50] Among women without a history of sexual violence *and* in a monogamous relationship or widowed, screening every 3 years beyond age 30 is appropriate.[50] Pelvic examinations, however, need not be performed on the first visit when establishing a relationship with a new healthcare provider, but it is vitally important for women after arrival to have ongoing cervical cancer screening.

## Biliary flukes

Two chronic parasite infections are associated with increased risk of liver cancer, presumably due to chronic inflammation caused by the biliary flukes *Opisthorchis* spp, and *Clonorchis sinensis*. They are acquired by eating raw freshwater fish, and in endemic areas infection rates may exceed 80% of the population. Infection with biliary flukes confers a 100-fold greater risk of cholangiocarcinoma. These infections predominate in Asia, particularly in northeast Thailand and in the lowland areas of Laos. This region was a site for many Hmong refugee camps in the 1980s and has the highest rate of cholangiocarcinoma in the world at 86 and 35 per 100 000 men and women, respectively.[51] In one small series, 25% of *Opisthorchis* infections were detected more than 5 years after immigration.[21]

## Schistosomiasis

Urinary schistosomiasis, principally caused by infection with *S. haematobium*, is associated with bladder cancer and intermittent, chronic hematuria. Asking whether an individual has ever had 'red urine' has a 67% sensitivity and 80% specificity for positive *S. haematobium* microscopy in Malawian school children.[52] Many immigrants from endemic areas are aware of the disease but will not know the disease by the term 'schistosomiasis,' but rather the term 'bilharzia.' Eosinophilia is present in about 60% of those chronically infected.[16,53] Seroprevalence rates are > 25% in many African countries but may exceed 80% in certain locales. Infection is highly regional.

Infection occurs when the cercarial form penetrates the skin during contact with freshwater. Prevalence rates are higher among refugees, and those living near lakes or slow moving rivers. Dams consistently exacerbate the problem of schistosomiasis.[54,55] Plans to dam the Mekong river may increase the rates of schistosomiasis among immigrants from Southeast Asia in the future. In addition, national health initiatives in many developing countries may decrease seroprevalence. Detection of ova is best on a freshly voided urine collected midday from a terminal urine specimen. Intestinal schistosomiasis is caused by *S. mansoni* or *S. japonicum*, neither associated with cancer but with cirrhosis. The available CDC IgG serology reportedly is very sensitive for *S. mansoni* (99%) and *S. haematobium* (95%) but insensitive (<50%) for *S. japonicum* found in Asia.[56] Commercial tests are slightly less sensitive, detecting between 80% and 88% dependent on species, and real-world performance may be less.[16,57]

## Human T-cell leukemia virus

Human T-cell leukemia virus (HTLV) type 1 is endemic in large regions of the tropics in the Caribbean, Latin America, and Africa. HTLV is unusual in most of Southeast Asia with the exception of southwestern Japan where 1–5% of the general populations is infected, with pockets of even higher prevalence.[58] Transmission of HTLV-1 is via breast feeding, sexual exposure, and blood and body fluid exposure. Acute adult T-cell leukemia and tropical spastic paraparesis occur in up to 10% of those infected, with a greater incidence with HIV coinfection. The tropical spastic paraparesis is characterized as a slow-onset degenerative disorder. From the onset of initial symptoms to the inability to walk is longer than 2 years in 80% of persons.[59] The predominant findings are lower lumbar pain, spastic paraparesis of the lower extremities with ankle clonus, hyperreflexia, positive Babinski reflex, variable impairment of superficial and deep sensation, and interference of bladder and bowel function.[60] In nonendemic countries, this may be a perplexing diagnosis unless HTLV is considered. In addition, HTLV coinfection with *Strongyloides* seems to predispose to *Strongyloides* hyperinfection.[61]

## Chronic End-Stage Disease

Classic manifestations of end-stage disease may occur years from initial exposure or emigration from

## Table 17.4 Chronic infection by system

| Process | Etiologic agent | Maximum latency | Geography |
|---|---|---|---|
| **Cardiovascular** | | | |
| Dilated cardiomyopathy, conduction defect | Chagas' disease | Chronic | Latin America |
| High output failure | Schistosomiasis with hepatic failure | ≈30 years | Worldwide |
| **Hematologic** | | | |
| Iron deficiency anemia | Hookworm | <3–5 years | Worldwide |
| Thrombocytopenia | Splenomegaly | Chronic | Worldwide |
| | May be a marker of liver disease from chronic hepatitis B/C, schistosomiasis, visceral leishmaniasis | | |
| **Pulmonary** | | | |
| Pulmonary fibrosis | Strongyloidiasis | Indefinite | |
| | Lung flukes | 20 years | |
| Tropical pulmonary eosinophilia | *Wuchereria bancrofti* | ≈12–15 years | Sub-Saharan Africa |
| | *Brugia malayi* | | South Asia |
| Reactive airway disease, chronic Loeffler's syndrome | Strongyloidiasis | Indefinite | |
| | Filaria (TPE) | | |
| | Hookworm | During acute infection only with an initial one-time pulmonary migration | Worldwide, prevalence inversely proportional to country income |
| | *Ascaris* | | |
| Castleman's disease | HHV-8 | Unknown | High seroprevalence in developing countries |
| Pulmonary cavity or nodules | Melioidosis | Indefinite | SE Asia |
| | TB | | Worldwide |
| | Paragonimiasis | | East Asia |
| Pulmonary hypertension | *Strongyloides* | Indefinite | Worldwide |
| **Gastrointestinal** | | | |
| Hepatitis | Hepatitis B | Chronic | Worldwide, endemic vertical transmission |
| Cirrhosis | Schistosomiasis | ≈30 years | Africa, SE Asia, Brazil |
| | Hepatitis B/C | | |
| Hepatocarcinoma | Hepatitis B/C | ≈10–30 years | |
| Peptic ulcer disease | *H. pylori* | Chronic | Near universal exposure in developing countries |
| Hepatosplenomegaly | Chronic malaria, visceral leishmaniasis schistosomiasis | Variable | |
| **Renal** | | | |
| Hematuria | Schistosomiasis | ≈30 years | Africa |
| Bladder cancer | | | |
| Glomerulosclerosis | Hepatitis B/C – cryoglobulininemia | Chronic | Worldwide, Asia |
| Nephrotic syndrome | Chronic *P. malariae* infection | | Sub-Saharan Africa |

**Table 17.4 Chronic infection by system—cont'd**

| Process | Etiologic agent | Maximum latency | Geography |
|---|---|---|---|
| ***Neurologic*** | | | |
| Seizure | Neurocysticercosis<br>S. Japonicum | 30+ years | Worldwide<br>South East Asia Pacific Rim |
| Neurosyphilis | Syphilis | | Worldwide |
| Degenerative, peripheral neuropathy | Arsenic toxicity (may mimic tabes dorsalis) | Traditional herbal therapies | |
| Subacute sclerosing panencephalitis | Measles | Unknown (~15 years) | Worldwide |
| Tuberculosis | *Mycobacterium tuberculosis* | 50% reactivation in <2 years | Worldwide |
| Ringlike enhancements | Toxoplasmosis | Unknown | Worldwide |
| Nodules | Paragonimiasis | | East Asia |
| Tropic spastic paraparis | | | |
| HTLV1 | | | |
| ***Musculoskeletal*** | | | |
| Cysts, weakness | Trichinella | | Worldwide |
| ***Miscellaneous*** | | | |
| Extrapulmonary TB | | May present in virtually any organ system | Worldwide |

an endemic country (Table 17.4). Importantly, among refugees, exposure to a pathogen may have occurred while as a refugee in a neighboring country (country of asylum), and not one's home country. For example, schistosomiasis has a relatively low prevalence in Somalia, but a much higher seroprevalence in Ethiopia and Kenya, sites of Somali refugee camps during the 1990s.[62,63]

## Chagas' disease

Chagas' disease, or American trypanosomiasis, is caused by infection with *Trypanosoma cruzi*. An estimated 16–18 million individuals in Latin America are infected, with approximately 50 000 deaths annually.[64] Approximately one-third of infected individuals will develop chronic disease 10–30 years later. Chronic manifestations of disease include dilated cardiomyopathy with congestive heart failure, heart block, megaesophagus, or megacolon. People who regularly sleep in poorly constructed houses found in the rural areas of Latin America are most likely to become infected. Houses constructed from mud, adobe, or thatch are more likely to be infested with triatomine (reduviid) bugs, the disease vector.

Approximately 100 million persons in Latin America live in such conditions and are at risk for Chagas' disease.[64] Screening Latin American immigrants by obtaining a history of living conditions prior to emigration is warranted. Having lived in a rural region with a house with a thatched roof has the highest association.[65] Diagnosis is rarely made outside of endemic regions, but in the US serology for *T. cruzi* is available from the CDC.[65] Testing should be targeted as testing a population with a low pretest probability may yield a 60–80% false-positive rate.[66] Newer techniques of nested-PCR and enzyme-linked immunoassays show improved diagnostic capabilities but do not have widespread availability.[67] The disease should be suspected when a patient who has resided in an endemic area and has an appropriate history presents with new-onset heart failure, dysphagia, or chronic gastrointestinal complaints. Chagas' disease is potentially transmissible by blood transfusion, and is not part of routine blood screening. Among blood donors in Miami and Los Angeles, the Chagas seroprevalence was 1 in 7700 donors.[68] Among blood donors in Mexico, the seroprevalence from 1999 to 2003 was 0.4% and was nearly equal to the prevalence of HIV, hepatitis B, and hepatitis C combined (0.5%).[69]

## Filarial infections

Subcutaneous filarial infections of *onchocerciasis* and *loaisis* have prepatent, asymptomatic periods that may last months to years from initial infection. These diseases are transmitted by the bites of flies in West and Central Africa. *Loa loa* presents in > 50% with localized areas of temporary angioedema that may be pruritic, red, or painful.[69] Adult *Loa loa* may be directly visualized during subconjunctival migration across the eye, and a history of such may be elicited in >66%.[70] In approximately 75% of infections, eosinophilia is present.[71] In primate studies, the average prepatent period before detection of microfilariae in the blood is 5–6 months; adult worms had a lifespan of at least 9 years.[72] In humans, adult worms may live up to 2 decades, and produce microfilariae in 6–12 months. Onchocerciasis (river blindness) may present with ocular complaints in two-thirds of infected persons or with chronic papular onchodermatitis in > 50% with living microfilariae detectable by skin snips.[73] Onchodermatitis is characterized by severe pruritus, and any patient from an endemic area presenting with severe pruritus should have this diagnosis considered. When the adult worm lives under the skin it may present as an onchocercoma, a subcutaneous nodule. When the adult worm dies, an acute inflammatory response may occur and a previously unnoticed nodule may become acutely swollen and inflamed and mistaken for a bacterial skin infection.

Lymphatic filariasis is caused by infection with *Wuchereria bancrofti* and *Brugia* spp. These parasites are transmitted by mosquito vectors principally in sub-Saharan Africa, India, Southeast Asia, and Oceania. *W. bancrofti* has a longer prepatent, asymptomatic period of up to 3 years before lymphatic scarring and elephantiasis develop. Development of lymphedema after leaving an endemic area, since ongoing exposure is ended, is unusual. However, filariasis may persist for years after exposure and present with recurrent urticaria, eosinophilia, or other non-specific symptoms. Tropical pulmonary eosinophilia (TPE) is a rare but serious manifestation of infection with the lymphatic filarial parasites that may present months to years after immigration and may mimic asthma. Filaria serologies are available but are non-specific; IgG tests or filarial antigen testing may offer more specific information (see Ch. 36).

## Chronic Diseases in Children

In pediatric patients, reductions in height and body mass index (BMI) correlate with chronic parasitic infections.[74] Chronic infection is prevalent in children less than 2 years of age with low height for age, whereas in older children low weight for age is more closely associated with chronic parasitic infections.[75] Cognitive impairments are two- to fourfold more frequent among children with parasitic infections and can be memory, learning, or verbal domain deficits, depending on the infecting species of helminth.[76]

There are several congenital infections that are noteworthy among the immigrant population. Firstly, congenital toxoplasmosis is a relatively rare, but devastating neonatal condition. The incidence among babies born to Southeast Asian immigrant mothers was eightfold higher between 1988 and 1999 than among mothers born in the United States.[77] The risk for mothers born in Laos was 33-fold higher at a prevalence of 22.3 per 100 000 live births. Secondly, transplacental passage of malaria can result in congenital malaria among very recent immigrants. In sub-Saharan Africa, malaria among pregnant women is extremely common (>40%) and up to 20% of *all* pregnancies may develop placental malaria.[78] Placental malaria is a risk for congenital malaria as well as low birth weight and preterm delivery. Diagnosis can be made postpartum via biopsy of the placenta or smear of umbilical cord blood. Fortunately, only 10% of cases of placental malaria result in congenital malaria with parasitemia present in cord blood.[78,79]

Vertical transmission of hepatitis B virus (HBV) from infected mothers who are HBsAg positive to infants results in establishment of chronic infection in nearly 80% of those congenitally exposed. In older children, particularly from Southeast Asia, asymptomatic HBV infection may go unrecognized for years. Among Latin American immigrants, Chagas' disease also can result in congenital infection. The prevalence of congenital Chagas infection is 5–10% among seropositive mothers.[80,81] The incidence of seropositivity among pregnant Hispanic women in Houston, Texas, was 0.4%.[82]

## Conclusion

Numerous latent infections may persist unrecognized in immigrants for decades. Most persons are either asymptomatic or have non-specific complaints from low-grade chronic infection. Often, diagnostic strategies for parasitic infections may need to reach beyond traditional stool O&P examination to other serologic or imaging techniques.

Guidance of testing is based on symptoms and geographic risk.

## References

1. World Health Organization. Tropical disease research: progress 2001–2002. The United Nations Development Programme/World Bank/WHO Special Programme for Research and Training in Tropical Diseases, programme report no. 16. Geneva: WHO, 2003. Available: http://www.who.int/tdr/publications/publications/pr16.htm October 25, 2005.
2. Gordin FM, Chaisson RE, Matts JP, et al. An international, randomized trial of rifampin and pyrazinamide versus isoniazid for prevention of tuberculosis in HIV-infected persons. JAMA 2000; 283:1445–1450.
3. Mohan AK, Cote TR, Block JA, et al. Tuberculosis following the use of etanercept, a tumor necrosis factor inhibitor. Clin Infect Dis 2004; 39:295–299.
4. CDC. Tuberculosis associated with blocking agents against tumor necrosis factor-alpha – California, 2002–2003. MMWR 2004; 53:683–686.
5. Wallis RS, Broder M, Wong J, et al. Reactivation of latent granulomatous infections by infliximab. Clin Infect Dis 2005; 41:S194–S198.
6. Verner E, Shteinfeld M, Raz R, et al. Diagnostic and therapeutic approach to Ethiopian immigrants seropositive for syphilis. Isr J Med Sci 1988; 24:151–155.
7. Bello CS. Treponemal antibodies in rural Gambian villagers: what significance? Afr J Sex Transmi Dis 1984; 1:19–20.
8. Buchwald D, Collier AC, Lukehart SA, et al. Evaluation of cerebrospinal fluid in Southeast Asian refugees with reactive serologic tests for syphilis. West J Med 1996; 165:289–293.
9. World Health Organization. Leishmaniasis: burden of disease. Available: http://www.who.int/leishmaniasis/burden/en/ October 27, 2005.
10. Van den Ende J, van Gompel A, Van den Ende E, et al. Hyperreactive malaria in expatriates returning from sub-Saharan Africa. Trop Med Int Health 2000; 5:607–611.
11. Schaefer KU, Khan B, Gachihi GS, et al. Splenomegaly in Baringo District, Kenya, an area endemic for visceral leishmaniasis and malaria. Trop Geogr Med 1995; 47:111–114.
12. De Cock KM, Hodgen AN, Lucas SB, et al. Chronic splenomegaly in Nairobi, Kenya. I. Epidemiology, malarial antibody and immunoglobulin levels. Trans R Soc Trop Med Hyg 1987; 81:100–106.
13. Torres-Rojas JR, Rothschild H, Krotoski WA. Tropical splenomegaly syndrome in a nontropical setting. Am J Trop Med Hyg 1981; 30:1–4.
14. Boulware DR, Stauffer W III, Hendel-Paterson BR, et al. Ten year case review of *Strongyloides stercoralis* infections in a non-endemic United States setting and an associated evaluation of medical resident knowledge of this parasitic infection. Am J Med, in press.
15. de Silva S, Saykao P, Kelly H, et al. Chronic *Strongyloides stercoralis* infection in Laotian immigrants and refugees 7–20 years after resettlement in Australia. Epidemiol Infect 2002; 128:439–444.
16. Bierman WF, Wetsteyn JC, van Gool T. Presentation and diagnosis of imported schistosomiasis: relevance of eosinophilia, microscopy for ova, and serology. J Travel Med 2005; 12:9–13.
17. Torres GB, Iwashita AT, Vargas CM, et al. Human fascioliasis and gastrointestinal compromise: study of 277 patients in the Cayetano Heredia National Hospital (1970–2002). Rev Gastroenterol Peru 2004; 24:143–157.
18. Osman MM, Ismail Y, Aref TY. Human fascioliasis: a study on the relation of infection intensity and treatment to hepatobiliary affection. J Egypt Soc Parasitol 1999; 29:353–363.
19. Cosme A, Ojeda E, Cilla G, et al. *Fasciola hepatica*: study of a series of 37 patients. Gastroenterol Hepatol 2001; 24:375–380.
20. Stauffer WM, Sellman JS, Walker PF. Biliary liver flukes (opisthorchiasis and clonorchiasis) in immigrants in the United States: often subtle and diagnosed years after arrival. J Travel Med 2004; 11:157–159.
21. Noyer CM, Coyle CM, Werner C, et al. Hypereosinophilia and liver mass in an immigrant. Am J Trop Med Hyg 2002; 66:774–776.
22. Kim YH, Kang KJ, Kwon JH. Four cases of hepatic fascioliasis mimicking cholangiocarcinoma. Korean J Hepatol 2005; 11:169–175.
23. Marcos L, Maco V, Samalvides F, et al. Risk factors for *Fasciola hepatica* infection in children: a case-control study. Trans R Soc Trop Med Hyg 2006; 100:158–166.
24. El-Shazly AM, El-Nahas HA, Abdel-Mageed AA, et al. Human fascioliasis and anaemia in Dakahlia Governorate. J Egypt Soc Parasitol 2005; 35:421–432.
25. von Bonsdorff B, Gordin R. Castle's test (with vitamin $B_{12}$ and normal gastric juice) in the ileum in patients with genuine and patients with tapeworm pernicious anaemia. Acta Med Scand 1980; 208:193–197.
26. Frisancho O, Ulloa V, Ruiz W, et al. Megaloblastic anemia associated with chronic diarrhea. A prospective and multicenter study in Lima. Rev Gastroenterol Peru 1994; 14:189–195.
27. Hoffner RJ, Kilaghbian T, Esekogwu VI, et al. Common presentations of amoebic liver abscess. Ann Emerg Med 1999; 34:351–355.
28. Ravdin J, Jackson T, Petri J, et al. Association of serum antibodies to adherence lectin with invasive amoebiasis and asymptomatic infection with *Entamoeba histolytica*. J Infect Dis 1990; 162:768–772.
29. Wynants H, Van den Ende J, Randria J, et al. Diagnosis of amoebic infection of the liver: report of 36 cases. Ann Soc Belg Med Trop 1995; 75:297–303.
30. CDC. Recommendations for prevention and control of tuberculosis among foreign-born persons. Report of the Working Group on Tuberculosis among Foreign-Born Persons. MMWR 1998; 47:1–26.
31. Vos AM, Meima A, Verver S, et al. High incidence of pulmonary tuberculosis persists a decade after immigration, The Netherlands. Emerg Infect Dis 2004; 10:736–739.
32. Dahle UR, Sandven P, Heldal E, et al. Genetic analysis of *Mycobacterium tuberculosis* in Norway 1994–98. Tidsskr Nor Laegeforen 2002; 122:697–700.
33. Dankner WM, Waecker NJ, Essey MA, et al. *Mycobacterium bovis* infections in San Diego: a clinicoepidemiologic study of 73 patients and a historical review of a forgotten pathogen. Medicine (Baltimore) 1993; 72:11–37.
34. Mfinanga SG, Morkve O, Kazwala RR, et al. Mycobacterial adenitis: role of *Mycobacterium bovis*, non-tuberculous mycobacteria, HIV infection, and risk factors in Arusha, Tanzania. East Afr Med J 2004; 81:171–178.
35. Hardie RM, Watson JM. *Mycobacterium bovis* in England and Wales: past, present and future. Epidemiol Infect 1992; 109:23–33.
36. Milian F, Sanchez LM, Toledo P, et al. Descriptive study of human and bovine tuberculosis in Queretaro, Mexico. Rev Latinoam Microbiol 2000; 42:13–19.
37. CDC. Human tuberculosis caused by *Mycobacterium bovis* – New York City, 2001–2004. MMWR 2005; 52:605–608.
38. Leelarasamee A. *Burkholderia pseudomallei*: the unbeatable foe? Southeast Asian J Trop Med Public Health 1998; 29:410–415.
39. Ip M, Osterberg LG, Chau PY, et al. Pulmonary melioidosis. Chest 1995; 108:1420–1424.
40. Currie BJ. Melioidosis: an important cause of pneumonia in residents of and travellers returned from endemic regions. Eur Respir J 2003; 22:542–550.

41. Sarmati L. HHV-8 infection in African children. Herpes 2004; 11:50–53.

42. Wundisch T, Thiede C, Morgner A, et al. Long-term follow-up of gastric MALT lymphoma after *Helicobacter pylori* eradication. J Clin Oncol 2005; 23:1–7.

43. Mwanda OW, Fu P, Collea R, et al. Kaposi's sarcoma in patients with and without HIV infection, in a tertiary referral centre in Kenya. Ann Trop Med Parasitol 2005; 99:81–91.

44. Caruana SR, Kelly HA, De Silva SL, et al. Knowledge about hepatitis and previous exposure to hepatitis viruses in immigrants and refugees from the Mekong Region. Aust NZ J Public Health 2005; 29:64–68.

45. Matsumoto A, Tanaka E, Rokuhara A, et al. Efficacy of lamivudine for preventing hepatocellular carcinoma in chronic hepatitis B: a multicenter retrospective study of 2795 patients. Hepatol Res 2005; 32:173–184.

46. Fattovich G, Stroffolini T, Zagni I, et al. Hepatocellular carcinoma in cirrhosis: incidence and risk factors. Gastroenterology 2004; 127:S35–S50.

47. Vatanasapt V, Sriamporn S, Vatanasapt P. Cancer control in Thailand. Jpn J Clin Oncol 2002; 32:S82–S91.

48. Proietti FA, Carneiro-Proietti AB, Catalan-Soares BC, et al. Global epidemiology of HTLV-1 infection and associated diseases. Oncogene 2005; 24:6058.

49. Yang RC, Mills PK, Riordan DG. Cervical cancer among Hmong women in California, 1988 to 2000. Am J Prev Med 2004; 27:132–138.

50. US Preventive Services Task Force. Screening for cervical cancer: recommendations and rationale. Am Fam Physician 2003; 67:1759–1766.

51. Vatanasapt V, Parkin DM, Sriamporn S. Epidemiology of liver cancer in Thailand. In: Vatanasapt V, Sripa B, eds. Liver cancer in Thailand, epidemiology, diagnosis and control. Khon Kaen: Siriphan Press; 2000:3–6.

52. Bowie C, Purcell B, Shaba B, et al. A national survey of the prevalence of schistosomiasis and soil transmitted helminths in Malawi. BMC Infect Dis 2004; 4:49.

53. Harris AR, Russell RJ, Charters AD. A review of schistosomiasis in immigrants in Western Australia, demonstrating the unusual longevity of *Schistosoma mansoni*. Trans R Soc Trop Med Hyg 1984; 78:385–388.

54. Malek EA. Effect of the Aswan High Dam on prevalence of schistosomiasis in Egypt. Trop Geogr Med 1975; 27:359–364.

55. Sow S, de Vlas SJ, Engels D, et al. Water-related disease patterns before and after the construction of the Diama dam in northern Senegal. Ann Trop Med Parasitol 2002; 96:575–586.

56. Tsang VC, Wilkins PP. Immunodiagnosis of schistosomiasis. Immunol Invest 1997; 26:175–188.

57. Van Gool T, Vetter H, Vervoort T, et al. Serodiagnosis of imported schistosomiasis by a combination of a commercial indirect hemagglutination test with *Schistosoma mansoni* adult worm antigens and an enzyme-linked immunosorbent assay with *S. mansoni* egg antigens. J Clin Microbiol 2002; 40:3432–3437.

58. De The G. Clinical and biological epidemiology of onco-retroviral HTLV-I and II infections. Bull Acad Natl Med 1991; 175:861–869.

59. Gotuzzo E, Cabrera J, Deza L, et al. Clinical characteristics of patients in Peru with human T cell lymphotropic virus type 1-associated tropical spastic paraparesis. Clin Infect Dis 2004; 39:939–944.

60. Beilke MA, Japa S, Moeller-Hadi C, et al. Tropical spastic paraparesis/human T cell leukemia virus type 1-associated myelopathy in HIV type 1-coinfected patients. Clin Infect Dis 2005; 41:e57–e63.

61. Lim S, Katz K, Krajden S, et al. Complicated and fatal *Strongyloides* infection in Canadians: risk factors, diagnosis and management. Can Med Assoc J 2004; 171:479–484.

62. Miller JM, Boyd HA, Ostrowski SR, et al. Malaria, intestinal parasites, and schistosomiasis among Barawan Somali refugees resettling to the United States: a strategy to reduce morbidity and decrease the risk of imported infections. Am J Trop Med Hyg 2000; 62:115–121.

63. Koura M, Upatham ES, Awad AH, et al. Prevalence of *Schistosoma haematobium* in the Koryole and Merca Districts of the Somali Democratic Republic. Ann Trop Med Parasitol 1981; 75:53–61.

64. Wanderley DM, Correa FM. Epidemiology of Chagas' heart disease. Sao Paulo Med J 1995; 113:742–749.

65. Rizzo NR, Arana BA, Diaz A, et al. Seroprevalence of *Trypanosoma cruzi* infection among school-age children in the endemic area of Guatemala. Am J Trop Med Hyg 2003; 68:678–682.

66. Barrett VJ, Leiby DA, Odom JL, et al. Negligible prevalence of antibodies against *Trypanosoma cruzi* among blood donors in the southeastern United States. Am J Clin Pathol 1997; 108:499–503.

67. Andersson J. Molecular diagnosis of experimental Chagas' disease. Trends Parasitol 2004; 20:52–53.

68. Leiby DA, Herron RM Jr, Read EJ, et al. *Trypanosoma cruzi* in Los Angeles and Miami blood donors: impact of evolving donor demographics on seroprevalence and implications for transfusion transmission. Transfusion 2002; 42:549–555.

69. Hernandez-Becerril N, Mejia AM, Ballinas-Verdugo MA, et al. Blood transfusion and iatrogenic risks in Mexico City. Anti-*Trypanosoma cruzi* seroprevalence in 43,048 blood donors, evaluation of parasitemia, and electrocardiogram findings in seropositive. Mem Inst Oswaldo Cruz 2005; 100:111–116.

70. Noireau F, Apembet JD, Nzoulani A, et al. Clinical manifestations of loiasis in an endemic area in the Congo. Trop Med Parasitol 1990; 41:37–39.

71. Carrillo Casas E, Iglesias Perez B, Gomez I, et al. Screening of microfilariasis in blood (*Loa loa*) among the immigrant population in endemic areas. Rev Esp Salud Publica 2004; 78:623–630.

72. Orihel TC, Eberhard ML. *Loa loa*: development and course of patency in experimentally-infected primates. Trop Med Parasitol 1985; 36:215–224.

73. Enk CD, Anteby I, Abramson N, et al. Onchocerciasis among Ethiopian immigrants in Israel. Isr Med Assoc J 2003; 5:485–488.

74. Zhou H, Ohtsuka R, He Y, et al. Impact of parasitic infections and dietary intake on child growth in the schistosomiasis-endemic Dongting Lake Region, China. Am J Trop Med Hyg 2005; 72:534–539.

75. Oberhelman RA, Guerrero ES, Fernandez ML, et al. Correlations between intestinal parasitosis, physical growth, and psychomotor development among infants and children from rural Nicaragua. Am J Trop Med Hyg 1998; 58:470–475.

76. Ezeamama AE, Friedman JF, Acosta LP, et al. Helminth infection and cognitive impairment among Filipino children. Am J Trop Med Hyg 2005; 72:540–548.

77. Jara M, Hsu HW, Eaton RB, et al. Epidemiology of congenital toxoplasmosis identified by population-based newborn screening in Massachusetts. Pediatr Infect Dis J 2001; 20:1132–1135.

78. Tako EA, Zhou A, Lohoue J, et al. Risk factors for placental malaria and its effect on pregnancy outcome in Yaounde, Cameroon. Am J Trop Med Hyg 2005; 72:236–242.

79. Bergstrom S, Fernandes A, Schwalbach J, et al. Materno-fetal transmission of pregnancy malaria: an immunoparasitological study on 202 parturients in Maputo. Gynecol Obstet Invest 1993; 35:103–107.

80. Nisida IV, Amato Neto V, Braz LM, et al. A survey of congenital Chagas' disease, carried out at three health institutions in Sao Paulo City, Brazil. Rev Inst Med Trop Sao Paulo 1999; 41:305–311.

81. Russomando G, de Tomassone MM, de Guillen I, et al. Treatment of congenital Chagas' disease diagnosed and followed up by the polymerase chain reaction. Am J Trop Med Hyg 1998; 59:487–491.

82. Di Pentima MC, Hwang LY, Skeeter CM, et al. Prevalence of antibody to *Trypanosoma cruzi* in pregnant Hispanic women in Houston. Clin Infect Dis 1999; 28:1281–1285.

# CHAPTER 18

# Emerging Infectious Diseases of Immigrant Patients

Jonathan Sellman and Patrick Pederson

## Introduction

Today, accounts of emerging infectious diseases spill from newspaper headlines and garner lead story status on the evening news. Just as globalization has brought humanity closer together in trade and culture, infections are transmitted rapidly across the globe. The public seems as interested in 'bird flu' in Asia or Ebola in central Africa as in an account of neisserial meningitis at the local high school. It now seems surprising that recognition of emerging infections is less than a few decades old.

It is understandable that a sense of complacency about infectious disease took hold of medicine and public health in the late twentieth century. Improvements in sanitation, nutrition, housing, and occupational health dramatically decreased infectious disease rates in the United States. Immunizations were effective against viral infections: smallpox was eradicated world-wide; rubella was eliminated from North America; and rates of other childhood viral diseases markedly reduced.[1,2] With the development of safe and effective vaccines and drugs to treat bacterial infections, bacteria appeared defeated. All these factors caused an inappropriate confidence that infectious diseases would be completely eradicated as a public health problem. In fact, in 1967, US Surgeon General William H. Stewart announced that it was 'time to close the book on infectious diseases, declare the war against pestilence won, and shift national resources to such chronic problems as cancer and heart disease.'[3] Despite this hubris, others began to sound the alarm. The term 'emerging dis-

eases' was first used by David J. Sencer in 1971.[4] In 1976, the Centers for Disease Control (CDC) investigated an outbreak of disease affecting attendees at the National American Legion Convention in Philadelphia, and the following year CDC isolated the causative agent, *Legionella pneumophila*, for what is now called Legionnaire's disease. In 1981, Richard M. Krause, director of the National Institutes of Allergy and Infectious Diseases, published an early clarion call with his book *The Restless Tide: The Persistent Challenge of the Microbial World*.[5] Shortly thereafter, the epidemic of AIDS was recognized and over the next 10 years a growing sense of unease arose as new infectious disease outbreaks were identified.

## Recognition and Surveillance for Emerging Infectious Disease

The Institute of Medicine triggered a landslide of interest in emerging infections when it addressed the issue in the early 1990s. In the seminal work on the topic, a 1992 Institute of Medicine report defined emerging infectious diseases as 'infections that have newly appeared in a population or have existed but are rapidly increasing in incidence or geographic range.'[6] Aside from numerous academic and lay-public publications, several landmark developments are notable in the history of emerging infections. The Centers for Disease Control and Prevention (CDC) started publication of the journal *Emerging Infectious Diseases* in January 1995. The journal continues to provide a venue for discussion of emerging diseases in human and animal populations.

ProMED-mail, the Program for Monitoring Emerging Diseases, (http://www.promedmail.org) is an internet-based reporting system established in 1994 with the support of the Federation of American Scientists and SatelLife. Since 1999, ProMED-mail has operated as a program of the International Society of Infectious Diseases. The electronic mail system provides subscribers with daily updates about emerging diseases from around the world. The importance and effectiveness of the system has been repeatedly documented. A notable example was an email sent by a travel medicine physician, Stephen O. Cunnion, on February 10, 2003.[7] He quoted an email that he had received, stating, 'Have you heard of an epidemic in Guangzhou? An acquaintance of mine from a teacher's chat room lives there and reports that the hospitals there have been closed and people are dying.' This email was an early warning of an outbreak of the previously unidentified human coronavirus causing severe acute respiratory syndrome (SARS).

The International Society of Travel Medicine (ISTM) provided seed money to establish GeoSentinel in July 1995. Initially, GeoSentinel was founded as a working group of nine US-based ISTM member travel clinics which agreed to collaborate as a sentinel emerging infections network by monitoring illness among returning international travelers. The following year the network was awarded funding from the CDC. GeoSentinel now incorporates a global network of providers at over 30 sites on all continents. A successful early recognition of disease emergence by GeoSentinel was the identification of leptospirosis among participants in the Borneo Eco-Challenge 2000 Adventure Race while many participants were still in the incubation period.[8]

## Historical Observations: Plagues, Pestilences, People, Immigration

As a focused field of study, interest in emerging infections grew out of observations of a number of new diseases that emerged in the last three decades of the twentieth century. These diseases included the worldwide pandemic of a newly recognized pathogen (HIV); reemergence of the old disease of tuberculosis; newly recognized infectious syndromes associated with known pathogens, such as toxic shock syndrome caused by group A *Streptococcus*; and introductions of known agents into naïve populations, such as West Nile virus.

The history of epidemic diseases involves the increasing interconnectedness of people. Early societies brought together humans in large enough concentrations that epidemic disease could take hold and spread within villages and city-states. Epidemic disease took advantage of contacts between early city states and then nations engaged in wars or trade. Multiple epidemics of plague spread out of China via the Silk Road.

The opening of the New World to European settlement led to an interchange of species, including pathogens, termed the Columbian exchange.[9] Measles and smallpox brought to the New World by immigrant Europeans devastated Native Americans. Meanwhile, syphilis, which is theorized to have arisen in the Americas, spread in epidemic fashion in Europe after 1492. The slave trade was responsible for the movement of HTLV (human T-cell lymphotropic virus)- I, HTLV-II, yellow fever virus and, importantly, its mosquito vector, *Aedes aegypti*, to the Americas. In the 1970s, *Aedes albopictus*, a mosquito vector competent for transmission of dengue was inadvertently imported into North America from Asia as a result of the international trade in used tires. Global air travel has connected distant corners of the planet like never before, offering pathogens unprecedented potential for rapid transmission to far-flung immunologically naïve populations.

## Epidemiology and Modeling of Emerging Infectious Diseases

Why do some diseases emerge and spread globally, while others sputter out locally? Disease occurs when a pathogen meets a host that is vulnerable to the agent in an environment that allows the agent and host to interact. Agent, host, and environment alone are not sufficient to cause an epidemic, however. For a pathogen to be successful in causing an epidemic, an unbroken chain of transmission must be present. Given a suitable mode of spread and a chain of transmission from one susceptible host to another, an outbreak can develop. The chain of transmission may be thought of categorically as a source for the agent, the presence of the agent (pathogen), a portal of exit from the source, a mode of transmission, a portal of entry into the host, and a susceptible host.

The first link in the chain, the source for the agent, is the place where the agent originates. This may be another infected human, or the animal reservoir in the case of zoonotic infections, or the environmental reservoir in the case of pathogens acquired from environmental sources, such as soil. Influenza, for example, circulates as a zoonotic infection with the principle reservoir being waterfowl.

The second link is the presence of the agent or pathogen. Even though a host may be in contact with the source, the agent must be present in order for transmission to occur. Certain characteristics of the pathogen are important to consider. Infectivity is the capacity to cause infection in a susceptible host. Not all infections result in symptomatic disease, however. The pathogenicity of the agent is the capacity to cause disease in a host. And finally, the virulence of the pathogen determines the severity of disease that the agent causes in the host. Pursuing influenza as an example, although humans who interact with poultry are likely frequently exposed, many avian influenza viruses are either not spread to humans (low infectivity) or, of those which are, they may infect a human but are unable to cause disease (low pathogenicity). However, with reassortment of the influenza genome, there is potential for influenza viruses to cause severe illness and death in humans (i.e. H5N1).

The third link, a portal of exit, is a pathway by which the agent can leave the source. This pathway is usually related to the place where the agent is localized. Influenza is spread from human to human primarily via respiratory secretions. Another example, the dimorphic fungus *Coccidioides immitis*, has an environmental reservoir. The organism is found in desert sands in the American southwest and its arthrospores are blown from the earth by winds.

Once the agent leaves the source, a mode of transmission, or means of carrying it to the host, is needed. Although in the case of influenza fomite spread plays a role, with humans carrying the virus from poultry farm to farm, the main route of transmissions from person to person tends to be droplet spread of infected respiratory material. Other modes of transmission are shown in Box 18.1.

Direct transmission occurs with direct transfer of the infectious agent from person to person. This category includes transmission spread by direct contact, including touching, kissing, and sexual interactions. Rabies is spread by direct transmission via the bite of a rabid animal, for example. Droplet spread in which there is direct projection of infectious droplets onto the mucus membranes of the host also is included in this category. Droplet transmission, such as with influenza, occurs via large particles (measuring 5 microns) expelled when a person coughs, sneezes, or talks. These particles are generally pro-

---

**Box 18.1**

**Modes of transmission**

**Direct transmission**
- Direct contact
- Sexual transmission
- Droplet

**Indirect transmission**
- Vehicle-borne
- Fomites (clothing, bedding, surgical instruments)
- Blood-borne
- Fecal–oral
- Vector-borne
- Mechanical
- Biological

**Airborne**
- Droplet nuclei
- Dust

---

pelled no more than 3 feet from the infected person in any direction. Indirect transmission may be vehicle-borne, in other words, spread via fomites, blood products (blood-borne transmission), or fecal contamination of water and food (fecal–oral transmission). Vector-borne diseases are transmitted indirectly by a live carrier, usually an arthropod, such as mosquitoes, fleas, or ticks. The transmission may be mechanical, in which the vector acts to transport the pathogen, but is not biologically necessary for replication, such as fecal coliform bacteria transported by a housefly, or biological transmission in which the vector is a site of replication of the pathogen, such as malarial parasites in mosquito species.

Airborne transmission is via droplet nuclei or dusts (measuring < 5 microns) that can remain suspended in air for long periods of time and may be carried by air currents for long distances. The classic example of a disease transmitted by the airborne route is measles. In some cases, the pathogen is not able to be transmitted effectively from one human host to another. In this case, the human is a 'dead-end host' and the chain of transmission is cut. Examples of dead-end infections in humans include those due to the dimorphic fungi, *Histoplasma*, *Blastomyces*, and *Coccidioides*.

There must be a pathway into the host, a portal of entry, which gives the agent access to tissue where it can multiply or act. Often, the agent enters the host in the same way that it left the source. This is the case with influenza or *Mycobacterium tuberculosis*, which leave the source through the respiratory tract and usually enter a new host through the respiratory tract.

And finally, there must be a susceptible host. The immune status of the host is generally classifiable as susceptible, immune, or infected. The susceptible host's response to exposure can vary widely, from manifesting subclinical infection, atypical symptoms, straightforward illness, severe illness, or death. Host susceptibility is extremely complex, with intensive infectious disease research currently directed at gaining an understanding of why certain hosts are susceptible, why infected hosts display variation in clinical manifestations, and why different hosts vary in their ability to transmit disease. This understanding is being greatly advanced through evolving applications of molecular genetic techniques.

Yet even when all of the above factors are present, some diseases do not become epidemics. Mathematical modeling of infectious disease outbreaks has led to the characterization of the basic reproduction number, $R_0$, which describes the average number of secondary cases of disease generated by each typical case in a susceptible population. For epidemic spread of a disease, the $R_0$ for the pathogen must be greater than one ($R_0 > 1$). In its most simplistic form, the SIR model divides the population into proportions corresponding to susceptible (S), infected (I), and removed (either recovered and immune, or dead) (R).[10] By definition:

$$S + I + R = 1$$

The uniform mixing assumption posits that epidemics depend only on the total number of infectives (I) and susceptibles (S). Even diseases with similar $R_0$ values can have different patterns of epidemic spread, with one turning into a pandemic and the other extinguishing locally. This highlights problems with the SIR model. Notably, it assumes a well-mixed, homogeneous population. Populations are frequently heterogeneous, however, with people interacting through networks of relationships. Disease transmission is facilitated between members of such networks more efficiently than outside these networks. Studies of sexually transmitted infections (STIs) highlight the important role of networks in disease transmission, but networks are equally important in diseases transmitted by other routes besides sexual transmission. Tuberculosis, for example, is much easier spread to family members because it requires prolonged, close contact. Additionally, the model does not take into account stochastic events which may have profound effects on the course of an epidemic. One infectious patient traveling on an intercontinental flight to an immunologically naïve population may have a profound impact on spread of a respiratory disease. Finally, the model fails to recognize the importance of host factors that lend to epidemic potential. For example, in some diseases, there are outliers of transmission potential in which an infected individual, a superspreader, may be more efficient at transmitting the disease than the observed average $R_0$ of the disease.

Although modeling is far from perfect, these basic concepts help guide the selection of public health strategies to interrupt infectious disease spread. Depending on which approach might be most effective, efforts may be directed to the specific agent (e.g. screwworm), host (e.g. immunization to prevent measles), or environment (e.g. sanitation improvements to prevent salmonella). We can also target a specific point in the chain of transmission, such as limiting fomite transmission.

## Recent Trends Notable for Emerging Infectious Diseases

Aside from the infectiousness of a pathogen to be spread person-to-person, what are the reasons some diseases newly appear in outbreaks or reappear after years of quiescence? A 2003 Institute of Medicine follow-up report on emerging infectious diseases identified 13 factors associated with the appearance of new and recurrent emerging infections (Box 18.2).[11]

By multiple health measures, immigrants and refugees are, in general, in poorer health than the average for citizens of their country of destination. Infectious diseases favor the poor and disenfranchised. It should not be surprising that emerging infectious diseases would be associated with social inequality.[12] Refugees frequently have fled their country of origin with little in the way of financial resources. If they were in a refugee camp prior to immigration they endured privations including crowding, malnutrition, poor sanitation, inadequate clothing, and poor access to basic health services. For example, patients may acquire tuberculosis that recrudesces later or is diagnosed after arrival in their new home country.[13] Multidrug resistant tuberculosis (MDRTB) is of particular concern because it is difficult to diagnose and treat. Tuberculosis should be considered in the differential diagnosis of any

## Box 18.2
### Factors associated with disease emergence

Microbial adaptation and change
Human susceptibility to infection
Climate and weather
Changing ecosystems
Human demographics and behavior
Economic development and land use
International travel and commerce
Technology and industry
Breakdown of public health measures
Poverty and social inequality
War and famine
Lack of political will
Intent to harm

Source: Smolinski MS, Hamburg MA, Lederberg J, eds. Microbial threats to health: emergence, detection, and response. Washington: Institute of Medicine National Academy Press; 2003.

immigrant presenting even years later with symptoms compatible with reactivated or disseminated disease. Alternatively, immigrants who have not received appropriate immunizations may serve as pockets of susceptible persons in countries that otherwise have low endemic rates of disease. Examples include measles and rubella.

## Emerging infectious diseases of note for immigrants and refugees

Though there is a broad literature of emerging infections, there is little documentation of emerging disease transmission or epidemic spread to the US attributable to refugees or immigrants. Although it is clear that refugee camp conditions lead to excessive outbreaks of diseases (i.e. measles, cholera, TB), controlled immigration, as occurs with refugees, greatly decreases the risk of the introduction of infectious diseases to the US in this population. This is true because under CDC protocols some refugees receive both overseas preventive therapy (antimalarials) as well as post-arrival medical screening. Some legal immigrants must also receive overseas preventive care and basic medical screening. Therefore, although immigrants (especially undocumented immigrants) and refugees may pose a potential reservoir for the spread of emerging infectious diseases to the US, they are significantly less likely than unregulated travelers to spark a true epidemic in the US. This stated, a number of emerg-

ing infections could theoretically expand their range because of the movement of immigrant and refugee populations.

### Influenza

Few other highly transmissible contagions carry the historic profile of pandemic influenza. While seasonal outbreaks of interpandemic influenza occur annually, they can generally be predicted using international surveillance and their impact blunted by mass vaccination and prophylactic antiviral treatment strategies. In contrast, the emergence of highly pathogenic strains, such as the 1918 'Spanish' flu which killed an estimated 50 million people worldwide, pose a substantially greater public health risk.[14] More recently, the discovery of the H5N1 avian strain has led to considerable government preparation for the possibility of a new pandemic.[15] Local physicians and state health departments remain on the forefront of such outbreaks. Special attention should be paid to infected foreign travelers and immigrants as one potential nidus for community-wide spread.

Influenza viruses are enveloped segmented RNA viruses of the Orthomyxoviridae family. Three of the five genera constitute the three individual species of influenza: influenza A, influenza B, and influenza C. Of the three, only influenza A has shown pandemic potential. Influenza A subtypes are classified according to two envelope glycoproteins, hemagglutinin, of which there are 16 variants (H1–H16), and neuraminidase, of which there are 9 variants (N1–N9).

The pandemic aptitude of influenza A stems from both its nonhuman reservoir and its potential for frequent genetic mutation. Influenza A viruses have been known to infect horses, whales, seals, mink, and humans, but are most abundant in wild waterfowl.[16] With few exceptions, wild avian hosts remain asymptomatic from infection, and, over centuries, have allowed the virus to enter evolutionary stasis, creating a stable platform from which numerous mutant variants have entered the human population.[17,18] These mutations are facilitated by years of *antigenic drift* induced by the influenza RNA polymerase, which lacks proofreading capacity, and *antigenic shift* which occurs via genetic reassortment when more than one strain coexist in a single host.

Achieving human-to-human transmissibility is most often a two-step process. Initially, antigenic drift allows an avian strain to infect a human host, but does not typically confer sufficient specificity to humans to allow for human-to-human transmission.

It is postulated that this initial step has been facilitated in the past by the ongoing practice of human–avian cohabitation in the rural regions of Southeast Asia. Domesticated ducks, in particular, are known to excrete high titers of influenza from their GI tracts, with influenza deposited into local ponds remaining active for weeks.[18] Next, individuals infected by both avian and human strains provide the opportunity for an antigenic shift to occur, whereby the virulent avian strain can gain characteristics that allow it to propagate human to human. Of note, both the 1957 H2N2 and the 1968 H3N2 pandemic strains were thought to develop along similar two-step pathways, while the 1918 H1N1 strain has more recently been shown to be a product of antigenic drift alone.[19] Of more concern to contemporary policy makers, the highly lethal H5N1 avian virus has been shown to need only minimal modification by either route to gain a foothold among humans.[20]

Recognition, treatment, and containment of pandemic influenza remain problematic. Influenza's primary mode of transmission, via aerosolization of respiratory secretions, allows for the rapid inoculation of multiple hosts, particularly during the initial asymptomatic 2–4-day incubation period.[16] Of the 10–20% of the US population who are infected annually, primary symptoms remain non-specific, typically comprising fever, myalgias, cough, and headache.[21,22] Symptoms of previously documented pandemic strains begin similarly, though may rapidly convert to a multilobar, hemorrhagic pneumonitis followed quickly by bacterial superinfection and/or death.[14,23] Strategies for containment at this time rely on respiratory isolation of infected individuals, and on the rapid development of new influenza vaccines to cover emerging strains. Treatment typically consists of the early administration of antiviral medications, notably oseltamivir and zanamivir, which have limited efficacy, and supportive care.[24]

## Multidrug resistant tuberculosis

Over 2 billion people internationally are currently infected with *Mycobacterium tuberculosis* which also infects 8–10 million more per year, and has an associated annual mortality of nearly 2 million individuals. Despite global eradication efforts, the re-emergence and spread of multidrug resistant tuberculosis (MDRTB), continues to threaten global eradication goals, and has again made the disease a public health threat. MDRTB is defined as a strain of tuberculosis that has developed resistance to both isoniazid and, most importantly, rifampin, the most

powerful bactericidal antituberculosis medications presently available. MDRTB strains originate from sites of poor tuberculosis-control infrastructure, where inadequate drug supplies, inconsistent treatment regimens, multistrain infections, and compliance failures lead to a vicious cycle of resistance build-up and reinfection.[25] Infectivity does not differ from nonresistant strains, with cough and aerosolization being the primary mode of transmission. Because of resistance, treatment of MDRTB requires the use of less potent and less tolerable second-line agents. In order to assure cure, treatment duration must be extended, typically to 18–24 months. Consequently, treatment failures are more common compared with non-MDRTB cases. Mortality rates for MDRTB presently range from 12% for persons not infected by the human immunodeficiency virus (HIV) to 90% for HIV-positive individuals.[26]

Control of MDRTB abroad and within the US requires a strong global eradication effort and the geographically sensitive screening of new immigrants.[27] Global efforts led by the World Health Organization's (WHO) Stop TB Partnership via the institution of directly observed therapy (DOT) programs among member countries has increased the number of individuals treated and slowed the annual incidence among most countries surveyed.[28] Despite this progress, however, MDRTB continues to comprise 2–4% of new infections, and has resulted in multiple serious urban outbreaks throughout the United States.[29-34] Though foreign-born individuals comprise only 10% of the US population, they also account for greater than 50% of tuberculosis cases, and consequently play an important role in spread of MDRTB.[27] Suspicion of drug-resistant TB can largely be based on origin of the immigrant. Though MDRTB has been identified in nearly every country surveyed, additional attention should be paid to immigrants from global 'hot spots' where the prevalence of MDRTB exceeds 5%, and include the countries of Kazakhstan, Uzbekistan, Israel, Estonia, Lithuania, Latvia, Ecuador, the Russian oblast Tomsk, and the Lianoning and Henan provinces of China.[35] Recently, an outbreak of MDRTB in Hmong refugees who were in the process of settling in the US from Thailand served as a reminder of the cost and threat of this infection and has led to enhanced refugee screening overseas.

## Pediatric HIV infection

An abundance of economic and social resources facilitates ease of treatment of HIV infection in the developed world. Women known to be HIV positive are offered therapy during pregnancy and their babies are offered formula rather than being breast fed, virtually eliminating mother-to-child transmission. However, in the developing world lack of public health resources has hampered efforts to control pediatric HIV/AIDS. In some countries with high rates of HIV, limited healthcare resources, social stigmatization, lack of safe alternative nutrition sources, and poor infrastructure hinder prevention efforts aimed at reducing perinatal HIV transmission. Although perinatal HIV infection in the US has become rare because of available interventions, it is worth noting that because of many disparities in healthcare, including lack of knowledge of the importance of prenatal care, immigrant women are much more likely to present for delivery with unknown or positive HIV status, placing the infant at greater risk. Also, some immigrants and refugees are coming from areas of the world where HIV is highly endemic. At the time of migration, existing children in the family may be infected. With the reduction in mother-to-child transmission in the US, the pediatric HIV-infected cohort is rapidly aging. Thus, access to a provider experienced in handling pediatric HIV infection and its concomitant complications may be more difficult, particularly if families resettle in smaller communities.

### Arthropod-borne disease

The viral mosquito-borne diseases, dengue and chikungunya, have emerged over the past several decades. There are competent vectors for both these diseases in the US, and, as with West Nile virus, there is a real possibility of the introduction of disease into the US. In fact, dengue fever has been transmitted within the continental US near the Mexican border and outbreaks have occurred in Hawaii and Puerto Rico. With international air travel, an infected traveler, immigrant, or refugee may travel to another continent during the incubation period of these diseases. As a result, ill patients may present to healthcare providers in locales without endemic disease, confounding the diagnostic skills of clinicians and acting as a potential nidus for introduction to the US.

Dengue is a flavivirus causing acute illness, classically presenting with fever, arthralgia, headache, retro-orbital pain, and rash, though clinical manifestations may vary from asymptomatic to undifferentiated viral syndrome to classic disease. Severe manifestations include dengue shock syndrome and dengue hemorrhagic fever. Although serologic tests for dengue are quite good, other flavivirus serologies

are notoriously non-specific, and may cross-react, further complicating diagnosis. False-positive test results may incorrectly suggest the diagnosis of yellow fever, West Nile, or St. Louis encephalitis, for example.

Chikungunya fever has a similar presentation to dengue, with symptoms of polyarthropathy, rash, and fever most common. As opposed to dengue, the articular manifestations are more severe and may persist for months. The maculopapular rash may be pruritic, although it is very difficult to distinguish from dengue on clinical grounds. It is caused by an alphavirus transmitted primarily by *Aedes aegypti*. *Aedes albopictus* and *Ae. vittatus* may also serve as vectors. The virus normally circulates in a sylvatic cycle similar to yellow fever, transmitted between primates in forests, with occasional epidemic urban spread. The incubation period is 2–10 days. Starting in late 2005, a very large outbreak of chikungunya was noted in the southwest Indian Ocean countries of Mauritius, the Seychelles, and Reunion Island and is currently ongoing in southern India.[36] The epidemic led to numerous imported cases to Europe, especially French-speaking nations, and a smaller number of cases to Canada, Martinique, French Guyana, and the US.

## Imported Products and Emerging Infectious Diseases

Aside from the movement of peoples, trade of products can serve as a mode of transmission of emerging infectious diseases. International trade in bushmeat (the meat of wild animals) and animal products may facilitate transmission of infectious agents across borders.[37,38]

## Prevention

The struggle to contain emerging infectious disease relies on public health investment and prevention efforts. As has been demonstrated over the last century, public health investment can achieve eradication of disease, improve standards of living, and increase life expectancy. Spread of infectious diseases by refugees and immigrants is prevented by the careful assessment of individuals prior to immigration and after arrival in the US. This includes general health assessment, testing for select infections, PPD placement and chest roentgenography, immunizations, and in some cases, antimicrobial presumptive therapy. The Centers for Disease

Control and Prevention may use quarantine and isolation procedures to prevent spread of disease from those suspected or documented with contagious disease.

## Conclusion

The threat of emerging infectious diseases will continue to cloud our future, with new and recurring infections ever present to wreck havoc on human populations. The pathogens that are the threat of the future may be ones that were previously thought contained or even eradicated. They may be diseases long ignored because they no longer afflict those living in comfort in the developed world despite continuing to exact their toll among the disenfranchised. Or they may be newly identified as they emerge from the crevices of an ever-shrinking world. The challenge to healthcare providers and public health workers is to continue to advocate for basic healthcare for all and to be ever vigilant to the smoldering outbreak poised to become the next headline emerging disease.

## Acknowledgements

Sincere appreciation is given to Dr. Christie Reed of the Centers for Disease Control and Prevention for her erudite comments and expert review of draft versions of this chapter.

## References

1. World Health Organization. The global eradication of smallpox: final report of the global commission for the certification of smallpox eradication. History of International Public Health, No. 4. Geneva: World Health Organization; 1980.
2. Achievements in Public Health: Elimination of Rubella and Congenital Rubella Syndrome – United States, 1969–2004. Vol 54, No MM11;279.
3. World Health Organization. Report on global surveillance of epidemic-prone infectious disease. Geneva, Switzerland: WHO; 2003.
4. Sencer DJ. Emerging diseases of man and animals. Ann Rev Microbiol 1971; 25:465–486.
5. Krause R. The restless tide: the persistent challenge of the microbial world. Washington, DC: National Foundation for Infectious Diseases; 1981.
6. Lederberg J, Shope RE, Oakes SC Jr. Emerging infections: microbial threats to health in the United States. Washington, DC: Institute of Medicine National Academy Press; 1992.
7. ProMED-mail. 2/10/2003. Archive number 20030210.0357. Available: http://www.promedmail.org/pls/askus/f?p = 2400:1001:::NO::F2400_P1001_BACK_PAGE,F2400_P1001_PUB_MAIL_ID:1000%2C20658 January 14, 2006.
8. Centers for Disease Control and Prevention. Update: outbreak of acute febrile illness among athletes participating in Eco-Challenge-Sabah 2000 – Borneo, Malaysia, 2000. MMWR 2001; 50(2):21–24.
9. Crosby AW Jr. The Columbian exchange: Biological and cultural consequences of 1492. Westport, CT: Greenwood press; 1972.
10. Kermack WO, McKendrick AG. Contributions to the mathematical theory of epidemics. R Statistical Soc J 1927; 115:700–721.
11. Smolinski MS, Hamburg MA, Lederberg J, eds. Microbial threats to health: emergence, detection, and response. Washington, DC: Institute of Medicine National Academy Press; 2003.
12. Farmer P. Social inequalities and emerging infectious diseases. Emerg Infect Dis 1996; 2(4):259–269.
13. Centers for Disease Control and Prevention. Increase in African immigrants and refugees with tuberculosis – Seattle–King County, Washington, 1998–2001. MMWR 2002; 51(39):882–883.
14. Johnson NPAS, Mueller J. Updating the accounts: global mortality of the 1918–1920 'Spanish' influenza pandemic. Bull Hist Med 2002; 76:105–115.
15. Fauci AS. Emerging and re-emerging infectious diseases [commentary]. Cell 2006; 124:665–670.
16. Kaye D, Pringle CR. Avian influenza viruses and their implication for human health. Clin Infect Dis 2005; 40:108–112.
17. Webster RG, Bean WJ, Gorman OT, et al. Evolution and ecology of influenza A viruses. Microbiol Rev 1992; 56(1):152–179.
18. Cox NJ, Subbarao K. Global epidemiology of influenza: past and present. Ann Rev Med 2000; 51:407–421.
19. Taubenberger JK, Reid AH, Lourens RM, et al. Characterization of the 1918 influenza virus polymerase genes. Nature 2005; 437:889–893.
20. Russell CJ, Webster RG. The genesis of pandemic influenza virus. Cell 2005; 123(3):368–371.
21. Call SA, Vollenweider MA, Hornung CA, et al. Does this patient have influenza? JAMA 2005; 293:987–997.
22. Thompson WW, Shay DK, Weintraub E, et al. Influenza-associated hospitalizations in the United States. JAMA 2004; 292:1333–1340.
23. Kobasa D, Takada A, Shinya K, et al. Enhanced virulence of influenza A viruses with the haemagglutinin of the 1918 pandemic virus. Nature 2004; 431:703–707.
24. Jefferson T, Demicheli V, Rivetti D, et al. Antivirals for influenza in healthy adults: systematic review. Lancet 2006; 367:303–313.
25. Mukherjee JS, Rich ML, Socci AR, et al. Programmes and principles in treatment of multidrug-resistant tuberculosis. Lancet 2004; 363:474–481.
26. Chan ED, et al. Treatment and outcome analysis of 205 patients with multidrug-resistant tuberculosis. Am J Resp Crit Care Med 2004; 169:1103–1109.
27. Khan K, Muennig P, Behta M, et al. Global drug-resistance patterns and the management of latent tuberculosis infection in immigrants to the United States. N Engl J Med 2002; 347:1850–1859.
28. Dye C, Watt CJ, Bleed DM, et al. Evolution of tuberculosis control and prospects for reducing tuberculosis incidence, prevalence, and deaths globally. JAMA 2005; 293:2767–2775.
29. Dye C, Espinal MA, Watt CJ, et al. Worldwide incidence of multidrug-resistant tuberculosis. J Infect Dis 2002; 185:1197–1202.
30. Granich RM, Oh P, Lewis B, et al. Multidrug resistance among persons with tuberculosis in California, 1994–2003. JAMA 2005; 293:2732–2739.
31. Ridzon R, Kent JH, Valway S, et al. Outbreak of drug-resistant tuberculosis with second-generation transmission in a high school in California. J Pediatr 1997; 131:863–868.
32. Centers for Disease Control and Prevention. Outbreak of multidrug-resistant tuberculosis – Texas, California, and Pennsylvania. JAMA 1990; 264:173–174.

33. Friedman CR, Stoeckle MY, Kreiswirth BN, et al. Transmission of multidrug-resistant tuberculosis in a large urban setting. Am J Respiratory Crit Care Med 1995; 152:355–359.

34. Frieden TR, Fujiwara PI, Washko IM, et al. Tuberculosis in New York City: Turning the Tide. N Engl J Med 1995; 333:229–233.

35. World Health Organization. Anti-tuberculosis drug resistance in the world, third global report. Publication WHO/HTM/TB/2004.343. Geneva: World Health Organization; 2004.

36. World Health Organization. Available: http://www.who.int/csr/don/2006_02_17a/en/ June 27, 2006.

37. Parliamentary Office of Science and Technology. 2005. The bushmeat trade. Postnote 236: 1–4. Available: http://www.parliament.uk/documents/upload/POSTpn236.pdf. June 27, 2006.

38. Centers for Disease Control and Prevention. Inhalation anthrax associated with dried animal hides – Pennsylvania and New York City. 2006 MMWR 55(10):280–282.

# CHAPTER 19

# Tuberculosis

John Bernardo

## Introduction

Tuberculosis (TB) remains a leading cause of morbidity and mortality in the world today. The disease is pandemic, with the highest per-capita rates now occurring in Africa, where disease incidence is increasing and a quarter of the world's new cases develop; another half occurs in six Asian countries. In 2003, 8.8 million people around the world became ill with TB, corresponding to case rates in many countries far in excess of 100 per 100 000 of population (Fig. 19.1). More than 2 million TB-related deaths are estimated to occur annually, worldwide. Tuberculosis is the most common cause of death among HIV-infected people, especially in Africa, being responsible for nearly 250 000 deaths annually, and the disease causes more deaths among women worldwide than all causes of maternal mortality combined. Most TB deaths occur among young adults during their most productive years, providing an additional, substantial burden for developing economies.

Widespread mismanagement of infectious cases and lack of adequate prevention efforts have contributed to the increasing disease incidence and the emergence of drug-resistant strains of the organism. Multidrug resistant (MDR) disease, defined by resistance to at least isoniazid and rifampin, remains a serious problem, with almost 500 000 cases occurring each year, most in the former USSR and in China. Furthermore, within many cultures, TB is highly stigmatized, adding additional complexities to diagnosis and management.[1]

The effects of this pandemic clearly are being seen in the United States where, despite overall declines in incidence, non-US-born persons are making up an ever increasing proportion of persons with the disease. In contrast to the world situation, US cases have been decreasing in overall number since 1992. The 14,093 domestic TB cases reported in 2005 represented a case rate of 4.8 per 100 000, a 3.8% decrease from 2004. Yet that rate of decline is slowing and in 2005, 20 states reported increases in disease incidence from 2004; furthermore, non-US-born persons accounted for 54% of cases, representing a majority of US cases for the fourth consecutive year (Fig. 19.2). Among these cases, most develop TB disease within 5 years of entering the United States.[2]

Patterns of immigration and resettlement therefore drive the epidemiology of TB in the US today. In the United States, the regions with highest disease incidence include those states on the southern border and states with 'port' cities, those cities where large numbers of people enter the country and settle. Screening of persons entering the United States from abroad for tuberculosis is limited to those entering as legal immigrants and those applying for legal status once in residence (see below). Countless others undergo no screening; these include visitors, students, business people, and other, undocumented entrants, who arrive daily, many from regions of the world where TB is endemic, and where exceedingly high rates of 'latent TB infection,' i.e. tuberculosis in its latent (or dormant) form, occur. While many persons may enter the US with undetected, active disease, TB is preventable in persons with latent infection, in whom disease has not developed. Persons with latent TB infection, if untreated, make up the reservoir of future cases of TB disease, and have a clear impact on the epidemiology of TB in the US today.

Tuberculosis is a preventable disease for which there is good treatment. However, strategies to control TB must include four elements: (1) *early diagnosis* of disease, to reduce morbidity and minimize

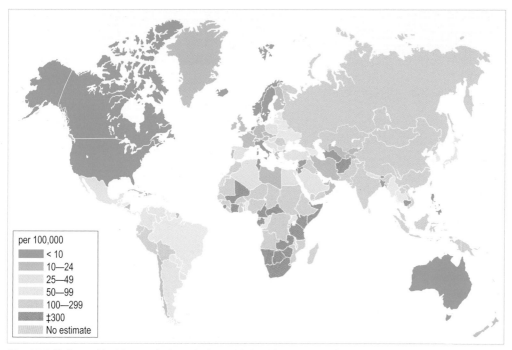

**Fig. 19.1** Estimated incidence of tuberculosis worldwide, World Health Organization, 2002.

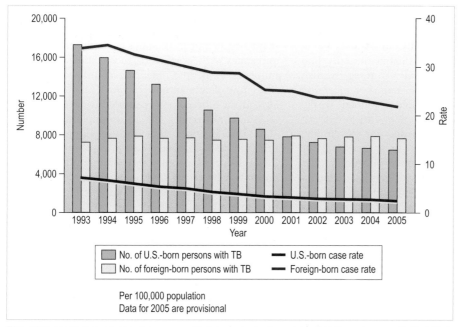

**Fig. 19.2** Number and rate of persons with tuberculosis, by origin of birth and year – United States, 1993–2000. (From: CDC. Trends in tuberculosis – United States. 2005; MMWR 55(11):305–308.)

disease transmission, (2) appropriate administration of a complete course of *multidrug treatment* to persons with active tuberculosis for a sufficient period of time (usually 6 months or longer) to cure the disease, (3) treatment of high-risk, *TB-infected* persons to prevent future cases, and (4) a program of *education and support* for healthcare providers and for people at risk, in order to destigmatize the disease and facilitate the previous three elements.[3] Many new arrivals have customs and beliefs that may be in conflict with these principles of TB control and may have limited resources and conflicting priorities; TB control must be made *accessible and acceptable* to them if the US health system is to have an impact on the disease in the United States. Furthermore, since many features of successful TB control reside outside the domain of the private healthcare sector, where many new arrivals turn for healthcare, implementation of successful TB control demands that public health resources be applied to support an infrastructure that now involves these private providers and prioritizes the effective management of TB infection and disease.

## Etiology

The natural history of the disease may make the detection of clinical tuberculosis difficult. Primary infection may not be clinically apparent; patients with active TB disease may be asymptomatic or may deny symptoms, but still may transmit the disease, and fears of social stigmatization and of government authority may deter patients who may be ill from seeking care until the disease has become advanced. Also, healthcare providers may not be considering TB in their evaluation of a patient with respiratory symptoms, unless TB is commonly seen in their patient populations.

*Mycobacterium tuberculosis* is transmitted in most cases by human-to-human spread of aerosolized respiratory secretions. Droplet nuclei generated by coughing or sneezing, suspended in the air, are dispersed from a source case by air currents.[4] During inhalation by a naïve host, droplet nuclei from an infectious patient that contain viable mycobacteria are small enough to penetrate the alveolar ducts of the tracheobronchial tree, where they are ingested by alveolar macrophages and establish a focus of infection, which may be subclinical. Infectiousness of the source varies from patient to patient, with virulence of the organisms that cause the disease, and with susceptibility of the new host. Patients with clinical TB who have a tuberculous cavity may dis-

charge millions of tubercle bacilli into the air with each cough, and usually are judged the most infectious.

*Primary infection* results when macrophages containing viable mycobacteria penetrate the alveolar wall and circulate via the blood and lymphatic systems to other regions of the body.[5] During this time, usually 4–12 weeks, lymphocytes become sensitized to TB antigens, in a process that may be documented as development of tuberculin sensitivity. This is measured by conversion of the tuberculin skin test from negative to positive. Following sensitization, healing usually begins with the formation of granulomas and fibrosis at the sites to which these macrophages have migrated, as originally described by Robert Koch in 1881. However, viable bacilli remain localized within these granulomas; they alter their metabolism and enter a period of *latency* (dormancy) in order to survive in the inhospitable environment at these sites.[6,7] Rarely, in some patients, such as children under the age of 5 and immunosuppressed HIV-infected persons, containment may not occur, and *progressive, primary tuberculosis* develops. This may involve primarily the lung, but usually it is a disseminated process that may involve multiple organs and may be rapidly fatal.

Latency usually persists for the life of the new host. However, in an estimated 10% of persons with latent TB infection (LTBI), sites of containment may break down at some later date, usually for poorly understood reasons, and *reactivation tuberculosis* develops. The greatest risk for reactivation disease appears to be within the first 2 years of acquiring the primary TB infection, also for unclear reasons. Several *medical conditions* favor development of reactivation disease; these include malnutrition, chronic corticosteroid use or use of certain immunologic-suppressant medications (such as *tumor necrosis factor-alpha* inhibitors), AIDS, insulin-dependent diabetes mellitus, and some hematologic/lymphoreticular malignancies. The lung apices are the most common sites of reactivation TB (70–85%), but the disease also may commonly appear in the lymphatic system, the kidneys and adrenal glands, or the central nervous system as isolated foci of disease. Reactivation pulmonary TB usually is the most infectious form of the disease; its development recapitulates the infection cycle, permitting spread to others via aerosolized respiratory droplets. Latency provides an opportunity for *prevention* of tuberculosis by treatment of latent infection with medications.

To healthy, non-TB-infected adults, tuberculosis generally is not highly infectious. Unlike influenza, where brief exposure may result in infection, it is believed that a relatively intense and prolonged exposure to an infectious patient, usually expressed as hours in a confined airspace where air is shared among individuals, is required for a primary infection to become established. In contrast, young children, especially those under the age of 5, or immunosuppressed persons have a greater risk of becoming infected, and then, as noted earlier, of developing disseminated primary disease, than do others. Racial and genetic predispositions to tuberculosis have never been proved; tuberculosis is a disease that does not discriminate by race.

Timely diagnosis and prompt initiation of treatment of persons with infectious TB is the best way to minimize spread to others; treatment with multiple antituberculosis medications renders most patients noninfectious within weeks. Although many cases may be treated as outpatients with appropriate case management, persons with infectious tuberculosis who may be a danger to the public's health should be kept in respiratory isolation until they are judged to be not infectious. Medications must be taken as recommended, medical and social conditions that might impair treatment must be addressed, and patients should be educated about their disease. Nonhospitalized patients early in treatment should avoid situations where others may be exposed; they also should be instructed in how to cover their mouth/nose when coughing/sneezing in order to minimize the spread of infectious respiratory droplets. Clearly, however, *prevention* of development of disease is effective in reducing the need to take these measures.[3]

## Primary tuberculosis

### Clinical presentation

Primary tuberculosis today in the US occurs most commonly in young *children*; often clinically silent, it usually is discovered during the investigation of contacts of an infectious case.[8] As described above, during the 4–12 weeks following inhalation of infected droplets, local tissue reactions develop in the lungs and lympho-hematogenous dissemination of tubercle bacilli occurs, along with immune sensitization. In young children, tubercle bacilli proliferate within the exudative parenchymal focus in the lung, usually located in its lower zones (middle or lower lobes, or lingula), and are carried to regional, draining lymph nodes, including those of the regional hilum (Fig. 19.3). These nodes become the site of a further inflammatory response, as sensitization

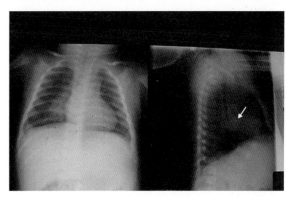

**Fig. 19.3** Primary tuberculosis, right lower lobe, in a child. Note hilar adenopathy, especially on lateral view (arrow).

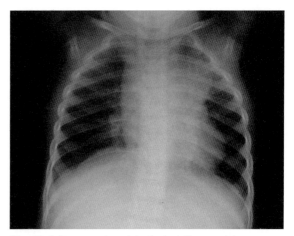

**Fig. 19.4** Compression atelectasis, left upper lobe. Primary tuberculosis in a child (different patient from Figure 19.3).

develops; they become enlarged and they may compress adjacent bronchi, causing segmental lobar atelectasis, often seen as a manifestation of primary tuberculosis in children (Fig. 19.4). Central necrosis within the parenchymal focus and regional lymph nodes may occur; this process is followed by eventual healing of the lesions and, in some cases, by subsequent calcification. If the disease process continues, caseation ('cheese-like') necrosis in enlarged nodes may erode into bronchi and result in endobronchial spread of infected, necrotic material. The calcified lesions seen on radiographic studies at sites of healed infection and in the local nodes are the classic lesions of primary tuberculosis, termed *Ghon complexes*.

Irritability or failure to thrive may be the only symptoms of primary TB disease in children; weight loss also is common. The symptoms of acute primary tuberculosis in children also may include abdominal pain as a manifestation of pulmonary or intra-abdominal disease, diarrhea, cough, and anorexia. Young children with primary TB usually are not infectious, despite symptoms. Low numbers of organisms contained in the lesions and poor generation of aerosol droplets usually are given as the reason for children being noninfectious.

Primary tuberculosis in *adults* usually also may be asymptomatic or non-specific in its presentation. Fever, a mild 'flu-like' syndrome, or a nonproductive cough may be noted; malaise, weight loss, anorexia, and fatigue also may occur, usually of several weeks' or months' duration. Regional and hilar adenopathy on the chest radiograph is not as prominent as in children with primary TB; the local pulmonary infection usually is contained more rapidly by cellular immune mechanisms than in young children and it often heals with few, if any, radiologic sequelae.

Persons at risk who present to medical care with persisting (generally greater than 3–4 weeks), non-specific complaints, fatigue, or cough should be evaluated clinically for TB. The risk assessment and evaluation generally should include a thorough history, including recent travel to an endemic area, inquiry for recent contact to a known case of TB, a physical examination, with particular attention to the lungs and lymphatic system, and a chest radiograph, to rule out tuberculosis. A single, frontal view (usually posterior–anterior) chest radiograph usually is sufficient in adults.[9] In children, addition of a lateral view permits visualization of hilar structures that may not be seen on the frontal projection. A positive tuberculin skin test or gamma-interferon release assay for TB (e.g. QuantiFERON-Gold®) may be helpful in supporting a diagnosis of TB, although a negative result does not exclude disease. Fifteen to 25% of patients with newly diagnosed tuberculosis fail to demonstrate a positive skin test or Quanti-FERON test; therefore, these should not be used as sole screening tests for disease. Importantly, a child or adult with TB risks, such as former residence in a TB-endemic country, and a respiratory illness that fails to respond to treatment in a timely fashion should be evaluated carefully for active tuberculosis.

## Other presentations

A localized, healed tuberculous pneumonia, a 'tuberculoma,' must be differentiated from other causes of solitary nodules (also called coin lesions), especially in persons at risk for other disorders, such as adults with risk factors for lung cancer, or children or adults

from regions where other pulmonary infections (e.g. fungal lesions, melioidosis, etc.) may be common. Likewise, hilar adenopathy may be striking in primary tuberculosis, especially in children, but it also may be attributable to other disorders, such as lymphoma, sarcoid, or other infections.

*Tuberculous pleurisy* usually is caused by inflammatory lesions ('tubercles') lying close to the pleural surface that rupture through the visceral pleura into the pleural space, creating a pleural effusion. This process may cause pleuritic pain, although it may be asymptomatic and first noted as an incidental finding during a medical evaluation. Spontaneous pneumothorax also may occur as a complication of pleural TB. Pleural fluid characteristically is exudative, lymphocytic, and has a very low glucose concentration; the chest radiograph also may show evidence of disease elsewhere. Tuberculous pleural effusion rarely demonstrates organisms on microscopy; a pleural biopsy often is required to establish the diagnosis. *Primary tuberculous pneumonia* may progress from the primary lesion, presenting with pulmonary infiltration on radiography in lower lung zones (i.e. middle lobe or lingula, or lower lobes) and physical findings similar to other, nontuberculous pneumonias, with which it may be confused.

*Miliary tuberculosis* may first be suspected when a fine nodular infiltration is noted on the chest radiograph or computed tomography (CT) scan. Other organs, such as the liver, spleen, kidney, bone marrow, and the central nervous system are often involved; patients may have high fever; weakness and prostration are common and cough and pulmonary findings may be absent. The tuberculin skin test usually is not reactive. Confirmation of a diagnosis of miliary TB requires a confirmatory laboratory test result (nucleic acid amplification or culture) from an involved organ or tissue (e.g. sputum, liver, lymph node, bone marrow, cerebrospinal fluid). However, once the diagnosis is suspected treatment must not be withheld; prompt initiation of multiple drug therapy is critical, since this form of tuberculosis is almost uniformly fatal if not treated.

## Latent tuberculosis

The vast majority of persons who become infected with *M. tuberculosis* are able to contain the organisms that become disseminated during the process of primary infection. These organisms remain in a latent state at sites of dissemination until the containment process breaks down and reactivation disease occurs – in about 10% of infected persons (see below). This period of latency offers an important opportunity to prevent reactivation TB disease from developing by treating the infection. Diagnosis is established by the *tuberculin skin test* or by new, blood cell *gamma-Interferon release assays*, such as *QuantiFERON-Gold®*.

## The tuberculin skin test

Tuberculin, discovered by Koch around 1890, was developed into a diagnostic test for identifying tuberculous infection by von Pirquet in 1907. The tuberculin antigen used in the United States is 'purified protein derivative' (PPD) of *M. tuberculosis*, stabilized by the addition of detergent (Tween 80) to the suspension; the antigen is standardized by bioassay and is stable in its bottle if refrigerated. Intracutaneous injection of 0.1 mL of 5 TU PPD is performed using a 1 mL calibrated syringe and a 25- or 26-gauge needle. Skin, by convention usually on the flexor surface of the forearm, is cleansed with alcohol, and the needle tip is inserted just beneath the surface so that the injection creates a slight wheal (termed *Mantoux technique*).[10,11] A tuberculin test is interpreted 48–72 hours after its application. Induration at the test site, transverse to the long axis of the arm, is palpated and is measured in millimeters; erythema is not relevant. A positive reaction, defined as a reaction greater than 5, 10, or 15 mm induration,

according to risk, identifies *M. tuberculosis* infection (Table 19.1).

The TB skin test is not ideal; its sensitivity and specificity are influenced by the integrity of the immune response to TB infection and to the test, and by prior sensitization to other mycobacterial antigens, such as environmental mycobacteria or prior vaccination with bacille Calmette-Guérin (BCG). Skin reactivity in a positive reactor may be lessened or completely suppressed by a number of factors; these include AIDS, recent live viral vaccination, current viral infection, extreme malnutrition, overwhelming TB disease, or concurrent use of immunosuppressive medications, such as corticosteroids.

The *BCG vaccine* uses an attenuated, live strain of bovine tuberculosis; it usually is administered to children in most countries outside the US for protection against tuberculosis, although protection conferred by the vaccine likely is limited to early childhood.[12] It is believed by many BCG-vaccinated people that prior BCG vaccination induces tuberculin skin test reactivity, and that a positive TB skin test in a vaccinated person is a sign of the vaccine's effectiveness. However, the cross-reacting response to tuberculin testing following BCG, if one occurs at all, usually is small and it decreases in size rapidly following vaccination. In addition, the degree of actual protection conferred by the vaccination is highly variable, and people who receive BCG usually

**Table 19.1 Criteria for positive tuberculin skin test, by risk**

| 5 mm | 10 mm | 15 mm |
|---|---|---|
| HIV-positive (known) | Recent (≤5 yr) immigration | No known risk |
| Recent close contact to infectious TB patient | Injection drug users | |
| Fibrotic changes on chest radiograph consistent with old active TB (not pleural thickening) | Residents/employees of high-risk settings (e.g. prisons/jails, long-term care facilities, nursing homes, healthcare facilities, homeless shelters, residences for HIV-infected persons) | |
| Other immunosuppression (e.g. organ transplant recipient, chronic corticosteroid therapy: equiv. of prednisone ≥15 mg/d for ≥1 mon | Mycobacterial laboratory staff<br>Children ≤4 yr of age; infants/children/adolescents exposed to high-risk adults | |
| | Persons with clinical conditions that place them at high TB risk: silicosis, diabetes mellitus, chronic renal failure, some lympho/hematologic disorders (e.g. leukemias, lymphomas), certain malignancies (e.g. carcinoma of head/neck, lung), weight loss of ≥10% ideal body weight, gastrectomy, jejuno-ileal bypass | |

arrive from regions of the world where TB is endemic and a large proportion of the adult population truly is infected with *M. tuberculosis*. For these reasons, a positive skin test response in a high-risk person who has received BCG in the past usually is interpreted in the US as signaling true infection with *M. tuberculosis*, often putting the patient in conflict with his or her US provider and the US healthcare system. These issues may be settled in the future as experience is gained with new tests for TB infection (see below).

## Gamma-Interferon release assays

Newer blood tests for tuberculosis infection, such as the gamma-Interferon release assays *QuantiFERON Gold®* (Cellestis, Ltd., Carnegie, Victoria, Australia), approved by the US Food and Drug Administration (FDA) in 2005, and the *T- SPOT.TB®* (Oxford Immunotech, Ltd., Abingdon, Oxon, UK), utilize antigens that are secreted by *M. tuberculosis*-complex organisms and a small number of other mycobacteria – *but not by BCG* or by common environmental mycobacteria. These tests demonstrate sensitivity similar to that of the tuberculin skin test in persons with active tuberculosis. In addition, they render greater specificity to testing for TB infection than does the skin test; this enhanced specificity has been shown in several recent studies,[13-15] suggesting that current recommendations for interpretation of the tuberculin skin test in people who have received BCG may classify many skin test positive persons incorrectly as TB infected. Yet, while specificity of these tests appears greater than that of the skin test, their sensitivity for TB infection and, more importantly, their ability to identify TB-infected persons at risk for developing active TB disease is not clear, and needs to be studied. Additional studies also are needed to define the sensitivity of these tests in selected populations, such as young children and immunocompromised persons.

Blood tests for TB infection also have other limitations. These tests rely on stimulation of live, blood mononuclear leukocytes with antigen, *in vitro*; therefore, and importantly, blood samples must reach the testing laboratory and begin processing within hours of being drawn (currently 12 hours for QuantiFERON Gold®; 8 for T- SPOT.TB®), in order to ensure viability of the cells. In addition, these tests require special equipment and procedures, and availability may be limited in some jurisdictions. Guidelines for the use and interpretation of QuantiFERON Gold® were published recently by CDC.[16] These tests have other potential benefits. They require only one visit

for the blood draw and test results are not subject to the subjectivity (e.g. in interpreting the margins of a skin test induration) that has plagued the skin test. Furthermore, many people who received BCG, while familiar with the skin test and its possible confounding by BCG, do not have a similar context in which to interpret a positive laboratory test result, such as QuantiFERON. Therefore, one might speculate that they may be more likely to accept a diagnosis of TB infection if indicated by a blood test rather than a skin test.

## Reactivation tuberculosis: *adult-type* tuberculosis disease

### Pulmonary tuberculosis

The lympho-hematogenous dissemination of organisms during the primary infection and their containment during the healing phase that follows sensitization create sites that contain viable, latent organisms in various organs; this includes the lungs. These are sites where latent infection may be 'reactivated,' during post-primary, *adult-type* reactivation tuberculosis. Several medical risk factors for reactivation are well known and have been mentioned previously; these include diabetes mellitus, immunosuppression, malnutrition or recent significant weight loss, or some hematologic or lymphatic malignancies. Reactivation most often occurs in the lungs, primarily involving the lung apices (apical or posterior segments of the upper lobes) or the superior segments of the lower lobes. However, in up to 30% of cases, the disease may present in other parts of the lung. The reactivation process usually is accompanied by respiratory symptoms; however, it may be indolent until extensive pulmonary infiltration has occurred. Some patients will be asymptomatic or deny symptoms.

The radiographic characteristics of acute tuberculous pneumonia generally are similar to pneumonia of many other etiologies, such as bacterial or fungal infections. The 'typical' location of pulmonary infiltrates, accompanied by risk factors for TB, immediately should raise one's suspicion for tuberculosis (Figs. 19.5 and 19.6) (for a review of the chest radiograph in tuberculosis, see: http://www.nationaltbcenter.edu/catalogue/epub/index.cfm?tableName=RMT).[17] Parenchymal infiltrates seen on a chest radiograph may be homogeneous and lobar, and may contain air-bronchograms. Tissue necrosis resulting from intense inflammation may accompany the infiltration, creating cavities within the parenchyma. A productive cough may render such patients highly infectious at this stage of their

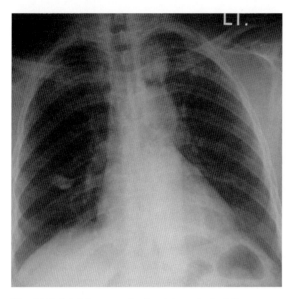

**Fig. 19.5** Adult-type reactivation tuberculosis, left upper lobe. This was the source case for the patient illustrated in Figure 19.4 (grandmother). Note calcified focus left-mid lung field, likely representing site of remote, primary infection (with accompanying hilar node representing Gohn complex).

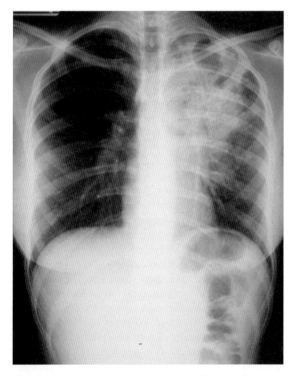

**Fig. 19.6** Left upper lobe tuberculosis, with cavitation.

illness. Many cases heal spontaneously, resulting in focal fibrosis and lung volume loss. This in turn may result in compensatory changes within adjacent lung, such as localized emphysema, and calcification of healed foci. While treatment may speed healing, untreated disease may progress to cause respiratory failure or fatal hemoptysis.

Typical symptoms include fevers and/or night sweats (described classically as 'drenching'), weight loss, as well as cough or chest pain. The patient may appear chronically ill, or the patient may be afebrile and appear well. Physical examination may reveal focal rales or signs of focal airways involvement (wheezes or rhonchi), or signs of a pleural effusion. Nevertheless, early diagnosis and initiation of effective multiple drug therapy minimizes destruction of lung and late consequences of disease.

### Extrapulmonary tuberculosis

Extrapulmonary tuberculosis still constitutes approximately 20% of new cases in the US and a greater proportion of cases overseas. Extrapulmonary TB may represent a sequel of primary infection or reactivation disease; it usually is not infectious, unless drainage from an active site of disease becomes aerosolized. The most common disease sites include lymph nodes, bones and joints, and the liver.

**Lymph nodes** Patients with lymphatic tuberculosis usually present with signs and symptoms related to their site of disease, although, as with TB anywhere, symptoms may be nonspecific ('constitutional') or they may be absent. Hilar and mediastinal lymphadenopathy are common features of primary tuberculosis infection, but they also may be present in reactivation TB. Enlarged intrathoracic lymph nodes may compress airways, creating focal wheezing or bronchial obstruction. Infected lymph nodes may enlarge further during treatment, in a phenomenon often attributed to a 'reconstitution' of the cellular immune response, as with TB/AIDS patients who are undergoing treatment for both diseases. Cervical lymph nodes are commonly the primary site of disease. Aspiration of infectious material or biopsy are often required to differentiate TB lymphadenitis from other causes of lymph node enlargement in the neck (Fig. 19.7). As with TB adenitis anywhere else, treatment with multiple drugs is effective, but enlargement of involved lymph nodes during treatment, especially early, is common.

**Bone/joint** Bone or joint tuberculosis occurs in adults and in children. Because of its protean and

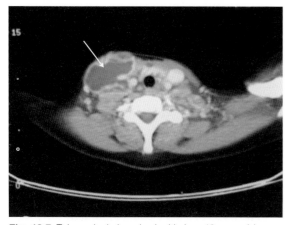

**Fig. 19.7** Tuberculosis lymphadenitis in a 13 year old child. CT scan of the neck demonstrating large, fluid-filled lymph node (arrow). Needle aspiration revealed pus, AFB stain positive.

nonspecific manifestations, the diagnosis often is delayed and may be difficult to establish. Tuberculosis should be considered in an at-risk child who presents with scoliosis or a limp, especially if other constitutional symptoms are present. In adults, reactivation of TB in bone or a joint may occur spontaneously or may be associated with trauma; the disease should be suspected in persons at risk for TB who present with bone or joint pain (including back pain) with or without swelling or fever. Radiographic findings typically include demineralization of involved bone with preservation of joint surfaces, especially in early stages of the disease. With chronic disease, complete destruction of bone may be seen. Vertebral body tuberculosis (Pott's disease) can be particularly devastating if bone destruction leads to vertebral instability and compression of the spinal cord. A diagnosis of tuberculosis usually is established by biopsy and culture of the affected tissue.

**Liver** The liver usually is involved in disseminated (miliary) tuberculosis. Granulomas on freshly cut sections have the appearance of millet seeds scattered throughout the liver. Serum alkaline phosphatase usually is elevated, and jaundice and hepatomegaly are rare.

**Peritoneum** Tuberculous peritonitis, usually the result of spread from adjacent organs, should be suspected whenever a patient at risk for tuberculosis has ascites and a positive tuberculin skin test. Constitutional symptoms, including fevers and malaise, or abdominal distension and pain, also are common. Often confused for malignancy, the diagnosis may be

missed or delayed. The peritoneal surface may reveal scattered miliary lesions with caseating granulomas demonstrated on biopsy; peritoneal fluid usually is characterized by an elevated protein concentration and markers of inflammation, with a lymphocytosis. These findings are not diagnostic, however, and culture of the peritoneal fluid or of the peritoneum usually is required to document the disease.

**Meninges** Tuberculous involvement of the central nervous system, including the meninges, may occur as a manifestation of progressive primary disease or of reactivation TB, as a result of impaired containment of latent infection. The disease may be elusive in its presentation; it may occur as an acute meningitis in a young child or in an immunocompromised adult, or as an indolent disease in an elderly person. Cerebrospinal fluid (CSF) examination usually reveals a high protein, with or without xanthochromia, and very low glucose; lymphocytosis is common, although polymorphonuclear leukocytes may be seen early in the disease. Isolation of *M. tuberculosis* by culture confirms the diagnosis, and nucleic amplification testing of the CSF may support the diagnosis, but treatment should be initiated as soon as tuberculosis is suspected. If unrecognized and untreated, the disease can be fatal.

**Kidney** Tuberculosis of the urinary tract may present indolently with hematuria, proteinuria, and 'sterile' pyuria. Typically, the major involvement with disease is localized to the renal papillae, where characteristic distortion of the collecting system may be seen on radiographic studies. Flank pain, hydronephrosis, and cystitis may signal more severe disease, and spread to the genitalia is not uncommon. Focal scarring of the kidneys and the collecting system may follow successful treatment. Diagnosis is established by culture of the organism from the urine; acid-fast microscopy generally is not performed on urine samples because of the presence of non-pathogenic, non-tuberculous organisms that may inhabit the urinary tract of normal persons.

**Genitalia** Tuberculosis of the female genital tract may result from progressive spread of a primary infection or from reactivation of latent infection. Tuberculous salpingitis may accompany untreated TB elsewhere, and a concordant history of menstrual abnormalities in a woman with TB should raise this possibility. Diagnostic evaluation should include ultrasonography or other radiographic studies, dilation and curettage, and colposcopy, with histologic examination and culture of biopsy materials.

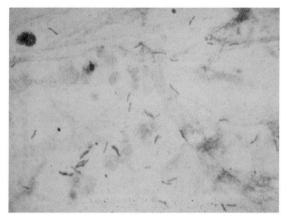

**Fig. 19.8** Acid-fast (Ziehl-Neelsen) stain demonstrating pleomorphic, acid-fast organisms. Clumping of organisms is common.

Scrotal pain and swelling, and tenderness in the epididymis or the prostate should prompt consideration of genital tuberculosis in a male patient who is at risk for TB. Urine culture and biopsy are required for diagnosis.

## Field and Laboratory Studies

### Sputum examination

Sputum microscopy should be the first test attempted in a person with suspected pulmonary tuberculosis. A sputum specimen, ideally produced by a deep cough, is digested and decontaminated in the laboratory and then is concentrated and examined by a mycobacterial stain, using either acid-fast (Ziehl-Neelsen or Kinyoun; requires approx. $10^4$ bacteria/mL sputum for a positive result) staining (Fig. 19.8) or the more sensitive fluorochrome technique (appoxr. $10^3$ bacteria/mL). Mycobacteria retain the red stain of carbol fuchsin after washing with acid alcohol, hence, the acid-fast designation.[18] Interpretation of this stain gives a *preliminary* indication of a bacteriologic diagnosis of TB if acid-fast organisms are seen; however, culture is required for confirmation. Organisms other than *M. tuberculosis* may be stained by this process, especially atypical mycobacteria, such as *M. avium*, making the smear relatively non-specific. When organisms are identified by microscopy in a sample in the proper clinical setting, a presumptive diagnosis of tuberculosis may be made. It should be noted that most patients with extensive cavitary lesions on chest X-ray will have positive results on sputum smear; however, many patients with less extensive disease will have negative smears. Negative sputum smears cannot 'rule out' a diagnosis of tuberculosis. A single sputum smear will be positive in only 20–40% of cases of pulmonary TB; three consecutive morning specimens, however, can raise the sensitivity of the smear to as high as 90%. Therefore, multiple samples should always be considered; the CDC/ATS/IDSA guidelines recommend that three sputum samples, taken at least 8 hours apart and with at least 1 early morning specimen, should be examined. Nevertheless, sputum culture is the gold standard for establishing a diagnosis of *M. tuberculosis* pulmonary disease.

Fluids and tissues obtained from sites of presumed disease also should be subjected to microscopy as an initial step in attempting to establish the diagnosis. As with sputum, however, staining is non-specific, and a positive or negative result must be interpreted in the clinical setting in which it was obtained. Here, also, culture is the gold standard.

## Culture of sputum and other specimens

### Specimens

As with microscopy, sputum obtained by deep coughing yields best results. If spontaneously produced sputum cannot be obtained, inhalation of aerosolized hypertonic (3–5%) saline may induce sputum production. Sputum induction should be performed utilizing appropriate precautions to prevent spread of infection, such as in a specialized booth or a negative-pressure room. Sputum culture should be obtained monthly during treatment in order to monitor the patient's response. In young children, gastric contents obtained by first-morning gastric aspiration following at least 9 hours of fasting, may be cultured. As with urine, discussed above, microscopy is not performed on gastric specimens.

In pleural tuberculosis, pleural fluid is positive on smear or culture in approximately 20% of cases; pleural biopsy, with culture of a specimen of parietal pleura, is positive in more than 90% of cases of pleural TB.

### Culture techniques

Mycobacterial culture methods using *liquid media* can identify mycobacterial growth in as few as 7–21 days. Culture using *solid media* usually requires up to 8 weeks to demonstrate growth; yet solid media culture remains the gold-standard. Identification of growth on cultures as *M. tuberculosis* complex usually requires additional steps, such as biochemical assays or the use of DNA/RNA probes. Growth in culture also is required to provide *drug susceptibility data* on an isolate; these may be performed using liquid or solid media, although, again, solid media-based assays are the standard.

## Other laboratory investigations

Urine, ascites, joint fluid, pus, or tissue biopsy samples should be cultured for *M. tuberculosis* when clinical disease is suspected. Instructions on appropriate handling of the sample should be obtained from consultants and/or the laboratory before an invasive procedure is performed, in order to ensure appropriate management of specimens.

## Rapid diagnostic tests

Nucleic acid amplification (NAA) assays are available (MTD®; Gen-Probe, San Diego, CA; Amplicor®, Roche Diagnostics, Alameda, CA) and are approved by the FDA for clinical use in limited settings to identify mycobacteria in sputum or respiratory secretions. In general, the use of these tests does not replace sputum microscopy and culture;[19-22] however, they may be particularly helpful in cases of smear-positive disease to provide rapid identification of the organism seen on microscopy. Nevertheless, even if NAA is performed, a culture is required for drug susceptibility testing of an isolate. Also, these tests are costly, and they generally require highly trained technical staff and specialized laboratory equipment.

## Drug susceptibility testing

Drug susceptibility testing should be performed on all initial specimens from each site of disease, and again at 3 months if cultures fail to convert to negative with appropriate treatment. This testing requires growth of organisms in culture, and it usually is performed using single drugs rather than drug combinations. Knowledge of the susceptibility of an isolate to anti-mycobacterial drugs is necessary in order to design and maintain an appropriate treatment regimen and to help assess reasons for treatment failures. Newer molecular methods, such as *molecular beacons*, are being used to detect genetic polymorphisms that confer drug resistance, such as the *rpoB* gene mutation associated with resistance to

rifampin. These tests are not approved by the FDA for clinical use at this time.

## Treatment of Tuberculosis

### Multidrug chemotherapy

The treatment of tuberculosis requires adherence to a somewhat complex regimen of multiple medications that must be taken as prescribed for a relatively lengthy time – at least 6 months, in most cases. Effective anti-tuberculosis treatment rapidly renders the patient noninfectious and reduces symptoms. However, medications must be continued for the required period in order to assure cure and prevent relapse. This may be difficult to achieve if a patient begins to feel well soon after starting treatment, if a patient is experiencing adverse side effects from the medications, or if the patient does not accept treatment.[23]

Treatment for active tuberculosis must include multiple drugs to which the patient's isolate is susceptible, in order to cover for primary drug resistance (in 2004, 10.4% of non-US-born cases were resistant to isoniazid on initial culture; 1.3% were resistant to isoniazid and rifampin[24]) and to prevent the development of secondary drug resistance. Single-drug therapy should never be used in a TB suspect, since use of a single drug in a patient with a high organism burden, as usually is seen in active disease, may select for drug resistance. Since drug susceptibility information rarely is known at the start of treatment, current CDC/ATS/IDSA treatment guidelines recommend an *initial four-drug regimen* for most patients; this regimen then is modified as bacteriology data become available. Prompt treatment, if started early in the course of the disease, reduces destruction of lung parenchyma and reduces the risk to the public health by minimizing spread to the community. More than 95% of patients receiving appropriate multidrug treatment will be sputum-culture negative within 3 months.

### Case management

Responsibility for successful completion of therapy for tuberculosis rests with the *provider* and the *public health-TB program – not* with the patient.[3,23]

In the US, a system of *patient-centered case management* for TB cases and suspects, using direct observation of medication ingestion by a healthcare worker (termed *DOT*) as a major strategy, has become the standard of care. True case management requires collaboration between the treating physician, the public health system and its laboratory infrastructure, and the patient to ensure that treatment is completed safely and achieves cure. Barriers to treatment, such as access to medications and clinic visits, and a lack of understanding of the disease and its treatment by patient and, in some cases, provider must be overcome. Medications must be made available to patients; medical care also must be provided for patients with insufficient resources to engage healthcare independently. This care must be acceptable to the patients in order to be successful. Among immigrant populations, community-based public health services that provide education to persons at risk and to patients serve to raise awareness of TB and reduce stigmatization of the disease. Such program efforts have been shown to improve acceptance of principles of TB control among difficult to reach populations.[25]

## Drug regimens

Treatment with at least two medications to which the organism is believed to be susceptible should be initiated as soon as tuberculosis is suspected. Isoniazid (INH), rifampin (RIF), pyrazinamide (PZA), and ethambutol (EMB) are the standard initial drugs used for treatment of most active TB cases or suspects in the US today.[23] The inclusion of PZA for 8 weeks in the initial regimen permits a 6-month course in most patients with drug-susceptible disease; EMB is added to cover for possible primary resistance to any of the other drugs. Pyridoxine (vitamin $B_6$; 50 mg) may be given to prevent neurologic side effects of INH, but may not be necessary if the patient's diet is adequate. Following an initial four-drug, 8-week regimen, PZA and EMB may be stopped in most patients with drug-susceptible disease who have responded to treatment and INH and RIF continued for an additional 16 weeks.

If drug susceptibility is known at the start of treatment and the isolate is susceptible, INH and RIF alone may be given for a total of 9 months, as an alternative. If cultures of respiratory tract secretions are negative in a pulmonary tuberculosis suspect, 16 weeks (4 months) of INH and RIF may be considered complete treatment. Specific drug regimens, including doses and schedules, and alternative treatment regimens are provided in detail in the CDC/ATS/IDSA treatment guidelines.[23]

During treatment of pulmonary TB, a sputum specimen must be obtained for culture *at least monthly* until at least two sequential samples are culture negative. Extending therapy beyond 6 months may be required if cultures remain positive at 2 months, especially if cavitary disease was present on the initial chest radiograph.[23] Sputum cultures that remain positive after 3 months' treatment should prompt a search for an explanation for delayed culture conversion. This investigation should include repeat drug susceptibility testing on the 3-month isolate.

Patients with INH- and/or RIF-resistant disease, with a delayed clinical response, or with delayed sputum conversion, should be managed with the assistance of an expert in tuberculosis.

## Monitoring: adverse effects of treatment

Patients, case managers, and physicians must understand the possible adverse effects of anti-tuberculosis medications in order to maximize the safety of treatment. Clinical monitoring for adverse effects of treatment should be conducted at least monthly; in some patients this may be supplemented by laboratory tests. Case managers and persons administering DOT should question the patient at each DOT session about possible side effects of the medications.

A small number of patients receiving INH will experience fatigue; this may be avoided if the patient takes the drug at night before bed. Isoniazid elevates hepatic enzymes mildly (up to $3–5 \times$ the upper limit of normal) in 10–20% of patients. These elevations usually are transient and subside during treatment. Drug-induced hepatitis is an uncommon but potentially serious, even fatal, side effect of INH; patients with INH hepatitis usually are older and use other hepatotoxic drugs or alcohol.[26] Also, an increased incidence has been reported in young black or Hispanic women, especially postpartum.[27] Liver function tests ('baseline' ALT and/or AST) should be obtained at the initiation of treatment in persons at risk for hepatitis (history of hepatitis B or C, alcohol or injecting drug abuse, co-ingestion of potentially hepatotoxic medications, age > 35, or Hispanic or black women, or pregnant and recent (3 months) postpartum women.

Monthly evaluations should include a symptom review for toxicity.[28] In persons older than 35 years or at risk for hepatitis, monthly liver function studies may be obtained.

Patients should be instructed to stop isoniazid *immediately* should symptoms of hepatitis develop (right-upper quadrant abdominal pain or discomfort, anorexia, nausea, vomiting, dark [like coffee or tea] urine, jaundice) and then consult the care provider. Isoniazid also must be stopped if serum ALT/AST rises to greater than three times the upper limit of normal if the patient has symptoms, or to greater than five times normal levels in the absence of symptoms. An increase in hepatic enzymes, prior to starting treatment or during therapy, should prompt the provider to search for a reason for this increase. A repeat set of liver function studies should include a bilirubin, alkaline phosphatase, and a prothrombin time, and a screen for viral hepatitis. The patient should be questioned about ingestion of other potentially hepatotoxic drugs or substances, and these should be discontinued. If the rise in the serum transaminases is accompanied by a rise in bilirubin or alkaline phosphatase or by an increase in prothrombin time, the INH should be stopped. Consultation with a TB expert or a hepatologist should be obtained before INH is restarted in these patients.

*Rifampin* is an inducer of hepatic enzymes that metabolize and clear many drugs and endogenous compounds, such as methadone or oral contraceptives. Doses of drugs affected must be adjusted in patients receiving rifampin. Oral or hormonal contraceptives must not be used as the sole method of birth control in women who may become pregnant; in such women, barrier methods should be used. Rifampin may cause leukopenia, thrombocytopenia, and orange discoloration of sweat, tears, semen, and urine that may stain clothing or soft contact lenses. The drug rarely causes a flu-like syndrome and renal failure. Rifampin-induced hepatitis is less common than INH-hepatitis.

*Pyrazinamide* may cause hepatitis or nausea. Asymptomatic elevation of serum uric acid is common among patients receiving PZA (as high as 40%), but it may cause gout. The safety of PZA in pregnancy has not been determined, and its use generally is avoided in this situation.

A dose-related optic neuritis is the major side effect of *ethambutol*. Since the drug is metabolized by the kidneys, its dosing must be adjusted (reduced) for patients with renal insufficiency. Color vision testing for red-green discrimination and visual acuity should be determined monthly in patients receiving EMB. In children where monthly determinations of visual acuity and color are not possible, or where monthly examinations for changes of optic neuritis by an ophthalmologist are not possible, the drug should be used with great caution.

# Prevention of Tuberculosis: Treatment of Latent Infection

Tuberculosis is a preventable disease. Studies using molecular epidemiologic methods have determined that most cases in the US today result from the reactivation of latent TB infection.[3] Persons who are infected with tuberculosis therefore represent the reservoir of future cases of active disease; these persons should be targeted for preventive efforts.

Unfortunately, the concept of disease prevention is not familiar to many immigrant and refugee populations. Furthermore, conflicting beliefs concerning TB skin testing, BCG vaccination, and protection against tuberculosis make many high-risk, non-US-born persons unwilling to accept a diagnosis of TB infection. Patients may seem confused, as well, when a provider informs them that a chest radiograph is 'negative,' but they are recommending treatment for a condition that the patient does not believe to be a threat, especially if the patient believes that a positive skin test reflects protection conferred by BCG. Community education by trusted agencies and individuals has been shown to improve acceptance of the principles of TB prevention among non-US-born communities;[29] such models must be replicated in high-risk communities in order to make an impact on future disease incidence.

Lifetime risk of developing clinical tuberculosis for persons infected with TB, as defined by tuberculin skin test reactivity, is approximately 10%, with the greatest risk occurring within the first 2 years following infection. Close contacts to active, infectious cases also are at increased risk for developing active disease, as well as persons with some medical conditions, such as HIV infection or diabetes mellitus; coinfection with HIV may carry a 7–10% annual risk of activation.[30] Similar information is not available for *gamma-Interferon* release assay-positive patients. Screening of high-risk persons for infection (TB skin test or *gamma-Interferon* release assay), followed by a clinical evaluation and chest radiograph to rule out active disease, and administration of INH to infected people, reduces the reservoir of infection and thereby has impact on future disease incidence.

*Contact investigation* is performed when a new case of potentially infectious tuberculosis, suspected or confirmed, is identified, in order to screen and to offer treatment to high-risk persons. Designing and conducting contact investigations are discussed in great detail in a recent CDC statement.[31] However configured, the contact investigation process must protect the confidentiality and privacy of the case as much as possible. This becomes especially important in communities where tuberculosis is stigmatized and identification of the patient could have adverse social and/or economic consequences for the patient, as well as for the patient's family.

## Isoniazid treatment for latent TB infection

Persons infected with tuberculosis should undergo a medical evaluation, which should include a chest radiograph, to exclude active disease, and be considered for treatment of LTBI. A 6–9 month course of INH, if taken as prescribed, is up to 90% effective in reducing risk of reactivation disease in persons with TB infection.[30] However, because of its possible toxicities, especially to the liver, INH should be administered only to infected persons at highest risk for reactivation. These include TB-infected new arrivals (within 5 years) from high-TB incidence regions of the world, persons who travel to such regions, recent skin test converters (within the past 2 years, with a change of > 10 mm induration), close contacts to active potentially infectious cases, children under the age of 5 years, persons with an abnormal chest radiograph demonstrating healed tuberculosis (fibrotic lesions), or persons with medical risk factors for active disease (including patients who require chronic corticosteroids or who demonstrate other types of immunosuppression, such as HIV infection or use of tumor necrosis factor inhibitor medications; patients with diabetes mellitus, end-stage renal disease, or silicosis; patients with recent significant weight loss; or patients with lympho-hematogenous malignancies, such as leukemia, lymphoma, or Hodgkin's disease).

Most experience is available for INH therapy for LTBI. Studies of liver function (AST and ALT) may be obtained before initiating therapy in persons at risk for hepatitis, with further consultation with a specialist considered should elevated baseline levels (see above) be encountered. Patients receiving INH should be given a 1-month supply at a time and be seen by a physician or nurse *at least monthly* to determine adherence and to inquire about possible adverse effects before the next month's supply of medication is given. Tests of liver function studies may be repeated monthly in high-risk persons, as they may be in persons receiving multidrug therapy for active disease (see above).

## Alternative drug regimens for treatment for latent TB infection

The administration of rifampin for 4 months is an alternative to 9 months of INH, although fewer data are available on its effectiveness.[30,32] While generally considered less hepatotoxic than INH, drug interactions (including those with hormonal contraceptives) and specific adverse effects should be considered when prescribing rifampin. Because of its lower cost, possibly greater safety, and greater convenience (i.e. 4 months of treatment rather than 9), some programs now use a 4-month regimen of rifampin as their standard treatment for LTBI. As with administration of INH, monitoring by a healthcare provider should occur at least monthly.

Originally recommended as another alternative for treatment of LTBI,[30] a 2-month regimen using daily rifampin and pyrazinamide was found to have been associated with excessive toxicity, including severe hepatotoxicity,[33,34] and the recommendation was withdrawn by CDC.[35] The mechanism(s) responsible for this excess toxicity is not known.

Persons known or presumed to be infected with multidrug resistant (i.e. resistant to at least both INH and rifampin) tuberculosis should receive at least two drugs to which the infecting organism has demonstrated susceptibility, for at least 6 months. Because of anecdotal reports of severe hepatotoxicity among persons receiving combinations of PZA and a fluoroquinolone or PZA and ethambutol, careful monitoring of persons receiving either of these regimens for toxicity should be performed. In countries where a high prevalence of primary resistance to INH is encountered, it has been suggested that rifampin or a rifampin-containing regimen be used for treatment of LTBI. In 2000, this included Vietnam, Haiti, and the Philippines, and the list is likely to expand.[36] Consultation with an expert in tuberculosis is recommended in such situations.

## Pregnancy

Pregnancy is not a risk factor for tuberculosis. Pregnant women who otherwise are at risk for tuberculosis should undergo standard screening with a tuberculin skin test or *QuantiFERON Gold*® test. Persons classified as reactive should undergo a medical evaluation to exclude active tuberculosis. If the woman is asymptomatic, a history and physical examination should be conducted to search for additional risk factors (historical/epidemiologic or medical, including a full symptom screen). If no high-risk situation is identified, the chest radiograph (frontal view only, with shielding of the abdomen) may be deferred until the second trimester. However, if the patient is a contact to an active case of possibly infectious TB, is a known skin test or *QuantiFERON Gold®* converter (2 years), has a medical condition associated with increased risk (such as diabetes mellitus, HIV, etc.), is a recent arrival from a TB-endemic community, or has symptoms suggestive of TB, the radiograph and full medical evaluation should proceed immediately. Once active TB is excluded, treatment of LTBI should be offered to high-risk women with isoniazid for 9 months (rifampin for 4 months is an alternative).[30] Women who are treated with INH in late pregnancy and the immediate (3 months) postpartum period are at increased risk for drug-induced hepatotoxicity.[27]

Tuberculosis disease during pregnancy is a hazard to the mother and the fetus; treatment should be initiated promptly if the probability of active disease is moderate to high.[23] The initial treatment regimen should include isoniazid, rifampin, and ethambutol, and should be adjusted according to clinical response and drug susceptibility testing of the isolate obtained by culture. Pyridoxine (vitamin $B_6$), 25 mg/day, should be administered with this regimen. Treatment should continue for at least 9 months. Pyrazinamide is *not* recommended for use during pregnancy in the US, since there are inadequate data on its safety to the fetus. However, the World Health Organization and the International Union Against Tuberculosis and Lung Disease endorse its use in pregnancy. Streptomycin (and presumably Kanamycin, Amikacin, and Capreomycin, also) should *not* be used, because of its potential to cause eighth cranial nerve injury with resulting hearing loss or deafness.

Pregnant women with drug-resistant tuberculosis should be counseled about the unknown risks to the fetus of second- and third-line drugs.

Breast-feeding is not contraindicated while a woman is receiving treatment. Small amounts of drug that appear in breast milk are not toxic to the infant, although the infant should receive pyridoxine (vitamin $B_6$) if the mother is receiving INH. The amounts of drugs in breast milk are not considered sufficient for treatment; infants being treated for LTBI or for active TB disease must receive oral (or parenteral) medications, even if they are being breast-fed by a woman who also is receiving therapy.

## Hospitalization

Most diagnostic procedures for tuberculosis and its treatment can be accomplished outside the hospital; yet hospitalization may be justified for an ill patient early in his/her illness or when the patient is a risk to the public's health. Early-morning gastric aspiration in young children is most easily performed during an inpatient stay. Hospitalization also may be desirable for other diagnostic procedures such as lung biopsy, bronchoscopy, or paracentesis.

A patient with infectious tuberculosis who cannot, or will not, adhere to treatment may require *involuntary hospitalization* to protect the health of the public.[3] Since involuntary hospitalization severely curtails personal liberties, its use is governed by law in most states. Involuntary hospitalization should be considered a measure of last resort; it should be invoked only when all other measures fail. Providing a potentially nonadherent patient with an enabler or an incentive (such as a public transportation pass) in return for appearing for DOT may avoid a costly hospital stay. However, when alternatives are considered, including development of drug resistance or disease relapse, in persons who do not take their medications properly, public safety must be considered more important than personal freedom.

## Immigrant Screening for Tuberculosis

The vast majority of persons entering the United States undergo no screening for tuberculosis at all. However, overseas screening for tuberculosis and for other disorders with public health importance is mandated by US immigration law for immigrants who are applying for permanent residence status and for selected refugees or asylees. The TB screening process is designed to exclude from entry persons with untreated, infectious tuberculosis who may be a danger to the public health; it relies on sputum microscopy and evaluations by approximately 400 worldwide 'panel physicians', appointed and licensed by US embassies and consulates that issue visas. Between 1992 and 2002, an estimated 400 000 to 500 000 persons were screened by this mechanism.

For persons 15 years of age and older, screening consists of a brief medical history and a frontal chest radiograph. Children (<15 years) are screened only if symptoms of TB are reported or if they are identified as a contact to an active case.

If the radiograph suggests *active tuberculosis*, three sputum smears are examined; cultures are not performed:

(a) Persons with *positive sputum smears* are designated *Class A TB*; they are excluded from entry until they either (1) complete a course of therapy and demonstrate sputum smear conversion and undergo reclassification, or (2) initiate treatment and apply for an immigration *waiver* after demonstrating sputum smear conversion to negative. A patient with a *Class A waiver* may enter the US only after a US provider and jurisdictional public health agency in the US destination agree to assume responsibility for the patient's completion of therapy.

(b) Persons with a radiograph suggestive of active TB and *negative sputum smears* are designated *Class B1 TB*, and are permitted entry.

If the chest radiograph suggests *inactive tuberculosis*, no sputum smears are obtained and the patient is designated *Class B2 TB*, and also is allowed to enter the US.

Immigrants classified as *Class A waiver* or *Class B1 or B2* status are reported on entry to CDC's *Division of Global Migration and Quarantine (DGMQ)* which, in turn, notifies state/local health departments of *A* or *B* classifications who are moving to their jurisdiction. *Class A waiver* designees are required to report to the state or local public health agency for follow-up evaluations or risk deportation; reporting for *B1* and *B2* immigrants for follow-up evaluations, however, is voluntary.

A relatively large proportion of *B1* and *B2* immigrants (est. 4–14% and 0.4–4%, respectively) who enter the United States with abnormal chest radiographs and negative sputum smears overseas are later discovered to have active TB at the time of entry, based on follow-up medical evaluations. Suggestions have been made to improve the screening and entry process, and collaborations between federal agencies responsible for screening of immigrants and refugees are continuously reviewing and updating procedures for screening, notification of arrivals, and follow-up once they reach the US.[3,37]

Currently, the Technical Instructions to Panel physicians for overseas examinations are being revised, and will likely increase active screening of children and induce sputum cultures overseas prior to arrival. If approved, implementation of revised procedures will be phased in, at specific sites, over time.

## Adjustment of Status

Non-immigrants who wish to adjust their immigration status after residing in the United States must undergo medical evaluation by one of the approximately 3000 US physicians designated by DGMQ as *civil surgeons*. Persons with a skin test reaction of > 5 mm induration) or a positive *QuantiFERON Gold®* test are required to have a chest radiograph; if this is suggestive of active TB, the person is referred to his or her public health agency for further evaluation and management. Referral for possible treatment of LTBI also is recommended for persons with skin test reactions of > 10 mm. In 2002, approximately 679 000 foreign-born persons applied for permanent residency and were screened by civil surgeons. While responsible for providing guidance to civil surgeons, CDC has no regulatory role in monitoring the quality or outcomes of adjustment-of-status examinations.

## Conclusion

Tuberculosis remains a prominent cause of morbidity and mortality around the world. The leading killer of people with AIDS, the disease is responsible for more deaths from infection than any other agent. People migrating to the United States bring with them high rates of TB infection and disease which reflect the environments from which they come. The greatest risk for active tuberculosis for most people from overseas TB-endemic regions occurs within the first 5 years of arrival in the US. Overseas screening reaches only a small proportion of new arrivals, and it is in great need of reform. Once in the US, many of those at-risk do not engage the healthcare system, for a variety of reasons. Free access to culturally appropriate and competent clinical services must be made available to people with symptoms of disease, in order to prevent further morbidity and spread within the community. Programs to provide prevention services must be available and acceptable to persons with divergent beliefs about tuberculosis, its prevention, and its treatment. In order to accomplish this, the healthcare system must engage at-risk communities to develop trust and to educate the people and their healthcare providers about tuberculosis. Barriers must be identified and addressed. Tuberculosis is preventable and treatable. People arriving from overseas endemic areas and their families deserve the same high-quality treatment that anybody else does.

# References

1. Corbett EL, Watt CJ, Walker N, et al. The growing burden of tuberculosis. Global trends and interactions with the HIV epidemic. Arch Intern Med 2003; 163:1009–1021.
2. Centers for Disease Control and Prevention. Trends in Tuberculosis – United States, 2005. MMWR 2006; 55(11):305–308.
3. Centers for Disease Control and Prevention. Controlling tuberculosis in the United States: Recommendations from the American Thoracic Society, CDC, and the Infectious Diseases Society of America. MMWR 2005; 54:RR-12. Available: http://www.cdc.gov/nchstp/tb/rtmcc.htm
4. Wells WF. Aerodynamics of droplet nuclei [Chapter 3]. In: Airborne contagion and air hygiene. Cambridge, MA: Harvard University Press; 1955.
5. Dannenberg AM. Immune mechanisms in the pathogenesis of pulmonary tuberculosis. Rev Infect Dis 1989; 11: S369–S378.
6. Flynn JL, Chan J. Tuberculosis: latency and reactivation. Infect Immun 2001; 69:4195–4201.
7. Schluger NW. Recent advances in our understanding of human host responses to tuberculosis. Respir Res 2001; 2:157–163.
8. Centers for Disease Control and Prevention/American Thoracic Society. Diagnostic standards/classification of TB in adults and children. Am J Respir Crit Care Med 2000; 161:1376–1395.
9. Meyer M, Clarke P, O'Regan AW. Utility of the lateral chest radiograph in the evaluation of patients with a positive tuberculin skin test result. Chest 2003; 124:1824–1827.
10. American Thoracic Society, Centers for Disease Control. The tuberculin skin test. Am Rev Respir Dis 1981; 124:356–363.
11. Lee E, Holzman RS. Evolution and current use of the tuberculin skin test. Clin Infect Dis 2002; 34:365–370.
12. Centers for Disease Control and Prevention. The role of BCG vaccine in the prevention and control of tuberculosis in the United States. (ACET and ACIP) MMWR 1996; 45: RR-4).
13. Pai M, Gokhale K, Joshi R, et al. *Mycobacterium tuberculosis* infection in healthcare workers in rural India. Comparison of a whole-blood interferon-gamma assay with tuberculin skin testing. JAMA 2005; 293:2746–2755.
14. Kang YA, Lee HW, Yoon HI, et al. Discrepancy between the tuberculin skin test and the whole-blood interferon gamma assay for the diagnosis of latent tuberculosis infection in an intermediate tuberculosis-burden country. JAMA 2005; 293:2756–2761.
15. Brock I, Weldingh K, Lillebaek T, et al. Comparison of tuberculin skin test and new specific blood test in tuberculosis contacts. Amer J Respir Crit Care Med 2004; 170:65–69.
16. Centers for Disease Control and Prevention. Guidelines for using the QuantiFERON-TB Gold test for detecting *Mycobacterium tuberculosis* infection – United States. MMWR 2005; 54:RR-15, 49–55.
17. Daley CL, Gotway MB, Jasmer RM. Radiographic manifestations of tuberculosis. A primer for clinicians. San Francisco, CA: The Francis J. Curry National Tuberculosis Center; 2003. Available: http://www.nationaltbcenter.edu/catalogue/epub/index.cfm?tableName=RMT)
18. Kent PT, Kubica GP. Public health mycobacteriology. A guide for the level III laboratory. Atlanta, GA: CDC; 1985.
19. Catanzaro A, Perry S, Clarridge JE, et al. The role of clinical suspicion in evaluating a new diagnostic test for active tuberculosis: results of a multicenter prospective trial. JAMA 2000; 283:639–645.
20. Conaty SJ, Claxton AP, Enoch DA, et al. The interpretation of nucleic acid amplification tests for tuberculosis: do rapid tests change treatment decisions? J Infect 2005; 50:187–192.
21. Lim TK, Mukhopadhyay A, Gough A, et al. Role of clinical judgment in the application of a nucleic acid amplification test for the rapid diagnosis of pulmonary tuberculosis. Chest 2003; 124:902–908.
22. Wiener RS, Della-Latta P, Schluger NW. Effect of nucleic acid amplification for *Mycobacterium tuberculosis* on clinical decision making in suspected extrapulmonary tuberculosis. Chest. 2005; 128:102–107.
23. Centers for Disease Control and Prevention. Treatment of tuberculosis. MMWR 2003; 52:RR-11.
24. Centers for Disease Control and Prevention. Reported tuberculosis in the United States, 2004. Atlanta, GA: US Department of Health and Human Services; 2005.
25. Goldberg SV, Wallace J, Jackson JC, et al. Cultural case management of latent tuberculosis infection. Int J Tuberc Lung Dis 2004; 8:76–82.
26. Mitchell JR, Zimmerman HJ, Ishak KG, et al. Isoniazid liver injury: clinical spectrum, pathology, and probable pathogenesis. Ann Intern Med 1976; 84:181–192.
27. Franks AL, Binkin NJ, Snider DE Jr, et al. Isoniazid hepatitis among pregnant and postpartum Hispanic patients. Pub Health Rep 1989; 104:151–155.
28. Nolan CM, Goldberg SV, Buskin SE. Hepatotoxicity associated with isoniazid preventive therapy: a 7-year survey from a public health tuberculosis clinic. JAMA 1999; 281:1014–1018.
29. Goldberg SV, Wallace J, Jackson JC, et al. Cultural case management of latent tuberculosis infection. Int J Tuberc Lung Dis 2004; 8:76–82.
30. Centers for Disease Control and Prevention. Targeted tuberculin testing and treatment of latent tuberculosis infection. MMWR 2000; 49:RR-6; 8, Table 2. Available: http://www.cdc.gov/mmwr/PDF/rr/rr4906.pdf. Accessed 2/13/07.
31. Centers for Disease Control and Prevention. Guidelines for the investigation of contacts of persons with infectious tuberculosis: recommendations from the National Tuberculosis Controllers Association and CDC. MMWR 2005; 54:RR-15, 1–37.
32. Polesky A, Farber HW, Gottlieb DJ, et al. Rifampin preventive therapy for tuberculosis in Boston's homeless. Am J Respir Crit Care Med 1996; 154:1473–1477.
33. Jasmer RM, Saukkonen JJ, Blumberg HM, et al. Short-course rifampin and pyrazinamide compared with isoniazid for latent tuberculosis infection: a multicenter clinical trial. Ann Intern Med 2002; 137: 640–647.
34. Centers for Disease Control and Prevention. Update: fatal and severe liver injuries associated with rifampin and pyrazinamide treatment for latent tuberculosis infection. MMWR 2002; 51:998–999.
35. Centers for Disease Control and Prevention. Update: Adverse event data and revised American Thoracic Society/CDC recommendations against the use of rifampin and pyrazinamide for treatment of latent tuberculosis infection MMWR 2003; 52(31):735–739.
36. Khan K, Muennig P, Behta M, et al. Global drug-resistance patterns and the management of latent tuberculosis infection in immigrants to the United States. N Engl J Med 2002; 347:1850–1859.
37. Centers for Disease Control and Prevention. Preventing and controlling tuberculosis along the US–Mexico Border; Work Group Report. MMWR 2001; 50:RR-1.

# CHAPTER 20

# Intestinal Parasites

Rajal Mody

## Intestinal Parasitosis at a Glance

- There is a high prevalence of intestinal protozoan and helminth infections among immigrants and refugees.
- Most of these infections are asymptomatic but some may have significant clinical and/or public health consequences.
- Several intestinal parasites can cause serious health consequences many years after immigration.
- The best way to prevent the potential complications of intestinal parasitosis among immigrants remains debated. The options include screening all immigrants and treating only those found to harbor parasites, or presumptively treating all immigrants.
- Effective treatments regimens are available for all intestinal parasites.

## Etiologic Agents of Intestinal Parasitosis

Intestinal parasitosis constitutes one of the most common types of human infections. One-third of the world's population is affected by these organisms, including people living in both tropical and temperate climates, and it has been shown that all immigrant groups are affected to some degree.[1] These infections often go unnoticed, but have the potential to cause serious health consequences. Therefore, familiarity with intestinal parasites is important for any healthcare provider caring for immigrant populations.

Parasites are broadly categorized as single-celled protozoa and multicellular helminths, or worms (Fig. 20.1). Both types frequently infect the human gastrointestinal system. The helminths consist of two phyla: the hermaphroditic platyhelminthes (flatworms) and the nemahelminthes (nematodes or roundworms), which consist of separate male and female worms. The platyhelminthes are further subdivided into two classes: the trematodes (flukes) and cestodes (tapeworms).

Nematodes are the parasites that most closely resemble common soil worms. Intestinal nematodes are transmitted to humans via two primary mechanisms: ingestion of soil contaminated with infective eggs (*Ascaris lumbricoides*, *Trichuris trichiura*) or by penetration of skin with infective larvae (hookworms, *Strongyloides stercoralis*). *Ascaris*, *Trichuris*, hookworms, and *Strongyloides* are all considered geohelminths, meaning at least part of their lifecycle takes place in the soil. *Strongyloides* is unique in that an alternative soil-independent cycle can occur in which affected individuals are repetitively autoinfected with infectious larvae. Consequently, immigrants may have *Strongyloides* infections for many years after leaving endemic areas. *Enterobius vermicularis*, pinworm, is a common intestinal nematode throughout the world, spread by fecal–oral transmission and does not involve a soil stage. Important nonintestinal nematodes include the tissue-dwelling filariae, are discussed in Chapter 36. There are many nematodes which are unable to develop into adult worms within humans. However, larval stages of many of these organisms can cause considerable morbidity by eliciting inflammatory responses in a variety of tissues. Some of these nonhuman nematodes of potential importance among immigrants include *Toxocara canis*, *Angiostrongylus* species, *Gnathostoma* species, and *Trichinella spiralis*.

Trematodes are a group of parasites that can cause chronic infections with many important long-term

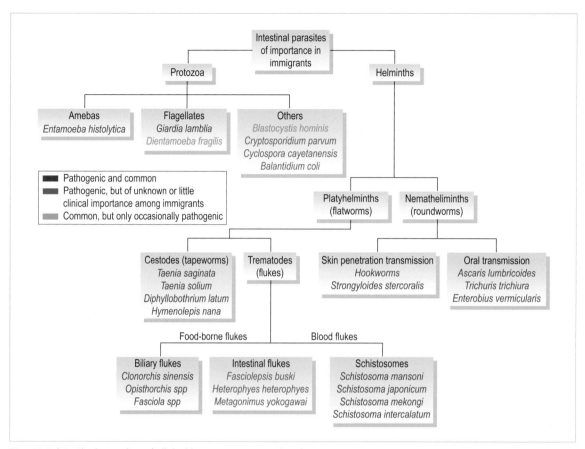

**Fig. 20.1** Intestinal parasites of clinical importance among immigrants.

consequences. All trematodes require intermediate snail hosts. The manner in which the infective larvae that exit the snail go on to enter humans defines two broad groups of trematodes, the blood flukes and the food-borne flukes. The blood flukes infect humans by direct skin penetration, while the food-borne flukes, fittingly, infect humans through the consumption of food. There are five blood flukes of human importance, all of which are part of the genus *Schistosoma*. For detailed information on schistosomiasis, see Chapter 39. Food-borne trematodes can be divided into the biliary liver flukes (*Opisthorchis* species, *Clonorchis sinensis*, and *Fasciola* species), intestinal flukes (*Fasciolepsis buski*, heterophyids, and echinostomes) and lung flukes (*Paragonimus* species). All food-borne trematodes are transmitted via consumption of raw fish, crustaceans, or aquatic plants that are contaminated with the infective stages.

The cestodes, or tapeworms, comprised of characteristic segments, or proglottides, are relatively benign. All, except the human dwarf tapeworm, are transmitted to humans through consumption of undercooked meats. When humans consume undercooked beef, pork, or fish with larvae-containing cysts, they become infected with the adult form of *Taenia saginata*, *Taenia solium*, and *Diphyllobothrium latum*, respectively. These three species can grow to impressive lengths within the intestines. If eggs, passed in the feces of individuals harboring an adult *Taenia solium* worm(s), are accidentally ingested by fecal–oral contact, humans become accidental hosts for the larval stages and cysticercosis may develop with potentially serious consequences, which are discussed in chapter 27. A similar process, reviewed in Chapter 28, occurs if humans accidentally ingest eggs of the *Echinococcus* tapeworms of carnivorous animals. *Hymenolepis nana*, the dwarf tapeworm, is the most commonly detected human cestode in nearly all immigrant groups. This likely is due to its simple fecal–oral means of transmission and its ability to persist in a cycle of autoinfection.

## Table 20.1 Nonpathogenic intestinal protozoa

| Never pathogenic | Occasionally pathogenic |
|---|---|
| Entamoeba hartmanni | Blastocystis hominis |
| Entamoeba coli | Dientamoeba fragilis |
| Entamoeba polecki | |
| Entamoeba dispar | |
| Entamoeba moshkovskii | |
| Endolimax nana | |
| Iodamoeba butschlii | |
| Chilomastix mesnili | |
| Trichomonas hominis | |

The pathogenic protozoa most likely to affect immigrants include the amoeba, *Entamoeba histolytica*, and the flagellate, *Giardia lamblia* (also known as *G. intestinalis* or *G. duodenalis*). Although many other protozoa are known to cause intestinal disease throughout the world, such as *Crypotosporidium parvum, Cyclospora cayetanensis, and Balantidium coli*, the importance of these organisms in immigrant populations remains unclear. Most protozoa detected in immigrants are considered nonpathogenic. However, two of these organisms, *Blastocystis hominis* and *Dientamoeba fragilis*, traditionally thought to be benign commensals, may actually cause disease in some individuals. *Blastocystis hominis* is the most commonly detected intestinal parasites in all refugee populations arriving to the US, affecting 20–40% of refugees from Africa, the Middle East, Southeast Asia, Eastern Europe, and Latin America.[2] However, since the pathogenic potential of this protozoan is debated, it is typically not reported in surveys of intestinal parasite prevalence.

## Nonpathogenic parasites

All intestinal helminths are potentially pathogenic. However, many protozoan parasites detected in screening stool ova and parasites (O&P) specimens are nonpathogenic (Table 20.1). These organisms should not be treated (except for symptomatic *Blastocystis hominis* and *Dientamoeba fragilis* infections). Further investigations are always indicated among symptomatic patients who have only nonpathogenic parasites detected. Their presence indicates time spent in areas where poor sanitation led to fecal–oral contact. As a group, these nonpathogenic protozoans account for the first or second most common type of intestinal parasite detected in immigrant populations, depending on whether one considers *Blastocystis hominis* to be a pathogen.[2]

## Epidemiology

Immigrants and refugees from every region of the world are at risk for harboring intestinal parasites. Although certain parasites are seen more often in those from tropical locations, even individuals from temperate climates are at risk. Except for *Giardia*, mandatory federal reporting of intestinal parasitic infections in the US was discontinued in 1994. Therefore, the primary sources of prevalence data for parasitic infections in immigrant groups in the US are individual state refugee screening programs and published series on parasitic infections in convenience samples of immigrants in specific areas.[1] Although current information is lacking on the prevalence of intestinal parasites in nonrefugee immigrant groups, several studies in the past describe the patterns of intestinal parasitosis in these populations.

This section will focus on the risk factors associated with intestinal parasitic infections among immigrants and refugees as well as a general overview of which types of parasites are seen most commonly in different groups. Details on the epidemiology of specific parasitic infections are included in the following section as well as in the parasite-specific chapters.

## Overall prevalence

The overall reported prevalence rates of pathogenic intestinal parasites among refugees, immigrants, and migrant workers in North America have ranged between 8.4% and 86%.[1,3–16] This wide range can be explained primarily by differences in the geographic origin and ages of the populations studied. Other determinants include education level and past occupational exposures. Additionally, for refugees, the implementation of pre-departure empiric treatment with albendazole in 1999 greatly altered the detection rates of certain parasites. Furthermore, methodological differences partially explain the wide range in reported prevalence. For example, intestinal parasitosis rates among a population of Cambodian refugees in New York varied from 31% to 86% depending on the method of stool examination.[14]

These past studies all utilized various methods of stool microscopy for ova and parasites (O&P) to determine prevalence. Relying on stool microscopy may underestimate the true prevalence of intestinal parasitic infections due to poor sensitivity for several organisms, especially *Strongyloides*.[17] On the other hand, despite the low sensitivity of stool O&P examinations to detect *Entamoeba histolytica*, all past surveys overestimated the prevalence of *E. histolytica* infections due to the inability to differentiate this organism morphologically from the more common nonpathogenic *Entamoeba dispar* and *Entamoeba moshkovskii*.[18]

## Geography

Country of origin is likely the strongest predictor of intestinal parasitosis.[3] Refugees of all ages from Southeast Asia have consistently been shown to have very high rates of intestinal parasitosis. Among refugees from this region resettling in North America in the 1970s and 1980s, prevalence ranged from 37% to 78%.[13] In more recent years, Southeast Asians have consistently been found to be the most highly affected refugees with 22–48% of individuals harboring pathogenic parasites. In the same studies, refugees from sub-Saharan Africa follow close behind with rates of 16–43%.[4,5,19] Those from the Middle East and Eastern Europe carry slightly lower burdens of intestinal parasites, ranging 13–32% and 8–22%, respectively.[5,19]

These geographic variations are explained primarily by differing rates of helminthic infections. For example, compared to refugees from the Middle East and Eastern Europe, those from Africa and South Central Asia (including Afghanistan, Bangladesh, Bhutan, India, Maldives, Nepal, Pakistan, and Sri Lanka) were 5.9 and 8.0 times more likely to have a helminthic infection, respectively. In contrast, there was no statistical difference in protozoan infections among refugees from these various regions.[1] This study did not include refugees from Southeast Asia.

Very little current information is available for Latin American refugees and immigrants. In a group of Latin American refugees to Sweden, 42% harbored pathogenic parasites.[19] Similar high levels were noted among Latin American refugee claimants within Montreal in 1987. In fact, among 1967 individuals originating from over 70 countries throughout the world, those from Central America had the highest odds of having an intestinal parasite in multivariate analysis (OR = 2.4, 95% CI 1.5–3.7).[3] Rates of helminthic carriage were as high as 65% in claimants from some Central American countries. Older data on Latin American immigrants to the US from the late 1970s to early 1990s reveal rates of pathogenic parasite carriage of 35–46%.[8-11]

## Age

In general, younger immigrants are more likely to harbor intestinal parasites than adults. Among 2129 refugees arriving in Minnesota in 1999, the prevalence of having at least one pathogenic parasite was 30% for those under 18 years of age, as compared to 15% among those 18 years of age or older ($p < 0.001$).[4] School-aged children, aged 7–17 years old, were most heavily affected. Most protozoan pathogens disproportionately affect immigrants under 10 years old, while helminthic infections tend to affect older children and young adults most frequently.[3] Young children actually have the lowest rates of helminthic infections of all age groups.[3] The type of helminths detected also varies by age. For example, among Southeast Asian refugees, school-aged children had the highest rates of *Trichuris*, *Strongyloides*, and *Hymenolepis nana* infections, while adults had the highest prevalence of hookworm and *Clonorchis* infections.[11,14]

Age may, in fact, be the only known predictor of the likelihood of protozoan infections among immigrants and refugees. Among refugee claimants to Montreal, the frequency of protozoan infections significantly increased with decreasing age. Protozoan infections, but not helminthic infections, were noted to be significantly more common in newly arrived refugees to California under the age of 18 years (OR = 2.2, 95% CI 1.2–4.2).[1] This age variation appears to be most likely explained by especially high rates of *Giardia* in children. *Entamoeba histolytica* is more evenly distributed by age.[14,15]

## Education

Among adult immigrants, the amount of past formal education has been strongly associated with the likelihood of helminthic infections. Half of all adult refugee claimants in Montreal with less than 5 years of schooling were found to have helminthic infections. This compared to 32%, 24%, and 12% of immigrants with 5–9, 10–14, and 15 or more years of education, respectively ($p < 0.0001$).[3] This is in agreement with recent information on refugees arriving in California, in which there was a trend for adult refugees with less than 12 years of education to be at increased risk for helminthic infections (OR = 2.2, 95% CI 0.93–5.1).[1] In both studies, level of education did not affect the likelihood of protozoan infections.

Parental education levels likely affect their immigrant children's likelihood of parasite carriage as well. Although this has never been reported for immigrants to North America, a study in Turkey revealed that children whose mothers have less than a primary school education were significantly more likely to harbor parasites.[20]

## Occupation

Immigrants who formerly worked in agriculture or fishing in their countries of origin may be more likely to harbor a variety of helminths as a result of occupational exposures.[21,22] Both farming and fishing may increase the likelihood of hookworm infection.[22,23] Chronic trematode infections can result from work exposures and may cause disease many years after immigration. For example, farming has been shown to increase the likelihood of *Schistosoma haematobium* infections in West Africa and *Schistosoma japonicum* infections in China.[24,25] Fishing increases the likelihood of *Schistosoma mansoni* infection among people in East Africa.[26] Individuals who have worked closely with sheep or cattle may be at risk for infection with *Fasciola* species.[27] Farming may also increase the risk of *Strongyloides stercoralis* infections.[28]

In addition to the occupational exposures in countries of origin, the types of work immigrants do after settling in their new countries may place them at increased risk of intestinal parasites. The prevalence of pathogenic parasites among migrant farm workers in the southeastern area of the US has been found to be very high. Even though workers born in Central America and Haiti have much higher rates of pathogenic parasite carriage compared to US-born workers, there is evidence to suggest that ongoing transmission occurs among all workers on farms.[16]

## Gender

Some of the occupational exposures described above may lead to higher rates of infection in men. This was noted for hookworm and *Schistosoma* infections in Africa.[22,24,26] Among refugee claimants in Montreal, hookworm infections were almost twice as common in men.[3] However, considering all pathogens detected in refugees entering the US and Canada, males have just a slight, often statistically nonsignificant, increased likelihood of harboring intestinal parasites.[1,3,4]

## Close contacts

Intestinal parasitosis in individual immigrants is more likely if family members have been found to harbor parasites. Among a group of Southeast Asian refugees, the percentage of families with more than one individual carrying a pathogen was 86%, while the overall prevalence in the study group was 61%.[12]

## Past living circumstances

Those who have lived in areas destroyed by wars may be at risk for parasites that otherwise are non-endemic to certain regions. For example, high rates of hookworm infections have been reported in refugees from Bosnia, an area with a typically low hookworm risk.[19] Also immigrants who have spent time in refugee or emigration camps are often more likely to harbor parasites than others from the same countries who have not lived in such camps.[29,30] However, in the case of refugees, this observation has been affected by the advent of pre-departure albendazole therapy.

### Pre-departure albendazole treatment

In 1997, the Centers for Disease Control and Prevention (CDC) and the International Organization for Migration conducted an enhanced screening for intestinal helminthic and protozoan infections in a group of Somali refugees living in refugee camps in Kenya. They found that 38% of those screened harbored pathogenic intestinal parasites and, therefore, decided to treat empirically all nonpregnant refugees over the age of 2 years with a single 600 mg dose of albendazole within 3 days prior to departure to the United States.[31] In May of 1999, the CDC extended this practice to refugees from locations throughout sub-Saharan Africa. At some point after 1999, individuals in Southeast Asian refugee camps relocating to the US also began receiving this same treatment regimen prior to departure.

Pre-departure albendazole treatment has dramatically decreased the prevalence of parasitic infections detected in stool samples in newly arrived refugees.[6,15] A reduction from 24% to 4% in the prevalence of intestinal helminth infections has been documented in African refugees arriving in Massachusetts before and after May 1999, respectively (OR = 0.15, 95% CI 0.09–0.24).[15] In this study, those who arrived after the initiation of pre-departure treatment had over a 90% lower odds of harboring

*Ascaris* (OR = 0.07, 95% CI 0.01–0.58), hookworm (OR = 0.03, 95% CI 0.00–0.29), or *Trichuris* (OR = 0.05, 95% CI 0.02–0.13) compared to those who arrived before 1999. Surprisingly, a decrease in *Entamoeba histolytica/dispar* prevalence was also detected (OR = 0.47, 95% CI 0.26–0.86).[15]

In Northern California, a relatively low overall pathogenic parasite prevalence of 14% was observed in a group of refugees arriving between 2001 and 2004, after implementation of universal pre-departure treatment. However, the investigators noted that the group with the highest prevalence of parasites, sub-Saharan Africans, came from the region of the world where pre-departure treatment is most highly enforced. This is likely explained by the relatively higher rates of *Strongyloides* and *Schistosoma* in this group.[1] Albendazole has no activity against *Schistosoma* and is not the most effective treatment for *Strongyloides*, especially when given as a single dose.

### Types of intestinal parasites commonly detected in different locations

There is very little effect of geography on the prevalence of protozoan infections. Excluding *Blastocystis hominis*, *Giardia* is the most or nearly the most common pathogenic parasite detected in all newly arrived immigrant populations.[1,5,7–9,15,19] It occasionally falls second behind *Trichuris* or hookworm infections. The other protozoan pathogens, including *Entamoeba histolytica* and *Dientamoeba fragilis*, also show little geographic variation.[1]

In contrast to protozoan infections, the epidemiology of helminthic infections varies more by region of origin. It is difficult to make broad generalizations

regarding the types of parasites most frequently encountered by people in different areas of the world. There can be significant variation in the ecology of parasitic infections even within a relatively small region of the world. For example, large differences have been noted in both the overall prevalence of parasitic infection and types of parasites detected among Cambodian, Hmong, Laotian, and Vietnamese refugees.[12] Nevertheless, it is important to have a general idea of which types of helminths are especially common in different populations. Geographic distributions of important intestinal parasites are listed in Table 20.2.

## Clinical Manifestations

In general, most individuals harboring pathogenic intestinal parasites are asymptomatic at the time of screening. Most investigators have failed to find correlations between symptoms and the presence of intestinal parasitosis. In a study of East African immigrants living in Minnesota, the presence of abdominal pain, nausea, vomiting, indigestion, or diarrhea had a sensitivity of 71% and a specificity of 24% for detecting the presence of pathogenic intestinal parasites. These values translate into a positive predictive value of only 26% and a negative predictive value of 69%, indicating the inability to base clinical decision-making on the presence or absence of gastrointestinal symptoms.[32] Other studies also have failed to find associations between gastrointestinal symptoms and intestinal parasites among Southeast Asian refugees[33] and Latin American immigrants.[8,9] The lack of correlation with symptoms, however, should not downplay the pathogenic

**Table 20.2 Geographic distributions of common intestinal parasites**

| Global | Africa | Asia | Latin America | Middle East | Eastern Europe |
|---|---|---|---|---|---|
| Ascaris<br>Trichuris<br>Hookworm<br>Strongyloides<br>Enterobius<br>Fasciola<br>Hymenolepis<br>All protozoa | Schistosoma<br>  mansoni<br>  haematobium<br>  intercalatum<br>Taenia saginata<br>  (especially Ethiopia<br>  & Eritrea) | Fasciolepsis buski<br><br>Southeast Asia:<br>Opisthorchis viverrini<br>Clonorchis sinensis<br>Schistosoma<br>  japonicum<br>  mekongi<br><br>South Asia:<br>Taenia solium | Taenia solium<br>Schistosoma<br>  mansoni<br><br>Opisthorchis<br>  guayaquilensis<br>  (Ecuador) | Echinococcus | Diphyllobothrium<br>  latum<br>  (especially Russia)<br><br>Opisthorchis<br>  felineus<br>  (especially Russia) |

Adapted with permission from Reference 73 with additional data from Reference 36.

potential of intestinal parasites. The following sections will review important clinical aspects of some of these organisms.

## Nematodes

### Box 20.1
### Case study 1

An actual email: "I am an English Language Learners teacher and have many students from Liberia. I had a student complain about coughing up a long white worm as he was eating a lemon at lunch (Fig. 20.2). I sent him to the nurse at school, as he said this was the second time it had happened to him. She sent him back to class saying there wasn't enough to tell anything at this point. Is there anything you can suggest, or anywhere I can direct his parents?"

**Etiology:** *Ascaris lumbricoides* is the largest intestinal nematode of humans, reaching lengths of 40 cm and diameters of 6 mm. The description of the worm in Box 20.1 is pathognomonic for ascariasis.

**Epidemiology:** *Ascaris lumbricoides* is estimated to affect a quarter of the world's human population.[34]

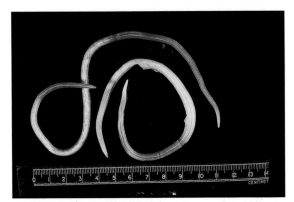

**Fig. 20.2** Adult *Ascaris lumbricoides*. After returning to the gut, the larvae mature into adult roundworms in the small intestine. The adult males are about 15–30 cm long, and females 20–35 cm. The adults, if sufficient in number, can cause bowel obstruction and individual worms can migrate up the bile duct, causing obstructive jaundice. Reproduced with permission from Peters W, Pasvol G. Tropical medicine and parasitology, 5th edn. London: Mosby; 2002:122.

*Ascaris* is a geohelminth, meaning that part of its lifecycle occurs in soil. Ova require warm, moist soil to embryonate into infective larvae. In ideal settings, *Ascaris* ova can persist for over 14 years. Therefore, this parasite flourishes in tropical areas where year-round transmission is possible. However, its distribution is global and it has been found in up to 4% of refugees from Eastern Europe.[19] Transmission is facilitated by crowded living conditions and breakdowns in sanitation. Worm burdens are highest in 5–15-year-olds.[34] Geophagia, the intentional consumption of soil, is a common behavior of children in endemic areas and has been shown to greatly increase both the risk of harboring any *Ascaris* worms and the risk of having large worm burdens.[35]

**Life cycle:** Humans are infected through ingestion of embryonated eggs in contaminated soil. The larvae hatch in the small intestines, penetrate the intestinal wall, and migrate to the lungs via blood or lymphatic vessels within 4 days after ingestion. While developing in the alveoli for approximately 10 days, the larvae can cause a transient respiratory syndrome, characterized by fever, cough, wheezing, and radiological pulmonary infiltrates, known as Loffler's syndrome. Loffler's syndrome can be caused by other intestinal nematodes with a similar transpulmonary migration, such as hookworms and *Strongyloides*. The pulmonary symptoms, if present, rapidly resolve as the larvae leave the lungs through the bronchi and then are swallowed. After returning to the intestines the larvae develop into adult worms. Within 2–3 months, gravid females start releasing 200 000 fertilized ova per day. Adult worms live for up to 2 years and then are passed in stool. In individuals infected with only male worms, no ova will be detected (Fig. 20.3). If the migrating larvae gain access to the systemic circulation, they may cause local symptoms resembling those of visceral larva migrans caused by *Toxocara canis*, the dog roundworm, which is discussed below.[36]

**Clinical manifestations:** The vast majority of infections go unnoticed. However, there is considerable evidence that even these apparently asymptomatic infections can lead to poor growth in children via decreased appetite and malabsorption.[34] A variety of other nonspecific symptoms may be caused by worms within the intestines (Table 20.3). Both children and adults may suffer from serious acute complications. Over half of these complications occur when a mass of worms within the small intes-

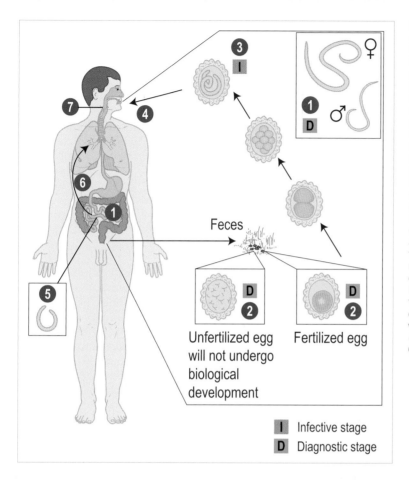

Feces

Unfertilized egg will not undergo biological development

Fertilized egg

**I** Infective stage
**D** Diagnostic stage

Fig. 20.3 *Ascaris* lifecycle. Adult worms (1) live in the lumen of the small intestine. A female may produce approximately 200,000 eggs per day, which are passed with the feces (2). Unfertilized eggs may be ingested but are not infective. Fertile eggs embryonate and become infective after 18 days to several weeks (3), depending on the environmental conditions (optimum: moist, warm, shaded soil). After infective eggs are swallowed (4), the larvae hatch (5), invade the intestinal mucosa, and are carried via the portal, then systemic circulation to the lungs (6). The larvae mature further in the lungs (10 to 14 days), penetrate the alveolar walls, ascend the bronchial tree to the throat, and are swallowed (7). Upon reaching the small intestine, they develop into adult worms (1). Between 2 and 3 months are required from ingestion of the infective eggs to oviposition by the adult female. Adult worms can live 1 to 2 years. (Adapted from Centers for Disease Control and Prevention DPDx.)

tines leads to intestinal obstruction.[34] This typically occurs in 1–5-year-old children with large worm burdens and may present with colicky abdominal pain and emesis. Occasionally, adult worms are seen in the vomitus. In some areas of the world, intestinal obstruction from *Ascaris* worms is the leading cause of acute abdominal emergencies (Fig. 20.4).[37] Other acute complications, including cholangitis, hepatic abscess, pancreatitis, and appendicitis, occur when adult worms migrate into various locations. Complications may arise many years after immigration if remnants of deceased worms or eggs remain in the biliary system and elicit the formation of calculi. For example, recurrent pyogenic cholangiohepatitis has been reported in a Vietnamese-American woman approximately 15 years after emigration.[38]

**Diagnosis:** Diagnosis is made by finding characteristic eggs in the stool, or passage of worms in vomitus or feces or via the nose or mouth. Diagnosis of the

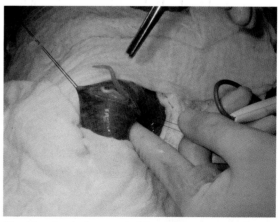

Fig. 20.4 Surgical removal of *Ascaris* worms in child with intestinal obstruction. Photo courtesy of Dr. Christian Blanc.

## Table 20.3 Intestinal nematodes

| Parasite | Distribution | Transmission | Potential Complications |
|---|---|---|---|
| *Ascaris* | Global | Ingestion of contaminated soil | Loffler's syndrome (during transpulmonary larval migration): cough, wheezing, dyspnea, substernal pain or burning, fever, eosinophilia<br>Aberrant larval migration: Rash, conjunctivitis, seizures<br>Adult worms in small intestines: abdominal pain or distention, nausea, vomiting, anorexia, malabsorption, malnutrition, growth and cognitive impairment<br>Aggregation of adult worms: intestinal obstruction, intussusception, volvulus and perforation<br>Migration of adult worms: cholangitis, hepatic abscess, pancreatitis, appendicitis, airway obstruction, emergence of worms from nose or mouth |
| *Trichuris* | Global | | Light to moderate worm burden: anemia, impaired growth and poor school performance, epigastric and right lower quadrant pain, vomiting, flatulence, anorexia, weight loss<br>Heavy worm burden: loose stools with blood and/or mucous, dysentery, rectal prolapse, digital clubbing, hypoproteinemia |
| *Enterobius* | Global | Fecal-oral | Pruritus ani, secondary bacterial infection, insomnia, restlessness, irritability, anorexia, enuresis, vulvitis |
| Hookworms | Global | Skin penetration | See Chapter 32 |
| *Strongyloides* | Global | Skin penetration | See Chapter 40 |

Data are from References 34, 35, and 36.

acute complications may be facilitated by imaging studies. Eosinophilia is commonly seen only during larval migration through the lungs.

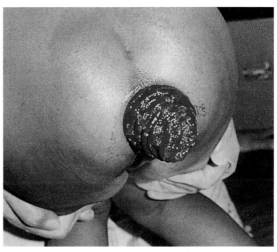

Fig. 20.5 Rectal prolapse. Heavy infections may cause rectal prolapse following chronic bloody diarrhea with abdominal pain in infants and children, especially if they are undernourished. Reproduced with permission from Peters W, Pasvol G. Tropical medicine and parasitology, 5th edn. London: Mosby; 2002:125.

**Etiology:** *Trichuris trichiura*, commonly called whipworm due to its unique morphology, is a ubiquitous geohelminth (Box 20.2; Fig. 20.6). These worms live in the cecum, but may cover the entire colon in heavy infections. The presence of visible worms on the mucosa of a prolapsed rectum is pathognomonic for trichuriasis.

**Epidemiology:** Like *A. lumbricoides*, *T. trichiura* thrives in climates with abundant rainfall, high humidity, and shade. However, it occurs in individuals throughout the world, including 8% of refugees

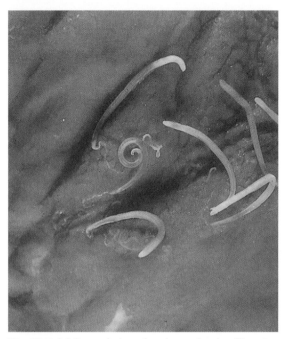

**Fig. 20.6** Adult morphology, females and males. Three to 10 days after the eggs are ingested, the young worms pass down to the cecum where the whip-like anterior portion becomes entwined in the mucosa. The adult worms are about 3–5 cm long, with the females being slightly larger than the males which are coiled. The adult worms (one male and several females) are seen in this figure of the cecal mucosa. (· 2) (AFIP No. 69–3583.) Reproduced with permission from Peters W, Pasvol G. Tropical medicine and parasitology, 5th edn. London: Mosby; 2002:125.

from Eastern Europe.[19] Over one billion people worldwide are estimated to be infected with this organism.[35] The highest worm burden is seen in school-aged children. Geophagia increases the risk of *Trichuris* infection.[35]

**Lifecycle:** Its method of transmission is similar to *A. lumbricoides*, the ingestion of mature eggs via fingers contaminated with infected soil. However, after the larvae hatch they remain in the intestine as they develop into adult worms, lacking a transpulmonary migration (Fig. 20.7). Given the similar mode of transmission, it is not surprising that children are often coinfected with *Ascaris*.

**Clinical manifestations:** Most *T. trichiura* infections involve relatively few worms and the vast majority of these light infections are thought to be asymptomatic. However, there is considerable evidence that,

even with light to moderate worm burdens, children may suffer from anemia, impaired growth, and poor school performance.[35] Several non-specific signs and symptoms may include abdominal distension and pain, especially in the epigastric and right iliac fossa areas, vomiting, flatulence, anorexia, and weight loss. These gastrointestinal symptoms may be more likely in individuals coinfected with *Ascaris* and/or hookworm.

Heavy infections can cause significant morbidity. Dysentery with mucus and blood in stools is a common presentation that is often accompanied by rectal prolapse. Dysentery can be made worse by coinfection with protozoa such as *Entamoeba histolytica* and *Balantidium coli* or by dysentery-associated bacterial pathogens. In severe infections, young children may develop digital clubbing and hypoalbuminemia.[36] Intermittent painless hematochezia has been reported in adult immigrants.[39] The differential diagnosis of the *Trichuris* dysentery syndrome includes amoebic colitis. Trichuriasis may also present similarly to acute appendicitis with right-lower quadrant abdominal pain (see Table 20.3).

**Diagnosis:** Trichuriasis is not associated with prominent eosinophilia since there is no tissue migration of the worms. Diagnosis can be made in heavy infections by visible worms on a prolapsed rectum or by proctoscopy. Colonoscopy has also diagnosed symptomatic infections.[39] Typically, diagnosis is made by detecting the eggs, with characteristic bipolar plugs, on stool O&P examination.

### Other nematodes

Hookworm and *Strongyloides* are covered in detail in separate chapters.

**Enterobius vermicularis:** *E. vermicularis*, commonly known as pinworm, is found throughout the world. It occurs more often in children and among individuals living in crowded living conditions, such as orphanages.[40] The prevalence among immigrant groups is unknown since screening stool O&P examinations have an extremely low sensitivity for detecting this organism (<5%).[36] It is primarily transmitted via fecal–oral contamination. Adult female worms live in the cecum and migrate to the anus at night to deposit eggs on the perineum. Adult worms only live for 1–3 months, but persistent infections are common due to repetitive infections resulting from ongoing fecal–oral spread among affected individuals, facilitated by the pruritic response to the deposited eggs. Other means of transmission include

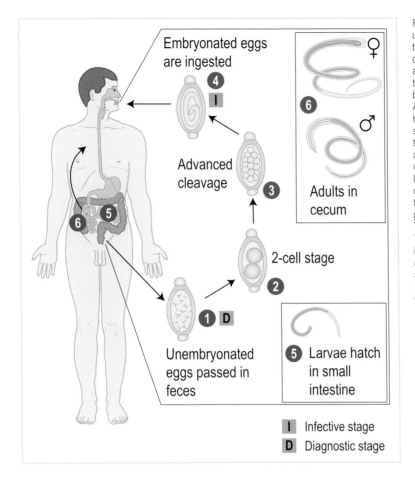

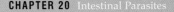

**Fig. 20.7** *Trichuris* lifecycle. The unembryonated eggs are passed with the stool (1). In the soil, the eggs develop into a 2-cell stage (2), an advanced cleavage stage (3), and then they embryonate (4); eggs become infective in 15 to 30 days. After ingestion (soil-contaminated hands or food), the eggs hatch in the small intestine, and release larvae (5) that mature and establish themselves as adults in the colon (6). The adult worms (approximately 4 cm in length) live in the cecum and ascending colon. The adult worms are fixed in that location, with the anterior portions threaded into the mucosa. The females begin to oviposit 60 to 70 days after infection. Female worms in the cecum shed between 3,000 and 20,000 eggs per day. The life span of the adults is about 1 year. (Adapted from Centers for Disease Control and Prevention DPDx.)

contact with soiled bed linens and inhalation of contaminated dust.[36]

The most common symptom is *pruritus ani* caused by the irritating effects of the deposited ova (see Table 20.3). Secondary bacterial infections may develop if excoriations are severe. Several nonspecific symptoms include insomnia, restlessness, irritability, anorexia, and enuresis. In females, *E. vermicularis* can occasionally cause vulvitis with associated mucoid discharge and itching. Diagnosis relies on detection of eggs on cellophane tape placed in the perianal area or by visualization of adult worms near the anus at night.[36]

### Larval nematode infections

***Toxocara canis:*** The dog roundworm has a global distribution, and has a similar lifecycle to *Ascaris*. Dogs ingest soil containing eggs, and puppies can become infected in utero by transplacental transmis-

sion. When humans, typically young children, accidentally ingest eggs, the larvae do not develop into adult worms. Instead, they wander throughout the body causing local inflammation in various tissues, especially the liver and eye, before becoming phagocytosed.[36] Most human infections are asymptomatic. However, children with heavy infections may present with findings of the visceral larva migrans (VLM) syndrome: fever, wheezing, hepatomegaly, and occasionally symptoms of heart failure, seizures and/or focal neurological deficits. Laboratory findings include marked eosinophilia, leukocytosis, and increased serum globulins. Ultrasonography may reveal hypoechoic liver lesions. Most VLM cases spontaneously resolve after 2 years, but some children may die without treatment. Another potential presentation is ocular toxocariasis. Affected children often present with strabismus or a white pupil, leukocoria, due to a retinal granuloma. Imaging studies should be performed to differentiate these granulomas from retinoblastomas. Occasionally, extensive intraocular inflammation can occur leading to retinal detachment. Detection of *Toxocara* antigens in the serum and/or vitreous fluid by enzyme-linked immunosorbent assay (ELISA) facilitates the diagnosis.[36]

*Angiostrongylus costaricensis:* This rare infection, seen in Central and South Americans, may cause a tender right-lower quadrant abdominal mass mimicking appendicitis, intussusception, inflammatory bowel disease, or ileocecal tuberculosis. Although rats are the definitive host and slugs are the intermediate hosts, humans may become accidentally infected after ingesting vegetation contaminated with the mucous secretions of slugs. The immune response to migrating larvae causes granulomatous lesions to form near the ileocecal region. Eosinophilia is often pronounced. Surgery is usually indicated.[41]

*Angiostrongylus cantonensis:* Larvae of this rat nematode can affect humans via consumption of undercooked snails, prawns, or crab from Southeast Asia or the Caribbean. It is the most common infectious cause of eosinophilic meningitis.[42] Affected individuals often present with headache, papilloedema, and cutaneous sensory alterations. The incubation period is relatively short, so it would most likely be seen in recently arrived immigrants or travelers. In an outbreak among travelers to Jamaica, the median time to presentation was 11 days after returning to the US. Peripheral eosinophilia or cerebrospinal fluid (CSF) eosinophilia may not be seen at the time of initial presentation.[43] Giemsa staining of CSF fluid is crucial to facilitate early diagnosis.[44] The diagnosis can be confirmed by detection of *A. cantonensis* antibodies in convalescent serum. Treatment consists of corticosteroids and repeat lumbar punctures to decrease intracranial pressure.

*Gnathostoma spinigerum:* This nematode is most frequently found throughout Southeast Asia, but it is also seen in India, East Africa, Central and South America, and Mexico. Increasing numbers of case reports of gnathostomiasis in international travelers have served to increase awareness of this obscure condition. The adult nematode lives in cats, dogs, and other carnivores. Eggs passed into water are picked up by *Cyclops*, a type of small crustacean. Infected *Cyclops* are then consumed by larger second intermediate hosts. Humans become infected with larvae by eating undercooked fish, shrimp, crab, crayfish, frogs, and even chicken. Patients typically present with episodic cutaneous, gastrointestinal, or neurological symptoms over a period of months to years. The classic skin lesion is an intermittent, migratory, erythematous swelling. These lesions are often pruritic and painful. Visceral involvement may lead to vague, nonspecific episodic gastrointestinal symptoms. Neurological involvement most frequently causes a radiculomyelopathy, presenting with episodic, severe, burning sensations. Occasionally paresis of one or more limbs develops, and urinary retention can also occur. Some individuals may develop severe eosinophilic meningitis with mortality rates of 7.7–25%. Eosinophilia is present in only about half of cases, but when present it can be used as a marker for treatment response and predictor of relapses. Diagnosis can be made by direct visualization of larvae or by serological testing.[45,46]

*Anisakis* species: Human infection with the larval stages of these nematodes of marine mammals occurs through consumption of raw or undercooked fish, often in the form of sushi or sashimi. In humans, the larvae may cause tissue invasion near the iliocecal region and mimic acute appendicitis. There is no diagnostic test for these larvae. They may be found incidentally during endoscopy or laparotomy.[36]

## Food-borne trematodes

**Etiology:** *Opisthorchis viverrini* is the most common biliary liver fluke of humans and has the strongest association with cholangiocarcinoma (Box 20.3).

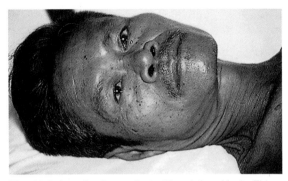

Fig. 20.8 Jaundice in a patient with opisthorchiasis. This adult Thai was heavily infected with *O. viverrini*. Reproduced with permission from Peters W, Pasvol G. Tropical medicine and parasitology, 5th edn. London: Mosby; 2002:151.

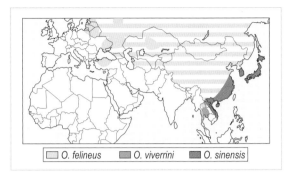

Fig. 20.10 Distribution map of *Opisthorchis* species in humans. Reproduced with permission from Peters W, Pasvol G. Tropical medicine and parasitology, 5th edn. London: Mosby; 2002:147.

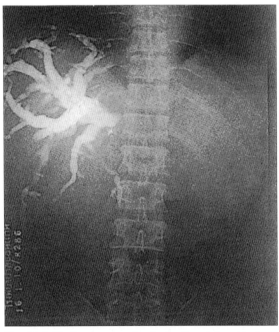

Fig. 20.9 Cholangiogram of patient with opisthorchiasis. This X-ray shows dilatation of the main bile ducts and disorganization of the biliary tree. Reproduced with permission from Peters W, Pasvol G. Tropical medicine and parasitology, 5th edn. London: Mosby; 2002:151.

**Epidemiology:** *Opisthorchis* species and *Clonorchis sinensis*, occasionally identified as *Opisthorchis sinensis*, are transmitted to humans through eating raw fish that contain infective metacercariae cysts (Table 20.4). An estimated 17 million people are infected throughout the world with these organisms; 9 million with *O. viverrini*, 7 million with *C. sinensis*, and 1.5

million with *O. felineus*.[47] The geographic distribution of these flukes depends on the range of the intermediate snail and fish hosts (Fig. 20.10). *O. viverrini* is endemic in Laos, Cambodia, and Thailand. *C. sinensis* is found in China, Taiwan, Vietnam, Korea, Hong Kong, and Japan. *O. felineus* is found in parts of Asia, Eastern Europe, and Siberia.

As opposed to *Ascaris* and *Trichuris*, both the prevalence and severity of biliary liver fluke infections increase with age. Traditional food preparation leads to a continual lifetime exposure. In Laos, Cambodia, and parts of northern Thailand people of all ages enjoy koi pla, a combination of pounded raw fish and spices.[47] In China, where many children catch and eat raw fish, the age distribution is skewed towards children.[36]

Although the vast majority of infected immigrants come from Southeast Asia, cases of *O. guayaquilensis* and *O. felineus* have been reported in immigrants from Ecuador and the former Soviet Union, respectively, in the United States.[47] In regions within Siberia, thinly sliced frozen cyprinoid fish is a popular dish.[36]

Biliary liver fluke infections are chronic and remain a concern in immigrants for many years after immigration. *C. sinensis* has been documented as causing pancreatitis in an individual 24 years after leaving an endemic area.[48] Prevalence of *Opisthorchis* infections was 5% among a group of Cambodian refugees after living in Canada for 6 years.[13] Detection of biliary liver fluke infections has a bimodal distribution in terms of time since immigration. In a series of 17 cases, approximately half of infections were diagnosed during initial arrival screening within 3 months of immigration. One-quarter of infections were diagnosed in immigrants living

**Table 20.4  Biliary liver flukes**

| Fluke | Distribution | Transmission | Potential complications | Diagnosis |
|---|---|---|---|---|
| *Clonorchis sinensis* | China, Taiwan, Vietnam, Korea, Hong Kong Japan | Ingestion of undercooked fish | Vague abdominal symptoms: abdominal fullness, right upper quadrant pain, diarrhea, anorexia | Clues:<br>– eosinophilia<br>– ultrasound findings: multiple nonshadowing foci, increased periductal echogenicity, floating foci in the gallbladder |
| *Opisthorchis viverrini* | Laos, Cambodia, Thailand | | Long-term consequences: hepatomegaly, gallbladder enlargement, biliary thickening, cholecystitis, cholangitis, cholelithiasis, intrahepatic stones, cirrhosis, pancreatitis, cholangiocarcinoma | Definitive:<br>– detection of eggs in stool<br>– serum antibody and/or stool antigen detection (if available) |
| *Opisthorchis felineus* | Eastern Europe and Siberia | | | |
| *Opisthorchis guayaquilensis* | Ecuador | | | |
| *Fasciola hepatica* | Global | Ingestion of raw aquatic plants | Acute fascioliasis: fever, night sweats, malaise, anorexia, weight loss, nausea, vomiting, right costal margin pain, hepatomegaly, splenomegaly, hepatic abscess, urticaria<br>Aberrant larval migration: symptoms of visceral larva migrans in heart, lungs, brain and intestinal wall | Acute fascioliasis: marked eosinophilia, imaging studies of liver and serological tests<br>Chronic fascioliasis: multiple stool specimens (stool O&P testing has very low sensitivity) and serological testing |
| *Fasciola gigantica* | South and Southeast Asia, Africa | | Chronic fascioliasis: choledocholithiasis, cholangitis, cholelithiasis, cholecystitis, jaundice, abdominal pain, hepatomegaly, and fatty food intolerance, ascites | |

Data are from References 17, 36, 47, 54, and 55.

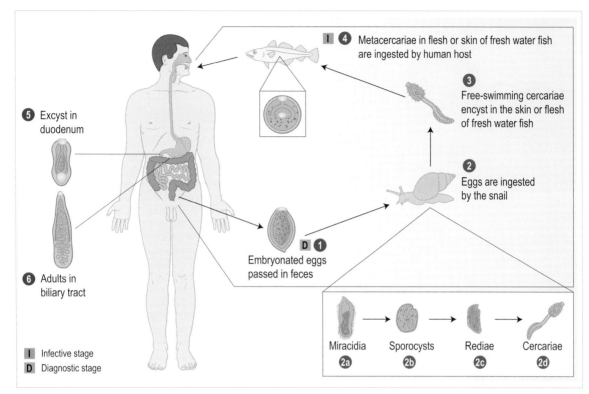

**Fig. 20.11** *Opisthorchis* lifecycle. The adult flukes deposit fully developed eggs that are passed in the feces (1). After ingestion by a suitable snail (first intermediate host) (2), the eggs release miracidia (2a), which undergo in the snail several developmental stages (sporocysts (2b), rediae (2c), cercariae (2d)). Cercariae are released from the snail (3) and penetrate freshwater fish (second intermediate host), encysting as metacercariae in the muscles or under the scales (4). The mammalian definitive host (cats, dogs, and various fish-eating mammals including humans) become infected by ingesting undercooked fish containing metacercariae. After ingestion, the metacercariae excyst in the duodenum (5) and ascend through the ampulla of Vater into the biliary ducts, where they attach and develop into adults, which lay eggs after 3 to 4 weeks (6). The adult flukes (*O. viverrini*: 5 mm to 10 mm by 1 mm to 2 mm; *O. felineus*: 7 mm to 12 mm by 2 mm to 3 mm) reside in the biliary and pancreatic ducts of the mammalian host, where they attach to the mucosa. (Adapted from Centers for Disease Control and Prevention DPDx.)

In the figure, the labels are:

5 Excyst in duodenum

6 Adults in biliary tract

I Infective stage

D Diagnostic stage

I 4 Metacercariae in flesh or skin of fresh water fish are ingested by human host

3 Free-swimming cercariae encyst in the skin or flesh of fresh water fish

2 Eggs are ingested by the snail

D 1 Embryonated eggs passed in feces

Miracidia (2a) Sporocysts (2b) Rediae (2c) Cercariae (2d)

in the US for over 5 years, with 12% occurring after 10 years. Several of those with late diagnoses had visited their countries of origin after emigrating, suggesting the possibility of travel-related infections.[47]

**Lifecycle:** The adult flukes reside in the intrahepatic ducts of humans, cats, dogs, and other fish-eating mammals. Eggs exit through the bile ducts into the intestines and are passed in stool. If fecal material enters water, snails may ingest the eggs. Within a snail, development of miracidiae into motile cercariae occurs. After exiting the snail, cercariae penetrate into and encyst within certain species of fish, typically carp of the Cyprinidae and Anabatidae families. When humans consume undercooked fish, metacercariae within the cysts are released and

migrate through the ampulla of Vater into the intrahepatic ducts where they develop into the long-lived adult flukes. One month after infection, eggs can be detected in stools (Fig. 20.11).[36] Fishing villages provide environments which foster maintenance of this cycle with humans as the primary definitive host (Fig. 20.12).

**Clinical manifestations:** As with all intestinal parasitic infections, most affected individuals are asymptomatic. However, even these apparently healthy individuals often have hepatomegaly and evidence of gallbladder enlargement, stones, or sludging on ultrasonography.[36] When present, symptoms classically include abdominal fullness, right-upper quadrant pain, diarrhea, and anorexia.[36] Among a series of affected immigrants in Minnesota, presenting

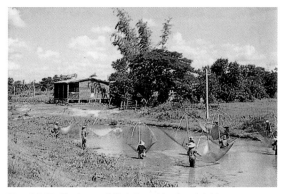

Fig. 20.12 Ecology of *Opisthorchis viverrini*. Humans are infected by ingesting the metacercariae in cyprinoid fish. The figure shows a typical village fishpond in north-east Thailand. Both the snail and fish populations of the ponds increase during the rainy season. Reproduced with permission from Peters W, Pasvol G. Tropical medicine and parasitology, 5th edn. London: Mosby; 2002:150.

complaints were commonly vague and nonspecific, including headaches, nausea, abdominal pain and cramping, rashes, pruritus, anorexia, facial swelling, insomnia, arthralgias, and dyspnea.[47]

Potentially severe long-term consequences include biliary thickening, cholecystitis, cholangitis, cholelithiasis, intrahepatic stones, cirrhosis, pancreatitis, and cholangiocarcinoma.[47,48] Among the liver flukes, *O. viverrini* infection carries the greatest risk of cholangiocarcinoma. In Thailand, a five fold increased risk of cholangiocarcinoma was found among individuals with any degree of *O. viverrini* infection and a 15-fold increased risk in individuals with a high fluke burden.[49] There is evidence that *C. sinensis* infection is associated with this malignancy as well.[50]

**Diagnosis:** Clinicians should consider *Opisthorchis* species and *C. sinensis* infections in patients from endemic areas presenting with right-upper quadrant abdominal pain or nonspecific complaints in association with eosinophilia. In the series of 17 immigrants in Minnesota with biliary liver fluke infections, 88% of cases had eosinophilia, defined as an absolute eosinophil count greater than 500/μL.[47] Diagnosis is typically made by stool O&P examinations. New serum tests for *O. viverrini* antibodies are promising, with reported 100% sensitivity and specificity.[51] Polymerase chain reaction (PCR) assays of stool samples are being developed for this organism, but currently have a low sensitivity.[52] In endemic areas, *Clonorchis* infections are often diagnosed by antigen detection in stool samples, with some assays having

a 92.5% sensitivity and 93.1% specificity.[53] Ultrasound studies that reveal multiple nonshadowing echogenic foci, increased periductal echogenicity, and floating echogenic foci in the gallbladder support the diagnosis.[17,54]

---

**Box 20.4**

**Case study 4**

A 26-year-old woman, who has emigrated from the Dominican Republic to the US 1 month earlier, presents to an emergency department with severe, right-upper quadrant pain of several hours duration. The pain radiates to the right shoulder. She denies any significant past history. On examination, she is anicteric, afebrile, and has mild right-upper quadrant tenderness without hepatosplenomegaly. Blood tests reveal peripheral eosinophilia (27%) and, on computed tomography (CT), a 6 × 5 × 4 cm heterogeneous necrotic mass is seen in the right hepatic lobe (Fig. 20.13). An IgG enzyme immunoassay is slightly positive for antibodies to *Echinococcus granulosus*. The patient denies any past exposure to farm animals, dogs, or fresh water. However, she does report frequent consumption of uncooked 'berro,' or watercress. One week after presentation, further testing is negative for *Entamoeba histolytica* and *Fasciola hepatica* antibodies, as well as *Echinococcus* western blot. Stool O&P examination reveals only nonpathogenic intestinal protozoa. Her eosinophilia peaks at 7000/mm³ (46%). Indirect immunofluorescence tests for antibodies to *Fasciola hepatica* performed 2 and 3 weeks after presentation reveal increased titers. After a single dose of triclabendazole, her symptoms, eosinophilia, and CT changes resolve.

The above text is adapted with permission from reference 55. Copyright © 2002 by The American Society of Tropical Medicine and Hygiene.

---

**Etiology:** *Fasciola hepatica*, the sheep liver fluke, can cause illness during both the acute, as in the case in Box 20.4, or chronic phase of infection.

**Epidemiology:** Human *F. hepatica* infection occurs globally and mirrors the prevalence of infection observed in sheep and cattle. The parasite is endemic in South and Central America, the Caribbean, and parts of Africa, the Middle East, Asia, China, and Australia. Outbreaks have also been reported in southern France and the Mediterranean.[36,55] The closely related *Fasciola gigantica* primarily affects

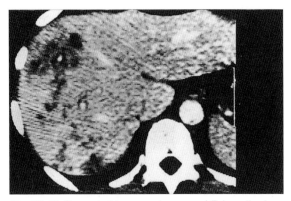

**Fig. 20.13** Computed tomography scan of *F. hepatica* in human liver. Using contrast, cystic filling defects suggestive of this trematode infection can be visualized. They usually disappear after therapy. Reproduced with permission from Peters W, Pasvol G. Tropical medicine and parasitology, 5th edn. London: Mosby; 2002:154.

cattle. *Fasciola gigantica* is found in South and Southeast Asia as well as Africa and Hawaii (see Table 20.4).[36]

**Lifecycle:** Unlike the other biliary liver flukes, *Clonorchis* and *Opisthorchis*, infection with *F. hepatica and F. gigantica* results from eating contaminated raw aquatic vegetation, especially watercress ('berro') and, in Asia, morning glory (Fig. 20.14). High infection rates in the Bolivian highlands stem from children eating kjosco, a raw water-plant salad, while in the wet pastures with grazing animals.[36] The free-swimming cercariae that exit the intermediate snail host deposit on the vegetation and encyst into metacercariae. After ingestion, the larval metacercariae excyst, penetrate the duodenum, and migrate through the liver parenchyma for several weeks before entering bile ducts and maturing into adults.[36]

**Clinical manifestations:** Both *F. hepatica* and *F. gigantica* cause human fascioliasis. Depending on the number of larval stages ingested, acute infection may be asymptomatic or associated with any combination of fever, night sweats, malaise, anorexia, weight loss, nausea, vomiting, right costal margin pain, hepatomegaly, splenomegaly, urticaria, and marked eosinophilia. These symptoms begin about 2 months after ingestion of the contaminated aquatic plants and may persist for several weeks to months while larvae are migrating through the liver.[36,55] Acute fascioliasis with an associated hepatic abscess may be differentiated from a hydatid cyst,

caused by *Echinococcus* larvae, by the absence of a capsule or calcification and by the presence of hemorrhage within the cavity on CT images.[55] Once larvae enter the bile ducts acute symptoms subside. Larvae can also migrate to aberrant locations, causing inflammation in heart, lungs, brain, and intestinal wall.[55]

Individuals with chronic fascioliasis are usually asymptomatic but may have symptoms of choledocholithiasis and cholangitis if the adult worms or eggs block the extrahepatic bile ducts, or cholelithiasis and cholecystitis if worms enter the gallbladder. Patients may develop jaundice, abdominal pain, hepatomegaly, and fatty food intolerance. If severe, ascites may develop. Although rare, death may result from hemorrhaging into bile ducts.[36]

**Diagnosis:** Acute fascioliasis should be considered in any immigrant from endemic areas presenting with eosinophilia, liver abscess, and history of raw aquatic plant ingestion.[55] Stool examinations will not reveal *F. hepatica* during acute infection, since only migrating larvae are present. Stool microscopy, even with use of multiple specimens, has a very low sensitivity to detect chronic-phase infections. Serological tests are almost always required to make the diagnosis. After treatment, antibody levels drop quickly.[36,55]

## Other food-borne trematodes

In addition to the biliary liver flukes discussed above, certain immigrant groups may be at risk for intestinal flukes. There are over 70 species of food-borne trematodes that may be found within human intestines. However, only a few are of clinical significance. These include *Fasciolepis buski* and some of the small intestinal flukes termed heterophyids, especially *Heterophyes heterophyes* and *Metagonimus yokagawai*. The key features of these intestinal flukes are listed in Table 20.5.

Other important trematode infections in immigrants are caused by *Paragonimus* species, or lung flukes. These flukes are seen throughout the world, but human infections are most common in Southeast Asia. Countries with substantial numbers of human infections include China, Taiwan, Thailand, Japan, Korea, Nigeria, Cameroon, Peru, Guatemala, and Ecuador.[36] Humans become infected by eating crustaceans, such as crabs, crayfish, or shrimp, that contain metacercariae cysts. After ingestion, the larvae excyst in the intestines, migrate through the diaphragm and mature into adults within the lungs. Adult lung flukes can live for 20 years. Eggs are

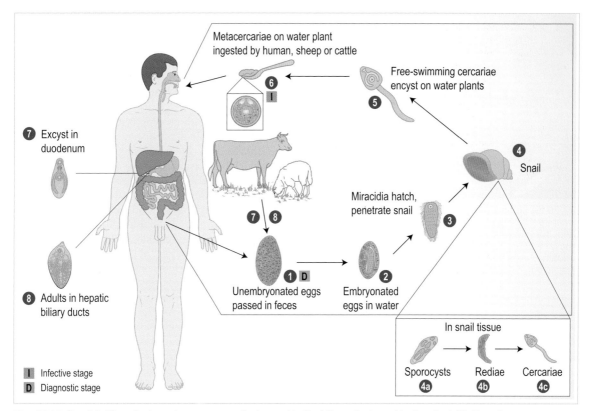

**Fig. 20.14** *Fasciola* lifecycle. Immature eggs are discharged in the biliary ducts and in the stool (1). Eggs become embryonated in water (2), eggs release miracidia (3), which invade a suitable snail intermediate host (4), including many species of the genus *Lymnae*. In the snail the parasites undergo several developmental stages (sporocysts (4a), rediae (4b), and cercariae (4c)). The cercariae are released from the snail (5) and encyst as metacercariae on aquatic vegetation or other surfaces. Mammals acquire the infection by eating vegetation containing metacercariae. Humans can become infected by ingesting metacercariae-containing freshwater plants, especially watercress (6). After ingestion, the metacercariae excyst in the duodenum (7) and migrate through the intestinal wall, the peritoneal cavity, and the liver parenchyma into the biliary ducts, where they develop into adults (8). In humans, maturation from metacercariae into adult flukes takes approximately 3 to 4 months. The adult flukes (*Fasciola hepatica*: up to 30 mm by 13 mm; *F. gigantica*: up to 75 mm) reside in the large biliary ducts of the mammalian host. *Fasciola hepatica* infect various animal species, mostly herbivores. (Adapted from Centers for Disease Control and Prevention DPDx.)

either coughed up and spit out in sputum or are swallowed and exit the body in feces. The remainder of the cycle is similar to the other food-borne flukes, involving intermediate snail hosts. Chronic cough is the primary clinical manifestation. Most species lead to the production of a brownish, blood-tinged, egg-containing sputum. Chest pain and night sweats are common. Chest X-rays or CT scans classically show patchy infiltrates and cavities. These symptoms and findings can lead to incorrect diagnoses of tuberculosis or bronchiectasis. Diagnoses can be made by serological testing or by detection of eggs in sputum, feces, or gastric washings. Eosinophilia is often seen. If the larvae migrate to the central nervous system instead of the lungs, eosinophilic meningitis or spastic paraplegia may develop.[36]

## Cestodes

**Box 20.5**

**Case study 5**

Parents of a 6-year-old Somali girl seen at a primary care clinic for well child care report that she has been complaining of occasional abdominal discomfort over the past few months. She and her family entered the US 3 months earlier after living in a refugee camp. Stool O&P revealed ova of *Hymenolepis nana*. She was treated with praziquantel, and follow-up stool examination showed no further ova. However, she continued to have occasional abdominal discomfort.

**Table 20.5 Intestinal flukes of clinical importance**

| Fluke | Distribution | Transmission | Potential complications | Diagnosis |
|---|---|---|---|---|
| *F. buski* | China, India, Bangladesh, Thailand, Malaysia, Borneo, Sumatra and Myanmar | Ingestion of metacercariae in water or attached to the seed pods of water plants (caltrops, hyacinth, bamboo, water chestnut, wild rice shoots, lotus roots) | If symptomatic, patients may have diarrhea, flatulence, decreased appetite, abdominal pain that may mimic peptic ulcers, and fever. If severe, may have generalized edema from intestinal protein loss | Eggs are easily detected by stool O&P testing |
| *M. yokogawai* | Korea, Eastern provinces of the former USSR, and Mediterranean basin | Ingestion of raw fish containing metacercariae | If symptomatic, may have mild abdominal pain, diarrhea, and lethargy that resolves spontaneously within 1 month | Difficult due to low egg output and similar appearance to *Opisthorchis* and *Clonorchis* eggs |
| *H. heterophyes* | Widely distributed | | Eggs may travel from the intestines to the heart (where myocarditis may develop), brain or spinal cord (and lead to transverse myelitis or other neurological deficits) | |

Data are from Reference 36.

**Etiology:** *Hymenolepis nana*, the human dwarf tapeworm, measures only up to 3–4 cm (Box 20.5).

**Epidemiology:** *H. nana* is ubiquitous in areas with both warm climates and poor sanitation. In these locations, often over 10% of children harbor these worms.[36] *H. nana* is routinely the most commonly detected tapeworm in refugees from throughout the world, with the possible exception of a higher risk of fish tapeworm in those from Russia.[5] Among Mexican immigrants aged 5–9 years old, 24% were found to harbor the dwarf tapeworm.[10]

**Lifecycle:** Unlike all other tapeworms, *H. nana* does not require an intermediate host. Rodents can harbor adult worms, but this is not essential for human transmission. It is spread in humans primarily via fecal–oral transmission. Although the lifespan of an adult worm is only 4–6 weeks, autoinfection by larvae released by the adult worm enables *H. nana* infections to persist for long periods of time in children (Fig. 20.15).[36] In adults, the infection is of limited duration due to acquired immunity.[56]

**Clinical manifestations:** Symptoms related to *H. nana* are rare except in those with very heavy worm burdens. In children with 1000–2000 adult worms, abdominal pain and diarrhea resulting from mucosal damage may occur.[56] Rare reports have linked recurrent itchy rashes to *H. nana*.[57] Death has occurred in an individual with AIDS due to aberrant larval migration.[58] It is unlikely that the abdominal pains experienced by the girl in case study 5 were related to *H. nana* infection.

**Diagnosis:** Diagnosis is made by detecting characteristic eggs on stool microscopic examination. Unlike individuals harboring other types of tapeworms, affected individuals will not see proglottids in their stool, since these degenerate while exiting the intestines. Eosinophilia is often seen with *H. nana* infections, but not in other adult tapeworm infections.

## Other cestodes

The other adult tapeworms that afflict humans are transmitted through eating undercooked beef, pork,

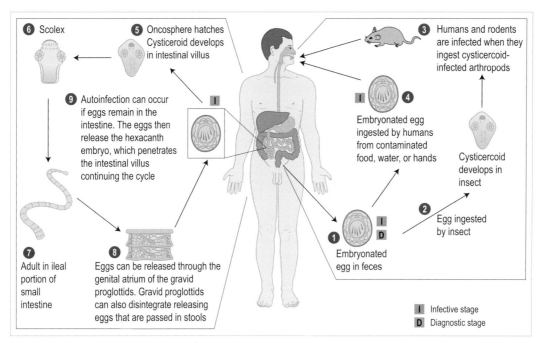

Fig. 20.15 *Hymenolepis nana* lifecycle. Eggs of *Hymenolepis nana* are immediately infective when passed with the stool and cannot survive more than 10 days in the external environment (1). When eggs are ingested by an arthropod intermediate host (2) (various species of beetles and fleas may serve as intermediate hosts), they develop into cysticercoids, which can infect humans or rodents upon ingestion (3) and develop into adults in the small intestine. A morphologically identical variant, *H. nana* var. *fraterna*, infects rodents and uses arthropods as intermediate hosts. When eggs are ingested (4) (in contaminated food or water or from hands contaminated with feces), the oncospheres contained in the eggs are released. The oncospheres (hexacanth larvae) penetrate the intestinal villus and develop into cysticercoid larvae (5). Upon rupture of the villus, the cysticercoids return to the intestinal lumen, evaginate their scoleces (6), attach to the intestinal mucosa and develop into adults that reside in the ileal portion of the small intestine producing gravid proglottids (7). Eggs are passed in the stool when released from proglottids through its genital atrium or when proglottids disintegrate in the small intestine (8). An alternate mode of infection consists of internal autoinfection, where the eggs release their hexacanth embryo, which penetrates the villus continuing the infective cycle without passage through the external environment (9). The life span of adult worms is 4 to 6 weeks, but internal autoinfection allows the infection to persist for years. (Adapted from Centers for Disease Control and Prevention DPDx.)

or fish. The adult worms residing in human intestines cause little morbidity, but can reach enormous lengths. The largest fish tapeworm recorded was 330 meters long, but lengths rarely exceed 15 meters (Fig. 20.16).[36,56] These organisms are reviewed in Table 20.6.

## Protozoa

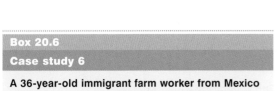

**Box 20.6**

**Case study 6**

A 36-year-old immigrant farm worker from Mexico presents to a community clinic for evaluation of high fevers that began suddenly 10 days earlier.

He reports a slight cough as his only other symptom. He has no significant past medical history. On physical examination, he is febrile (39°C), with a pulse of 90 and blood pressure of 110/70 mmHg. He has decreased breath sounds in his right lower lung fields, with dullness to percussion. He is tender to palpation in the right upper quadrant of his abdomen, but has no hepatosplenomegaly. A chest X-ray is interpreted as a right-lower lobe consolidation and he is sent home with levofloxacin for pneumonia. He returns 2 days later with continued fevers and new pleuritic chest pain. He is admitted to a local hospital where the radiologist reads the original chest X-ray as showing an elevated right hemidiaphragm with no consolidation and on his admission X-ray a new right pleural effusion is seen. An abdominal CT reveals a round homogeneous lesion with a well-defined border near the superior surface of the right hepatic lobe (Fig. 20.17). Antibodies to *Entamoeba histolytica* are detected in his blood. His symptoms resolve quickly after starting metronidazole and drainage of the pleural effusion.

**Etiology:** *Entamoeba histolytica* has been described as a 'macrophage on steroids with pumped-up phagocytic, proteolytic, and cytolytic capabilities invading the colonic mucosa, and occasionally penetrating through the portal circulation, reaching the liver and causing fatal abscesses' (Box 20.6).[59]

**Epidemiology:** *E. histolytica* is found throughout the world wherever there are breakdowns in public sanitation. The true prevalence of amoebiasis throughout the world remains a matter of debate since past prevalence studies were based on stool microscopy which is unable to distinguish nonpathogenic *E. dispar* and *E. moshkovskii* from *E. histolytica*.[18] This has

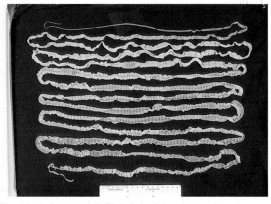

**Fig. 20.16** Intact adult *Diphyllobothrium latum*. A mature adult may reach 10 m in length. The head and mature proglottids are readily distinguished from those of *Taenia* in humans. Mature worms may produce 1 million eggs daily. Several other species of *Diphyllobothrium* occur in humans but all are rare except *Diphyllobothrium dalliae* (in western Alaska), *Diphyllobothrium pacificum* (in Peru) and the related *Diplogonoporus grandi*, of which several hundred have been recorded in Japan. Reproduced with permission from Peters W, Pasvol G. Tropical medicine and parasitology, 5th edn. London: Mosby; 2002:202.

**Table 20.6 Tapeworms**

| Parasite | Distribution | Potential complications | Diagnosis |
|---|---|---|---|
| *Taenia saginata* (beef tapeworm) | Global, especially in resource-poor settings where people commonly eat raw or undercooked beef. Most common in sub-Saharan Africa and the Middle East. Highland areas of Ethiopia are especially affected | Common: Usually asymptomatic, but may have distress caused by awareness of motile proglottids emerging from anus Rare: vomiting of worm segments, non-specific GI upset | Detection of eggs in stool Patient may see motile proglottides in feces No eosinophilia |
| *Taenia solium* (pork tapeworm) | Global. Most common in rural areas of Mexico, South and Central America, Africa, India, and parts of Southeast Asia | Common: development of cysticercosis Rare: non-specific GI upset. Patients are less likely to notice proglottids since they are less motile. | Detection of eggs in stool No eosinophilia |
| *Diphyllobothrium latum* (fish tapeworm) | Global, but most common in Russia | Common: asymptomatic. Up to 50% may have low vitamin $B_{12}$ levels. Patients may notice passage of proglottid segments Rare: spontaneous expulsion of entire worm. Only 2% of carriers have pernicious anemia | Detection of eggs in stool No eosinophilia |
| *Hymenolepis nana* (dwarf tapeworm) | Global, especially in warm areas with poor sanitation | Common: Asymptomatic Rare: Abdominal pain and diarrhea in heavy infections, pruritic rash | Detection of eggs in stool Eosinophilia is common |

Data are from References 36, 56, and 57.

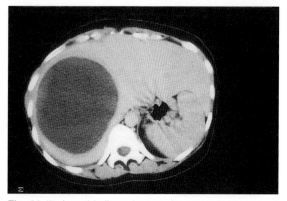

**Fig. 20.17** Amoebic liver abscess. An amoebic abscess of the liver is usually single and the volume of the contents of the lesion can vary from 500–1500 ml. The diagnosis is greatly facilitated by visualization of the abscess on a CT scan. A massive abscess is seen here in the right lobe of the liver. Such lesions are usually associated with right upper quadrant pain and fever. Reproduced with permission from Peters W, Pasvol G. Tropical medicine and parasitology, 5th edn. London: Mosby; 2002:177.

led to overestimations of asymptomatic carriage, but estimations of morbidity and mortality are more accurate. Of the approximately 50 million individuals who suffer from invasive disease annually, an estimated 100 000 die,[18] making *E. histolytica* the second leading cause of parasitic-related death, behind malaria.[59] Amoebic liver abscess occurs most frequently in men aged 18–50 years. Amoebic dysentery has traditionally been thought to affect all individuals equally, regardless of age or gender. However, recent reports suggest that males may be more prone to develop dysentery as well.[59] *E. histolytica* can spread easily between families. Therefore, contacts of patients with amoebiasis should be screened for intestinal colonization.[59] In 1993, 2970 cases of amoebiasis occurred in the US, with one-third occurring in immigrants from Latin America and 17% occurring in immigrants from Asia or the Pacific Islands.[59]

**Lifecycle:** Humans are the only significant reservoir of *E. histolytica*. Infection typically occurs via ingestion of cyst-containing water or food that has been contaminated with human feces. The cysts turn into the mobile trophozoite stage in the terminal ileum or colon. The trophozoites replicate by binary fission and then eventually revert back to the infectious cyst form that is excreted within feces (Fig. 20.18).[59]

**Clinical manifestations:** Although most individuals with *E. histolytica* infection are asymptomatic,

each year 4–10% of these individuals will develop clinical disease.[59] Amoebic colitis, or dysentery, presents with diarrhea and abdominal pain. The diarrhea is often bloody and even if gross blood is not visible, stools are nearly always heme-positive. Rectal bleeding, in the absence of diarrhea, may be seen and is more common in children. Loss of appetite and weight loss may occur. The onset of symptoms is usually gradual and patients may not present until several weeks into the illness. Fever is uncommon, unless the severe form of the illness, fulminant amoebic colitis, develops. Fulminant disease is associated with colonic perforation, marked leukocytosis, fever, severe bloody diarrhea, and generalized abdominal pain with peritoneal signs. Mortality of those with fulminant disease is over 40%.[59]

Amoebic liver abscesses (ALA) result from hematogenous spread of trophozoites that have penetrated the colonic mucosa. Patients have presented with ALA up to 12 years after being in an endemic area.[60] Usually, patients present with acute onset of fever and right-upper quadrant pain. Cough and rales in the right lung base are frequently observed and are likely related to atelectasis from elevation of the hemidiaphragm. Laboratory investigations often reveal leukocytosis, mild anemia, and elevations in the erythrocyte sedimentation rate and alkaline phosphatase level. Eosinophilia is not seen. Although amoebic liver abscess may occur at the same time as amoebic colitis, especially when fulminant colitis is present, most patients with liver abscesses have no symptoms of colitis.[59]

Clinicians may mistakenly diagnose an ALA as pneumonia due to the presence of respiratory symptoms and examination findings. In addition, 7–20% of patients develop fistulas from the liver abscess to the pleural space or lung. In these individuals empyemas may form, causing pleuritic pain, and if a hepatobronchial fistula forms, patients may expectorate large amounts of trophozoite-containing brownish sputum.[59] Extension of the abscess can also penetrate the peritoneum (2–7% of patients) and, more rarely, the pericardium. In less than 0.1% of ALA cases, abscesses may also form in the brain.[59]

**Diagnosis:** Diagnosis of amoebic colitis by fecal microscopy is complicated by a very low sensitivity using standard stool O&P techniques and the inability to differentiate *E. histolytica* from nonpathogenic amoebae. Sensitivity of microscopy can be increased by examining freshly purged stools.[14] Erythrophagocytosis, the presence of ingested red blood cells inside trophozoites, is supportive of amoebic colitis,

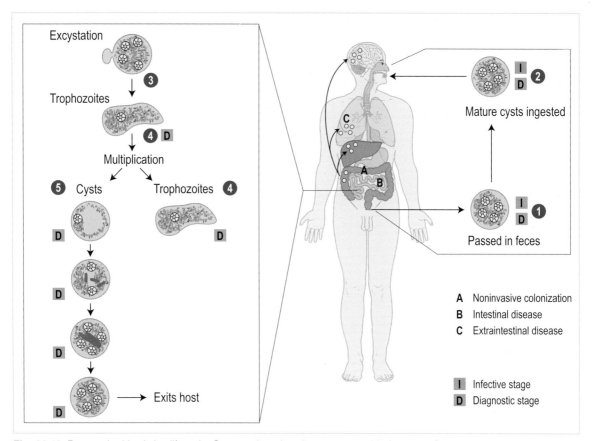

**Fig. 20.18** *Entamoeba histolytica* lifecycle. Cysts and trophozoites are passed in feces (1). Cysts are typically found in formed stool, whereas trophozoites are typically found in diarrheal stool. Infection by *Entamoeba histolytica* occurs by ingestion of mature cysts (2) in fecally contaminated food, water, or hands. Excystation (3) occurs in the small intestine and trophozoites (4) are released, which migrate to the large intestine. The trophozoites multiply by binary fission and produce cysts (5), and both stages are passed in the feces (1). Because of the protection conferred by their walls, the cysts can survive days to weeks in the external environment and are responsible for transmission. Trophozoites passed in the stool are rapidly destroyed once outside the body, and if ingested would not survive exposure to the gastric environment. In many cases, the trophozoites remain confined to the intestinal lumen (A: noninvasive infection) of individuals who are asymptomatic carriers, passing cysts in their stool. In some patients the trophozoites invade the intestinal mucosa (B: intestinal disease), or, through the bloodstream, extraintestinal sites such as the liver, brain, and lungs (C: extraintestinal disease), with resultant pathologic manifestations. It has been established that the invasive and noninvasive forms represent two separate species, respectively *E. histolytica* and *E. dispar*. These two species are morphologically indistinguishable unless *E. histolytica* is observed with ingested red blood cells (erythrophagocystosis). Transmission can also occur through exposure to fecal matter during sexual contact (in which case not only cysts, but also trophozoites could prove infective). (Adapted from Centers for Disease Control and Prevention DPDx.)

but it is now controversial whether this should be considered diagnostic. If all positive stool microscopy tests are considered diagnostic, then amoebic colitis may be overdiagnosed, and other dysentery causing pathogens will go untreated.[59] New sensitive ELISA tests are available that can accurately distinguish *E. histolytica* from *E. dispar*, but are not always widely available to clinicians.

The diagnosis of ALA is made by imaging studies in conjunction with positive *E. histolytica* serology. Both CT and ultrasound are sensitive imaging

studies. Positive serology is >94% sensitive and >95% specific for ALA, but false-negative results may occur during the first 10 days of infection. New PCR diagnostic assays are being developed.[59]

**Treatment:** Amoebic colitis and liver abscesses are treated with either metronidazole or tinidazole. However, it is important to follow treatment with administration of agents that eradicate colonic colonization (Table 20.7). Drainage of abscesses confined to the liver typically is not required, but it may be

**Table 20.7 Treatment regimens for intestinal parasites**

| Parasite | Drug | Pediatric dosage | Adult dosage |
|---|---|---|---|
| **Protozoa** | | | |
| *Entamoeba histolytica* | | | |
| Invasive Disease: | Metronidazole | 30–50 mg/kg/day ÷ tid × 7–10 days | 500–750 mg tid × 7–10 days |
| | Tinidazole* | 50 mg/kg daily (max. 2 g) × 3–5 days | 2 g daily × 3–5 days |
| Asymptomatic: | | | |
| Drug of choice: | Paromomycin | 25–35 mg/kg/day ÷ tid × 7 days | 25–35 mg/kg/d ÷ tid × 7 days |
| Alternative: | Diloxanide furoate | 30–40 mg/kg/day (max. 2 g) ÷ tid × 20 days | 650 mg tid × 20 days |
| | Iodoquinol | 20 mg/kg/day ÷ tid × 10 days | 500 mg tid × 10 days |
| *Giardia lamblia* | (see Giardia chapter for treatment regimens) | | |
| *Cryptosporidium parvum** (non-HIV-infected) | Nitazoxanide | 1–3 years old: 100 mg bid × 3 days; 4–11 years old: 200 mg bid × 3 days | 500 mg bid × 3 days |
| *Blastocystis hominis* (optimal treatment regimens for symptomatic patients remains unclear)* | Nitazoxanide | 1–3 years-old: 100 mg bid × 3 days; 4–11 years-old: 200 mg bid × 3 days | 500 mg bid × 3 days |
| | Metronidazole | | 750 mg tid × 10 days |
| | Iodoquinol | | 650 mg tid × 20 days |
| | TMP-SMX | | 1 double strength tab bid × 7 days |
| *Dientamoeba fragilis** | | | |
| Drugs of Choice: | Iodoquinol | 30–40 mg/kg/day (max. 2 g) ÷ tid × 20 days | 650 mg tid × 20 days |
| | Paromomycin | 25–35 mg/kg/day ÷ tid × 7 days | 25–35 mg/kg/d ÷ tid × 7 days |
| Alternatives: | Tetracycline | 40 mg/kg/day (max 2 g) ÷ qid × 10 days | 500 mg qid × 10 days |
| | Metronidazole | 20–40 mg/kg/day ÷ tid × 10 days | 500–750 mg tid × 10 days |
| **Nematodes** | | | |
| *Enterobius vermicularis** | Pyrantel pamoate | 11 mg/kg base × 1 dose | 11 mg/kg base × 1 dose |
| | Mebendazole | 100 mg × 1 dose | 100 mg × 1 dose |
| | Albendazole | 400 mg × 1 dose | 400 mg × 1 dose |
| *Ascaris lumbricoides* | Albendazole | 400 mg × 1 dose | 400 mg × 1 dose |
| | Mebendazole | 100 mg bid × 3 day, or 500 mg once* | 100 mg bid × 3 day, or 500 mg once* |
| | Ivermectin | 150–200 µg/kg × 1 dose | 150–200 µg/kg × 1 dose |
| *Trichuris trichiura* | | | |
| Drug of choice: | Mebendazole | 100 mg bid × 3 days, or 500 mg × 1 dose* | 100 mg bid × 3 days, or 500 mg × 1 dose* |
| Alternatives: | Albendazole | 400 mg daily × 3 days | 400 mg daily × 3 days |
| | Ivermectin | 200 µg/kg daily × 3 days | 200 µg/kg daily × 3 days |
| Hookworm: *Necator americanus* and *Ancylostoma duodenale* | Albendazole | 400 mg × 1 dose | 400 mg × 1 dose |
| | Mebendazole | 100 mg bid × 3 days, or 500 mg × 1 dose* | 100 mg bid × 3 days, or 500 mg × 1 dose* |
| | Pyrantel pamoate | 11 mg/kg daily × 3 days | 11 mg/kg daily × 3 days |

| | | | |
|---|---|---|---|
| *Strongyloides stercoralis* *Toxocara canis* | (see *Strongyloides* chapter for treatment regimens) | | |
| | Albendazole | 400 mg bid × 5 days | 400 mg bid × 5 days |
| | Mebendazole | 100–200 mg bid × 5 days | 100–200 mg bid × 5 days |
| *Angiostrongylus costaricensis* and *A. cantonensis*\* | There is no evidence that anthelmintic therapy is effective for these infections. | | |
| | *A. costaricensis* infection often requires surgery. | | |
| | *A. cantonensis* infection may respond to corticosteroids and repeat lumbar punctures. | | |
| | (All cases should be treated with medications, and surgery may be required in some cases)\* | | |
| *Gnathostoma spinigerum* | Albendazole | 400 mg bid × 21 days | 400 mg bid × 21 days |
| | Ivermectin | 200 µg/kg/day × 2 days | 200 µg/kg/day × 2 days |
| *Anisakis species*\* | Surgical or endoscopic removal | | |
| **Trematodes** | | | |
| *Clonorchis sinensis* and *Opisthorchis species* | | | |
| Drug of choice: | Praziquantel | 75 mg/kg/day ÷ tid × 1 day | 75 mg/kg/day ÷ tid × 1 day |
| Alternative: | Albendazole | 10 mg/kg daily × 7 days | 10 mg/kg daily × 7 days |
| *Fasciola species* | | | |
| Drug of choice: | Triclabendazole§ | 10 mg/kg × 1 dose | 10 mg/kg × 1 dose |
| Alternative: | Bithionol\* | 30–50 mg/kg every other day × 10–15 doses | 30–50 mg/kg every other day × 10–15 doses |
| *Fasciola buski, Heterophyes heterophyes,* and *Metagonimus yokogawa* | Praziquantel | 75 mg/kg/day ÷ tid × 1 day | 75 mg/kg/day ÷ tid × 1 day |
| *Schistosoma* | Praziquantel | (see Schistosomiasis chapter for species-specific dosing) | |
| **Cestodes** | | | |
| *Taenia solium* and *Taenia saginata, Diphyllobothrium latum* | | | |
| Drug of choice: | Praziquantel | 5–10 mg/kg × 1 dose | 5–10 mg/kg × 1 dose |
| Alternative: | Niclosamide | 50 mg/kg × 1 dose | 2 g × 1 dose |
| *Hymenolepis nana* | | | |
| Drug of choice: | Praziquantel | 25 mg/kg × 1 dose | 25 mg/kg × 1 dose |
| Alternative: | Nitazoxanide\* | 1–3 years-old: 100 mg bid × 3 days 4–11 years-old: 200 mg bid × 3 days | 500 mg daily × 3 days |

Unless specifically indicated as an alternative, all medications listed are considered first-line choices.
Adapted with permission from References 73 and 96 with additional data from Reference 55 (§) and Reference 84 (\*).
bid = twice daily, tid = three times per day, qid = four times per day.

considered in certain types of patients: those in which diagnostic uncertainty remains, those who have not responded after 4 days of therapy, those who are very ill with accelerated courses or have very large abscesses that may rupture, and for those with left-lobe abscesses that may rupture into the pericardium. Aspiration or drainage of amoebic empyemas improves outcomes in those whose abscesses have penetrated the diaphragm.[59]

### Other protozoa

The most frequently detected protozoan in immigrant groups, *Giardia*, is covered in detail in Chapter 29. Although *Cryptosporidum parvum* is distributed widely throughout the world, this organism likely does not pose a significant health risk for newly arrived immigrants. In Massachusetts, screening of these populations for *Cryptosporidium* is routinely performed using antigen detection tests on stool samples. *Cryptosporidium* was detected in 3 individuals of 5975 newly arrived refugees screened with antigen testing and microscopic examination of stool. Clinicians should, however, consider ordering *C. parvum* antigen detection tests on stool samples of newly arrived immigrants and those who have returned from travel abroad who present with persistent diarrhea.

*Blastocystis hominis* is generally considered a benign commensal. Several studies have found no correlation between this organism and clinical symptoms or pathological findings on endoscopy.[61,62] However, other studies have found possible associations with illness. In a retrospective review of 515 patients in Saudi Arabia who had stool specimens that contained large numbers of *B. hominis* either as the only parasite or in coinfections with other commensal organisms, 239 (46%) had symptoms, with the most common being abdominal pain, constipation, diarrhea, alternating diarrhea and constipation, vomiting, and fatigue. Forty-three of these symptomatic patients were treated with metronidazole and after 7–10 days of therapy all patients had recovered and their stool no longer contained *B. hominis*.[63] Significant associations between irritable bowel syndrome (IBS) and *B. hominis* infections have been found in Pakistan and Italy, while no association was detected in Thailand.[64–66]

The only study that has looked specifically at the consequences of *B. hominis* in immigrants found no association between the presence of gastrointestinal symptoms and *B. hominis* detection in 146 adult immigrants from developing countries in Italy.[67] Thus, the pathogenic potential of *B. hominis* remains unresolved. Clearly, some individuals appear to experience gastrointestinal illness. For individuals with symptoms that cannot be explained by other etiologies, treatment of *B. hominis* is reasonable. Asymptomatic individuals, however, have little to gain from treatment.

A second ubiquitous protozoan that classically has been labeled as nonpathogenic, but may in fact cause illness, is *Dientamoeba fragilis*. Its pathogenicity has been questioned since it is often seen in asymptomatic individuals. In addition, when isolated from symptomatic patients, coinfection with known pathogens is often present. However, several studies have shown that, in some patients, symptoms of abdominal pain, diarrhea, nausea, vomiting, and fatigue only subside after this organism is successfully treated. It has also been associated with IBS, urticaria, biliary infections, pruritus, and diarrhea.[68]

## Diagnosis

Any immigrant or refugee presenting with symptoms potentially attributable to an intestinal parasite should undergo testing which includes collection of stool for O&P examination on 3 consecutive days and a complete blood count with differential to evaluate for eosinophilia.[69] If no parasites are detected by stool O&P examinations, specific serologic or stool antigen testing should be performed if eosinophilia is present or if clinical suspicion for a parasitic infection remains high. The choice of testing in this situation is determined by the type of organisms suspected by the individual's symptoms and region of origin.[69]

The standard stool O&P technique to detect intestinal parasites involves preserving each individual stool sample in two different preservatives, usually formalin and either mercuric or zinc-polyvinyl alcohol (PVA).[70] A concentrate is prepared from the formalin-fixed material by adding ethyl acetate and then centrifuging the mixture to separate denser material containing any parasitic cysts, ova, and larvae from debris and fats. This concentrate is then stained with iodine and examined by light microscopy, enabling the detection of most intestinal parasites, although it is less sensitive for protozoan trophozoites. The mercuric- or zinc-PVA-preserved material is concentrated and the sediment is stained with trichrome to provide optimal detection and identification of protozoan trophozoites and cysts. The sensitivities of these methods are primarily dependent on the patient's parasite burden and the number of specimens examined. The specificity of these techniques is primarily dependent on the skill of the microscopist.[70]

## Treatment

Ideally, treatment for intestinal parasites should be provided directly to patients in clinics, especially if treatment can be accomplished with just one dose, to maximize adherence.[69] The treatment regimens for intestinal parasitic infections are listed in Table 20.7 and potential side effects are listed in Table 20.8.

## Special Considerations for Immigrants

How best to address the issue of intestinal parasitosis in immigrant groups remains uncertain. Clearly, given the high prevalence, asymptomatic nature of most infections, the potential for significant health consequences, and availability of effective, safe, and inexpensive therapies, all immigrants and refugees would benefit from routine screening for, or empiric treatment of, intestinal parasites. Screening has been estimated to decrease disability, hospitalizations, and mortality among immigrant groups in the US from throughout the world.[71] In addition, screening may decrease public health risks. Ideally, all immigrants would receive screening consisting of stool O&P examinations, absolute eosinophil count determination, and possibly serological tests for *Strongyloides* and *Schistosoma* species. However, cost considerations and limited sensitivity of screening methods for some pathogens have generated interest in replacing screening with presumptive treatment of all new immigrants with broad-spectrum antiparasitic medications.[71] Furthermore, the effect of universal pre-departure treatment of refugees may significantly alter their screening needs. Finally, the duration of time since emigration at which screening can be discontinued may depend on immigrants' areas of origin. These issues are discussed individually.

### Optimal screening protocols

#### Stool O&P examinations

The ideal number of stool specimens needed to screen asymptomatic immigrants remains a subject of debate. Some states recommend obtaining only one specimen while others encourage collection of three stool specimens on consecutive mornings.[72,73] Findings from a population comprised of primarily asymptomatic immigrants from Southeast Asia, East Africa, and Eastern Europe suggest that two samples may be ideal. The overall prevalence of pathogenic intestinal parasites in this group was 20%. Of 237 individuals with at least one out of three stool specimens positive for a pathogen, the first specimen was positive only 74.3% of the time. Examination of a second specimen increased the yield to 92.8%. The third specimen added additional information for 7% of the individuals. Furthermore, in only 5 (1.2%) out of all 546 individuals from which three specimens were received was the presence of a pathogenic parasite detected only in the third specimen. The investigator concluded that for populations with a high prevalence of parasites, which describes almost all immigrant groups, examination of two specimens is necessary and sufficient for screening asymptomatic individuals and that a third specimen does not add enough additional sensitivity to warrant the expense.[74] Ultimately, individual sites should assess the ratio of costs and benefits when deciding how many samples to collect.[69]

Since patients collect their stool specimens at home and are required to return them to the clinic or laboratory, there is a high likelihood that some or all of the specimens will not be returned. For example, in California, 31% of refugees who agreed to return stool specimens did not. Compared to those that did return specimens, those that did not were younger and less educated.[1] Among 73 newly arrived refugee children in Maine asked to return three stool specimens, 30 (41%) returned just one, 8 (11%) returned two, 11 (15%) returned all three, and one-third of children did not return any.[7] To help optimize compliance with this screening test, patients and parents should receive clear information in their own languages on the rationale for screening and how to collect, store, and deliver the specimens.[73]

#### Absolute eosinophil counts

Eosinophilia, typically defined as an absolute eosinophil count (AEC) of $\geq 450$ cells/$\mu$L, in immigrants and refugees from locations throughout the world is most often caused by helminthic infections.[75] Measuring the AEC of immigrants can add considerable ability to detect asymptomatic infections. In asymptomatic immigrants from Southeast Asia with eosinophilia and initially negative stool O&P examinations, 95% were found to have pathogenic intestinal para-

**Table 20.8 Side effects of drugs used to treat parasitic infections**

| Drug | Common side effects | Rare side effects (<1%) | Contraindications and interactions |
|---|---|---|---|
| Albendazole (data are based on longer treatment regimens used for neurocysticercosis [8–30 days] and hydatid cysts [three 28 day cycles]) | Abdominal pain 6%, nausea or vomiting 6%, headache 11%, dizziness 1.2%, reversible alopecia 1.6%, reversible liver transaminase elevation in those being treated for hydatid cysts (16%), *Ascaris* migration out of nostrils and mouth | Leukopenia: either mild reversible depression in white blood cell counts or, more rarely, profound granulocytopenia, thrombocytopenia or pancytopenia<br>Urticarial rash<br>Acute renal failure | Contraindications:<br>Pregnancy or > 7 days after start of last menstrual period. Pregnancy test should be obtained in women of child-bearing age before administering therapy, and pregnancy is not advised until 1 month after therapy ceases (teratogenic and embryotoxic in animals).<br>Unknown safety while breastfeeding.<br>Not extensively tested in children under the age of 2 years.<br>Interactions:<br>Increased albendazole levels when co-administered with dexamethasone, praziquantel, and cimetidine.<br>In prolonged courses, theophylline levels should be monitored closely. |
| Mebendazole | Abdominal pain and diarrhea (especially in those with large worm burdens), *Ascaris* migration out of nostrils and mouth | Agranulocytosis or neutropenia<br>Hepatoxicity (reported in prolonged treatment courses with higher than recommended doses)<br>Seizures<br>Rash, urticaria, angioedema | Contraindications:<br>Pregnancy or >7 days after start of last menstrual period. Pregnancy test should be obtained in women of child bearing age before administering therapy, and pregnancy is not advised until 1 month after therapy ceases (teratogenic and embryotoxic in animals).<br>Unknown safety while breastfeeding.<br>Not extensively tested in children under the age of 2 years.<br>Interactions:<br>Increased albendazole levels when co-administered with dexamethasone, praziquantel, and cimetidine.<br>In prolonged courses, theophylline levels should be monitored closely. |

| Drug | Common adverse effects | Notable reactions / complications | Contraindications / Special considerations |
|---|---|---|---|
| Pyrantel | Mild gastrointestinal discomfort, headache, dizziness, drowsiness, insomnia and rash | | Contraindications:<br>Pregnancy class C<br>Limited data in children under 2 years-old.<br>Use with caution in those with hepatic dysfunction.<br>Interactions:<br>Antagonized by piperazine. |
| Nitazoxanide | Abdominal pain 7–8%, diarrhea 2–4%, nausea 3%, vomiting 1.1%, headache 1–3% | Notable rare reactions include: flu-like syndrome, insomnia, urine and eye discoloration, tachycardia, hypotension, amenorrhea, metrorrhagia, elevated SGPT | Pregnancy class B<br>Diabetic children and their caregivers should be notified that each 5 mL of the liquid oral suspension (100 mg/5 mL) contains 1.48 grams of sucrose. |
| Ivermectin | Dizziness 2.8%, pruritus 2.8%, nausea 1.8%, elevated liver transaminases 2%, decreased WBC 3% | Fatigue, vertigo, abdominal pain, anorexia, constipation, diarrhea, vomiting, urticaria<br>Mazzotti-type reactions in patients with onchocerciasis, (fever, rash, pruritus, lymphadenopathy, arthralgias) | Pregnancy class C (teratogenic in mice)<br>Safety profile unknown for children <15 kg |
| Praziquantel | In decreasing order of severity: malaise, headache, dizziness, abdominal discomfort, fever | Pruritus, urticarial rash<br>Cardiac arrythmias<br>Seizures<br>May cause serious complications in those with ocular cysticercosis | Pregnancy class B<br>Should not breastfeed for 72 hours after treatment<br>Safety profile unknown for children < 4 years old.<br>Those with cardiac problems should be monitored during therapy.<br>Those with neurocysticercosis should be hospitalized when treated.<br>Patients should not drive vehicles for 48 hours after treatment.<br>May need to decrease dose in those with Child-Pugh class B and C liver disease.<br>Cimetidine, ketoconazole and itraconazole may increase drug levels.<br>Rifampin, chloroquine, phenytoin and carbamazepine may decrease drug levels. |

301

**Table 20.8 Side effects of drugs used to treat parasitic infections—cont'd**

| Drug | Common side effects | Rare side effects (<1%) | Contraindications and interactions |
|---|---|---|---|
| Niclosamide | Mild gastrointestinal disturbances | Lightheadedness, dizziness, pruritus, unpleasant taste | Pregnancy class B<br>Not available in the United States |
| Metronidazole | Headache 5%, dizziness 2%, abdominal discomfort 7%, nausea and vomiting 4%, anorexia, metallic taste, disulfuram-like reaction with alcohol, vaginal discharge 12%, cervicitis or vaginitis 10% | Seizures<br>Peripheral neuropathy<br>Dizziness, confusion, irritability<br>Neutropenia<br>Pseudomembranous colitis | Likely safe during pregnancy (Class B)<br>Minimal risk while breastfeeding.<br>Caution in those with history of neurological disease, blood dyscrasias, and those on anticoagulation.<br>Contraindicated in those taking ergotamines. |
| Tinidazole | Similar to metronidazole | Similar to metronidazole | Pregnancy (Class C) |
| Paromomycin | Diarrhea, nausea, vomiting, abdominal cramps | | Unknown safety during pregnancy and breastfeeding.<br>Contraindicated in intestinal obstruction.<br>Caution in those with ulcerative intestinal lesions, due to risk of renal toxicity from increased absorption. |
| Iodoquinol | Nausea, vomiting, diarrhea, abdominal pain, urticaria, anal pruritus, goiter, shivering, and muscle cramps | Long-term high doses may cause: optic neuritis/atrophy, loss of vision, peripheral neuropathy | Pregnancy and breastfeeding risks are unknown.<br>Contraindicated in those with hepatic or renal impairment, iodine allergy, or chronic diarrhea.<br>Caution in those with thyroid or neurological disease. |
| Diloxanide furoate | Flatulence, nausea, vomiting, pruritus, urticaria | | |

Data are from References 36, 72, 96, and 97.

sites upon additional testing (hookworm 55%, *Strongyloides* 38%, and *Entamoeba histolytica* 2%).[76] These findings indicate that an elevated AEC has a very high positive predictive value for helminthic infections in populations with a high burden of these parasites. Despite the strong association between eosinophilia and intestinal parasites, using AEC as the sole method of screening is inadequate. For example, among a group of Southeast Asian refugees only 58% with proven intestinal parasitosis had eosinophilia.[77] Thus, the negative predictive value of AEC is relatively low.

Some laboratories report only the eosinophil percentage when white blood cell differentials are ordered. It is important to calculate the absolute eosinophil count even when the eosinophil percentage falls in the normal range. In a study of *Clonorchis* and *Opisthorchis* infections among immigrants, approximately half of all infected patients with an elevated AEC had a normal white blood cell differential by percentage. Unless the AEC is calculated by clinicians in these circumstances, the important diagnostic clue of eosinophilia may be missed.[47]

### Serological testing

Presently, the universal use of serology or specific stool antigen testing of all asymptomatic immigrants and refugees is not done. As discussed in the following chapter, the use of these tests adds important diagnostic information in individuals with eosinophilia.[78] It remains unknown if testing all individuals at risk for certain parasites, regardless of their AEC, would improve screening. In a small study of 135 East African refugee children, serological testing of all children for *Strongyloides* and *Schistosoma* improved the detection of *Schistosoma* infection 3-fold compared to using only a single stool O&P specimen. While no children had *Strongyloides* detected in their stool samples, one child had a positive and 14 had equivocal *Strongyloides* serologies.[79]

Carriage of *Entamoeba histolytica* cysts would not be expected to cause eosinophilia and standard stool O&P techniques have a relatively low sensitivity for detection of these cysts. It remains unknown whether screening all immigrants for *E. histolytica* through stool antigen testing would significantly decrease illness in immigrants and reduce public health risks.[18]

### Treatment of asymptomatic infections

The uncertainty involved in predicting future complications leads most experts to treat all asymp-

tomatic patients harboring potentially pathogenic parasites.[80] In addition, possible public health ramifications have been included as justification for treatment. There are very limited data looking at the transmissibility of these infections. Parasites transmitted by fecal–oral contamination including *Hymenolepis nana* and *Giardia* have been reported in US-born children of immigrants living in California.[9] However, the prevalence of *Giardia* in this population was not considerably higher than the baseline prevalence in the state. Perhaps the most significant public health risk is the development of cysticercosis through fecal contamination of foods prepared by immigrants harboring the adult pork tapeworm, *T. solium*.[81-83]

Treatment guidelines are presented in Table 20.7. If *Entamoeba histolytica/dispar* is detected by stool microscopy, it is important to order an *E. histolytica* stool antigen test, if available, and only treat those who truly harbor *E. histolytica*. No treatment is necessary if only nonpathogenic species are reported. The following chapter discusses empiric treatment of asymptomatic individuals with eosinophilia of unknown etiology.

The effectiveness of the screen and treat approach to intestinal parasitosis was examined among a group of Cambodian refugees that had resettled in Montreal.[13] Using two stool specimens collected on consecutive days for both initial arrival screening and repeat screening 6 years later, prevalence of pathogenic intestinal parasites decreased by 41.8%, but still remained 21.9%. A control group that arrived in Canada at the same time but had not gone through the new arrival screening and treatment program was found to have a prevalence of 39.2% 6 years after arrival. The prevalences of various pathogens at time of arrival (baseline) and 6 years after arrival in refugees who had either been previously screened and treated (rescreened) or had not undergone screening (controls) were:

- *Ascaris*: baseline 10%, rescreened 0%, control 0%;
- Hookworm: baseline 49%, rescreened 12%, control 34%;
- *Strongyloides*: baseline 15%, rescreened 11%, controls 12%; and
- *Giardia*: baseline 18%, rescreened 3%, controls 4%. The prevalence in neither the rescreened nor control groups differed considerably from the level considered endemic to Canada or the US.

Although the rescreened group had a significantly lower overall prevalence of intestinal parasitosis, the observed effectiveness was less than ideal, especially for *Strongyloides*. Possible limitations to screening programs include: limited sensitivity of screening tests, suboptimal adherence to prescribed treatment regimens by patients, limited efficacy of antiparasitic medications, and repeat infections while visiting countries of origin.[13] Sensitivity of screening can be improved by including AEC determination and targeted use of serological testing. Adherence to treatment can be optimized through directly observed administration of medications. In this study *Strongyloides* was treated with thiabendazole. With the use of ivermectin, the current first-line agent, higher efficacy would be expected.

## Presumptive treatment

Given the lack of an ideal screening test, especially for some of the most clinically important parasites, such as *Strongyloides*, the idea of presumptively treating all asymptomatic immigrants with a high pre-test probability of intestinal parasitosis has been suggested for many years.[14] In some locations, such as the state of New Mexico, this is currently being done.[73] Compared to universal screening with a single O&P specimen, presumptive treatment of all immigrants to the US with a 5-day course of albendazole has been suggested to be more efficacious in preventing disability, hospitalizations, and deaths. In addition, presumptive treatment has been estimated to cost millions of dollars less.[71]

There are significant limitations to this approach, including lack of efficacy against *Schistosoma* and *Fasciola* species and less than optimal efficacy against *Strongyloides*, *Giardia*, and *Entamoeba histolytica*.[15,69,78,83] Although not considered first line, albendazole may be effective against tapeworms, *Clonorchis*, and *Opisthorchis* species.[71,84] The lack of optimal efficacy may lead to a false sense of assurance that immigrants who have been treated presumptively are free of any risk for future parasite-related complications. There is also a hypothetical risk of neurological complications with treatment of immigrants who unknowingly have neurocysticercosis.[71] In addition, although albendazole is relatively safe and inexpensive, when hundreds of thousands of immigrants are treated just a few serious reactions may minimize cost savings[85] and low-income immigrants with limited insurance coverage are unlikely to be interested in purchasing medications for an entire family of asymptomatic individuals.[86] Additional studies

are needed, especially among young children who do not have as high a prevalence of intestinal helminth carriage. Although the use of albendazole is likely safe in children under 2 years of age, the side effect profiles have not been studied as well in this young age group.[87] A more recent study suggests that ivermectin, in place of albendazole, is a more cost-effective presumptive treatment approach for populations with a prevalence of *Strongyliodes* of 10%.[88]

## Effects of pre-departure treatment

The same limitations of albendazole apply to universal treatment of refugees prior to departure. Therefore, unless pre-departure treatment is modified, such as by administering ivermectin to those at highest risk for strongyloidiasis and praziquantel for those at high risk for schistosomiasis, screening refugees on arrival is still indicated. However, even if current pre-departure treatment practices are unchanged, screening protocols for these groups could potentially be changed. Studies looking at replacing or augmenting stool O&P examinations with targeted serological testing among albendazole-treated refugees are needed.

## Duration of residence

Screening should not be limited to newly arrived immigrants. Even those who have lived outside of endemic areas for many years may be at risk of carrying several pathogenic organisms that may cause serious morbidity, especially *Strongyloides*, *Schistosoma*, *Opisthorchis*, *Clonorchis*, and *Entamoeba histolytica*. In a report from Australia, 23% of Laotians who had settled there 7–20 years earlier had chronic *Strongyloides* infections.[89] In Minnesota, eight out of nine cases of complicated *Strongyloides* hyperinfections occurred in Southeast Asian immigrants who had been living in the US for longer than 3 years.[90] Six years after settlement in Canada, 5% of asymptomatic Cambodian refugees were found to harbor *Opisthorchis* organisms.[13] Some have suggested targeted screening for these long-lived organisms among at-risk groups, such as biliary liver fluke infections in those of Laotian and Cambodian descent, regardless of the individual's duration of residence outside of endemic areas.[47] Pathogenic intestinal parasites have also been documented in East African immigrants living in the US for more than 3 years.[32]

In groups at lower risk of harboring long-lived helminthic infections, such as Latin American refugees, screening asymptomatic individuals with stool O&P examinations can reasonably be limited to those who have lived outside of endemic areas for less than 3 years.[9] All immigrants with eosinophilia should be assessed for the presence of helminths, especially those about to receive immunosuppressive therapies, including corticosteroids.[17]

## Other considerations for immigrants

- The carriage of intestinal parasites may alter the course of other important infections. For example, large helminthic burdens may impair cellular immune responses to both *Mycobacterium tuberculosis* and the human immunodeficiency virus through chronic immune-system activation characterized by an exaggerated helper T-cell subset 2 response. Among Ethiopian immigrants, helminthic burden was found to correlate with HIV plasma viral load as well as impaired immune responses to HIV and tuberculin skin testing. Anthelmintic therapy may improve these immune responses.[91]

- Food preferences may place certain immigrant groups at risk for certain nonintestinal parasitic infections. For example, consumption of raw or undercooked pork has led to both isolated cases and outbreaks of trichinosis, caused by *Trichinella spiralis*, among Southeast Asian immigrants.[92,93]

- Although very little information has been published on the management of intestinal parasites in pregnant women, reports suggest that, in the absence of severe anemia, treatment can be delayed until after delivery.[94,95]

## Prevention

Primary prevention of intestinal parasite infections in immigrants' countries of origin is beyond the scope of this chapter. By using routine screening programs as described above, clinicians in the areas where immigrants resettle can decrease the likelihood of morbidity and mortality due to parasitic infections. Universal pre-departure treatment has led to dramatic reductions in parasite burden among refugees. If improvements can be made to target gaps in albendazole coverage, perhaps screening

will no longer be needed for refugees. Presumptive treatment of nonrefugee immigrants after arrival may lead to similar changes in current prevention strategies for these groups as well. Clinicians should reinforce the importance of hand washing and avoiding undercooked meats as simple additional measures. Ongoing surveillance of parasitic infections among all immigrant groups is essential for determining prevention needs and monitoring the effectiveness of any prevention strategy.

## References

1. Garag PK, Perry S, Dorn M, et al. Risk of intestinal helminth and protozoan infection in a refugee population. Am J Trop Med Hyg 2005; 73(2):386–391.
2. Peterson MH, Konczyk MR, Ambrosino K, et al. Parasitic screening of a refugee population in Illinois. Diagnost Microbiol Infect Dis 2001; 40:75–76.
3. Godue CB, Gyorkos TW. Intestinal parasites in refugee claimants: a case study for selective screening? Can J Public Health 1990; 81:191–195.
4. Lifson AR, Thai D, O'Fallon A, et al. Prevalance of tuberculosis, hepatitis B, and intestinal parasites among refugees to Minnesota. Pub Health Reports 2002; 117:69–77.
5. Minnesota Department of Health. Refugee Health Program. Personal communication. 2005.
6. Swanson, S. Personal communication. 2006
7. Hayes EB, Talbot SB, Matheson ES. Health status of pediatric refugees in Portland, ME. Arch Pediatr Adolesc Med 1998; 152;564–568.
8. Safarty M, Rosenberg Z, Siegel, et al. Intestinal parasites in immigrant children from Central America. West J Med 1983; 139:329–331.
9. Salas SD, Heifetz R, Barrett-Connor E. Intestinal parasites in Central American immigrants in the United States. Arch Intern Med 1990; 150:1514–1516.
10. Arfaa F. Intestinal parasite among Indochinese refugees and Mexican immigrants resettled in Contra Costa County, California. J Fam Pract 1981; 12:223–226.
11. Bass JL, Mehta KA, Eppes B. Parasitology screening of Latin American children in a primary care clinic. Pediatrics 1992; 89:279–283.
12. Cantanzaro A, Moser RJ. Health status of refugees from Vietnam, Laos and Cambodia. JAMA 1982; 247:1303–1308.
13. Gyorkos TW, MacLean JD, Viens P, et al. Intestinal parasite infection in the Kampuchean refugee population 6 years after resettlement in Canada. J Infect Dis 1992; 166:413–417.
14. Lurio J, Verson H, Karp S. Intestinal parasites in Cambodians: comparison of diagnostic methods used in screening refugees with implications for treatment of populations with high rates of infestation. J Am Board Fam Pract 1991; 4:71–78.
15. Geltman PL, Cochran J, Hedgecock C. Intestinal parasites among African refugees resettled in Massachusetts and the impact of an overseas pre-departure treatment program. Am J Trop Med. Hyg 2003; 69(6):657–662.
16. Ciesielski SD, Seed JR, Ortiz JC, et al. Intestinal parasites among North Carolina migrant farmworkers. Am J Public Health 1992; 82:1258–1262.
17. Walker PF, Jaranson J. Refugee and immigrant health care. Med Clin N Am 1999; 83:1103–1120.
18. Stauffer W, Ravdin JI. *Entamoeba histolytica*: an update. Curr Opin Infect Dis 2003; 16:479–485.
19. Benzeguir AK, Capraru T, Aust-Kettis A, et al. High frequency of gastrointestinal parasites in refugees and asylum seekers upon arrival in Sweden. Scand J Infect Dis 1999; 31:79–82.

20. Okyay P, Ertug S, Gultekin B, et al. Intestinal parasites prevalence and related factors in school children, a western city sample – Turkey. BMC Public Health 2004; 4:64.

21. Marnell F, Guillet A, Holland C. A survey of the intestinal helminths of refugees in Juba, Sudan. Ann Trop Med Parasitol 1992; 86:387–393.

22. Xu LQ, Yu SH, Jiang ZX, et al. Soil-transmitted helminthiases: nationwide survey in China. Bull World Health Organ 1995; 73(4):507–513.

23. Udonsi JK, Amabibi MI. The human environment, occupation, and possible water-borne transmission of the human hookworm, *Necator americanus*, in endemic coastal communities of the Niger Delta, Nigeria. Public Health 1992; 106:63–71.

24. Okoli CG, Iwuala MO. The prevalence, intensity and clinical signs of urinary schistosomiasis in Imo state, Nigeria. J Helminthol 2004; 78:337–342.

25. Spear RC, Seto E, Liang S, et al. Factors influencing the transmission of *Schistosoma japonicum* in the mountains of Sichuan Province of China. Am J Trop Med Hyg 2004; 70:48–56.

26. Kabatereine NB, Kemijumbi J, Ouma JH, et al. Epidemiology and morbidity of *Schistosoma mansoni* infection in a fishing community along Lake Albert in Uganda. Trans R Soc Trop Med Hyg 2004; 98:711–718.

27. Adachi S, Kotani K, Shimizu T, et al. Asymptomatic fascioliasis. Intern Med 2005; 44:1013–1015.

28. Roman-Sanchez D, Pastor-Guzman A, Moreno-Guillen S. High prevalence of *Strongyloides stercoralis* among farm workers on the Mediterranean coast of Spain: analysis of the predictive factors of infection in developed countries. Am J Trop Med Hyg 2003; 69(3):336–340.

29. Diaz T, Achi R. Infectious diseases in a Nicaraguan refugee camp in Costa Rica. Trop Doct 1989; 19:14–17.

30. Huh S, Ahn C, Chai J. Intestinal parasitic infections in the residents of an emigration camp in Tijuana, Mexico. Korean J Parasitol 1995; 33:65–67.

31. Miller JM, Boyd HA, Ostrowski SR. Malaria, intestinal parasites and schistosomiasis among Barwan Somali refugees resettling to the United States: a strategy to reduce morbidity and decrease the risk of imported infections. Am J Trop Med Hyg 2000; 62:115–121.

32. Sachs WJ, Adair R, Kirchner V. Enteric parasites in East African immigrants: symptoms and duration of US residence are not predictive. Minnesota Med 2000; 83:25–28.

33. Buchwald D, Lam M, Hootan TM. Prevalence of intestinal parasites and association with symptoms in Southeast Asian refugees. J Clin Pharm Ther 1995; 20:271–275.

34. O'Lorcain P, Holland CV. The public health importance of *Ascaris lumbricoides*. Parasitology 2000; 121:S51–S71.

35. Stephenson LS, Holland CV, Cooper ES. The public health significance of *Trichuris trichiura*. Parasitology 2000; 121: S73–S95

36. Cook G, Zumla A. Manson's tropical diseases. 21st edn. London: WB Saunders; 2003.

37. Leder K, Weller PF. Ascariasis. UpToDate. Available with a subscription: http://www.uptodate.com November 18, 2005.

38. Hurtado RM, Sahani DV, Kradin RL. Case 9–2006: A 35-year-old woman with recurrent right-upper-quadrant pain. N Engl J Med 2006; 354:1295–1303.

39. Chandra B, Long J. Diagnosis of *Trichuris trichiura* (Whipworm) by colonoscopic extraction. J Clin Gastroenterol 1998; 27:152–153.

40. Peters W, Pasvol G. Tropical medicine and parasitology. 5th edn. London: Mosby; 2002.

41. Harries JR, Harries AD, Cook CG. Clinical problems in tropical medicine. 2nd edn. London: WB Saunders; 1998.

42. Slom T, Johnson S. Eosinophilic meningitis. Curr Infect Dis Rep 2003; 5:322–328.

43. Slom TJ, Cortese MM, Gerber SI, et al. An outbreak of eosinophilic meningitis caused by *Angiostrongylus cantonensis* in travelers returning from the Caribbean. N Engl J Med 2002; 346(9):668–675.

44. Bartschi E, Bordmann G, Blum J, et al. Eosinophilic meningitis due to *Angiostrongylus cantonensis* in Switzerland. Infection 2004; 32:116–118.

45. Gorgolas M, Santos-O'Connor F, Unzu AL, et al. Cutaneous and medullar gnathostomiasis in travelers to Mexico and Thailand. J Travel Med 2003; 10:358–361.

46. Moore DA, McCroddan J, Dekumyoy P, et al. Gnathostomiasis: an emerging imported disease. Emerg Infect Dis 2003; 9:647–650.

47. Stauffer WM, Sellman JS, Walker PF. Biliary liver flukes (opisthorchiasis and clonorchiasis) in immigrants in the United States: often subtle and diagnosed years after arrival. J Trav Med 2004; 11:157–160.

48. Shugar RA, Ryan JJ. *Clonorchis sinensis* and pancreatitis. Twenty-five after endemic exposure. Am J Gastroenterol 1975; 64(5):400–403.

49. Haswell-Elkins MR, Mairiang E, Mairiang P, et al. Cross-sectional study of *Opisthorcis viverrini* infection and cholangiocarcinoma in communities within a high risk area in Northeast Thailand. Int J Cancer 1994; 58:1–5.

50. Watanapa P, Watanapa WB. Liver-fluke-associated cholangiocarcinoma. Br J Surg 2002; 89:962–970.

51. Wongsaroj T, Sakolvaree Y, Chaicumpa W, et al. Affinity purified oval antigen for diagnosis of *Opisthorchiasis viverrini*. Asian Pac J Allergy Immunol 2001; 19:245–258.

52. Stensvold CR, Saijuntha W, Sithithaworn P, et al. Evaluation of PCR based coprodiagnosis of human opisthorchiasis. Acta Trop 2006; 97:26–30.

53. Choi MH, Park IC, Li S, et al. Excretory–secretory antigen is better than crude antigen for the serodiagnosis of clonorchiasis by ELISA. Korean J Parasitol 2003; 41:35–39.

54. Choi D, Hong ST, Lim JH, et al. Sonographic findings of active *Clonorchis sinensis* infection. J Clin Ultrasound 2004; 32:17–23.

55. Noyer CM, Coyle CM, Werner C, et al. Hypereosinophilia and a liver mass in an immigrant. Am J Trop Med Hyg 2002; 66:774–776.

56. Raether W, Hanel H. Epidemiology, clinical manifestations and diagnosis of zoonotic cestode infections: an update. Parsitol Res 2003; 91:412–438.

57. Di Lernia V, Ricci C, Albertini G. Skin eruption associated with *Hymenolepis nana* infection. Int J Dermatol 2004; 43(5):357–359.

58. Olson PD, Yoder K, Fajardo L-G, et al. Lethal invasive cestodiasis in immunosuppressed patients. J Infect Dis 2003; 187:1962–1966.

59. Stanley SL. Amoebiasis. Lancet 2003; 361:1025–1034.

60. Wells CD, Arguedas M. Amoebic liver abcess. South Med J 2004; 97:673–682.

61. Senay H, MacPherson D. *Blastocystis hominis*: epidemiology and natural history. J Infect Dis 1990; 162:987–990.

62. Chen TL, Chan CC, Chen HP, et al. Clinical characteristics and endoscopic findings associated with *Blastocystis hominis* in healthy adults. Am J Trop Med Hyg 2003; 69:213–216.

63. Qadri SMH, Al-Okaili GA, Al-Dyael F. Clinical significance of *Blastocytis hominis*. J Clin Microbiol 1989; 27:2407–2409.

64. Yakoob J, Jafri W, Jafri N. Irritable bowel syndrome: in search of an etiology: role of *Blastocystis hominis*. Am J Trop Med Hyg 2004; 70:383–385.

65. Giacometti A, Cirioni O, Fiorentini A, et al. Irritable bowel syndrome in patients with *Blastocystis hominis* infection. Eur J Clin Microbiol Infect Dis 1999; 18:436–439.

66. Tungtrongchitr A, Manatsathit S, Kositchaiwat C, et al. *Blastocystis hominis* infection in irritable bowel syndrome patients. Southeast Asian J Trop Med Pub Health 2004; 35:705–710.

67. Cirioni O, Giacometti A, Drenaggi D, et al. Prevalence and clinical relevance of *Blastocystis hominis* in diverse patient cohorts. Eur J Epidemiol 1999; 15(4):389–393.

68. Johnson EH, Widsor JJ, Clark CG. Emerging from obscurity: biological, clinical, and diagnostic aspects of *Dientamoeba fragilis*. Clin Microbiol Rev 2004; 17:553–570.

69. Barnett ED. Infectious disease screening for refugees resettled in the United States. CID 2004; 39:833–841.

70. Personal communication with Cartwright CP. Department of Laboratory Medicine and Pathology. Hennepin County Medical Center, Minneapolis, Minnesota.

71. Muennig P, Pallin D, Sell RL, et al. The cost effectiveness of strategies for the treatment of intestinal parasites in immigrants. N Engl J Med 1999; 340:773–779.

72. Commonwealth of Massachusetts, Department of Public Health. Refugee Health Assessment: a guide for health care clinicians. Available: http://www.mass.gov/dph/cdc/rhip/rha/index.htm Accessed 3/6/07.

73. Stauffer WM, Kamat D, Walker PF. Screening of international immigrants, refugees, and adoptees. Prim Care Clin Office Pract 2002; 29:879–905.

74. Cartwright CP. Utility of multiple-stool-specimen ova and parasite examinations in a high-prevalence setting. J Clin Microbiol 1999; 37:2408–2411.

75. Nutman TB. Asymptomatic peripheral blood eosinophilia redux: common parasitic infections presenting frequently in refugees and immigrants. CID 2006: 42:368–369.

76. Nutman TB, Ottesen EA, Leng S, et al. Eosinophilia in Southeast Asian refugees: evaluation at a referral center. J Infect Dis 1987; 155(2):309–312.

77. Hoffman SL, Barrett-Connor E, Norcross W, et al. Intestinal parasites in Indochinese immigrants. Am J Trop Med Hyg 1981; 30:340–343.

78. Seybolt LM, Christiansen D, Barnett ED. Diagnostic evaluation of newly arrived asymptomatic refugees with eosinophilia. CID 2006; 42:363–367.

79. Rice JE, Skull SA, Pearce C, et al. Screening for intestinal parasites in recently arrived children from East Africa. J Paediatr Child Health 2003; 39:456–459.

80. Barrett-Connor E. Natural history of intestinal parasites in asymptomatic adults. J Fam Pract 1984; 9:635–639.

81. Mody R, Nield LS, Stauffer W, et al. Seizures in a 20-month-old native of Minnesota: a case of neurocysticercosis. Pediatr Emerg Care 2006; 21:860–862.

82. Kruskal BA, Moths L, Teele DW. Neurocysticercosis in a child with no history of travel outside the continental United States. Clin Infect Dis 1993; 16:290–292.

83. Centers for Disease Control. Locally acquired neurocysticercosis – North Carolina, Massachusetts, and South Carolina, 1989–1991. MMWR1992; 41:1–4.

84. Drugs for parasitc infections. The Medical Letter. 2004. Available: http://www.medletter.com/freedocs/parasitic.pdf Accessed 3/6/07.

85. Mitre E. Treatment of intestinal parasites in immigrants. N Engl J Med 1999; 34:377.

86. Geltman P, Meyers A. Treatment of intestinal parasites in immigrants. N Engl J Med 1999; 34:377–378.

87. Montresor A, Awasthi S, Crompton DWT. Use of benzimidazoles in children younger than 24 months for treatment of soil-transmitted helminthiasis. Acta Tropica 2003; 86:223–232.

88. Muennig P, Pallin D, Challah C, et al. The cost-effectiveness of ivermectin vs. albendazole in the presumptive treatment of strongyloidiasis in immigrants to the United States. Epidemiol Infect 2004; 132:1055–1063.

89. de Silva S, Saykao P, Kelly H, et al. Chronic *Strongyloides stercoralis* infection in Laotian immigrants and refugees 7–20 years after resettlement in Australia. Epidemiol Infect 2002; 128:439–444.

90. Newberry AM, Williams DN, Stauffer WM, et al. *Strongyloides* hyperinfection presenting as acute respiratory failure and Gram-negative sepsis. Chest 2005; 128:3681–3684.

91. Borkow G, Weisman Z, Leng Q, et al. Helminths, human immunodeficiency virus and tuberculosis. Scand J Infect Dis 2001; 33:568–571.

92. Graves T, Harkess J, Crutcher JM. Case report: locally acquired trichinosis in an immigrant from Southeast Asia. J Okla State Med Assoc 1996; 89:402–404.

93. McAuley JB, Michelson MK, Hightower AW, et al. A trichinosis outbreak among Southeast Asian refugees. Am J Epidemiol 1992; 135:1404–1410.

94. King PA, Duthie SJ, Ma HK. Intestinal helminths in pregnant Vietnamese refugees. Trans R Soc Trop Med Hyg 1990; 84:723.

95. D'Alauro F, Lee RV, Pao-In K, et al. Intestinal parasites and pregnancy. Obstet Gynecol 1985; 66:639–643.

96. Moon TD, Oberhelman RA. Antiparasitic therapy in children. Pediatr Clin N Am 2005; 52:917–948.

97. Micromedex. Accessed on March 14, 2006 at http://www.micromedex.com

# CHAPTER 21

# Eosinophilia

Yae-Jean Kim and Thomas B. Nutman

## Introduction

Eosinophils are known to be associated with many conditions including parasitic infections, allergic or autoimmune diseases, and several primary hematologic disorders. In immigrant or refugee populations – newly arrived from developing countries and/or from tropical areas – most of the eosinophilia identified with or without symptoms can be considered a reflection of parasitic infection (particularly helminth [worm] infections).

## Definition of eosinophilia

Eosinophilia can be defined as an absolute eosinophil count greater than $450/mm^3$ in the peripheral blood. Physiologically, eosinophil levels in the peripheral blood have a diurnal variation with a peak in the morning, a time at which endogenous steroids are the lowest. Eosinophil levels are relatively high at birth, decrease during childhood, and can decline further during pregnancy.[1] Eosinophils are more abundant in tissues, particularly in those tissues with a mucosal–environmental interface such as the respiratory, gastrointestinal, and genitourinary tracts.

## Epidemiology

Among immigrant and refugee populations, the prevalence of peripheral blood eosinophilia defined as $> 450/mm^3$ or $> 500/mm^3$ has been shown to range from 12% to 53% of those screened.[2–10]

Although immigrants and refugees may have parasitic helminth infection, the absence of eosinophilia does not exclude parasitic infection.[3] It is known that eosinophilia has a relatively poor predictive value (both negative and positive)[4,11,12] for parasitic infection in returning travelers. However, eosinophilia in asymptomatic refugees and/or immigrants should draw attention to possible parasitic infections, as those with lifelong exposure to parasitic infections are more often asymptomatic compared to short-term travelers. In one study of Southeast Asian refugees with persistent eosinophilia and a negative initial screening evaluation, 95% were found to have gastrointestinal parasites with one or multiple organisms (55% with hookworm and 38% with *Strongyloides*).[6] Indeed, many of the tissue-invasive helminth infections (strongyloidiasis, filariasis, schistosomiasis) are associated with clinically asymptomatic conditions in chronic infections.[13-16] Moreover, in a study from a parasite-endemic region of Brazil, high-grade eosinophilia was more likely to be associated with parasite infection, and higher eosinophil counts were associated with having more than one infecting species of parasites in the same host (polyparasitism).[17]

Even in immigrant populations that have emigrated in the distant past, it must be remembered that some parasites (filarial parasites) have life spans that can exceed 10–15 years, and others have autoinfective cycles (*Strongyloides*) that enable lifelong parasite persistence. Indeed, the chronicity of infection, one of the hallmarks of helminth parasites, has been well documented, as can be seen in Table 21.1. Immigrants can also acquire new infections from visits back to their home country (so-called 'visiting friends and relatives').

## Pathophysiology

It has been suggested that eosinophils play an important role in the immune response to helminth infec-

## Table 21.1 Documented length of infection in selected parasites

| Pathogen (disease) | Length of infection (years) |
|---|---|
| S. stercoralis (strongyloidiasis) | 60+ |
| Schistosoma spp. (schistosomiasis) | 32 |
| E. granulosis (hydatid disease) | >20 |
| T. spiralis larvae in muscle (trichinellosis) | 18 |
| T. solium (cysticercosis) | >15 |
| W. bancrofti (lymphatic filariasis) | 5–10 |
| L. loa (loiasis) | 16–24 |
| O. volvulus (onchocerciasis) | 10–15 |
| N. americanus (hookworm disease) | 3–5 |
| A. lumbricoides (ascariasis) | 1–1.5 |

tion, based on the observation of eosinophils surrounding dying parasites in an animal infection model of *Nippostrongylus brasiliensis*.[18] Eosinophilia and increased serum IgE levels are characteristic of helminth infection which reflects the production of cytokines such as interleukins (IL-4 and IL-5) from CD4+ lymphocytes. In addition to IL-5 – the main cytokine responsible for the specific development of eosinophils – other cytokines (e.g. IL-4 and IL-13) and chemokines (e.g. RANTES and eotaxin) are important for the recruitment of eosinophils from the blood to the tissues.[19]

The degree of eosinophilia may also vary based on the parasites' tissue distribution pattern, their migration route, the maturation stage of the parasites and the actual parasite burden.[20,21] Eosinophilia is often particularly pronounced in the early phase of infection, when developing larvae migrate through the lungs (e.g. *Ascaris* or *Strongyloides*) or through other tissues (as in hookworm and *Trichinella* infection). Because of the long prepatent period characteristic of some helminth infections, eosinophilia may occur at a time when parasitologic diagnosis is difficult (prior to egg secretion or antibody positivity). In most instances, eosinophil levels from helminth parasites gradually diminish over time (even without anthelmintic treatment), although they rarely return to normal levels.

The kinetics of parasite infection-associated eosinophilia varies widely depending on the particular species of infecting parasite. In a human volunteer study with *Necator americanus*, it was shown that blood eosinophil counts began to rise from baseline 2–3 weeks after infection and reached a peak between 38 and 64 days.[22] In several experimental human filarial infections, peak eosinophil counts occurred 11–30 weeks after the initiation of infection.[23] In both types of infections there was a natural modulation (diminution) of the eosinophil levels over time.

Therefore, in immigrants or refugees who have been chronically exposed to helminth infection for an extended period of time, eosinophilia may be less prominent than in travelers infected from relatively recent exposure.[13]

## Etiology

Many of the causes of eosinophilia resulting from infectious and noninfectious processes are detailed in Table 21.2.

### Infectious causes

Major episodes of eosinophilia in immigrants or refugees from tropical or subtropical countries are induced by infections with multicellular helminthic worms that include nematodes (roundworms), cestodes (tapeworms), and trematodes (flukes). Accompanying localizing symptoms associated with eosinophilia can provide insights into the potential underlying diagnosis associated with the eosinophilia (see Table 21.2).

The parasitic diseases associated with peripheral blood eosinophilia include: angiostrongyliasis, anisakiasis, ascariasis, capillariasis, clonorchiasis, cysticercosis, dicrocoeliosis, echinococcosis, echinostomiasis, enterobiasis, fascioliasis, fasciolopsiasis, filariasis, gnathostomiasis, heterophyiasis, hookworm infection, hymenolepiasis, metagonimiasis, opisthorchiasis, paragonimiasis, schistosomiasis, sparganosis, strongyloidiasis, toxocariasis (e.g. visceral larval migrans), trichinellosis, and trichuriasis. Among these, those most commonly identified among immigrant or refugee populations in association with eosinophilia are ascariasis, filarial infections, hookworm infections, schistosomiasis, strongyloidiasis, trichuriasis, and toxocariasis.[2,6,10,11,24,25]

In general, protozoan infection does not cause eosinophilia, with the exception of isosporiasis, known to cause diarrhea associated with eosinophilia in both immunocompetent and immunocompromised patients.[26,27] Infection with *Blastocystis*

**Table 21.2 Symptoms and etiologies associated with eosinophilia**

| Anatomic compartment or symptom | Causes of eosinophilia |
| --- | --- |
| Ocular | Subconjunctival worm migration: loiasis<br>Subconjunctival/retinal hemorrhage: trichinellosis, cysticercosis<br>Retinitis/blindness: onchocerciasis<br>Other: visceral larva migrans (VLM, due to toxocariasis and baylisascariasis (raccoon roundworm)), gnathostomiasis, fascioliasis, sparganosis |
| Pulmonary | Migratory infiltrates (Loeffler's syndrome): ascariasis (most common), hookworm infection, strongyloidiasis<br>Eosinophilic pleural effusion: parasites: toxocariasis, filariasis, paragonimiasis, anisakiasis, echinococcosis, strongyloidiasis<br>    Other infections: Coccidioidomycosis, tuberculosis, histoplasmosis, paracoccidioidomycosis<br>    Other causes: Malignancy, hemothorax, pneumothorax, drug reactions, pulmonary infarct, rheumatologic disease, allergic bronchopulmonary aspergillosis<br>Parenchymal invasion with or without cavitation: paragonimiasis, tuberculosis, echinococcosis<br>Pulmonary infiltration and painful myositis of diaphragm: trichinellosis (predisposes to bacterial pneumonia)<br>Pulmonary embolism due to eggs through portal-systemic vascular shunts: chronic schistosomiasis (heavy infection by *S. mansoni* and *S. japonicum*)<br>Tropical pulmonary eosinophilia (filariasis)<br>Others: VLM |
| Gastrointestinal | Abdominal pain/diarrhea: angiostrongyliasis (*A. costaricensis*), anisakiasis, ascariasis, capillariasis, hookworm infection, strongyloidiasis, tapeworm infection, schistosomiasis, trichinellosis, isosporiasis, VLM<br>Upper GI bleeding: chronic schistosomiasis (portal hypertension and esophageal varices)<br>Duodenal ulcer: Echinostomiasis<br>Worm-bolus obstruction: ascariasis<br>Intussusception: ascariasis, schistosomiasis<br>Bloody diarrhea and rectal prolapse: trichuriasis (heavy infection)<br>Hepatobiliary disease<br>    Liver abscess or cyst: echinococcosis, fascioliasis<br>    Bile duct obstruction: ascariasis, capillariasis (rare), clonorchiasis and other liver flukes, echinococcosis, strongyloidiasis<br>    Hepatitis/hepatomegaly: fascioliasis, capillariasis, schistosomiasis, VLM, drugs<br>Pancreatitis: anisakiasis (perforating the stomach posteriorly into pancreas), ascariasis (acute hemorrhagic pancreatitis), clonorchiasis, fascioliasis |
| Genitourinary | Hematuria: schistosomiasis (*S. haematobium*)<br>Chyluria: lymphatic filariasis<br>Hydatiduria (grape like material) with/without hematuria: echinococcosis<br>Proteinuria and nephritic syndrome: lymphatic filariasis, loiasis<br>Hydrocele, groin mass: lymphatic filariasis (filarial dance sign by ultrasound), onchocerciasis<br>Seminal vesicle/ testis mass: schistosomiasis<br>Renal cyst/mass: echinococcosis<br>Enuresis (children), tubo-ovarian abscess (women): enterobiasis |
| Skin and soft tissue | Urticaria: ascariasis, fascioliasis, loiasis, onchocerciasis, hookworm infection, trichinellosis, gnathostomiasis, paragonimiasis, strongyloidiasis (larva currens), VLM, schistosomiasis<br>Serpiginous eruptions: cutaneous larva migrans, hookworm infection, strongyloidiasis (larva currens), gnathostomiasis<br>Migratory angioedema: loiasis (calabar swelling), gnathostomiasis, sparganosis<br>Subcutaneous nodules/mass: coenurosis (usually single) cysticercosis (often multiple), echinococcosis, fascioliasis, dirofilariasis, onchocerciasis (onchocercoma nodules on bony prominence), sparganosis, paragonimiasis, myiasis, mycosis (coccidioidomycosis, basidiobolomycosis) |

**Table 21.2 Symptoms and etiologies associated with eosinophilia—cont'd**

| Anatomic compartment or symptom | Causes of eosinophilia |
|---|---|
| | Dermatitis: cutaneous larva migrans, dracunculiasis, hookworm infection, gnathostomiasis, onchocerciasis, strongyloidiasis, schistosomiasis<br>Pruritis Ani: enterobiasis, strongyloidiasis<br>Myositis: trichinellosis<br>Lymphedema: filariasis |
| Peripheral or central nervous system | Eosinophilic meningitis : angiostrongyliasis (*A. cantonensis*, most common), neurocysticercosis, toxocariasis, schistosomiasis, coccidioidomycosis, cryptococcosis, baylisascariasis<br>Focal neurologic findings/seizures<br>  Cystic and/or calcified lesions: cysticercosis, echinococcosis, paragonimiasis<br>  Mass lesions: schistosomiasis, trichinellosis, toxocariasis, gnathostomiasis, baylisascariasis<br>Other (peripheral neuropathy, myelitis): schistosomal myeloradiculopathy (SMR) |
| Fever | Angiostrongyliasis, clonorchiasis, fascioliasis, filariasis (filarial fever), schistosomiasis (Katayama fever), echinococcosis (intermittent cystic content spillage), gnathostomiasis, strongyloidiasis (hyperinfection), trichinellosis, VLM |
| No focal symptoms | Drug reactions: drug reactions may be asymptomatic or associated with characteristic signs and symptoms<br>Drug rash, eosinophilia and systemic symptoms (DRESS): sulfasalazine, hydantoin, carbamazepine, cyclosporine, d-penicillamine, allopurinol, hydrochlorothiazide<br>Asymptomatic: quinine, penicillins, cephalosporins, quinolones<br>Pulmonary infiltrates: NSAIDs, sulfas, nitrofurantoin<br>Hepatitis: tetracyclines, semisynthetic penicillins<br>Eosinophilia myalgia syndrome (EMS): contaminated L-tryptophan and 5-hydroxy-L-tryptophan (5HTP)<br>Interstitial nephritis: cephalosporins, semisynthetic penicillins |

VLM, visceral larva migrans.

*hominis* has also been shown to present with chronic urticaria or diarrhea associated with mild eosinophilia in rare cases.[28,29] In general, most patients with *B. hominis* do not require treatment provided they are asymptomatic. Moreover, typically the presence of the *B. hominis* should not be considered an explanation of the peripheral blood eosinophilia. Eosinophilia can be caused by ectoparasites. Scabies can cause eosinophilia, presumably due to hypersensitivity reactions to the mites and their eggs.[30] Myiasis – a condition caused by infestation of fly larvae in the skin, subcutaneous tissue, and/or other internal organs – has also occasionally been associated with eosinophilia.[31]

Most acute bacterial and viral diseases are associated with eosinopenia, the exceptions being resolving scarlet fever, chronic indolent tuberculosis[32] and HIV infection.[33] Occasionally, fungal infections such as coccidioidomycosis,[34] paracoccidioidomycosis,[35–39] aspergillosis (allergic bronchopulmonary aspergillosis), and basidiobolomycosis[40,41] have been associated with eosinophilia. Coccidioidomycosis and aspergillosis usually present with pulmonary symptoms, and basidiobolomycosis is a rare form of fungal infections that presents with skin manifestations as well as gastrointestinal symptoms. Paracoccidioidomycosis usually presents with pulmonary symptoms in adults; most children demonstrate reticuloendothelial system involvement characterized by a febrile lymphoproliferative syndrome, anemia, and hypergammaglobulinemia associated with eosinophilia.[38,39,42]

## Noninfectious causes

Noninfectious etiologies for eosinophilia should be always considered even in immigrant and refugee populations. The major causes are drug hypersensitivity, atopy and atopic asthma, connective tissue disorders (such as Churg-Strauss syndrome, systemic lupus erythematosus, rheumatoid arthritis), neoplasms (lymphomas, leukemias, certain solid tumors), hypereosinophilic syndromes, eosinophilic gastrointestinal disorders, hypoadrenalism, sarcoidosis, inflammatory bowel disease, and some congenital immune deficiencies.

Immigrants have also been shown to develop allergic diseases after resettlement as reported in immigrants moved from the rural hills of Ethiopia to the more urban and industrialized setting of Israel.[9]

Drug reactions are another important cause of eosinophilia to consider in immigrant populations. Immigrants or refugees often have other preexisting health conditions,[43] and as a consequence are often placed on antibiotic treatment, analgesics, or other relevant medicines. It is also important to get information about traditional remedies or imported medications only accessible from their countries of origin. In addition, information should be obtained about healthcare practices carried out in the immigrant community after resettlement.[43] Drug reactions associated with peripheral eosinophilia may present without accompanying symptoms or may be associated with specific signs and symptoms. Asymptomatic eosinophilia has been associated most often with quinine, penicillins, cephalosporins, or quinolones. Pulmonary infiltrates with peripheral eosinophilia have been particularly associated with NSAIDs, sulfas, and nitrofurantoin. Hepatitis with eosinophilia can be induced by the tetracyclines or the semisynthetic penicillins. Interstitial nephritis with eosinophilia has been associated with cephalosporins (cefotaxime being the most commonly reported) and semisynthetic penicillins. Drug reaction with eosinophilia and systemic symptoms (DRESS) can occur with sulfasalazine, hydantoin, carbamazepine, d-penicillamine, allopurinol, hydrochlorothiazide, and cyclosporin, or can be associated with viral infection (human herpesvirus-6, Epstein-Barr virus, cytomegalovirus). Patients with DRESS present with fever, rash, systemic involvement, and an appropriate medication history. This syndrome often must be differentiated from acute infectious diseases.

## Approaches to Recent Immigrant Patients with Eosinophilia

The geographic region of the immigrants' home country can provide useful clues to the identification of the underlying cause of eosinophilia. In some cases, eosinophilia may be the only clue to a helminth infection in an asymptomatic patient. An algorithm for the approach to the assessment of eosinophilia for immigrant patients is illustrated in Figure 21.1.

> **Pearls in evaluation and management of eosinophilia in immigrants**
>
> - Eosinophilia should be considered a marker for pathogenic helminth infections in the vast majority of immigrants.
> - Negative stools for ova and parasites are not sufficient to exclude some important parasitic causes of eosinophilia.
> - Some parasites may persist many years after immigration.

## History and Physical Examination

To evaluate a patient with eosinophilia, a careful history should be taken, directed specifically at the nature of the symptoms (if present), previous eosinophil counts (if available), exposure history including the home country before immigration and including all countries the individuals has traveled through and lived in after departure from the country of origin, duration, and type of exposures (water contact, dietary habits, medication), allergy, and pertinent past medical history. Patients should be asked about diseases commonly found in their family or former community, thereby providing an epidemiologic benchmark for a particular region. It should also be noted that immigrants or refugees may have been displaced to different parts of their home country (due to civil conflict, economic conditions, or natural disaster such as drought, earthquake, flood, etc.) or have had intermediate stays in other countries (after having left their own country) where the acquisition of infections (or other conditions) responsible for the eosinophilia occurred. Therefore, consideration of the time of exposure should be also taken into account for the home country and departure port (refugee camp) and during the journey. Additionally, inquiring about any recent travel history back to their home country should be done. A list of specific exposures that could be asked about during the process of obtaining a medical history is presented in Table 21.3.

The duration of eosinophilia can also provide clues to narrow the diagnostic possibilities. The temporal relationships between potential exposure to a parasitic pathogen and the onset of eosinophilia or specific features of the eosinophilia can be helpful as

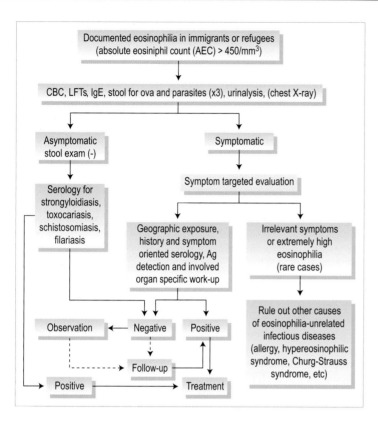

**Fig. 21.1** Algorithm to assess eosinophilia in immigrant and refugee patients.

Table 21.3 **Specific exposure history associated with eosinophilia and parasite infection**

| Exposure | Parasitic infection/disease |
|---|---|
| Meat | |
|   Pork, proximity to slaughterhouse or butchering activity | *Taenia solium* |
|   Wild boar/bear, pork/walrus | Trichinellosis |
| Raw freshwater fish/seafood consumption | Gnathostomiasis<br>Anisakiasis<br>Diphyllobothriasis<br>Clonorchiasis |
| Freshwater crab consumption | Paragonimiasis |
| Raw snake or frog consumption | Sparganosis |
| Watercress consumption | Fascioliasis |
| Snails or slime-contaminated vegetable consumption | Angiostrongyliasis |
| Swimming in fresh water | Schistosomiasis |
| Proximity to sheep-raising area | Echinococcosis |
| Soil, history of pica | Cutaneous larva migrans<br>Hookworm<br>Strongyloidiasis<br>Trichuriasis<br>Visceral larva migrans (toxocariasis) |
| Exposure to dogs and cats (esp. lactating mother animals, puppies, and kittens) | Visceral larva migrans (toxocariasis) |

well. Intermittent eosinophilia is characteristic of echinococcosis and cysticercosis and reflects the occasional inflammatory response toward released material from the cysts. Eosinophilia occurs early in infection with ascariasis, clonorchiasis, fascioliasis, fasciolopsiasis, hookworm infection, paragonimiasis, schistosomiasis, strongyloidiasis, and trichinellosis. Chronic, long-standing eosinophilia may occur in some cases of clonorchiasis, cysticercosis, echinococcosis, fascioliasis, filarial infections, gnathostomiasis, hookworm infection, paragonimiasis, strongyloidiasis, and schistosomiasis.

Physical examination should be performed with special attention to skin, soft tissues, liver, and spleen as well as an additional directed examination based on the patient's specific symptoms or chief complaints.

# Diagnostic Evaluation

## Initial evaluation

Ideally, the evaluation of eosinophilia in immigrant/refugee patients should include stool examinations, serologic assessments, antigen-detection assays (if available), liver function tests, urinalysis, IgE levels, and chest radiographs. In a resource-poor setting, urinalysis, stool examination, or blood smear (filariasis) may be the only available diagnostic options.

It is important to remember that when eosinophilia occurs during the early stages of infection, egg or larval excretion may be absent, in that the infection may be in the prepatent phase (before the adult female worms mature and reproduce). In some chronic infections, because egg excretion in the stool can be intermittent, multiple stool examinations may increase the diagnostic yield. And it is of note that stool examinations (while useful if a pathogen is identified) will miss a majority of the pathogens associated with eosinophilia either because the pathogen is not found in the stool (filarial species, *Schistosoma haematobium*) or is hard to find (*Strongyloides stercoralis*). Moreover, in some refugee/immigrant populations, pre-departure treatment with albendazole can reduce the parasite burden in certain infections (such as hookworm or *T. trichiura*) and thereby the ability to detect parasites in the stool.[44] Antibody-based serologies can remain positive indefinitely and do not distinguish between active and prior infection. Furthermore, as these tests tend to remain positive despite treatment, it is difficult to use them to identify reinfection unless a patient has

pathognomonic symptoms. In this situation, using antigen detection or molecular diagnosis can be useful, if available. For an initial serologic evaluation of eosinophilia with or without symptoms, tests for filariasis, strongyloidiasis, schistosomiasis, and toxocariasis (particularly in children) would be a reasonable screen depending on the exposure (and geographic) history, with further testing being an option if a particular serology were positive.

## Symptom-directed work-up

If localized signs or symptoms are present, a directed evaluation can be initiated. A list for causes of eosinophilia with associated symptoms is found in Table 21.2. Further information on specific evaluations for each disease and involved organ system can be found in Chapters 14, 20, and other chapters in Section 3.

**Eye involvement:** A migrating worm can be observed and extracted from its subconjunctival location under local anesthesia in loiasis. Slit lamp and fundoscopic examination may be needed to evaluate the extent of pathology of onchocerciasis or ocular larva migrans (toxocariasis).

**Respiratory system:** For those patients who present with pulmonary involvement and peripheral eosinophilia, sputum examination (fungi, acid-fast bacilli, helminth larvae, ova), and culture (*Mycobacterium tuberculosis* and fungi) can provide important insights into the etiology. High-resolution computed tomography (CT) can be performed to define the nature of the pulmonary lesions. In cases of tropical pulmonary eosinophilia (TPE), it is important to note that chest radiographic findings can be normal in up to 20% of cases. In some cases, the nature of the sputum (e.g. rust-colored sputum in paragonimiasis, salty/sandy sputum in echinococcosis), microscopic examination of sputum (for larvae of *Strongyloides* in disseminated infection), and stool findings with appropriate serological testing (for filarial infections, echinococcosis, strongyloidiasis, or paragonimiasis) will provide helpful insights into the diagnosis.

**Gastrointestinal and hepatobiliary system:** For eosinophilia associated with involvement of the gastrointestinal tract or the hepatobiliary axis, imaging studies (abdominal ultrasound, CT), endoscopy (including endoscopic retrograde cholangiopancreatography [ERCP]), and biopsies of appropriate tissues including rectal biopsies (for cases of schistosomiasis and isosporiasis to improve the diagnostic yield) when stool examinations or serology tests are unrevealing may be needed for diagnosis.

In some cases, during the diagnostic evaluation, therapy may be delivered as well. Anisakiasis can present acutely with abdominal or chest pain but typically will not have peripheral eosinophilia unless it is chronic; endoscopic diagnosis and removal of the parasite will provide both a diagnosis and treatment. Echinostomiasis can also cause duodenal ulcer and be diagnosed and treated endoscopically.[45,46] *Ascaris* worms can be removed by endoscopy from the biliary tree during ERCP.[47,48]

If echinococcosis is suspected, caution should be exercised not to perform aspiration or biopsy in the absence of albendazole pretreatment to prevent seeding of the cystic contents should spillage occur during the biopsy. Additional testing for muscle enzyme (creatine phosphokinase, aldolase, and lactate dehydrogenase) elevations or muscle biopsy (deltoid muscle) can be done if trichinellosis is suspected, typically associated with other abdominal symptoms and history of specific food consumption (e.g. pork, wild boar, walrus, or bear meat).[49,50] For enterobiasis, since the eggs of *Enterobius vermicularis* are not commonly seen in the stool, the tape test to sample the perianal region in the early morning should be considered.

**Genitourinary system:** For eosinophilia associated with genitourinary symptoms, urinalysis for hematuria (*Schistosoma haematobium*), chyluria (lymphatic filariasis), or proteinuria (seen occasionally in each of the filarial infections) will be helpful. If urinary schistosomiasis is a consideration, a midday or early afternoon urine to look for ova is useful. Physical examination for scrotal/testicular abnormalities should be performed in male patients. Ultrasound for bladder abnormalities (schistosomiasis) or for hydrocele or the filarial dance sign[51] (*Wuchereria bancrofti* infection) is an important adjunct for the diagnostic evaluation.

**Skin and soft tissue:** Skin snips, skin biopsy, or excision of masses or nodules can be performed (typically skin snips and nodulectomy should be done when onchocerciasis is suspected but any skin lesions with eosinophilia should prompt this approach). Occasionally, worms (or vermiform eruptions) can be seen; these can be carefully extracted (e.g. gnathostomiasis, loiasis). Lymphoscintigraphy can be performed to evaluate the lymphatic system dysfunction in patients with lymphedema due to filariasis.[52]

**Nervous system:** Various parasitic infections can cause central nervous system infection with eosinophilia in the peripheral blood and/or in the cerebrospinal fluid (CSF). For nervous system involvement with helminth parasites, CT or magnetic resonance imaging (MRI), lumbar puncture (with examination for parasites and eosinophils) or CSF serologies (e.g. *Angiostrongylus*, *Toxocara*) may provide diagnostic clues. Serologic tests are typically performed on acute and convalescent serum (1 month apart) but testing for *Angiostrongylus*, can be performed any time CSF is available. CSF may show pleocytosis with eosinophilia (more than 10%) with increased protein (and usually normal glucose levels).[53-55] Under certain circumstances (e.g. *Toxocara*) where it is difficult to exclude a brain tumor, biopsies (either stereotactic or open) may be required to reach a definite diagnosis.

## Can the level of eosinophilia help to narrow the differential diagnosis?

Although the role of eosinophil counts is limited in screening asymptomatic patients, and eosinophilia has poor positive predictive value for parasite infection,[4,11,12] having moderately to markedly elevated eosinophil counts will more likely be associated with parasite infection.[6,10] Marked eosinophilia ($>3000/mm^3$) tends to be associated with tissue invasion and can be seen in certain infections, such as angiostrongyliasis, ascariasis, clonorchiasis, fascioliasis, fasciolopsiasis, filariasis, gnathostomiasis, hookworm infection, opisthorchiasis, paragonimiasis, schistosomiasis, toxocariasis, and trichinellosis.

Extremely marked eosinophilia ($>10\,000/mm^3$) is uncommon in helminth infection, but rarely it can occur in TPE, localized onchocercal dermatitis (Sowda), and acute schistosomiasis; however, when the eosinophilia is extraordinarily high grade and extensive parasitic infection evaluation is negative, special attention must be made in consulting with hematologists or allergy/immunologists to exclude other hypereosinophilic conditions.[56]

## Special considerations in children and pregnant women

Physiologically, eosinophil counts are higher in neonates and young infants than those in older children and adults, and levels decrease with advancing age. Children are more likely to have eosinophilia and have multiple parasite infections and more recent infections due to young age and their behavior (e.g. playing on the ground, close contact with animals).[17] In a recent study of refugees who had asymptomatic eosinophilia, almost 30% were less than 10 years of age.[57] Congenital immune deficiency is a rare cause of eosinophilia in children and may be associated with recurrent bacterial infections and atopic or allergic diseases. After relocating to more hygienic environments, immigrants have been shown to acquire allergic diseases relatively soon after resettlement.[9] Eosinophil counts are low during pregnancy, reaching their nadir around delivery. Thus, pregnant women may have falsely low numbers of eosinophils in response to parasitic infection.

## Treatment

Pathogen-directed treatment should be initiated once the diagnosis is confirmed. Pathogen-specific treatment options are discussed in other sections of this book.

Typical first-line therapies directed at a specific underlying cause of helminth-induced eosinophilia include albendazole, mebendazole, diethylcarbamazine, ivermectin, and praziquantel and, for fascioliasis, triclabendazole.[58]

With the treatment of many systemic helminth infections (filariasis, schistosomiasis in particular),[59,60] there is a marked increase in circulating eosinophil levels 7–14 days after initiation of therapy. This increase in peripheral blood eosinophilia following anthelmintic therapy is preceded by an increase in serum levels of IL-5.[59] Corticosteroid treatment can be used to reduce host inflammatory response to the death of (or release of antigens by) the parasite in angiostrongyliasis, filariasis, neurocysticercosis, or trichinellosis.

Interventional procedures may be required in addition to the medical treatment: endoscopic removal of the *Anisakis* worm from the gastric mucosa, *Ascaris* and *Fasciola* parasites from the biliary system during ERCP, surgery for masses (e.g. hydatid cysts, ventricular cysts in neurocysticercosis, intestinal obstruction from *Ascaris* infection) or for acute abdomen in *Angiostrongylus costaricensis*, or intermittent lumbar punctures in angiostrongyliasis. Percutaneous aspiration and irrigation (termed puncture, aspiration, injection, and re-aspiration, PAIR) for echinococcosis in conjunction with preoperative albendazole therapy can often give better results than albendazole alone.[61,62] In filarial infections (particularly in loiasis when the number of microfilariae is extremely high), apheresis may

be performed to reduce the microfilarial burden in order to decrease post-treatment response to medication-induced parasite killing.[63]

Were there no financial constraints, the ideal approach to identify the underlying cause of eosinophilia would be an extensive but selective evaluation. However, in reality, despite reasonable evaluation, in asymptomatic patients with eosinophilia, there is up to a 50% failure rate in the identification of an etiologic cause. Therefore, empiric anthelmintic therapy has been advocated on the basis of cost-effectiveness.[64] In specific refugee populations with well-known parasitic infection epidemiology such as the Southeast Asian population in which *Strongyloides* and hookworm are most common,[6] single-dose therapy with ivermectin and/or albendazole has been suggested as a reasonable approach.[65]

## Conclusion

The evaluation and management of eosinophilia and associated conditions in immigrants from tropical and subtropical regions of the world requires a comprehensive approach consisting of a detailed exposure history, understanding of each helminth infection and its disease course, a diligent diagnostic work-up, and targeted treatment.

## References

1. Fleming AF, Akintunde EA, Harrison KA, Dunn D. Leucocyte counts during pregnancy and the puerperium and at birth in Nigerians. East Afr Med J 1985; 62(3):175–184.
2. Godue CB, Gyorkos TW. Intestinal parasites in refugee claimants: a case study for selective screening? Can J Public Health 1990; 81(3):191–195.
3. Lerman D, Barrett-Connor E, Norcross W. Intestinal parasites in asymptomatic adult Southeast Asian immigrants. J Fam Pract 1982; 15(3):443–446.
4. Libman MD, MacLean JD, Gyorkos TW. Screening for schistosomiasis, filariasis, and strongyloidiasis among expatriates returning from the tropics. Clin Infect Dis 1993; 17(3):353–359.
5. Lopez-Velez R, Huerga H, Turrientes MC. Infectious diseases in immigrants from the perspective of a tropical medicine referral unit. Am J Trop Med Hyg 2003; 69(1):115–121.
6. Nutman TB, Ottesen EA, Ieng S, et al. Eosinophilia in Southeast Asian refugees: evaluation at a referral center. J Infect Dis 1987; 155(2):309–313.
7. Parenti DM, Lucas D, Lee A, Hollenkamp RH. Health status of Ethiopian refugees in the United States. Am J Public Health 1987; 77(12):1542–1543.
8. Roca C, Balanzo X, Sauca G, et al. [Imported hookworm infection in African immigrants in Spain: study of 285 patients]. Med Clin (Barc) 2003; 121(4):139–141.
9. Rosenberg R, Vinker S, Zakut H, et al. An unusually high prevalence of asthma in Ethiopian immigrants to Israel. Fam Med 1999; 31(4):276–279.

10. Tittle BS, Harris JA, Chase PA, et al. Health screening of Indochinese refugee children. Am J Dis Child 1982; 136(8):697–700.
11. Huerga H, Lopez-Velez R. Infectious diseases in sub-Saharan African immigrant children in Madrid, Spain. Pediatr Infect Dis J 2002; 21(9):830–834.
12. Whitty CJ, Carroll B, Armstrong M, et al. Utility of history, examination and laboratory tests in screening those returning to Europe from the tropics for parasitic infection. Trop Med Int Health 2000. 5(11):818–823.
13. Klion AD, Massougbodji A, Sadeler BC, et al. Loiasis in endemic and nonendemic populations: immunologically mediated differences in clinical presentation. J Infect Dis 1991. 163(6):1318–1325.
14. Roca C, Balanzo X, Gascon J, et al. Comparative, clinico-epidemiologic study of Schistosoma mansoni infections in travellers and immigrants in Spain. Eur J Clin Microbiol Infect Dis 2002; 21(3):219–223.
15. Sudarshi S, Stumpfle R, Armstrong M, et al. Clinical presentation and diagnostic sensitivity of laboratory tests for Strongyloides stercoralis in travellers compared with immigrants in a non-endemic country. Trop Med Int Health 2003; 8(8):728–732.
16. Whitty CJ, Mabey DC, Armstrong M, et al. Presentation and outcome of 1107 cases of schistosomiasis from Africa diagnosed in a non-endemic country. Trans R Soc Trop Med Hyg 2000; 94(5):531–534.
17. Heukelbach J, Poggensee G, Winter B, et al. Leukocytosis and blood eosinophilia in a polyparasitised population in north-eastern Brazil. Trans R Soc Trop Med Hyg 2006; 100(1):32–40.
18. Taliaferro W, Sarles M. The cellular reactions in the skin, lungs, and intestine of normal and immune rats after infection with Nippostrongylus brasiliensis. J Infect Dis 1939; 64:157–192.
19. Klion AD, Nutman TB. The role of eosinophils in host defense against helminth parasites. J Allergy Clin Immunol 2004; 113(1):30–37.
20. Leder K, Weller PF. Eosinophilia and helminthic infections. Baillieres Best Pract Res Clin Haematol 2000; 13(2):301–317.
21. Mawhorter SD. Eosinophilia caused by parasites. Pediatr Ann 1994; 23(8):405, 409–413.
22. Maxwell C, Hussain R, Nutman TB, et al. The clinical and immunologic responses of normal human volunteers to low dose hookworm (Necator americanus) infection. Am J Trop Med Hyg 1987; 37(1):126–134.
23. Nutman TB. Experimental infection of humans with filariae. Rev Infect Dis 1991; 13(5):1018–1022.
24. Ryan N, Plackett M, Dwyer B. Parasitic infections of refugees. Med J Aust 1988; 148(10):491–494.
25. Huerga H, Aramburu H, Lopez-Velez R. Comparative study of infectious diseases in immigrant children from various countries. An Pediatr (Barc) 2004; 60(1):16–21.
26. Junod C. Isospora belli coccidiosis in immunocompetent subjects (a study of 40 cases seen in Paris). Bull Soc Pathol Exot Filiales 1988; 81(3):317–325.
27. Marcial-Seoane MA, Serrano-Olmo J. Intestinal infection with Isospora belli. P R Health Sci J 1995; 14(2):137–140.
28. Pasqui AL, Savini E, Saletti M, et al. Chronic urticaria and Blastocystis hominis infection: a case report. Eur Rev Med Pharmacol Sci 2004; 8(3):117–120.
29. Sheehan DJ, Raucher BG, McKitrick JC. Association of Blastocystis hominis with signs and symptoms of human disease. J Clin Microbiol 1986; 24(4):548–550.
30. Roberts LJ, Huffman SE, Walton SF, Currie BJ. Crusted scabies: clinical and immunological findings in seventy-eight patients and a review of the literature. J Infect 2005; 50(5):375–381.
31. Starr J, Pruett JH, Yunginger JW, et al. Myiasis due to Hypoderma lineatum infection mimicking the hypereosinophilic syndrome. Mayo Clin Proc 2000; 75(7):755–759.
32. Sharma OP, Bethlem EP. The pulmonary infiltration with eosinophilia syndrome. Curr Opin Pulm Med 1996; 2(5):380–389.
33. Cohen AJ, Steigbigel RT. Eosinophilia in patients infected with human immunodeficiency virus. J Infect Dis,1996; 174(3):615–618.
34. Case records of the Massachusetts General Hospital. Weekly clinicopathological exercises. Case 21–1994. A 20-year-old Mexican immigrant with recurrent hemoptysis and a pulmonary cavitary lesion. N Engl J Med 1994; 330(21):1516–1522.
35. Igarashi T, Kurose T, Itabashi K, et al. A case of chronic pulmonary paracoccidioidomycosis. Nihon Kokyuki Gakkai Zasshi 2004; 42(7):629–633.
36. Iralu JV, Maguire JH. Pulmonary infections in immigrants and refugees. Semin Respir Infect 1991; 6(4):235–246.
37. Tresoldi AT, Pereira RM, Castro LC, et al. [Hypercalcemia and multiple osteolytic lesions in a child with disseminated paracoccidioidomycosis and pulmonary tuberculosis]. J Pediatr (Rio J) 2005; 81(4):349–352.
38. Pereira RM, Bucaretchi F, Barison Ede M, et al. Paracoccidioidomycosis in children: clinical presentation, follow-up and outcome. Rev Inst Med Trop Sao Paulo 2004; 46(3):127–131.
39. Pereira RM, Tresoldi AT, da Silva MT, et al. Fatal disseminated paracoccidioidomycosis in a two-year-old child. Rev Inst Med Trop Sao Paulo 2004; 46(1):37–39.
40. Al Jarie A, Al-Mohsen I, Al Jumaah S, et al. Pediatric gastrointestinal basidiobolomycosis. Pediatr Infect Dis J 2003; 22(11):1007–1014.
41. Mathew R, Kumaravel S, Kuruvilla S, et al. Successful treatment of extensive basidiobolomycosis with oral itraconazole in a child. Int J Dermatol 2005; 44(7): 572–575.
42. Brummer E, Castaneda E, Restrepo A. Paracoccidioidomycosis: an update. Clin Microbiol Rev 1993; 6(2):89–117.
43. Stauffer WM, Kamat D, Walker PF. Screening of international immigrants, refugees, and adoptees. Prim Care 2002; 29(4):879–905.
44. Geltman PL, Cochran J, Hedgecock C. Intestinal parasites among African refugees resettled in Massachusetts and the impact of an overseas pre-departure treatment program. Am J Trop Med Hyg 2003; 69(6):657–662.
45. Chang YD, Sohn WM, Ryu JH, et al. A human infection of Echinostoma hortense in duodenal bulb diagnosed by endoscopy. Korean J Parasitol 2005; 43(2):57–60.
46. Cho CM, Tak W, Kweon Y, et al. A human case of Echinostoma hortense (Trematoda: Echinostomatidae) infection diagnosed by gastroduodenal endoscopy in Korea. Korean J Parasitol 2003; 41(2):117–120.
47. Pereira-Lima JC, Jakobs R, da Silva CP, et al. Endoscopic removal of Ascaris lumbricoides from the biliary tract as emergency treatment for acute suppurative cholangitis. J Gastroenterol 2001; 39(9):793–796.
48. Saowaros V. Endoscopic retrograde cholangio-pancreatographic diagnosis and extraction of massive biliary ascariasis presented with acute pancreatitis: a case report. J Med Assoc Thai 1999; 82(5):515–519.
49. Dupouy-Camet J, Kociecka W, Bruschi F, et al. Opinion on the diagnosis and treatment of human trichinellosis. Expert Opin Pharmacother 2002; 3(8):1117–1130.
50. Schellenberg RS, Tan BJ, Irvine JD, et al. An outbreak of trichinellosis due to consumption of bear meat infected with Trichinella nativa, in two northern Saskatchewan communities. J Infect Dis 2003; 188(6):835–843.
51. Mand S, Marfo-Debrekyei Y, Dittrich M, et al. Animated documentation of the filaria dance sign (FDS) in bancroftian filariasis. Filaria J 2003; 2(1):3.
52. Moore TA, Reynolds JC, Kenney RT, et al. Diethylcarbamazine-induced reversal of early lymphatic dysfunction in a patient with bancroftian filariasis: assessment with use of lymphoscintigraphy. Clin Infect Dis 1996; 23(5):1007–1011.

53. Batmanian JJ, O'Neill JH. Eosinophilic meningoencephalitis with permanent neurological sequelae. Intern Med J 2004; 34(4):217–218.

54. Lindo JF, Escoffery CT, Reid B, et al. Fatal autochthonous eosinophilic meningitis in a Jamaican child caused by *Angiostrongylus cantonensis*. Am J Trop Med Hyg 2004; 70(4):425–428.

55. Tsai HC, Lee SS, Huang CK, et al. Outbreak of eosinophilic meningitis associated with drinking raw vegetable juice in southern Taiwan. Am J Trop Med Hyg 2004; 71(2):222–226.

56. Kim YJ, Nutman TB. Eosinophilia: causes and pathobiology in persons with prior exposures in tropical areas with an emphasis on parasitic infections. Curr Infect Dis Rep 2006; 8(1):43–50.

57. Seybolt L, Christiansen D, Barnett ED. Diagnostic evaluation of newly arrived asymptomatic refugees with eosinophilia. Clin Infect Dis 2006; 42(3):363–367.

58. Graham CS, Brodie SB, Weller PF. Imported *Fasciola hepatica* infection in the United States and treatment with triclabendazole. Clin Infect Dis 2001; 33(1):1–5.

59. Gopinath R, Hanna LE, Kumaraswami V, et al. Perturbations in eosinophil homeostasis following treatment of lymphatic filariasis. Infect Immun 2000; 68(1):93–99.

60. Kimani G, Chunge CN, Butterworth AE, et al. Eosinophilia and eosinophil helminthotoxicity in patients treated for *Schistosoma mansoni* infections. Trans R Soc Trop Med Hyg 1991; 85(4):489–492.

61. Smego RA Jr, Bhatti S, Khaliq AA, et al. Percutaneous aspiration-injection-reaspiration drainage plus albendazole or mebendazole for hepatic cystic echinococcosis: a meta-analysis. Clin Infect Dis 2003; 37(8):1073–1083.

62. Smego RA Jr, Sebanego P. Treatment options for hepatic cystic echinococcosis. Int J Infect Dis 2005; 9(2):69–76.

63. Ottesen EA. Filarial infections. Infect Dis Clin North Am 1993; 7(3):619–633.

64. Muennig P, Pallin D, Sell RL, et al. The cost effectiveness of strategies for the treatment of intestinal parasites in immigrants. N Engl J Med 1999; 340(10):773–779.

65. Muennig P, Pallin D, Challah C, et al. The cost-effectiveness of ivermectin vs. albendazole in the presumptive treatment of strongyloidiasis in immigrants to the United States. Epidemiol Infect 2004; 132(6):1055–1063.

# CHAPTER 22

# Hepatitis B: Global Epidemiology, Diagnosis, and Prevention

Gregory L. Armstrong and Susan T. Goldstein*

## Hepatitis B: Clinical Pearls in Refugees and Immigrants

- Many immigrants come from countries with intermediate or high hepatitis B virus (HBV) prevalence.
- Perinatal and early childhood infection accounts for most cases of chronic hepatitis B among immigrants. In addition, lack of access to vaccination, unsafe medical procedures, and percutaneous exposures during traditional cultural practices also contribute to the high prevalence of HBV infection.
- Screening for hepatitis B surface antigen (HBsAg) should be done irrespective of length of time residing in the United States.
- Persons with chronic HBV infection are at substantial lifetime risk for cirrhosis and hepatocellular carcinoma.
- Chronically infected immigrants should be counseled on the means of reducing further liver damage and on ways to prevent transmission of the virus to others.
- Referral of the chronically infected immigrant to a specialist in the management of hepatitis B is appropriate.
- Hepatocellular carcinoma is a vaccine-preventable cancer.

---

* Drs. Armstrong and Goldstein contributed equally to this chapter.

## Virology

Hepatitis B virus (HBV) is an enveloped, partially double-stranded DNA virus of the Hepadnaviridae family. The virus replicates in the liver, where viral DNA often incorporates into the host genome, an important factor in HBV's capacity to induce liver cancer. In the blood, the complete 42 nm HBV particle, known as the 'Dane particle,' includes an inner capsid made from hepatitis B core antigen (HBcAg) and containing hepatitis E antigen (HBeAg), a marker of infectivity. The core is enclosed within a lipid envelope containing the hepatitis B surface antigen (HBsAg). In patients with acute or chronic hepatitis B, envelope is produced in great excess and self-assembles into small spherical or tubular structures. These 22 nm particles do not contain core protein or DNA and are typically present in much higher numbers than Dane particles.

In the blood of infected individuals, HBV is present in extremely high concentrations, often in viral loads exceeding $10^7$ per milliliter. On environmental surfaces, HBV is highly stable, remaining infectious for at least 1 week.[1] Nonetheless, the virus is susceptible to commonly used disinfectants.[2]

HBV has been sub-classified by two separate classification systems: serotype and genotype. Nine serotypes of HBV have been described on the basis of serologic heterogeneity of HBsAg (adrq+, adrq−, ayr, ayw1, ayw2, ayw3, ayw4, adw2, adw4).[3] At least

**Table 22.1 Annual number of hepatitis B-related deaths, by World Health Organization region[6]**

| Region | Number of deaths | Proportion of deaths from chronic infection |
|---|---|---|
| Africa | 69 000 | 90% |
| Americas | 12 000 | 92% |
| Eastern Mediterranean | 21 000 | 90% |
| Europe | 51 000 | 94% |
| Southeast Asia | 143 000 | 92% |
| Western Pacific | 325 000 | 95% |
| **Global** | **621 000** | **94%** |

eight genotypes of HBV have been described, designated A through H, on the basis of an 8% difference in nucleotide sequence. HBV serotypes and genotypes vary geographically.[4,5]

# Global Epidemiology

## Burden of disease from hepatitis B

Worldwide, hepatitis B virus infection is one of the leading causes of infectious disease-related morbidity and mortality. An estimated two billion people – one-third of the world's population – have serologic evidence of past or present HBV infection and 350 million people are chronically infected. Each year, an estimated 621 000 people die from HBV-related liver disease (Table 22.1).[6] The majority (95%) of these deaths result from the chronic sequelae of infection, cirrhosis, and hepatocellular carcinoma (HCC). Although most of these deaths occur in adulthood, 21% result from HBV infection acquired in the perinatal period and another 48% from infection acquired in early childhood. Infection acquired after 5 years of age accounts for only 31% of deaths.

The world can be divided into areas of high, intermediate, and low HBV endemicity based on the prevalence of chronic HBV infection (i.e. the prevalence of HBsAg-positive individuals) in the general population (Fig. 22.1). Approximately 45% of the world's population lives in countries of high endemicity where > 60% of the population has ever been infected with HBV and > 8% is chronically infected. Most of these countries are in Africa and Asia. In countries of intermediate endemicity, which include 43% of the world's population, 20–60% of the popula-

tion has evidence of prior infection and 2–7% is HBsAg-positive. Only 12% of the population lives in countries of low endemicity where the lifetime risk of infection is < 20% and the prevalence of chronic infection is < 2%.

## Transmission of hepatitis B virus

Hepatitis B virus is transmitted from person to person through exposure to infected blood or body fluids, including semen and vaginal fluid. Modes of transmission include percutaneous and permucosal exposures to infectious body fluids, sexual contact with an infected person, and perinatal transmission from an infected mother to her infant. Rare instances of transmission of HBV through saliva have been reported.[7]

Perinatal transmission of HBV occurs from blood exposure during labor and delivery. In utero transmission is relatively rare, accounting for < 3% of perinatal infections in most studies.[8–12] The risk of transmission from an infected mother to her infant depends on the HBeAg status of the mother, being 70–90% for infants born to HBsAg-positive/HBeAg-positive mothers and 5–20% for infants born to HBsAg-positive/HBeAg-negative mothers.[13–18] Although HBV is found in low concentrations in breast milk, transmission of HBV has not been documented through breast-feeding.[19]

Horizontal transmission, also known as intrafamilial or household transmission, refers to percutaneous transmission of HBV within the household, from infected family members – most often mothers and older siblings – to young children.[20–28] Horizontal transmission is most important in countries of high HBV endemicity, but its occurrence in the United States has also been well documented.[29–32] Horizontal transmission of HBV to adult members of households has also been reported, including in families of children adopted from overseas.[32–34]

Sexual transmission of HBV is most common among persons at increased risk for other sexually transmitted infections, including those with many sexual partners or a history of other sexually transmitted infections. Sexual intercourse with a known infected person puts one at risk and engaging in certain sexual practices, such as anal intercourse, may facilitate transmission of HBV.[35] Men who have sex with men are at particularly high risk for HBV infection, with up to 60% having serologic markers of past or current infection.[35,36]

Percutaneous and permucosal transmission of HBV can result from transfusion of unscreened blood, injection drug use, occupational exposure

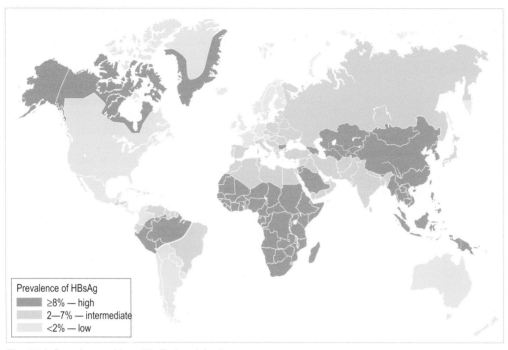

**Fig. 22.1** Prevalence of hepatitis B virus infection.

Prevalence of HBsAg
≥8% — high
2—7% — intermediate
<2% — low

(e.g. needle stick injuries) and nosocomial exposures (e.g. unsafe injection and other unsafe medical practices). In the United States, blood transfusion has not been an important mode of transmission since the institution of routine screening for markers of HBV in the early 1970s. However, blood transfusion remains an important source of infection in many less developed countries.

In recent years, unsafe injection and other unsafe medical practices have become increasingly recognized as major routes of HBV transmission, particularly in developing and transitional countries.[37] Unsafe injections, which account for an estimated 32% of new HBV infections annually,[38] are a consequence of both the reuse of injection equipment without proper sterilization and the overuse of injections where oral therapy would be indicated. The burden of disease from other unsafe medical practices is not known. Nosocomial transmission of HBV is not limited to less developed countries. In the United States and other developed countries, transmission of HBV in healthcare settings – both inpatient and outpatient – continues to occur.[39–42] Traditional healing practices that involve breaches in the skin barrier, such as piercing and scarification, have also been documented to transmit HBV. These practices may continue once immigrants and refugees have migrated to a host country.[30]

In healthcare settings, most transmission of HBV occurs from patient to patient, although transmission from patient to provider and provider to patient also occurs. Before widespread vaccination of healthcare workers, the prevalence of HBV infection in this group was three- to fivefold higher than that of the general US population.[43] Currently, an estimated 75% of healthcare workers in the United States are vaccinated.[44]

Illicit injection drug use is another common mode of transmission among adults worldwide and accounts for a substantial fraction of HBV infections in developing and transitional countries, including, or especially in, the countries of the former Soviet Union.[45–47] Drug users often share injection equipment, including needles and syringes as well as other paraphernalia such as cotton and cookers. This sharing, together with the stability of HBV outside the body, provides an easy route for the transmission of the virus. In the United States, approximately 64% of injection drug users have been infected with HBV.[48]

## Global patterns of HBV transmission

In highly endemic countries, the patterns of HBV transmission are very different from those seen in developed, low endemicity countries (Table 22.2). In

**Table 22.2 Differences in the epidemiology of hepatitis B virus infection by endemicity**

| Endemicity | Most common age at infection | Most common modes of transmission |
|---|---|---|
| High | Infancy<br>Early childhood | Perinatal<br>Horizontal<br>Unsafe injections and other medical practices<br>Unscreened blood |
| Intermediate | All age groups | Perinatal<br>Horizontal<br>Unsafe injections and other medical practices<br>Sexual<br>Injection drug use |
| Low | Adolescents<br>Adults | Sexual<br>Injection drug use |

particular, perinatal and early childhood transmission play key roles, both because they are common and because infections acquired early in life frequently lead to chronic infection (see below). Because most (>60–70%) residents of highly endemic countries are exposed to HBV during childhood, transmission during adulthood is relatively less important.

In developed countries with a low endemicity of HBV infection, hepatitis B is known predominantly as a disease of adulthood. Nonetheless, perinatal and childhood infections in these settings, although commonly clinically silent, do occur and may account for 50% or more of all chronic infections.

## Epidemiology in the United States

Before the introduction of hepatitis B vaccination, there were approximately 300 000 new HBV infections annually in the United States, including 24 000 among infants and children.[49] Beginning in the 1980s, the United States adopted a series of measures designed primarily to prevent chronic HBV infection and its long-term complications, cirrhosis and liver cancer. Since 1990, the incidence of hepatitis B has decreased by 90% among children and 63% among adults.[50]

The success of the US hepatitis B immunization program has highlighted the importance of hepatitis B prevention among immigrants. In a 2001–2002 study of US cases among children born after 1990, 8 of 19 cases were among children born outside of the United States. Many of these children were international adoptees.[51]

The decline in incidence of HBV infection in the United States has led to an increase in the proportion of new chronic HBV infections attributable to immigration. From 2000 to 2004, over 900 000 persons immigrated to the United States each year. Taking into account their countries of origin, an estimated 42 000 were chronically infected with hepatitis B (CDC, unpublished data). During the same time period, there were approximately 75 000 new infections annually in the United States, of which 5000 were chronic (CDC, unpublished data and ref. 49). Thus, almost 90% of new cases of chronic hepatitis B in the United States are now attributable to immigration.

## Epidemiologic features of immigrants and refugees in the United States

Most immigrants, refugees, and international adoptees come from countries of high and intermediate HBV endemicity where the prevalence of HBV infection is substantially higher than in the United States (see Fig. 22.1). Surveys among these migrant populations have generally shown HBsAg prevalence rates similar to those of their region of origin (Table 22.3).[30,52–68] However, among their US-born children, even before the widespread use of hepatitis B vaccine, HBsAg prevalence was substantially lower.[69,70]

The prevalence of chronic HBV infection varies by region and country of origin, with the highest prevalence among persons coming from East Asia, Southeast Asia and the Pacific (12–18% in most studies; see Table 22.3). The prevalence of anti-HBc among adults in these populations ranges 63–93%. The prevalences of HBsAg and anti-HBc among children and adolescents shown in Table 22.3, which are generally lower than among adults, do not reflect the impact of hepatitis B immunization, as few of the countries had implemented immunization before 2000.

In a population-based study in a community in Minnesota with a large immigrant population, the prevalence of chronic HBV infection was 2.1% among Asians, 1.9% among Africans, and 0.02% among Caucasians. The overwhelming majority (99%) of Asians were immigrants, mainly from Vietnam, Cambodia, China, and Laos; 91% of Africans were immigrants from Somalia.[71]

Chronic HBV infection is one of the most important causes of hepatocellular carcinoma (HCC).

**Table 22.3 Prevalence of HBV infection among immigrants and refugees in North America**

| Country/ethnic group (study period) | Age group/population | n | HBsAg positive | Anti-HBc positive |
|---|---|---|---|---|
| **Asia/Southeast Asia/Pacific** | | | | |
| Cambodian, Hmong (1984–1989)[30] | <20 | 339 | 14% | 54% |
| | ≥20 | 323 | 24% | 89% |
| Cambodia, Vietnam (1980s)[52] | 11 to 19; Mean: 14 | 74 | 14% | |
| Cambodia, Laos, Vietnam (1982)[53] | ≤20 | 1392 | 5–15% | |
| | >20 | 453 | 9–21% | |
| Cambodia, Laos, Vietnam (1985)[54] | Pregnant women | 338 | 7–13% | |
| Cambodia, Hmong, Laos, Vietnam (1980–1981)[55] | <1 to >50 | 301 | 14% | |
| Hmong, Laos, Vietnam (not given)[56] | | 446 | 18% | |
| Hmong (1994–1995)[57] | <20 | 162 | 16% | 26% |
| | ≥20 | 232 | 17% | 88% |
| Southeast Asia (1979–1980)[58] | <1 to 60 | 14,347 | 12% | 63% |
| Southeast Asia (1999)[59] | <6 to >50; Mean: 23 | 83 | 3% | |
| Southeast Asia (1980–1981)[60] | <20 | 333 | 9% | 54% |
| | ≥20 | 516 | 13% | 76% |
| Vietnam (1994–1996)[61] | 19 to 71; Mean: 34 | 96 | 14% | 73%–93% |
| Vietnam (1991–1999)[62] | <1 to >30 | 743 | 14% | |
| Philippines (1985)[54] | Pregnant women | 59 | 3% | |
| China (1982)[63] | Mean male: 57 Mean female: 49 | 243 | 14% | 75% |
| China (1985)[54] | Pregnant women | 55 | 19% | |
| China, Taiwan, Vietnam (1987)[64] | Median: 26 | 163 | 13% | |
| Tonga (1985)[54] | Pregnant women | 38 | 21% | |
| **Eastern Europe/Former Soviet Union** | | | | |
| Bosnia (1999)[65] | | 544 | 3% | |
| Bulgaria (1979–1991)[66,*] | | 38 | 5% | |
| Czechoslovakia (1979–1991)[66,*] | | 168 | 1% | |
| Hungary (1979–1991)[66,*] | | 94 | 1% | |
| Poland (1979–1991)[66,*] | | 903 | 2% | |
| Romania (1979–1991)[66,*] | | 754 | 4% | |
| Eastern Europe (1999)[59] | <6 to >50; Mean: 23 | 585 | 4% | |
| Former Soviet Union (1990–1993)[67] | <1 to >50 | 496 | 0.4% | 22% |
| Former Soviet Union (1979–1991)[66,*] | | 4504 | 2% | |
| **Africa** | | | | |
| Angola (1979–1991)[66,*] | | 14 | 7% | |
| Ethiopia (1979–1991)[66,*] | | 944 | 9% | |
| Somalia (1999)[65,†] | | 275 | 7% | |
| Sub-Saharan Africa (1999)[59] | <6 to >50; Mean: 23 | 1869 | 9% | |

**Table 22.3** Prevalence of HBV infection among immigrants and refugees in North America—cont'd

| Country/ethnic group (study period) | Age group/population | n | HBsAg positive | Anti-HBc positive |
|---|---|---|---|---|
| **Middle East** | | | | |
| Afghanistan (1979–1991) [66,*] | | 418 | 4% | |
| Iran (1979–1991) [66,*] | | 293 | 2% | |
| Iraq (1999)[65,†] | | 104 | 3% | |
| **Americas/Caribbean** | | | | |
| Cuba (1999)[65,†] | | 5061 | <1% | |
| Caribbean (1984–1985)[68] | 14 to 44; Mean: 26 | 18 | 6% | |
| Central and South America (1984–1985)[68] | 14 to 44; Mean: 26 | 24 | 13% | |
| Central and South America (1987)[64] | Median: 26 | 195 | 1% | |
| Dominican Republic (1984–1985)[68] | 14 to 44; Mean: 26 | 237 | 5% | |
| Haiti (1999)[65,†] | | 387 | 14% | |

* Did not differentiate time periods for each of the specific countries.
† Year of study not specified. Data provided to author by CDC in 1999.

Globally, HCC accounts for an estimated 6% of all cancer deaths, with the highest incidence in countries of high HBV endemicity, especially in Asia and sub-Saharan Africa.[72] In the United States, HCC mortality is highest among persons of Asian race/ethnicity, followed by Blacks and Hispanics.[73] It is lowest among whites. Although whites have the lowest age-adjusted incidence rates, they account for the largest proportion of the US population and thus they account for largest number of HCC cases.

In a study of cases of newly diagnosed liver cancer conducted in California, Hawaii, and Washington using data from a national cancer registry, the Surveillance, Epidemiology and End Results (SEER) program, the incidence of HCC was substantially higher among Asians (from China, Japan, Philippines) compared to whites. HCC incidence was also higher among foreign-born Asians compared to Asians born in the United States.[74]

## Clinical Manifestations

The manifestations of acute HBV infection range from asymptomatic infection to acute hepatitis to fulminant, life-threatening liver failure. If the virus is not cleared during this acute phase, a chronic, lifelong infection ensues.

The clinical presentation and long-term outcome of acute HBV infection are dependent on the immune response elicited by the infection. This immune reaction is responsible both for clearance of the virus and, because HBV is not cytopathic by itself, for the clinical presentation of acute hepatitis. In general, a more vigorous immune response will lead to more severe hepatitis and a lower likelihood of chronic HBV infection.

The characteristic age dependency of clinical outcomes from acute HBV infection[75,76] is probably at least partly due to age-dependent differences in the robustness of this immune response. In general, the younger the person at the time of infection, the less likely the person is to have symptoms of acute hepatitis and the more likely he or she is to develop chronic infection. Children infected at birth through perinatal transmission rarely develop signs of acute hepatitis but almost always (>90%) proceed to chronic infection. Children aged 1–5 years occasionally develop signs of acute hepatitis but have a lower risk (25–50%) of developing chronic infection. Adults more commonly develop acute hepatitis and are even less likely (less than 5–10%) to progress to chronic infection.

Acute hepatitis B presents after an incubation period of 6 weeks to 6 months, generally lasts 1–2 weeks, and is followed by a prolonged convalescent period that may last for weeks or months. Symptoms during the acute phase are clinically indistinguishable from those of other acute viral hepatitides and include fever, jaundice, dark urine, fatigue, and abdominal pain. Malaise and anorexia commonly precede jaundice by a few days. Fulminant hepatitis B occurs in less than 1% of cases and is frequently fatal if liver transplantation is not possible.

Chronic HBV infection is defined as the continued presence of HBsAg 6 months after acute illness or HBsAg in the absence of any clinical or serologic evidence of acute hepatitis B. Risk factors for progression to chronic infection, in addition to infection at a young age, include immunosuppression, and chronic, underlying illness.[77] Chronic hepatitis B is generally asymptomatic, although circulating immune complexes occasionally result in extrahepatic manifestations such as membranous or membranoproliferative glomerulonephritis or polyarteritis nodosa.

## Natural History of Chronic Hepatitis B

The greatest burden of disease attributable to hepatitis B is from the long-term complications of chronic infection, cirrhosis and HCC, which typically occur years to decades after the initial infection. The persistent, low-level hepatitis that occurs in persons with chronic hepatitis B results in a slowly progressive fibrosis of the liver.[78] The rate of progression of this fibrosis varies largely from individual to individual and is greater in those with additional risk factors for fibrosis such as alcohol use or coinfection with hepatitis C virus or hepatitis D virus. The end stage of fibrosis is hepatic cirrhosis. Cirrhosis is initially asymptomatic in many patients or may be associated with mild, non-specific symptoms such as fatigue. However, each year about 5% of persons with HBV-related cirrhosis will develop decompensated cirrhosis, with classic manifestations of cirrhosis such as ascites, esophageal varices, and encephalopathy.[79] Decompensated cirrhosis carries a poor prognosis, with high 5-year mortality rates.

HCC is particularly characteristic of chronic hepatitis B and is believed to be due to the regenerative hyperplasia associated with chronic fibrosis as well as insertional mutagenesis. Because of the latter, hepatitis B-associated HCC may occur in the absence of cirrhosis, which is distinctly different from hepatitis C-associated HCC, which generally occurs only after the development of cirrhosis.

HCC is the fourth leading cause of cancer deaths worldwide, and in countries where hepatitis B is highly endemic, liver cancer is generally the most common cause of cancer death or the second most common cause after lung cancer.[80] In a classic study

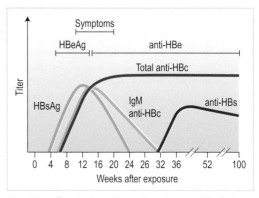

**Fig. 22.2** Serologic pattern of acute hepatitis B virus infection with resolution.

of chronically HBV-infected Taiwanese civil servants, most of whom had probably been infected in infancy or childhood, the incidence of HCC ranged from 2 per 1000 per year among men in their 30s to almost 10 per 1000 among men in their 60s.[81] Using the estimates from this study, 20% of men with chronic hepatitis B could expect to develop liver cancer before the age of 70 years. The incidence of liver cancer among women with chronic hepatitis B is approximately half that among men.[82] In addition to male sex, other risk factors for HCC among persons with chronic hepatitis B include alcohol use, cigarette smoking, and the presence of HBeAg, which is associated with a sixfold increase in risk.[83]

## Serologic Diagnosis

### Acute infection

After infection, the first detectable serologic markers are HBsAg and antibody of the IgM subclass to hepatitis B core antigen (IgM anti-HBc). Both appear within 1–2 months after infection and are present at symptom onset (Fig. 22.2; Table 22.4). IgM anti-HBc is diagnostic of acute HBV infection. There are no commercially available tests for HBcAg; thus, this marker is not included in diagnostic algorithms. HBeAg is also detectable in acute infection and its presence is associated with viral replication and high viral load.

### Resolution of acute infection

During resolution of infection (see Fig. 22.2), IgM anti-HBc is replaced by antibody of the IgG subclass (IgG anti-HBc). Around the same time, there is clearance of HBsAg followed by the appearance of antibody to

**Table 22.4 Interpretation of serologic markers for HBV infection**

| Serologic marker* | | | | |
|---|---|---|---|---|
| HBsAg | Anti-HBs | IgM anti-HBc | Total anti-HBc | Interpretation |
| – | – | – | – | Never infected; also may be seen in persons vaccinated in the remote past |
| + | – | – | – | Acute infection, early incubation, transient post-vaccination antigenemia (may be present for up to 3 weeks after vaccination) |
| + | – | + | + | Acute infection |
| – | – | + | + | Acute infection, resolving |
| – | + | – | + | Past infection, recovered and immune |
| + | – | – | + | Chronic infection |
| – | – | – | + | False positive (i.e. susceptible), past infection, or 'low level' chronic infection |
| – | + | – | – | Immune from vaccination if concentration ≥10 mL$^u$/mL |

\* HBsAg, hepatitis B surface antigen; anti-HBs, antibody to hepatitis B surface antigen; IgM anti-HBc, IgM antibody to hepatitis B core antigen; total anti-HBc, total antibody to hepatitis B core antigen.
\*\* Milli – International units per milliliter.

HBsAg (anti-HBs), a protective, neutralizing antibody whose presence indicates recovery from acute infection and immunity from reinfection. There may be a brief 'window period' between the clearance of HBsAg and the appearance of anti-HBs during which neither HBsAg nor anti-HBs is detectable. IgM anti-HBc may be the only serologic marker present during this time. During resolution, there is also loss of HBeAg and the appearance of anti-HBe. In persons with resolved HBV infection, IgG anti-HBc usually remains detectable throughout life but anti-HBs may become undetectable after many years.

## Chronic infection

In chronic infection, HBsAg persists for > 6 months and anti-HBs does not develop (Fig. 22.3; also see Table 22.4). As with acute infection with resolution, IgM anti-HBc disappears and is replaced by IgG anti-HBc. HBeAg, when present in chronic infection, indicates viral replication, high viral titers, increased infectivity, and higher probability of progression to HCC.[83] Conversely, the absence of HBeAg and presence of anti-HBe correlates with a lower viral load.

## Perinatal infection

Because HBsAg does not cross the placenta, the presence of HBsAg in the serum of an infant is diagnostic

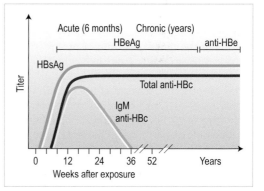

**Fig. 22.3** Serologic pattern of acute hepatitis B virus infection with progression to chronic infection.

of perinatal HBV infection. Both IgG anti-HBc and anti-HBs cross the placenta and thus neither is a useful diagnostic marker of infection in young infants. Passively acquired maternal anti-HBc antibody usually disappears within the first 1–2 years of an infant's life.[84-87]

## Special serologic patterns

**Isolated anti-HBs:** The presence of anti-HBs, with no other serologic marker of infection, is seen after hepatitis B vaccination (see Table 22.4).

**Isolated HBsAg:** The presence of HBsAg alone, with no other markers of infection, may be seen very early in infection, before the development of IgM anti-HBc, or immediately after hepatitis B vaccination (see Table 22.4). This transient presence of HBsAg within the first 3 weeks after vaccination has been documented in infants, adolescents, and adults.[88–90]

**Isolated anti-HBc:** Detection of anti-HBc without any other marker of infection, may occur in three situations: (1) false-positive result; (2) remote, past infection with the loss of detectable levels of anti-HBs; and (3) chronic infection in which HBsAg level is below level of detection of commercial assays. In this latter situation, person-to-person transmission of HBV rarely, if ever, occurs.[91]

**Persistent or recurring IgM anti-HBc:** Certain persons with chronic HBV infection test intermittently or consistently positive for IgM anti-HBc. The appearance of IgM anti-HBc in these individuals may be associated with exacerbations of their underlying hepatitis.

## Molecular Laboratory Methods

HBV DNA can be detected in the serum and tissues of persons with acute and chronic HBV infection through the use of a variety of hybridization and polymerase chain reaction (PCR) assays, some of which are commercially available. Detection of HBV DNA is not used for routine diagnostic purposes but may be useful for following the response to treatment. Subtyping and genotyping are useful only within the context of epidemiologic investigations.

## Prevention of Hepatitis B

### Hepatitis B vaccines

Hepatitis B vaccines are composed of HBsAg adsorbed to an adjuvant of aluminum hydroxide. HBsAg elicits production of anti-HBs, which confers protection from infection. Historically, two types of vaccine, one with plasma-derived HBsAg and the other with recombinant HBsAg, have been used. Recombinant vaccines are now almost exclusively used. Plasma-derived vaccines are manufactured from HBsAg purified from the plasma of persons with chronic HBV infection. Recombinant vaccines are produced through the insertion of the gene for

HBsAg into yeast cells (*Saccharomyces cerevisiae*, or baker's yeast) or, less commonly, mammalian cells (Chinese hamster ovary cells). Hepatitis B vaccines are formulated to contain 5–40 µg of HBsAg protein per dose of vaccine. In the United States, hepatitis B vaccines do not contain the preservative thimerosal, and are sold under the trade names Engerix-B® (GlaxoSmithKline Biologicals) and Recombivax® HB (Merck & Co., Inc.). Plasma-derived and recombinant vaccines are considered equivalent in their immunogenicity and effectiveness.

### Vaccination schedule

Hepatitis B vaccines are typically given as a three-dose series and there are a variety of vaccination schedules. In the most common schedule in the United States, the second and third doses of vaccine are administered 1–2 months and 6–12 months after the first dose (i.e. 0, 1–2, 6–12 month schedule, Table 22.5).[92] For routine infant immunization, the first

**Table 22.5 Hepatitis B vaccination schedule for children, adolescents, and adults**

| Age | Schedule |
|---|---|
| Children (1–10 years)* | 0, 1, 6 months[†]<br>0, 2, 4 months[†]<br>0, 1, 2, 12 months[††¶] |
| Adolescents (11–19 years)* | 0, 1, 6 months[†]<br>0, 1, 4 months[†]<br>0, 2, 4 months[†]<br>0, 12, 24 months[†]<br>0, 4–6 months[§]<br>0, 1, 2, 12 months[††¶] |
| Adults (≥20 years)* | 0, 1, 6 months**[††]<br>0, 1, 4 months**<br>0, 2, 4 months**<br>0, 1, 2, 12 months[¶] ** |

* Children, adolescents, and adults may be vaccinated according to any of the schedules indicated, except as noted. Selection of a schedule should consider the need to optimize compliance with vaccination.
[†] Pediatric/adolescent formulation.
[§] A two-dose schedule of Recombivax-HB adult formulation (10 µg) is licensed for adolescents aged 11–15 years. When scheduled to receive the second dose, adolescents aged > 15 years should be switched to a three-dose series, with doses 2 and 3 consisting of the pediatric formulation administered on an appropriate schedule.
[¶] A four-dose schedule of Engerix B is licensed for all age groups.
** Adult formulation.
[††] Twinrix may be administered to persons aged ≥18 years at 0, 1, and 6 months.

dose of vaccine should be administered within the first 24 hours after birth and the third dose should be given after 6 months of age.[92] Other schedules, including a two-dose series for adolescents 11–15 years old[93] and a four-dose series, are also approved for use in the United States.[92]

## Vaccine dosage

The dosage of vaccine varies by manufacturer and age of vaccine recipient: The typical dosage for infants, children, and adolescents ranges from 5–10 μg, and for adults from 10–20 μg.[92] A dosage of 40 μg is recommended for adults on hemodialysis or who are immunocompromised.[94] Vaccines from different manufacturers may be used interchangeably, provided that each vaccine is given at the dosage recommended by the manufacturer. If a low dosage of vaccine is administered, the dose should be repeated with the appropriate dosage.

## Administration of hepatitis B vaccines

Hepatitis B vaccine should be administered intramuscularly, in the anterior thigh in children < 2 years old and in the deltoid in older children, adolescents, and adults. The needle used for vaccination must be sufficiently long to reach the muscle mass and prevent seepage into the subcutaneous tissue.[92] Administration of vaccine intradermally or in the buttock has been associated with decreased immune response. If a dose of vaccine is missed, the vaccination series should not be restarted; the missed dose should be given as soon as possible, and the vaccination series continued. Hepatitis B vaccines may be given with other vaccines commonly given in infancy or childhood, including vaccines against diphtheria, pertussis, and tetanus (DTP), *Haemophilus influenzae* type B (Hib), poliovirus (IPV or OPV), hepatitis A, measles, varicella, and pneumococcus.

## Vaccination of preterm infants weighing less than 2000 grams

Vaccination of preterm infants (<2000 grams) of HBsAg-negative mothers should be delayed until 1 month of age or hospital discharge.[92]

If the mother of a preterm infant is HBsAg positive or her HBsAg status is unknown, the infant should receive both vaccine and hepatitis B immune globulin (HBIG) within 12 hours of birth, but the vaccine should not count as part of a series. A complete series should then be given beginning at 1–2 months of age.[92]

**Table 22.6** Hepatitis B-containing combination vaccines available on the global market and under development

| Vaccine formulation |
| --- |
| DTaP–hepatitis B |
| DTwP–hepatitis B |
| DTaP–hepatitis B–Hib |
| DTwP–hepatitis B–Hib |
| DTaP–hepatitis B–IPV |
| DTaP–Hib–IPV–hepatitis B |
| DTaP–Hib–IPV–hepatitis B–hepatitis A |
| Hepatitis B–Hib |
| Hepatitis B–hepatitis A |

## Combination vaccines

Various combination vaccines that contain a hepatitis B component are available on the global market or are being evaluated in clinical trials (Table 22.6).[95,96] In the United States, hepatitis B-Hib (Comvax®; Merck & Co., Inc.), DTaP-HepB-IPV (Pediarix®; GlaxoSmithKline Biologicals), and HepA-Hep B (Twinrix®; GlaxoSmithKline Biologicals) are currently licensed for use.[97–99] Only Comvax® and Pediarix® are licensed for use in infants and children < 10 years of age. Combination vaccines cannot be administered to infants < 6 weeks of age because of concerns about the decreased immunogenicity of the pertussis and Hib components of these vaccines. Therefore, only monovalent hepatitis B vaccine may be used for the birth dose.[92]

## Vaccine immunogenicity

A seroprotective immune response to hepatitis B vaccine is defined as development of an anti-HBs concentration of > 10 milli-international units per milliliter (mIU/mL) at 1–2 months after completion of the vaccination series. Hepatitis B vaccines are highly immunogenic, with seroconversion rates of > 95% after a licensed series in healthy infants, children, adolescents, and adults.[100] Concurrent administration of HBIG does not reduce seroconversion rates. Lower rates of seroconversion have been observed among vaccine recipients who are older (>40 years) or immunosuppressed.[101,102] In studies among infants and children infected with the human immunodeficiency virus, only 20 to 78% attained anti-HBs levels > 10 mIU/mL after a full vaccination series.[103-108] Among HIV-infected adults, the seroconversion rates ranged from 7% to 88%, with lower rates among persons with lower CD4 cell counts (<500/mL) and higher HIV viral loads (>1000 copies/mL).[109]

## Pre-vaccination and post-vaccination testing

Pre-vaccination testing for immunity is not indicated before routine vaccination of infants, children, and adolescents.[92] For immigrant and refugee adults resettling to the United States, a relatively high proportion will be HBV infected, and pre-vaccination testing may be cost-effective. If pre-vaccination testing is performed, consideration should be given to administering the first dose of vaccine while awaiting the test results, so as not to miss an opportunity for vaccination. There is no harm in vaccinating people with existing immunity, either natural or vaccine-induced, or with chronic HBV infection.

Because hepatitis B vaccines are highly immunogenic, routine post-vaccination serologic testing to confirm vaccine response is only indicated for the following groups: (1) infants born to HBsAg-positive mothers; (2) healthcare workers; (3) persons with immunosuppressive conditions, including those undergoing long-term hemodialysis; and (4) sex partners of HBsAg-positive persons.[92,94,110] Testing to determine adequate response to vaccine should be performed 1–2 months after administration of the last dose of vaccine. In persons who do not respond to the primary series (i.e. anti-HBs concentration <10 mIU/mL) revaccination with another, three-dose series is recommended. Persons who do not respond to a second series may be chronically infected and should be tested for HBsAg. Those not responding to two full vaccination series are unlikely to respond to further vaccination.

## Vaccine safety

The safety of the hepatitis B vaccine has been demonstrated in a large, prospective clinical trial[111] and in post-licensure safety analyses.[112] Pain at the injec-

tion site (3–29%) and increased temperature > 37.7°C (1–6%) are the most frequently reported side effects.[111] The incidence of anaphylaxis to hepatitis B vaccine is estimated to be 1 case per 1.1 million doses of vaccine distributed.[113] Several case reports of demyelinating or other neurologic disease temporally associated with hepatitis B vaccination have been reported. Although one study found that hepatitis B vaccine was associated with a small proportion of cases of multiple sclerosis among nurses in the United Kingdom,[114] no association has been observed in several other large, controlled studies,[115-118] and comprehensive reviews have favored rejection of a causal association between hepatitis B and multiple sclerosis.[119,120]

## Hepatitis B immune globulin

Hepatitis B immune globulin (HBIG) is prepared from plasma containing high concentrations of anti-HBs and provides short-term (i.e. 3–6 months) protection from infection. Before hepatitis B vaccines were available, HBIG was the only product available for post-exposure prophylaxis. Currently, HBIG, administered in conjunction with hepatitis B vaccine, is recommended for: (1) infants born to HBsAg-positive mothers; (2) unvaccinated sexual contacts of a person known or at high risk to be HBsAg-positive; and (3) unvaccinated persons with a percutaneous exposure (e.g. needle stick injury or injection drug use) to someone who is known or at high risk to be HBsAg positive. HBIG administration alone is the primary means of protection after exposure to HBV in known nonresponders to hepatitis B vaccination.[92]

When used for post-exposure prophylaxis, HBIG should be given as soon as possible after exposure, ideally within 12 hours after birth for infants born to HBsAg-positive mothers or within 24 hours after other exposures. Limited data suggest that the efficacy of HBIG is reduced if administered more than 7 days after a percutaneous exposure or 14 days after a sexual exposure.[92]

## Vaccine efficacy

**Prevention of perinatal infection:** Hepatitis B vaccines are highly efficacious in preventing perinatal transmission of HBV. Perinatal efficacy studies are difficult to compare because they differ by vaccine dosage, number of doses of vaccine, vaccination schedule, and concurrent administration of HBIG.

However, in most studies, the efficacy of hepatitis B vaccine alone and in combination with HBIG in preventing perinatal HBV infection was 90–95%.[100]

Although HBV is found in breast milk, breast-feeding has not been shown to increase the risk of HBV transmission from HBV-infected mothers to their infants.[19] Hepatitis B vaccination at birth, with or without HBIG, eliminates any theoretical risk of virus transmission through breast-feeding.[121,122]

In the United States, the program to prevent peri-natal HBV infection consists of two components: (1) routine vaccination of all infants beginning at birth; and (2) screening of all pregnant women for HBsAg and administration of HBIG along with hepatitis B vaccine to infants born to HBsAg-positive mothers.[92]

The hepatitis B vaccination schedule for newborn infants depends on the HBsAg status of the mother (Table 22.7). For infants born to mothers whose HBsAg status is positive or unknown, the third dose of vaccine should be administered at 6 months of age. For infants born to mothers who are HBsAg negative, the third dose may be administered between 6 and 18 months of age. Additionally, infants born to HBsAg-positive mothers should receive a dose of HBIG within 12 hours after birth.

In less developed countries, where resources are more limited and public health infrastructures weak, screening women for HBsAg and provision of HBIG is not recommended[123] because of the high cost of HBIG (approximately US$100 per dose), the high

**Table 22.7** Hepatitis B vaccination for newborn infants, by maternal hepatitis B surface antigen (HBsAg) status*

| Maternal HBsAg status | Single-antigen vaccine | | Single-antigen and combination vaccine | |
|---|---|---|---|---|
| | Dose | Age | Dose | Age |
| Positive | 1[†] | Birth (≤12 hrs) | 1[†] | Birth (≤12 hrs) |
| | HBIG[§] | Birth (≤12 hrs) | HBIG[§] | Birth (≤12 hrs) |
| | 2 | 1–2 months | 2 | 2 months |
| | 3[¶] | 6 months | 3 | 4 months |
| | | | 4[¶] | 6 months (Pediarix®) or 12–15 months (Comvax®) |
| Unknown** | 1[†] | Birth (≤12 hrs) | 1[†] | Birth (≤12 hrs) |
| | 2 | 1–2 months | 2 | 2 months |
| | 3[¶] | 6 months | 3 | 4 months |
| | | | 4[¶] | 6 months (Pediarix®) or 12–15 months (Comvax®) |
| Negative | 1[†,††] | Birth (before discharge) | 1[†,††] | Birth (before discharge) |
| | 2 | 1–2 months | 2 | 2 months |
| | 3[¶] | 6–18 months | 3 | 4 months |
| | | | 4[¶] | 6 months (Pediarix®) or 12–15 months (Comvax®) |

* For preterm infants weighing < 2000 grams, see 'Pre-term Infants' section in text.[92]
[†] Monovalent hepatitis B vaccine (Recombivax HB® or Engerix-B®) should be used for the birth dose. Combination vaccines (Comvax® and Pediarix®) cannot be administered before 6 weeks of age.
[§] Hepatitis B immune globulin (0.5 mL) administered intramuscularly in a separate site from vaccine.
[¶] The final dose in the vaccine series should not be administered before age 24 weeks (164 days).
** Mothers should have blood drawn and tested for HBsAg as soon as possible after admission for delivery; if the mother is found to be HBsAg positive, the infant should receive HBIG as soon as possible but no later than age 7 days.
[††] On a case-by-case basis and only in rare circumstances, the first dose may be delayed until after hospital discharge for an infant who weighs ≥2000 g and whose mother is HBsAg negative, but only if a physician's order to withhold the birth dose and a copy of the mother's original HBsAg-negative laboratory report are documented in the infant's medical record.

**Table 22.8 Recommendations for postexposure immunprophylaxis of unvaccinated persons**

| Exposure description | Intervention |
|---|---|
| **Discrete exposure to an HBsAg-positive source** | |
| Percutaneous (e.g. bite, needle stick) or mucosal exposure to HBsAg-positive blood or body fluids that contain blood | Hepatitis B vaccine and hepatitis B immune globulin (HBIG) |
| Sexual or needle-sharing contact of an HBsAg-positive person | Hepatitis B vaccine and HBIG |
| Victim of sexual assault/abuse by a perpetrator who is HBsAg-positive | Hepatitis B vaccine and HBIG |
| **Discrete exposure to a source with unknown HBsAg status** | |
| Percutaneous (e.g. bite, needle stick) or mucosal exposure to blood or body fluids that contain blood from a source with unknown HBsAg status | Hepatitis B vaccine |
| Victim of sexual assault/abuse by a perpetrator with unknown HBsAg status | Hepatitis B vaccine |

cost of routine screening for HBsAg, and because vaccination with hepatitis B vaccines alone, without concurrent administration of HBIG, is highly effective.

**Pre-exposure prophylaxis:** Hepatitis B vaccines are highly efficacious in preventing HBV infection when administered before exposure to HBV. Many of the early vaccine efficacy trials were conducted among adults at high risk for HBV infection, including healthcare workers and men who have sex with men. In these placebo-controlled trials, hepatitis B vaccines were found to be > 90% efficacious in preventing chronic HBV infection.[124–127] In studies among infants living in areas of high HBV endemicity who were not infected in the perinatal period, the protective efficacy of hepatitis vaccines against chronic infection was 90–100%.[100]

**Post-exposure prophylaxis:** Recommendations for post-exposure prophylaxis of persons with a discrete identifiable percutaneous, permucosal, or sexual exposure to HBV are given in Table 22.8.

**Long-term protection and the need for booster doses of vaccine:** Hepatitis B vaccines provide long-term protection against HBV infection and, except in immunocompromised persons (see below), booster doses of vaccine are not currently recommended. Follow-up studies published to date, most of which have been conducted 10–15 years after vaccination, have consistently shown continued protection against hepatitis B among participants who had been successfully vaccinated (Table 22.9).[92,94,110,128–143] Although breakthrough infection (i.e. anti-HBc seroconversion) has been observed in a small proportion

of participants in some studies, chronic infection (i.e. development of HBsAg) has occurred rarely and there have been no reports of clinically apparent acute hepatitis B.

Immune memory is thought to play a key role in protection against HBV infection among individuals who have lost detectable levels of anti-HBs years after successful vaccination against the virus.[129,131] Such individuals, upon challenge with HBsAg in the form of a booster dose of hepatitis B vaccine, generally show a rapid, very high increase in anti-HBs levels characteristic of an 'anamnestic response.'[134–136,140,142,143]

In persons with immunosuppressive conditions, vaccine-induced protection may persist only as long as antibody levels remain > 10 mIU/mL. In these persons, anti-HBs levels should be tested annually and booster doses given when antibody levels are <10 mIU/mL.[92]

## Management of Persons with Chronic HBV Infection

Management of chronic HBV infection has advanced substantially in recent years and should, whenever possible, be supervised by a clinician with experience in the care of persons with chronic hepatitis B. The principles of chronic HBV infection management are covered in more detail in a separate chapter (see Ch. 23) and include counseling to reduce further liver damage, regular screening for HCC, and evaluation for possible antiviral therapy.

In addition, anyone with chronic HBV infection should also be counseled on ways to reduce the risk of HBV transmission to sexual and household con-

**Table 22.9 Long-term protection after vaccination against hepatitis B**

| Study location by age group of vaccinees | n | Years of follow-up | Anti-HBs-positive (%) | HBsAg-positive (%) | Anti-HBc-positive (%) |
|---|---|---|---|---|---|
| **Infants[a]** | | | | | |
| Taiwan[b,134] | 78 | 15 | 70 | 1.2 | 33 |
| England[b,135] | 64 | 14 | 50 | 0 | 1.5 |
| Alaska[b,136] | 16 | 12 | 24 | 0 | 0 |
| Alaska[c,136] | 17 | 12 | 24 | 0 | 0 |
| Taiwan[b,137] | 805 | 10 | 85 | 0.4 | 14 |
| Taiwan[b,142] | 118 | 10 | 67 | 0 | 12 |
| Italy[b,143] | 53 | 10 | 68 | 0 | 0 |
| Alaska[b,c, 138] | 350 | 2–10 | 8–45 | 2 | 2 |
| **Older infants and children** | | | | | |
| Hong Kong[139] | 88 | 18 | 61 | 0 | 3 |
| China[141] | 52 | 15 | 50 | 2 | 6 |
| United States[140] | 18 | 13 | 83 | 0 | 0 |
| **Adults** | | | | | |
| United States[d,e,132] | 783 | 15 | 41–77 | 0.2 | 2 |
| Italy[133] | 310 | 10 | 85 | 0 | 0 |

[a] Vaccinated beginning at birth.
[b] Born to HBsAg-positive mothers.
[c] Born to HBsAg-negative mothers.
[d] Includes children and adolescents.
[e] Includes individuals who did not respond to the initial vaccination series (i.e. nonresponders).

tacts. Prevention messages should include using condoms, covering cuts and skin lesions, and refraining from sharing household articles that could become contaminated with blood, including toothbrushes, razors, or personal injection equipment.[92] Injection drug users should not share any drug-using equipment, including needles, syringes, cotton, or cookers. People with chronic HBV infection should not donate blood, plasma, tissue, or semen. When seeking medical or dental care, HBsAg-positive people should inform their healthcare providers of their HBsAg status.

## Hepatitis B Immunization Programs in the United States

The US strategy to eliminate transmission of HBV consists of four components: (1) routine screening of all pregnant women and appropriate postexposure prophylaxis with hepatitis B vaccine and HBIG for infants born to HBsAg-positive mothers; (2) routine vaccination of all infants beginning at birth; (3) vaccination of children and adolescents who were not previously vaccinated; and (4) vaccination of unvaccinated adults at increased risk for infection.[92]

Healthcare settings in which hepatitis B vaccine should be offered to all unvaccinated children and adolescents include primary care clinics, substance abuse treatment facilities, family planning clinics, institutions for the developmentally disabled, correctional facilities, nonresidential daycare facilities for the developmentally disabled, sexually transmitted disease (STD) clinics, and school-based clinics.[92] Adults seeking services in the following settings may be assumed to be at increased risk for HBV infection and should be offered vaccination: STD clinics, HIV testing and counseling facilities, correctional healthcare facilities, drug treatments and prevention facilities, and any healthcare settings serving primarily men who have sex with men.[144]

In the United States, underinsured persons under 20 years of age, including immigrants and refugees, are eligible to receive vaccine free of charge through the Vaccines for Children (VFC) program. VFC is a state-operated federal entitlement program to supply private and public healthcare providers with federally purchased vaccines at no cost to be administered to eligible children and adolescents in accordance with the recommended childhood and adolescent immunization schedule.[145] Eligible children include those who receive Medicaid, lack health insurance, and have American Indian and/or Alaska Native ethnicities. In addition, children who have health insurance that does not cover vaccination are eligible for the VFC program if they are served through a federally qualified healthcare center or rural health clinic.

In 2004, coverage with the hepatitis B vaccination series among children aged 19–35 months was 92%.[146] Among adolescents aged 13–15 years old in 2003, vaccination coverage was 52%.[147] Other than healthcare workers in whom coverage is estimated to be 75%, coverage among adult high-risk groups is low because there are currently no comprehensive, federally funded adult hepatitis B vaccination programs.[44]

For both clinicians and patients, an excellent source of information, including translated health materials, is the Immunization Action Coalition (www.immunize.org). Information on hepatitis may also be found at www.cdc.gov/hepatitis.

## Global Status of Hepatitis B Immunization Programs

Routine infant vaccination is the basis for a global hepatitis B prevention program. An important rationale for this strategy is that the majority (69%) of HBV-related deaths result from infection acquired in the perinatal and early childhood periods. In addition, the Expanded Programme for Immunizations provides an existing healthcare infrastructure for infant vaccination. In countries with strong infant hepatitis B immunization programs, hepatitis immunization can be expanded to include catch-up vaccination of older children and adolescents as well as vaccination of people in high-risk groups. In addition, hepatitis B prevention programs should include a safe blood and safe injection/safe medical practices component, including vaccination of healthcare workers.

Globally, over 150 countries and territories include hepatitis B vaccination in their national infant or childhood immunization programs.[148] Because many of these countries have just recently implemented vaccination and programs are not yet fully functional, global coverage with the vaccination series in 2004 was estimated to be 48% among young children.

Declines in HBV-related morbidity and mortality have already been demonstrated in countries with longstanding routine infant and childhood hepatitis B immunization programs. A decrease in the prevalence of chronic HBV infection among vaccinated children and adolescents has been documented throughout the world, including in China,[141] Hong Kong,[149] Taiwan,[137,142,150] the Gambia,[151] Senegal,[152] Alaska,[132] and Italy.[153] In the United States, which implemented routine hepatitis B vaccination in 1991, the incidence of acute hepatitis B among children and adolescents has decreased by 89%.[50] In Taiwan, where routine infant hepatitis B vaccination commenced in 1984, there has been a 75% decrease in the incidence of HCC among children, as well as a decrease in fulminant hepatitis among infants.[154-156] As countries continue to add hepatitis B vaccine to their immunization programs and as coverage increases in countries that have already implemented vaccination, HBV-related morbidity and mortality will continue to decline.

## Recommendations for Screening and Vaccinating Immigrants and Refugees

### Children (ages 0 to 18 years)

**Screening for chronic HBV infection:** All immigrant and refugee children *from countries of intermediate or high HBV infection prevalence* (see Fig. 22.1) should be screened for HBsAg upon entry to the United States to identify those with chronic HBV infection. This includes children who have completed or received part of the hepatitis B vaccination series. Children with chronic HBV infection (i.e. HBsAg-positive) need not be vaccinated. Because hepatitis B vaccine can cause a transiently positive HBsAg test, testing for HBsAg should not be done within 1 month after receipt of a dose of hepatitis B vaccine.

**Pre-vaccination testing for anti-HBc and anti-HBs:** Pre-vaccination screening for evidence of prior HBV infection using anti-HBc testing is generally not

**Table 22.10 Summary of screening and vaccination recommendations for immigrants and refugees**

*Children (ages 0 to 18 years)*
- All children from countries of intermediate or high endemicity for HBV infection (see Fig. 22.1) should be screened for HBsAg.
- All children who are HBsAg–negative, regardless of country of origin, should receive the hepatitis B vaccination series unless they have written documentation of having already completed the series according to current ACIP recommendations. The initiation of hepatitis B vaccination should not be delayed while awaiting the results of HBsAg testing.
- Post-vaccination testing for anti-HBs is only recommended for the following persons (see 'Pre-vaccination and post-vaccination testing' in text): infants born to HBsAg-positive mothers; persons on hemodialysis; immunocompromised persons; and sex partners of persons with chronic hepatitis B infection.

*Adults (ages 19 years and older)*
- All adults from countries of intermediate or high endemicity for HBV infection (see Fig. 22.1) should be screened for HBsAg.
- For adults in whom vaccination is indicated, pre-vaccination testing for anti-HBc may be cost-effective. Pre-vaccination anti-HBc testing is most likely to be cost-effective in adults from highly endemic countries and may or may not be cost-effective in adults from countries of intermediate endemicity.
- Susceptible adults living in households with a chronically infected household member should receive the hepatitis B vaccination series according to current ACIP recommendations. The initiation of hepatitis B vaccination should not be delayed while awaiting the results of HBsAg or anti-HBc testing.
- For adults, post-vaccination testing for anti-HBs is only recommended for persons on hemodialysis, immunocompromised persons, and sex partners and needle-sharing partners of persons with chronic hepatitis B infection (see 'Pre-vaccination and post-vaccination testing' in text). Post-vaccination testing is also recommended for certain healthcare and public safety workers.

cost-effective among children, including children from countries of high HBV endemicity. Anti-HBs testing should not be used to assess a child's vaccination status. Anti-HBs titers decline after vaccination and children who have been successfully vaccinated may, over time, lose detectable levels of anti-HBs.

**Vaccination:** All immigrant and refugee children, *regardless of country of origin*, should receive the hepatitis B vaccination series in accordance with current Advisory Committee on Immunization Practices (ACIP) recommendations for vaccinating children in the United States (Table 22.10).[92] Children with written, reliable documentation of vaccination before entry into the United States need not be revaccinated. Children without written documentation should be considered unvaccinated and the first dose of vaccine should be administered as soon as possible after arrival in the United States. Vaccine may be administered at the same time as screening for HBsAg is done. Children found to be chronically infected do not need to continue the vaccination series.

Children with written documentation of having received an incomplete series of hepatitis B vaccine should complete the series in the United States.

There is no need to restart the series if more than the recommended time has elapsed between doses of vaccine. However, there is limited evidence that the effectiveness of infant hepatitis B vaccination is reduced when the final dose is administered before the age of 24 weeks. For children with documentation of having received the final dose before age 24 weeks, an additional dose should be given after 24 weeks of age.

Hepatitis B vaccine is not harmful if given to someone who has been previously infected (i.e. has resolved or chronic infection) or previously received a complete or partial hepatitis B vaccination series.

**Post-vaccination testing for antibody response:** Post-vaccination testing for anti-HBs to assess response to the vaccination series is not indicated for most children but may be indicated in specific clinical situations (see 'Pre-vaccination and post-vaccination testing' above).

## Adults (ages 19 years and higher)

**Screening for chronic HBV infection:** All immigrant and refugee adults *from countries of intermediate or* *high HBV infection prevalence* (see Fig. 22.1) should be screened for HBsAg to identify those with chronic HBV infection (see Table 22.10). This includes adults who have received a full or partial hepatitis B vaccination series. Persons with chronic HBV infection (i.e. HBsAg positive) need not be vaccinated.

**Pre-vaccination testing for anti-HBc and anti-HBs:** For adults from countries of intermediate and high endemicity, the prevalence of HBV infection is likely to be high enough to make pre-vaccination screening for immunity (i.e. anti-HBc) cost-effective. As with children, serologic screening for anti-HBs should not be used to assess vaccination status.

**Vaccination:** All susceptible adults > 18 years old living in households with a chronically infected (i.e. HBsAg-positive) person should receive the hepatitis B vaccination series according to current ACIP recommendations.[92] Adults with documentation of a three-dose vaccination series or with serologic evidence of current or prior HBV infection (i.e. anti-HBc positive or HBsAg positive) do not need to be vaccinated. Neither pregnancy nor lactation is considered a contraindication to vaccination. Other adults at increased risk for hepatitis B should receive a licensed hepatitis B vaccination series, in accordance with current ACIP recommendations.

**Post-vaccination testing:** Routine post-vaccination testing for anti-HBs to document a protective serologic response is not indicated for household contacts of persons with chronic HBV infection unless the person being vaccinated is on hemodialysis, is immunocompromised, or is a sex partner of the HBV-infected person (see 'Pre-vaccination and post-vaccination testing' above).

# Conclusion

Hepatitis B virus infection is very common among immigrants. Clinicians should appropriately screen for chronic infection and offer immunization according to current guidelines. Chronically infected immigrants should receive education regarding self-care and means for preventing transmission to others; family members of chronically infected persons should be screened for HBsAg and, if negative, vaccinated against hepatitis B. Chronically HBV-infected immigrants should be referred to a specialist for evaluation, periodic HCC screening, and consideration of antiviral therapy.

# References

1. Bond WW, Favero MS, Petersen NJ, et al. Survival of hepatitis B virus after drying and storage for one week. Lancet 1981; 1:550–551.
2. Bond WW, Favero MS, Petersen NJ, et al. Inactivation of hepatitis B virus by intermediate-to-high-level disinfectant chemicals. J Clin Microbiol 1983; 18:535–538.
3. Magnius LO, Norder H. Subtypes, genotypes and molecular epidemiology of the hepatitis B virus as reflected by sequence variability of the S-gene. Intervirology 1995; 38:24–34.
4. Verschuere V, Yap PS, Fevery J. Is HBV genotyping of clinical relevance? Acta Gastroenterol Belg 2005; 68:233–236.
5. Kramvis A, Kew M, Francois G. Hepatitis B virus genotypes. Vaccine 2005; 23:2409–2423.
6. Goldstein ST, Zhou F, Hadler SC, et al. A mathematical model to estimate global hepatitis B disease burden and vaccination impact. Int J Epidemiol 2005; 34:1329–1339.
7. Hui AY, Hung LC, Tse PC, et al. Transmission of hepatitis B by human bite – confirmation by detection of virus in saliva and full genome sequencing. J Clin Virol 2005; 33:254–256.
8. Tang JR, Hsu HY, Lin HH, et al. Hepatitis B surface antigenemia at birth: a long-term follow-up study. J Pediatr 1998; 133:374–377.
9. Stevens CE, Taylor PE, Tong MJ, et al. Yeast-recombinant hepatitis B vaccine. Efficacy with hepatitis B immune globulin in prevention of perinatal hepatitis B virus transmission. JAMA 1987; 257:2612–2616.
10. Wong VC, Ip HM, Reesink HW, et al. Prevention of the HBsAg carrier state in newborn infants of mothers who are chronic carriers of HBsAg and HBeAg by administration of hepatitis-B vaccine and hepatitis-B immunoglobulin. Double-blind randomised placebo-controlled study. Lancet 1984; 1:921–926.
11. Lee CY, Huang LM, Chang MH, et al. The protective efficacy of recombinant hepatitis B vaccine in newborn infants of hepatitis B e antigen-positive-hepatitis B surface antigen carrier mothers. Pediatr Infect Dis J 1991; 10:299–303.
12. Poovorawan Y, Sanpavat S, Pongpunlert W, et al. Protective efficacy of a recombinant DNA hepatitis B vaccine in neonates of HBe antigen-positive mothers. JAMA 1989; 261:3278–3281.
13. Ding L, Zhang M, Wang Y, et al. A 9-year follow-up study of the immunogenicity and long-term efficacy of plasma-derived hepatitis B vaccine in high-risk Chinese neonates. Clin Infect Dis 1993; 17:475–479.
14. Xu ZY, Liu CB, Francis DP, et al. Prevention of perinatal acquisition of hepatitis B virus carriage using vaccine: preliminary report of a randomized, double-blind placebo-controlled and comparative trial. Pediatrics 1985; 76:713–718.
15. Okada K, Kamiyama I, Inomata M, et al. E antigen and anti-e in the serum of asymptomatic carrier mothers as indicators of positive and negative transmission of hepatitis B virus to their infants. N Engl J Med 1976; 294:746–749.
16. Stevens CE, Beasley RP, Tsui J, et al. Vertical transmission of hepatitis B antigen in Taiwan. N Engl J Med 1975; 292:771–774.
17. Beasley RP, Hwang LY, Stevens CE, et al. Efficacy of hepatitis B immune globulin for prevention of perinatal transmission of the hepatitis B virus carrier state: final report of a randomized double-blind, placebo-controlled trial. Hepatology 1983; 3:135–141.
18. Beasley RP, Trepo C, Stevens CE, et al. The e antigen and vertical transmission of hepatitis B surface antigen. Am J Epidemiol 1977; 105:94–98.
19. Beasley RP, Stevens CE, Shiao IS, et al. Evidence against breast-feeding as a mechanism for vertical transmission of hepatitis B. Lancet 1975; 2:740–741.

20. Martinson FE, Weigle KA, Royce RA, et al. Risk factors for horizontal transmission of hepatitis B virus in a rural district in Ghana. Am J Epidemiol 1998; 147:478–487.

21. Craxi A, Tine F, Vinci M, et al. Transmission of hepatitis B and hepatitis delta viruses in the households of chronic hepatitis B surface antigen carriers: a regression analysis of indicators of risk. Am J Epidemiol 1991; 134:641–650.

22. Ko YC, Li SC, Yen YY, et al. Horizontal transmission of hepatitis B virus from siblings and intramuscular injection among preschool children in a familial cohort. Am J Epidemiol 1991; 133:1015–1023.

23. Whittle H, Inskip H, Bradley AK, et al. The pattern of childhood hepatitis B infection in two Gambian villages. J Infect Dis 1990; 161:1112–1115.

24. Davis LG, Weber DJ, Lemon SM. Horizontal transmission of hepatitis B virus. Lancet 1989; 1:889–893.

25. Marinier E, Barrois V, Larouze B, et al. Lack of perinatal transmission of hepatitis B virus infection in Senegal, West Africa. J Pediatr 1985; 106:843–849.

26. Botha JF, Ritchie MJ, Dusheiko GM, et al. Hepatitis B virus carrier state in black children in Ovamboland: role of perinatal and horizontal infection. Lancet 1984; 1:1210–1212.

27. Beasley RP, Hwang LY. Postnatal infectivity of hepatitis B surface antigen-carrier mothers. J Infect Dis 1983; 147:185–190.

28. Beasley RP, Hwang LY, Lin CC, et al. Incidence of hepatitis B virus infection in preschool children in Taiwan. J Infect Dis 1982; 146:198–204.

29. Mahoney FJ, Lawrence M, Scott C, et al. Continuing risk for hepatitis B virus transmission among Southeast Asian infants in Louisiana. Pediatrics 1995; 96:1113–1116.

30. Hurie MB, Mast EE, Davis JP. Horizontal transmission of hepatitis B virus infection to United States-born children of Hmong refugees. Pediatrics 1992; 89:269–273.

31. Franks AL, Berg CJ, Kane MA, et al. Hepatitis B virus infection among children born in the United States to Southeast Asian refugees. N Engl J Med 1989; 321:1301–1305.

32. Friede A, Harris JR, Kobayashi JM, et al. Transmission of hepatitis B virus from adopted Asian children to their American families. Am J Public Health 1988; 78:26–29.

33. Van Damme P, Cramm M, Van der Auwera JC, et al. Horizontal transmission of hepatitis B virus. Lancet 1995; 345:27–29.

34. Sokal EM, Van Collie O, Buts JP. Horizontal transmission of hepatitis B from children to adoptive parents. Arch Dis Child 1995; 72:191.

35. Alter MJ, Margolis HS. The emergence of hepatitis B as a sexually transmitted disease. Med Clin North Am 1990; 74:1529–1541.

36. MacKellar DA, Valleroy LA, Secura GM, et al. Two decades after vaccine license: hepatitis B immunization and infection among young men who have sex with men. Am J Public Health 2001; 91:965–971.

37. Quddus A, Luby SP, Jamal Z, et al. Prevalence of hepatitis B among Afghan refugees living in Balochistan, Pakistan. Int J Infect Dis 2006; 10(3):242–247.

38. Hauri AM, Armstrong GL, Hutin YJ. The global burden of disease attributable to contaminated injections given in healthcare settings. Int J STD AIDS 2004; 15:7–16.

39. Henderson DK. Healthcare behaviors and risky business: first, do no harm. Infect Control Hosp Epidemiol 2005; 26:739–742.

40. Tugwell BD, Patel PR, Williams IT, et al. Transmission of hepatitis C virus to several organ and tissue recipients from an antibody-negative donor. Ann Intern Med 2005; 143:648–654.

41. Williams IT, Perz JF, Bell BP. Viral hepatitis transmission in ambulatory healthcare settings. Clin Infect Dis 2004; 38:1592–1598.

42. Centers for Disease Control and Prevention. Transmission of hepatitis B and C viruses in outpatient settings – New York, Oklahoma, and Nebraska, 2000–2002. MMWR 2003; 52:901–906.

43. Shapiro CN. Occupational risk of infection with hepatitis B and hepatitis C virus. Surg Clin North Am 1995; 75:1047–1056.

44. Simard EP, Miller JT, George PA, et al. Hepatitis B vaccination coverage levels among healthcare workers in the United States, 2002–2003. Abstracts of the Infectious Diseases Society of America, 43rd Annual Meeting, San Francisco, 2005.

45. Atlani L, Carael M, Brunet JB, et al. Social change and HIV in the former USSR: the making of a new epidemic. Soc Sci Med 2000; 50:1547–1556.

46. Abdala N, Carney JM, Durante AJ, et al. Estimating the prevalence of syringe-borne and sexually transmitted diseases among injection drug users in St Petersburg, Russia. Int J STD AIDS 2003; 14:697–703.

47. Isralowitz RE, Straussner SL, Rosenblum A. Drug abuse, risks of infectious diseases and service utilization among former Soviet Union immigrants. A view from New York City. J Ethn Subst Abuse 2006; 5:91–96.

48. Murrill CS, Weeks H, Castrucci BC, et al. Age-specific seroprevalence of HIV, hepatitis B virus, and hepatitis C virus infection among injection drug users admitted to drug treatment in 6 US cities. Am J Public Health 2002; 92:385–387.

49. Coleman PJ, McQuillan GM, Moyer LA, et al. Incidence of hepatitis B virus infection in the United States, 1976–1994: estimates from the National Health and Nutrition Examination Surveys. J Infect Dis 1998; 178:954–959.

50. Shepard CW, Finelli L, Fiore AE, et al. Epidemiology of hepatitis B and hepatitis B virus infection in United States children. Pediatr Infect Dis J 2005; 24:755–760.

51. Centers for Disease Control and Prevention. Acute hepatitis B among children and adolescents – United States, 1990–2002. MMWR 2004; 53:1015–1018.

52. Fitzpatrick S, Johnson J, Shragg P, et al. Healthcare needs of Indochinese refugee teenagers. Pediatrics 1987; 79:118–124.

53. McGlynn KA, Lustbader ED, London WT. Immune responses to hepatitis B virus and tuberculosis infections in Southeast Asian refugees. Am J Epidemiol 1985; 122:1032–1036.

54. Klontz KC. A program to provide hepatitis B immunoprophylaxis to infants born to HBsAg-positive Asian and Pacific Island women. West J Med 1987; 146:195–199.

55. Catanzaro A, Moser RJ. Health status of refugees from Vietnam, Laos, and Cambodia. JAMA 1982; 247:1303–1308.

56. Hill LL, Hovell M, Benenson AS. Prevention of hepatitis B transmission in Indo-Chinese refugees with active and passive immunization. Am J Prev Med 1991; 7:29–32.

57. Gjerdingen DK, Lor V. Hepatitis B status of Hmong patients. J Am Board Fam Pract 1997; 10:322–328.

58. Chaudhary RK, Nicholls ES, Kennedy DA. Prevalence of hepatitis B markers in Indochinese refugees. Can Med Assoc J 1981; 125:1243–1246.

59. Lifson AR, Thai D, O'Fallon A, et al. Prevalence of tuberculosis, hepatitis B virus, and intestinal parasitic infections among refugees to Minnesota. Pub Health Rep 2002; 117:69–77.

60. Goodman RA, Sikes RK. Hepatitis B markers in Southeast Asian refugees. JAMA 1984; 251:2086.

61. Nelson KR, Bui H, Samet JH. Screening in special populations: a 'case study' of recent Vietnamese immigrants. Am J Med 1997; 102:435–440.

62. Patel PA, Voigt MD. Prevalence and interaction of hepatitis B and latent tuberculosis in Vietnamese immigrants to the United States. Am J Gastroenterol 2002; 97:1198–1203.

63. Tong MJ, Yu M, Co R, et al. Hepatitis B virus markers in the foreign-born Chinese population of Los Angeles, California. J Infect Dis 1984; 149:475.

64. Arevalo JA, Arevalo M. Prevalence of hepatitis B in an indigent, multi-ethnic community clinic prenatal population. J Fam Pract 1989; 29:615–619.

65. Walker PF, Jaranson J. Refugee and immigrant healthcare. Med Clin North Am 1999; 83:1103–1120, viii.

66. Centers for Disease Control and Prevention. Screening for hepatitis B virus infection among refugees arriving in the United States, 1979–1991. MMWR 1991; 40:784–786.
67. Hurie MB, Gennis MA, Hernandez LV, et al. Prevalence of hepatitis B markers and measles, mumps, and rubella antibodies among Jewish refugees from the former Soviet Union. JAMA 1995; 273:954–956.
68. Friedman SM, DeSilva LP, Fox HE, et al. Hepatitis B screening in a New York City obstetrics service. Am J Public Health 1988; 78:308–310.
69. Stevens CE, Toy PT, Tong MJ, et al. Perinatal hepatitis B virus transmission in the United States. Prevention by passive–active immunization. JAMA 1985; 253:1740–1745.
70. Tong MJ, Hwang S. Hepatitis B virus infection in Asian Americans. Gastroenterol Clin North Am 1994; 23:523–536.
71. Kim WR, Benson JT, Therneau TM, et al. Changing epidemiology of hepatitis B in a US community. Hepatology 2004; 39:811–816.
72. El Serag HB. Hepatocellular carcinoma: an epidemiologic view. J Clin Gastroenterol 2002; 35:S72–S78.
73. El Serag HB. Epidemiology of hepatocellular carcinoma. Clin Liver Dis 2001; 5:87–107, vi.
74. Rosenblatt KA, Weiss NS, Schwartz SM. Liver cancer in Asian migrants to the United States and their descendants. Cancer Causes Control 1996; 7:345–350.
75. McMahon BJ, Alward WL, Hall DB, et al. Acute hepatitis B virus infection: relation of age to the clinical expression of disease and subsequent development of the carrier state. J Infect Dis 1985; 151:599–603.
76. Edmunds WJ, Medley GF, Nokes DJ, et al. The influence of age on the development of the hepatitis B carrier state. Proc R Soc Lond B Biol Sci 1993; 253:197–201.
77. Hyams KC. Risks of chronicity following acute hepatitis B virus infection: a review. Clin Infect Dis 1995; 20:992–1000.
78. Lok AS, Heathcote EJ, Hoofnagle JH. Management of hepatitis B: 2000 – summary of a workshop. Gastroenterology 2001; 120:1828–1853.
79. Fattovich G, Giustina G, Schalm SW, et al. Occurrence of hepatocellular carcinoma and decompensation in Western European patients with cirrhosis type B. The EUROHEP Study Group on Hepatitis B Virus and Cirrhosis. Hepatology 1995; 21:77–82.
80. Pisani P, Parkin DM, Bray F, et al. Estimates of the worldwide mortality from 25 cancers in 1990. Int J Cancer 1999; 83:18–29.
81. Beasley RP. Hepatitis B virus – the major etiology of hepatocellular carcinoma. Cancer 1988; 61:1942–1956.
82. Kirk GD, Lesi OA, Mendy M, et al. The Gambia Liver Cancer Study: infection with hepatitis B and C and the risk of hepatocellular carcinoma in West Africa. Hepatology 2004; 39:211–219.
83. Yang HI, Lu SN, Liaw YF, et al. Hepatitis B e antigen and the risk of hepatocellular carcinoma. N Engl J Med 2002; 347:168–174.
84. Stevens CE, Taylor PE, Tong MJ, et al. Prevention of perinatal hepatitis B virus infection with hepatitis B immune globulin and hepatitis B vaccine. In: Zuckerman AJ (ed). Viral hepatitis and liver disease. New York: Wiley; 1988:982–988.
85. Poovorawan Y, Sanpavat S, Chumdermpadetsuk S, et al. Long-term hepatitis B vaccine in infants born to hepatitis B e antigen positive mothers. Arch Dis Child Fetal Neonatal Ed 1997; 77:F47–F51.
86. Lee PI, Lee CY, Huang LM, et al. Long-term efficacy of recombinant hepatitis B vaccine and risk of natural infection in infants born to mothers with hepatitis B e antigen. J Pediatr 1995; 126:716–721.
87. Lo KJ, Lee SD, Tsai YT, et al. Long-term immunogenicity and efficacy of hepatitis B vaccine in infants born to HBeAg-positive HBsAg-carrier mothers. Hepatology 1988; 8:1647–1650.
88. Lunn ER, Hoggarth BJ, Cook WJ. Prolonged hepatitis B surface antigenemia after vaccination. Pediatrics 2000; 105:E81
89. Weintraub Z, Khamaysi N, Elena H, et al. Transient surface antigenemia in newborn infants vaccinated with Engerix B: occurrence and duration. Pediatr Infect Dis J 1994; 13:931–933.
90. Bernstein SR, Krieger P, Puppala BL, et al. Incidence and duration of hepatitis B surface antigenemia after neonatal hepatitis B immunization. J Pediatr 1994; 125:621–622.
91. Silva AE, McMahon BJ, Parkinson AJ, et al. Hepatitis B virus DNA in persons with isolated antibody to hepatitis B core antigen who subsequently received hepatitis B vaccine. Clin Infect Dis 1998; 26:895–897.
92. Mast EE, Margolis HS, Fiore AE, et al. A comprehensive immunization strategy to eliminate transmission of hepatitis B virus infection in the United States: recommendations of the Advisory Committee on Immunization Practices (ACIP) part 1: immunization of infants, children, and adolescents. MMWR Recomm Rep 2005; 54:1–31.
93. Centers for Disease Control and Prevention. Notice to readers: Alternate two-dose hepatitis B vaccination schedule for adolescents aged 11–15 years. MMWR 2000; 49:261.
94. Centers for Disease Control and Prevention. Recommendations for preventing transmission of infections among chronic hemodialysis patients. MMWR 2001; 50:1–43.
95. Greenberg DP. Considerations for hepatitis B as part of a combination vaccine. Pediatr Infect Dis J 2001; 20:S34–S39.
96. Decker MD. Principles of pediatric combination vaccines and practical issues related to use in clinical practice. Pediatr Infect Dis J 2001; 20:S10–S18.
97. Centers for Disease Control and Prevention. Combination vaccines for childhood immunization. MMWR Recomm Rep 1999; 48:1–14.
98. Centers for Disease Control and Prevention. FDA approval for infants of a *Haemophilus influenzae* type b conjugate and hepatitis B (recombinant) combined vaccine. MMWR 1997; 46:107–109.
99. Centers for Disease Control and Prevention. FDA licensure of diphtheria and tetanus toxoids and acellular pertussis adsorbed, hepatitis B (recombinant), and poliovirus vaccine combined, (PEDIARIX) for use in infants. MMWR 2003; 52:203–204.
100. Andre FE, Zuckerman AJ. Review: protective efficacy of hepatitis B vaccines in neonates. J Med Virol 1994; 44:144–151.
101. Averhoff F, Mahoney F, Coleman P, et al. Immunogenicity of hepatitis B vaccines. Implications for persons at occupational risk of hepatitis B virus infection. Am J Prev Med 1998; 15:1–8.
102. Roome AJ, Walsh SJ, Carter ML, et al. Hepatitis B vaccine responsiveness in Connecticut public safety personnel. JAMA 1993; 270:2931–2934.
103. Arrazola MP, de Juanes JR, Ramos JT, et al. Hepatitis B vaccination in infants of mothers infected with human immunodeficiency virus. J Med Virol 1995; 45:339–341.
104. Rutstein RM, Rudy B, Codispoti C, et al. Response to hepatitis B immunization by infants exposed to HIV. AIDS 1994; 8:1281–1284.
105. Zuccotti GV, Riva E, Flumine P, et al. Hepatitis B vaccination in infants of mothers infected with human immunodeficiency virus. J Pediatr 1994; 125:70–72.
106. Diamant EP, Schechter C, Hodes DS, et al. Immunogenicity of hepatitis B vaccine in human immunodeficiency virus-infected children. Pediatr Infect Dis J 1993; 12:877–878.
107. Zuin G, Principi N, Tornaghi R, et al. Impaired response to hepatitis B vaccine in HIV infected children. Vaccine 1992; 10:857–860.
108. Watanaveeradej V, Samakoses R, Kerdpanich A, et al. Antibody response to hepatitis B vaccine in infants of HIV-positive mothers. Int J Inf Dis 2002; 6:240–241.

109. Laurence JC. Hepatitis A and B immunizations of individuals infected with human immunodeficiency virus. Am J Med 2005; 118(Suppl 10A):75S–83S.

110. Centers for Disease Control and Prevention. Updated US Public Health Service guidelines for the management of occupational exposures to HBV, HCV, and HIV and recommendations for postexposure prophylaxis. MMWR 2001; 50:1–42.

111. McMahon BJ, Helminiak C, Wainwright RB, et al. Frequency of adverse reactions to hepatitis B vaccine in 43 618 persons. Am J Med 1992; 92:254–256.

112. Niu MT, Rhodes P, Salive M, et al. Comparative safety of two recombinant hepatitis B vaccines in children: data from the Vaccine Adverse Events Reporting System (VAERS) and Vaccine Safety Datalink (VSD). J Clin Epidemiol 1998; 51:503–510.

113. Bohlke K, Davis RL, Marcy SM, et al. Risk of anaphylaxis after vaccination of children and adolescents. Pediatrics 2003; 112:815–820.

114. Hernan MA, Jick SS, Olek MJ, et al. Recombinant hepatitis B vaccine and the risk of multiple sclerosis: a prospective study. Neurology 2004; 63:838–842.

115. Ascherio A, Zhang SM, Hernan MA, et al. Hepatitis B vaccination and the risk of multiple sclerosis. N Engl J Med 2001; 344:327–332.

116. Confavreux C, Suissa S, Saddier P, et al. Vaccinations and the risk of relapse in multiple sclerosis. Vaccines in Multiple Sclerosis Study Group. N Engl J Med 2001; 344:319–326.

117. Sadovnick AD, Scheifele DW. School-based hepatitis B vaccination programme and adolescent multiple sclerosis. Lancet 2000; 355:549–550.

118. Zipp F, Weil JG, Einhaupl KM. No increase in demyelinating diseases after hepatitis B vaccination. Nature Med 1999; 5:964–965.

119. Stratton K, Almario DA, McCormick MC, eds. Hepatitis B vaccine and central nervous system demyelinating disorders. Washington, DC: Institute of Medicine; 2002.

120. Halsey NA, Duclos P, Van Damme P, et al. Hepatitis B vaccine and central nervous system demyelinating diseases. Viral Hepatitis Prevention Board. Pediatr Infect Dis J 1999; 18:23–24.

121. Hill JB, Sheffield JS, Kim MJ, et al. Risk of hepatitis B transmission in breast-fed infants of chronic hepatitis B carriers. Obstet Gynecol 2002; 99:1049–1052.

122. Wang JS, Zhu QR, Wang XH. Breastfeeding does not pose any additional risk of immunoprophylaxis failure on infants of HBV carrier mothers. Int J Clin Pract 2003; 57:100–102.

123. World Health Organization. WHO position on the use of hepatitis B vaccines. Weekly Epidemiological Record 2004; 79:253–264.

124. Szmuness W, Stevens CE, Harley EJ, et al. Hepatitis B vaccine: demonstration of efficacy in a controlled clinical trial in a high-risk population in the United States. N Engl J Med 1980; 303:833–841.

125. Francis DP, Hadler SC, Thompson SE, et al. The prevention of hepatitis B with vaccine. Report of the centers for disease control multi-center efficacy trial among homosexual men. Ann Intern Med 1982; 97:362–366.

126. Coutinho RA, Lelie N, Albrecht-Van Lent P, et al. Efficacy of a heat inactivated hepatitis B vaccine in male homosexuals: outcome of a placebo controlled double blind trial. Br Med J (Clin Res Ed) 1983; 286:1305–1308.

127. Crosnier J, Jungers P, Courouce AM, et al. Randomised placebo-controlled trial of hepatitis B surface antigen vaccine in French haemodialysis units: II, Haemodialysis patients. Lancet 1981; 1:797–800.

128. Fitzsimons D, Francois G, Hall A, et al. Long-term efficacy of hepatitis B vaccine, booster policy, and impact of hepatitis B virus mutants. Vaccine 2005; 23:4158–4166.

129. Banatvala J, Van Damme P, Oehen S. Lifelong protection against hepatitis B: the role of vaccine immunogenicity in immune memory. Vaccine 2000; 19:877–885.

130. European Consensus Group on Hepatitis B Immunity. Are booster immunisations needed for lifelong hepatitis B immunity? European Consensus Group on Hepatitis B Immunity. Lancet 2000; 355:561–565.

131. West DJ, Calandra GB. Vaccine induced immunologic memory for hepatitis B surface antigen: implications for policy on booster vaccination. Vaccine 1996; 14:1019–1027.

132. McMahon BJ, Bruden DL, Petersen KM, et al. Antibody levels and protection after hepatitis B vaccination: results of a 15-year follow-up. Ann Intern Med 2005; 142:333–341.

133. Floreani A, Baldo V, Cristofoletti M, et al. Long-term persistence of anti-HBs after vaccination against HBV: an 18-year experience in healthcare workers. Vaccine 2004; 22:607–610.

134. Lu CY, Chiang BL, Chi WK, et al. Waning immunity to plasma-derived hepatitis B vaccine and the need for boosters 15 years after neonatal vaccination. Hepatology 2004; 40:1415–1420.

135. Boxall EH, Sira A, El Shuhkri N, et al. Long-term persistence of immunity to hepatitis B after vaccination during infancy in a country where endemicity is low. J Infect Dis 2004; 190:1264–1269.

136. Petersen KM, Bulkow LR, McMahon BJ, et al. Duration of hepatitis B immunity in low-risk children receiving hepatitis B vaccinations from birth. Pediatr Infect Dis J 2004; 23:650–655.

137. Wu JS, Hwang LY, Goodman KJ, et al. Hepatitis B vaccination in high-risk infants: 10-year follow-up. J Infect Dis 1999; 179:1319–1325.

138. Dentinger CM, McMahon BJ, Butler JC, et al. Persistence of antibody to hepatitis B and protection from disease among Alaska natives immunized at birth. Pediatr Infect Dis J 2005; 24:786–792.

139. Yuen MF, Lim WL, Chan AO, et al. 18-year follow-up study of a prospective randomized trial of hepatitis B vaccinations without booster doses in children. Clin GastroenterolHepatol 2004; 2:941–945.

140. Watson B, West DJ, Chilkatowsky A, et al. Persistence of immunologic memory for 13 years in recipients of a recombinant hepatitis B vaccine. Vaccine 2001; 19:3164–3168.

141. Liao SS, Li RC, Li H, et al. Long-term efficacy of plasma-derived hepatitis B vaccine: a 15-year follow-up study among Chinese children. Vaccine 1999; 17:2661–2666.

142. Huang LM, Chiang BL, Lee CY, et al. Long-term response to hepatitis B vaccination and response to booster in children born to mothers with hepatitis B e antigen. Hepatology 1999; 29:954–959.

143. Resti M, Azzari C, Mannelli F, et al. Ten-year follow-up study of neonatal hepatitis B immunization: are booster injections indicated? Vaccine 1997; 15:1338–1340.

144. Advisory Committee on Immunization Practices (ACIP). A comprehensive immunization strategy to eliminate transmission of hepatitis B virus infection in the United States: recommendations of the Advisory Committee on Immunization Practices (ACIP) part 2: immunization of Adults. MMWR Recomm Rep 2006; (in press).

145. Santoli JM, Rodewald LE, Maes EF, et al. Vaccines for Children program, United States, 1997. Pediatrics 1999; 104: e15.

146. Barker L, Luman E, Zhao Z, et al. National, state, and urban area vaccination coverage levels among children aged 19–35 months – United States, 2001. MMWR 2002; 51:664–666.

147. Stokley S, McCauley M, Fitzgerald MA, et al. Adolescent vaccination coverage levels: results from the 1997–2003 National Health Interview Survey. 2006. 40th National Immunization Conference, March 6–9,2006, Atlanta, GA.

148. Centers for Disease Control and Prevention. Global progress toward universal childhood hepatitis B vaccination, 2003. MMWR 2003; 52:868–870.

149. Yuen MF, Lim WL, Cheng CC, et al. Twelve-year follow-up of a prospective randomized trial of hepatitis B recombinant DNA yeast vaccine versus plasma-derived vaccine without booster doses in children. Hepatology 1999; 29:924–927.

150. Lin HH, Wang LY, Hu CT, et al. Decline of hepatitis B carrier rate in vaccinated and unvaccinated subjects: sixteen

years after newborn vaccination program in Taiwan. J Med Virol 2003; 69:471–474.

151. Whittle H, Jaffar S, Wansbrough M, et al. Observational study of vaccine efficacy 14 years after trial of hepatitis B vaccination in Gambian children. Br Med J 2002; 325:569.

152. Coursaget P, Leboulleux D, Soumare M, et al. Twelve-year follow-up study of hepatitis B immunization of Senegalese infants. J Hepatol 1994; 21:250–254.

153. Mele A, Tancredi F, Romano L, et al. Effectiveness of hepatitis B vaccination in babies born to hepatitis B surface antigen-positive mothers in Italy. J Infect Dis 2001; 184:905–908.

154. Chang MH, Chen CJ, Lai MS, et al. Universal hepatitis B vaccination in Taiwan and the incidence of hepatocellular carcinoma in children. N Engl J Med 1997; 336:1855–1859.

155. Kao JH, Hsu HM, Shau WY, et al. Universal hepatitis B vaccination and the decreased mortality from fulminant hepatitis in infants in Taiwan. J Pediatr 2001; 139:349–352.

156. Kao JH, Chen DS. Global control of hepatitis B virus infection. Lancet Infect Dis 2002; 2:395–403.

# CHAPTER 23

# Management of Chronic Hepatitis B

Paola Ricci

## Introduction

The understanding of hepatitis B, one of the most challenging conditions affecting the liver, has greatly expanded over the past 20 years. During this time the use of improved laboratory diagnostic methods has helped increase our knowledge of its natural history. New, excellent drugs have become available in the past 3 years. However, management of hepatitis B remains challenging for the physician at both diagnostic and therapeutic levels because its clinical issues are complex. One general, important concept regarding chronic hepatitis B is that it may be 'suppressed' rather than 'cured' by the available treatments. Unfortunately, current treatment guidelines help only partially with decision-making. Very often, the decision-making process of the hepatologist is one of a very careful individualized patient approach that goes beyond the current available guidelines. The primary care physician has a central role in identifying the patients who may need screening, biochemical and clinical monitoring, and referral to a specialist for consideration of treatment.

## Natural History of Chronic Infection

As stated in the previous chapter by Drs. Armstrong and Goldstein, risk of progression from acute to chronic infection differs according to the age of the subject at the time of infection: less than 1% in immunocompetent adults who contract hepatitis B virus (HBV) as opposed to 90% in newborns and 20% in childhood.[1,2,3]

Chronic HBV infection develops because the immune response fails to clear or completely control virus replication. Infected hepatocytes are persistently attacked by the immune response, resulting in mild to severe liver disease. Chronic infection is linked to increased rates of fibrosis, cirrhosis, and hepatocellular carcinoma (HCC).

Once chronic HBV infection is established, its course is considered to consist of 5 phases (Table 23.1):

- Immune tolerance;
- Immune clearance ('HBeAg-positive chronic hepatitis');
- Inactive carrier;
- Reactivation ('HBeAg-negative chronic hepatitis'); and
- Resolved hepatitis B.

It is important to point out that:

- Not all patients go through every phase; and
- The HBeAg status of a patient only helps to determine the 'phase' of chronic hepatitis B infection, not the 'replicative' state of the hepatitis B virus.

Both HBeAg-positive and HBeAg-negative patients may replicate HBV, the former in higher degree than the latter. Most HBeAg-negative patients have detectable HBV DNA serum levels and may fluctuate above and below detectable thresholds (current available HBV DNA assays may detect <50 IU/mL, that is, <250 copies/mL). HBeAg-negative patients cannot produce HBeAg because of a viral mutation in the pre-core or core-promoter regions of the pre-genomic RNA.

**Table 23.1  Natural history of chronic hepatitis B**

| Disease phase | Duration | HBsAg status | HBeAg status | HBV-DNA level (IU/mL) by PCR | ALT level | Liver histology |
|---|---|---|---|---|---|---|
| Immune tolerance | 1–4 decades in patients with perinatal infection; short lived or absent in childhood-/adult-acquired infection | HBsAg positive | HBeAg positive | High (>20000) | Normal | Normal or minimal inflammation and/or fibrosis |
| Immune clearance | Duration and severity of flares correlate with risk of cirrhosis and HCC | HBsAg positive | HBeAg positive followed by HBeAg-negative (so-called 'HbeAg seroconversion') | High (>20000) or fluctuating | Abnormal, flares of transaminases | Chronic inflammation |
| Inactive HBsAg carrier state | Indefinite | HBsAg positive | HBeAg negative, HBeAb positive | Low (<2000) or undetectable | Normal | Normal or minimal inflammation; may have advanced fibrosis or cirrhosis |
| Reactivation of HBV replication | | HBsAg positive | HBeAg negative, HBeAb positive | Detectable on serial testing | Abnormal,'fluctuating' | Chronic inflammation |
| Resolved | | HBsAg negative ± HBsAb positive | HBeAg negative, HBeAb positive | Undetectable | Normal | Normal or minimal inflammation, stage of fibrosis variable and depends on the activity of disease before resolution |

Modified and Adapted from: McMahon BJ. Clin Gastro and Hepatology. October 2005 Sem Liver Dis 2004; 24(suppl 1):17–21.
ALT, alanine aminotransferase; HBeAg, hepatitis B early antigen; HBsAg, hepatitis B surface antigen; PCR, polymerase chain reaction.
*4–20% of inactive carriers have one or more reversions back to HBeAg-positive status.

**Table 23.2 Commercially available tests for HBV DNA quantification**

| Test | Units | Conversion |
|---|---|---|
| Liquid hybridization (Abbott) | Pg/mL | 1 pg HBV DNA = 383 000 copies/mL (≈3 × $10^5$ copies) |
| Hybrid capture (Digene) | Pg/mL | 1 pg HBV DNA = 383 000 copies/mL |
| Branched DNA (Bayer) | Copies/mL | |
| PCR-amplicor (Roche) | Copies/mL | |
| TaqMan PCR | IU/mL | 1 IU = 5.1 copies ($10^5$ copies = 20 000 IU) |

## Molecular testing in assessment and management of hepatitis B

This testing consists of two groups of assays:

1. HBV DNA quantification assays which measure the amount of HBV DNA in peripheral blood, which reflects the level of HBV replication in the liver (Table 23.2).
2. Assays which identify sequences or motifs of clinical or pathophysiological importance in the HBV genome.

### HBV DNA quantification

Hybridization and/or signal amplification methods have been used to quantify HBV DNA for many years, and are of lower sensitivity. The development of more sensitive HBV quantification molecular assays (polymerase chain reaction [PCR]) revealed that HBeAg-negative patients may replicate HBV. In addition, a more recent technique based on 'real time' PCR technology has allowed accurate quantification over a broad range of HBV DNA levels. This in turn has made it possible to accurately identify HBV DNA values in the untreated patient, as well as to better monitor the antiviral efficacy of highly potent antiviral drugs. The current real-time PCR assays, however, raise some technical issues: for very high DNA levels above 7–8 logs the range of quantification may be insufficient, different genotypes may not be equally quantified, and HBV DNA levels lack standardized reporting units. Besides technical issues specific to any particular new technology,

there are issues related in general to the use of HBV DNA assays in the assessment of HBV disease and monitoring of therapy. For example, precise thresholds to guide medical decisions need to be established; different therapies are associated with different endpoints in HBeAg-positive and -negative patients; response to therapy can be assessed by different means; 'undetectable HBV DNA' is difficult to standardize in clinical practice; and assays must be sensitive enough to detect a virologic breakthrough early enough to allow the decision to modify therapy, i.e. before the patient experiences an ALT flare. Once these issues are resolved, real-time PCR technology should become the standard technology for monitoring hepatitis B therapy.

### HBV DNA sequence analysis

Various assays can be used to determine genotype, assess pre-core and core mutations, and to determine resistance mutations. At present, these tests are not yet routinely used in clinical practice.

### The five phases of chronic hepatitis B infection

The first phase of chronic hepatitis B (*immunotolerance*) may last 2–4 weeks in healthy adults. In subjects infected at birth or in early childhood it may persist several decades.

In the immune tolerance phase spontaneous and treatment-induced HBeAg seroconversion (that is, loss of the HBeAg and production of HBeAb) is infrequent (<5% per year). HBV DNA levels are high, usually >20 000 IU/mL, transaminases are normal, and liver histology is benign. Prognosis is generally favorable for patients who are in this phase. A study of 240 patients in this phase from Taiwan (mean age 27.6 years) found that only 5% progressed to cirrhosis and none to HCC during a follow-up period of 10.5 years.[4]

The *immune clearance* phase ('HBeAg-positive chronic hepatitis') is characterized by flares of transaminases, believed to be manifestations of immune-mediated lysis of infected hepatocytes secondary to increased T-cell responses to hepatitis B core antigen (HBcAg) and HBeAg.[5,6] These flares may precede HBeAg seroconversion, but many flares only result in transient decreases in serum HBV DNA levels without loss of HBeAg. Some flares may lead to hepatic decompensation.[7,8] The duration of this phase and the frequency/severity of flares correlate with the risk of cirrhosis and HCC.[9] So-called 'seroconversion' is the outcome of this phase; factors associated with higher rates of spontaneous HBeAg seroconversion include older age,[10] higher transaminases levels,[11,12] and HBV genotypes (B > C).[13,14] In particular, genotype B is associated with a lower prevalence of HBeAg, HBeAg seroconversion at an earlier age, and more sustained virological and biochemical remission after HBeAg seroconversion.

In the *inactive HBsAg carrier state* prognosis is generally favorable, especially if this state is reached early. However, inactive cirrhosis may be observed in patients who had developed severe liver injury during the preceding 'immune clearance' phase. Some inactive carriers have reactivation of HBV replication (either spontaneously or as a result of immunosuppression). Reversion back to HBeAg positive status is also possible.

Most patients who are in the fourth phase ('*reactivation* of HBV replication/HBeAg-negative chronic hepatitis B') come from a state of inactive carrier lasting a variable period of time. However, some patients progress directly from HBeAg-positive chronic hepatitis to HBeAg-negative chronic hepatitis. This phase is characterized by a fluctuating course both in terms of transaminases levels and HBV DNA levels. HBV DNA levels are usually lower than in the HbeAg-positive patients but may reach 20 or 200 million IU/ml. Transaminases were reported intermittently normal in 44% of 164 HBeAg-negative/HBeAb-positive patients followed for 21 months.[15]

This finding is important because it implies that a single HBV DNA level determination and a single transaminases level are not sufficient to differentiate patients in the inactive HBsAg carrier state from those with HBeAg-negative chronic hepatitis. Given the fluctuating course of the fourth phase, serial testing is more reliable than a single test.[16]

Recent studies in Europe, Asia, and the United States have all reported an increased prevalence of HBeAg-negative and a decreased prevalence of HBeAg-positive chronic hepatitis.[17,18] This may be related to aging of existing carriers, decrease in new HBV infections, and increased awareness. This finding has important impact on treatment strategies.

The *resolved phase* of HBV infection is characterized by HBsAg seroclearance, which occurs at the rate of 0.5–1.0% per year in patients with chronic HBV infection.[10,19]

## Factors influencing the natural history of chronic hepatitis B

The following risk factors have been implicated in the progression of chronic hepatitis B to cirrhosis and HCC:

### Host factors

- Age at infection.
- Older age.
- Male gender.
- Alpha fetoprotein (AFP).
- NAFLD (nonalcoholic fatty liver disease).

### Exogenous factors

- Alcohol consumption.
- HIV/HCV/HDV coinfection.
- Aflatoxin.

### Viral factors

- Genotype.
- HBeAg/anti-HBe status.
- HBsAg seroclearance and occult HBV infection.
- Viral load.
- cccDNA.

AGE AT INFECTION/OLDER AGE: A Taiwanese study reported significant correlation between incidence of cirrhosis and patient's age at study entry ($p < 0.001$).[20] Peak age for symptomatic cirrhosis and HCC is 50–60 years.

MALE GENDER: Males are more susceptible to development of liver complications,[21] and the male:female ratio for development of HCC is 5:1 in some populations.[22] Crude mortality rate for HCC in Chinese males is 207 per 100 000 patient-years and 42.5 per 100 000 patient-years in females.

ALPHA FETOPROTEIN: A Taiwanese study reported cirrhosis to be more common in patients experiencing repeated episodes of severe acute exacerbations of chronic hepatitis B with AFP levels >100 ng/mL (57.1%, $p < 0.001$).[20]

In a Hong Kong study, acute exacerbations of chronic hepatitis B with AFP >100 ng/mL were associated with cirrhosis complications and HCC.

NAFLD (nonalcoholic fatty liver disease): While there are no studies yet that address the potential effect of NAFLD on the progression of fibrosis in hepatitis B, this effect has been shown in hepatitis C.[25]

ALCOHOL CONSUMPTION: Alcohol abuse increases the risk of HCC 2–4-fold relative to alcohol abstinence.[24] Heavy use of alcohol is also a risk factor for the development of cirrhosis in chronic hepatitis B.

This corresponds to >20 grams/day in women and >30 grams/day in men.

COINFECTION: HIV is associated with more rapid onset of cirrhosis and incidence of HCC.[10] HCV is associated with 2–6-fold increased risk of HCC in cirrhotic patients when compared to monoinfection.[24] HDV is associated with 3-fold increased risk of HCC in cirrhotic patients compared to monoinfection.[24]

EXPOSURE TO AFLATOXIN: Aflatoxin is present in grains and in developing countries is known to contribute to the development of HCC. Some authors have proposed a synergism of action between aflatoxin and HBV in producing HCC.[96]

GENOTYPE: Evidence is currently emerging for a role of genotype in the progression of chronic HBV hepatitis.[26] Genotype D is associated with more severe liver disease and higher incidence of HCC at a younger age (<40 years) than genotype A.[27-29] Conflicting data exist for genotypes B and C.[27-29]

HBeAg/anti-HBe STATUS: There is conflicting evidence in regards to a possible association between HBeAg positivity and the risk of HCC. In a prospective study of 684 Taiwanese HBsAg-positive patients with histologically proven chronic hepatitis, those who were anti-HBe positive were equally at risk for the development of cirrhosis as those who were HBeAg positive.[21] Another prospective Taiwanese study of >11 000 men[30] found that the relative risk of developing HCC was much higher for HBeAg-positive/HBsAg-positive men than for HBeAg-negative/HBsAg-positive men and higher than for HBeAg-negative/HBsAg-negative men. However, because HBeAg/HBeAb status was recorded only upon study entry, it is likely that during the long follow-up (10 years) a substantial proportion of the HBeAg-positive patients seroconverted to HBeAb before developing HCC. For this reason it is difficult to conclude that HBeAg positivity is associated with an increased risk of HCC.

HBsAg SEROCLEARANCE: This produces favorable biochemical, virological, and histologic parameters, but may not reduce the risk of HCC in patients when seroclearance occurs after the age of 50 years and/or after development of cirrhosis.[31-33]

VIRAL LOAD: Prolonged low-level viremia is probably more influential in the development of cirrhosis and HCC than short-lived, high-level viremia.[31] Recom-

mendations of the American Association for the Study of Liver Diseases (AASLD) state that HBeAg-positive patients with serum HBV DNA levels above 20 000 IU/mL should be considered for treatment. However, there is evidence that active disease occurs at lower levels of HBV DNA, particularly in HBeAg-negative patients who have lower levels of HBV DNA than those with HBeAg-positive disease. In a Chinese retrospective study, 45% of HBeAg-negative patients with evidence of inflammation (raised ALT levels) had HBV DNA levels below 20 000 IU/mL.[34] These findings suggest that using a threshold value of HBV DNA 20 000 IU/mL to differentiate active and inactive disease in HBeAg-negative patients will exclude a substantial proportion of patients with active hepatitis. For this reason HBeAg-negative patients with lower HBV DNA levels (2 000–20 000 IU/mL) undergo liver biopsy and be treated if significant inflammation of fibrosis are present.

cccDNA (= COVALENTLY CLOSED CIRCULAR DNA): Infection of hepatocytes with HBV is followed by conversion of the relaxed circular viral DNA genome (rcDNA) into covalently closed circular DNA (cccDNA). cccDNA is localized to the nucleus, where it is transcribed to form the viral mRNA. cccDNA is an important pool of viral DNA that acts as a template for viral replication but *is relatively resistant to existing therapies*. Two Hong Kong studies have investigated the changes in cccDNA levels as chronic hepatitis B progresses.[31,35]

One study quantified total HBV DNA and cccDNA levels in sera and liver biopsies from 16 HBeAg-positive patients and 36 anti-HBe-positive patients. Intrahepatic and serum HBV DNA and cccDNA levels were significantly lower in subjects with anti-HBe-positive disease. In the early replicative phase, during which total intrahepatic HBV DNA levels were high, only a small proportion was present in the form of cccDNA. As the disease progressed, total viral load decreased and cccDNA became the predominant form of intrahepatic HBV DNA. In the second study, on 92 patients who had undergone HBsAg clearance, intrahepatic total and cccDNA were qualitatively measured in 16 patients. Of these, 37.5% had detectable intrahepatic DNA, predominantly in the form of cccDNA. The results of these two studies demonstrate that as chronic hepatitis B progresses and viral load decreases, cccDNA becomes the principal form of HBV DNA in the liver. This represents a stable pool of intrahepatic viral DNA that has impacts for successful antiviral therapy and may explain the viral exacerbations often reported in anti-HBe-positive patients.

## Screening High-Risk Populations for Chronic Hepatitis B Virus Infection By the Primary Care Physician

Table 23.3 lists the subject groups who are at risk for developing chronic hepatitis B. If an HBsAg-positive person is identified in a first-generation immigrant family, then screening should include second- and third-generation family members. Individuals found to be seronegative should then be vaccinated.

In high-risk subjects, serologic testing can be performed with either HBsAg and anti-HBs antibodies (HBsAb), or with anti-HBc antibodies (HBcAb). If HBcAb is used, further testing of those individuals positive for HBcAb is necessary with both HBsAg and HBsAb. Individuals found to be HBsAg positive should be evaluated for chronic HBV infection (see next section). Subjects who are negative for HBsAg and HBsAb, or who are negative for HBcAb, should receive a full three-dose immunization schedule of HBV vaccine.

---

### Table 23.3 High-risk groups who should be screened for HBV infection and vaccinated if seronegative

- Pregnant women
- Healthcare workers
- Hemodialysis patients
- Recipients of clotting factor concentrates
- Individuals from areas where there are high prevalence rates of HBV, including immigrants and adopted children:
  Asia
  Sub-Saharan Africa
  South Pacific islanders (Samoans, Tongans, etc.)
  Middle East, European, Mediterranean
  Indigenous populations of the Arctic
  Amazon delta of South America
  Eastern Europe including Russia
- Household and sexual contacts of persons who are HBsAg positive
- Injection drug users
- Sexually active men, women, adolescents, and adults, with multiple partners
- Inmates of correctional facilities
- Individuals with abnormal ALT or AST of unknown cause
- Individuals infected with HCV or HIV
- Homosexual men who are sexually active

---

## General evaluation of the HBsAg-positive patient by the primary care physician

At the initial consultation, patients with chronic hepatitis B infection (that is, HBsAg positive for >6 months) should undergo a thorough physical examination and a comprehensive patient history should be taken to identify risk factors for coinfection, alcohol use, and any family history of HBV infection and/or liver cancer. Laboratory tests should be undertaken to assess liver disease (complete blood count with platelets, hepatic panel including ALT, AST, total bilirubin, and prothrombin time/INR), markers of HBV replication (HBeAg/HBeAb, HBV DNA), hepatitis A (HAV) total antibodies, and at-risk patients should be tested for coinfection with hepatitis C virus (HCV), hepatitis D virus (HDV), and/or HIV. Patients should also be screened for HCC (alpha fetoprotein, abdominal ultrasound or computed tomography [CT] scanning of the liver). It is common practice to test alpha fetoprotein every 6 months and perform ultrasonography of the liver every 6 months. The reliability of ultrasound studies is operator dependent, thus the capabilities of the sonographer should be taken into consideration. HCC surveillance is recommended for high-risk patients: Asian men over the age of 40, Asian females over the age of 50, all patients with cirrhosis, and patients with a family history of HCC, among others. A recent AASLD guideline specifically addresses this issue in relation to level of HCC risk for different patient groups (Table 23.4).[36]

It is recommended that all individuals with chronic hepatitis B who are not immune to hepatitis A should be vaccinated, because of the higher risk of clinically severe hepatitis A in patients coinfected with hepatitis B. Both primary care physician and specialist should counsel patients with chronic hepatitis B in regard to lifestyle modifications, such as

---

### Table 23.4 In all HBsAg-positive patients the primary care physician should assess the following at initial evaluation

- Transaminases (ALT, AST)
- Total bilrubin and prothrombin time/INR
- Replicative status (HBeAg/HBeAb, HBV-DNA)
- Viral serologies for Hepatitis A, Hepatitis C, Hepatitis D and HIV
- Alphafetoprotein
- Abdominal ultrasound

---

reducing alcohol intake, and the risk of transmission to others. It is important to counsel them regarding screening and vaccination of sexual partners and second- and third-generation relatives, as well as regarding precautions to avoid exposing others to their blood and body fluids.[1]

## Special situations encountered by the primary care physician

HBsAg testing should be performed in subjects at high risk of HBV infection who need cancer chemotherapy or immunosuppressive treatment. HBsAg-positive subjects undergoing chemotherapy for malignancies or treatment with TNF-alpha inhibitors for inflammatory bowel disease or rheumatoid arthritis have a significant 50% risk of developing an exacerbation of hepatitis. They should be treated regardless of transaminases elevation and HBV DNA level, at the onset of chemotherapy or immunosuppressive therapy. Treatment should be maintained for at least 6 months after the end of the immunosuppressive therapy. Lamivudine or Telbivudine can be used if treatment duration is short (≤12 months) otherwise Adefovir or Entrecavir may be preferred when longer duration of treatment is anticipated.

### HBsAg-positive pregnant women

Vaccination breakthrough has been reported in newborns of mothers carrying HBV DNA $>1.2 \times 10^9$ copies/mL (N $>2.4 \times 10^8$ IU/mL). Lamivudine administered in the third trimester of pregnancy has been shown to be effective in reducing vertical transmission.[37] Although the use of prophylactic lamivudine in pregnant women to prevent maternal–fetal transmission is still a matter of controversy, these patients should be evaluated case by case in conjunction with a specialist.

### Further evaluation by the specialist

Defining any individual patient's own phase within the natural history of HBV is the next step; this is best accomplished by referring the patient to a specialist (gastroenterologist/hepatologist) who will obtain serial monitoring of serum HBV DNA and transaminases over some time, eventually followed by liver biopsy. A liver biopsy may become indicated after the laboratory values obtained throughout the monitoring period (which may vary widely) are reviewed. Recommendations for monitoring patients

chronically infected with HBV (inactive HBsAg carrier state, HBeAg-positive HBV infection, HBeAg-negative HBV infection) are included in AASLD, AGA, and ACG guidelines.[39,70]

Monitoring of serum transaminases and viral load (HBV DNA) over time is used by the gastroenterologist/hepatologist together with a liver biopsy in order to indicate the need for treatment. The different methods commercially available for measuring HBV DNA levels report results in international units 'IU'. This is also the unit used in the most recently published medical guidelines.[38,70]

A liver biopsy is necessary to determine the 'ongoing' *activity* of liver disease (= degree of necro-inflammatory activity or histologic *grade*) and the 'long-term' *progression* of liver disease (= degree of fibrosis or histologic *stage*).

Liver biopsy is recommended in patients who show intermittent or persistent elevation of transaminases in addition to a significant level of HBV replication. However, liver biopsy may be reasonable also in patients who have persistently elevated levels of HBV DNA but normal transaminases and are HBeAg negative.

## Hepatoma Prevention and Screening

Chronic hepatitis B infection can lead to cirrhosis and hepatocellular carcinoma. HCC develops as a result of both indirect and direct mechanisms. Chronic disease secondary to HBV infection is associated with a prolonged host-versus-virus interaction, which induces continuous or recurrent phases of hepatic necroinflammation. This indirectly facilitates the progression of chronic hepatitis to cirrhosis and ultimately to HCC.[40,41] HCC may also develop as the result of a direct carcinogenic mechanism, whereby the HBV genome integrates into oncogenic sites in the hepatocyte genome and produces proteins with potential transforming properties.[42,43] The cirrhotic process facilitates this random integration. A recent interesting theory supports a major role of the immune response in the emergence of HCC by inducing selection of hepatocytes clones that have lost the ability to replicate the virus.[44] These clones would have a selective growth advantage in that they would not be recognized and attacked by antiviral cytotoxic T lymphocytes.

An increased risk of hepatoma after years of follow-up has been shown to be associated with active viral replication and active liver disease.[30,45] In some studies, the presence of HBeAg years prior to the development of HCC imparts a greater risk of

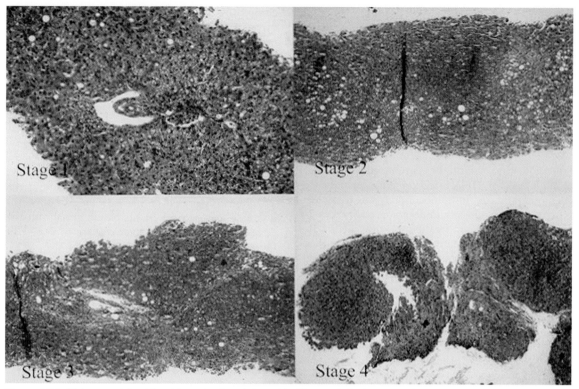

**Figure 23.1** Trichrome stain of liver biopsy in chronic hepatitis. Most pathologists use a four-point system for staging fibrosis in chronic hepatitis, based on the amount of fibrosis seen in relation to the portal tract (Desmet VJ et al. Hepatology 1994; 19:1513).
In stage 1, an increased amount of collage expands the portal area.
In stage 2, strands of fibrosis extend out from portal areas but do not interconnect.
In stage 3, strands of fibrosis begin to connect from one portal tract to another, forming septa.
In stage 4, or cirrhosis, the septa have formed a network of interconnecting bands surrounding nodules of liver cells. At this point, the original architecture of the liver has been completely transformed.

HCC than that in HBeAg-negative patients.[30] It may make sense that a treatment effective in suppressing inflammation and decreasing viral load would in turn prevent cirrhosis and reduce the risk of HCC. Published studies on the effectiveness of interferon in preventing HCC have produced conflicting results, at least partially due to the different genotypes and natural history of HBV in different parts of the world.[46-48] Treatment with lamivudine reduced risk of HCC in HBV cirrhotics in comparison to placebo, after a median follow-up period of 32 months.[49]

Should all hepatitis B carriers be screened? The risk of HCC in a 50-year-old man is much higher than in a 30-year-old female; however, there are no published data that clearly define age-specific incidence rates. Also, there are no experimental data to indicate what level of risk or what incidence of HCC should trigger surveillance.

HBV-related HCC occurs most commonly in men above the age of 50 and in those with cirrhosis. However, HBV-related HCC is also found in women and in children. In countries that are endemic for HBV, HCC is one of the most common childhood tumors. Risk for HCC varies with ethnicity and family history of HCC, besides age and cirrhosis. For example, risk of HCC persists in long-term carriers from Asia who lose HBsAg and Africans get HCC at a younger age. Unlike with HCV-related HCC, up to 40% of HBV-related HCCs are found in carriers who do not have cirrhosis.[50] This may be related to integration of HBV DNA into the host genome at an early stage of HBV infection. To maximize cost-effectiveness, practice guidelines have recommended HCC surveillance for carriers above 40–50 years of age, those with cirrhosis, and those with a family history of HCC.[51,52] The most recent AASLD guideline is summarized in Table 23.5.[36]

## Box 23.1

## Case study 1

A 37-year-old female was admitted to the hospital in April 2005 with 3 weeks' h/o fatigue, dyspnea on mild exertion, and progressive abdominal pain associated with nausea and heartburn. During her first pregnancy in 2003 she had been told that she was an HbsAg carrier. No other HBV serologies were available in her old medical records. She was of Korean descent and was adopted as a child together with her sister by Caucasian parents. On physical examination she had hepatomegaly, a palpable epigastric mass, and a hard and irregular inferior liver margin

Labs on admission were: ALP 214 U/L, ALT 74 U/L, AST 67 U/L, total bilirubin 1.3 mg/dL, HBsAg-pos, HBsAb-neg, HBeAg-pos, HBeAb-neg, HBV DNA 4 270 000 IU/mL, HCV Ab-neg, INR 1.2, Hgb 12.1 g/dL, WBC 5,800, platelets 138 000, alpha fetoprotein >10 000 IU/mL.

A triphasic CT of the abdomen showed multiple hepatic masses, with the largest in the left lobe measuring 6.4 × 5 × 9 cm, ascites, portal vein thrombus extending in both right and left portal vein branches, splenomegaly, and varices (Fig. 23.2).

The clinical diagnosis was multifocal hepatocellular carcinoma. The patient underwent chemotherapy and chemoembolization.

### Discussion

This patient had HBeAg-positive status associated with high serum HBV DNA; baseline transaminases levels prior to her time of presentation were not available and their mildly elevated levels on admission to the hospital may have been a consequence of her hepatoma. As well reported in

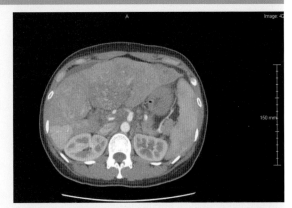

Figure 23.2 'Multifocal Hepatocellular carcinoma' CT of abdomen: multfocal.

the literature, it is unusual for a patient to progress to cirrhosis and HCC during the immune tolerance phase. It is plausible that this patient had multiple flares of hepatitis B as part of an immune clearance phase, but these were not effective in inducing seroconversion.

### Take-home message

Any patient who is HBsAg positive should have an assessment of the HBV replicative status, which includes HBeAg, HBeAb, and HBV DNA; obtaining a baseline abdominal ultrasound is also appropriate. Ethnicity and country of origin associated with high HBV endemicity and infection at time of birth point to a high probability of chronicity of infection. This patient's sister should be invited to undergo HbsAg screening and further evaluation as necessary.

## Box 23.2

## Case study 2

A 40-year-old Cambodian male presented to his primary care physician on November 2005 with progressive fatigue, epigastric distress/nausea, and intermittent flu-like symptoms for 5 weeks and jaundice for 4 days. PMH was relevant for h/o 'hepatitis B carrier state;' 2 months prior to the current illness he had been seen for a 'general check-up' by his primary care physician: labs had shown a normal blood cell count, INR, and only mildly elevated ALT (66 U/L, with upper limit of normal being 55). AFP and abdominal ultrasound were normal. He had no other risk factor for chronic liver disease. His mother died 'of some type of liver disease' soon after developing ascites.

The current labs ordered by his primary care physician were as follows: ALT 721 U/L, AST 412 U/L, total bilirubin 6.4mg/dL (direct 3.0), alk phosphatase 90 U/L, platelets 163 000. An urgent consult to the liver clinic was requested. On physical examination, the patient was jaundiced with spider nevi, and had a smooth and nontender liver edge and a barely palpable inferior spleen pole. Labs were: HBeAg-negative, HBeAb-positive, HBV DNA 16 400 000 IU/mL. Abdominal CT scan showed mild splenomegaly. An upper GI endoscopy revealed portal hypertensive gastropathy and grade I esophageal varices. A careful review of his past medical history revealed a cholestatic syndrome in 1999 with symptoms very

## Box 23.2

### Case study 2—cont'd

similar to the current ones, and an unremarkable ERCP. A liver biopsy had shown a subacute hepatitis with extensive focal unicellular necrosis and piecemeal necrosis but no fibrosis. He was HBeAg negative and HBeAb positive at that time; he was believed to have a flare of hepatitis B; lamivudine was prescribed but the patient took it only 'for few months.' A repeat liver biopsy this time showed chronic hepatitis B with bridging fibrosis (stage 3–4) and moderate portal inflammatory infiltrate and mild piecemeal necrosis.

He was started on lamivudine; his HBV DNA decreased to 48 200 IU/mL. Because of his current degree of fibrosis with early cirrhosis, it was decided to add tenofovir in an attempt to decrease his future potential for development of lamivudine resistance and, in turn, the potential for clinically significant acute flares. The patient's symptoms completely abated in 8 weeks from the beginning of therapy and the hepatic biochemical panel improved dramatically after 7 weeks of treatment (AST 50 U/L, ALT 56 U/L and total bilirubin 3.3 mg/dL).

### Discussion

This is a case of chronic HBeAg-negative hepatitis B characterized by recurrent flares with progressive development of severe fibrosis over a relatively short period of time (6 years). The presence of bridging fibrosis associated with gastric varices and portal hypertensive gastropathy means that this patient has actually developed cirrhosis. Given his family history and his country of origin, he probably contracted the same HBV genotype that affected his mother. He will hopefully benefit from long-term anti-HBV therapy with the goal to prevent further acute flares. The recent data about association of HCC with viral load support the concept of an additional benefit of therapy in preventing HCC development in this patient.

### Take-home message

Only the viral load, that is, the serum HBV DNA, can inform the physician about the replication status of HBV in any given patient. Consultation with a specialist followed by close monitoring of the patient over time (by clinic visits, hepatic biochemistries, and viral serologies) is necessary in patients with chronic hepatitis B, including those with HBeAg-negative status, especially if they already have had a serious flare with cholestatic features. Also, a mother dying of decompensated liver disease in a patient's family history points out that the HBV genotype of the patient may be the same and cause a clinical course in the future similar to the one of the mother.

## Box 23.3

### Case study 3

**A 27-year-old Asian female presented to her primary care physician to review blood work done by her obstetrician. She was 19 weeks pregnant; she moved to the United States 5 months earlier and was just found to be HBsAg positive. Her 3-year-old son was also HBsAg positive, although she states that he 'was vaccinated at birth.'**

The laboratory had automatically generated a full HBV serology panel (as it usually does at our institution for every positive HBsAg test) with the following results: HBeAg-positive, HBeAb-negative, HBV DNA 37 600 000 IU/mL. Her HBV DNA had been fluctuating between 248 000 000 IU/mL and 100 200 000 IU/mL in the previous 2 months, while her transaminases had been just above the upper limit of normal. Her transaminases this time were mildly elevated: ALT = 108 U/L (nl < 55), AST = 90 U/L (nl < 45). Alkaline phosphatase, total bilirubin, cell blood count, and INR were normal. She complained of fatigue, decreased appetite, weight loss, mild nausea and vomiting, and insomnia. Physical examination was unremarkable. Her primary care physician asked a gastroenterologist to evaluate the patient. The patient's symptoms improved spontaneously and transaminases remained stable on the earlier values. Laboratory tests obtained at about 7.5 months of pregnancy showed HBV DNA = 120 000 000 IU/mL, ALT 118 U/L, AST 113 U/L. The patient was started on oral lamivudine 100 mg a day which was continued until delivery. Transaminases and HBV serologies were monitored after delivery.

### Discussion

This patient's initial symptoms and increasing transaminases raised the concern that she might be experiencing an acute flare of HBeAg-positive hepatitis and was appropriately referred to a specialist. After her symptoms abated and her transaminases stabilized, there was no indication for HBV treatment. She was, however, noticed to have a viral load >$10^8$ IU/mL during her last trimester of pregnancy and she reported her son being HBsAg positive in spite of passive/active immunization. High maternal viremia has been associated with vaccination breakthrough in the newborn. Use of antiviral therapy in the mother during the last trimester of pregnancy has been effective in preventing perinatal transmission of hepatitis B virus infection when the maternal HBV DNA level was >2.4 × $10^8$ IU/mL (=1.2 × $10^9$ copies/mL).[37] Current treatment guidelines do not yet address this issue and large, controlled trials are awaited.

The published literature about safety of antihepatitis B medications in pregnancy is very limited. The available information is derived from pregnancy registries, case reports, and inadvertent exposures reported to the manufacturer. Lamivudine crosses the placenta and accumulates in the amniotic fluid.[97] Clinical experience has demonstrated no increased incidence of congenital anomalies among infants following intrauterine exposure to lamivudine.[95,98]

**Take-home message**

Transaminases and HBV serology should be tested in pregnant women who are found to be HBsAg positive during prenatal screening.

The implementation by the local laboratory of an 'HBsAg-cascade,' that is, the automatic reflex testing of HBeAg, HbeAb and HBV DNA following a positive HBsAg test, facilitates the medical care of such subjects, in that both obstetrician and primary care physician are provided together with both HBsAg screening test result and those HBV serologies necessary to indicate whether or not consultation with a hepatologist is necessary.

Transaminases should be periodically (possibly monthly) checked in pregnant women who have evidence of active HBV replication. Symptoms and known previous transaminases values may dictate individual intensity of monitoring.

Treatment of HBV infection during pregnancy may be necessary in cases of an acute flare of chronic hepatitis B.

While waiting for large clinical trials, a case-by-case approach is reasonable to address the issue of as possible newborn vaccination breakthrough by use of prophylactic lamivudine in the last trimester of pregnancy.

---

**Table 23.5 Surveillance for hepatocellular carcinoma is recommended for the following groups of patients**

Hepatitis B carriers
- Asian males ≥40 years
- Asian females ≥50 years
- All cirrhotic hepatitis B carriers
- Family history of HCC
- Africans over age 20

For noncirrhotic hepatitis B carriers not listed above the risk of HCC varies depending on the severity of the underlying liver disease, and current and past hepatic inflammatory activity. Patients with high HBV DNA concentrations and those with ongoing hepatic inflammatory activity remain at risk for HCC.

Several studies have shown that periodic testing for alpha fetoprotein (AFP) and ultrasound can lead to earlier detection of HCC and an increased likelihood of eligibility for 'curative' treatment.[53-56] An improvement in survival has also been reported among patients whose tumors were detected through surveillance as opposed to those who presented with symptomatic tumors. In the only randomized, con-trolled trial of screening in hepatitis B carriers,[57] subjects were screened with 6-monthly ultrasound and AFP: the screened group experienced a signifi-cantly lower mortality than the control group.

The most common regimen for HCC surveillance includes 6-monthly testing for AFP and abdominal ultrasound. However, both AFP and ultrasound have limitations.

AFP has a low sensitivity (40–65%) and variable specificity (75–90%) for the detection of HCC, depend-ing on the cutoff value used.[58] AFP values more than 500 ng/mL are highly suggestive of HCC, but these values have also been reported in patients with ex-acerbations of chronic hepatitis B. This was illus-trated in a study involving 290 patients in Hong Kong screened for HCC using AFP.[59] Forty-four patients had elevated AFP during a follow-up of up to 4 years, only six (14%) had HCC; most of the remaining patients with AFP increase (up to 1934 ng/mL) had flares in underlying chronic hepatitis B. High AFP levels can also be seen during pregnancy and in association with gonadal tumors. Conversely, AFP can be normal in 30–40% of HCC patients with small tumors.[60] Thus, AFP is useful in defining high-risk groups and establishing a diagnosis, but not as useful for surveillance.

Ultrasound can detect tumors that are not AFP secreting, but the technique is operator dependent and its accuracy in detecting diffuse HCC and in differentiating regenerative/dysplastic nodules from HCC in a cirrhotic liver is limited. Spiral (= triphasic) CT scanning is more sensitive than ultrasound, but is associated with a significant amount of radiation when used every 6 months for many years. In the cirrhotic liver ultrasound is more difficult; however, it should be possible to identify nodules larger than 1 cm which may be amenable to either biopsy or more intensive follow-up. Alternating ultrasound and CT scanning may be preferable for cirrhotic and/or obese subjects. Contrast ultrasonography is a new and promising technique, which is being studied as a screening tool.[61] The optimal frequency of HCC surveillance has not been determined; 6-monthly surveillance has been suggested in most guidelines.[51,52] This interval is based on a study of HCC in Chinese patients, in which the most rapidly growing tumors required 4–5 months to reach a size of 3 cm.[62]

## Hepatitis B Treatment

The immediate goals of treatment of chronic hepatitis B are sustained viral suppression, normalization of transaminases, and improvement of hepatic histology. The long-term goals are decreased risk of cirrhosis and hepatoma.

The following is a brief summary of the AASLD recommendations.[38]

Subjects in the immune tolerant phase, in the inactive HBsAg-positive state, and in the resolved HBV infection phase should not be treated. Individuals in the immune tolerant phase very rarely seroconvert when treated, while the risk of developing resistance increases with time in those patients treated with nucleos(t)ide inhibitors. Individuals in the other two phases have very low (<2000 IU/mL) or undetectable HBV DNA level.

HBeAg-positive patients in the immune clearance phase should be monitored first with serologies every 3–6 months to look for spontaneous seroconversion if they have well compensated liver disease (that is, if they have no indirect evidence of cirrhosis and/or hepatic synthesis dysfunction).

HBeAg-positive patients in the immune tolerance phase with a rise of their transaminases to >2 ULN and patients in the immune clearance phase who have not seroconverted after 3–6 months should be considered for treatment. HBeAg-negative patients whose transaminases are increased and HBV DNA is >20 000 IU/mL should be treated. Patients with HBeAg-negative chronic hepatitis B (2000 to 20 000 IU/mL HBV DNA) should have a liver biopsy and be considered for treatment if they have moderate inflammation and/or moderate fibrosis.

Long-term therapy is usually required in persons with HBeAg-negative chronic HBV, as withdrawal of therapy frequently results in relapse; periodic HBV DNA level testing is required in these patients to monitor response and detect emergence of resistance.

The AASLD's 2007 guidelines recommend PegIFN-alpha adefovir[2a], or entecavir as first line treatments. However, all six licensed drugs may be used as first-line treatments for both chronic HBeAg-positive and HBeAg-negative hepatitis (Table 23.5). Once treatment is initiated (see Medical Societies Guidelines) monitoring of serum HBV DNA level (in both HBeAg-positive and HBeAg-negative patients) and HbeAg status (in the HBeAg-positive patients) is used to evaluate treatment response. Tables 23.6 and 23.7 summarize treatment recommendations for HBeAg-positive and HBeAg-negative patients, respectively. For HBeAg-positive patients, the goals include loss of HBeAg with or without seroconversion to anti-HBe, suppression of HBV DNA to low or undetectable levels, and normalization of ALT. For HBeAg-negative patients the end points are as much suppression of HBV DNA replication as possible and normalization of ALT; treatment should be continued until the patient has achieved HBsAg clearance.

### Interferon-alpha

Interferon-alpha has antiviral and immunomodulatory activity. Its advantages are its finite duration of therapy (16–48 weeks), lack of emergence of resistance, and durability of response. Its disadvantages include a response less durable in HBeAg-negative chronic hepatitis B, side effects profile, and the mode of administration (subcutaneous). Side effects include flu-like symptoms, psychiatric effects, and bone marrow toxicity. In HBeAg-positive patients the standard is to treat for 16 weeks; following discontinuation of therapy, the rate of HBeAg seroconversion often increases with duration of follow-up. Review of the literature shows that when compared to placebo and given for at least 3 months, HBeAg loss is obtained in 33% versus 12% of patients, HBV DNA is decreased to below the quantifiable limit in

**Table 23.6 Summary of licensed agents for chronic hepatitis B infection**

| | Interferon | Lamivudine | Adefovir | Entecavir | Peginterferon alpha-2a* | Telbivudine |
|---|---|---|---|---|---|---|
| Dose | 5 MU qd or 10 MU t.i.w. | 100 mg qd | 10 mg qd | Nucleoside naive: 0.5 mg daily Lamivudine-resistant patients 1.0 mg daily | 180 µg qw | 600 mg qd |
| Route Duration of treatment | Subcutaneous | Oral | Oral | Oral | Subcutaneous | Oral |
| HBeAg-positive patients | 4 months | ≥1 yr | ≥1 yr | ≥1 yr | 48 wk | ≥1 yr |
| HBeAg-negative patients | 48 wk | >1 yr | >1 yr | >1 yr | 48 wk | >1 yr |
| Drug resistance | None | Year 1: ~20% Year 5: ~70% | Year 1: 0% Year 5: ~29% | Year 1: 0% in nucleos(t)ide naïve 7% in lamivudine-resistant cases | None | ~25% up to year 2 |

**Table 23.7 Treatment recommendations for HBeAg-positive patients**

| HBV DNA | ALT | Treatment strategy |
|---|---|---|
| >20 000 IU/mL | ≤2 × ULN (upper limit of normal) | Observer q 3 mo ALT; 6 mo HBeAg Consider biopsy in persons >40 years, ALT hight nl-2 × ULN or with family h/o HCC; treat if disease is evident |
| >20 000 IU/mL | >2 × ULN | Observe for 3–6 months and treat if no spontaneous HBeAg loss. Consider liver biopsy before treatment if compensated. Otherwise treat immediately if decompensated or jaundiced. |

**Table 23.8 Treatment recommendations for HBeAg-negative patients**

| HBV DNA | ALT | Treatment strategy |
|---|---|---|
| ≤2 000 IU/mL | Normal | No treatment; monitor HBV DNA & ALT;* treat if HBV DNA or ALT becomes higher |
| >2 000 IU/mL | 1–2 × ULN | q 3 mo ALT & HBV DNA Consider biopsy; treat if disease is evident |
| >20 000 IU/mL | >2 ULN | Long-term treatment required; liver biopsy optional |

* Upon initial diagnosis and every 3 months for 1 year to ensure stability, then every 6–12 months.

37% versus 17%, and HBsAg loss occurs in 8% versus 2%.[63] In HBeAg-negative patients prolonged treatment beyond 16 weeks may be needed to achieve optimal response. Twenty-eight to 69% of patients reach undetectable HBV DNA and ALT normaliza-tion at end of therapy; sustained response at end of follow-up was 6–33 %; loss of HBsAg at end of follow-up was 4.5–13%.[64-68]

Interferon-alpha is contraindicated in patients with decompensated cirrhosis because of the risk of inducing a flare leading to liver failure;[69] in compensated cirrhosis prolonged treatment carries a risk of decompensation.[70,71]

## Pegylated interferon (peg-ifn-alpha)

Two forms exist, with improved pharmacokinetics over standard interferon: alpha-2a and alpha-2b. In HBeAg-positive patients both forms have been studied in separate trials in comparison to lamivudine monotherapy and/or to combination therapy with lamivudine. Sustained anti-HBe seroconversion at 24 weeks after end of therapy is around 30% in HBeAg-positive patients, and 48-week HBV DNA suppression to less than 20 000 IU/mL is about 30% in HBeAg-negative patients.[72-76]

## Lamivudine

Lamivudine (LAM) is an oral nucleoside analogue that inhibits HBV DNA polymerase activity and hence viral replication. It is well tolerated and safe. One year of therapy in HBeAg-positive patients is associated with HBeAg loss in 17–33% of patients and HBeAg seroconversion rates of 16–18%. Full seroconversion was found to occur only in patients with decreased HBV DNA to <2000 IU/mL.[77-81] Continuing therapy beyond a year is associated with an increased rate of HBeAg seroconversion from 18% at 1 year to 47% at 4 years. Unfortunately, longer therapy is accompanied by a concomitant increase in the rate of virologic resistance from 25% at 1 year to 74% at 5 years; usually, the appearance of resistance abrogates most of the clinical benefit of extended therapy. A common LAM-resistant HBV strain is M204V/I.

In HBeAg negative patients a significant proportion of patients (72–73%) achieves undetectable HBV DNA levels by PCR at the end of 48 weeks of therapy, but the relapse rate is extremely high (90%) 6 months after the end of therapy.[82,83] Long-term therapy seems to be necessary for this group of patients (until either loss of HBsAg or the development of resistance occurs). Patients on LAM should be followed periodically (preferably every 3 months) with quantitative HBV DNA assays and transaminases to assess viral and biochemical response. In addition, HBeAg and HBeAb should be checked in HBeAg-positive patients.

## Adefovir

Adefovir (ADV) is an oral nucleotide analogue that is converted to the active metabolite, adefovir diphosphate. In HBeAg-positive patients 48 weeks of ADV achieve undetectable HBV DNA by a very sensitive PCR assay (400 copies/mL) in 28% of treated patients, HBeAg loss in 21%, and HBeAg seroconversion in 12%.[84] The rates of HBeAg loss and seroconversion doubled after 144 weeks of therapy.[85] After 48 weeks of therapy HBV DNA was undetectable in 51% of HBeAg-negative patients[86] and after 96 weeks it was undetectable in 71%.[87]

Incidence of genotypic resistance to ADV is delayed and much less frequent when compared to lamivudine, being 18% at 4 years.[88] Two resistance mutations have been observed after 1 year of ADV therapy: N236T and A181V. In LAM-resistant patients with compensated chronic hepatitis B it is appropriate to 'add' long-term ADV treatment to LAM. There is increasing evidence that this strategy (as opposed to simply switching drugs) avoids the appearance of ADV resistance later.

Patients on ADV should be followed periodically as those on LAM, but monitoring at less frequent intervals may be reasonable for the first 2–3 years, especially after virologic response has been obtained, because of the lower frequency of emergent resistance.

ADV is nephrotoxic only at higher doses than those used for treatment of hepatitis B. Periodic follow-up of creatinine is recommended in all patients during treatment.

## Entecavir

Entecavir (ETV) is a nucleoside analogue which inhibits HBV DNA polymerase with a very potent antiviral activity possibly accounted for by the capacity to inhibit HBV replication at three steps (DNA priming, DNA synthesis, and reverse transcription). ETV has shown to be superior to LAM for multiple end points in HBeAg-positive, HBeAg-negative and LAM-resistant patients. At the end of 2 years of therapy 81% of HBeAg-positive patients,[89] 96% of HBeAg-negative patients,[90] and 40% of LAM-resistant patients[91] reached undetectable levels of HBV DNA. At 2 years of treatment no genotypic or phenotypic resistance to entecavir occurred. On the other hand, genotypic resistance to ETV was detected in 7% of LAM-resistant patients at 1 year of treatment while viral rebound due to resistance was detected in 1% of patients at 1 year of treatment and in 9% at 2 years of treatment.[92] ETV is as well tolerated as LAM in comparative studies.

## Telbivudine

Telbivudine (LdT) is an L-nucleoside analogue more potent than Lamivudine in suppressing HBV replication, but with resistant mutations that are cross resistant with Lamivudine.

## Table 23.9 Treatment guidelines

The following three sets of guidelines (developed by medical liver specialty societies, evidence-based, and updated every 2–3 years) are not meant to represent 'standards of care.' They are meant to be used by clinicians as a tool by which a rational but individualized care plan may be carried out for specific patients with chronic hepatitis B.

- AASLD (American Association for the Study of Liver Disease)[38]
- EASL (European Association for the Study of Liver Disease)[93]
- APASL (Asian Pacific Association for the Study of Liver Disease)[94]

Additional HBV treatment recommendations have been published by the AGA (American Gastroenterological Association)[70] and the ACG (American College of Gastroenterology)[39]

In a clinical trial comparing Telbivudine versus Lamivudine in HBeAg-positive patients, undetectable HBV DNA by PCR was found in 60% vs 40% and in 54% vs 38% after 1 and 2 years of treatment, respectively.[99,100] In the same study, HBeAg-negative subjects had undetectable HBV DNA by PCR after 1 and 2 years of treatment in a larger proportion when tested with Telbivudine as opposed to Lamivudine: 88% vs 71% and 79% vs 53%.[99,100] However, the rate of HBeAg loss at the end of 1 and 2 years of treatment did not differ (26% vs 23% and 34% vs 29% for Telbivudine and Lamivudine respectively).

## Conclusion

Ethnicity and immigration patterns influence strongly the incidence and prevalence of HBV infection in the USA. Chronic HBV infection is life long, due to perinatal acquisition, in most infected immigrants from highly endemic areas of the world. The primary care physician has a key role in the detection of undiagnosed HBV-infected individuals by screening persons at high-risk and in the vaccination of those who are found to be seronegative. The initial work-up of HBV-infected individuals (that is, who are HBsAg positive) should include a viral serology panel comprised of HBeAg, HBeAb, and HBV DNA followed by a consultation with a gastroenterologist/hepatologist. HBV-infected persons need life-long monitoring to determine when/if treatment is needed and surveillance to detect hepatoma at an early, treatable stage. Excellent antiviral treatment

that can suppress (but not eradicate) HBV is available and should be offered to those individuals who might benefit from treatment (Table 23.8).

## References

1. Tassopoulos NC, Papaevangelou GJ, Sjogren MH, et al. Natural history of acute hepatitis B surface antigen-positive hepatitis in Green adults. Gastroenterology 1987; 92(6):1844–1850.
2. Beasley RP, Hwang LY, Lin CC, et al. Incidence of hepatitis B virus infections in preschool children in Taiwan. J Infec Dis 1982; 146(2):198–204.
3. Beasley RP, Trepo C, Stevens CE, et al. The e antigen and vertical transmission of hepatitis B surface antigen. Am J Epidemiol. 1977 Feb;105(2):94–98.
4. Chu CM, Hung SJ, Lin J, et al. Natural history of hepatitis B e antigen to antibody seroconversion in patients with normal serum aminotransferase levels. Am J Med 2004; 116(12):829–834.
5. Tsai SL, Chen PJ, Lai MY, et al. Acute exacerbations of chronic type B hepatitis are accompanied by increased cell responses to hepatitis B core and e antigens. Implications for hepatitis B e antigen seroconversion. J Clin Invest 1992; 89(1):87–96.
6. Chu CM, Liaw YF. Intrahepatic distribution of hepatitis B surface and core antigens in chronic hepatitis B virus infection. Hepatocyte with cytoplasmic/membranous hepatitis core antigen as a possible target for immune hepatocytolysis. Gastroenterology 1987; 92(1):220–225.
7. Liaw YF, Chu CM, Su IJ, et al. Clinical and histological events preceding hepatitis B e antigen seroconversion in chronic type B hepatitis. Gastroenterology 1983; 84(2):216–219.
8. Sheen IS, Liaw YF, Tai DI, et al. Hepatic decompensation associated with hepatitis B e antigen clearance in chronic type B hepatitis. Gastroenterology 1985; 89(4):732–735.
9. Liaw YF, Tai DI, Chu CM, et al. The development of cirrhosis in patients with chronic type B hepatitis: a prospective study. Hepatology 1988; 8(3):493–496.
10. McMahon BJ, Holck P, Bulkow L, et al. Serologic and clinical outcomes of 1536 Alaska Natives chronically infected with hepatitis B virus. Ann Intern Med 2001; 135(9):759–768.
11. Yuen MF, Yuan HJ, Hui CK, et al. A large population study of spontaneous HBeAg seroconversion and acute exacerbation of chronic hepatitis B infection: implications for antiviral therapy. Gut 2003; 52(3):416–419.
12. Liaw YF. Hepatitis flares and hepatitis B e antigen seroconversion: implication in antihepatitis B virus therapy [review]. J Gastroenterol Hepatol 2003; 18(3):246–252.
13. Kao JH, Chen PJ, Lai MY, et al. Hepatitis B virus genotypes and spontaneous hepatitis B e antigen seroconversion in Taiwanese hepatitis B carriers. J Med Virol 2004; 72(3):363–369.
14. Chu CJ, Hussain M, Lok AS. Hepatitis B virus genotype B is associated with earlier HBeAg seroconversion compared with hepatitis B virus genotype C. Gastroenterology 2002; 122(7):1756–1762.
15. Brunetto MR, Oliveri F, Coco B, et al. Outcome of anti-HBe-positive chronic hepatitis B in alpha-interferon treated and untreated patients: a long-term cohort study. J Hepatol 2002; 36(2):263–270.
16. Chu CJ, Hussain M, Lok AS. Quantitative serum HBV DNA levels during different stages of chronic hepatitis B infection. Hepatology 2002; 36(6):1408–1415.
17. Funk ML, Rosenberg DM, Lok AS. World-wide epidemiology of HBeAg-negative chronic hepatitis B and associated precore and core promoter variants [review]. J Viral Hepatol 2002; 9(1):52–61.
18. Chu CJ, Keeffe EB, Han SH, et al. Prevalence of HBV precore/core promoter variants in the United States. Hepatology 2003; 38(3):619–628.

19. Manno M, Camma C, Schepis F, et al. Natural history of chronic HBV carriers in northern Italy: morbidity and mortality after 30 years. Gastroenterology 2004; 127(3):756–763.

20. Liaw YF, Tai DI, Chu CM, et al. The development of cirrhosis in patients with chronic type B hepatitis: a prospective study. Hepatology 1988; 8(3):493–496.

21. Beasley RP. Hepatitis B virusas the etiologic agent in hepatocellular carcinoma – epidemiologic considerations. Hepatology 1982; 2(2):21S–26S.

22. Evans AA, Chen G, Ross EA, et al. Eight-year follow-up of the 90 000 person Haimen City cohort. I. Hepatocellular carcinoma mortality, risk factors and gender differences. Cancer Epidemiol Biomarkers Prev 2001; 11:369–376.

23. Keeffe EB, Dieterich DT, Han SB, et al. A treatment algorithm for the management of chronic hepatitis B virus infection in the United States. Clin Gastroenterol Hepatol 2004; 2:87–106.

24. Fattovich G, Stroffolini T, Zaqni I, et al. Hepatocellular carcinoma in cirrhosis: incidence and risk factors. Gastroenterology 2004; 127(5 supp.1):S35–S50.

25. Castera L, Hezode C, Roudot-Thoroval F, et al. Worsening of steatosis is an independent factor of fibrosis progression in untreated patients with chronic hepatitis C and paired liver biopsies. Gut 2003; 52: 288–292

26. Sanchez T, Costa J, Mas A, et al. Influence of hepatitis B virus genotype on the long-term outcome of chronic hepatitis B in Western patients. Gastroenterology 2002; 123(6):1848–1856.

27. Kao JH, Chen PJ, Lai MY, et al. Hepatitis B genotypes correlate with clinical outcomes in patients with chronic hepatitis B. Gastroenterology 2000; 118(3):554–559.

28. Orito E, Ichida T, Sakugawa H, et al. Geographic distribution of hepatitis B virus (HBV) genotype in patients with chronic HBV infection in Japan. Hepatology 2001; 34(3):590–594.

29. Sumi H, Yokosuka O, Seki N, et al. Influence of hepatitis B virus genotype on the progression of chronic type-B liver disease. Hepatology 2003; 37(1):19–26.

30. Yang HI, Lu SN, Liaw YF, et al. Hepatitis B e antigen and the risk of hepatocellular carcinoma. N Engl J Med 2002; 347(3):168–174.

31. Yuen NF, Wong DKH, Sablon E, et al. HBsAg seroclearance in chronic hepatitis B in the Chinese: virological, histological, and clinical aspects. Hepatology 2004; 39(6):1694–1701.

32. Brechot C, Degos F, Lugassy C, et al. Hepatitis B virus DNA in patients with chronic liver disease and negative tests for hepatitis B surface antigen. N ENgl J Med 1985; 312(5):270–276.

33. Pollicino T, Squadrito G, Cerenzia G, et al. Hepatitis B virus maintains its pro-oncogenic properties in the case of occult HBV infection. Gastroenterology 2004; 126(1):102–110.

34. Chu CM, Hussain M, Lok ASF, et al. Quantitative serum HBV-DNA levels during different stages of chronic hepatitis B infection. Hepatology 2002; 36(6):1408–1415.

35. Wong DKH, Yuen MF, Yuan HJ, et al. Quantitation of covalently closed circular hepatitis B virus DNA in chronic hepatitis B patients. Hepatology 2004; 40(3):727–737.

36. Bruix J, Sherman M, Llovet J, et al. Management of hepatocelluair carcinoma. AASLD practice guideline. Hepatology 2005; 42:5.

37. van Zonneveld M, van Nunnen AB, Niesters HG, et al. Lamivudine treatment during pregnancy to prevent perinatal transmission of hepatitis B virus infection. J Viral Hepat 2003; 10 (4):294–297.

38. Lok ASF, McMahon BJ. American Association for the study of Liver Disease Practice Guidelines. Chronic Hepatitis B. Hepatology 2007; 45:507–539.

39. Proceedings from the Roundtable. A cross-disciplinary discussion on chronic hepatitis B. Am J Gastroenterol 2006; 101:S1–S39.

40. Lau GKK, Lai CL, et al. Hepatocarcinogenesis. Trop Gastroenterol 1990; 11(1):9–24.

41. Bruix J, Sherman M, Llovet JM, et al. Clinical management of hepatocellular carcinoma. Conclusions of the Barcelona 2000 EASL conference. European Association for the Study of the Liver. J Hepatol 2001; 35(3):421–430.

42. Buendia MA. Hepatitis B viruses and carcinogenesis. Biomed Pharmacother 1998; 52(1):34–43.

43. Brechot C, Gozuacik D, Murakami Y, et al. Molecular bases for the development of hepatitis B virus (HBV)-related hepatocellular carcinoma. Semin Cancer Biol 2000; 10(3):211–231.

44. Mason WS, Jilbert AR, Summers J. Clonal expansion of hepatocytes during chronic woodchuck hepatitis virus infection.Proc Natl Acad Sci USA 2005; 102:1139–1144.

45. Ohata K, Hamasaki K, Toriyama K. High viral load is a risk factor for hepatocellular carcinoma in patients with chronic hepatitis B virus infection. J Gastroenterol Hepatol 2004; 19:670–675.

46. Niederau C, Heintges T, Lange S, et al. Long-term follow-up of HBeAg-positive patients treated with interferon alfa for chronic hepatitis B. N Engl J Med 1996; 334:1422–1427.

47. Lin SM, Tai DI, Chien RN, et al. Comparison of long-term effects of lymphoblastoid interferon alpha and recombinant interferon alpha-2a therapy in patients with chronic hepatitis. Br J Viral Hepatol 2004; 11:349–357.

48. Yuen MF, Hui CK, Cheng CC, et al. Long-term follow-up of interferon alfa treatment in Chinese patients with chronic hepatitis B infection: the effect of hepatitis B e Ag seroconversion and the development of cirrhosis-related complications. Hepatology 2001; 34:139–145.

49. Liaw YF, Sung JJY, Chow WC, et al. Lamivudine for patients with chronic hepatitis B and advanced liver disease. N Engl J Med 2004; 351:1521–1531.

50. Zhou XD, Tang ZY, Yang BH, et al. Experience of 1000 patients who underwent hepatectomy for small hepatocellular carcinoma. Cancer 2001; 91:1479–1486.

51. Lok AS, McMahon BJ. Chronic hepatitis B. Hepatology 2001; 34(6):1225–1241.

52. Bruix J, Llovet JM. Hepatitis B virus and hepatocellular carcinoma. J Hepatol 2003; 39:S59–S63.

53. McMahon BJ, Bulkow L, Harpster A, et al. Screening for hepatocellular carcinoma in Alaska Natives infected with chronic hepatitis B: a 16-year population-based study. Hepatology 2000; 32:842–846.

54. Sherman M, Peltekian KM, Lee C, et al. Screening for hepatocellular carcinoma in chronic carriers of hepatitis B virus: incidence and prevalence of hepatocellular carcinoma in a North American urban population. Hepatology 1995; 22:432–438.

55. Yang HI, Zhang B, Xu Y, et al. Prospective study of early detection for primary liver cancer. J Cancer Res Clin Oncol 1997; 123:357–360.

56. Yuen MF, Cheng CC, Lauder IJ, et al. Early detection of hepatocellular carcinoma increases the chance of treatment: Hong Kong experience. Hepatology 2000; 31:330–335.

57. Zhang BH, Yang BH, Tang ZY, et al. Randomized controlled trial of screening for hepatocellular carcinoma. J Cancer Res Clin Oncol 2004; 130(7):417–422.

58. Trevisani F, D'Intino PE, Morselli-Labate AM, et al. Serum alfa-fetoprotein for diagnosis of hepatocellular carcinoma in patients with chronic liver disease: influence of HBsAg and anti-HCV status. J Hepatol 2001; 34:570–575.

59. Lok AS, Lai CL. Alfa-fetoprotein monitoring in Chinese patients with chronic hepatitis B virus infection: role in the early detection of hepatocellular carcinoma. Hepatology 1989; 9:110–115.

60. Chen DS, Sung JL, Sheu JC, et al. Serum alfa-fetoprotein in the early stage of hepatocellular carcinoma. Gastroenterology 1984; 86:1404–1409.

61. Gaiani S, Celli N, Piscaglia F, et al. Usefulness of contrast-enhanced perfusional sonography in the assessment of hepatocellular carcinoma hypervascular at spiral computed tomography. J Hepatol 2004; 41(3):421–426.

62. Sheu JC, Sung JL, Chen DS, et al. Growth rate of asymptomatic hepatocellular carcinoma and its clinical implications. Gastroenterology 1985; 90:259–266.

63. Wong DKH, Cheung AM, O'Rourke K, et al. Effect of alpha-interferon treatment in patients with hepatitis B e antigen-positive chronic hepatitis B. A meta-analysis. Ann Int Med 1993; 19(4):312–323.

64. Lampertico P, Del Ninno E, Manzin A, et al. A randomized, controlled trial of a 24-month course of interferon alfa 2b in patients with chronic hepatitis B who had hepatitis B virus DNA without hepatitis B e antigen in serum. Hepatology 1997; 26:1621–1625.

65. Olivieri F, Santantonio T, Bellati G, et al. Long-term response to therapy of chronic anti-HBe-positive hepatitis B is poor independent of type and schedule of interferon. Am J Gastroenterol 1999; 94:1366–1372.

66. Brunetto MR, Olivieri F, Coco B, et al. Outcome of anti-HBe positive chronic hepatitis B in alpha-interferon treated and untreated patients: A long-term cohort study. J Hepatol 2002; 36:263–270.

67. Manesis EK, Hadziyannis SJ. Interferon-a treatment and re-treatment of hepatitis B e antigen-negative chronic hepatitis B. Gastroenterology 2001; 121:101–109.

68. Papatheodoridis GV, Manesis E, Hadziyannis SJ. The long-term outcome of interferon-alpha treated and untreated patients with HBeAg-negative chronic hepatitis B. Hepatology 2001; 34:306–313.

69. Lee WM. Hepatitis B virus infection. N Engl J Med 1997; 337:1733–1745.

70. Keeffe EB, Dieterich DT, Han SHB, et al. A treatment algorithm for the management of chronic hepatitis B virus infection in the United States. Clin Gastroenterol Hepatol 2006; 4(8):936–962.

71. Perrillo RP, Mason AL. Therapy for hepatitis B virus infection. Gastroenterol Clin North Am 1994; 23:581–601.

72. Cooksley WBE, Piratvisuth T, Lee S-D, et al. Peginterferon alfa 2a (40KD): an advance in the treatment of hepatitis B e antigen-positive chronic hepatitis B. J Viral Hepat 2003; 10:298–305.

73. Lau GKK, Piratvisuth T, Luo K, et al. Peginterferon alfa 2qa, lamivudine, and the combination for HBeAg-positive chronic hepatitis B. N Engl J Med 2005; 352:2682–2695.

74. Janssen HLA, van Zonnaveld M, Senturk H, et al. Pegylated interferon alfa 2b alone or in combination with lamivudine for HbeAg-positive chronic hepatitis B: a randomized trial. Lancet 2005; 365:123–129.

75. Marcellin P, Lau GKK, Bonino F, et al. Peginterferon alfa 2a alone, lamivudine alone, and the two in combination in patients with HBeAg-negative chronic hepatitis B. N Engl J Med 2004; 351:1206–1217.

76. Van Zannoveld M., Flink HJ, Verhey E, et al. The safety of pegylated interferon alfa 2b in the treatment of chronic hepatitis B: predictive factors for dose reduction and treatment discontinuation. Ailment Pharmacol 2005; 21:1163–1171.

77. Lai CL, Chien RN, Leung NWY, et al. A one-year trial of lamivudine for chronic hepatitis B. N Engl J Med 1998; 339:61–68.

78. Dienstag JL, Schiff ER, Wright TL, et al. Lamivudine as initial treatment for chronic hepatitis B in the United States. N Engl J Med 1999; 341:1256–1263.

79. Schalm SW, Heathcote J, Cianciara J, et al. Lamivudine and alpha interferon combination treatment of patients with chronic hepatitis B infection: A ramdonised trial. Gut 2000; 46:562–568.

80. Schiff ER, Dienstag JL, Karayalcin S, et al. Lamivudine and 24 weeks of lamivudine/interferon combination therapy for hepatitis B e antigen-positive chronic hepatitis B in interferon nonresponders. J Hepatol 2003; 38:818–826.

81. Gauthier J, Bourne EJ, Lutz MW, et al. Quantitation of hepatitis B viremia and emergence of YMDD variants in patients with chronic hepatitis B treated with lamivudine. J Infec Dis 1999; 180:1757–1762.

82. Marcellin P, Lau GK, Bonino F, et al. Peginterferon Alfa-2a HBeAg-Negative Chronic Hepatitis B Study Group. Peginterferon alfa-wa alone, lamivudine alone, and the two in combination in patients with HBeAg-negative chronic hepatitis B. N Engl J Med 2004; 351(12):1206–1217.

83. Lai CL, Shouval D, Lok AS, et al. Entecavir versus lamivudine for patients with HBeAg-negative chronic hepatitis B. N Engl J Med 2006; 354(10):1011–1020.

84. Marcellin P, Chang TT, Lim SG, et al. Adefovir dipivoxil for the treatment of hepatitis B e antigen-positive chronic hepatitis B. N Engl J Med 2003; 348:808–816.

85. Marcellin P, Chang TT, Lim S, et al. Long-term efficacy and safety of adefovir dipivoxil (ADV) 10 mg in HBeAg+ chronic hepatitis B (CHB) patients: increasing serologic, virologic and biochemical response over time. Hepatology 2004; 40(suppl1):A655.

86. Hadziyannis S, Tassopoulos N, Heathcote E, et al. Long-term (96 weeks) adefovir dipivoxil in HBeAg negative chronic hepatitis results in significant virological, biochemical and histological improvement. Hepatology 2003; 38(suppl1):273A.

87. Hadziyannis S, Tassoupoulos N, Chang TT, et al. Long-term adefovir treatment induces regression of liver fibrosis in patients with HBeAg-negative chronic hepatitis B: results after 5 years of therapy. Hepatology 2005; 42(suppl1):754A.

88. Qi X, Snow A, Thibault V, et al. Long-term incidence of adefovir, dipivoxil (ADV) resistance in chronic hepatitis B (CHB) patients after 144 weeks of therapy. J Hepatol 2004; 40(suppl 1):A57.

89. Gish RG, Chang TT, DeMan RA, et al. Entecavir results in substantial virologic and biochemical improvement and HBeAg seroconversion through 96 weeks of treatment in HBeAg(+) chronic hepatitis B patients (Study ETv-022). Hepatology 2005; 42:267A.

90. Lai CL, Chang TT, Chao YC, et al. Continued virologic and biochemical improvement through 96 weeks of entecavir treatment in HBeAg(−) chronic hepatitis B patients (Study ETV-027), 16th Conference of the Asian Pacific Association for the Study of the Liver, March 5–8, 2006, Manila, Philippines.

91. Sherman M, Martin P, Lee WA, et al. Entecavir results in continued virologic and biochemical improvement and HBeAg seroconversion through 96 weeks of treatment in lamivudine-refractory, HBeAg(+) chronic hepatitis B patients (ETV-026. Digestive Disease Week 2006, May 14–19, Chicago, IL (accepted as oral presentation).

92. Colonno R, Rose R, Levine S, et al. Entecavir two year resistance update: no resistance observed in nucleoside naïve patients and low frequency resistance emergence in lamivudine refractory patients. Hepatology 2005; 452 (Suppl1):573A.

93. The EASL Jury. EASL International Consensus Conference on Hepatitis B, 13–14 September, 2002, Geneva, Switzerland. Consensus statement (short version). J Hepatol 2003; 38:533–540.

94. Liaw YF, Leung N, Guan R, et al. Asian-Pacific consensus statement on the management of chronic hepatitis B: a 2005 update. Liver Internat 2005; 25:472–489.

95. Micromedex. Available: http://www.thomsonhc.com

96. Lunn RM, Zhang YJ, Wang LY, et al. p53 Mutations, chronic hepatitis B infection, and alphatoxin exposure in hepatocellular carcinoma in Taiwan. Cancer Research 1997; 57:3471–3477.

97. Mandelbrot, Peytavin G, Firtion G, et al. Maternal – fetal transfer and amniotic fluid accumulation of lamivudine in human immunodeficiency virus – infected pregnant women. Am J Obstet Gynecol 2001; 184(2):153–158.

98. Antiretroviral Pregnancy Registry Interim Report: http://www.apregistry.com

99. Lai GL, Gane E, Liaw YF, et al. Telbivudine (LdT) vs Lamivudine for chronic Hepatitis B: first-year results from the international phase III globe trial (Abs). Hepatology 2005; 42(suppl):748A.

100. Lai CL, Gane E, Hsu CW, et al. Two-year results from the Globe Trial in patients with hepatitis B: greater clinical and antiviral efficacy for Telbivudine (LdT) vs Lamivudine (Abs). Hepatology 2006; 44(suppl):222A.

CHAPTER 24

# HIV Infection

Sondra S. Crosby, Linda A. Piwowarczyk,
and Ellen R. Cooper

## Introduction

Little published information is available to inform the best model of care for human immunodeficiency virus (HIV) type 1-infected immigrants in the United States. Some of the issues that make caring for immigrants with HIV especially challenging include: the impact of immigration law and its implications for HIV counseling and testing; cultural beliefs relating to general healthcare; gender dynamics; use of interpreters when dealing with sensitive issues; stigma regarding HIV; and widespread misinformation concerning HIV pathogenesis and current treatment possibilities. This chapter will address those issues related to HIV infection that are unique to immigrants, but is not intended to provide comprehensive information about management of HIV infection. Readers are referred to other comprehensive sources or local experts for this information.

## Background

Many immigrants to the United States come from countries with a high seroprevalence of HIV, including those in Africa, Asia, and Eastern Europe. There are few data concerning the prevalence of HIV infection among specific immigrant populations residing in the US since The Centers for Disease Control and Prevention (CDC) report surveillance data by race and ethnicity only, rather than by country of origin. Regional and state-specific data, however, reveal that immigrant communities are disproportionately affected by the HIV/AIDS epidemic. People born outside of the United States are estimated to make

up 12% of the general population of Massachusetts, yet of the 15 289 people living with HIV/AIDS in that state at the end of 2004, 2699 (18%) were foreign born. Twenty-six percent of those newly diagnosed and 41% of newly diagnosed females in 2004 were foreign born. In addition, the proportion of non-US-born individuals among annual AIDS diagnoses in Massachusetts increased from 9% in 1994 to 29% in 2003.[1] The incidence of HIV/AIDS has also been reported to be increasing among Minnesota's African-born communities. Less than 1% of Minnesota's population is African-born, yet in 2004 19% of newly reported cases of HIV were among African-born individuals. Actual numbers may be higher, as fear and stigma prevent many individuals from being tested.[2] As demonstrated by the above statistics, immigrants from countries with higher prevalence of HIV infection may have a large impact on healthcare systems, especially when they settle in states with a relatively low prevalence of HIV infection, such as Minnesota. The effect of immigration on prevalence of HIV infection within communities in the US is important to consider when strategizing AIDS services at local levels.

Hispanics living in the US are also affected disproportionately by HIV/AIDS. Although Hispanics made up 14% of the population of the United States through 2002, they accounted for more than 18% of AIDS cases since the beginning of the epidemic.[3] At the end of 2004, Hispanics accounted for 17% of all people in the United States living with HIV/AIDS in the 35 areas with confidential name-based HIV infection reporting since 2000, and accounted for 20% of persons in the United States living with AIDS.[4] Risk factors for HIV may vary with country of origin for Hispanics living in the US. Sexual contact among men is the primary cause of HIV infections among men born in Mexico and Central/South America. Hispanic women are most likely to be infected with HIV as a result of sex with men. Social and behavioral factors driving the HIV epidemic in Hispanic communities include poverty, denial, substance abuse, and sexually transmitted diseases.[3]

There are no data concerning the prevalence of HIV infection in asylees or asylum seekers, since HIV testing is not required as part of the asylum process.

## Immigration Law and HIV

The basic body of United States immigration law is contained in the Immigration and Nationality Act.[5] In 1993, the Immigration and Naturalization Act required testing, and specifically barred individuals with HIV from admission to the United States. In 1999, the policy was revised, and HIV-infected refugees were allowed to enter the US with a waiver. Waivers are available to refugees entering the US, as well as for asylees and individuals who are the parent, spouse, or unmarried child of a US citizen or lawful permanent resident (LPR). The number of refugees that have entered the US through this waiver program remains small: 179 in 2000, 323 in 2001, 33 in 2002, 98 in 2003, and 360 in 2004 (personal communication, Department of State, Bureau of Population, Migration and Refugees).

Asylum may be claimed because of persecution based on belonging to a social group. In 1996, the INS officially stated that: 'Aliens with HIV who are seeking asylum or withholding of deportation may be able to qualify for recognition as members of a "particular social group" if the evidence in the individual case supports such a conclusion.' Clinicians may be asked to provide documentation of their positive HIV status or evidence of mental or physical sequelae of torture in the form of an affidavit as part of the applicant's asylum application. Further information regarding clinician advocacy and the writing of medical and psychological affidavits has been published previously by Physicians for Human Rights.[6] Information on the preparation of the clinician as an expert witness in immigration court can be found on the Boston Center for Refugee Health and Human Rights website.[7]

Further details on the Immigration and Naturalization Act can be found at the United States Citizenship and Immigration Services website: http://www. uscis.gov/portal/site/uscis Professionals familiar with these rules and regulations should be consulted as necessary for advocacy.

## Eligibility to enter the US and risk for deportation

HIV infection is a reason for inadmissibility to the United States, with the exception of the waiver program discussed above. INA Sec 237(a) (1) (A) makes individuals deportable if they were 'inadmissible at the time of entry;' hence if someone was inadmissible for having HIV/AIDS at the time of entry, she or he is also deportable. An immigrant who has entered the US unlawfully after April 1, 1997, can be removed for being HIV infected. Public charge is also a deportation ground, so if someone becomes a public charge by virtue of receiving benefits for HIV/AIDS treatment within 5 years of entry, that person is deportable (INA 237 (a) (5). It is understandable, therefore, that fear of deportation may discourage undocumented immigrants from being tested or treated for HIV (Box 24.1).

## Eligibility to gain legal status

Except for refugees who have undergone HIV testing prior to entering the country, noncitizens applying for lawful permanent residency in the US must be tested for HIV. Those who do not qualify for a waiver and are found to be HIV infected may risk deportation. The type of waiver an applicant must obtain

---

**Box 24.1**

**Case study 1**

**A 37-year-old woman who has been tortured is seeking political asylum.**

She is extremely paranoid, which worsened after the events of September 11, 2001. She does not want to fill out any personal information on registration forms or free care forms. She does not pick up her HIV medications in the pharmacy because she has heard in her community that the INS is monitoring pharmacy records.

The belief that health professionals report to the Immigration Service may be held by many individuals in immigrant communities. Specific education about the confidentiality of health and pharmacy records and the lack of reporting of health information to Immigration may be needed in order to avoid potential interruption of HIV treatment.

depends on the status for which the applicant is applying. Because of the complexity of immigration law for individuals with HIV, referral to an immigration expert is recommended.

The requirements for HIV-infected noncitizens to obtain legal permanent residence include a three-part waiver, as well as overcoming the immigration law 'public charge' condition. The three parts to the waiver stipulate: minimal danger to public health, minimal possibility of the spread of HIV, and no cost to the government agency without that agency's consent. To overcome the minimal danger to public health requirement, a medical clinician may be asked to provide documentation that the applicant understands prevention of HIV transmission, and is not a public health threat in the clinician's opinion. The waiver may also require a statement of consent from the local or state health department accepting care for the applicant. A noncitizen who becomes primarily dependent on the government for subsistence is a public charge. Noncitizens 'who are likely at any time to become a public charge' are inadmissible, and this can present a real obstacle. This may require an affidavit of support from a sponsor/family member and proof of medical insurance or adequate resources to pay for projected medical care costs. A distinction of some import is that the use of public benefits does not in and of itself constitute becoming a public charge, and DHS considers all circumstances in such cases. This is relevant to applicants with HIV infection, because of the projected costs of lifelong medical care. Since 1999, DHS eliminated the public charge criteria for HIV-infected refugees, and asylees should be entitled to the same benefits as refugees. This is not, however, clearly stated in the law, and expert advocacy assistance may be needed in such situations. In spite of the fact that asylees and refugees with HIV do not have to overcome the public charge element, they must still apply for a waiver when applying to become lawful permanent residents

Clinicians should encourage HIV-positive asylum applicants to discuss their HIV status with their immigration attorney, who might be better positioned to decide if HIV status is relevant to the asylum case. It has been documented by the Boston Center for Refugee Health and Human Rights that stigma and fear of repercussions have in the past prevented this information from being shared with immigration attorneys, even when it might have benefited the asylum claim.

Additional sources of information about HIV and immigration law include: http://www.national immigrationproject.org/HIVPage/HIVPage.html and

National Immigration Project of the National Lawyers Guild, 14 Beacon Street, Suite 602, Boston, MA 02108 (617) 227-9727 http://www.nationalimmigrationproject.org

## HIV Counseling and Testing of Immigrants

### Preconceived beliefs regarding HIV

Education about health in general and HIV in particular is crucial and should be individualized for each patient during the process of HIV counseling and testing. In some cases, this may take considerable time, and occur over many visits, once trust has been established and other basic needs met.

Beliefs as to the causes of HIV may need to be explored in order to gain an understanding of the patient. Kalichman and Simbaya studied the associations between the belief that AIDS is caused by spirits, AIDS-related knowledge, and AIDS-related stigmas in South Africa.[8] The results of this study showed that people who believed HIV/AIDS is caused by spirits had more misinformation about AIDS and were more likely to endorse repulsion and stigmatizing beliefs about people with AIDS. This association, however, was not significant when knowledge about AIDS was included as a variable, suggesting that AIDS-related traditional beliefs and stigmas are mediated by knowledge.

Preconceived beliefs about HIV are not limited to immigrants, but identifying and addressing these beliefs may be complicated by discordance in culture between health professional and patient and exaggerated further by language barriers. Some of these beliefs include: medications 'cure' the virus; HIV is a death sentence (many have witnessed family and friends who have died from AIDS); without symptoms, one cannot be ill and cannot transmit the virus; HIV can be transmitted by handling money or by touching an infected person; and those with HIV cannot legally marry or have children. Discussions about HIV may call attention to cultural taboos such as premarital sex, rape, homosexuality, or injection drug use. Disclosure of HIV infection which may have occurred as a result of these situations may be very difficult to elicit.

Cultural beliefs and taboos may impair implementation of risk-reduction behaviors. Use of condoms or other forms of birth control may not be culturally acceptable. Virility may be linked to manhood and sense of self-worth. Insistence of condom use may indicate to a partner that one is HIV

---

**Box 24.2**

**Case study 2**

**A 21-year-old male refugee has had a marriage arranged for him by his family, who raised a bridal payment of 100 cattle.**

He is to return to Sudan for the wedding, and is concerned about condom use. Condoms are not used in his village. His wife and family will not approve, and think something is wrong.

Safe sexual practices and condom use require dedicated time to education and counseling in a way that is nonjudgmental and respectful. It can be helpful to use examples that are understandable in a patient's cultural context. For young men, the idea of protecting women from harm may be helpful. It is critically important to target men for HIV education, as in some cultures women have limited decision-making power in the sexual relationship.

---

**Box 24.3**

**Case study 3**

**A 35-year-old man from Africa is married and has five children ranging in age from 2 to 14. He has not disclosed his HIV status to his wife and is evasive about condom use.**

When counseled about protection and getting his wife and children tested, he changes his family's healthcare to a different hospital.

This case underscores some of the challenges involved in protecting sexual partners from HIV transmission and addressing the healthcare needs of children of HIV-infected individuals. The process of developing trust in order to provide reassurance about confidentiality may be a lengthy one, requiring nonjudgmental support from the healthcare team.

---

positive and may trigger domestic violence. In some cultures, women may not hold decision-making power in the sexual relationship (Box 24.2). Tomkins et al surveyed an immigrant and refugee Sudanese population in Nebraska about HIV knowledge, attitudes and beliefs about HIV, as well as risk behavior. Their results demonstrated that a significant number of this population are poorly educated about HIV, and exhibit attitudes and beliefs about HIV/AIDS that may increase risk for disease and create barries to provision of care, and engage in high risk sexual behavior.[9]

## Barriers to HIV testing

Foley[10] published a qualitative study describing the experience of African immigrants and HIV/AIDS in Philadelphia. Barriers to HIV testing and treatment that African women faced included legal status, linguistic barriers, fear of the American health system, and misunderstandings about modes of transmission of HIV and antiretroviral treatment. Lack of disclosure to partners and social risks associated with disclosure were main themes. Privacy and confidentiality were more important to African immigrant women than overall health status. Through interviews with African women, these investigators found that African women have limited power to negotiate condom use or testing of partners. Service providers reported frustration and insufficient resources to care adequately for this population. These findings underscore the need for culturally appropriate HIV education for African immigrants.

Additional resources may be needed if these needs are to be addressed adequately.

Other examples of barriers to acceptance of HIV testing include stigma and fear of being ostracized by families and communities, fear of deportation, or the belief that a diagnosis itself will lead to illness. Liddicoat et al. characterized reasons for refusal of HIV testing at an HIV testing program in four Massachusetts urgent-care centers. Non-English-speaking patients who were Hispanic, Haitian, or 'other' were more likely to refuse HIV testing than their English-speaking counterparts. Immigration concerns, and/or language barriers in the HIV counseling and testing process could have contributed to the higher levels of HIV test refusal among the non-English-speakers in this study.[11] When counseling undocumented immigrants to undergo HIV testing in the clinical setting, it is important to reassure them of confidentiality, and provide assurance that test results will not be reported to immigration officials. The CDC now recommends HIV testing for patients in all healthcare settings, unless the patient declines ('opt out' screening[12]), and it is hoped that the stigma of merely being asked to test will eventually diminish (Box 24.3).

## Approach to counseling

The procedures used in the counseling and testing of immigrants for HIV should be the same as those for any US-born individual, but complicating factors should be considered. There are specific challenges to be addressed when caring for immigrant patients that go well beyond those related to privacy and immigration issues.

Developing trust with foreign-born patients is essential for the development of a therapeutic alliance in which frank discussion of HIV infection is possible. This can be a difficult process for those who have suffered trauma and betrayal, and may require extra time, much effort, empathy, and respect. HIV pretest counseling may be time consuming, requiring an individualized exploration of each patient's beliefs and knowledge about HIV. It must include an awareness of the individual's potential fear of stigmatization in their families and/or communities. It is also important to be aware that talking about HIV may elicit painful recollections of family or friends who have died from HIV. Providers should be aware of some patients' concerns regarding meeting another individual from their country in the waiting room of an HIV Clinic. A person's frame of reference may be that HIV-infected friends or family members were ostracized or expelled by families and the community. Spending time explaining confidentiality is critical to relationship building.

Talking about HIV may also trigger memories or flashbacks of violence in patients who may have been exposed to HIV in the context of torture.[13]

## Situations where testing should be prioritized

In general, testing for HIV is important, although seldom an emergency. There are, however, certain exceptions to this that should be recognized. Because of the current ability to reduce significantly the risk of perinatal transmission of HIV to infants, pregnant women should be prioritized for HIV testing. Appropriate referrals for prophylactic antiretroviral medication and planning for mode of delivery and infant feeding should be implemented as soon as possible. Referral to a center expert in the care of the HIV-infected pregnant woman is advisable.[12] In addition, mothers who recently delivered and are still breastfeeding their infants should also be prioritized for testing since duration of breastfeeding remains an important risk factor in the transmission of the virus from mother to baby. Other individuals for whom HIV testing should be obtained as early as feasible are those who may be experiencing a seroconversion illness. Symptoms of viral illness including headache, fever, lymphadenopathy, and pharyngitis within 2 months (average 2–3 weeks) after an exposure should alert the provider to this possibility.[15] Testing for HIV during seroconversion requires simultaneous antibody as well as specialized viral load testing, and consultation with experts may be

beneficial when interpreting the results. Diagnosis of acute HIV seroconversion is of paramount importance since prompt antiretroviral therapy during this time has been shown to have a beneficial effect on the long-term outcome of infection.[16–19]

Other immigrants for whom special consideration to early testing should be given are infants and young children. Children experience a much more rapid disease progression compared to adults, and statistics in Africa and other resource-limited areas document a 50% mortality by age 2 years, with a 75% mortality by 3 years of age unless appropriate management and treatment are instituted. This underscores the importance of early testing and evaluation for eligibility for antiretrovirals and prophylactic medications. Referral to specialists in the care of the pediatric patient may be necessary for both testing and treatment, since antibody testing cannot be relied upon under the age of 18 months, and qualitative DNA PCR testing may be required.

## Other testing considerations for the HIV-infected immigrant

### Non-B clades of HIV

HIV-1 can be divided into a number of clades which broadly represent families of viral types. Clade B is by far the most common clade seen in the US, but other clades may be more common in other parts of the world. Non-B clades of HIV may be present in immigrants from Africa and Asia, and viral load testing might not be accurate on standard Amplicor assays for HIV RNA often used in the US, resulting in underestimation of true viral load. Testing for non-B clades should be considered in appropriate immigrant populations when clinically indicated, such as when viral load is unexpectedly low given clinical manifestations, or when CD4 lymphocyte counts decrease in the face of 'undetectable' viral RNA levels.[20,21]

### HIV-2

HIV-2 infection is uncommon in the United States, but testing for HIV-2 should be considered in certain immigrant populations. HIV-2 is found predominantly in West Africa. As of mid-2006, West African nations with a prevalence of HIV-2 of more than 1% in the general population are Cape Verde, Côte d'Ivoire, Gambia, Guinea-Bissau, Mali, Mauritania, Nigeria, Sierra Leone, Angola, and Mozambique. Other West African countries reporting HIV-2, but at a lower prevalence, are Benin, Burkina Faso, Ghana, Guinea, Liberia, Niger, São Tomé, Senegal, and Togo.[22] In some areas, the testing for HIV-2 is incorporated into the routine screening of all patients. Where testing for HIV-2 is not included routinely, it should be requested specifically when suspected.

HIV-2 is transmitted by the same routes as HIV-1, though the efficiency of transmission is lower than that of HIV-1, probably due to a lower viral load in most infected individuals.[23] The clinical manifestations of HIV-2 are similar to those of HIV-1, though disease progression is much slower.[24] Some differences in disease manifestations have been observed. In the Côte d'Ivoire, encephalitis was shown at autopsy to occur more frequently in individuals with HIV-2-related cause of death compared to those with HIV-1 (18% versus <1%).[25] Kaposi's sarcoma has been observed to occur less often in HIV-2 versus HIV-1 infected Gambians.[24] It is important to note that some patients may be coinfected with HIV-1 and HIV-2, and generally these have a more rapid progression.

## Medical Care of HIV-Infected Immigrants

### Medical care may require more than medicine

The Boston Center for Refugee Health and Human Rights (BCRHHR) conducted a needs assessment to gain understanding of the healthcare needs of this vulnerable population. Respondents included a BCRHHR case manager, a psychiatrist with HIV/AIDS agencies, resettlement staff, health providers, mutual assistance association leaders, and case managers in the Boston area who have served refugees, including those who are HIV positive. Results indicated that after arrival in the US, immigrants are confronted with a number of competing priorities including hunger, lack of safe housing or appropriate clothing, safety, and challenges related to acculturation. Individuals who arrive without their families face some of the most difficult situations; the pain and anxiety of being separated from children may be of great concern, and there may be pressure to send financial support to family members who remain in the country of origin. HIV diagnosis and medical care may not seem like a high priority when compared to these other issues. Healthcare professionals taking care of immigrants must be able to assess these priorities in order to achieve optimal success with engaging the patient in HIV care.

### Optimizing care

Published literature suggests that minority populations in the United States have not enjoyed equal benefit from highly active antiretroviral therapy (HAART), in terms of improved outcomes and decreased mortality from HIV/AIDS, as have nonminority populations. There is a higher HIV-related death rate in minorities, and HIV infection is reported to be a major cause of decreased life expectancy in minorities.[4,26] In addition, minority patients in the US are less satisfied with their HIV care than nonminority patients.[27] It is reported that minorities have a longer delay after diagnosis until receipt of care, and once into care, they are still less likely to receive HAART than nonminority patients.[28–30] Although these studies invariably include immigrants, there are no stratified data that compare outcomes of HIV treatment in immigrants to nonimmigrants in the US. Clinicians and researchers working in settings where immigrants with HIV are cared for will need to develop methods of data collection and analysis in order to broaden descriptions of health disparities in HIV care and inform programs to address these disparities.

### Obtaining a history

Medical history should include careful inquiry about antiretroviral exposure prior to arriving in the United States, and possibly knowledge of commonly available antiretrovirals in the country of origin. History of opportunistic infections (OIs) or treatment of OIs should be sought, as this will help determine urgency for antiretrovirals and will help direct choice of regimen and prophylaxis. Patients should be asked about history of hepatitis or jaundice, as hepatitis B is endemic in many countries and coinfection with hepatitis B or C has important implications for treatment. History should also include past history of tuberculosis and treatment. Any traditional treatments or medications should be recorded. Additional history should include trauma, childbearing history, whether or not children have been tested, methods of birth control used, and disclosure to spouses or sexual partners. A full mental health history is also important to obtain, and is discussed more fully later in this chapter.

### Baseline testing in HIV-infected immigrants

Screening of immigrants with HIV infection presenting for medical care should include standard screening recommended in newly diagnosed HIV infection, plus screening specific to immigrants. Resources for baseline testing in newly diagnosed HIV infection have been published widely,[31] and include those available from the Infectious Disease Society of America Guidelines,[32] and the Department of Health and Human Services Guidelines for the Use of Antiretroviral Agents in HIV-1-Infected Adults and Adolescents.[19]

Screening of new immigrants is discussed in Chapter 12. Few studies of results of screening tests of new immigrants stratify results by HIV status. A single small study described a cohort of 34 HIV-infected refugees and identified 15 (44%) with positive tuberculin skin test, 15 (47%) with positive toxoplasma antibodies, 7 (28%) with intestinal parasites, 31 (97%) with positive hepatitis A IgG antibodies, 22 (67%) with positive hepatitis B core or surface antibodies, 4 (12%) with positive hepatitis C

antibodies, and 1 (3%) with positive rapid plasma reagent.[33]

Recommended screening tests in newly diagnosed HIV infection in immigrants compared with those for non-HIV-infected immigrants are included in Table 24.1. HIV serology should be repeated and verified when patients come into care with positive tests from outside the US, as these tests are generally limited to antibody tests and may represent screening without Western blot confirmation. Additional testing related to HIV should include CD4 lymphocyte count and percentage, HIV viral load, and viral resistance testing per current standard recommendations using either genotype or phenotype methodology if available.[19,34] Although surveillance data about prevalence of drug-resistant virus by geographic region are not available, there are reports of highly resistant virus in immigrants, even without prior antiretroviral therapy. Some patients may have

**Table 24.1 Screening tests in HIV-infected immigrants**

| Test | Standard HIV screening | Standard immigrant screening | Comments |
|---|---|---|---|
| HIV serology | X | X | Confirmation of overseas exam |
| CD4 and percentage | X | | |
| Plasma HIV RNA | X | | |
| HIV resistance testing | X | | Per current standards |
| PPD | X | X | Unless known to be PPD positive |
| CXR | X | If clinically indicated or if + PPD | |
| RPR or VDRL | X | X | False positives may occur in HIV infection, need confirmatory test |
| Hepatitis B serology | X | X | |
| Hepatitis A and C serology | X | When indicated according to standard recommendations | |
| CBC with differential | X | X | Evaluate for concomitant parasitic infections in patients with eosinophilia |
| Chemistry panel LFTs | X | | |
| PAP smear | X | X | After appropriate preparation for pelvic examination |
| Toxoplasmosis serology | X | | |
| Stool for ova and parasites | X | X | |
| G6PD | X | When indicated clinically or by race/ethnicity | |
| Cytomegalovirus (by serology or culture) | X | | |

been on antiretroviral therapy, but with medications in inconsistent supply. This produces viral pressure towards the development of resistance.

All new immigrants should be tested for tuberculosis with a tuberculin skin test or other approved test if available. A positive test for tuberculosis is ≥5 mm of induration for HIV-infected individuals. Those with signs or symptoms consistent with tuberculosis should receive a diagnostic evaluation that is appropriate for the clinical situation. If negative, the PPD should be repeated annually. In those coinfected with HIV, there is a high rate of reactivation of 5–10% per year. In addition, there are high rates of primary tuberculosis and high rates of drug resistance.[35] Persons with latent or active TB should be referred for treatment. A chest radiograph is indicated routinely in HIV-infected patients for detection of asymptomatic tuberculosis and to serve as a baseline study, especially before antiretroviral therapy is initiated, since immune reconstitution inflammatory syndrome in the setting of untreated tuberculosis can be life threatening.[36]

A screening serologic test for syphilis is recommended with VDRL or reactive plasma reagin (RPR),[37] with confirmatory testing of positive samples with FTA-ABS or other similar test.[38] False-positive and false-negative tests may be more likely in HIV-infected individuals.

Screening for hepatitis B should include testing for hepatitis B surface antigen, surface antibody, and core antibody.[39] The CDC recommends postvaccination serology for anti-HBsAg at 1–6 months after the final dose of hepatitis B vaccine in patients with HIV infection to assess response. Testing for hepatitis A and C is important, as those without antibody to hepatitis A can be immunized, and identifying hepatitis C infection is important because of the interaction of hepatitis C and HIV and the need for specialized monitoring and care for these patients.

A complete blood count will identify lymphopenia or neutropenia, anemia, thrombocytopenia, and eosinophilia. Eosinophilia is common in persons with HIV infection, and in immigrants parasitic infection is a likely cause. It has also been associated with eosinophilic folliculitis, atopic dermatitis, and prurigo nodularis in those with HIV, and may be a marker of advanced HIV disease.[40] The differential diagnosis of eosinophilia in immigrants with HIV/AIDs may be particularly challenging and should include investigation for concomitant parasitic diseases, such as strongyloidiasis, schistosomiasis, or filariasis. This requires knowledge of parasites specific to the country of origin and intermediate countries prior to arrival to the United States. Kaminsky et al. reported that of

133 HIV-infected individuals in Honduras, 67% were coinfected with pathogenic and nonpathogen parasites, including *Trichuris trichiura*, *Ascaris lumbricoides*, hookworm, and *Strongyloides stercoralis*.[41]

Toxoplasma serology is indicated routinely in the initial screening of HIV-infected individuals to identify those in need of prophylaxis and should prompt preventive counseling for seronegative patients.[42] Cytomegalovirus (CMV) serology or viral urine culture, though not recommended routinely for non-HIV-infected immigrants, is recommended for those with HIV to detect latent CMV infection that may become clinically significant with worsening immunosuppression or during the period of immune reconstitution.[39]

All patients should be screened for glucose-6-phosphate dehydrogenase (G6PD) deficiency, since this may be more clinically significant in HIV infection because of depressed bone marrow reserve and preexisting anemia. In addition, drugs commonly used during the care of the infected individual such as sulfonamides, dapsone, and primaquine may cause hemolysis in the setting of G6PD deficiency.[43]

Papanicolaou screening is recommended in all women soon after their initial evaluation. This may be challenging for providers of new immigrants, since some immigrant women have never had vaginal or pelvic examinations, and may not understand the rationale for such exams. Special sensitivity may be required when examining women who have experienced sexual trauma and/or rape. In accordance with the Agency for Health Care Policy and Research, the PAP smear should be performed twice during the first year after diagnosis of HIV infection, and annually thereafter if the results are normal. Cervical squamous intraepithelial lesions are increased 8–10-fold in HIV infection and close follow up is recommended according to the Interim Guidelines for Management of abnormal Cervical Cytology, published by the National Cancer Institute Consensus Panel.[44,45] There are reports of rapidly progressive cervical cancer in women infected with HIV.[46,46a]

## Special psychiatric considerations

Depression is common for those learning of a new diagnosis of HIV[49a], and this may be further exaggerated by the stress of recent immigration. Some immigrants also bear the additional burden of having been tortured. A small study assessing the historical, clinical, and psychological characteristics of a cohort of 34 HIV-infected refugees found that 23 of the 30

(77%) patients who agreed to discuss their trauma history had been tortured according to the definition of the World Medical Association's Declaration of Tokyo. Mechanisms of torture included beatings, threats, use of handcuffs/shackles, forced witnessing of killing, and rape. Fifty-six percent of these individuals were diagnosed with major depression, 32% were diagnosed with post-traumatic stress disorder, and 35% had been exposed to HIV high-risk situations as a result of torture.[33]

Some immigrants are tested for HIV before arrival to the United States and are aware of the diagnosis, but many may first learn of an HIV diagnosis after arrival in the United States. Sadness and anxiety can relate to images of HIV infection from home. Moreover, the decision to come to the United States can also be associated with many losses, including family, occupation, social supports, communities of faith, and that which is familiar. Consequently, it is important to have included questions regarding depressive symptoms in the general history obtained. These include sadness, disturbances of memory and concentration, difficulties of sleep, energy or appetite, guilt feelings, difficulty experiencing pleasure, and suicidal preoccupation or past attempts. It is also important to screen for alcohol or substance abuse, as substance abuse may increase risky sexual behavior. Substance abuse may also be a form of self-medication.[47] In addition, immigrants may be suffering from post-traumatic stress disorder, other anxiety disorders, mood disorders, psychotic symptoms, or cognitive impairment.

Refugees and asylum seekers have fled their countries due to persecution or fear of persecution on the basis of race, religion, nationality, political opinion, or membership in a particular social group. It is important to ask about trauma exposure using a chronological approach: events during the country of origin, during flight, within a refugee camp or country of first asylum, and since living in the United States. Psychological consequences of torture can include depressive and anxiety symptoms, depression, bipolar disorder, cognitive problems, and psychotic symptoms.[48] Although many survivors are resilient, being exposed to torture or trauma can place someone at risk for development of mental health symptoms that compound the difficulty of coping with an HIV diagnosis.

Because immigrants may be reluctant to seek care from mental health professionals due to perceptions of stigma associated with mental illness, HIV providers may be required to provide mental health treatment. In some cultures, disclosure of personal information to a stranger may be culturally foreign or taboo. In many societies, there are family and community solutions to dealing with emotional distress such as working things out with the rest of the family, the use of traditional healers, spiritual healers, herbal remedies, and the traditional role of elders. It should also be remembered that people may come from countries in which limited words exist to describe emotional experience. Various beliefs about causality of mental health symptoms must be taken into account. The presence of somatic symptoms may be indicative of underlying emotional distress. It is also necessary to be knowledgeable about the idioms of distress present in other cultures. Sometimes, patients do not make the connection between how they are currently feeling and the difficult things they have passed through. The use of screening tools can be used, though with the awareness that they require cross-cultural validity, and cannot be purely translated and back-translated.

As noted in the Practice Guideline for the Treatment of Patients with HIV/AIDS by the American Psychiatric Association (APA) (2000),[49] there are unique treatment issues with HIV patients including: disclosure of HIV status; assessment of danger of HIV transmission and risk reduction; legacy planning for familes with dependent children; treatment of HIV-infected children who have developmental delays resulting from prenatal drug exposure or from HIV infection; negotiating disability status and, for some patients, returning to work; bereavement and loss; and treatment adherence.

The APA notes that people with HIV infection have higher rates of most psychiatric conditions when compared with the general population. They suggest using similar principles as when working with the elderly or patients with comorbid illness. Psychiatric disorders increase the risk of acquiring HIV as well as increasing its morbidity by diminishing treatment.[50]

Certain medications used to treat HIV have similar effects on the cytochrome P450 metabolic system as some psychotropic medications. When using psychotropics, the APA suggests to: (1) use starting doses and slowly titrate; (2) simplify dosing regimens as much as possible; (3) focus on side effect profiles; and (4) maintain awareness of drug metabolism and clearance. Drug–drug interactions may affect levels of psychotropic effectiveness, and also reduce the antiviral effectiveness by reducing levels.[49,49a] It is important to consult with an HIV specialist and pharmacist as drug regimens continue to evolve, as good communication between providers is key to provision of excellent care across disciplines (Box 24.4).

**Box 24.4**

**Case study 4**

A 39-year-old woman with neurovegetative symptoms and disabling PTSD symptoms refuses a mental health referral or pharmacologic therapy because she is 'not crazy.' She does not want to use the hospital's Arabic interpreter, because he is in her community and goes to her mosque.

This case highlights the potential stigma of mental health diagnoses and treatment, underscores the need of primary care providers to be equipped to treat mental health disorders in the primary care setting, and the importance of a multidisciplinary team approach. It can be helpful in some situations for the mental health provider to see the patient in the primary care clinic setting. Concerns by patients when needing to use an interpreter can sometimes be alleviated by using an anonymous phone interpreter, and assuring the patient that the interpreter is part of a national interpreter bank and so is unlikely to be from the patient's state or community.

**Box 24.5**

**Case study 5**

A 20-year-old male refugee becomes angry during a clinic visit after he is told he doesn't need HIV medications because of his high absolute CD4 count and low viral load. He accuses the provider of withholding medications because he is African. The interpreter explains that the patient thinks the medications can 'cure' HIV.

This illustrates the critical need to explore each patient's baseline beliefs and knowledge about HIV and treatment, and to work with patients from an individual vantage point to develop a successful treatment plan. Patients may have unrealistic expectations about treatment, or may believe that treatment is being withheld because they are immigrants.

## Immunizations in HIV-infected immigrants

The United States Public Health Service and the Infectious Disease Society of America published recommendations for immunization of those infected with HIV.[51] Need for immunizations should be addressed early. In general, better immunological responses are achieved when the vaccines are administered early after infection when immune function is relatively preserved (in those whose CD4 lymphocyte count is >200 cells/$\mu$L). Efficacy is less with advanced immunosuppression when humoral response may be impaired. Most live virus vaccines can be administered safely to HIV-infected individuals who are not severely immunocompromised.[52] Immunizations for immigrants are discussed in detail in Chapter 13. Differences in immunization recommendations for HIV-infected immigrants include the additional recommendation of pneumococcal immunization in all age groups, annual influenza vaccine, hepatitis A vaccine if not already immune, and the precautions associated with live virus vaccines in immunosuppressive states. Current CDC recommendations can be found at http://www.cdc.gov/nip/recs/adult-specinfo.htm and http://www.cdc.gov/nip/recs/adult-schedule.pdf

Guidelines for the immunization of children with HIV differ from those of adults, as do the risks for various vaccine-preventable diseases. Routine child-hood and catch-up immunizations are discussed in Chapter 13; consultation with experts in the care of pediatric HIV may be helpful in specific situations when interpretation of the child's level of immune suppression is needed.

## Antiretroviral therapy

Antiretroviral (ARV) treatment should follow current guidelines.[19] For infected adults, experts recommend therapy for all patients with a history of an AIDS-defining illness regardless of absolute CD4 lymphocyte cell count, and patients with absolute CD4 lymphocyte counts below 200 cells/mm[19]. The decision to treat asymptomatic patients with absolute CD4 lymphocyte cell counts between 200 cells/mm$^3$ and 350 cells/mm$^3$ should be considered on an individual basis. It is reasonable to initiate therapy at the upper end of this range if the patient is willing and committed to lifelong adherence.[31,32] Morbidity and mortality are increased, however, when treatment is delayed until absolute CD4 lymphocyte counts drop below 200 cells/mm$^3$.[53,54] There are inconsistent data regarding the benefit of starting treatment before the count falls below 350 cells/mm$^3$ and some experts recommend deferring treatment if the HIV RNA is <100 000 copies/mL of plasma. Treatment may be considered in those with absolute CD4 counts greater than 350 cells/mm$^3$ and plasma HIV RNA >100 000 copies/mL of plasma (Box 24.5).

The criteria for ARV initiation are different in children, and rely more on CD4 percentage than on absolute CD4 count since baseline absolute CD4 cell counts are generally higher in children under the age of 6 years. HIV-infected infants and children ideally should be referred to an expert in pediatric HIV medicine, or managed in collaboration with such experts.[54]

## Medication adherence in the HIV-infected immigrant

A high degree of medication adherence is needed with all ARV regimens to prevent the selection of drug resistance. Successful ARV therapy requires a realistic treatment plan that is understandable and acceptable to the patient given the individual circumstances, and a trusting patient–provider relationship. Language and cultural barriers may present unique challenges, which require increased time and effort on the part of the healthcare team. For example, providers should ensure that patients fully understand the refill process, or whom to call if difficulties arise. For non-English-speaking patients, the plan will need to include a trusted interpreter. For patients with limited English literacy, understandable diagrams or illustrations can be used to explain side effects and indications of when to seek medical care. Patients should be reassured of confidentiality when utilizing the pharmacy. Assessment of readiness to commit to therapy should include reassurance that patients' other priorities are being met, including food, housing, children's needs, legal matters, and potentially discussion about other family members back home who are infected with HIV, and who may not have access to treatment (Box 24.6). In general, ARV care for the recent immigrant should be a collaborative effort on the part of experienced ARV providers and the staff most sensitive to the general issues of the immigrant (Box 24.7).

Many immigrants live with family members or community members who do not know their HIV

---

**Box 24.6**

**Case study 6**

A 30-year-old woman is failing her antiretroviral therapy. It is finally discovered that she is sending a portion of her medications home to a family member who is unable to get therapy for HIV.

It is important to discuss the ramifications of family members back home with HIV who might not have access to treatment, and address the complications of sending medicines home.

---

**Box 24.7**

**Case study 7**

A 22-year-old man from Africa feels that having his blood drawn, as is required frequently to monitor the status of his HIV disease, makes him feel very weak and unable to enjoy playing soccer. He believes giving blood is fundamentally wrong. The subspecialty consultant, who is irritated by the patient's refusal of venipuncture, notifies the primary care doctor that 'the patient is refusing blood drawing and is noncompliant.'

It is important to work with patients and be respectful of cultural beliefs, while providing education to both the patient and others on the healthcare team about factors affecting adherence to recommendations. Arrangements were made to minimize phlebotomy, not schedule blood draws before soccer games, and educate the patient on biomedical theories of blood regeneration.

---

status and may hide their HIV medication from family. It should also be kept in mind that immigrants may work multiple jobs or have rotating shifts. For these reasons, simplified drug regimens are often preferred, and drugs requiring refrigeration may be problematic, since refrigeration may either be unavailable or shared. Efavirenz may cause exacerbation of PTSD,[55] and also should be avoided in women with childbearing potential due to teratogenicity. Adherence counseling and assessment should be done at each visit, and potential problems detected early. Patients should understand that the first antiviral regimen is the best chance for long-term success due to the relative absence of already resistant mutants.[17] In some cases, traditional treatment modalities such as cupping, coining, and Somali black seed can be integrated successfully into treatment plans, and may increase the level of trust between patient and provider.

## Travel preparation for HIV-infected individuals

Travel medicine for immigrants is discussed in Chapter 58; special issues related to HIV-infected travelers are discussed briefly here and are available at: http://www2.ncid.cdc.gov/travel/yb/utils/ybGet.asp?section=special&obj=hivtrav.htm&cssNav=browseoyb[56]

Providing appropriate travel advice to HIV-infected travelers depends on knowledge and understanding of the degree of immunosuppression. Ability to provide live virus vaccines, such as yellow fever vaccine, will depend on the immune status. Risk of food- and water-borne illness is even greater when immune status is compromised; appropriate prophylaxis and teaching about food and water precautions are critical. Antibiotics for presumptive treatment of traveler's diarrhea should be prescribed; the threshold for beginning treatment may be lower in the severely immunocompromised individual. Malaria prophylaxis should be provided as indicated by current recommendations for the specific destination. Malaria in the HIV-infected woman can be very severe. The use of quinidine and quinine are contraindicated in patients on some antiretrovirals such as the protease inhibitors; patients for whom this would be relevant should be counseled about treatment alternatives for malaria and how to advocate for them. As with any traveler, insect bite prevention measures are important and should include a combination of effective insect repellents, bed nets, and window screens or air-conditioned environment.

Infections that may have more severe consequences in immunocompromised individuals include visceral leishmaniasis and some of the inhaled fungal infections.

Other issues to consider in preparing HIV-infected travelers include travel insurance, making sure all medications are available and there is a way to replace medications that might be lost, educating about the fact that some countries may restrict entry of those with HIV infection, and discussing when it is appropriate to seek medical attention during travel.

Legal issues may arise when HIV-infected immigrants travel to either their country of origin or to a third country where family members live. Noncitizens with HIV who wish to travel outside of the United States need to be aware that DHS may try to prevent them from re-entering the country. In general, noncitizens should be referred to an immigration advocate prior to departing, to determine if they might benefit from 'advance parole.' This may prevent problems upon re-entrance to the country.

## Conclusion

A multidisciplinary approach is valuable in addressing the multiple spheres in which the HIV-infected immigrant lives. Providing medical care to HIV-infected immigrants requires not only knowledge of HIV medicine, but also knowledge of tropical medicine, a willingness to explore cultural beliefs, an understanding of mental health issues affecting immigrants and those with HIV, and knowledge of legal issues affecting immigrants with HIV.

## References

1. Commonwealth of Massachusetts Department of Public Health. HIV/AIDS in Massachusetts: an epidemiologic profile FY 2006. Available: http://www.mass.gov/dph/aids
2. A growing crisis: a funder's response to HIV/AIDS in the African community in Minnesota. Available: http://www.phillipsfnd.org/documents/FinalHIVAfricanReport.pdf
3. CDC Division of HIV/AIDS Prevention. HIV/AIDS among Hispanics. Available: http://www.cdc.gov/hiv/resources/Factsheets/PDF/hispanic.pdf
4. Centers for Disease Control and Prevention. HIV/AIDS surveillence report. Available: http://www.cdc.gov/hiv/topics/surveillance/resources/reports/2004report/default.htm
5. United States Citizenship and Immigration Services website. Available: http://uscis.gov/graphics/lawsregs/INA.htm
6. Physicians for Human Rights. Available: http://www.phrusa.org/
7. The Boston Center for Refugee Health and Human Rights. Available: http://www.bcrhhr.org
8. Kalichman SC, Simbayi L. Traditional beliefs about the cause of AIDS and AIDS related stigma in South Africa. AIDS Care 2004; 16:572–580.
9. Tompkins M, Smith L, Jones K, Swindells S. HIV education needs among Sudanese immigrants and refugees in the Midwestern United States. AIDS and Behavior 2006; 10:319–323.
10. Foley EE. HIV/AIDS and African immigrant women in Philadelphia: structural and cultural barriers to care. AIDS Care 2005; 17:1030–1043.
11. Liddicoat RV, Losina E, Kang M, et al. Who refuses HIV testing in an urgent care setting? AIDS Patient Care and STDs 2006; 20:84–92.
12. Revised Recommendations for HIV Testing of Adults, Adolescents, and Pregnant Women in Health Care Settings. MMWR 2006; 55(RR14):1–17 http://www.cdc.gov/mmwr/preview/mmwrhtml/rr5514a1.htm
13. Coping with Traumatic Stress Reactions. U.S. Department of Veteran Affairs. National Center for PTSD. Available: http://www.ncptsd.va.gov/ncmain/ncdocs/fact_shts/fs_coping_stress.html
14. World Health Organization. Prevention of mother-to child transmission of HIV. Available: http://www.who.int/docstore/hiv/PMTCT/001.htm#1.1
15. Schacker T, Collier AC, Hughes J, et al. Clinical and epidemiological features of primary HIV infection. Ann Intern Med 1996; 125:257–264.
16. Pope M, Haase AT. Transmission, acute HIV-1 infection and the quest for strategies to prevent infection. Nature Med 2003; 9:847–852.
17. Quinn TC, Wawer MJ, Serwankambo N, et al. Viral load and heterosexual transmission of human immunodeficiency virus type 1. Rakai Project Study Group. N Engl J Med 2000; 342:921–929.
18. Hecht F, Wang L, Collier A, et al. Outcomes of HAART for acute/early HIV-1 infection after treatment discontinuation. Presented at the 12th Conference on Retroviruses and Opportunistic Infections; 2005. Abstract # 568.
19. Guidelines for the use of antiretroviral agents in HIV-1 infected adults and adolescents. Panel on clinical practices for treatment of HIV-1 infection (Department of Health and Human Services). Available: http://aidsinfo.nih.gov/guidelines/adult/AA

20. Treadwell TL, Fleisher J. Underestimation of HIV-1 plasma viral burden in patients who acquire infection abroad: the experience in a community hospital clinic. Arch Intern Med. 2003; 163:1613–1614.
21. Thomson MM, Najera R. Travel and the introduction of human immunodeficiency virus type 1 non-B subtype genetic forms into Western countries. Clin Infect Dis 2001; 32:1732–1737.
22. CDC Division of HIV/AIDS Prevention. Human immunodeficiency virus type 2. Available: http://www.cdc.gov/hiv/resources/factsheets/hiv2.htm
23. Reeves JD, Doms RW. Human immunodeficiency virus type 2. J Gen Virol 2002; 83:1253–1265.
24. Jaffar S, Grant AD, Whitworth J, et al. The natural history of HIV-1 and HIV-2 infections in adults in Africa: a literature review. Bull World Health Org 2004; 82(6):462–469.
25. Lucas SB, Hounnou A, Peacock C, et al. The mortality and pathology of HIV infection in a West African city. AIDS 1993; 7:1569–1579.
26. Wong MD, Shapiro MF, Boscardin WJ, et al. Contribution of major diseases to disparities in mortality. N Engl J Med 2002; 347:1585–1592.
27. Stone VE, Weissman JS, Cleary P. Satisfaction with ambulatory care of persons with AIDS: predictors of patient ratings of quality. J Gen Intern Med 1995; 10:239–245.
28. Stone VE, Stegar KA, Hirschhorn LR, et al. Access to treatment with protease inhibitor (PI) containing regimens: is it equal for all? [Abstract 42305]. In: Program and abstracts of the 12th International Conference on AIDS (Geneva). Stockholm: International AIDS Society, 1998.
29. Shapiro MF, Morton SC, McCaffrey DF et al. Variations in the care of HIV-infected adults in the United States. JAMA 1999; 281:2305–2315.
30. Turner, BJ, Cunningham WE, Dunan N, et al. Delayed medical care after diagnosis in a US national probability sample of persons infected with HIV. Arch Intern Med 2000; 160:2614–2622.
31. Hammer SM. Management of newly diagnosed HIV infection. N Engl J Med 2005; 353:1702–1710.
32. Aberg JA, Gallant JE, Anderson J, et al. Primary care guidelines for the management of persons infected with human immunodeficiency virus: recommendations of the HIV Medicine Association of the Infectious Diseases Society of America. Clin Infect Dis 2004; 39:609–629.
33. Moreno A, Crosby S, LaBelle C, et al. Health assessment of HIV infected refugees. J Acquir Immune Defic Syndr 2003; 34:251–254.
34. Hirsch MS, Brun-Vezinet F, Clotet B, et al. Antiviral drug resistance testing in adults infected with human immunodeficiency virus type 1: 2003 recommendations of an International AIDS Society-USA Panel. Clin Infect Dis 2003; 37:113–128.
35. Markowitz N, Hansen NI, Hopewell PC, et al. Incidence of tuberculosis in the United States among HIV-infected persons. The Pulmonary Complications of HIV Infections Study Group. Ann Intern Med 1997; 126:123.
36. Breen RA, Smith CJ, Cropley I, et al. Does immune reconstitution syndrome promote active tuberculosis in patients receiving highly active antiretroviral therapy? AIDS 2005; 19:1201–1207.
37. Centers for Disease Control and Prevention. Recommendations for diagnosing and treating syphilis in HIV-infected patients. MMWR 1988; 37:600.
38. Augenbraun MH, DeHovitz JA Feldman J, et al. Biological false positive syphilis test results for women infected with human immunodeficiency virus. Clin Infect Dis 1994; 19:1040.
39. Kaplan JE, Masur H, Holmes KK, et al. USPHS/IDSA guidelines for the prevention of opportunistic infections in persons infected with human immunodeficiency virus: an overview. USPHS/IDSA Prevention of Opportunistic Infections Working Group. Clin Infect Dis 1995; 21 (Suppl 1):S12.
40. Skeist DJ, Keiser P. Clinical significance of eosinophilia in HIV-infected individuals. Am J Med 1997; 102:449–553.
41. Kaminsky RG, Soto RJ, Campa A, et al. Intestinal parasitic infections and eosinophilia in a human immunodeficiency virus positive population in Honduras. Mem Inst Oswaldo Cruz 2004; 99:773–778.
42. Bearman MH, Luft BJ, Remington JS, et al. Prophylaxis for toxoplasmosis in AIDS. Ann Intern Med 1992; 117:163.
43. Beutler E. G6PD deficiency. Blood 1994; 84:3613–3636.
44. Guidelines for the Prevention of Opportunistic Infections Among HIV-Infected Persons – 2002. http://aidsinfo.nih.gov/contentfiles/OIpreventionGL.pdf
45. Kurman RJ, Henson DE, Herbst AL, et al. Interim Guidelines for the management of abnormal cervical cytology. 1992. National Cancer Institute Workshop. JAMA 1999; 281:1822–1829.
46. Maiman M, Tarricone N, Vieira J, et al. Colposcopic evaluation of human immunodeficiency virus-seropositive women. Obstet Gynecol 1991; 78:84.
46a. Vernon SD, Holmes KK, Reeves WC. Human papillomavirus infection and associated disease in persons infected with human immunodeficiency virus. Clin Infect Dis. 1995; 21(Suppl 1):S121–124.
47. Leigh BC, Stall R. Substance use and risky sexual behavior for exposure to HIV. Am Psychologist 1993; 48:1035–1045.
48. The Istanbul Protocol. Available: http://www.physiciansforhumanrights.org/library/istanbul-protocol.html
49. American Psychiatric Association for the Treatment of Patients with HIV/AIDS (2000). Available: http://www.psych.org
49a. American Psychiatric Association. Guideline Watch: Practice Guidelines for the Treatment of Patients with HIV/AIDS. April 2006. http://www.psych.org
50. Angelino AF, Treisman. Management of psychiatric disorders in patients infected with human immunodeficiency virus. Clin Infect Dis 2001; 33:847–856.
51. Centers for Disease Control and Prevention. Guidelines for preventing opportunistic infections among HIV-infected persons; 2002 recommendations of the US Public Health Service and the Infectious Diseases Society of America. MMWR 2002; 51(RR-8):1.
52. Glesby MJ. Immunization during HIV infection. Curr Opin Infect Dis 1998; 11:17.
53. Palella FJ Jr, Deloria-Knoll M, Chmiel JS, et al. Survival benefit of initiating antiretroviral therapy in HIV-infected persons in different CD4+ cell strata. Ann Intern Med 2003; 138:620–626.
54. Sterling TR, Chaisson RE, Keruly J, et al. Improved outcomes with earlier initiation of highly active antiretroviral therapy among human immunodeficiency virus-infected patients who achieve durable virologic suppression: longer follow-up of an observational cohort study. J Infect Dis 2003; 188:1659–1665.
55. Guidelines for the use of anitiretroviral agents in pediatric HIV infection. Available: http://aidsinfo.nih.gov
56. Moreno A, LaBelle C, Samet JH. Recurrence of post-traumatic stress disorder symptoms after initiation of antiretrovirals including efavirenz: A report of two cases. HIV Med 2003; 4:302–304.
57. Centers for Disease Control and Prevention – Yellow Book: [9] The immunocompromised traveler- CDC Travelers' Health, 2005–2006. Available: http://www2.ncid.cdc.gov/travel/yb/utils/ybGet.asp?section=special&obj=hivtrav.htm&cssNav=browseoyb Accessed 2/16/07.

CHAPTER 25

# Skin Problems

Jay S. Keystone

## Introduction

Health problems in immigrants from developed to developing countries are very much a reflection of the endemicity of infectious diseases in the country of origin, the living conditions and socioeconomic status of the immigrant, ethnic differences concerning noninfectious diseases, and the time elapsed between departure from the country of origin and arrival in the country of destination. This chapter will cover only those skin diseases that are imported into developed countries from the developing world. A number of the conditions mentioned in this chapter are more fully covered in other chapters of this book and therefore will not be covered in detail. This chapter is not intended to be a comprehensive review of dermatological problems in immigrants, but rather an approach to the diagnosis of skin lesions based on their morphology, anatomical location, and associated symptoms.

There is a remarkable paucity in the medical literature concerning skin problems in immigrants from developing countries compared with those born in industrialized nations. One of the few reviews of immigrant dermatological problems was carried out in the late 1980s by five European hospital-based dermatology clinics, one each in the Netherlands and Germany, and three in the UK.[1] In the Dutch clinic, the top diagnoses among immigrants, mostly from Surinam, Turkey, Indonesia, Morocco, and the Caribbean, were contact dermatitis, alopecia, dermatophytosis, psoriaisis, herpes simplex, vitiligo and pityriasis versicolor. In hospitalized patients in Germany, made up mostly of Turks and Yugoslavs, idiopathic urticaria and sexually transmitted diseases (STDs) were the primary diagnoses. In a South London clinic, made up mostly

of Afro-Caribbeans, the major disorders were those of pigmentation and hair. Curly hair was associated with folliculitis of the scalp, ingrown hairs of the beard, abscess formation, and keloid scarring. Traction alopecia was seen with changes in hair fashion. On the other hand, in the Asian population of South London, eczema, warts, dermatomycosis, and acne were the primary presenting diagnoses and were similar to the non-immigrant population. The middle-class Asian population reviewed in Leicester, England, were most likely to complain of pigmentary disorders (vitiligo, postinflammatory pigmentary alterations, and facial hyperpigmentation), idiopathic pruritus, and atopic eczema, compared with the non-Asian population. Among both Asian populations surveyed, there was considerable social stigma attached to vitiligo and other skin conditions that leave visible marks, especially those found in young women (Table 25.1).

Although dermatological problems among newly arrived immigrants are not well documented, several reviews have focused on skin problems in ethnic communities of which the majority would be immigrants.[2] A survey of 75 589 patients seen over 2 years at the National Skin Centre in Singapore documented the spectrum of disease in its Asian population.[3] The majority of its patients were Chinese with 5–10 % each of Indian, Malay, and others. The 11 most common diagnoses were: dermatitis (34.1%), acne (10.9%), viral infections (5.7%), fungal infections (5.4%), contact dermatitis (4.0%), psoriasis (3.3%,) bacterial infection (3.0%), alopecia (2.4%), nonvenomous insect bites (2.3%), and postinflammatory hyperpigmentation (1.9%).

Sanchez recently reported his findings on dermatological problems in 2000 Latinos in a large hospital based clinic.[4] The top 10 diagnoses included: eczema/

**Table 25.1 Disorders of pigmentation**

| Lesion | Cause | Geography | Incubation period | Site of lesions | Clinical features | Diagnosis |
|---|---|---|---|---|---|---|
| Vitiligo | Unknown | Worldwide | None | Symmetric, genitalia | Achromia, leukotrichia, well defined | Wood's lamp, biopsy |
| Pityriasis alba | Unknown | Worldwide, especially in tropics | None | Face, especially around mouth; extremities | Scaling, ill-defined | Clinical |
| Pityriasis (tinea) versicolor | Malassezia furfur | Worldwide | | Upper trunk, neck | Hyperpigmentation or hypopigmentation; scaling, well defined, occasionally pruritic | Fungal culture, KOH preparation |
| Tinea nigra | Exophilia werneckii Cladosporium mansoni | Americas Asia | | Palms, rarely soles | Well defined, hyperpigmentation symptomatic | Fungal scraping and culture |
| Phytophotodermatitis | Furocoumarins in plant sap with ultraviolet A | Worldwide | 24 hr | Contact site with sap (e.g. lime juice) | Resembles sunburn plus intense prolonged hyperpigmentation | Clinical |
| Leprosy | Mycobacterium leprae | Tropical, subtropical | 6 mon–12 yr | All except scalp and intertriginous | Sensory loss, nerve thickening, loss of sweating | Biopsy, slit skin smears plus AFB stain |
| Pinta | Treponema carateum | Central and South America (rural) | 1–3 mon | Bony prominences and extremities | Polychromia in children, hyperpigmentation and hypopigmentation | VDRL, slit skin smears, darkfield, and phase contrast |

KOH, potassium hydroxide; AFB, acid-fast bacilli; VDRL, Venereal Disease Research Laboratory.

contact dermatitis (20.1%), condyloma/warts (17.5%), acne (12.3%), tinea/onychomycosis (9.3%), pyoderma (8.8%), hyperpigmentation (7.5%), seborrheic dermatitis (7.2%), psoriasis (5.5%), facial melasma (4.1%), and pruritus (2.3%).

Infectious skin problems in immigrants are often very much different from those found in returned travelers and immigrants returning home to visit friends and relatives (VFRs). In the latter, insect bites, secondarily infected bites, skin abscesses, cutaneous larva migrans, and myiasis are most common. On the other hand, immigrants, especially refugees, are more likely to present with more exotic diseases such as cutaneous leishmaniasis, scabies, and filariasis. A recent review of the geosentinel database showed that tourists made up 57% of the database, and accounted for the majority (47%) of the skin problems. On the other hand, 16% of the geosentinel database were made up of immigrants but only 8% of the dermatological problems were found in this group ($p < 0.001$) (Edie Lederman, personal communication [2006]).

In a recent study from France of 622 ill returned travelers, dermatological problems were the most frequent reason for consultation, making up 23.4% of all the medical conditions found in these travelers.[5] Immigrants accounted for one-third of the 149 travelers with skin problems, only slightly less than tourists.

## History

The approach to the diagnosis of skin problems in immigrants begins with a detailed epidemiological and exposure history. The history should begin with a review of the patient's travel history, beginning with the country of origin, as well as any stops en route to the final destination. It is not unusual for an immigrant or refugee to have spent time in one or more countries, sometimes in refugee camps, before arriving in the destination country. This information is particularly important with respect to possible exposures to infectious diseases as well as in the determination of the incubation period of the skin problem. The history should also include information concerning the specific region within the country that has been visited, as well as that of the country of origin. Many infectious skin problems are confined to rural areas only or to specific regions within a country.

The type of activities or work in which immigrants were involved while in their country of origin or asylum affects the infectious diseases, vectors, and environmental hazards to which they might have been exposed. One has to assume that they are exposed to almost everything since they are less likely to remember or be aware of specific exposures. Unlike the history in returned travelers, who are often knowledgeable about their potential exposure during travel, immigrants will have been exposed to infections over many years, and therefore may be less certain about this history. It is important to take a detailed occupational history since, for example, farmers, mineworkers, and animal handlers will potentially have an entirely different set of infections than will urban workers. Similarly, immigrants who have been in transit through refugee camps in remote areas of developing countries will be exposed to the diseases of that region as well as to infections that might be transmitted from person to person within the refugee camps.

Immigrants are more likely than returned travelers to be knowledgeable about infectious diseases in the areas where they have lived in their country of origin. Although they may not know the medical terminology for a particular infection, they will often know about the symptoms, such as the swelling of the eye in the case of *Loa loa* or Chagas' disease, limb enlargement in bancroftian filariasis, the skin ulcer of leishmaniasis, or of the deformities seen in leprosy. In addition, they will often be able to tell the healthcare provider whether they have come from an area where there are tsetse flies, ticks, or reduviid (Vinchuca, assassin) bugs. In the case of the latter, it will be important to know whether an individual has lived in a residence which was adobe-style or had a thatched roof.

The dietary history, with an emphasis on culturally diverse foods, is particularly important. For example, the eating of uncooked pork, raw fish, watercress, or shellfish may be an important clue to the diagnosis of tapeworm (or cysticercosis), gnathostomiasis, fascioliasis, or paragonimiasis, respectively.

Finally, it will be important to know the family history, both present and past, to assess whether the patient might have been in contact with family members with infectious diseases such as scabies, head lice, body lice, tuberculosis, or leprosy.

## Physical Examination

Unlike many other aspects of infectious disease, where the history is the most important element in diagnosis, the physical examination is paramount in those presenting with a skin problem. One of the cardinal rules of the physical examination involving a dermatological complaint is that the physical examination must be complete and comprise all areas of skin, including the breasts, buttocks, and scalp. In patients with suspected leprosy, superficial cutaneous nerves must be examined as well (see Ch. 34). For some immigrant populations, it might be necessary for a different examiner of the same gender as the patient to carry out the examination in order to examine the skin thoroughly.

The location of lesions (extremities versus trunk, unexposed versus exposed skin), their morphology (maculopapular, nodules, ulcers, vesicular, verrucous, pigmented), pattern (grouping, linear), progression of lesions (rapidity, lymphocuticular spread), and associated symptoms (pruritus, pain, sensory loss, fever), combined with the exposure and epidemiologic history, are especially useful in establishing the correct diagnosis.

## Laboratory Investigations (General Principles)

Laboratory investigations may be non-specific, such as a complete blood count, or specific, such as disease serology or biopsy and culture of a lesion. It is important to understand that alterations in the white blood count, such as eosinophilia, may or may not be related to the clinical problem under investigation (see Ch. 21). Not infrequently, immigrants from developing countries have eosinophilia due to a cryptic helminth infection; therefore, eosinophilia in the presence of skin lesion may be completely unrelated to the clinical problem. Along the same lines, serological tests for infectious diseases, particularly when the disease is chronic, cannot distinguish between an active infection and one that has been treated and cured. For example, a patient who has leishmania antibodies and a skin ulcer may not have active cutaneous leishmaniasis but rather evidence of a previous, silent infection.

The gold standard for the diagnosis of a cutaneous skin problem is the skin biopsy. The biopsy should be carried out at the most active portion of the lesion and include a portion of normal skin. In the case of leprosy, normal skin is not required and the biopsy should include subcutaneous fat in order that cutaneous nerves may be visualized. If there is a possibility that the cutaneous lesion has an infectious etiology, the biopsy should always be sent for bacterial, mycobacterial, and fungal cultures, and stains for these infections should be performed. In specific situations, special

cultures, stains or polymerase chain reaction (PCR) for viruses or *Leishmania* may be required.

In leprosy, in addition to the skin biopsy, slit skin smears are often used to detect mycobacteria, while in onchocerciasis skin snips are used for the detection of microfilariae.

It would be impossible for one to cover all of the possible infectious skin disorders found in immigrants and refugees. Febrile illnesses associated with rash have been covered in the tabular approach to differential diagnosis. In this chapter, cutaneous infectious diseases that are most common among immigrants, or that are rare, but less likely to be recognized by practitioners have been selected for a more detailed discussion. Other diseases, including some found in other chapters, have been included in table form according to their clinical appearance (Table 25.2).

## Papular Lesions

### Scabies

Although scabies has been a scourge of humans for thousands of years, it has enjoyed a resurgence recently because of the HIV epidemic and its association with a form of disease which is highly infectious due to the large numbers of mites present. Scabies is caused by the mite *Sarcoptes scabei var. hominis*, an ectoparasite requiring an appropriate host on which to feed. Symptoms of scabies usually begin 10–30 days after the onset of the infection, but may occur within 48 hours of a repeat infection because of host hypersensitivity.[6,7]

Human scabies is transmitted mainly by direct personal or sexual contact, and less often by contact with infested bedding or clothing. The gravid female mite burrows into the skin. Mature adults lay eggs at the rate of two or three per day, and a new cycle of replication will occur. At any given time, the average infected human has approximately 10–15 adult female mites. Scabies is characterized by severe pruritus. The characteristic primary lesion is the burrow. It appears as a white or gray linear, raised papule with a small vesicle at one end. These primary lesions are found in the web spaces of the fingers, on the flexor surfaces of the wrists and the elbows, on the penis, the scrotum, umbilicus, beltline and on the areola of the breasts in women. Secondary papules, pustules, vesicles, and excoriations may be present. The secondary lesions, often more numerous and more spread out than the burrows,

## Table 25.2 Tropical dermatology quick reference: differential diagnosis

### Macules
Hyperpigmented
  Tinea versicolor
  Phytophotodermatitis, postinflammatory
Hypopigmented
  Leprosy
  Onchocerciasis
  Pinta
  Pityriasis alba
  Postinflammatory
  Post-kala azar dermal leishmaniasis
  Tinea corporis
  Pityriasis (tinea) versicolor
  Vitiligo
Vesiculobullous
  Blister beetle dermatitis
  Bullous impetigo
  Butterfly moth dermatitis
  Cutaneous larva migrans
  Herpes simplex
  Herpes zoster
  Photodermatitis
  Phytophotodermatitis
  Sunburn

### Subcutaneous swellings or nodules
Cysticercosis
Gnathostomiasis
Leprosy
Loa loa
Maduromycosis
Mycobacterium marinum
Myiasis
Onchocerciasis
Paracoccidioidomycosis
Sea urchin spines
Tungiasis

### Vegetating and verrucous
Bartonellosis
Chromomycosis
Histoplasmosis
Leishmaniasis
Leprosy
Maduramycosis
M. marinum
Paracoccidioidomycosis
Pinta
Schistosomiasis
Syphilis
Tuberculosis
Yaws

### Migratory lesions
Cutaneous larva migrans
Fascioliasis
Gnathostomiasis
Larva currens (strongyloidiasis)
Loiasis
Myiasis

Paragonimiasis
Sparganosis

### Papules
Cercarial dermatitis
Dermatophytosis
Drug reaction
Dyshidrotic eczema
Insect bites
Miliaria
Myiasis
Onchocerciasis
Photodermatitis
Scabies
Sea bather's eruption
Seaweed dermatitis
Streptocerciasis
Tungiasis
Blister beetle dermatitis
Cutaneous larva migrans
Flea bites
Gnathostomiasis
Larva currens (strongyloidiasis)
Leishmaniasis
M. marinum
Myiasis
Phytodermatitis
Phytophotodermatitis
Sporotrichosis

### Ulcers
Anthrax
Diphtheria
Ecthyma
Leishmaniasis
M. marinum
Buruli ulcer
Pyoderma gangrenosum
Syphilis
Tick eschar
Tropical phagedenic
Tuberculosis
Yaws

### Pruritic lesions
Cercarial dermatitis
Cutaneous larva migrans
Drug reaction
Enterobiasis
Gnathostomiasis
Insect bites
Larva currens (strongyloidiasis)
Loiasis
Onchocerciasis
Phytodermatitis
Scabies
Sea bather's eruption
Seaweed dermatitis
Streptocerciasis

likely represent an immune response to the infection. While scabies lesions are very uncommon on the head and neck area, infants not infrequently have involvement of the face and may have widespread, extensive lesions.

Norwegian or crusted scabies occurs in those patients who are immunocompromised, particularly among homeless individuals and those with AIDS. In this infection, the individual has severe cutaneous crusting due to hundreds to thousands of adult mites.[8] In contrast to scabies in the immunocompetent host, papules and burrows may be limited or absent and pruritus may not occur. Crusted lesions may be found in the head and neck region and are found around the buttocks and perianal region.

Scabies should be one of the first diagnoses to be considered in any immigrant who presents with generalized pruritus. It is important to remember that one family member may have scabies while others may not be infected or symptomatic. The diagnosis of scabies can be confirmed by finding mite ova or excreta using a skin scraping with an oil-covered scalpel blade. Scrapings can then be placed on a slide for a microscopic examination. Because so few mites are present, multiple examinations are often necessary.

Treatment of scabies includes management of the pruritus, treatment of secondary bacterial infection, eradication of the scabies mite, and prevention of secondary transmission.[9] Topical antiscabetic treatments include sulfur compounds, benzyl benzoate, crotamiton oil, lindane, malathion, permethrin, and ivermectin. Currently, the drugs of choice include 5% permethrin and ivermectin. The former should be applied from the neck down at bedtime and washed off in the morning and repeated in 1 week. All household members should be treated and all bedding and clothing of the symptomatic case should be washed in hot water. Ivermectin, in a single dose of 150–200 µg per kg, is a very safe avermectin derivative that is taken orally.[10,11] It is the treatment of choice for Norwegian scabies and in the case of an institutional outbreak. It is a convenient oral medication, but may be costly when a large family requires treatment. The pruritus of scabies may take 6–8 weeks to resolve after successful treatment because of the hypersensitivity reaction to parasite antigen in the skin.

## Lice

Pediculosis, infection with blood-sucking lice, comprises three clinical conditions: pediculosis capitis (head lice) caused by *Pediculus humanus var. capitis*, pediculosis corporis (body lice) caused by *Pediculus humanus var. corporis*, and phthiriasis pubis (pubic lice) caused by *Phthirus pubis*.[12] Lice range 1.5–4.5 mm in length and can live off the host for up to 2 days. Head lice are transmitted by direct contact or from combs, hats, bedding, or other materials that come in contact with infected hair.[13] The major symptom is scalp itching. Eggs, that are cemented onto hair (nits), can easily be seen while the adult louse, usually found near the scalp, is less easily visualized. Treatment consisting of 1% permethrin cream rinse is applied to the scalp and left on for 10 minutes. Nits should be removed by careful combing with a fine-toothed comb. Resistance is not uncommon; in such cases 0.5% malathion has been shown to be effective. Recent studies show that ivermectin works; adult lice feed on human blood, taking up the drug.[14]

Body lice are most likely to be seen in refugees who have not changed their clothing for prolonged periods.[15] They live in the seams of clothing and are seen only when they take a blood meal. In addition to severe pruritus, a papular rash may appear as groups of papules, often on the neck, underarms, shoulders, and flanks. Bluish-brown hemosiderin-laden macules (*maculae ceruleae*) due to intradermal hemorrhage occur at sites where lice feed. Body lice may be eliminated by washing clothes in hot water or drying them at high temperatures. Recent studies suggest that ivermectin may be useful in the management of body lice infestations.[16]

## Bedbugs

The bedbug (*Cimex lectularis*), dorsoventrally flat and 3–6 mm in length, hides in cracks and crevices of furniture, floorboards, beds, baggage, and even clothing.[17] The bug is a nocturnal feeder that comes out of hiding when the victim is asleep, bites for a few minutes, and then returns to its hiding place. The bites themselves are usually painless and are found in groups or a linear distribution, often on the neck or extremities that are not covered by blankets or sheets. However, papular, bullous, or urticarial reactions to bites with a hemorrhagic punctum at the center are not uncommon. An important clue to the infection is the finding of blood spots on the sheets corresponding to the bite sites on the patient. In addition to symptomatic treatment with topical steroids or antihistamines, the source of the bedbugs must be determined and eliminated.

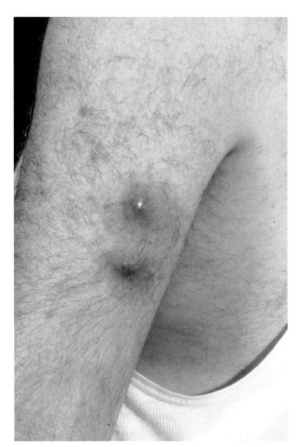

**Figure 25.1** Myiasis.

## Nodular Lesions

Nodular lesions are summarized in Table 25.3.

### Myiasis

Cutaneous myiasis is the term applied to the infestation of the skin of live humans and vertebrate animals with larvae (maggots) of a dipterous (two winged) fly (Fig. 25.1). When an open wound is involved, the myiasis is known as traumatic and when boil-like, the lesion is termed furuncular. Although furuncular myiasis is much more likely to be found in travelers, it may be found in newly arrived immigrants or refugees. There are two forms of tropical cutaneous myiasis. The most frequent one seen in travelers is *Dermatobium hominis*, the botfly.[6,18] The less common form, due to *Anthropophaga* species, is the tumbu or mangoe fly. Although both species produce identical lesions, the epidemiology and clinical presentation are different.

The botfly is endemic throughout Central and South America and Mexico where it is found predominantly in warm, humid, lowland forests. Adult females cement 10–50 eggs on the abdomen of a mosquito or other blood-sucking arthropod. When the arthropod feeds on a human or mammal, the eggs drop off and penetrate the skin through the bite site or hair follicle. Within 24 hours a pruritic papule develops and gradually enlarges to 1–3.5 cm. Clues to the diagnosis are the central punctum through which serosanguinous fluid may drain and/or the visualization of a white threadlike structure that moves intermittently in and out of the hole. In most cases, a single larva is found within each lesion. Patients may complain of sharp, stabbing pains and the sensation of movement within the boil-like lesion. Botfly lesions are found on exposed surfaces such as the scalp, forearms, and legs. If left untreated, the larva (maggot) matures over 5–12 weeks to up to 2 cm in length and emerges from the opening of the furuncle and drops into the soil where it pupates and molts into an adult fly.

Diagnosis is clinical, based on the appearance of a furuncular lesion containing a central aperture. Although some authors recommend surgical extraction of the larva using local anesthesia, suffocation by occluding the orifice with Vaseline, butter, uncooked bacon or other viscous material is a much less invasive approach. The larva is either forced to the surface where it can be removed by forceps, or it is weakened to the point where lateral pressure on the furuncle allows it to be squeezed out easily. When occlusion of the aperture is not practical, such as on the scalp, a drop of 'Krazy glue' or nail polish has been shown to be effective in sealing off the aperture permanently, allowing the host to eliminate the dead larva. Lidocaine injection into the base of the cavity also forces the larva to the surface.

The tumbu fly, found throughout sub-Saharan Africa, lays its eggs directly on the clothing left to dry out-of-doors.[19,20] In this case, lesions are found in unexposed areas of the trunk, particularly the buttocks. Unlike botfly myiasis where one or several lesions are present, in tumbu fly myiasis numerous furuncular lesions are usually found. Treatment is by suffocation or extraction of the larvae.

### Tungiasis

Tungiasis, an infestation with the human flea, *Tunga penetrans* (Figure 25.2), is known in various locations as chigger flea, sand flea, chigoe, jigger, nigua, pigue, and le bicho de pe. The infestation is very common

**Table 25.3 Subcutaneous swellings and nodules**

| Lesion | Cause | Pathogenesis | Geography | Incubation period | Site of lesion | Clinical features | Diagnosis |
|---|---|---|---|---|---|---|---|
| **Fixed and painful** | | | | | | | |
| Myiasis | *Dermatobia hominis, Cordylobia anthropophaga* | Mosquito-borne; clothing drying on ground | Central and South America, Africa | Several days | Trunk and extremities | Painful, indurated, erythematous papule or furuncle with central opening and sensation of movement inside; some *Diptera* sp. migrate in tissue | Extraction of fly maggot |
| Tungiasis | *Tunga penetrans* (jigger flea) | Barefoot walking, including sandals | Africa, Central America, India | 1–2 wk | Feet and legs | Painful nodule approximately 1 cm with central black dot | Extraction of flea |
| **Fixed and painless** | | | | | | | |
| Cysticercosis | *Cysticerca cellulose* | Eating uncooked pork or raw vegetables | Worldwide, tropics/subtropics | Several months | Limbs and trunk | Painless fixed nodules about 1 cm long | Biopsy, soft tissue X-ray, serology |
| Onchocerciasis | *Onchocerca volvulus* | Black fly bite | Rural Africa, Central and South America | 12 mon | Bony prominences, especially iliac crests in Africa | Painless fixed nodules | Biopsy, skin snips for microfilaria, serology |
| **Migratory** | | | | | | | |
| Loiasis | *Loa loa* | Deer fly bite | Rural West Africa | 6–12 mon | Limbs, especially wrist and forearms | Migratory, transient, pruritic, edematous, erythematous; ±worm migration across conjunctiva or eyelid lasting hours-days | Microfilariae in daytime blood counts, marked eosinophilia, worm extraction from eye |
| Gnathostomiasis | *Gnathostoma spinigerum* | Eating uncooked freshwater fish, crabs, frogs, and snakes | Asia, Southeast Asia | 3–12 mon | Trunk and extremities | Painless, pruritic, migratory, edematous swelling, especially eyelid | Marked eosinophilia, worm extraction |

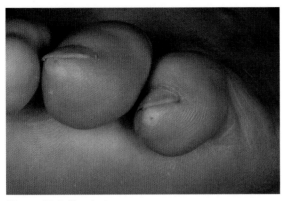

**Figure 25.2** Tungiasis.

in Central America, South America, India, and tropical Africa.[21] In some areas up to 50 % of the population may be affected.

The pregnant flea burrows into the skin of the host near the plantar surfaces of the foot, in the webbing between the toes, and around the periungual region. Clinically, a painful, whitish-colored nodule with a central dark spot develops at the site and measures approximately 1 cm in diameter. Uncomplicated infestation results in pain, swelling, tenderness, and some limitation in mobility.

Squeezing the lesion may cause the discharge of a whitish material containing hundreds of eggs, each measuring 1 mm in length. Enucleation of the lesion using a sterile needle or curette cures the infestation.[22] Since surgical intervention may be complicated by secondary infection, the use of an antibiotic cream after extraction may be prudent. Without treatment, the lesion usually resolves following discharge of the eggs and the death of the female.

## Macular Lesions

### Pityriasis versicolor

This is a chronic, benign skin infection of *Malessezia* yeasts that is characterized by scaly hypo- or hyperpigmented macules, primarily affecting the upper trunk, neck, or upper arms.[23] The lesions may coalesce over large areas of the body. Most patients are asymptomatic; if there is a concern, it is cosmetic. It occurs much more frequently in the tropics (affecting up to 40% of the population at some time), in young adults and in the summer months. Genetic and/or immunologic factors likely play a role in determining which individuals develop disease. The

diagnosis is easily made when fluorescence is detected by Wood's lamp or the 'meatballs and spaghetti' (spores and hyphae respectively) are found microscopically on a methylene blue-stained piece of clear cellulose acetate tape onto which superficial skin scales have adhered.

Systemic or topical treatments are effective.[24] The classical nonspecific selenium sulfide approach using Selsun shampoo is effective but requires the shampoo to be on the skin for 10 minutes twice weekly for several weeks. The azole antifungals (itraconazole, fluconazole, or ketoconazole) are the most widely used and are effective in both topical and oral formulations. For convenience, the oral form is the most popular, albeit somewhat expensive.

### Tinea capitis

Tinea capitis, also called ringworm, is the most frequent superficial fungal infection in the pediatric population, occurring almost exclusively in young children and disappearing after puberty.[25] *Trichophyton* species are the most frequent mycoses detected and thrive in warm, moist areas. Susceptibility to tinea infection is increased by poor hygiene and prolonged wetness of the skin (such as from sweating). Tinea infections are contagious and may be passed by direct contact with affected individuals or by contaminated items such as combs, hats, or clothing. They may be acquired by contact with pets such as cats or dogs that carry the fungus.

Lesions on the scalp may be itchy and appear as round, scaly, gray or reddened bald patches where hair is broken off. Infection may be complicated by the formation of a pus-filled lesion (kerion) or scarring with permanent baldness. The diagnosis is usually made clinically or by Wood's lamp. Systemic antifungals such as griseofulvin and terbinafine or the azoles, itraconazole and fluconazole, are very effective.[26]

### Tinea corporis and pedis

Tinea corporis, or ringworm, acquired from contact with infected humans or animals, is a common skin condition found in any non-hair-bearing area of skin.[27] Initially, pruritic annular lesions develop with a central clearing and surrounding ring of vesicles. With the rupture of these vesicles, the rings become scaly and erythematous. An initial lesion may spread peripherally or multiple annular lesions may coalesce to form one large area that may be several centimeters in diameter. Autoinoculation may lead to spread to other parts of the body.

Tinea pedis is confined to the feet and is acquired from direct contact with contaminated surfaces, especially in warm, moist environments such as showers, bathrooms, and locker room floors. It presents with pruritus, burning, cracking, and maceration of the skin in web spaces of the toes. Vesicular lesions and desquamation may occur, especially in the areas outside of the web spaces on the instep and dorsum of the foot.

Diagnosis is usually clinical. It can be confirmed by scraping a few scales from the margins of the lesion and examining them for fungal hyphae under low power after fixing them with 20% potassium hydroxide.

Treatment of tinea is usually by the application of topical antifungal creams and ointments such as clotrimazole, ketoconazole, or terbinafine.[28] Systemic therapy may be necessary for multiple lesions or a severe inflammatory reaction.

## Capsaicin dermatitis

In many cultures chili peppers are used extensively for cooking. Those who peel chili peppers may develop erythema and edema of the hands and fingers.[29] Depending on the duration of contact, symptoms may consist of burning, prickling, or throbbing, and may be mild or intense. Symptoms may be delayed and often last for hours to days. The mechanism of capsaicin dermatitis appears to be nerve depolarization leading to vascular dilatation, smooth muscle contraction, and sensory nerve activation. The condition may be managed by washing affected hands with soap and large amounts of cold water and then immersing them in vegetable oil for 1 hour. Topical anesthetics and potent corticosteroids may also be helpful. Prevention of the condition may be accomplished by the use of rubber gloves by those handling chili peppers.

## Coining

'Coining' is a common form of indigenous medicine found in Southeast Asian communities (Fig. 25.3).[30] Traditionally, coining is used for conditions associated with 'wind illness,' a wide variety of febrile illnesses, as well as stress-related symptoms in adults such as headaches, muscle aches and pain, and fatigue. The practice involves the rubbing of the skin with a coin in symmetrical bands producing linear petechiae and ecchymosis on the chest and back

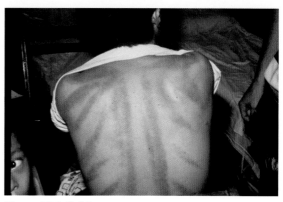

**Figure 25.3** Coining.

which resolve over several days. Instances have been reported in which parents have been accused of 'child abuse' as a result of their children have been subjected to coining.

## Cupping

Cupping is one of the oldest methods of traditional Chinese medicine.[31,32] Today, most acupuncturists use cups made of thick glass or plastic, although bamboo, iron, and pottery cups are still used in other countries. In China, cupping is used primarily to treat respiratory conditions such as bronchitis, asthma, and congestion, arthritis, gastrointestinal disorders, and certain types of pain. Some practitioners also use cupping to treat depression and reduce swelling. Fleshy sites on the body, such as the back and stomach (and, to a lesser extent, the arms and legs), are the preferred sites for treatment.

In a typical cupping session, glass cups are warmed using a cotton ball or other flammable substance, which is soaked in alcohol, lit, then placed inside the cup. Burning a substance inside the cup removes all the oxygen, which creates a vacuum. As the substance burns, the cup is turned upside-down so that the practitioner can place the cup over a specific area. The vacuum created by the lack of oxygen anchors the cup to the skin and pulls the skin upward on the inside of the glass as the air inside the jar cools. Drawing up the skin is believed to open up the skin's pores, which helps to stimulate the flow of blood, balances and realigns the flow of *qi*, breaks up obstructions, and creates an avenue for toxins to be drawn out of the body. Depending on the condition being treated, the cups will be left in place for 5–10 minutes. Several cups may be placed on a patient's body at the same time.

In addition to the traditional form of cupping described above, which is known as 'dry' cupping, some practitioners also use what is called 'wet' or 'air' cupping. In 'air' cupping, instead of using a flame to heat the cup, the cup is applied to the skin, and a suction pump is attached to the rounded end of the jar. The pump is then used to create the vacuum. In 'wet' cupping, the skin is punctured before treatment. When the cup is applied and the skin is drawn up, a small amount of blood may flow from the puncture site, which is believed to help remove harmful substances and toxins from the body.

While cupping is considered relatively safe (especially air cupping, which does not include the risk of fire and heat), it can cause some swelling and bruising on the skin. As the skin under a cup is drawn up, the blood vessels at the surface of the skin expand. This may result in small, circular bruises on the areas where the cups were applied. These bruises are usually painless, however, and disappear within a few days of treatment.

## Plaques or Verrucous Lesions

### Chromomycosis

In Latin America, a chronic skin infection is found frequently among farmers infected with one of several species of dematiacious (pigmented) fungi (*Fonsecaea pedrosi, Phialophora verrucosa, Cladosporium carrionii*, etc) which live as saprophytes in soil and decaying vegetation (Fig. 25.4).[33,34] The vast majority of cases are caused by traumatic inoculation of a wood splinter contaminated with *Fonsecaea pedrosi*.

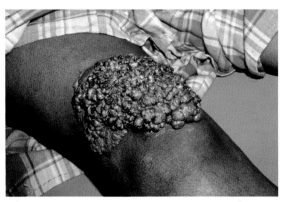

**Figure 25.4** Chromomycosis.

Typically, a pink, scaly papule develops at the inoculation site, most often on the lower extremity. The lesion enlarges slowly into a scaly or verrucous plaque or nodule. In the nodular form, firm, reddish, smooth, moist nodules break down leaving purulent, malodorous ulcers with vegetating borders. The initial lesion may spread along lymphatics or by autoinoculation.

The diagnosis is made by skin biopsy and culture of tissue in Sabouraud glucose agar. Histological examination shows pseudoepitheliomatous hyperplasia and microabscesses in the epidermis, along with acute and chronic granulomatous inflammation, vascular proliferation, and fibrosis. The diagnosis is confirmed by the finding of dematiacious hyphae and sclerotic bodies ('copper penny' bodies).

Small, localized lesions may be treated with excision, cryotherapy, curettage, or electrodessication. More advanced lesions are best treated with a combination of drugs chosen by the results of antifungal susceptibility testing. Prolonged courses of itraconazole and terbinafine are usually effective, but fluconazole is not. Amphotericin B and fluocytocine have been used with some success.[35]

### Maduramycosis

Mycetoma is an infection involving cutaneous and subcutaneous tissues, fascia, and bone caused by soil-inhabiting bacteria (actinomyces) or fungi (eumycetes).[36,37] Approximately 50% of all cases of mycetoma are caused by aerobic actinomycetes, primarily *Actinomadura madurae* and *Nocardia brasiliensis*, and the other half by true fungi, most commonly *Madurella mycetomatis* and *Madurella grisea*. These fungi gain entrance to the host through penetrating trauma with sharp objects or abrasions. Maduramycosis is most common as an occupational risk in middle-aged males in tropical and subtropical areas, especially in India and several countries of Africa, and South America that have a prolonged hot and dry season (Fig. 25.5).[38]

Clinically, maduramycosis is most often found on the lower extremity and is characterized by subcutaneous induration and painless cutaneous papules or nodules which are later associated with draining sinus tracks with visible grains. The infection gradually extends into deep tissues, spreading along fascial planes to involve bone. Although initially painless, tissue destruction and swelling may produce considerable pain, especially in the foot during walking.

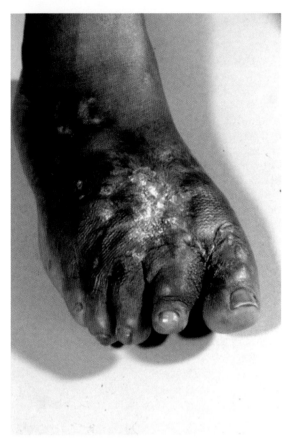

**Figure 25.5** Maduramycosis.

The diagnosis may be confirmed by examining exudate, pus, and biopsy tissue grossly for the presence of grains which are characteristic of both forms of mycetoma. This material should be mixed with potassium hydroxide on a slide and crushed under a coverslip to view the filaments of actinomycetoma and the hyphae of eumycetoma. Isolation of the etiologic agent often requires a deep biopsy with tissue cultured in both bacterial and mycologic media, the latter held for 6 weeks because of the slow growth of some eumycetes.

Treatment of mycetoma is invariably prolonged (many months to years), and is often unsatisfactory when osteomyelitis is involved. In very early cases, excision along with chemotherapy is most effective. However, chronic, longstanding infections are best managed with appropriate antibiotics (based on culture and sensitivity results) for actinomycetes. Itraconazole and terbinafine have become the drugs of choice for eumycetes, although small case series have shown the newer azoles, posaconazole and voriconazole, to be effective in resistant cases.[39] In late stages when drug therapy has failed, amputation of the whole or part of the foot or extremity may be the only way to stop the inexorable spread of the infection.

## Verruga peruana

*Bartonella bacilliforme* can produce a febrile systemic infection or cutaneous eruptive disease. The infection is endemic to Andean areas of Peru, Ecuador, and Colombia although recently it has been reported in areas of the Amazon basin. Infection is transmitted to humans by the bite of *Lutzomya* sandflies.[40]

The febrile illness (Carrion's disease) is characterized by a febrile illness associated with hepatosplenomegaly, severe hemolytic anemia and, in some cases, superinfection with nontyphoidal *Salmonella* species.[41] The eruptive phase, known as verruga peruana, which usually occurs independently of the systemic illness, is characterized by the presence of angiomatous nodules usually located on the legs, arms, and face, and less commonly elsewhere on the body. The lesions may be single or numerous, and clinically are identical to bacillary angiomatosis.

Skin biopsy shows histicytic and endothelial proliferation with capillary vessel formation and granulomatous changes. In contrast with bacillary angiomatosis, bacteria are rarely found on H&E stain but are readily visible with silver staining.

Treatment is always indicated for the systemic illness, whereas the cutaneous disease may resolve spontaneously within 4–6 months or may remain indefinitely. Chloramphenicol along with a betalactam (to cover secondary infections) or a fluoroquinolone is indicated for severe systemic disease, whereas rifampin, azithromycin, and fluoroquinolones may be used for mild systemic illness and skin manifestations.[42]

## Paracoccidioidomycosis

Paracoccidioidomycosis, or South American blastomycosis, is a chronic, progressive, systemic mycosis that is primarily a pulmonary and lymph node disease associated with mucocutaneous disease (Fig. 25.6).[43,44] The etiologic agent, *Paracoccidiodes brasiliensis*, a dimorphic fungus, is unique to parts of Central and South America, stretching from Mexico to Argentina. Chile is the only country in which the disease has not been reported. The organism is found in soil, although animals are a possible natural

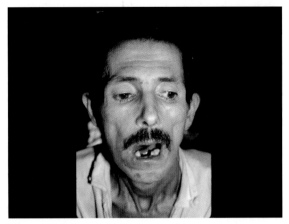

**Figure 25.6** Paracoccidioidomycosis.

reservoir. Adult men who work outdoors, especially farmers and hunters, are at highest risk for infection.

The incubation period may be as long as several years. Inhalation of the fungus causes a primary lung infection that is characterized by productive cough, fever, and weight loss. Approximately 50% of clinical cases subsequently develop pharyngeal and nasal lesions, usually accompanied by ulcerations, and a similar percentage have adrenal involvement. Typically, the ulcerations have a punctate vascular pattern over a granulomatous base. Hoarseness, dysphagia, and perioral crusted plaques are common. Unlike mucocutaneous leishmaniasis, the mucosal lesions are painful. The oral manifestations are followed by bilateral sub-mental and cervical adenopathy. Other remote lymph node sites may be involved as well. Facial lesions are common and vary in appearance, with ulcers, crusted papules, plaques, nodules and verrucous lesions. Untreated disease may be fatal as a result of pulmonary fibrosis, central nervous system involvement, or adrenal insufficiency. However, subclinical, asymptomatic infection is probably the most frequent sequela of the infection.

The diagnosis is confirmed by means of tissue culture or histological examination of skin, lymph nodes, or sputum in which budding yeasts are found. Serological diagnosis by immunodiffusion (ELISA) may also be helpful. Treatments of choice include long-acting sulfonamides such as sulfamethoxine, and azole compounds (itraconazole, ketoconazole, fluconazole) administered for 4–6 months.[45] In severe cases, amphotericin B alone or in combination with sulfonamides is effective.

## Prayer calluses

In areas of the world where conservative Catholicism remains, very devout practitioners, often elderly women who kneel during prayer for hours every day, may develop calluses on their knees because of repeated pressure and friction from kneeling during prayer.[4] This leads to skin thickening and hyperkeratosis and often to hyperpigmentation. Devout Muslims may also develop calluses on their knees, and in addition on their forehead, as a result of their form of worship.

## Migratory Subcutaneous Swellings

### Gnathostomiasis

Gnathostomiasis is an infection of the nematode *Gnathostoma spinigerum* that traditionally had been found in Southeast Asia, particularly Thailand and Japan, but which has become an increasingly recognized problem in Central and South America and Mexico due to the ingestion of raw fish in ceviche.[46] Infection is acquired by eating uncooked food infected with the larval third stage in such foods as fish, shrimp, crab, crayfish, frog, or chicken. Cats and dogs serve as important reservoirs in endemic areas.

Since the larva cannot mature into the adult form in humans, it wanders through host tissues causing an inflammatory reaction and the clinical syndromes involve the skin and subcutaneous tissues, eye, viscera and, rarely, the central nervous system.[47] Skin manifestations are usually those of migratory subcutaneous swellings lasting for several days each or, less commonly, cutaneous larva migrans. The latter is a very pruritic linear, serpiginous rash that progresses within the dermis, and which is less likely to be found on the foot than is the dog or cat hookworm acquired from walking on a beach. The incubation period of gnathostomiasis is variable but usually presents within several months of ingestion of contaminated food. The main differential diagnoses for gnathostomiasis, depending on the geographic history, include loiasis (*Loa loa*), fascioliasis, myiasis, and paragonimiasis, and in the case of dermal involvement, strongyloidiasis and cutaneous larva migrans from dog or cat hookworms (see Table 25.3).

The clinical diagnosis can be confirmed by serology, available at Mahidol University in

**Table 25.4 Tropical ulcers**

| Ulcers | Cause | Geography | Incubation period | Site of lesion | Clinical features | Diagnosis |
|---|---|---|---|---|---|---|
| Pyoderma | *Staphylococcus aureus*, beta-hemolytic streptococcus | Worldwide | Several days | Lower limbs | Vesicle or pustule, crusted ulcer | Bacterial culture, Gram stain |
| Leishmaniasis | *Leishmania* spp. | Rural Asia, Middle East, Northeast Africa, Central and South America, Southern Europe | 2–8 wk (up to 3 yr) | Exposed skin (face, limbs) | Painless, rolled edge, slow healing 6 mon– 2 yr | Scraping of base, slit skin smear, or aspiration of rolled edge for smear and culture; biopsy for touch preparation and culture |
| Boutonneuse fever or tick typhus | *Rickettsia conorii* | Southern Europe, Northeast and Southern Africa, Middle East, India | 5–7 d | Lower limbs | 2–5 mm ulcer with black center, red areola; regional lymph node enlargement | Serology |
| South African tick typhus | *Rickettsia africae* | Southern Africa | 5–7 d | Exposed skin, lower limbs | Eschar plus enlarged lymph nodes | Serology |
| Rickettsial pox | *Rickettsia akari* | US and Russia | 9–17 d | Bite site | Initial eschar-like lesion | Serology |
| Scrub typhus | *Orientia tsutsugamushi* | East and South Asia, Western and Southern Pacific | 9–18 d | Bite site | Central necroses with eschar | Serology |
| Swimming pool granuloma | *Mycobacterium marinum* | Worldwide, usually temperate | 1–6 wk | Hands, elbows, and knees | Violaceous nodule–ulceration, occasional proximal lymphatic spread | Biopsy, AFB stain and culture (30°C) |
| Cutaneous tuberculosis | *Mycobacterium tuberculosis* | Worldwide | | | | |

| Disease | Organism | Distribution | Incubation | Location | Clinical features | Diagnosis |
|---|---|---|---|---|---|---|
| Ulcerous tuberculosis | | | | Usually around body orifices and limbs | Ragged, painful shallow ulcer in patient with advanced tuberculosis | Biopsy, AFB stain and culture |
| Lupus vulgarus | | | | Usually neck as extension of scrofula | Reddish plaque that ulcerates, apple-jelly nodules or lupomas | |
| Papulonecrotic tuberculid | | | | Hypersensitivity response to tuberculosis; posterior lower limbs, | Papules to pustules | PPD positive, response to tuberculosis treatment |
| Buruli ulcer | *Mycobacterium ulcerans* | Tropics—focal, Southern Australia | Approximately 1–8 wk | Limbs | Painless undetermined borders, extensive necrosis | Biopsy, AFB stain, and culture (32°C) |
| Cutaneous amoebiasis | *Entamoeba histolytica* | Worldwide | 7–21 d | Perianal, penile, fistulous site | Painful, necrotic ulcer; erythematous halo | Scraping and smear of ulcer base; biopsy |
| Anthrax | *Bacillus anthracis* | Worldwide | 12 hr–7 d | Face, neck, hands, and arms | Papule, vesicle, painless black eschar, nonpitting gelatinous edema | Wright or Giemsa smear, culture, serology |
| Tropical phagedenic ulcer | *Fusobacterium ulcerans* and other anaerobes, *Treponema vincenti* | Humid, tropics | 3–7 d | Below knees (extremities); malnourished | Rapid early spread; slow chronic deep tissue destruction | Bacterial culture |
| Cutaneous diphtheria | *Corynebacterium diphtheriae* | Worldwide | 1–7 d | Limbs | Slow healing superficial painful ulcer | Gram stain and culture; toxin determination |
| Yaws | *Treponema pertenue* | Tropics and subtropics | 2–8 wk | Anywhere, especially lower limbs | Single 'mother' yaw | Darkfield |
| | | | | | Multiple 2° lesions | VDRL |
| | | | | | Gumma and plantar keratoderma | FTA-ABS |

AFB, acid-fast bacilli; PPD, purified protein derivative; VDRL, Veneral Disease Research Laboratory; FTA-ABS, fluorescent treponemal antibody absorption.

Thailand. Eosinophilia is found in more than 50% of cases and is often of low grade. The treatment of choice of gnathostomiasis is a 3-week course of albendazole. Ivermectin, in a single dose of 200 µg/kg, is less effective.

## Ulcers

Tropical ulcers are listed in Table 25.4.

### Buruli ulcer

Buruli ulcer, caused by infection with *Mycobacterium ulcerans*, is common among children in rural tropical areas of west Africa, Uganda, Australia and, more recently, South America.[48,49] The mechanism of transmission has not been completely elucidated but it is likely that a wound or abrasion is the portal of entry for organisms found in contaminated rivers, ponds, or mud.

The infection begins as a painless nodule that breaks down and the ulcer spreads rapidly or slowly. It undermines the skin, invading subcutaneous tissues and underlying fascia, and produces marked tissue destruction leading to deformity and large, disfiguring scars. Clinically, the Buruli ulcer can often be differentiated from other ulcers by its lack of pain and presence of deep undermining ulceration and destructiveness.

The diagnosis is made by growing the organism in mycobacterial culture media.

In the early stages the infection can be cured by excision of the ulcer. However, in later stages a 4–8-week course of rifampicin and streptomycin has been shown to be highly effective.[50]

The major differential diagnosis for any chronic ulcer in immigrants is leishmaniasis, tuberculosis, atypical mycobacteriosis, paracoccidioidomycosis, pyoderma gangrenosa, syphilis, sickle cell ulcer, and yaws (see Table 25.4).[51]

## Additional Sources of Information

For those without a background in geographic medicine, making a diagnosis of an exotic infection in an immigrant may be quite challenging. Several excellent reviews have been written on skin problems in the returned traveler, but very few recent reviews have focused on skin diseases in the immigrant.[52-54] Several tropical disease textbooks have specific sections devoted to tropical skin disorders[55,56] and

contain detailed information on classical tropical skin diseases such as leprosy, leishmaniasis, and onchocerciasis. Wilson's remarkable textbook on the geographic distribution of infectious diseases provides information on disease location according to geographic region and excellent tables of skin disorders based on morphology and associated symptoms.[57] In addition, there are a number of websites with a focus on dermatological problems and global infectious diseases. One of the most comprehensive web-based programs on the differential diagnosis, epidemiology, and treatment of infectious diseases is the Global Infectious Disease and Epidemiology Network (GIDEON).[58-60] Although the site is being updated to add clinical material such as photographs of dermatological lesions, a major focus is on ranked differential diagnosis based on country of travel, activities and clinical symptoms including rashes. Its major strength is the generation of a differential diagnosis of infectious diseases presenting with fever and rash. GIDEON is a fee-based service that is updated on-line regularly; it is the most comprehensive on-line site available for current information on global infectious disease epidemiology. Another recent addition to web-based programs is Logical Images, a site that specializes in dermatological information and images.[61] This site, also fee-for-service, has a module dedicated to tropical skin disorders.

## References

1. Graham-Brown RA, Berth-Jones J, Dure-Smith B, et al. Dermatologic problems for immigrant communities in a Western environment. Int J Dermatol 1990; 29(2):94–101.
2. Taylor SC. Epidemiology of skin diseases in ethnic populations. Dermatol Clin 2003; 21(4):601–607.
3. Chua-Ty G, Goh CL, Koh SL. Pattern of skin diseases at the National Skin Centre (Singapore) from 1989–1990. Int J Dermatol 1992; 31(8):555–559.
4. Sanchez MR. Cutaneous diseases in Latinos. Dermatol Clin 2003; 21(4):689–697.
5. Ansart S, Perez L, Vergely O, et al. Illnesses in travelers returning from the tropics: a prospective study of 622 patients. J Travel Med 2005; 12(6):312–318.
6. Orion E, Matz H, Wolf R. Ectoparasitic sexually transmitted diseases: scabies and pediculosis. Clin Dermatol 2004; 22(6):513–519.
7. Huynh TH, Norman RA. Scabies and pediculosis. Dermatol Clin 2004; 22(1):7–11.
8. Roberts LJ, Huffam SE, Walton SF, et al. Crusted scabies: clinical and immunological findings in seventy-eight patients and a review of the literature. J Infect 2005; 50(5):375–381.
9. Johnston G, Sladden M. Scabies: diagnosis and treatment. Br Med J. 2005; 331(7517):619–622.
10. Dourmishev AL, Dourmishev LA, Schwartz RA. Ivermectin: pharmacology and application in dermatology. Int J Dermatol 2005; 44(12):981–988.
11. Elgart GW, Meinking TL. Ivermectin. Dermatol Clin 2003; 21(2):277–282.

12. Ko CJ, Elston DM. Pediculosis. J Am Acad Dermatol 2004; 50(1):1–12.

13. Leung AK, Fong JH, Pinto-Rojas A. Pediculosis capitis. J Pediatr Health Care 2005; 19(6):369–373.

14. Elston DM. Drugs used in the treatment of pediculosis. J Drugs Dermatol 2005; 4(2):207–211.

15. Badiaga S, Menard A, Tissot Dupont H, et al. Prevalence of skin infections in sheltered homeless. Eur J Dermatol 2005; 15(5):382–386.

16. Foucault C, Ranque S, Badiaga S, et al. Oral ivermectin in the treatment of body lice. J Infect Dis 2006; 193(3):474–476.

17. Thomas I, Kihiczak GG, Schwartz RA. Bedbug bites: a review. Int J Dermatol 2004; 43(6):430–433.

18. Maier H, Honigsmann H. Furuncular myiasis caused by *Dermatobia hominis*, the human botfly. J Am Acad Dermatol 2004; 50(2 Suppl):S26–S30.

19. Tamir J, Haik J, Schwartz E. Myiasis with Lund's fly (*Cordylobia rodhaini*) in travelers. J Travel Med 2003; 10(5):293–295.

20. Jelinek T, Nothdurft HD, Rieder N, et al. Cutaneous myiasis: review of 13 cases in travelers returning from tropical countries. Int J Dermatol 1995; 34(9):624–626.

21. Heukelbach J, de Oliveira FA, Hesse G, et al. Tungiasis: a neglected health problem of poor communities. Trop Med Int Health 2001; 6(4):267–272.

22. Heukelbach J. Revision on tungiasis: treatment options and prevention. Expert Rev Anti Infect Ther 2006; 4(1):151–157.

23. Thoma W, Kramer HJ, Mayser P. Pityriasis versicolor alba. J Eur Acad Dermatol Venereol 2005; 19(2):147–152.

24. Schwartz RA. Superficial fungal infections. Lancet 2004; 364(9440):1173–1182.

25. Mohrenschlager M, Seidl HP, Ring J, et al. Pediatric tinea capitis: recognition and management. Am J Clin Dermatol 2005; 6(4):203–213.

26. Roberts BJ, Friedlander SF. Tinea capitis: a treatment update. Pediatr Ann 2005; 34(3):191–200.

27. Gupta AK, Chaudhry M, Elewski B. Tinea corporis, tinea cruris, tinea nigra, and piedra. Dermatol Clin 2003; 21(3):395–400.

28. Huang DB, Ostrosky-Zeichner L, Wu JJ, et al. Therapy of common superficial fungal infections. Dermatol Ther 2004; 17(6):517–522.

29. Fett DD. Botanical briefs: capsicum peppers. Cutis 2003; 72(1):21–23.

30. Buchwald D, Panwala S, Hooton TM. Use of traditional health practices by Southeast Asian refugees in a primary care clinic. West J Med 1992; 156(5):507–511.

31. Yoo SS, Tausk F. Cupping: East meets West. Int J Dermatol 2004; 43(9):664–665.

32. http://www.acupuncturetoday.com/abc/cupping.php February 13, 2007.

33. Queiroz-Telles F, McGinnis MR, Salkin I, et al. Subcutaneous mycoses. Infect Dis Clin North Am 2003; 17(1):59–85.

34. Brandt ME, Warnock DW. Epidemiology, clinical manifestations, and therapy of infections caused by dematiacious fungi. J Chemother 2003; 15(Suppl 2):36–47.

35. Bonifaz A, Paredes-Solis V, Saul A. Treating chromoblastomycosis with systemic antifungals. Expert Opin Pharmacother 2004; 5(2):247–254.

36. Ahmed AO, van Leeuwen W, Fahal A, et al. Mycetoma caused by *Madurella mycetomatis*: a neglected infectious burden. Lancet Infect Dis 2004; 4(9):566–574.

37. Fahal AH. Mycetoma: a thorn in the flesh. Trans R Soc Trop Med Hyg 2004; 98(1):3–11.

38. Bravo F, Sanchez MR. New and re-emerging cutaneous infectious diseases in Latin America and other geographic areas. Dermatol Clin 2003; 21(4):655–668.

39. Loupergue P, Hot A, Dannaoui E, et al. Successful treatment of black-grain mycetoma with voriconazole. Am J Trop Med Hyg 2006; 75:1106–1107.

40. Huarcaya E, Maguina C, Torres R, et al. Bartonelosis (Carrion's disease) in the pediatric population of Peru: an overview and update. Braz J Infect Dis 2004; 8(5): 331–339.

41. Kosek M, Lavarello R, Gilman RH, et al. Natural history of infection with *Bartonella bacilliformis* in a nonendemic population. J Infect Dis 2000; 182(3):865–872.

42. Rolain JM, Brouqui P, Koehler JE, et al. Recommendations for treatment of human infections caused by *Bartonella* species. Antimicrob Agents Chemother 2004; 48(6):1921–1933.

43. Lupi O, Tyring SK, McGinnis MR. Tropical dermatology: fungal tropical diseases. J Am Acad Dermatol 2005; 53(6):931–951.

44. Pang KR, Wu JJ, Huang DB, et al. Subcutaneous fungal infections. Dermatol Ther 2004; 17(6):523–531.

45. Miyaji M, Kamei K. Imported mycoses: an update. J Infect Chemother 2003; 9(2):107–113.

46. Ligon BL. Gnathostomiasis: a review of a previously localized zoonosis now crossing numerous geographical boundaries. Semin Pediatr Infect Dis 2005; 16(2):137–143.

47. Rusnak JM, Lucey DR. Clinical gnathostomiasis: case report and review of the English-language literature. Clin Infect Dis 1993; 16(1):33–50.

48. van der Werf TS, Stienstra Y, Johnson RC, et al. *Mycobacterium ulcerans* disease. Bull World Health Organ 2005; 83(10):785–791.

49. Wansbrough-Jones M, Phillips R. Buruli ulcer. Br Med J. 2005; 330(7505):1402–1403.

50. Etuaful S, Carbonnelle B, Grosset J, et al. Efficacy of the combination rifampin-streptomycin in preventing growth of *Mycobacterium ulcerans* in early lesions of Buruli ulcer in humans. Antimicrob Agents Chemother 2005; 49(8):3182–3186.

51. Wagner D, Young LS. Nontuberculous mycobacterial infections: a clinical review. Infection 2004; 32(5):257–270.

52. Caumes E, Carriere J, Guermonprez G, et al. Dermatoses associated with travel to tropical countries: a prospective study of the diagnosis and management of 269 patients presenting to a tropical disease unit. Clin Infect Dis 1995; 20(3):542–548.

53. Wilson ME, Chen LH. Dermatologic infectious diseases in international travelers. Curr Infect Dis Rep 2004; 6(1): 54–62.

54. Kain KC. Skin lesions in returned travelers. Med Clin North Am 1999; 83(4):1077–1102.

55. Mawhorter SD, Longworth D. Cutaneous Lesions chapter 126. In: Guerrant RL, Walker DH, Weller PF, eds. Tropical infectious diseases. 2nd edn. London: Churchill Livingstone; 2005.

56. Kain KC, Keystone JS. Skin lesions in travelers. In: Strickland T, ed. Hunter's tropical medicine and emerging infectious diseases. 8th edn. Philadelphia: WB Saunders; 2000.

57. Wilson ME. A world guide to infectious diseases. New York: Oxford University Press; 1991.

58. Luo RF, Bartlett JG. Use of the computer program GIDEON at an inpatient infectious diseases consultation service. Clin Infect Dis 2006; 42(1):157–158.

59. Berger SA. GIDEON: a comprehensive web-based resource for geographic medicine. Int J Health Geogr 2005; 4(1):10.

60. http://www.gideononline.com February 13, 2007.

61. http://www.logicalimages.com February 13, 2007.

# CHAPTER 26

# Chagas' Disease (American Trypanosomiasis)

James H. Maguire

## Chagas' Disease at a Glance

- An estimated 10–12 million persons in Latin America and tens of thousands of immigrants living outside of Latin America are infected with *Trypanosoma cruzi*.
- Chagas' disease is a major cause of mortality and cardiac disease among young and middle-aged adults in Latin America.
- Vector-borne transmission by blood-sucking triatomine bugs occurs in poorly constructed houses in Central and South America and Mexico.
- Persons remain infected for life and can transmit the parasite through blood or organ donation or transplacentally.
- Most infections are subclinical.
- Twenty to thirty percent of persons develop chronic disease after decades of infection:
  1. Progressive dilated cardiomyopathy with ventricular conduction defects, arrhythmias, heart block, congestive heart failure, sudden death;
  2. Denervation and motility disorders of esophagus (megaesophagus) and colon (megacolon);
  3. Reactivation of chronic infection with acute meningoencephalitis or myocarditis among persons receiving immunosuppressive therapy or with advanced HIV infection.
- Serological screening is indicated for persons with a history of exposure regardless of symptoms.
- Treatment with nifurtimox or benznidazole is indicated for all infected children, congenitally infected infants, and persons with reactivated or acute infection; treatment of chronically infected adults should be on a case-by-case basis.

## Epidemiology

The flagellate protozoan *Trypanosoma cruzi* is the cause of Chagas' disease (American trypanosomiasis), a zoonotic infection of approximately 10–12 million persons and over 100 species of wild and domestic animals in the Americas.[3,8] Most infected persons living today acquired infection from the triatomine vector, which in different countries is called by such names as *vinchuca, barbeiro, chinche*, kissing bug, or cone-nosed bug. Triatomine bugs transmit the parasite when they take a blood meal from sleeping persons. As a rule, bugs colonize only poorly constructed houses such as those made of mud and stick, thatch, or adobe. For this reason, Chagas' disease traditionally has been a disease of poor persons living in rural areas or urban slums in Latin America.

Highly successful control programs in the past 10–15 years have interrupted or greatly reduced vector-borne transmission in several countries, most dramatically in the Southern Cone and Venezuela.[3] The Andean and Central American countries and Mexico recently initiated vector control programs with the goal of interrupting transmission within a decade.

*Trypanosoma cruzi* can also be transmitted from an infected pregnant mother to her developing fetus or from an infected donor of blood products or organ transplant to the recipient. Congenital infection occurs in 1% to greater than 7% of pregnancies among women with chronic infection.[2,9] In the early 1980s, over 20 000 cases of transfusion-associated infections occurred each year in South America. The incidence of such infections has declined dramatically, because serological screening of donors is now required by law throughout Latin America.[9] However, screening tests may not be reliable in some blood donation centers, and several countries instituted mandatory screening only in recent years.

Millions of immigrants from countries where Chagas' disease is endemic are living in the United States, Canada, Europe, and other industrialized countries. Based on serological surveys of blood donors and immigrant populations, estimates of the number of immigrants with *T. cruzi* infection living in the United States range from 50 000 to over 120 000.[5,7,9] The majority of infected persons are asymptomatic, and few are aware that they are infected.[4] Not surprisingly, there have been six reports of transfusion-associated transmission and three episodes of transplant-associated transmission in the United States. Universal screening of blood and organ donors for *T. cruzi* infection is not mandatory in the United States and other nonendemic countries but the United States Red Cross began screening in January 2007. As screening becomes routine healthcare providers will need to learn how to care for the large numbers of asymptomatically infected immigrants who will be detected.

## Etiology and Pathogenesis

Infective trypanosomes shed in the feces of triatomine bugs during or shortly after taking a blood meal enter the body through the bite wound or conjunctiva. After invading host cells locally and replicating intracellularly, they exit the cell and destroy it in the process. Parasites then invade nearby cells or travel via the bloodstream to other tissues. Widespread intracellular replication and circulation of high numbers of parasites continues for approximately 6–8 weeks, at which time the host immune response markedly curtails intracellular replication, and circulating parasites become difficult to detect on blood smears. Numbers of parasites in the blood and within cells remain at low levels as long as cellular immunity remains intact.

Without treatment, infection persists for life. For most persons there is little or no further damage to tissue, but for unknown reasons, approximately 20–30% of persons develop overt disease of the heart and gastrointestinal system after an asymptomatic interval averaging 2–3 decades. In the heart, widespread inflammation and progressive destruction of cardiac muscle and conducting tissue result from direct parasite-mediated injury and possibly an autoimmune reaction. In the gastrointestinal tract, destruction of autonomic ganglia in the wall of hollow organs causes motility disturbances and eventual dilation, especially in the esophagus and colon.

## Clinical Manifestations

It would be exceedingly unusual for a recently arrived immigrant to present with manifestations of acute Chagas' disease. Coincidental acquisition of infection within a few months of departure has become increasingly improbable because of effective control programs in many endemic countries. Moreover, most acute infections are subclinical.[8] During the acute stage of infection, less than 10% of persons experience a febrile illness, and less than 1% becomes seriously ill with acute myocarditis or meningoencephalitis.

The acute stage resolves within 1–3 months, and thereafter infection remains asymptomatic for at least several decades. While the majority of infected persons never become ill, 20–30% of persons with chronic *T. cruzi* infection eventually develop clinically significant cardiac or gastrointestinal disease. The electrocardiogram of those with heart disease frequently shows right bundle branch block or anterior fascicular block for a decade or more before the first symptoms appear. Progression of disease leads to a dilated cardiomyopathy with involvement of all chambers. Because the right ventricle fails soon after the left, clear lung fields, peripheral edema, and congestive hepatomegaly are prominent findings. Progression of the myocarditis is rapid and relentless, and patients may develop ascites and cardiac cachexia before dying of congestive heart failure within 2–3 years of the onset of symptoms. Others die suddenly from high-grade ventricular arrhythmias, sometimes before other symptoms of heart disease develop. Strokes, pulmonary embolism, other thromboembolic events, complete heart block, and profound sinus bradyarrhythmias are not uncommon and may be fatal.

The manifestations of Chagas' esophageal disease are identical to those of idiopathic achalasia: progressive dysphagia and dilation of the esophagus that can reach massive dimensions. Persons with Chagas' megaesophagus experience repeated episodes of aspiration pneumonia and become severely malnourished. Those with Chagas' megacolon, which resembles Hirschsprung disease, go weeks to months between bowel movements and are at risk of developing volvulus of the colon.

Intracellular replication and levels of parasitemia increase when chronically infected persons develop AIDS, receive immunosuppressive medications, or suffer from other conditions that compromise cellular immunity.[9] The most common manifestation of reactivated infection is meningoencephalitis, with fever, headache, seizures, focal neurological signs, and enhancing hypodense lesions on computed tomography (CT) or magnetic resonance imaging (MRI) similar to those of central nervous system toxoplasmosis. Other presentations include acute myocarditis and subcutaneous nodular lesions.

## Diagnosis

Any Latin American immigrant who may have been exposed to *T. cruzi* infection should undergo serological or parasitological evaluation, regardless of symptoms. Persons at risk include those who have lived in substandard housing in rural areas or urban slums in parts of Latin America where Chagas' disease is endemic, have received inadequately screened blood products in Latin America, or whose mother is infected with *T. cruzi*. In assessing risk, the age of the immigrant in relation to the implementation of Chagas' disease control in the country of origin should be considered. Because of successful interventions in previously endemic areas, young persons have grown up with no risk of infection, even though a large number of older persons in the same area are infected.

The approach to laboratory diagnosis of Chagas' disease depends on the stage of infection and the presence or absence of symptoms. In cases of suspected acute, congenital, or reactivated infection, wet mounts or Giemsa-stained smears of peripheral blood and buffy coat are examined microscopically for trypanosomes. Parasites occasionally can be found in cerebrospinal fluid, bone marrow, or other tissues. When microscopic examinations are negative, parasites frequently can be isolated after several weeks of incubation of blood or other specimens on special culture media such as NNN or Schneider's. Serological tests for IgM antibodies to *T. cruzi* may be positive, but reliable assays are not widely available. Serial IgG tests for antibodies to *T. cruzi* demonstrate seroconversion in acute cases, and persistence of IgG antibodies beyond age 6–9 months supports the diagnosis of congenital Chagas' disease.

Because direct examination of the blood is always negative during chronic infection, diagnosis relies on detection of IgG antibodies to *T. cruzi*. In competent laboratories, the sensitivity of the most commonly employed serological assays, the indirect fluorescent antibody test (IFAT) and enzyme-linked immunoassay (ELISA), approaches 99%; the hemagglutination inhibition test (IHAT) does not perform as well.[6] To improve sensitivity and specificity, at least two different assays should be employed. Blood culture and polymerase chain reaction (PCR)-based assays that detect parasite DNA in the blood are useful for diagnosis of acute infection, for confirmation of infection when serological results are equivocal, and for monitoring response to therapy. However, the sensitivity of PCR-based assays also falls short of 100%, and cultures are even less sensitive. In the United States, several serological assays are available commercially, and IFAT, ELISA, and blood cultures for *T. cruzi* are performed at the Centers for Disease Control and Prevention.

## ICD-9 Codes

- 086.0 Chagas' disease (American trypanosomiasis, infection with *Trypanosoma cruzi*) with heart involvement
- 086.1 Chagas' disease with other organ involvement
- 086.2 Chagas' disease without mention of organ involvement
- V75.3 trypanosomiasis (Chagas' disease or sleeping sickness).

## Treatment

At present, there are two drugs for treating *T. cruzi* infection. Benznidazole is available in endemic countries, and in the US, CDC's Parasitic Drug Service provides nifurtimox. Both drugs are administered orally for at least 60 days (Table 26.1). Children tolerate treatment better than adults, who may have to interrupt treatment to allow serious side effects to resolve.

All patients with acute, congenital, or reactivated infections should receive benznidazole or nifurtimox in order to lower the level of parasitemia and decrease the duration and severity of infection. In up to 70% or more cases of acute and congenital infection, early treatment results in cure as docu-

**Table 26.1 Drugs for treatment of Chagas' disease**

| Drug | Adult dose | Pediatric dose | Administration | Efficacy | Adverse events | Comments |
|---|---|---|---|---|---|---|
| Nifurtimox (Lampit®) | 8–10 mg/kg/day | 11–16 years: 12.5–15 mg/kg/day ≤11 years: 15–20 mg/kg/day | 3–4 divided oral doses daily for 60–90 days | Parasitological cure in 75% or more if given in early acute stage Data limited for chronic infections, but may effect parasitological cure and reduce or prevent progression of heart disease in children and adults | Abdominal pain, nausea, anorexia, weight loss, insomnia, seizures, peripheral neuropathy, rashes, leukopenia | Contraindicated for use during pregnancy Tolerated better by children than adults Not recommended for persons with advanced heart disease |
| Benznidazole (Rochagan®) | 5 mg/kg/day | <40 kg: 5–7.5 mg/kg/day ≥40 kg: 5 mg/kg/day | 2–3 divided oral doses daily for 60 days | Parasitological cure in 75% or more if given in early acute stage and in >60% of chronically infected children Data limited for chronic infections, but may effect parasitological cure in adults and reduce or prevent progression of heart disease in children and adults | Rash, peripheral neuropathy, ageusia, bone marrow depression, gastrointestinal disturbances | Contraindicated for use during pregnancy Tolerated better by children than adults Not recommended for persons with advanced heart disease |

mented by negative parasitological and serological tests. Although treatment of reactivated infection can be life saving, it does not eliminate all parasites, and intermittent suppressive therapy is necessary to prevent recrudescence.

Recent studies of children with chronic *T. cruzi* infection have shown that 60 days of benznidazole therapy can eliminate parasites in over 60% of cases. While similar data are not available for adults[1], several studies suggest that treatment of chronically infected adults without heart failure can prevent or retard the progression of cardiac disease.[10] Currently, treatment is recommended for all infected children, but until further data are available, the decision to treat older persons should be left to the discretion of the patient and the physician. Following treatment of chronic cases, cure of infection should be regarded as certain only if culture and PCR-based assays remain negative, and all serological tests have become negative, a process that may require years.

Persons with chronic infection should be screened for evidence of cardiac and gastrointestinal disease with a resting electrocardiogram, and, for persons with symptoms suggestive of gastrointestinal disease, barium contrast or motility studies. Any suggestion of heart disease on screening should prompt a careful cardiac evaluation, including an echocardiogram. Treatments of congestive heart failure, arrhythmias, and heart block improve quality of life and prolong survival, but do not prevent progression of the cardiomyopathy. Cardiac transplantation may be the only means of preserving life. *T. cruzi* infection is not a contraindication to transplantation because reactivated infections respond promptly to chemotherapy, and survival is similar or superior to that following transplantation for other conditions. Symptoms of megaesophagus or megacolon may respond to dietary modifications and medications, but in more advanced cases, esophageal dilatation or surgical procedures such as cardiomyotomy and fundoplasty, esophagectomy, or bowel resection may be required.

## Prevention

National control programs that focus on vector control, house improvement, and screening of blood and organ donors will continue to decrease the risk of transmission of *T. cruzi* in endemic countries. Nevertheless, immigrants visiting their homes or traveling elsewhere in Latin America should avoid overnight stays in poorly constructed houses that may be infested with triatomine bugs. These travelers should also avoid camping or sleeping outdoors in areas where natural cycles of transmission exist. They should be aware that blood donors are not adequately screened for *T. cruzi* in all parts of Latin America. No vaccine to prevent *T. cruzi* infection is available.

Treatment of chronically infected pregnant women to prevent transplacental transmission is not recommended because of the toxicity and teratogenicity of nifurtimox and benznidazole. Their newborns, however, should be evaluated for congenital infection

## Infection Control Measures

Prevention of transmission of *T. cruzi* in the clinical setting is achieved through implementation of universal precautions as for other blood-borne pathogens. Measures include use of barriers such as gloves and protective eye wear for potential contact with blood or other body fluids, washing hands and other skin surfaces after contact with blood or body fluids, and careful handling of sharp instruments during and after use.

---

### Clinical Pearls

- Most persons with *T. cruzi* infection are asymptomatic, but all remain infected for life and are at risk for developing severe cardiac and gastrointestinal disease.
- Persons infected during childhood who as adults have a normal resting electrocardiogram are extremely unlikely to develop Chagas' heart disease.
- Tip-offs for recognizing Chagas' disease in Latin Americans include: right bundle branch block or combinations of conduction defects and complex arrhythmias on electrocardiogram; apical aneurysm on echocardiogram; motility disorders of the esophagus or colon; enhancing central nervous system lesions by CT or MRI in immunocompromised persons.
- Two or more different serological tests are necessary to rule in or rule out Chagas' disease in persons in whom the diagnosis is suspected.
- Antitrypanosomal drugs are most effective in children and persons with recent infections.
- Chagas' disease is not a contraindication to cardiac transplantation.

## Special Considerations for Immigrants

- Thousands of immigrants from Latin America with undiagnosed infection with *T. cruzi* live in the United States, Canada, Europe, and other nonendemic areas.
- Because there is effective treatment for Chagas' disease, all immigrants from Latin America (not the Caribbean), including those without symptoms, should be questioned about potential exposure to *T. cruzi* and undergo serological testing if there is a history of exposure.
- Serological screening is especially important in children, pregnant women, and women of child-bearing age, HIV-infected or other immunocompromised persons.
- Children of mothers with *T. cruzi* infection may be infected despite never having lived in an endemic area.
- Persons with a history of Chagas' disease or persons with exposure to *T. cruzi* and unknown serological status should not donate blood.

## References

1. Andrade AL, Martelli CM, Oliveira RM, et al. Short report: benznidazole efficacy among *Trypanosoma cruzi*-infected adolescents after a six-year follow-up. Am J Trop Med Hyg 2004; 71:594–597.
2. Carlier Y, Torrico F. Congenital infection with *Trypanosoma cruzi*: from mechanisms of transmission to strategies for diagnosis and control. Rev Soc Bras Med Trop 2003; 36:767–771.
3. Dias JCP, Silveira AC, Schofield CJ. The impact of Chagas' disease control in Latin America – a review. Mem Inst Oswaldo Cruz 2002; 97:603–612.
4. Haggar JM, Rahimtoola SH. Chagas' heart disease in the United States. N Engl J Med 1992; 326:492–493.
5. Leiby DA, Herron RM Jr, Read EJ, et al. *Trypanosoma cruzi* in Los Angeles and Miami blood donors: impact of evolving donor demographics on seroprevalence and implications for transfusion transmission. Transfusion 2002; 42:549–555.
6. Malan AK, Avelar E, Litwin SE, et al. Serological diagnosis of *Trypanosoma cruzi*: evaluation of three enzyme immunoassays and an indirect immunofluorescent assay. J Med Microbiol 2006; 55:171–178.
7. Nowicki MJ, Chinchilla C, Corado L, et al. Prevalence of antibodies to *Trypanosoma cruzi* among solid organ donors in Southern California: a population at risk. Transplantation 2006; 81:477–479.
8. Prata A. Clinical and epidemiological aspects of Chagas' disease. Lancet Infect Dis 2001; 1:92–100.
9. World Health Organization. Control of Chagas' disease. Second report of the WHO expert committee. WHO Technical Report Series. Geneva: World Health Organization; 2002.
10. Viotti R, Vigiliano C, Lococo B, et al. Long-term cardiac outcomes of treating chronic Chagas' disease with benznidazole versus no treatment. Ann Intern Med 2006; 144:724–733.

# CHAPTER 27

# *Taenia Solium* and Neurocysticercosis

Linda Siti Yancey and A. Clinton White, Jr.

---

### Neurocysticercosis at a Glance

- Neurocysticercosis includes a diverse spectrum of diseases with varying clinical manifestations, pathophysiology, and treatment.
- Neurocysticercosis should be suspected in all patients with neurological disease and a history of exposure.
- Diagnosis is based upon neuroimaging and serological studies.
- Treatment varies by the form of the disease and may involve symptomatic therapy, antiparasitic drugs, anti-inflammatory treatment, and surgical interventions.

## Introduction

Neurocysticercosis was originally recognized by the ancient Greeks, who termed parasites in meat cysticerci (meaning cyst-tail). By the end of the nineteenth century, European investigators had identified the major parasite forms and their relationship. By the early twentieth century, large case series had been published which described infection in hundreds of patients, identifying nearly all of the major clinical manifestations of disease.

Prior to 1980, cysticercosis was regarded as a fairly rare disease found in endemic areas. Subsequent advances in neuroimaging and serological assays are facilitating the diagnosis of patients with both cysticercosis and taeniasis. Neurocysticercosis is now recognized as a critical public health problem in endemic countries and among immigrants from resource-limited countries.[1-3]

## Epidemiology

Neurocysticercosis is endemic in areas where pigs are raised under conditions that allow them access to human fecal material.[3] In these endemic areas, the majority of pig rearing is done on small farms. The pigs are generally not penned and are allowed to forage freely, enabling even small farms to raise animals without the expense of having to feed them. Meat inspection, improved sanitation, and improved animal husbandry led to the eradication of cysticercosis in Western Europe (an area highly endemic as late as the nineteenth century). However, these approaches have generally failed in developing countries. Currently, porcine cysticercosis remains widespread throughout Latin America, sub-Saharan Africa, South and Southeast Asia, as well as parts of Korea, China, Indonesia, and Papua New Guinea. In these areas, human tapeworms and cysticercosis are common. There are few good data upon which to base estimates of global prevalence or burden of disease. Around 2.5 million people worldwide are thought to carry the pork tapeworm. The estimated prevalence of neurocysticercosis ranges from 20 to 100 million cases with 50 000 deaths each year attributed to the infection. Case series employing neuroimaging studies find neurocysticercosis in 20–50% of adults with seizures and a similar portion of patients with chronic epilepsy.

In the United States, neurocysticercosis is primarily a disease of immigrants. It was rarely diagnosed prior to 1980. The numbers of cases, however, had increased fourfold by the early 1980s. An investigation by the Centers for Disease Control and Prevention concluded that most of the increase was attributable to improved diagnosis due to the introduction and increased use of computed tomography (CT) scanning.[4] In the 1980s and 1990s, large case series were reported from California, Colorado, Texas, New York, and Chicago. The vast majority of cases were diagnosed in Hispanic immigrants, mainly from Mexico and Central America. However, cases were also seen among immigrants from Asia (especially India, Korea, and Southeast Asia), and, less frequently, Africa. These proportions are similar to the percentage of the foreign-born population from those areas. Most case series also include US-born cases, most associated with travel to endemic areas. However, there have been over 70 well-documented cases of local transmission in the US. Most of these cases can be tied to tapeworm carriers. For example, four Orthodox Jews in New York City were documented to have neurocysticercosis.[5]

More recently, prospective and population-based studies have been applied to the epidemiology of neurocysticercosis in the US. After neurocysticercosis was made a reportable disease in California it was noted that among the first 138 cases, 19 were US born, but only 10 did not report travel outside of the US.[6] A study of family contacts identified tapeworm carriers among the contacts of US-born cases. Among 57 cases seen in Oregon, 72% were born in Mexico and 5% in Guatemala, but 18% were born in the US, some of whom denied travel to endemic areas.[7] In patients presenting with seizures to emergency rooms, neurocysticercosis was felt to be the cause in 38/1801 (2.1%) patients, and 13.5% among Hispanics.[8] All of the cases in which information was available were either born in or traveled to an endemic region and most were Hispanic or immigrants. In a series from Houston, Texas,[9] most of the cases were immigrants, primarily from Central Mexico or Central America. Among six US-born cases, all had traveled frequently to villages in Latin America. Again, 2% of all seizures and 16% of seizures among Hispanics were thought to be due to neurocysticercosis.

Sorvillo and colleagues reviewed death certificates from California from 1988 until 2000.[10] Of the 124 deaths attributed to neurocysticercosis most were among Hispanics (115/124), primarily immigrants from Mexico. In a survey of seroprevalence of cysticercosis and taeniasis,[11] the seroprevalence for antibody to the tapeworm stage was 1.7%, but none of the children was seropositive.

In summary, neurocysticercosis is a common neurologic infection among immigrants to the US. Most patients are Hispanic immigrants. Whether this is due to the high proportion of immigrants to the US from Latin America or due to a higher incidence in this group is not known. While eating pork does not transmit cysticercosis, most of the cases have significant exposure to pig-raising villages and, in many cases, their families raise pigs. Tapeworm infections are also common among immigrants. While local transmission undoubtedly does occur, it is rare compared to imported infection.

## Etiology and Pathogenesis

*Taenia solium*, the pork tapeworm, is a cestode parasite that causes two different and highly distinct forms of infection in the human host. Taeniasis (or taeniosis) refers to infestation of the intestinal tract by the adult tapeworm (Fig. 27.1). The term cysticercosis refers to infection of tissues such as muscle and brain with the larval cysticercus form. The term neurocysticercosis refers to cysticercosis involving the central nervous system (CNS) (including the subarachnoid space, spinal cord, and eyes).

Humans are the definitive hosts of *T. solium*, harboring the adult tapeworm in the intestines. The tapeworms reach lengths of several meters. The worm sheds eggs and/or gravid proglottids intermittently into the feces. In areas where pigs have access to the infected human waste, foraging pigs ingest the eggs or proglottids. Once ingested, the eggs hatch to release the larval oncospheres, which attach to and penetrate the wall of the gut. The larvae enter the bloodstream and migrate to the tissues, where they develop into cysticerci over a period of a few weeks. The cysticerci have an invaginated scolex (poised to develop into a tapeworm when ingested), a bladder wall, and cyst fluid (which contains a mixture of parasite and host material). They actively suppress the host inflammatory response and are able to survive in the porcine tissues for periods of a few years. When infected pork is eaten, the scolex evaginates, attaches to the intestinal wall, and develops segments termed proglottids. The proglottids mature as they are displaced from the scolex by newer proglottids. As they mature, they develop testes and ovaries that form eggs. The mature, gravid proglottids and eggs are shed intermittently. The eggs are not only shed into the environment, but also contaminate the hand and fingernails of the tapeworm carriers. These eggs can then autoinfect the tapeworm carrier or other people in close contact

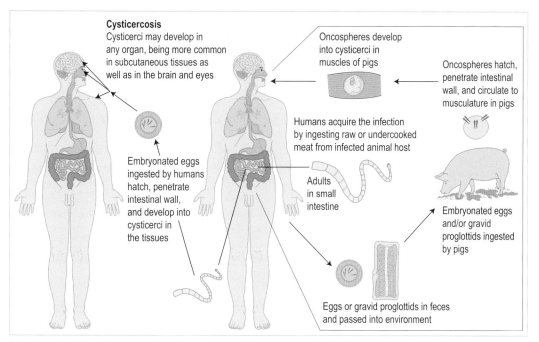

**Fig. 27.1** The life cycle of *Taenia solium*. (Adapted from Centers for Disease Control and Prevention DPDx.)

with the carrier. Thus, human cysticercosis requires no contact with pigs or pork, as illustrated by cases described in vegetarians in India and orthodox Jews in the United States. When these eggs are ingested by humans they hatch and release the enclosed larvae, called oncospheres, which migrate through the blood and develop into cysticerci in a wide range of tissues. In most tissues, the cysticerci cause few symptoms and their survival is limited. By contrast, infection of the central nervous system often lasts for years and can cause severe symptoms.

Cysticerci reach their mature size within a few weeks of infection. However, studies of British subjects who developed neurocysticercosis after working in India, and of US immigrants, reveal that there is typically an incubation period of several years between infection and clinical presentation.[9] Laboratory studies have identified a complex array of parasite molecules that suppress the host inflammatory response.[12] Thus, the quiescent phase is thought to result from the parasite's ability to evade the host immune system. Over time, the cysticerci age and lose the ability to evade immune attack. A brisk cell-mediated response ensues, during which the cysticerci are surrounded by and infiltrated with a granulomatous reaction composed primarily of mononuclear cells, with variable numbers of eosinophils and neutrophils. In an animal model, the gran-

ulomatous host response to the degenerating cysts rather than the parasite per se produces seizure activity, the characteristic clinical presentation of parenchymal neurocysticercosis. Over a period of months, the inflamed parasite passes through a series of stages of inflammation until it either resolves radiographically or is replaced by a small calcified granuloma (which appears as a small nodule on imaging studies). If the lesions resolve, seizure activity usually also resolves. Persistent seizure activity has been associated with the presence of calcifications. While the pathophysiology is not clear, periodic release of persistent parasitic antigen from the calcification is thought to lead to recurrent seizures.

The pathogenesis of extra-parenchymal neurocysticercosis is somewhat different.[12] Cysticerci in the cerebral ventricles often cause obstructive hydrocephalus. Pathologic studies show that most of these cysticerci are viable. Thus, the obstructive hydrocephalus is thought to result from mechanical obstruction of cerebrospinal fluid (CSF) flow by the cysticerci. Cysticerci in the subarachnoid space are often accompanied by an inflammatory response. In this case, the inflammation may lead to meningeal inflammation (with headache and nuchal rigidity) and chronic arachnoiditis. The latter may cause vasculitis and strokes or communicating hydrocephalus. Occasionally, cysticerci in the sub-arachnoid space may enlarge and cause mass effect. In patients with multiple cysticerci, several forms of the disease can be present at the same time.

## Clinical Manifestations

*T. solium* can cause a wide range of clinical manifestations depending on the form of the parasite involved, the number of parasites, the location, and the degree of host inflammation.[1-3]

### Taeniasis

Taeniasis results from the adult worm dwelling in the lumen of the intestine. Some patients note the passage of proglottids in the stool. Some patients also complain of minor gastrointestinal complaints, but, for the most part, there are no significant ill effects.

### Cysticercosis

Cysticerci have been observed in a wide range of tissues including all groups of skeletal muscles as well as in the myocardium. Cysticerci in muscle are usually asymptomatic; however, massive infection may result in weakness and/or pseudo-hypertrophy. In muscle, the cysticerci form elongated structures parallel to the muscle fibers. In most cases, the cysticerci progress to calcified granulomas without causing significant symptoms. Thus, muscle involvement is typically identified via cigar-shaped calcifications found as an incidental finding on X-rays (Fig. 27.2A).

When located close to the skin surface, cysticerci present as small, firm nodules (similar in appearance to a sebaceous cyst). As they undergo degeneration, these nodules can become transiently painful and inflamed. Subcutaneous cysticercosis appears to be more common among patients infected in Africa and Asia than in those infected in Latin America. Cysticerci can also involve the eye (including subconjunctival, aqueous or vitreous humor, or subretinal locations).

### Neurocysticercosis

Most clinical presentations of cysticercosis are associated with involvement of the central nervous system, and termed neurocysticercosis. Historically, neurocysticercosis has been viewed as a single disease entity. Recent studies, however, have emphasized that neurocysticercosis presents with a spectrum of clinical forms, all or none of which may be present in a given patient. Neurocysticercosis can be broadly divided into parenchymal and extra-parenchymal manifestations, which differ in pathophysiology, clinical presentation, treatment, and prognosis.

### Parenchymal neurocysticercosis

Parenchymal neurocysticercosis is caused by cysticerci located within the parenchyma of the brain or within the folds of the gyri. These cysts are limited in size by the surrounding brain parenchyma. They cause few symptoms until their degenerative phase, when they can cause seizures.

The most common presentation of neurocysticercosis in the United States is that of a solitary degenerating parenchymal lesion (Fig. 27.2B). These patients tend to present with new-onset seizures or headaches. Neurocysticercosis patients are less likely to report generalized seizures than other seizure patients. The seizures are typically focal with secondary generalization. However, they are often initially described as generalized.

Patients from endemic areas may also present with multiple parenchymal lesions (Fig. 27.2C). In such cases, seizure activity is also the most common presenting symptom.

Cysticercal encephalitis is a rare presentation primarily seen in children and young women. These patients are infected with large numbers of parasites, which induce a brisk inflammatory response and associated diffuse cerebral edema. They present with symptoms of cerebral edema, including headache, altered mental status, and focal neurologic findings.

### Extra-parenchymal neurocysticercosis

Extra-parenchymal neurocysticercosis includes cysts within the ventricles of the brain (either freely floating or attached to the ventricular wall) (Fig. 27.2D), in the subarachnoid space, in the eye, or in the spine. The presentation of extra-parenchymal disease varies depending on the location of the cysts.

Ventricular cysticercosis characteristically presents with increased intracranial pressure from obstructive hydrocephalus. Headache, nausea, papilledema and altered level of consciousness can all

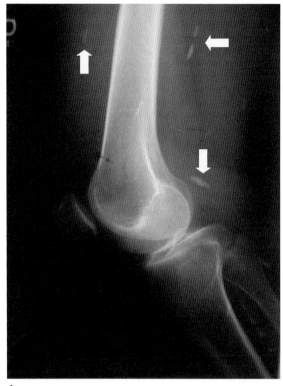

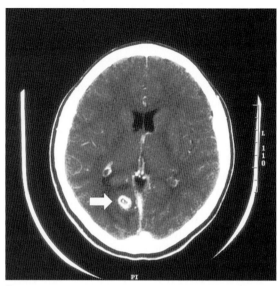

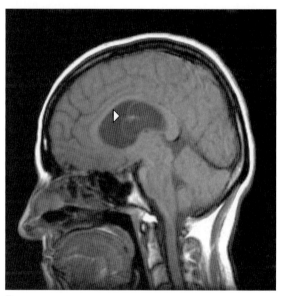

Fig. 27.2 **(A)** Calcified cysticerci in the large muscles surrounding the knee (arrows). Note the classic cigar shape that aligns with the direction of the muscle fibers. **(B)** Solitary enhancing parenchymal lesion (arrow) in the occipital lobe of child presenting with new-onset seizures. **(C)** Multiple parenchymal cysticerci (arrows) some with visible scolices (small arrowheads). **(D)** Cysticercus within the lateral ventricle causing obstructive hydrocephalus. Note the visible scolex (arrowhead).

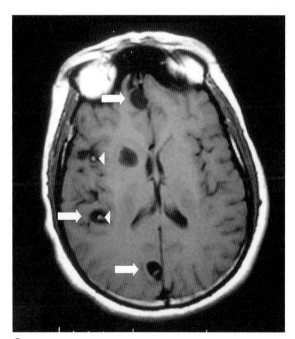

be seen. The onset is quite variable and may range from mild intermittent headaches to sudden loss of consciousness. In some cases, symptoms may vary with head position from ball-valve effects of the parasites.

Subarachnoid cysticercosis is quite variable in presentation. Most of these patients are infected with large numbers of parasites and they frequently have ventricular and/or parenchymal as well as subarachnoid disease. Subarachnoid cysticerci in the basilar cisterns typically cause arachnoiditis. This may present as meningitis (headache, stiff neck, and CSF pleocytosis), stroke (usually associated with vasculitis), or communicating hydrocephalus. Cysticerci that form in the basilar cisterns or fissures (particularly in the sylvian fissure) are not enclosed by surrounding tissue. They can grow unchecked to a diameter of over 5 cm. These cysts often lack identifiable parasitic components and appear as a cluster of cystic lesions (termed racemose cysticercosis). Giant cysticerci may be associated with mass effect (either directly or, more often, from associated edema), seizures, or arachnoiditis.

## Diagnosis

### Taeniasis

Because of the paucity of symptoms present in tapeworm carriers, testing generally occurs when a case of neurocysticercosis has been detected and the patient, as well as household contacts, is being screened for tapeworm carriage.

The traditional method of diagnosing taeniasis has been serial stool studies for ova and parasites. Tapeworms shed eggs and proglottids intermittently. Furthermore, collection of an adequate amount of stool for study can be challenging. Thus, overall sensitivity of stool microscopy is thought to be only 26%.[13] Furthermore, stool studies cannot distinguish between carriers of *T. solium* and *T. saginata*.

Antigen-detection assays and recent serologic tests have improved the diagnosis. Coproantigen testing has been found to have a specificity of 99.2% and a sensitivity of 70–92%.[13] *T. solium* tapeworm-stage antigens have been employed in serum ELISAs to identify tapeworm carriers.[14] These assays may be more sensitive than stool-based tests and they seem to be quite specific but are so far only available as research tools. However, the antibody continues to be detected after treatment. Thus, some assays

will detect prior rather than active tapeworm infection.

## ICD-9 Codes

- 123.1 Cysticercosis; cysticerciasis; infection by the larval form of *Taenia solium* (formerly called *Cysticercus cellulosae*); neurocysticercosis
- 123.0 *Taenia solium* infection, intestinal form; pork tapeworm (adult, infection)

### Neurocysticercosis

Neurocysticercosis presents with neurologic syndromes such as seizures, symptoms of increased intracranial pressure, headaches, and/or meningeal signs. Thus, neuroimaging remains the primary means of diagnosis.[15,16] Anyone presenting from an endemic area with new-onset seizures or symptoms of increased cranial pressure should undergo CT or magnetic resonance imaging (MRI) of the head.

Cysticerci can be seen on both CT and MRI. CT is better at detecting calcifications, while MRI has better success in detecting cysts in extra-parenchymal locations such as the ventricles and basilar cisterns. The better resolution available in MRI scans enables subtle areas of edema to be recognized and more often allows the visualization of the scolex. CT still is the primary initial imaging study employed in most areas. This may lead to underdiagnosis; hence, MRI is the modality of choice for imaging cysticerci.

Viable cysts can be seen on neuroimaging as 1–2 cm round fluid collections. On CT and $T_1$ MRI scans, the cyst fluid is hypodense compared to the brain parenchyma, and isodense with CSF. A small internal nodule is sometimes seen, which represents the invaginated scolex. The wall of the cysticercus is usually isodense with the parenchyma and not easily visualized. On $T_2$ and FLAIR images, the fluid is seen as hyperintense, which facilitates visualization of the cyst cavity in brain parenchyma. As the cysticercus becomes inflamed, perilesional edema and contrast enhancement appear, which are often more easy to distinguish on FLAIR images. Subsequently, the cyst fluid increases in density as it is infiltrated by host inflammatory cells. The cyst fluid eventually collapses, forming a solid area of focal enhancement. At that point, the granulomatous inflammation either resolves or leads to the formation of calcified granulomas, which appear as nodular calcifications usually 2–6 mm in diameter. Inflammatory cysticerci in the basilar cisterns can be quite variable in presentation. As the inflammation destroys the cysticercus, imaging studies may only reveal basilar meningitis.

Neuroimaging studies can identify abnormalities in almost all cases, but the findings are rarely pathognomonic. The finding of a typical cysticercus containing a clearly defined scolex is thought to be diagnostic, but this is only rarely seen. More frequently, patients present with one or more ring-enhancing lesions which have a radiographic appearance similar to that of a metastatic tumor or infection. Rajshekhar and Chandy developed clinical criteria to distinguish neurocysticercosis from other causes among patients with single enhancing CT lesions.[17] The criteria for cysticercal granuloma included having a single round CT lesion 2 cm or less in diameter without midline shift. By history and examination, patients with cysticercosis lacked systemic symptoms or signs of disease outside of the CNS. For example, they should not have fever, night sweats, or adenopathy. On neurologic examinations, cysticercosis patients lacked focal neurologic signs or evidence of increased intracranial pressure. In a prospective study of 401 patients with seizures and a single enhancing lesion, 215 met criteria for cysticercal granulomas and only two were subsequently found to have another cause. By contrast, the vast majority of those not meeting criteria were subsequently found to have either tumors or tuberculosis.

Serologic tests also can play an important role in diagnosis of neurocysticercosis. Serologic testing for cysticercosis using crude antigens has been hampered by poor sensitivity and specificity.[14] Although laboratories in developing countries continue to use assays with crude antigens (derived from cysticerci obtained from infected pork), several studies have demonstrated poor performance characteristics, even when CSF is used as a source of antibody. Tsang and colleagues (in Garcia et al.[14]) developed an immunoblot assay using parasite glycoprotein antigen to detect specific antibody in serum and CSF to one or more of seven glycoprotein antigens. The assay has proven to be highly specific and performs better with serum samples than with CSF, although recent reports have noted rare false-positive results in patients with only antibody to the gp50 band. However, the sensitivity of this assay is poor in patients with single lesions or just calcifications. Hancock and colleagues noted that most of the immunogenic glycoproteins belong to a family of 8 kD proteins and have cloned several members of this family.[14] The sensitivity and specificity of ELISA

using recombinant antigens was between 97% and 100% compared to the EITB test. One particular protein sequence (TsRS1) is 100% sensitive and specific for the studied sera but these tests are not yet commercially available.

Assays to detect parasite antigens, rather than antibody, could potentially improve diagnosis because their results should only be positive with active parasite infection. In a recent study using CSF samples, the sensitivity was better with inflamed than with noninflamed lesions, and with multiple rather than single cysticerci. This parallels results with the EITB assay but, again, the assays are not yet widely available.

Other studies may be helpful in diagnosing cysticercosis. If patients have subcutaneous nodules, biopsies can be performed to document cysticercosis. Also, typical cigar-shaped calcifications may be visualized in muscle by X-rays or CT scanning. Lumbar puncture and studies of cerebrospinal fluid are mainly helpful for excluding alternative diagnoses. The cerebrospinal fluid in neurocysticercosis can be quite variable. It can be completely normal, or have marked abnormalities of protein, glucose, and cell counts. When CSF pleocytosis is present, the cell counts display variable numbers of mononuclear cells such as lymphocytes, neutrophils, and eosinophils.

## Treatment

Symptomatic therapy is the cornerstone of management in neurocysticercosis.[18] Seizures should be treated with antiepileptic medications, hydrocephalus should be treated surgically, and cerebral edema should be managed with corticosteroids (Tables 27.1 and 27.2).

### Seizures

In patients presenting with seizures attributed to neurocysticercosis, the initial emphasis must be on control of the seizure activity. Most seizures can be easily controlled with any of a number of antiepileptic drugs. Usually a single drug is adequate. Most published experience is with phenytoin, phenobarbital, or carbamazepine. Newer agents (e.g. valproate, lamotrigine, levitiracetam, topiramate, or oxcarbazepine) are likely at least as effective. Breakthrough seizures usually occur when antiepileptic drug levels are sub-therapeutic such as during periods of poor medication adherence.[19]

**Table 27.1 Treatment recommendations for different forms of neurocysticercosis**

| Form of Disease | Recommendations |
|---|---|
| **Parenchymal lesions** | |
| Calcified lesions only | Symptomatic therapy (e.g. antiepileptic medications[a]) |
| | Antiparasitic agents not recommended |
| Single enhancing lesions | Symptomatic therapy (e.g. antiepileptic medications[a]) |
| | Corticosteroids should be continued 5–7 days after completion of antiparasitic drugs |
| | Minimal benefit of antiparasitic drugs (e.g. albendazole for 8 days may hasten resolution) |
| Multiple enhancing lesions | Symptomatic therapy (e.g. antiepileptic medications[a]) |
| | Corticosteroids should be continued 5–7 days after completion of antiparasitic drugs |
| | Antiparasitic drugs for 8–28 days |
| Cysticercal encephalitis (diffuse cerebral edema with multiple lesions) | Symptomatic therapy (e.g. antiepileptic medications[a]) |
| | Corticosteroids until resolution of cerebral edema |
| | Antiparasitic drugs contraindicated |
| Nonenhancing lesions[b] | Symptomatic therapy (e.g. antiepileptic medications[a]) |
| | Corticosteroids should be continued 5–7 days after completion of antiparasitic drugs |
| | Antiparasitic drugs for 8–28 days |
| **Extra-parenchymal lesions** | |
| Ventricular | Removal of the cyst(s) if possible (If available, removal via endoscopy is preferred over open surgical procedures) |
| | Antiparasitic drugs should *not* be given prior to endoscopic removal of cysts as dying cysts can adhere to the wall of the ventricle complicating removal and are not needed when completely removed |
| | Symptomatic therapy (e.g. ventriculoperitoneal shunt or endoscopic surgery) to relieve increased intracranial pressure |
| | **Alternative approach:** |
| | Ventriculoperitoneal shunt placement followed by: |
| | Antiparasitic drugs for 8–28 days |
| | Corticosteroids should be continued 5–7 days after completion of antiparasitic drugs |
| Subarachnoid | Ventriculoperitoneal shunting in cases of hydrocephalus |
| | Corticosteroids should be continued at least 5–7 days after completion of antiparasitic drugs |
| | Antiparasitic drugs for ≥28 days |
| Giant subarachnoid cysts (lesions >5 cm in diameter) | Ventriculoperitoneal shunting in cases of hydrocephalus or surgical decompression if mass effect |
| | Corticosteroids should be continued 5–7 days after completion of antiparasitic drugs |
| | Antiparasitic drugs for ≥28 days |

[a] The first line of therapy in any patient with active seizures is control of the seizure activity. Any patient with seizure activity should be evaluated as soon as possible by a physician with experience in seizure management.
[b] Limited to symptomatic presentation.

The duration of antiepileptic therapy is the subject of ongoing study and debate. Several studies have indicated that patients can be tapered off seizure medications after at least a year of symptom-free maintenance therapy if radiographic resolution of the lesion is seen. This approach should always be undertaken with care as the rate of seizures after withdrawal of medications has been shown to be as high as 40% in some populations. The presence of a residual inflamed or calcified lesion correlates with continued seizure risk. Some authorities continue antiepileptic drugs indefinitely if patients develop calcifications. Thus, antiepileptic drugs should probably be continued for at least a year after neuroradio-

**Table 27.2 Medications commonly used in the treatment of neurocysticercosis**

| Class | Drug | Dose | Common Side Effects |
|---|---|---|---|
| Antiparasitic medications (adult and pediatric doses) | Albendazole | 15 mg/kg/day in 2–3 doses | Headache, liver function test elevation, nausea/vomiting |
| | Praziquantel | 50–100 mg/kg/day divided into 3 doses | Headache, dizziness, diaphoresis, nausea/vomiting |
| Anti-inflammatory corticosteroids | Dexamethasone | 12–24 mg/day in 1–4 doses | Insomnia, elevated blood sugar, leukocytosis |
| | Prednisolone | 30–40 mg/day | Insomnia, elevated blood sugar, leukocytosis |

logic resolution of the lesions. For patients who go on to develop calcifications, it is unclear whether antiepileptic drugs should ever be tapered.

## Hydrocephalus

Patients with neurocysticercosis frequently present with increased intracranial pressure. In some cases, elevated pressures are the result of cerebral edema. This can usually be managed with corticosteroids. Patients with obstructive hydrocephalus usually require surgery. If symptoms are mild or intermittent (e.g. a cysticercus in the lateral ventricles not associated with midline shift), management may be delayed until elective endoscopic removal of the cysticercus (see below). However, many cases require CSF diversion procedures. Emergency diversion can be accomplished via a ventriculostomy. In the authors' center, however, most cases are initially managed with placement of a ventriculoperitoneal shunt. There is a high rate of shunt failure if shunting is not followed by antiparasitic and anti-inflammatory therapy. Patients with arachnoiditis may develop communicating hydrocephalus. This usually requires placement of a ventriculoperitoneal shunt as well. In some patients, cysticerci and associated edema may lead to mass effects. If the symptoms are life threatening or if the cysticercus is easily approachable (e.g. in the sylvian fissure), surgical decompression of the cysticercus is the preferred approach.

## Antiparasitic drugs

The role of antiparasitic drugs in the treatment of neurocysticercosis has been controversial.[18] Praziquantel and later albendazole were recognized as antiparasitic agents that could kill the parasites. Praziquantel was approved for use in the US in the early 1980s and albendazole became available in the early 1990s. However, the first controlled trial on their use in neurocysticercosis was published in 1995 and it showed no effect. Subsequent trials and expert meetings are beginning to clarify the role of antiparasitic therapy in cysticercosis. Much of the controversy has stemmed from poor study design, including grouping patients with markedly different forms of disease and failure to account for the natural history. There is an emerging consensus among experts about the proper role of antiparasitic drugs in management of neurocysticercosis. All experts agree that neurocysticercosis represents a spectrum of diseases that not only differ in clinical manifestations, but also differ in pathogenesis and optimal management.[18] Thus, the major different forms will be discussed separately, as parenchymal and extra-parenchymal.

### Parenchymal neurocysticercosis

**Single enhancing lesions** The most common presentation of neurocysticercosis among immigrants to the US is with seizures and a single enhancing lesion on neuroimaging studies. Overall, the seizures usually respond to a single antiepileptic medication.[20] In the absence of antiparasitic therapy, the lesions usually resolve over months to years. Controlled trials of antiparasitic therapy in patients with single enhancing lesions have given variable results. However, most studies show more rapid radiologic resolution with antiparasitic drugs. Recurrent seizures tend to occur at the time of resolution. Thus, they occur earlier in patients receiving antiparasitic medications. By contrast, the proportion of patients who go on to develop chronic calcifications does not appear to be affected. The role of steroids in reducing inflammation around lesions is better defined with several recent studies showing clear benefit in reduction of seizure activity and faster resolution of lesion on CT when steroids were used in conjunction with antiepileptic medications.

Overall, the major focus of management of patients with seizures and single enhancing lesions should be on optimizing antiseizure medications. There is also likely a small benefit from antiparasitic drugs (e.g. albendazole 15 mg/kg/day for 8 days, as listed in Tables 27.1 and 27.2) and a short course of corticosteroids.

**Multiple parenchymal lesions** Patients presenting with seizures with multiple cysticerci will usually have at least one cysticercus in the process of degenerating (e.g. edema or contrast enhancement on imaging studies). Other cysticerci may be in the viable stage. Thus, patients are at risk for sequential degradation of the cysticerci and prolonged seizure risk. A recent placebo-controlled trial from Peru showed a small but statistically significant reduction in generalized seizures in patients treated with albendazole.[19] The difference was most dramatic after tapering of antiseizure medications. However, there was no decrease in development of chronic calcifications. While this trial mainly focused on patients with at least one cysticercus thought to be viable, most experts also extend this result to patients with only enhancing lesions. Thus, patients with multiple parenchymal cysticerci should usually be treated with a course of an antiparasitic (albendazole 15 mg/kg/day for 8 days or praziquantel 50–100 mg/kg/day for 28 days, see Tables 27.1 and 27.2). They should also generally receive a short course of corticosteroids at the same time.

**Cysticercal encephalitis (numerous cysticerci with cerebral edema)** A minority of patients with multiple cysticerci will develop diffuse cerebral edema from the inflammatory response to the parasites.[18] These patients should be treated with anti-inflammatory drugs such as corticosteroids. Antiparasitic drugs are contraindicated because of the potential to exacerbate the host inflammatory response and cerebral edema. In most cases, the cysticerci will resolve spontaneously with anti-inflammatory medications. However, some authorities would treat these patients with antiparasitic drugs after the cerebral edema has resolved.

**Calcifications** Parenchymal calcifications caused by neurocysticercosis can be seen in more than 10% of residents of some endemic areas. The presence of

intraparenchymal calcifications is a significant risk factor for continued seizure activity.[21] Patients with seizures associated with a calcified lesion should be treated as those with any other focal epilepsy. Treatment of a calcification with antiparasitic medications is not indicated. Anti-inflammatory drugs have been used in some cases but there is no clear evidence whether they provide any benefit. Surgical removal of the calcified focus has been used in some cases of intractable seizures. Most cases, however, are easily managed with a single antiepileptic medication.

### Extra-parenchymal neurocysticercosis

**Ventricular neurocysticercosis** When hydrocephalus due to obstruction occurs, the first priority must be to relieve the intracranial pressure. Historically, ventricular cysticerci have been removed via open craniotomy, but this was associated with substantial postoperative morbidity. With advances in the use of neuroendoscopic devices, cysticercus removal can now be carried out using minimally invasive procedures, with significantly decreased morbidity. The method of choice at this time is endoscopic removal of the cysts. Endoscopic foramenotomy can often be used to treat residual hydrocephalus. Antiparasitic medications should not be given prior to the procedure as they can cause the cysticerci to be friable or to adhere to the ventricular wall. The cysticerci often rupture during removal, but this has not been associated with any sequelae when accompanied by intraprocedural irrigation to remove parasitic debris.[22]

Neuroendoscopy is not available in all centers and some patients may need to be treated emergently. These patients can usually be managed with emergent CSF diversion (usually via placement of a ventriculoperitoneal shunt). The rate of shunt failure is high in patients treated only with ventriculoperitoneal shunting. This failure rate appears to be lowered by the addition of corticosteroids and antiparasitic drugs. Case series have identified some patients treated with only chemotherapy and steroids. However, this approach should generally be discouraged since it carries a substantial risk of development of acute hydrocephalus from cysticerci and/or accompanying inflammation causing obstruction of the foramina.

**Subarachnoid neurocysticercosis** Cysticerci in the basilar cistern can cause arachnoiditis leading to CSF outflow obstruction, communicating hydrocephalus, vasculitis, and strokes.[14] In the era before antiparasitic drugs were available, this form carried a high case fatality rate. By contrast, more recent case series have been characterized by low case fatality rates.[14,18,23] Expert consensus recommendations are to treat with antiparasitic drugs, anti-inflammatory drugs and, in most cases, CSF diversion procedures. Nevertheless, there are few good data on optimal doses or durations for medication. Most experts recommend treatment with albendazole (typically 15 mg/kg/day in divided doses for at least 28 days), but cure is rare with a single course of albendazole. Repeated courses, prolonged therapy, higher doses, or switching to praziquantel have been tried in some cases. There are anecdotal reports of improved responses with endoscopic debulking of the number of parasites, but this approach has not yet been systematically studied.

In some cases, however, the residual symptoms may reflect the chronic inflammatory response to cysticercal antigens rather than ongoing viable cysticerci. Thus, inflammation seems to drive much of the pathogenesis, but optimal management has not been defined. Prednisone (doses up to 60 mg per day) or dexamethasone (doses up to 24 mg per day) should be used along with the antiparasitic drugs. After 2–4 weeks, the dose can often be tapered. In cases that require more prolonged steroid therapy, methotrexate has been used as a steroid-sparing agent.

**Giant subarachnoid neurocysticercosis** Some cysticerci, particularly in the sylvian fissure or basilar cisterns, may enlarge to over 5 cm in diameter. In contrast to most other cysticerci, these large cysticerci can cause mass effect and midline shift, either directly or via surrounding edema. If the mass effect cannot be quickly reversed by corticosteroids and even mannitol, surgical decompression may be required. This can take the form of puncture and aspiration of the cyst fluid or removal of the cysticercus. If the patients are not symptomatic from mass effect, however, giant cysticerci can be treated similarly to other subarachnoid cysticerci.

## Prevention

Endemic porcine cysticercosis was eliminated from Western Europe with improvements in sanitation and meat inspection. Inspection of meat and animals at time of slaughter has been used to prevent acquisition of tapeworms. However, the greatest burden of taeniasis occurs in rural areas where animal slaugh-

ter and meat processing take place informally, and the general poverty of the regions makes the economic loss of condemned pork unacceptable. Thus, regulation of meat processing, while necessary, is not sufficient to address the problem.

Improved sanitation and pig husbandry can interrupt the lifecycle by preventing porcine cysticercosis. Economic barriers, however, pose a major obstacle. Mass chemotherapy to cure tapeworm carriers and of pigs to eliminate porcine cysticercosis can have a temporary effect on prevalence. Finally, vaccines have been developed, which can effectively prevent infection with larval cestodes. These are in development for porcine cysticercosis. Even when they become available there remain major obstacles to their effective use in endemic areas.

## Infection Control Measures

Patients with cysticercosis alone are not able to transmit any of the taenial diseases to others. However, patients with taeniasis, tapeworm carriage, have the potential to spread cysticercosis. Carriers of the pork tapeworm should be treated as soon as they are identified and should observe strict hygiene measures including hand washing and refraining from the preparation of food until completion of therapy.

---

### Clinical Pearls

- The first line of treatment in a patient with seizures is antiepileptic medications.
- The first line of treatment in a patient with hydrocephalus is surgery.
- Seizures in the parenchymal form of neurocysticercosis are caused by the host immune reaction to the dying parasite.
- Calcified cysts have already died and there is no benefit to treatment of this form of the disease with antiparasitic agents.
- Patients with subarachnoid cysticercosis should be treated with prolonged courses of antiparasitic and anti-inflammatory drugs.
- In heavily parasitized patients (>20 cysts), consider screening of the patient and their household contacts for the presence of a tapeworm carrier.

## Special Considerations for Immigrants

- New-onset seizures or hydrocephalus in a patient from an endemic area should prompt the consideration of neurocysticercosis as a possible etiology.
- In cases of neurocysticercosis, contact with pigs or pork, though commonly noted, is not necessary for acquisition of the disease.
- The importance of close neurological follow-up should be stressed to patients with seizures as a result of neurocysticercosis.

## References

1. Garcia HH, Gonzalez AE, Evans CA, et al. *Taenia solium* cysticercosis. Lancet 2003; 362:547–556.
2. White AC Jr. Neurocysticercosis: updates on epidemiology, pathogenesis, diagnosis, and management. Ann Rev Med 2000; 51:187–206.
3. Singh G, Prabhakar S. *Taenia solium* cysticercosis: From basic to clinical science. New York: CABI Publishing; 2002.
4. Richards FO, Schantz PM, Ruiz-Tiben E, et al. Cysticercosis in Los Angeles county. JAMA 1985; 254:3444–3448.
5. Moore AC, Lutwick LI, Schantz PM, et al. Seroprevalence of cysticercosis in an orthodox Jewish community. Am J Trop Med Hyg 1995; 53:439–442.
6. Sorvillo FJ, Waterman SH, Richards FO, et al. Cysticercosis surveillance: locally acquired and travel-related infection and detection of intestinal tapeworm carriers in Los Angeles. Am J Trop Med Hyg 1992; 47:365–371.
7. Townes JM, Hoffmann CJ, Kohn MA. Neurocysticercosis in Oregon, 1995–2000. Emerg Infect Dis 2004; 10:508–510.
8. Ong S, Talan DA, Moran GJ, et al. Neurocysticercosis in radiographically imaged seizure patients in US emergency departments. Emerg Infect Dis 2002; 8:608–613.
9. del la Garza Y, Graviss EA, Daver NG, et al. Epidemiology of neurocysticercosis in Houston, Texas. Am J Trop Med Hyg 2005; 73:766–770.
10. Sorvillo FJ, Portigal L, DeGiorgio C, et al. Cysticercosis-related deaths, California. Emerg Infect Dis 2004; 10:465–469.
11. DeGiorgio C, Pietsch-Escueta S, Tsang V, et al. Seroprevalence of *Taenia solium* cysticercosis and *Taenia solium* taeniasis in California, USA. Acta Neurol Scand 2005; 111:84–88.
12. White AC Jr, Robinson P, Kuhn R. Taenia solium cysticercosis: host–parasite interactions and the immune response. In: Freedman DO, ed. Immunopathogenetic aspects of disease induced by helminth parasites. Vol. 66. Basel: Karger; 1997:209–230.
13. Allan JC, Velasquez-Tohom M, Torres-Alvarez R, et al. Field trial of the coproantigen-based diagnosis of *Taenia solium* taeniasis by enzyme-linked immunosorbent assay. Am J Trop Med Hyg 1996; 54:352–356.
14. Garcia HH, Del Brutto OH, Nash TE, et al. New concepts in the diagnosis and management of neurocysticercosis (*Taenia solium*). Am J Trop Med Hyg 2005; 72:3–9.
15. Del Brutto OH, Rajshekhar V, White AC Jr, et al. Proposed diagnostic criteria for neurocysticercosis. Neurology 2001; 57:177–183.
16. Garcia HH, Del Brutto OH. Neurocysticercosis: updated concepts about an old disease. Lancet Neurol 2005; 4:653–661.
17. Rajshekhar V, Chandy MJ. Validation of diagnostic criteria for solitary cerebral cysticercus granuloma in patients presenting with seizures. Acta Neurol Scand 1997; 96:76–81.
18. Garcia HH, Evans CA, Nash TE, et al. Current consensus guidelines for treatment of neurocysticercosis. Clin Microbiol Rev 2002; 15:747–756.
19. Garcia HH, Pretell EJ, Gilman RH, et al. A trial of antiparasitic treatment to reduce the rate of seizures due to cerebral cysticercosis. N Engl J Med 2004; 350:249–258.
20. Rajashekhar V. Solitary cerebral cysticercus granuloma. Epilepsia 2003; 44 (Suppl 1):25–28.
21. Nash TE, Del Brutto O, Butman JA, et al. Calcific neurocysticercosis and epileptogenesis. Neurology 2004; 62:1934–1938.
22. Psarros TG, Krumerman J, Coimbra C. Endoscopic management of supratentorial ventricular neurocysticercosis: case series and review of the literature. Minim Invasive Neurosurg 2003; 46:331–334.
23. Proano JV, Madrazo I, Avelar F, et al. Medical treatment for neurocysticercosis characterized by giant subarachnoid cysts. N Engl J Med 2001; 345:879–885.

# CHAPTER 28

# Echinococcosis

Pedro L. Moro and Peter M. Schantz

## Echinococcosis at a Glance

- Worldwide distribution in association with domestic livestock populations.
- In endemic areas, prevalence can be as high as 4–6% for cystic echinococcosis and 4% for alveolar echinococcosis.
- Tumor-like or cystlike lesions develop most commonly in the liver followed by the lung. Other organs affected less frequently.
- Screening for echinococcosis in immigrants coming from endemic areas is not cost effective.
- Most common treatment is surgery but chemotherapy with benzimidazoles is indicated if surgery is contraindicated, if cysts are small, and as adjunct to surgery to prevent secondary hydatidosis due to accidental spillage of protoscoleces in peritoneal cavity.

## Etiology

Hydatid disease (echinococcosis) is the infection of humans by the larval stages of taeniid cestodes of the genus *Echinococcus*. Four species of *Echinococcus* are currently recognized, of which three cause distinct forms of disease: *E. granulosus* (cystic hydatid disease), *E. multilocularis* (alveolar hydatid disease), and *E. vogeli* (polycystic hydatid disease). The fourth species, *E. oligarthrus*, has only rarely (fewer than five cases) been identified as a cause of human disease. Diverse subpopulations of *E. granulosus*, distinguished by morphologic and biologic characteristics, have long been recognized; the taxonomic significance of these differences remains unresolved and controversial. However, recent demonstrations of

consistent genetic differences has prompted calls for splitting this species.[1] As a cause of morbidity in humans, *Echinococcus* species rank high among the helminths.

## Life cycle

The life cycles of *Echinococcus* species involve carnivores as final hosts and herbivores or omnivores as intermediate hosts (Fig. 28.1). In their adult stage, these cestodes are small, ranging about 2–12 mm in length, with three to six segments. They typically localize in the lower duodenum and jejunum of the final host. Embryophores containing infective embryos are expelled in large numbers in the feces of the final carnivorous host. After ingestion by the intermediate host, the embryo is released into the small intestine, which it penetrates, and enters the portal circulation. The site of localization and development of the embryo to the larval or hydatid stage differs with species of *Echinococcus* and may be influenced as well by species of the intermediate host. Humans are an incidental intermediate host, since further development of these cestodes depends on ingestion of their larvae (hydatids) by a carnivore. The microscopic structure of a hydatid cyst is shown in Figure 28.2.

## Epidemiology

### Distribution and transmission patterns

Cystic hydatid disease (CHD) is caused by the larval stage of *E. granulosus*. Molecular studies using mitochondrial DNA sequences have identified nine

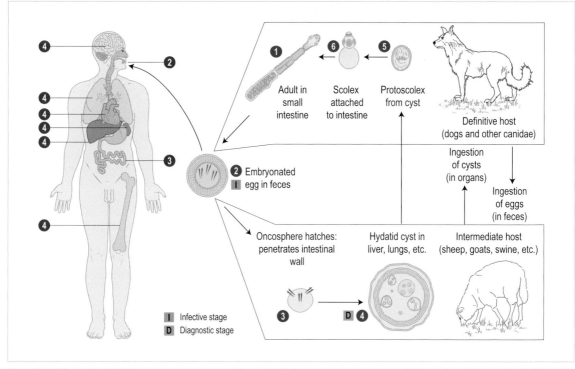

**Fig. 28.1** Life cycle of *Echinococcus granulosus*. The adult *Echinococcus granulosus* (3–6 mm long) (1) resides in the small bowel of the definitive hosts, dogs or other canids. Gravid proglottids release eggs (2) that are passed in the feces. After ingestion by a suitable intermediate host (under natural conditions: sheep, goat, swine, cattle, horses, camel), the egg hatches in the small bowel and releases an oncosphere (3) that penetrates the intestinal wall and migrates through the circulatory system into various organs, especially the liver and lungs. In these organs, the oncosphere develops into a cyst (4) that enlarges gradually, producing protoscoleces and daughter cysts that fill the cyst interior. The definitive host becomes infected by ingesting the cyst-containing organs of the infected intermediate host. After ingestion, the protoscoleces (5) evaginate, attach to the intestinal mucosa (6), and develop into adult stages (1) in 32–80 days. The same life cycle occurs with *E. multilocularis* (1.2–3.7 mm), with the following differences: the definitive hosts are foxes, and to a lesser extent dogs, cats, coyotes and wolves; the intermediate hosts are small rodents; and larval growth (in the liver) remains indefinitely in the proliferative stage, resulting in invasion of the surrounding tissues. With *E. vogeli* (up to 5.6 mm long), the definitive hosts are bush dogs and dogs; the intermediate hosts are rodents; and the larval stage (in the liver, lungs and other organs) develops both externally and internally, resulting in multiple vesicles. *E. oligarthrus* (up to 2.9 mm long) has a life cycle that involves wild felids as definitive hosts and rodents as intermediate hosts. Humans become infected by ingesting eggs (2), with resulting release of oncospheres (3) in the intestine and the development of cysts (4) in various organs. (Adapted from Centers for Disease Control and Prevention DPDx.)

distinct genetic types (G1–9) within *E. granulosus*.[2,3] These include two sheep strains (G1, G2), two bovid strains (G3, G5), a horse strain (G4), the camelid strain (G6), a pig strain (G7), and the cervid strain (G8). A ninth genotype (G9) has been described in swine in Poland.[2] The sheep strain (G1) is the most cosmopolitan form that is most commonly associated with human infections. The other strains appear to be genetically distinct, suggesting that the taxon *E. granulosus* is paraphyletic and may require taxonomic revision.[2,3] The 'cervid,' or northern sylvatic genotype (G8), is maintained in cycles involving wolves and dogs and moose and reindeer in northern North America and Eurasia. Human infection with this strain is characterized by predominantly pulmonary localization, slower and more benign growth, and less frequent occurrence of clinical complications than reported for other forms.[2] The presence of distinct strains of *E. granulosus* has important implications for public health. The shortened maturation time of the adult form of the parasite in the intestine of dogs suggests that, where echinococcidal drugs are used for controls, the period for administering antiparasite drugs to dogs will have to be

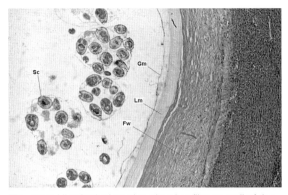

**Fig. 28.2** Histological section showing fibrous wall of the host (Fw) and parasite's laminated membrane (Lm), germinal membrane (Gm), and scoleces (Sc).

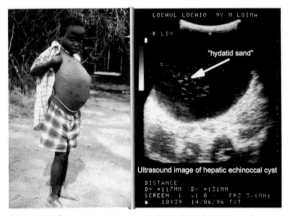

**Fig. 28.3** Boy with abdominal distention due to cystic echinococcosis of the liver as shown by ultrasound imaging.

shortened in those areas where the G2, G5, and G6 strains occur.[4]

*E. granulosus* is prevalent in broad regions of Eurasia, in several South American countries, and in Africa (Fig. 28.3). Humans become infected through association with dogs that have been fed viscera from slaughtered animals or have had access to carcasses or discarded offal of domestic ungulates in which the larvae are present.

Most cases of cystic echinococcosis reported in North America continue to be diagnosed in immigrants who acquired their infections in their countries of origin;[5] historically, this was mainly Icelanders, Italians, and Greeks, but in more recent years increasing numbers of cases are diagnosed in persons of Middle Eastern and Asian origin [Schantz, unpublished].

Hospital record reviews indicate that local transmission continues to occur in Native American communities in Arizona and New Mexico states [J. Cheek, Indian Health Service, USPHS, Albuquerque, NM, 2005, personal communication].

*E. granulosus* is highly endemic in Argentina, southern Brazil, Chile, Peru, and Uruguay. In endemic areas the prevalence of infection in humans can be as high as 3–6%; 89% of adult livestock may be infected and 46% of dogs.[6] Practices that facilitate transmission of the parasite include feeding dogs with infected offal or discarding infected offal in the field where dogs can have easy access to it. In areas with no control programs, livestock is commonly slaughtered in open areas where there is no veterinary supervision.[7]

Alveolar hydatid disease is caused by *E. multilocularis*, which has an extensive geographical range in the northern hemisphere. The natural cycle involves foxes and small rodents as final and intermediate hosts, respectively. *E. multilocularis* is endemic in the central part of Europe, parts of the Near East, Russia, and the central Asian republics, China, northern Japan, and Alaska.[6] Recent surveys in central Europe have extended the known distribution of *E. multilocularis* from four countries at the end of the 1980s to 11 countries in 1999, although the annual incidence of disease in humans remains low.[9] There is evidence of parasites spreading from endemic to previously nonendemic areas in North America and on the north island, Hokkaido, of Japan, due principally to the movement or relocation of definitive hosts, foxes and coyotes. In North America the parasite has been recorded in two distinct geographic regions: the north tundra zone (western Alaska) and central North America.[9,10] Despite the presence of infected definitive and intermediate hosts in 12 of the states in central North America, only one human case of alveolar echinococcosis has been described in Minnesota.[11]

China is a newly recognized focus of alveolar echinococcosis (AE) in Asia. *E. multilocularis* occurs in three areas: northeastern China including Inner Mongolia Autonomous region and Heliongjiang Province; central China including Gansu Province, Ningxia Hui Autonomous Region, Sichuan Province, Qinghai Province and Tibet Autonomous Region; northwestern China including Xingjian Uygur Autonomous Region.[12] The highest prevalence of AE in the world was found in Qinghai Province with 800 infections per 100 000 inhabitants.[13]

The infection of humans by the larval *E. multilocularis* is often the result of association with dogs and perhaps cats that have eaten infected rodents. Until recently, certain villages within the zone of tundra were hyperendemic foci because of the close interaction between dogs and wild rodents that live as commensals in and around dwellings; however, transmission has declined as a result of improved housing and control measures. In central Europe, rodents inhabiting cultivated fields and gardens become infected by ingesting embryophores expelled by foxes and, in turn, may be a source of infection for dogs and cats. A recent case-control study demonstrated a higher risk of alveolar hydatidosis among individuals who owned dogs that killed game, dogs that roamed outdoors unattended, individuals who were farmers, and individuals who owned cats.[14] In rural regions of central North America, the cycle involves foxes and rodents of the genera *Peromyscus* and *Microtus*. Allowing pet dogs and cats in these regions to prey on local rodents may be hazardous.

Polycystic hydatid disease, caused by *E. vogeli*, has been reported infrequently from Central and South America. The natural hosts of this cestode are the bush dog, *Speothos venaticus*, and the paca, *Cuniculus paca*.[1] The larval stage occurs occasionally in rodents or other species. Little is known of the epidemiology of polycystic hydatid disease. The natural final host of *E. vogeli*, the bush dog, is a wary and rarely seen animal that is an unlikely source of infection for humans. The intermediate host, the paca, is widely hunted for food in northern South America and local hunters routinely feed the viscera of pacas to their dogs; thus, infected dogs may be the primary source of infection for humans.[15]

## Clinical Manifestations

### Cystic hydatid disease

In humans, hydatid cysts of *E. granulosus* are slowly enlarging masses comparable to benign neoplasms; most human infections remain asymptomatic. Hydatid cysts are frequently observed as incidental findings at autopsy at rates much higher than the reported local morbidity rates. The clinical manifestations are variable and are determined by the site, size, and condition of the cysts.[16] Hydatid cysts in the liver and the lungs together account for 90% of affected localizations. The average liver-to-lung infection ratio varies from 2.1:1 in clinical cases to 6:1 and 12:1 in asymptomatic individuals with hydatid disease.[17] The chronic signs of hepatic cystic echinococcosis include hepatomegaly with or without the

presence of a mass in the upper right quadrant (see Fig. 28.3). Obstructive jaundice accompanied by symptoms such as mild epigastric pain, indigestion, and nausea may occur occasionally. Cysts may also become secondarily infected with bacteria and manifest as an abscess. Features of lung involvement include coughing, hemoptysis, dyspnea, and fever. In about 10% of cases the cysts occur in organs other than the lungs and liver. Other known complications include anaphylaxis, secondary spread following rupture, pathological fracture of bones and formation of hepatopulmonary fistulae.[18] The northern form (G7 genotype) causes a milder form of the disease with cysts usually localized in the lungs.

### Alveolar hydatid disease

The embryo of *E. multilocularis* seems to localize invariably in the liver of the intermediate host. Development of the larval *E. multilocularis* is inhibited in humans, so that it persists indefinitely in the proliferative phase. As a result, the hepatic parenchyma is gradually invaded and replaced by fibrous tissue in which great numbers of vesicles, many microscopic, are embedded. Proliferation continues peripherally, with the result that an entire hepatic lobe may be replaced over a period of years. As the lesion enlarges, it usually undergoes degenerative changes that lead to central necrosis, often with liquefaction, and abscesses with a volume of several liters may be produced. Uneven calcification of necrotic tissues is typical in lesions of long standing. Hepatomegaly is characteristic and may be extreme. The disease takes a chronic course, with deterioration of health often occurring around middle age. Patients eventually succumb to hepatic failure, invasion of contiguous structures, or, less frequently, metastases to the brain.[19] However, instances of spontaneous death of the cyst during its early stage of development have been reported in people with asymptomatic infection.

### Polycystic hydatid disease

In human cases, hepatomegaly or tumor-like masses in the liver have been typical findings. Proliferation of vesicles may lead to destruction of much of the liver, and involvement of adjacent structures by extension does not appear to be unusual. The prognosis in polycystic hydatid disease is poor. The known cases have been described by D'Alessandro and associates.[15]

# Diagnosis

## Who should be tested?

Routine diagnostic screening of immigrants for echinococcosis is not recommended.

Individuals with a cystlike mass in liver or lungs from areas in which *E. granulosus* is endemic should be screened for cystic hydatid disease.[17] Alveolar echinococcosis is very rare in North America as only two cases have been reported in central North America. Alveolar echinococcosis mimics hepatic carcinoma and cirrhosis.

## Differential diagnosis

Echinococcal cysts must be differentiated from benign cysts, cavitary tuberculosis, mycoses, abscesses, and benign or malignant neoplasms. Alveolar hepatic lesions may be confused with hepatic carcinoma or cirrhosis.

## Diagnosis

A noninvasive confirmation of the diagnosis can usually be accomplished with the combined use of radiologic imaging and immunodiagnostic techniques. Chest roentgenography permits the detection of echinococcal cysts in the lungs; this is the most common means of diagnosis of the northern form that most commonly localizes in the lungs (Fig. 28.4). In other sites, calcification is necessary for roentgenographic visualization by X-ray. Computerized axial tomography (CT), magnetic resonance, and ultrasound imaging are useful for diagnosing deep-seated lesions in the liver and other organs and are further useful for defining the extent and condition of avascular fluid-filled cysts. The CT image of *E. granulosus* larval cysts typically shows sharply contoured cysts (sometimes with internal daughter cysts) and marginal calcifications.[20,21] Portable ultrasonography machines have been used for field surveys with excellent results.[22,23]

Serologic tests are useful to confirm presumptive radiologic diagnoses, although some patients with cystic echinococcosis do not develop a detectable immune response.[16] Hepatic cysts are more likely to elicit an immune response than pulmonary cysts; however, it appears that, regardless of location, the sensitivity of serologic tests is inversely related to the degree of sequestration of the echinococcal antigens inside cysts. Enzyme-linked immunosorbent assay

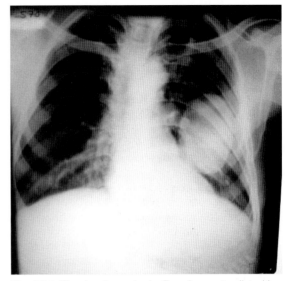

**Fig. 28.4** Chest radiograph of a Peruvian pastoralist with a hydatid cyst in the left lung field detected as part of an imaging survey in an endemic area. The patient was asymptomatic as is often the case in echinococcosis.

(ELISA) or the indirect hemagglutination test are highly sensitive procedures for the initial screening of sera; specific confirmation of reactivity can be obtained by immunodiffusion (arc 5) procedures or immunoblot assays (8/12 kDa band).[24] Eosinophilia is present in fewer than 25% of infected persons.

In seronegative patients, a presumptive diagnosis may be confirmed by demonstrating protoscoleces or hydatid membranes in the liquid obtained by percutaneous aspiration of the cyst. Although previously considered taboo because of the potential for anaphylaxis or dissemination of protoscoleces, with certain precautions percutaneous aspiration for purposes of diagnosis or treatment is now standard procedure. Ultrasound guidance of the puncture, anthelmintic coverage, and anticipation of the possible need to treat an allergic reaction now minimize risks. Protoscoleces can sometimes be demonstrated in sputum or bronchial washings; identification of hooklets is facilitated by acid-fast stains.

Diagnosis of alveolar echinococcosis (AE) may be difficult, particularly in regions where its possible occurrence is not known to clinicians and pathologists, as in central North America; the disease is typically seen in persons of advanced age in whom it closely mimics hepatic carcinoma or cirrhosis. Plain roentgenography shows hepatomegaly and characteristic scattered areas of radiolucency outlined by calcified rings 2–4 mm in diameter. The usual CT image of *E. multilocularis* infection is that of indistinct solid tumors with central necrotic areas and perinecrotic plaquelike calcifications.[25] Serologic tests are usually positive at high titers; highly specific antigens have been identified and synthesized that, when used in serologic assays, are highly sensitive and specific for diagnosis of AE and can distinguish this infection from CE (*E. granulosus*) and other forms of echinococcosis.[26] Needle biopsy of the liver may confirm the diagnosis if larval elements are demonstrated. Exploratory laparotomy is often done for diagnosis and delineation of the size and extent of the invasion.

Polycystic echinococcosis has characteristics intermediate between those of the cystic and alveolar forms.[15] The relatively large cysts are filled with liquid and contain brood capsules with numerous protoscoleces. The primary location is the liver, but cysts may spread to contiguous sites or occur in other primary locations. Immunodiagnostic and other techniques useful for diagnosing cystic or alveolar hydatid disease are also of value in diagnosing polycystic hydatid disease. The hydatid cysts of *E. vogeli* can be differentiated from those of other species based on differences in the dimensions of the hooks of the protoscoleces.[15]

## ICD-9 Codes

- 122.0 *E. granulosus* infection of liver
- 122.1 *E. granulosus* infection of lung
- 122.2 *E. granulosus* infection of thyroid
- 122.3 *E. granulosus* infection, other
- 122.4 *E. granulosus* infection, unspecified
- 122.5 *E. multilocularis* infection of liver
- 122.6 *E. multilocularis* infection, other
- 122.7 *E. granulosus* infection, unspecified
- 122.8 Echinococcosis, unspecified, of liver
- 122.9 Echinococcosis, other and unspecified

## ICD-10 Codes

- B67.0 *E. granulosus* infection of liver
- B67.1 *E. granulosus* infection of lung
- B67.2 *E. granulosus* infection of bone
- B67.3 *E. granulosus* infection, other and multiple sites
- B67.4 *E. granulosus* infection, unspecified
- B67.5 *E. multilocularis* infection of liver
- B67.6 *E. multilocularis* infection, other and multiple sites

- B67.7 *E. multilocularis* infection, unspecified
- B67.8 Echinococcosis, unspecified, of liver
- B67.9 Echinococcosis, other and unspecified

## Treatment

Until recently, surgery was the only option for treatment of hydatid cysts; however, in the past 15 years chemotherapy has been introduced and evaluated and, more recently, combinations of cyst puncture, aspiration and drainage, with or without injection of chemicals (called percutaneous aspiration, injection, re-aspiration, or PAIR), have been evaluated and, increasingly, are seen to supplement or even replace surgery as the preferred treatment.[27] Surgery remains the preferred treatment when cysts are large (>10 cm diameter), secondarily infected, or located in certain organs, i.e. the brain or heart. The aim of surgery is total removal of the cyst while avoiding the adverse consequences of spilling its contents. Pericystectomy is the usual procedure, but simple drainage, capitonnage, marsupialization, and resection of the involved organ may be used, depending on the location and condition of the cyst(s). Preoperative albendazole or mebendazole is indicated to prevent secondary recurrences following leakage or even rupture of cyst and spillage of its content and should begin at least 4 days before surgery and last for 1 month (albendazole) or 3 months (mebendazole) (Table 28.1).[27]

### Management of patients who fail initial treatment or in whom surgery is contraindicated

At times, surgery may be impossible because of the patient's general condition and the extent and location of the cysts. Under such conditions, treatment with benzimidazole drugs may be tried; approximately one-third of patients treated with benzimidazole drugs have been cured of their disease (e.g. complete and permanent disappearance of cysts) and an even higher proportion have responded with significant regression of cyst size and alleviation of symptoms.[28] Both albendazole (10–15 mg per kg body-weight per day) and mebendazole (40–50 mg/kg) have demonstrated efficacy; however, albendazole, because of its superior pharmacokinetic profile, which favors intestinal absorption and penetration into the cyst(s), is slightly more efficacious. Similar adverse reactions (neutropenia, liver toxicity, alope-

**Table 28.1 Treatment of Echinococcosis**

| Drug | Adult Dose | Efficacy | Adverse events | Comments |
|------|-----------|----------|----------------|----------|
| Albendazole | 10–15 mg/kg orally two times a day<br>Should be taken in courses of 28 days each with 2 weeks of rest between courses for 3–6 months or longer<br>Prophylactic use: 1 week before surgery and 1 month after surgical procedure | Cure in ⅓ of patients<br>30–50% show significant regression and alleviation of symptoms<br>20–40% do not respond<br>No response in ⅓ of patients | Neutropenia, hepatotoxicity (transient increases of aminotransferases), transient alopecia | Not to be used in pregnancy or in patients with chronic liver disease and bone marrow depression.<br>Leukocyte counts and liver enzymes should be assayed during treatment<br>Imaging examinations should be carried out at intervals of about 3–6 months for 1–3 years after termination of treatment |
| Mebendazole | 40–50 mg/kg daily for 3–6 months or longer<br>Prophylactic use: 1 week before surgery and 3 months after surgical procedure | Less efficacious than albendazole | Nausea, vomiting, abdominal pain and diarrhea | Not to be used in pregnancy or in patients with chronic liver disease and bone marrow depression<br>Not as readily absorbed as albendazole |
| Praziquantel | 50 mg/kg per day<br>Once daily or once weekly | No clinical trials conducted but cure reported in case series when combined with albendazole[31] | Mild symptoms such as dizziness, headache, malaise, abdominal pain, nausea | Better results obtained if used with albendazole |

cia, and others), reversible upon cessation of treatment, have been noted in most patients treated with both drugs. A minimum of treatment is 3 months. The long-term prognosis in individual patients is difficult to predict; therefore, prolonged follow-up with ultrasound or other imaging procedures is needed to determine the eventual outcome. The combination of praziquantel and albendazole has been used successfully in the treatment of hydatid disease.[29,30] Praziquantel used at 50 mg/kg in different regimens (once daily, once weekly or once every 2 weeks) in combination with albendazole produced very effective and rapid results compared with albendazole therapy alone.[29] Further research is needed to determine the optimum dosage and length for this form of therapy. A third option for the treatment of echinococcosis cysts in the liver is PAIR which is based on percutaneous puncture using ultrasound guidance; aspiration of cyst fluid; injection of protoscolecidal substances (20% sodium chloride or 95% ethanol) for at least 15 minutes; and re-aspiration of the cyst fluid content. PAIR is indicated for univesicular hepatic cysts of >5 cm in diameter, for cysts with daughter cysts, for cysts with detached membranes and for multiple cysts if accessible to puncture.[31] PAIR is contraindicated for inaccessible or superficially located liver cysts and lung cysts. It is also contraindicated for honeycomb-like cysts, cysts with echogenic lesions, inactive cysts or calcified lesions, and cysts communicating with the biliary tree. To avoid sclerosing cholangitis, cysts should be inspected for bilirubin prior to injection of protoscolecidal substances. Presence of bile indicates direct communication between cyst contents and biliary ducts. Concomitant drug treatment should be provided in the form of benzimidazoles before the procedure and should last for 1 month (albendazole) or 3 months (mebendazole) after the procedure. Risks include those associated with any puncture; anaphylactic shock or allergic reactions caused by leakage of cyst fluid; and secondary echinococcosis due to spillage.

Favorable results have been reported from more than 2000 PAIR interventions. A meta-analysis comparing the clinical outcomes for 769 patients with hepatic cystic echinococcosis treated with PAIR plus albendazole or mebendazole with 952 era-matched historical control subjects undergoing surgical intervention found greater clinical and parasitological efficacy, lower rates of morbidity and mortality and disease recurrence, and shorter hospital stays than surgical treatment.[32] A policy of conservative management has been adopted generally in the treatment of infections by the relatively benign northern form of *E. granulosus*, and surgical intervention is considered only in cases of uncertain diagnosis (i.e. possible neoplasms) or in rare cases of symptomatic disease.

Until recently, surgery has offered the only possibility for treatment of alveolar echinococcosis. The usual procedure has involved removal of the lesion with part of or the entire affected hepatic lobe. Cases of advanced disease and those involving multiple lesions often are inoperable. With or without surgery, alveolar hydatid disease has a very high mortality rate. With metastases to the brain, death occurs within a few months after onset of neurologic disorders. Long-term treatment for several years with mebendazole (50 mg/kg per day) or albendazole (10 mg/kg per day) inhibits growth of larval *E. multilocularis*, reduces metastasis, and enhances both the quality and length of survival; prolonged therapy may eventually be larvicidal in some patients.[27] Liver transplantation has been employed successfully on otherwise terminal cases.[33] In a Swiss study, therapy for nonresectable alveolar echinococcosis with mebendazole and albendazole resulted in an increased 10-year survival rate of approximately 80% (versus 29% in untreated historical controls) and a 16- to 20-year survival rate of approximately 70% (versus 0% in historical controls).[9]

Experience in treatment of polycystic echinococcosis is limited.[15] Because the lesions are so extensive, surgical resection may be difficult and usually incomplete. A combination of surgery with albendazole is most likely to be successful.

## Information for patients and providers

Centers for Disease Control and Prevention: http://www.cdc.gov/ncidod/dpd/parasites/alveolarechinococcosis/default.htm

## Prevention

Infection of humans by larval cestodes of the genus *Echinococcus* is contingent on ingestion of eggs distributed in the feces of dogs and perhaps other carnivores that harbor the adult worms. Control of hydatid disease in humans depends on the means to prevent or to eliminate infection of dogs.

Programs have been based on public education combined with strict regulations directed particularly toward control of dogs and regulated slaughter of livestock. Nearly complete control of *E. granulosus* in the Greek-controlled area of Cyprus was accomplished during the period between 1971 and 1975 through elimination of excess dogs, destruction of all dogs found to be infected, and regulation of slaughter. Development of the effective echinococcicidal drug, praziquantel, permitted the effective use of an anthelmintic in conjunction with other measures for the control of hydatid disease. The mass treatment of dogs and strict control of slaughter is effective under some conditions but of little value where early reinfection is probable. A promising advance has been the development of a recombinant vaccine (EG95) which seems to confer 96–98 % protection against challenge infection.Further research is needed to assess the costs and benefits of this intervention as part of control programs.

Control of *E. multilocularis* presents a difficult problem of potentially increasing importance. Since infection in dogs appears to be the most important source of infection in humans, educational measures aimed at preventing dogs from preying on rodents should be implemented in endemic areas. Measures for control of the cestode have involved anthelmintic treatment of dogs and destruction of stray animals. In Alaska, the general reduction of numbers of dogs and improvements in housing probably have had some effect on the prevalence of *E. multilocularis*. In endemic areas, strict controls on the movement of pet dogs and cats as pets is necessary to prevent ingestion of infected rodents. Regular anthelmintic treatment of such animals might be practicable under some conditions.

## Clinical Pearls

- Asymptomatic infection is frequent.
- Presence of a mass in the upper-right quadrant of the abdomen in an individual coming from an endemic area is suggestive of hydatid disease.
- Individuals who report expectoration of a salty fluid ('hydatid vomit') and who come from an endemic area probably harbor a ruptured hydatid cyst in the lung.

## Special Considerations for Immigrants

- It is not cost effective to screen immigrants from endemic countries for echinococcosis.
- Hydatidosis should be considered if a tumor or cystlike lesion in the liver or lung with or without symptoms in an individual coming from an endemic area (Middle East, South America, Africa) is observed.

## General References

Eckert J, Deplazes P. Biological, epidemiological, and clinical aspects of echinococcosis, a zoonosis of increasing concern. Clin Microbiol Rev 2004; 17:107–135.

El-On J. Benzimidazole treatment of cystic echinococcosis. Acta Trop 2003; 85:243–252.

Craig PS, Rogan MT, Campos-Ponce M. Echinococcosis: disease, detection and transmission. Parasitology 2003; 127:S5–S20.

McManus DP, Zhang W, Li J, et al. Echinococcosis. Lancet 2003; 362:1295–1304.

Smego RA, Bhatti S, Khaliq AA, et al. Percutaneous aspiration-injection-reaspiration drainage plus albendazole or mebendazole for hepatic cystic echinococcosis: a meta-analysis. Clin Infect Dis 2003; 37:1073–1083.

## References

1. Rausch RL. Life-cycle patterns and geographic distribution of Echinococcus species. In: Thompson RCA, Lymbery AJ, eds. Echinococcus and hydatid disease. Wallinggford, UK: CAB International; 1995:89–134.
2. McManus DP, Thompson RCA. Molecular epidemiology of cystic echinococcosis. Parasitology 2003; 127:S37–S51.
3. Thompson RCA, McManus DP. Towards a taxonomic revision of the genus Echinococcus. Trends Parasitol 2002; 18:452–457.
4. Rosenzvit MC, Zhang LH, Kamenetzky L, et al. Genetic variation and epidemiology of Echinococcus granulosus in Argentina. Parasitology 1999; 118:523–530.
5. Donovan SM, Mickiewicz N, Meyer RD, et al. Imported echinococcosis in southern California. Am J Trop Med Hyg 1995; 53:668–671.
6. Moro PL, McDonald J, Gilman RH, et al. Epidemiology of Echinococcus granulosus infection in the central Peruvian Andes. Bull World Health Organ 1997; 75:553–561.
7. Moro PL, Lopera L, Bonifacio N, et al. Risk factors for canine echinococcosis in an endemic area of Peru. Vet Parasitol 2005; 130:99–104.
8. McManus DP, Zhang W, Li J, et al. Echinococcosis. Lancet 2003; 362:1295–1304.
9. Eckert J, Deplazes P. Biological, epidemiological, and clinical aspects of echinococcosis, a zoonosis of increasing concern. Clin Microbiol Rev 2004; 17:107–135.
10. Eckert J, Conraths FJ, Tackmann K. Echinococcosis: an emerging or re-emerging zoonosis? Int J Parasitol 2000; 30:1283–1294.
11. Gamble WB, Segal M, Schantz PM, et al. Alveolar hydatid disease in Minnesota: first human case acquired in the contiguous United States. JAMA 1979; 241:904–907.
12. Vuitton DA, Zhou H, Bresson-Hadni S, et al. Epidemiology of alveolar echinococcosis with particular reference to China and Europe. Parasitology 2003; 127(Suppl):S87–S107.
13. Schantz PM, Wang H, Qiu J, et al. Echinococcosis on the Tibetan Plateau: prevalence and risk factors for cystic echinococcosis in Tibetan populations in Qinghai Province, China. Parasitology 2003; 127(Suppl):S109–S120.
14. Kern P, Ammon A, Kron M, et al. Risk factors for alveolar echinococcosis in humans. Emerg Infect Dis 2004; 10:2088–2893.
15. D'Alessandro A. Polycystic echinococcosis in tropical America: Echinococcus vogeli and E. oligarthrus. Acta Trop 1997; 67:43–65.
16. Kammerer WS, Schantz PM. Echinococcal disease. Infect Dis Clin North Am 1993; 7:605–618.
17. Pawlowski ZS, Eckert J, Vuitton DA, et al. In: WHO/OIE manual on echinococcosis in humans and animals: a public health problem of global concern. Echinococcosis in humans: clinical aspects, diagnosis and treatment. Paris, France, World Health Organization Office International des Epizooties. World Organization for Animal Health, 2001:20–66.
18. Wilson JF, Diddams AC, Rausch RL. Cystic hydatid disease in Alaska. A review of 101 autochthonous cases of Echinococcus granulosus infection. Am Rev Respir Dis 1968; 98:1–15.
19. Wilson JF, Rausch RL. Alveolar hydatid disease: a review of clinical features of 33 indigenous cases of Echinocccus multilocularis infection in Alaskan Eskimos. Am J Trop Med Hyg 1980; 29:340–349.
20. Morris DL, Richards KS. Hydatid disease: current medical and surgical management. Oxford: Butterworth-Heineman; 1992.
21. Craig PS, Rogan MT, Campos-Ponce M. Echinococcosis: disease, detection and transmission. Parasitology 2003; 127(Suppl):S5–S20.
22. MacPherson CNL, Bartholomot B, Frider B. Application of ultrasound in diagnosis, treatment, epidemiology, public health and control of Echinococcus granulosus and Echinococcus multilocularis. Parasitology 2003; 127(Suppl):S21–S35.
23. Larrieu E, Del Carpio M, Salvitti JC, et al. Ultrasonographic diagnosis and medical treatment of human cystic echinococcosis in asymptomatic school age carriers: 5 years of follow-up. Acta Trop 2004; 91:5–13.
24. Maddison SE, Slemenda SB, Schantz PM, et al. A specific diagnostic antigen of Echinococcus granulosus with an apparent molecular weight of 8 kDA. Am J Trop Med Hyg 1989; 40:337–383.
25. Didier D, Weiler S, Rohmer P, et al. Hepatic alveolar echinococcosis: Correlative US and CT study. Radiology 1985; 154:179–186.
26. Ito A, Sako Y, Yamasaki H, et al. Development of Em18-immunoblot and Em18-ELISA for specific diagnosis of alveolar echinococcosis. Acta Trop 2003; 85:173–182.
27. Anon. Guidelines for treatment of cystic and alveolar echinococcosis in humans. Bull World Health Org 1996; 74:231–243.
28. Davis A, Pawlowski ZS, Dixon H. Multicentre clinical trials of benzimidazole carbamates in human echinococcosis. Bull World Health Organ 1986; 64:383–387.
29. Mohamed AE, Yasawy MI, Al Karawi MA. Combined albendazole and praziquantel versus albendazole alone in

the treatment of hydatid disease. Hepatogastroenterology 1998; 45:1690–1694.

30. Cobo F, Yarnoz C, Sesma B, et al. Albendazole plus praziquantel versus albendazole alone as a pre-operative treatment in intra-abdominal hydatidosis caused by *Echinococcus granulosus*. Trop Med Int Health 1998; 3:462–466.

31. World Health Organization Informal Working Group of Echinococcosis. 2001. Puncture, aspiration, injection, re-aspiration. An option for the treatment of cystic echinococcosis. Document WHO/CDS/CSR/APH/2001.6. Geneva, Switzerland: World Health Organization; 1–40.

32. Smego RA, Bhatti S, Khalij AA, et al. Percutaneous aspiration-injection-reaspiration-drainage plus albendazole or mebendazole for hepatic cystic echinococcosis: a meta-analysis. Clin Infect Dis 2003; 27:1073–1083.

33. Koch S, Bresson-Hadni S, Miguet JP, et al. European collaborating clinicians. Experience of liver transplantation for incurable alveolar echinococcosis: a 45-case European collaborative report. Transplantation 2003; 75:856–863.

# CHAPTER 29

# Giardiasis

Elizabeth D. Barnett

## Giardiasis at a Glance

- Giardiasis occurs worldwide.
- Prevalence rates may be as high as 15–20% in children under 10 years of age in developing countries.
- *Giardia intestinalis* (also known as *lamblia* or *duodenalis*) is the most commonly identified intestinal parasite in the US, with prevalence rates as high as 16% in some areas.
- Diarrhea is the most common symptom; foul-smelling stools may be accompanied by flatulence, abdominal distension, and poor appetite.
- Screening of all new immigrants with possible exposure to contaminated water is warranted.
- Successful treatment will result in clearance of parasites from stool in 3–5 days, and resolution of symptoms in 5–7 days.
- Refractory cases may require longer treatment at higher dose, change of agent, or combination therapy.

## Clinical Manifestations

Clinical symptoms of *Giardia* infection range from asymptomatic cyst passage to acute, self-limited diarrhea, to prolonged diarrheal disease.[1-3] Asymptomatic infection is common. Symptoms of acute illness include watery diarrhea with abdominal pain; stools may be foul-smelling with accompanying flatulence, abdominal distension, and poor appetite. A small proportion of patients will develop a prolonged diarrheal syndrome with intermittent diarrhea, abdominal and epigastric discomfort exac-

erbated by eating, malaise, fatigue, and occasional headache, often leading to weight loss (a distinguishing feature) and anemia. Lactose intolerance is common (20–40% of cases), may persist for weeks after infection, and may be mistaken for relapse or reinfection.[4] *Giardia* has been implicated in growth failure in children in the developing world who are chronically infected or frequently reinfected. Catch-up growth has been shown to occur when *Giardia* is eliminated.

Manifestations of *Giardia* infection in children may be non-specific and include anorexia, irritability, flatulence, chronic abdominal pain, behavioral changes, or poor weight gain. Eosinophilia is rare and should prompt a search for other diagnoses.

Fever and vomiting occur in a minority of patients. Gross blood or polymorphonuclear cells in the stool and tenesmus do not occur. Rarely, there may be an association with urticaria, and reactive arthritis has been reported.

The disease is transmitted by ingestion of cysts. Onset of symptoms occurs 1–2 weeks after cyst ingestion, though the period of time to detection of cysts in the stool may be longer than the incubation period. The disease is communicable for as long as cyst passage occurs (may be as long as 6 months).[1]

Individuals with humoral immunodeficiencies are at increased risk of chronic disease if infected.

## Etiology

*Giardia* is a flagellate protozoan. The two stages in the life cycle are the free living trophozoite form, and the infectious form, the cyst. Acquisition of disease is by ingestion of as few as 10–25 cysts, occurring most frequently by drinking contaminated water,

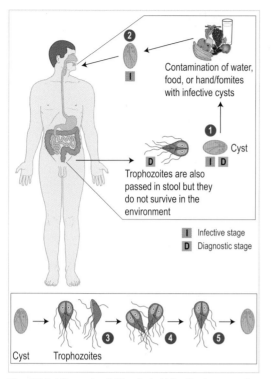

**Fig. 29.1** Life cycle of *Giardia lamblia*. Cysts are resistant forms and are responsible for transmission of giardiasis. Both cysts and trophozoites can be found in the feces (diagnostic stages)(1). The cysts are hardy and can survive several months in cold water. Infection occurs by the ingestion of cysts in contaminated water, food, or by the fecal–oral route (hands or fomites)(2). In the small intestine, excystation releases trophozoites (each cyst produces two trophozoites) (3). Trophozoites multiply by longitudinal binary fission, remaining in the lumen of the proximal small bowel where they can be free or attached to the mucosa by a ventral sucking disk (4). Encystation occurs as the parasites transit toward the colon. The cyst is the stage found most commonly in nondiarrheal feces (5). Because the cysts are infectious when passed in the stool or shortly afterward, person-to-person transmission is possible. While animals are infected with *Giardia*, their importance as a reservoir is unclear. (Adapted from Centers for Disease Control and Prevention DPDx.)

but also by person-to-person transmission. Under the influence of gastric acid, excystation releases trophozoites which colonize and multiply in the upper small bowel and biliary tract (Fig. 29.1).[2]

## Epidemiology

Giardiasis occurs worldwide, in both temperate and tropical climates. *Giardia* is one of the first parasites to infect children in the developing world; prevalence rates may be as high as 15–20% in children under 10 years of age. Over 60% of children may be infected at some point during childhood.[1] In the US, it is the most commonly identified intestinal parasite, with prevalence rates as high as 16% in some areas. Outbreaks have been associated with contamination of water supplies, exposure to water contaminated by animal feces containing cysts infectious for humans, and person-to-person transmission in settings such as childcare centers. Food-borne transmission also occurs. Exposure to infected feces may also occur during sexual contact.

## ICD-9 Codes

- 007.1 Giardiasis

## Diagnosis

### Who should be tested?

Screening of all new immigrants with possible exposure to contaminated water is warranted given the widespread distribution of *Giardia*. Testing should also be considered for individuals with chronic diarrhea or malabsorption syndromes, those who have acute diarrhea accompanied by a potential exposure (children in day care, men who have sex with men, foreign travel, drinking possibly contaminated water, such as on a camping trip), and those exposed to infected individuals. Individuals with growth failure, unexplained anemia, or chronic abdominal or epigastric pain are also candidates for testing.

### Differential diagnosis

The differential diagnosis includes other protozoan infections (including cryptosporidiosis, isosporiasis, cyclosporiasis), lactose intolerance, Whipple's disease, Crohn's disease, tropical or nontropical sprue, and lymphoma.

### Diagnostic evaluation

Evaluation for *Giardia* in new immigrants should be carried out with both standard stool evaluation for ova and parasites (O&P), because of the possibility of identifying other organisms, and with assays that detect *Giardia* antigen, because they are more sensitive than standard O&P for detection of *Giardia* infection.[3]

Antigen detection uses a polyclonal or multiclonal antibody directed against cyst or trophozoite antigens. Either an immunofluorescence or enzyme-linked immunosorbent assay (ELISA) is used. These assays have a sensitivity of 91–98% and specificity of nearly 100%. Both assays appear superior to stool examination for ova and parasites, and increased sensitivity may be obtained by testing three separate stool samples.[1]

Examination of stool can be performed on a fresh specimen or on preserved samples. Detection rates of 50–70% can be obtained by examination of a single specimen, and rates as high as 90% can be achieved by examining three specimens of fresh or preserved stool. Convenience to patients (most specimens will be collected at home and placed immediately into preservative solution) limits opportunity to examine fresh samples.

Duodenal aspiration, biopsy, or the string test (duodenal sampling obtained by having the patient swallow a string ending in a gelatin capsule which dissolves in the stomach, allowing the string to pass into the duodenum and become saturated with duodenal fluid; the string is removed after several hours and the fluid examined for presence of the organism) have greater sensitivity than examination of stool.[3] As they are more invasive than other currently available techniques, they are at this time reserved for patients with chronic symptoms when other diagnostic tests have been inconclusive, or when biopsy of the small bowel or duodenum is necessary for other diagnostic considerations.

Serodiagnosis is available but is used primarily in epidemiologic studies. Lack of ability to distinguish between current and past infection, unpredictability of serologic response to infection in individual patients, and availability of other diagnostic tests limit the usefulness of serology.

Radiography is not generally indicated, and culture of isolates is limited to research laboratories.

## Treatment

Symptomatic patients should be treated, using one of the available drugs (Table 29.1). Management of asymptomatic cyst passers is controversial; most experts recommend treatment for food handlers, and suggest consideration of treatment for asymptomatic individuals residing in households with patients with hypogammaglobulinemia or cystic fibrosis.[3,5] Though treatment is not required for asymptomatic children, it seems reasonable to treat immigrant children, especially those with growth delay, anemia, nonspecific abdominal pain, or other symptoms potentially attributable to *Giardia* infection. Treatment of pregnant women is controversial; treatment of disease severe enough to compromise hydration or nutritional status is warranted, using agents available for use during pregnancy.

Successful treatment will result in clearance of parasites from stool in 3–5 days, and resolution of symptoms in 5–7 days.

## Management of patients who fail initial treatment

The first step is to document persistence of infection by examining the stool and sending *Giardia* antigen. If reinfection is possible, treatment with the same agent is appropriate, though some experts would favor treating at a higher dose of metronidazole or furazolidone or increasing the length of treatment to 10–14 days. Treatment of family members may be effective in reducing the rate of reinfection. Reviewing methods of reducing transmission (hand hygiene, reducing possible exposures) is helpful. If reinfection is unlikely, treatment with a drug from a different class is most appropriate. Other alternatives include drug combinations such as metronidazole–albendazole or metronidazole–quinacrine.[1-3,5,6]

Infection with *Giardia* is associated with damage to the intestinal epithelium and resulting inability to digest lactose. A lactose-free diet for several weeks may result in improvement of diarrhea. In highly refractory cases, other diagnoses such as immunoglobulin deficiency or other immunodeficiency should be considered.

## Information for patients and providers

A fact sheet prepared by the CDC is available at: http://www.cdc.gov/ncidod/dpd/parasites/giardiasis/factsht_giardia.htm

## Prevention

Ability to prevent spread of infection in the developing world is limited where there is limited ability to provide for adequate sewage disposal and sufficient potable water. Breast-feeding is associated with lower infection rates. There are no vaccine candidates on the horizon currently.

**Table 29.1 Treatment of giardiasis**

| Drug | Adult dose | Pediatric dose | Formulation | Efficacy | Adverse events | Comments; use in pregnancy |
|------|-----------|----------------|-------------|----------|----------------|----------------------------|
| Metronidazole | 250 mg orally 3 times a day for 5–7 days | 15 mg/kg/day orally divided three times a day for 5–7 days | | 80–95% | GI, metallic taste, headache, disulfiram-like effect | Drug of choice; Probably safe in last two trimesters; advisable to take with food |
| Furazolidone | 100 mg orally 4 times a day for 10 days | 6 mg/kg/day orally four times a day for 7–10 days | | 80% | GI, allergic reaction, headache rarely; mild hemolysis in G6PD deficiency; ? carcinogenic | Available in liquid form; not recommended for use in pregnancy |
| Paromomycin | 25–35 mg/kg/day orally in three doses for 7 days | Same as adult dose | | 60–70% | GI | Not absorbed; recommended for treatment of symptomatic infection in pregnancy |
| Tinidazole | 2 g orally, given as a single dose | 50 mg/kg orally, given as a single dose (max 2 gm) | 250 mg and 500 mg tablets | 90–98% | GI, metallic taste, headache, disulfiram-like effect | Not approved for children under 3 years of age in the US; advisable to take with food |
| Quinacrine | 100 mg orally three times a day for 5 days | 6 mg/kg/day divided three times a day for 5 days (max 300 mg/day) | | 90–95% | GI, headache, yellow discoloration; rarely toxic psychosis | No longer produced in the US |
| Nitazoxanide[7] | 500 mg orally twice daily for 3 days | 12–47 months: 100 mg twice daily for 3 days; 4–11 years: 200 mg twice daily for 3 days | 500 mg tablets and 100 mg/5mL oral suspension | 71–94% | Abdominal pain, diarrhea, nausea | |

Prevention of *Giardia* infections is accomplished by avoiding exposure to contaminated feces. Most often, exposures occur via contaminated water, including recreational water and untreated water from shallow wells or other bodies of water. Water can be made safer for drinking by bringing to a rolling boil for at least 1 minute, filtering water using a filter with a pore size of one micron or smaller or that has been NSF rated for 'cyst removal,' or treating water with chlorine or iodine preparations.[1,2] Because *Giardia* cysts are resistant to routine levels of chlorination, levels in municipal water supplies may be inadequate alone to prevent transmission; addition of flocculation, sedimentation, and filtration techniques may be necessary.[1]

Personal hygiene (hand washing) is the mainstay of protection against person-to-person transmission.

## Infection Control Measures

Contact precautions, in addition to standard precautions, are recommended for diapered and incontinent hospitalized patients with symptomatic giardiasis for the duration of the illness. Symptomatic children should be excluded from childcare settings until asymptomatic (as should caregivers). Testing or treatment of asymptomatic children in childcare facilities in the setting of an outbreak is not recommended, and asymptomatic carriers should not be excluded. Improved sanitation and personal hygiene, especially hand washing, should be emphasized.

*Giardia* is reportable to state and local health departments and individuals. New immigrants, who may be frightened by involvement of the health department, should be informed of this requirement when the diagnosis is made.

**Clinical Pearls**

- Asymptomatic infection with *Giardia* is common.
- Prolonged diarrhea and weight loss are cardinal features of giardiasis.

**Special Considerations For Immigrants**

- Diagnosis of *Giardia* is accomplished by *Giardia* antigen testing (more sensitive than microscopic examination of stool) in combination with stool examination for ova and parasites (because of the possibility of multiple parasitic infections).
- *Giardia* is a reportable communicable disease; preparation of families for contact with the health department may allay anxiety.
- Treatment of asymptomatic patients, especially children, is encouraged, especially in settings of poor nutrition, growth failure, or anemia, as catch-up growth may occur, and reinfection is less likely once the child has left the endemic area.

## References

1. Hill DR, Nash TE. Intestinal flagellate and ciliate infections. In: Guerrant RL, Walker DH, Weller PF, eds. Tropical infectious diseases: principles, pathogens, and practice 2nd ed. Philadelphia: Churchill Livingstone; 2006.
2. Ortega YR, Adam RD. *Giardia*: overview and update. Clin Infect Dis 1997; 25:545–550.
3. American Academy of Pediatrics. *Giardia intestinalis* infections (Giardiasis). In: Pickering LD, ed. Red Book: 2006 report of the committee on infectious diseases. 27th edn. Elk Grove Village: IL: American Academy of Pediatrics; 2006:296–301.
4. Farthing MJ. Giardiasis. Gastroenterol Clin N Am 1996; 25:493–515.
5. Gardner TB, Hill DR. Treatment of giardiasis. Clin Microbiol Rev 2001; 14:114–128.
6. Miller LC. Intestinal parasites and other enteric infections. In: Miller LC, ed. The Handbook of International Adoption Medicine. Oxford University Press, New York, 2005.
7. Fox LM, Saravolatz LK. Nitozoxanide: a new thiazolide antiparasitic agent. Clin Infect Dis 2005; 40:1173–1180.

# CHAPTER 30

# Helicobacter Pylori

Roger L. Gebhard and Kristin H. Gebhard

## Helicobacter Pylori at a Glance

- Fifty percent or more of immigrants from endemic, underdeveloped countries may harbor gastric *H. pylori*.
- *H. pylori* infection is associated with gastric and duodenal ulcers, gastritis, and gastric cancer. It has not been associated with acid reflux, esophagitis, or esophageal cancer.
- However, most infected persons appear to have no consequences of their infection.
- *H. pylori* infection is diagnosed (in order from least to most expensive testing) by serology, stool antigen, urea breath testing, or endoscopic biopsy.
- Patients with documented ulcers, MALT lymphoma, or at risk for gastric cancer should be tested and treated if positive. Universal testing for asymptomatic individuals is not currently recommended.
- Standard treatment typically consists of two effective antibiotics plus one non-antibiotic (bismuth or a proton pump inhibitor).
- Testing should be done only if treatment of a positive test is intended. Treatment should only be undertaken if adherence to the therapeutic regimen may reasonably be expected.
- Persons having high-stakes infections (documented ulcer, MALT lymphoma, or high risk for gastric cancer) should be tested for successful eradication 6–12 weeks after treatment. Eradication testing methods include stool antigen, urea breath tests, or endoscopic biopsy. (Serology is not useful for eradication testing.)

The 2005 Nobel Prize for medicine was given to Robin Warren and Barry Marshall for their isolation, identification, and recognition of the pathophysiologic consequences of a bacterium that is able to chronically infect gastric mucosa. Beginning in 1983, these investigators reported the unexpected observation that the *Helicobacter pylori* bacterium is a principal cause of gastric and duodenal ulcers.[1] Subsequently, *H. pylori* gastric infection has also been convincingly implicated as a risk factor for acute and chronic gastritis, dyspepsia, gastric carcinoma, and a form of gastric lymphoma known as 'mucosa-associated lymphoid tissue' (MALT) B-cell lymphoma. Since colonization and/or infection with *H. pylori* are particularly common in immigrant populations, it is important for physicians involved in the care of immigrant patients to be knowledgeable about the organism. In this chapter, we will first discuss the disease states associated with *H. pylori* and management considerations for patients in general. Then we will discuss special management considerations for immigrant populations.

## Bacteriology

A spiral-shaped, Gram-negative, motile bacillus with multiple flagella, *H. pylori* is able to survive and thrive in the harsh acidic environment of the stomach (Fig. 30.1). *H. pylori* produces a protective urease enzyme that is able to convert urea to ammonia. The ammonia produced then serves as a buffering base to protect the organism from high gastric acidity. The organism is difficult to culture, but it can be demonstrated by histologic staining or by detection of its urease activity. Once the organism establishes itself in an individual's gastric mucosa, it typically persists and becomes a long-term colonization or

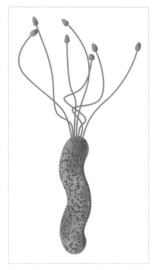

Fig. 30.1 H. pylori image (Courtesy of www.hpylori.com. au).

### Table 30.1 Worldwide *H. pylori* prevalence and gastric cancer deaths

| Country/region | *H. pylori* prevalence (%) | Gastric cancer mortality (deaths/100 000/yr) |
|---|---|---|
| **Americas** | | |
| USA/Canada | 20–40 | <10 |
| Mexico | 70 | 10–20 |
| Andean So. Am. | 80–90 | >30 |
| So. Am. (other) | 80–90 | 10–20 |
| **Europe** | | |
| Western | 10–50 | 10–20 |
| Eastern | 70 | 20–30 |
| Russia | 70–80 | >30 |
| China/ East Asia | 60–80 | 20–30 |
| India/SE Asia | 70 | 10–20 |
| Japan | 50 | >30 |
| Africa | 80–90 | <10* |
| Australia | 20–30 | 10 |

Data derived from reference 27 and the Helicobacter Foundation website at www.helico.com
* Data not reliable.

chronic infection. *H. pylori* elicits an inflammatory and immune response, with antibody production, but the organism is generally not eliminated from the host by this response. Chronic infection then ensues, typically with chronic gastritis. Initial gastric mucosal infection and persistence of infection are enabled by the bacteria's motility, its production of urease, and its production of a variety of virulence proteins such as *VacA* and *CagA* (reviewed in reference 2).

## Epidemiology

More than half of the world's population is colonized with *H. pylori*! (This may beg the question; 'What is "normal:" to be colonized or to be free of the organism?') As shown in Table 30.1, the prevalence of 'infection' is 70–90% in less developed areas such as Asia, Africa, South and Central America, and Eastern Europe. Prevalence is much lower (though still in the range of 20%) in developed countries of Western Europe, North America, and Australia. It appears that the incidence in developed countries has decreased substantially since World War II, probably as a result of better sanitation and safe water supplies.

In developing countries, infection typically occurs at an early age (by age 5–10 years), and then persists throughout life. In developed countries such as the US, Finland, and Japan, *H. pylori* prevalence is high in older individuals (presumably a cohort infected early in their life), but is much lower in younger persons (presumably benefiting from improvements in sanitation). The organism can be found in feces, dental tartar, and gastric juice. From polymerase chain reaction (PCR) studies, it can apparently survive for several days in contaminated water. Thus, transmission of *H. pylori* may be by fecal–oral, oral–oral, or gastro–oral routes, or via contaminated water. Person-to-person spread is considered most likely. Presence of the bacteria in the mucus layer of gastric mucosa correlates with lower socioeconomic status, overcrowding, greater number of siblings, sharing a bed, and a lack of running water. Infection is shown to cluster within close household/family members, consistent with person-to-person transmission. Genetic predisposition to infection has also been suggested.

## Pathogenesis and Symptoms

It is important to recognize that, while a majority of the world's population is infected (or colonized) with *H. pylori*, the vast majority of these infected persons will have no significant symptoms or medical consequences of the infection! Nevertheless, *H. pylori* infection is associated with several serious potential diseases. Why some individuals develop disease, while most do not, is unclear. However, proteins produced by various *H. pylori* subspecies, and not by others (such as *VacA* and *CagA*) may be important virulence factors that may favor the development of mucosal ulceration or cancer. Additional environmental or genetic cofactors, as yet unrecognized, may also be involved. The following conditions have been associated with gastric *H. pylori* infection.

## Peptic ulcer disease (duodenal ulcer/gastric ulcer)

It has been said that most duodenal and gastric ulcers are a result of *H. pylori* infection. In the US, and other developed countries where the prevalence of *H. pylori* has fallen, overall prevalence of ulcer disease has also fallen. Meanwhile, in the US, there has been a great increase in the use of nonsteroidal anti-inflammatory drugs (NSAIDs), which are themselves an independent risk factor for ulcers. Consequently, NSAID use has become an important ulcer risk factor in the US, particularly for gastric ulcers.

In the US, it has been estimated that peptic ulcers may occur in 10–20% of *H. pylori*-infected individuals, or a risk of 1% per year.[3] Other estimates suggest a lifetime risk for ulcers of 3% for infected persons in the US, up to 25% for infected persons in Japan.[2] Barry Marshall, in his *Helicobacter pylori Foundation* website, gives a figure of 30% lifetime risk for ulcer in infected persons. Thus, risk estimates for duodenal and gastric ulcer range from 3–30%. However, in some other countries where *H. pylori* prevalence is very high (such as Africa), reported ulcer incidence appears to be lower than would be expected from *H. pylori* infection prevalence data. This seeming contradiction may be explained by differing production of bacterial virulence proteins (including *VacA* and *CagA*) in regional *H. pylori* subspecies, by under-recognition/under-reporting of ulcers, or by additional environmental and ethnic factors involved in ulcer genesis.

Classic ulcer symptoms include epigastric pain, food-related abdominal symptoms (discomfort relieved by eating or elicited by meals), 'dyspepsia,' nausea, and vomiting, as well as symptoms caused by ulcer complications. Complications include gastrointestinal (GI) bleeding (melena, hematemesis, or even occult blood loss with anemia), obstruction (emesis), and perforation (acute abdomen). However, many ulcers are asymptomatic, particularly in older individuals. All current medical guidelines call for

*H. pylori* testing of patients with active ulcer disease, or history of ulcer disease, and treatment of individuals who test positive. Eradication of *H. pylori* is proven to facilitate ulcer healing and to substantially reduce the very high rate of ulcer recurrence (90%) that is seen in the absence of eradication.

The possibility of interactions between *H. pylori* and NSAIDs with respect to ulcer risk and complications is somewhat controversial. However, it is clear that both NSAIDs and *H. pylori* are independent risk factors for gastric and duodenal ulcers. Up to 20–30% of chronic NSAID users develop ulcer disease, and 1–1.5% of chronic NSAID users have bleeding per year. NSAID use is associated with 10 000–20 000 deaths from ulcer bleeding per year in the US.[4] Risk for NSAID ulcer complications is increased for individuals older than 60 years, individuals with prior history of ulcer or ulcer complications, persons taking high-dose or multiple types of NSAIDs (such as NSAID plus cardioprotective aspirin), and persons concurrently taking prednisone or anticoagulants.[4] Because of these added risks, it has been suggested that testing and treating *H. pylori* may reduce the chance for bleeding ulcer in such higher-risk persons who receive high-dose or long-term NSAIDs.[5,6]

## Gastritis

Initial infection with *H. pylori* appears to produce an acute neutrophilic gastritis with hypochlorhydria. Patients may have no symptoms, or they may experience acute dyspepsia – as described by Barry Marshall when he induced infection in himself.[7] Typically, chronic infection or colonization of the gastric antrum (and to a lesser extent the gastric body and ectopic gastric mucosa in the duodenal bulb) ensues. Chronic infection is associated with the histologic appearance of chronic gastritis (Fig. 30.2). Mucosal gastritis may be appreciated visually during upper GI endoscopy, or the gastric mucosa may appear visually normal. Some subjects will develop more severe chronic gastritis that can progress to histologic atrophic gastritis and intestinal metaplasia. Intestinal metaplasia appears to be the histologic risk factor for development of distal gastric adenocarcinoma. Treatment of *H. pylori* may be able to cause regression[8] or, at least, a reduced rate of progression of the histologic sequence.[9] Patients with chronic gastritis from *H. pylori* also have subnormal acid production, and gastric acid production may actually increase after *H. pylori* infection has been eradicated.

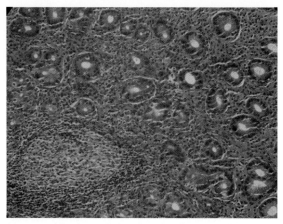

**Fig. 30.2** Histology of chronic active (lymphocytic) gastritis with lymphoid follicle, in *H. pylori* infection.

## Dyspepsia

'Dyspepsia' is an imprecise term that has been used to refer to a vague, but extremely common, constellation of abdominal and digestive symptoms. Complaints of pain, burning, gas, bloating, fullness after eating, nausea/vomiting, heartburn, etc. all may fall under this heading. Dyspepsia has been classified into three main categories: pain ('ulcer-type') symptoms, motility-type symptoms (such as postprandial fullness, nausea, and bloating), and reflux-type symptoms. While *H. pylori* has been associated with dyspeptic symptoms and eradication of the organism has been reported to relieve some symptoms in some patients, most dyspeptic patients – with or without *H. pylori* infection – do not appear to benefit from *H. pylori* treatment. This is probably related to the broad range of potential physical and psychological causes, including irritable bowel syndrome, which may create 'dyspepsia' symptoms. Initial enthusiasm for a generalized *H. pylori* 'test and treat' algorithm for dyspeptic patients has diminished. A review by Moayyedi et al. is illustrative: they report that 36% of chronic dyspeptics improved naturally, 57% continued to have chronic symptoms, and only 7–9% improved as a consequence of an *H. pylori* test-and-treat strategy.[2,10,11]

Nevertheless, *H. pylori* infection may be considered in selected patients with chronic dyspepsia. Careful elucidation of the symptoms and good history taking are important. Reflux-type symptoms (such as heartburn, regurgitation, or esophageal reflux) do not generally correlate with *H. pylori* infection (see below), so that 'test-and-treat' is not useful for patients having these symptoms. Individuals with a history of ulcer or typical ulcer symptoms are more likely to benefit from a 'test-and-treat' strategy. Symptomatic individuals who have gastritis observed on endoscopic examination should be biopsied (or otherwise tested) for *H. pylori* and treated if positive. Typical symptoms of irritable bowel syndrome, with prominent features of disordered bowel function, are less likely to be related to *H. pylori*. In addition, *H. pylori* screening in a population having low prevalence of *H. pylori* (such as younger citizens of the US) may result in false-positive tests – with no potential benefit, and risk for adverse side effects from subsequent antibiotic treatment.

## Distal gastric cancer (body and antrum)

Worldwide, gastric cancer is one of the top three causes of cancer-related deaths – with 870 000 new cases and nearly 650 000 deaths per year.[12] One report estimated that up to 70% of distal (body and antrum) gastric cancers could be attributed to *H. pylori*.[13] The International Agency for Research on Cancer (IARC) estimated that 47% of all gastric cancers could be attributed to *H. pylori* infection in developing countries, and 36% attributed in developed countries. In the US, the incidence of distal gastric cancer has fallen markedly since 1930. It has been suggested that this reduction correlates with the increase in number of home refrigerators (with resultant decrease in food spoilage and use of salt as a preservative), but the reduction in gastric cancer incidence has also occurred during a time of reduction in *H. pylori* prevalence in developed countries. As seen in Table 30.1, worldwide gastric cancer prevalence is highest in Andean South America, Central America, Japan, Russia and Eastern Europe, and Eastern Asia – areas having high prevalence of *H. pylori*. Nevertheless, discrepancies in the *H. pylori*: gastric cancer relationship exist: cancer risk in Japan is high while *H. pylori* prevalence is reportedly moderate at 50%; cancer risk in Andean South America and Central America (e.g. Columbia and Costa Rico) is higher than in other parts of South America having similar high *H. pylori* prevalence; gastric cancer incidence in Africa and Southeast Asia is reported to be lower than *H. pylori* prevalence might predict. Possible explanations for such discrepancies include the bacterial production of potential cancer virulence factors (including *CagA*) in *H. pylori* subspecies endemic to high cancer regions,[13,14] under-recognition and under-reporting of gastric cancer in low cancer incidence regions, and the role of other local environmental and dietary factors in gastric cancer pathogenesis.

Immigration affects gastric cancer risk. Studies indicate that when persons from a region of high gastric cancer incidence (e.g. Japan) migrate to regions of low incidence (e.g. the US), gastric cancer risk in the immigrants is reduced, particularly for second- and third-generation immigrants.[15,16] The studies suggest that environmental factors, perhaps including *H. pylori* as well as dietary factors, have a greater impact than genetic factors on gastric cancer risk.

There is a clear relationship between *H. pylori* infection and distal gastric cancer and there is an identified histologic progression from *H. pylori* chronic gastritis or atrophic gastritis to intestinal metaplasia to dysplasia to cancer. As a result, the IARC has listed *H. pylori* as a group 1 human carcinogen. It must be remembered, however, that only a very small fraction of the enormous population of *H. pylori*-infected individuals will ever have this histologic progression and develop cancer! In addition, there is as yet no conclusive evidence that eradication of *H. pylori* will ameliorate the risk for distal gastric cancer. Such a study would need to be very large and very long term. Two recent critiques[12,17] discuss the limited evidence for reduced progression of intestinal metaplasia following *H. pylori* treatment and the mixed results of studies with respect to whether gastric cancer risk can be substantially reduced or eliminated by *H. pylori* eradication.

Gastric cancer symptoms include abdominal pain with weight loss, as well as upper GI obstructive symptoms (nausea, vomiting) and GI blood loss (melena or occult loss). Unfortunately, symptoms in the pre-cancer state are typically absent or nonspecific.

## MALT Lymphoma

Gastric lymphoma accounts for only 3% of gastric cancers and 10% of lymphomas. The immune activation and development of gastric mucosal lymphoid follicles (follicular gastritis; see Fig. 30.2) precipitated by chronic *H. pylori* infection has been associated with B-lymphocyte 'mucosa-associated lymphoid tissue' (MALT or MALToma) lymphoma.[18] Furthermore, antibiotic treatment with eradication of *H. pylori* has been shown to cause resolution and complete remission of MALT lymphoma in patients with lymphoma localized to mucosa – that is, without lymph node spread, metastases, or bulky disease.[19] Chemotherapy, radiation, and/or surgery certainly

must be considered in MALToma, but *H. pylori* eradication is an important component of the treatment for patients with this type of lymphoma when patients have evidence for *H. pylori* infection.

## *H. Pylori* Non-Relationships

As alluded to above, esophageal reflux and reflux symptoms and complications are not associated with gastric *H. pylori* infection. A dramatic increase in the prevalence of gastroesophageal reflux disease (GERD), particularly Barrett's esophagus and esophageal adenocarcinoma, has appeared in the US and other developed Western countries during the past three decades, a time of dramatic decrease in *H. pylori* prevalence. The possibility that eradication of *H. pylori* may lead to worsening of esophageal acid reflux consequences has been suggested.[20] Mechanistically, *H. pylori* infection (with chronic gastritis) reduces gastric acid secretion, so that eradication of the infection may result in increased gastric acid production. Some investigators have emphasized the negative correlation between *H. pylori* infection and Barrett's esophagus and esophageal adenocarcinoma, and suggest that the infection may actually be protective for these diseases.[20,21] Concurrently, the incidence of adenocarcinoma in the gastric cardia ('proximal gastric cancer') has increased in the US (while distal – or *H. pylori* linked – gastric cancer has decreased). Adenocarcinoma of the gastric cardia also may be negatively correlated with *H. pylori* infection. In summary, these concerns give caution to the concept that *all H. pylori* infections warrant detection and eradication.

## Diagnosis

Diagnostic *H. pylori* infection testing methods include invasive (endoscopic) and noninvasive tests. The most common tests and their characteristics are listed in Table 30.2.[2,22-25] The typical serology test uses serum to detect IgG antibody to *H. pylori* by ELISA methodology. Chronic *H. pylori* infection elicits an antibody response that persists during chronic infection. After eradication of *H. pylori*, antibody persists for up to 6–12 months, or even longer. Thus, serology tests are a simple and reasonably reliable method to identify infected patients, but they are not useful for demonstrating eradication (unless one waits to re-test 6–12 months after treatment). Antibody tests are not affected by a patient's use of antibiotics, bismuth, or proton pump inhibitors

**Table 30.2 Characteristics of *H. pylori* diagnostic tests**

| Test | Availability | Cost | Sensitivity (%) | Specificity (%) | Comments |
|---|---|---|---|---|---|
| *H. p.* serology (IgG) | Yes | $ | 90–93 | 95–96 | Good for screening, not for follow-up |
| *H. p.* stool antigen | Yes | $$ | 89–98 | 92–95 | Good for follow-up |
| Urea breath tests<br>C14<br>C13 | <br>Yes<br>Limited | $$$ | 90–100 | 95 | Good for follow-up |
| Endoscopy<br>Histology | <br>Yes | $$$$ | <br>82–95 | <br>99–100 | Biopsy is done if endoscopy is needed |
| Urease | Yes | | 85–90 | 92–100 | Biopsy is done if endoscopy is needed |
| Culture | Limited | | 70–80 | 100 | Generally not needed. |

Data derived from references 2, 22, 23, 25.

(PPIs, such as omeprazole). In a population having a low prevalence of *H. pylori*, some 'positive' samples may actually be 'false positives,' and not represent infection.

*H. pylori* protein can be found in stool, so that the stool antigen test is also a reasonably simple, available, and reliable test. Patients collect a small amount of stool, which is kept refrigerated until brought to the lab for testing. The test can be used to detect infected patients, and then used to check for eradication. Current or recent use of antibiotics, bismuth, or PPIs may reduce bacteria numbers and cause a false-negative result. For this reason, patients should be off these medications for at least 2, and preferably 4, weeks prior to testing or re-testing.

*H. pylori* breath tests make use of the abundant urease enzyme activity produced by the organism. A dose of labeled (radioactive $C^{14}$ or the non-radioactive $C^{13}$ isotope) urea is given by mouth. *H. pylori* urease, if present, will quickly metabolize urea to ammonia and labeled $CO_2$, which is then detected in breath samples. $C^{14}$ labeled $CO_2$ is measured by means of scintillation counters, which are readily available and simple. This test does expose the patient to a small quantity of radioactivity. $C^{13}O_2$ detection requires mass spectrometry measurement, which is less available but avoids patient exposure to radioactivity. Breath tests may be used for initial diagnosis of *H. pylori* infection, but have a greater utility for re-testing to assure eradication. Like the stool antigen test, breath tests may give a false-negative result if patients have taken antibiotics, bismuth, or PPIs within 2–4 weeks of testing.

Invasive tests for *H. pylori* involve mucosal biopsy during upper GI endoscopy, and are therefore substantially more expensive as well as invasive. If the patient is undergoing endoscopy anyway (e.g. in order to diagnose the presence of ulcer or to evaluate upper GI symptoms), it may be reasonable to request or perform biopsy testing. The biopsy tissue may be placed in contact with urea and a pH indicator – in a gel or impregnated paper. For infected patients, urease will release ammonia and raise the pH, causing the indicator to change color. Biopsies can also be examined histologically. Most pathologists can recognize *H. pylori* organisms on the gastric mucosal surface, particularly when special stains are applied (Fig. 30.3). Finally, mucosa can be cultured for detection of *H. pylori* bacteria. *H. pylori* culture allows for the ability to test antibiotic sensitivities of the individual patient's *H. pylori* species (see below), but culture of this organism is a difficult process and is not done in most standard labs. All of these mucosal biopsy tests may give false-negative results if the patient has recently taken antibiotics, bismuth, or PPIs. Again, it is advised to have the patient avoid these drugs for at least 2–4 weeks before testing.

## Treatment

Drugs that have activity against *H. pylori* include antibiotics and nonantibiotics. The antibiotics most commonly used include amoxicillin, tetracycline, metronidazole, and clarithromycin. Nonantibiotics include bismuth (bismuth subsalicylate in the US) and PPIs (PPIs having US FDA approved indications for treatment of *H. pylori* include omeprazole, esomeprazole, lansoprazole, and rabeprazole). Unfortunately, *H. pylori* infection is difficult to eradicate and most regimens that have shown efficacy have required two (or more) antibiotics given concurrently with one (or more) nonantibiotic drug(s), given in rather high dose. The most commonly used, proven regimens are shown in Table 30.3.[2,23] For all of these regimens, adherence to dose and duration of therapy (typically 10–14 days in the US) is critical for efficacy. Patients who do not rigorously adhere to the rather complicated treatment regimen will have diminished chance of eradication, and risk development of resistant organisms. Reported treatment strategies include 3–4 drugs taken for 7, 10, and 14 days. In general, eradication success is somewhat greater for longer-duration therapy.

Regimen 1 'triple therapy' (bismuth/metronidazole/amoxicillin – or tetracycline for penicillin allergic patients) is the least expensive regimen, but has a somewhat lower reported eradication rate. Regimen 2 (PPI/amoxicillin/clarithromycin) is the most common regimen currently used in the US. Metronidazole (500 mg b.i.d.) may be used instead of clarithromycin for cost reduction. Patients allergic to amoxicillin may substitute tetracycline (500 mg q.i.d.) or use Regimen 3, which incorporates both clarihromycin (500 mg b.i.d.) and metronidazole (500 mg b.i.d.). Regimen 4 'quadruple therapy' may be used for patients who have failed one or two courses of treatment or where antibiotic resistance is proven or felt to be likely. Additional 'salvage' regimens have been reported, using norfloxacin (250–500 mg b.i.d.) or rifabutin (150–200 mg b.i.d.) plus amoxicillin (1 g b.i.d.) and b.i.d. PPI.[24] Czinn[25] reviews treatment regimens and doses for pediatric patients.

The *H. pylori* bacterium appears to be frustratingly prone to develop antibiotic resistance. Patients

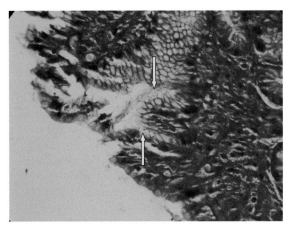

**Fig. 30.3** Giemsa stain histology of gastric mucosa infected with *H. pylori* (arrows).

**Table 30.3 Four popular *H. pylori* treatment regimens in the US**

| Regimen | Drugs | Dosing | Duration | Comments |
|---|---|---|---|---|
| 1 | Bismuth subsalicylate 525 mg (2 tablets) | q.i.d. | 10–14 d | Original regimen. Least expensive. |
| | Metronidazole 250 mg | q.i.d. | | 16 tablets per day. |
| | Amoxicillin 500 mg | q.i.d. | | Lower eradication rate. |
| | (or tetracycline 500 mg) | (q.i.d.) | | (if penicillin allergic) |
| 2 | PPI* | b.i.d. | 7–14 d | Standard Rx in US |
| | Amoxicillin 1000 mg | b.i.d. | | |
| | Clarithromycin 500 mg | b.i.d. | | |
| 3 | PPI | b.i.d. | 7–14 d | For patients allergic to penicillin |
| | Metronidazole 500 mg | b.i.d. | | |
| | Clarithromycin 500 mg | b.i.d. | | |
| 4 | Bismuth subsalicylate 525 mg (2 tablets) | q.i.d. | 10–14 d | May be used for rescue after failed Rx |
| | Metronidazole 500 mg | t.i.d. | | |
| | Tetracycline 500 mg | q.i.d. | | |
| | PPI | b.i.d. | | |

Data derived from references 2, 23, 24, 25.
* Proton pump inhibitor.

who do not adhere to the treatment regimen run the risk of developing resistant – and then more difficult to treat – organisms. Metronidazole resistance is especially common, particularly in the immigrant population, since this very inexpensive antibiotic is widely used for a variety of purposes in developing countries. In spite of metronidazole resistance, there are reports of successful eradication with the use of metronidazole-containing regimens. Amoxicillin and clarithromycin resistance also develop, and these resistances do reduce therapeutic efficacy.

The success of treatment for these regimens is reported to be in the range of 80–95%. These rates, given treatment with 3–4 high-dose drugs, are a bit discouraging, and attest to the resilience of the organism. Again, it should be emphasized that likelihood of eradication relates to adherence or compliance. In general, re-testing to demonstrate eradication has not been recommended for most treated patients. However, 'high-stakes' patients (e.g. those with history of bleeding ulcer, MALT lymphoma, or at higher risk for gastric cancer, such as those with gastric body intestinal metaplasia) should be considered for re-testing in order to assure that the organism has been eradicated. Patients treated for dyspepsia, and having persisting dyspeptic symptoms after treatment, may also be offered re-testing. As noted above, *H. pylori* serology is not useful for demonstrating eradication, unless a year has passed since treatment. Although antibody may convert from positive to negative as early as 6 months after *H. pylori* eradication, the authors recommend a 1-year interval between treatment and serologic testing in order to avoid false-positive tests due to the fact that some patients may not convert for as long as 12 months after successful treatment.

Once *H. pylori* has been eradicated, it is reported that the risk for re-infection, in adults, is generally quite low at 0.44–2.3% per year.[26] Risk is higher in the pediatric age group. The greatest re-infection risk appears to come from close household members. Because of this, some have advocated that close household/family members be tested and treated if positive, particularly when *H. pylori* infection is felt to be a high-stakes issue (see above). The strategy of testing and treating family members may be particularly important for such high-risk patients in the immigrant population, given the likely high infection prevalence and the possibility of crowding and poverty living conditions. If stakes are high, new immigrants entering a close household may also need to be considered for test-and-treat in order to protect the treated patient from re-infection.

# Pearls in the Management of Immigrant Patients

## Who is at risk?

It is clear from Table 30.1 that the vast majority of immigrants to the US will come from countries of very high *H. pylori* prevalence. Infection is particularly likely for immigrants who have grown up in poverty, crowding, or poor sanitation (e.g. refugee camps). Immigrants with high socioeconomic background are likely to have lower *H. pylori* prevalence. As with non-immigrants, it is recommended that practitioners limit testing and treating to clinical situations in which there is evidence to support benefit.

## Who should be tested and treated in immigrant populations?

The authors would like to preface this answer with these three caveats: First, we suggest that testing should only be done if there is intention to treat a positive result. Second, since the eradication rate is primarily related to adherence to the dose and duration of the treatment regimen, we suggest that treatment only be initiated if the practitioner is reasonably confident that the regimen can be communicated and that compliance is likely. Finally, since most infected persons will never suffer medical consequences of their infection, it should be recognized that indiscriminate mass screening has the potential to create needless cost and may expose healthy persons to adverse side effects of antibiotic treatment.

Having said this, *H. pylori* testing and treatment should be undertaken using the same indications as for non-immigrant patients:[2]

- Persons with documented ulcer disease (especially when associated with complications of bleeding/obstruction/perforation).
- Persons with MALT lymphoma. *H. pylori* treatment *alone* may result in 'cure' in selected cases and *H. pylori* treatment is clearly part of any comprehensive management. MALT lymphoma requires management by a specialist.
- Persons with atrophic gastritis or recent surgical resection of distal gastric carcinoma.

- First-degree relatives of persons with distal gastric carcinoma.
- Test-and-treat should be considered for persons expected to require long-term or high-dose NSAIDs, in order to reduce the risk for gastroduodenal ulcer.[5,6]
- A test-and-treat strategy may be considered for persons with (non-reflux) chronic dyspepsia, although evidence here is less compelling. This issue is discussed above. For patients having upper GI symptoms or signs (such as GI blood loss or iron deficiency anemia) that affect their health or quality of life, upper GI endoscopy should be considered. At time of endoscopy, mucosal biopsy for *H. pylori* testing can be undertaken. If the biopsy or other *H. pylori* test is positive, treatment should be provided. (It is our opinion that if the physician decides to look for the organism, a positive result should be treated.)

## Additional special considerations in the immigrant population

- Consideration may be given for testing and treating immigrants having ethnic, dietary, and/or familial high risk for gastric cancer. High-risk regions of origin would include Japan, Eastern Europe/Russia, Western Asia, Andean South America, and Central America, and particularly immigrants who also have family history or personal symptoms.
- Close household members of a 'high-stakes' person identified as being in need of effective and durable eradication should be considered for test-and-treat in order to reduce re-infection of the at-risk patient. This strategy may also include 'new' immigrant household members arriving in the US.

## Cautions

- Treatment failure and resistance: This problem is greatest for patients who do not fully comply with or adhere to their (admittedly complicated) treatment regimen. Antibiotic resistance will reduce the success rate, but eradication is still possible for patients where treatment is important.

- Re-infection: This is felt to be low for most US adults, but may be a problem in the immigrant population, particularly in a setting of crowding and many small children in the household.
- Antibiotic therapy side effects: The antibiotics used have all been associated with allergic reactions, postantibiotic diarrhea, and *Clostridium difficile* diarrhea and colitis. The latter has even been associated with disease severe enough to cause death or require colectomy.
- The potential for emergence or worsening of acid reflux, including the possibility of Barrett's esophagus and esophageal/cardia adenocarcinoma after *H. pylori* eradication. This is a controversial area, as discussed above, but warrants consideration.
- Cost for the individual: Serologic testing for *H. pylori* is relatively inexpensive. Treatment regimens for positive patients may be expensive, and are somewhat complicated (3–4 drugs, taken 2–4 times daily, for 7–14 days). If patients are re-tested to assure eradication, follow-up tests are more expensive than the original serology. Induction of side effects and anxiety in treated patients may also create additional costs.
- Cost for society: The magnitude of the *H. pylori* issue must be taken into account. A majority of the world's population is *H. pylori* 'infected,' and yet the majority of them will have no health consequences. Over-exuberant screening may result in creation of more problems with antibiotic side effects and antibiotic resistance than benefits. Furthermore, antibiotic resistance may be induced in bacteria other than *H. pylori*. Even in the case of risk for the serious consequence of gastric cancer there is not yet clear proof for risk reduction by the *H. pylori* test-and-treat strategy.[12] It is suggested that practitioners individualize their decisions regarding whom to test and treat, based upon region of origin, family history, and patient symptoms. It is reassuring to know that gastric cancer risk reduction appears to occur spontaneously for high-risk immigrants and their progeny after relocation to a low-risk country such as the US.

# References

1. Marshall B. Unidentified curved bacilli on gastric epithelium in active chronic gastritis [letter]. Lancet,1983; 1:1273–1274.

2. Suerbaum S, Michetti P. *Helicobacter pylori* infection. N Engl J Med 2002; 347:1175–1186.

3. Sipponen P, Varis K, Fraki O, et al. Cumulative 10-year risk of symptomatic duodenal and gastric ulcer in patients with or without chronic gastritis: a clinical follow-up study of 454 outpatients. Scand J Gastroenterol 1990; 25:966–973.

4. Wolfe MM, Lichtenstein DR, Singh G. Gastrointestinal toxicity of nonsteroidal anti-inflammatory drugs. N Engl J Med 1999; 340:1888–1899.

5. Chan FK, To K, Wu JC, et al. Eradication of *Helicobacter pylori* and risk of peptic ulcers in patients starting long-term treatment with non-steroidal anti-inflammatory drugs: a randomized trial. Lancet 2002; 359:9–13.

6. Huang J-Q, Sridhar S, Hunt RH. Role of *Helicobacter pylori* infection and non-steroidal anti-inflammatory drugs in peptic-ulcer disease: a meta-analysis. Lancet 2002; 359:14–22.

7. Marshall BJ, Armstrong JA, McGechie DB, et al. Attempt to fulfill Koch's postulates for pyloric *Campylobacter*. Med J Aust 1985; 142:436–439.

8. Correa P, Fontham E, Bravo LE, et al. Chemoprevention of gastric dysplasia: randomized trial of antioxidant supplements and anti-*Helicobacter pylori* therapy. J Natl Cancer Inst 2000; 92:1881–1888.

9. Leung WK, Lin S-R, Ching JYL, et al. Factors predicting progression of gastric intestinal metaplasia: results of a randomized trial on *Helicobacter pylori* eradication. Gut 2004; 53:1244–1249.

10. Moayyedi P, Soo S, Deeks J, et al. Systematic review and economic evaluation of *Helicobactor pylori* eradication treatment for non-ulcer dyspepsia. Brit Med J 2000; 321:649–664.

11. Laine L, Schoenfeld, Fennerty B. Therapy for *Helicobacter pylori* in patients with nonulcer dyspepsia: A meta-analysis of randomized, controlled trials. Ann Intern Med 2001; 134:361–369.

12. Correa P. Is gastric cancer preventable? Gut 2004; 53:1217–1219.

13. Ekstrom AM, Held M, Hansson L-E, et al. *Helicobacter pylori* in gastric cancer established by *CagA* immunoblot as a marker of past infection. Gastroenterology 2001; 121:784–791.

14. Huang JQ, Zheng GF, Sumanac K, et al. Meta-analysis of the relationship between *CagA* seropositivity and gastric cancer. Gastroenterology 2003; 125:1636–1644.

15. Haenszel W, Kurihara M. Studies of Japanese immigrants. I. Mortality from cancer and other diseases among Japanese in the United States. J Natl Cancer Inst 1968; 40:43–68.

16. Haenszel W, Kurihara M, Segi M, et al. Stomach cancer among the Japanese in Hawaii. J Natl Cancer Inst 1972; 49:969–998.

17. Malfertheiner P, Sipponen P, Naumann M, et al. *Helicobacter pylori* eradication has the potential to prevent gastric cancer: a state-of-the-art critique. Am J Gastroenterol 2005; 100:2100–2115.

18. Farinha P, Gascoyne RD. *Helicobacter pylori* and MALT lymphoma. Gastroenterology 2005; 128:1579–1605.

19. Steinbach G, Ford R, Glober G, et al. Antibiotic treatment of gastric lymphoma of mucosa-associated lymphoid tissue. Ann Intern Med 1999; 131:88–95.

20. Blaser MJ. Not all *Helicobacter pylori* strains are created equal: should all be eliminated? Lancet 1997; 349:565–568.

21. Blaser MJ, Atherton JC. *Helicobacter pylori* persistence: biology and disease. J Clin Invest 2004; 113:321–333.

22. Cutler AF, Havstad S, Ma CK, et al. Accuracy of invasive and noninvasive tests to diagnose *Helicobacter pylori* infection. Gastroenterology 1995; 109:136–141.

23. Meurer LN, Bower DJ. Management of *Helicobacter pylori* infection. Am Fam Physician 2002; 65:1327–1336.

24. Gisbert JP, Pajares JM. *Helicobacter pylori* 'rescue' therapy after failure of two eradication treatments. Helicobacter 2005; 10:363–372.

25. Czinn SJ. *Helicobacter pylori* infection: Detection, investigation, and management. J Pediatr 2005; 146:S21–S26.

26. Archimandritis A, Balatsos V, Delis V, et al. 'Reappearance' of *Helicobacter pylori* after eradication: implications on duodenal ulcer recurrence: a prospective 6 year study. J Clin Gastroenterol 1999; 28:345–347.

27. Koh TJ, Wang TC. Tumors of the Stomach. In: Feldman M, Friedman LS, Sleisenger MH, eds. Sleisenger and Fordtran's Gastrointestinal and Liver Disease, ed 7. Philadelphia, 2002, WB Saunders. p. 830.

# CHAPTER 31

# Hepatitis C

Gregory L. Armstrong and Ian T. Williams

## Hepatitis C at a Glance

- Two percent of the world's population has been infected with hepatitis C virus (HCV).
- In developed countries, injection drug use is the predominant mode of transmission. In developing countries, unsafe medical procedures and blood transfusions may be the predominant source of infection.
- Chronic hepatitis C is usually asymptomatic.
- In the long term, chronic hepatitis C can lead to cirrhosis and liver cancer.
- Everyone with hepatitis C should be counseled on means to avoid transmission and to reduce the risk of disease progression.
- Treatment is evolving. Current regimens require several months of therapy, are associated with high rates of adverse effects, and have overall success rates of 40–90%, depending on the genotype of virus.

## Epidemiology

An estimated 123 million people, or 2% of the world's population, have been infected with hepatitis C virus.[1] Few population-based prevalence studies have been published and many of the available data are from surveys of blood donors, outpatients, and other specific subpopulations that are not representative of the general population. These data show a substantial variation from country to country within a region and large differences within individual countries. Prevalence is relatively low (<2%) in the Americas, Europe, and Australia, and intermediate or high (≥ 2%) in developing or transitional countries in Asia and Africa (Fig. 31.1). Prevalence is perhaps highest in Egypt (12% nationally, 40% in some villages),[2] where HCV may have been inadvertently spread during schistosomiasis control campaigns that used parenteral therapy with sometimes inadequate infection control measures.[2]

HCV is chiefly spread via percutaneous routes. Two distinct epidemiologic patterns exist: that of developed countries, where injection drug use is the predominant risk factor, and that of developing and transitional countries, where unsafe medical practices, particularly unsafe therapeutic injections, account for most infections.

Injection drug use is an especially strong risk factor for HCV infection because of the high prevalence of chronic infection among injection drug users, frequent sharing of injection equipment among users, and the ease with which HCV is spread by parenteral exposures. In a study in Baltimore in the 1980s, 80% of drug users were infected with the virus within the first year of initiating injection drug use.[3] More recent studies have found a lower (10–40% per year) but still substantial rate of infection.[4,5] Despite the lower incidence, studies of patients presenting with acute hepatitis C show that injection drug use remains the source of most infections in the United States.

In developing countries, unsafe injection practices may account for most HCV infections.[6,7] Surveys in sub-Saharan Africa, for example, have found that 15–20% of injections given for therapeutic purposes within the formal medical system are administered with reused injection equipment that has not been sterilized. In addition, in many developing countries there is a large, informal medical sector where injection practices are undoubtedly worse. There is also a substantial overuse of therapeutic injections where

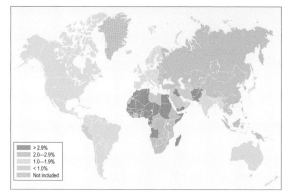

**Figure 31.1** Estimated prevalence of anti-HCV. In this map, prevalences have been estimated for 14 regions of the world defined in the World Health Organization's *The Comparative Quantification of Health Risks* (Reference 7). The map has been modified from Reference 1, with permission of the author.

oral therapies could be used or where no pharmacologic therapy is indicated. Household surveys in Romania and Moldova, for example, have found that participants received an average of 5–11 injections per year. Fortunately, injection practices are generally safe in vaccination programs, which are careful to provide adequate supervision and adequate numbers of sterile needles and syringes.

Exposure to HCV through blood transfusion has been extremely rare in developed countries since the implementation of sensitive assays for antibody to HCV (anti-HCV). However, blood banks in developing countries may not test for HCV or may use relatively insensitive rapid diagnostic tests. For this reason, transfusion-transmitted HCV remains a problem. Nosocomial exposure to HCV through needle-stick injuries also occurs and accounts for a relatively small number of infections. For an HCV-contaminated needle-stick injury, the risk of infection (around 1.8%) is intermediate between that for human immunodeficiency virus (HIV) (0.3%) and hepatitis B virus (HBV) (37–62% if the source patient is hepatitis B e-antigen positive).[8] The prevalence of anti-HCV among healthcare workers is not demonstrably different from that among the general population.

HCV is also sexually transmitted, but much less easily than, for example, hepatitis B virus. Epidemiologic studies have consistently found high-risk sexual practices to be risk factors for both acute and chronic hepatitis C. However, these associations are not nearly as strong as associations with percutaneous exposures, particularly injection drug use. Furthermore, the prevalence of HCV infection among long-term monogamous partners of HCV-infected individuals is less than 3% and the annual incidence of transmission has been too low to be measured.

Perinatal transmission from HCV RNA-positive mothers occurs at a rate of approximately 6% and is higher if the mother is also infected with HIV.[9] There is no clear, consistent evidence that elective cesarean section decreases the rate of transmission. Although HCV can be demonstrated in breast milk, breast-fed infants are at no higher risk of HCV infection than bottle-fed infants.

## Etiology

Hepatitis C virus is an enveloped, single-stranded RNA virus of the Flaviviridae family. On environmental surfaces, the virus may remain viable for at least 16 hours but less than 4 days.[10] Six genotypes are recognized. Genotype 1 is the most common in many developed countries such as the United States. Certain genotypes have specific geographic distributions, such as genotypes 4 (Egypt), 5 (southern Africa) and 6 (southeast Asia). For patients infected with HCV, the genotype has clinical implications: genotypes 1 and 4 are more difficult to treat and generally require longer courses of therapy than genotypes 2 and 3.[11] There are few data on treatment response of other genotypes.

## Clinical manifestations and natural history

Acute infection with HCV occurs after a 2-week to 6-month incubation period and is often either asymptomatic or mildly symptomatic and thus not recognizable as acute hepatitis C. For the minority of people who experience symptoms in the acute phase, the presentation is indistinguishable from that of the other acute viral hepatitides. Symptoms include jaundice, dark urine, nausea, fever, malaise, anorexia, and abdominal pain. The acute illness often lasts 1–3 weeks and may be followed by a prolonged convalescent phase. Fulminant acute hepatitis C has been reported but is rare. For the 15–30% who clear the infection during the acute phase, recovery is complete but may not protect against future infections should the patient be re-exposed to the virus.

The other 70–85% of persons with acute HCV infection progress to chronic infection. In long-term follow-up studies of adults with chronic infection, spontaneous clearance of the virus is rare. Chronic infection is generally asymptomatic, although studies have found that it is associated with a lower perceived quality of life.[12] Alanine aminotransferase (ALT) levels fluctuate, often between two and five times the upper limit of normal. In some HCV-infected individuals, ALT levels are persistently normal despite the presence of hepatitis.

A chronic, low-grade hepatic inflammation occurs in most chronically infected persons. Over years, this inflammation results in progressive fibrosis, the end stage of which is cirrhosis. The course of this disease is highly variable: many patients never develop significant fibrosis while a small number develop cirrhosis within a few years. Long-term studies suggest that in the first 20 years, cirrhosis will develop in 5–20% of patients with chronic hepatitis C. There are few data on the progression beyond 20 years.[13] Chronic hepatitis C can lead to hepatocellular carcinoma. The latter generally occurs in the setting of cirrhosis and is probably due to fibrosis and regenerative hyperplasia.

Several factors may accelerate the progression of chronic hepatitis C, particularly heavy alcohol use.[13]

There is no consensus as to whether light and moderate alcohol use are also risk factors for cirrhosis. Infection at an older age and coinfection with HIV are also associated with faster progression. In Egypt, schistosomiasis has been associated with more severe disease.

## Diagnosis

### Who should be tested?

Recommendations for anti-HCV screening were first published in the United States in 1998 (Table 31.1) and continue to be applicable to the United States.[14] As there are currently no formal recommendations for screening immigrants and refugees, at a minimum these recommendations should be applied. In addition, the following should be taken into consideration:

---

**Table 31.1 US Hepatitis C virus screening recommendations**

***Persons who should be tested routinely for hepatitis C virus (HCV) infection based on their risk for infection***
 Persons who ever injected illegal drugs, including those who injected once or a few times many years ago and do not consider themselves to be drug users
 Persons with selected medical conditions, including:
  Persons who received clotting factor concentrates produced before 1987;
  Persons who were ever on chronic (long-term) hemodialysis; and
  Persons with persistently abnormal alanine aminotransferase levels
 Prior recipients of transfusions or organ transplants, including:
  Persons who were notified that they received blood from a donor who later tested positive for HCV infection;
  Persons who received a transfusion of blood or blood components before July 1992; and
  Persons who received an organ transplant before July 1992

***Persons who should be tested routinely for HCV infection based on a recognized exposure***
 Healthcare, emergency medical, and public safety workers after needle sticks, sharps, or mucosal exposures to HCV-positive blood
 Children born to HCV-positive women

***Persons for whom routine HCV testing is of uncertain need***
 Recipients of transplanted tissue (e.g. corneal, musculoskeletal, skin, ova, sperm)
 Intranasal cocaine and other noninjecting illegal drug users
 Persons with a history of tattooing or body piercing
 Persons with a history of multiple sex partners or sexually transmitted diseases
 Long-term steady sex partners of HCV-positive persons

***Persons for whom routine HCV testing is not recommended***
 Healthcare, emergency medical, and public safety workers
 Pregnant women
 Household (nonsexual) contacts of HCV-positive persons
 The general population

Adapted from Reference 14.
These recommendations are based on risk factors for hepatitis C in the United States.

- *Illicit injection drug use*: Because injection drug use is such an efficient transmitter of HCV, anyone who has ever used illicit injection drugs, even if many years ago and for a short period of time, should be tested for anti-HCV.

- *Blood and blood product transfusions*: The US recommendations call for anti-HCV testing of anyone transfused before July 1992, when second-generation anti-HCV testing was implemented nationwide in blood banks. This rule clearly does not apply to persons transfused outside the United States. In other developed countries, sensitive testing was implemented around the same date, but in developing countries, testing procedures vary widely. Therefore, immigrants who have received blood transfusions, regardless of the date of the transfusion, should consider anti-HCV testing, particularly if they received a transfusion in a developing country. For similar reasons, immigrants who have ever received blood products (e.g. clotting factor concentrates) should also consider anti-HCV testing.

- *Unsafe medical procedures*: There are no formal recommendations about anti-HCV testing of persons subjected to unsafe medical procedures and there are few published data to guide such recommendations. Nonetheless, clinicians should be aware that infection control procedures in many parts of the world are poor. In addition, in many countries there is an informal, unregulated, and generally illegal medical sector in which injection practices may be highly unsafe.

- *Persons with unexplained liver function test abnormalities*: Clinicians should offer counseling and anti-HCV testing to anyone, regardless of his or her risk factor history, with an unexplained and persistent serum transaminase elevation. Similarly, because there is often a reluctance to disclose certain risk factors, anyone requesting anti-HCV testing should be offered counseling and testing.

## Differential diagnosis

There are many etiologies of chronic, low-grade hepatitis, including the hepatitis viruses (hepatitis B,

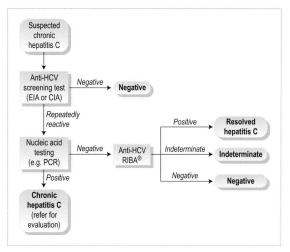

**Figure 31.2** Algorithm for HCV testing. HCV, hepatitis C virus; EIA; enzyme immunoassay; CIA, chemiluminescence immunoassay; PCR, polymerase chain reaction; RIBA, recombinant immunoblot assay.

C, and D viruses), autoimmunity, alcoholism, medications, other hepatotoxins, and storage diseases (e.g. iron overload, Wilson's disease). Nonalcoholic steatohepatitis (NASH, or 'fatty liver') is a common and increasingly recognized cause of chronic hepatitis, particularly among obese patients.

## Diagnostic evaluation

Persons for whom HCV testing is indicated should be offered anti-HCV testing, and if positive, testing for HCV RNA (Fig. 31.2). Those who are RNA positive should be referred to a physician experienced in HCV treatment for counseling and consideration of liver biopsy.

Anti-HCV testing is a two-step process, involving screening with a highly sensitive and moderately specific enzyme immunoassay (EIA) or chemiluminescence immunoassay (CIA), followed by supplemental testing. Specimens nonreactive by EIA or CIA are reported as negative while those testing positive are generally reported as 'repeatedly reactive,' although some laboratories may report strongly positive samples as 'positive' based on data that such results are almost always true positives. Repeatedly reactive specimens should be subjected to supplemental testing such as the recombinant immunoblot (RIBA®) assay or nucleic acid testing.

Nucleic acid testing, such as reverse transcriptase polymerase chain reaction (RT-PCR) assay, is indicated for anyone positive for anti-HCV and, if positive, may be used instead of RIBA testing to confirm a repeatedly reactive EIA or CIA. Persons testing positive for HCV RNA should be considered chronically infected and referred for evaluation. Persons testing RNA negative have almost always cleared their infection, although there are rare reports of individuals with intermittent viremia.

Liver biopsy is the only reliable method for assessing the degree of liver inflammation and fibrosis in patients positive for HCV RNA. Although there is a correlation between serum liver function tests and liver histology, the correlation is poor; persons with normal liver function tests may have significant fibrosis on biopsy.

For patients considering therapy, HCV genotyping is indicated.

## ICD-9 Codes

- 070.41 Acute hepatitis C with hepatic coma
- 070.44 Chronic hepatitis C with hepatic coma
- 070.51 Acute hepatitis C without mention of hepatic coma
- 070.54 Chronic hepatitis C without mention of hepatic coma
- 070.70 Unspecified viral hepatitis C without hepatic coma
- 070.71 Unspecified viral hepatitis C with hepatic coma

## Treatment

Treatment for hepatitis C is a specialized and evolving field that is beyond the scope of this chapter. Anyone considering therapy for hepatitis C should be referred to a clinician experienced in its management.

The current standard for the treatment of hepatitis C involves weekly injections of pegylated interferon (interferon with covalently attached polyethylene glycol to prolong its half-life) and daily oral ribavirin for a period of 24 to 48 weeks.[11,15] The treatment has high rates of adverse effects, including fatigue, flu-like symptoms, and anemia. Depression is common during treatment and a history of major depression was once considered a contraindication to interferon therapy. However, paroxetine has been shown to prevent interferon-induced depression.[16] Ribavirin is teratogenic; both men and women should be counseled to use at least two forms of contraception while on therapy and for 6 months afterwards.

The goal of therapy is to obtain a 'sustained virologic response,' generally defined as a lack of detectable HCV 24 weeks after the end of treatment. Patients who achieve a sustained virologic response rarely relapse but are susceptible to reinfection if exposed to hepatitis C again. Response to current regimens depends greatly on the genotype, with better responses among patients with HCV genotype 2 or 3 (70–90%) than among those with genotype 1 (40–60%).

Follow-up studies of patients newly diagnosed with chronic hepatitis C have shown that most either do not pursue or do not complete therapy. Many have mild disease and choose not to undergo treatment or to postpone treatment until better alternatives are available. Others have one or more of the many contraindications to treatment or are unable to follow through with treatment.

For the rare patient presenting with acute hepatitis C, recent studies suggest that early treatment may be highly effective at preventing progression to chronic infection. Such patients should be immediately referred for evaluation by an experienced clinician.[17]

## Prevention

Hepatitis C virus is not spread by sneezing, hugging, coughing, food or water, sharing eating utensils or drinking glasses, or casual contact. Therefore, persons should not be excluded from work, school, play, childcare, or other settings on the basis of their HCV infection status.

Anyone who uses illicit injection drugs should be encouraged to seek counseling and to quit using drugs. Those unable to quit should be counseled to avoid sharing needles, syringes, and other injection equipment with other users.

There are no data on the usefulness of safe sex practices (e.g. barrier condoms) in preventing HCV infection, but such practices are always prudent and are clearly effective at preventing other infections such as HIV and HBV infection. For HCV-discordant, long-term, monogamous couples, the risk of transmission is extremely low. For this reason, there is no need to counsel such couples to change their sexual practices. However, these couples should be informed of available data regarding the risk of transmission by sexual activity. Because this risk is not zero, some couples may wish to take additional precautions.

For HCV-infected patients, counseling is of key importance, both to reduce the risk of transmission to others and to decrease the likelihood of progressive liver disease. All HCV-infected patients should be counseled against the use of alcohol. Available data suggest that even modest amounts of alcohol use may be detrimental to persons with chronic hepatitis C. In addition, patients should consult their physicians before starting new medications, including over-the-counter medications.

## Infection Control Measures

Standard Precautions (formerly known as 'Universal Precautions') are adequate to prevent transmission of hepatitis C in clinical settings.

### Clinical Pearls

- Think of hepatitis C in anyone with an unexplained, persistently elevated ALT level.
- Chronic hepatitis C is asymptomatic and slowly progressive.
- Young, otherwise healthy persons with acute hepatitis C have a low risk (probably 5% or lower) of progressing to cirrhosis within 20 years of their infection. Older persons and persons with other risk factors, particularly alcohol use, are at higher risk of progression.
- Anyone with *chronic* HCV infection (i.e. anyone positive for HCV RNA) should be counseled on the means of preventing progression of disease and avoiding transmission to others. Persons with chronic HCV infection should also be evaluated for possible treatment by an experienced clinician.
- Anyone with *acute* HCV infection should be immediately referred for evaluation and possible treatment.

### Special Considerations for Immigrants

- Unsafe medical procedures, particularly unsafe injections, may be the most common risk factor for HCV infection in developing countries.
- Recommendations for HCV testing of US residents are based on risk factors. No such recommendations exist for immigrants or refugees, for whom risk factors may be very different.
- Coinfection with HIV or coexistence of schistosomiasis may accelerate the progression of hepatitis C.

## References

1. Shepard CW, Finelli L, Alter MJ. Global epidemiology of hepatitis C virus infection. Lancet Infect Dis 2005; 5:558–567.
2. Rao MR, Naficy AB, Darwish MA, et al. Further evidence for association of hepatitis C infection with parenteral schistosomiasis treatment in Egypt. BMC Infect Dis 2002; 2:29.
3. Garfein RS, Vlahov D, Galai N, et al. Viral infections in short-term injection drug users: the prevalence of the hepatitis C, hepatitis B, human immunodeficiency, and human T-lymphotropic viruses. Am J Public Health 1996; 86:655–661.
4. Hahn JA, Page-Shafer K, Lum PJ, et al. Hepatitis C virus seroconversion among young injection drug users: relationships and risks. J Infect Dis 2002; 186:1558–1564.
5. Hagan H, Thiede H, Des J. Hepatitis C virus infection among injection drug users: survival analysis of time to seroconversion. Epidemiology 2004; 15:543–549.
6. Hutin YJ, Hauri AM, Armstrong GL. Use of injections in healthcare settings worldwide, 2000: literature review and regional estimates. Br Med J 2003; 327:1075–1078.
7. Hauri AM, Armstrong GL, Hutin YJF. Contaminated injections in healthcare settings. In: Ezzati M, Lopez AD, Rodgers A, et al., eds. Comparative quantification of health risks. Geneva: World Health Organization; 2004:1803–1850.
8. Centers for Disease Control and Prevention. Updated US Public Health Service guidelines for the management of occupational exposures to HBV, HCV, and HIV and recommendations for postexposure prophylaxis. MMWR Recommendations and Reports 2001; 50:1–42.
9. England K, Thorne C, Newell ML. Vertically acquired paediatric coinfection with HIV and hepatitis C virus. Lancet Infect Dis 2006; 6:83–90.
10. Krawczynski K, Alter MJ, Robertson BH, et al. Environmental stability of hepatitis C virus (HCV): viability of dried/stored HCV in chimpanzee infectivity studies. In: Proceedings of the 54th Annual Meeting of the American Society for the Study of Liver Disease. Alexandria, VA: American Society for the Study of Liver Disease; 2003.
11. Strader DB, Wright T, Thomas DL, et al. Diagnosis, management, and treatment of hepatitis C. Hepatology 2004; 39:1147–1171.
12. Teixeira MC, Ribeiro MF, Gayotto LC, et al. Worse quality of life in volunteer blood donors with hepatitis C. Transfusion 2006; 46:278–283.
13. Thomas DL, Seeff LB. Natural history of hepatitis C. Clin Liver Dis 2005; 9:383–398.
14. Centers for Disease Control and Prevention. Recommendations for prevention and control of hepatitis C virus (HCV) infection and HCV-related chronic disease. MMWR Recommendations and Reports 1998; 47:1–39.
15. Heathcote J, Main J. Treatment of hepatitis C. J Viral Hepat 2005; 12:223–235.
16. Musselman DL, Lawson DH, Gumnick JF, et al. Paroxetine for the prevention of depression induced by high-dose interferon alfa. N Engl J Med 2001; 344:961–966.
17. Craxi A, Licata A. Acute hepatitis C: in search of the optimal approach to cure. Hepatology 2006; 43:221-224.

# CHAPTER 32

# Hookworm Infection

Peter J. Hotez

## Hookworm at a Glance

- Hookworm infection, ascariasis, and trichuriasis comprise the three major soil-transmitted helminth infections of humans.
- It is estimated that 15% of the world's population is infected with hookworm.[1]
- Both *Necator americanus* and *Ancylostoma duodenale* are considered the major etiologic agents of hookworm infection, with the former accounting for a majority of the cases.
- Rural areas of sub-Saharan Africa and Southeast Asia exhibit the highest prevalence of hookworm infection, though transmission also occurs in tropical areas of the Americas, India and Nepal, and South China.
- Hookworm occurs almost exclusively among the poor.
- Immigrants at highest risk for hookworm infection are refugees from the poorest rural areas of Africa, Southeast Asia, South Asia, South China, and the Americas, especially Central America and Brazil.

## Epidemiology

The transmission of human hookworm infection occurs in poor and rural areas of the developing world. Sub-Saharan Africa and Southeast Asia exhibit the highest prevalence (Table 32.1), although areas of high hookworm transmission also occur in tropical areas of the Americas (e.g. Central America, the Caribbean, and Brazil), India and Nepal, and South China.[1] Hookworm is found predominantly in the rural areas of these regions because the infective

larval stages that live in the soil depend on precise environmental conditions for their survival. Coastal areas are also notorious for endemic hookworm infection,[2] probably because the sandy soils there facilitate the larval migrations required for transmission to humans.[3] Finally, there is a very strong relationship between the prevalence of hookworm and poverty.[1] Hookworm occurs almost exclusively among the poor, including the estimated 2.7 billion people who live on less than US $2 per day.[4]

These demographic and epidemiologic features of hookworm infection are useful for assessing the risk of hookworm in immigrants. Hookworm would not be expected to be a significant health problem in immigrants from urban areas or among the middle and upper classes even if they are from developing countries. Instead, the immigrant patient populations at highest risk for hookworm infection are refugees from the poorest rural areas of Africa,[5] Southeast Asia,[6] South Asia, South China, and the Americas, especially Central America and Brazil.

## Pathogenesis

Hookworm infection occurs when third-stage larvae penetrate the skin, usually through the hands and feet (especially between the toes). Repeated episodes of larval skin invasion result in a pruritic, papular rash known as 'ground itch.'[3] *A. duodenale* hookworm infection can also result from ingestion of the larvae. Subsequently, the larvae enter the venous circulation and reach the lungs within 10 days. Larval migration through the lungs can result in hookworm pneumonitis, which is characterized by a mild to moderate cough and sore throat. However, because it is associated with only recent infections, hookworm

**Table 32.1 Global distribution (by World Bank region) and prevalence of hookworm infection**

| World Bank region | Number of infections (millions) | Infection prevalence (%) |
|---|---|---|
| Latin America and the Caribbean | 50 | 10 |
| Sub-Saharan Africa | 198 | 29 |
| Middle East and North Africa | 10 | 3 |
| South Asia | 59 | 16 |
| India | 71 | 7 |
| East Asia and the Pacific Islands | 149 | 26 |
| China[a] | 203 | 16 |
| Total | 740 | 15 |

Modified from de Silva et al.[1]

[a] A new survey for intestinal parasites in China has been completed and there are indications that the prevalence of hookworm and other soil-transmitted helminths is lower than previous estimates might suggest.

pneumonitis would not be expected to be common among refugees.

After leaving the lungs, hookworm larvae pass over the epiglottis and are swallowed. Within 5–9 weeks after initial infection the larvae molt twice to the adult stage. The appearance of adult hookworms in the intestine coincides with the onset of eosinophilia.[7] Eosinophilia is a useful indicator for hookworm infection among refugees. For example, hookworm was detected in 55% of Southeast Asian refugees with persistent eosinophilia.[6]

## Clinical Features

The presence of hookworms in the small intestine can result in nausea, as well as recurrent epigastric pain and tenderness.[8] However, the greatest morbidity from hookworm infection results from intestinal blood loss as a consequence of hookworm blood ingestion.[3] There is a strong association between the magnitude of the blood loss and the number of hookworms present,[9] and infection with *A. duodenale* produces more blood loss than *N. americanus* infection.[10] Chronic blood loss from moderate and heavy hookworm infection results in hookworm disease, which is characterized by iron deficiency anemia (IDA) and hypoalbuminemia.[3] Severe hookworm disease can

result in profoundly low hemoglobin concentrations[11] and, consequently, extreme pallor as well as clinically evident protein malnutrition.[3]

The development of hookworm disease depends significantly on the underlying nutritional state of the host and whether the number of hookworms present in the intestine is sufficient to deplete those reserves.[9] It is not commonly appreciated that heavy hookworm infection and disease occurs in both children and adults. Children and women in their reproductive years typically have low iron reserves and are therefore are especially susceptible to developing IDA from their hookworm infections.[3,9] As a result, chronically infected children can experience delays in growth, physical fitness, and intellectual and cognitive development, and infected pregnant women are at risk for severe anemia that leads to increased maternal mortality, prematurity, and low birth weights.[12]

## Diagnosis

Because adult female hookworms produce thousands of eggs per day, it is relatively easy to diagnose hookworm through fecal examination. Therefore, a fecal examination should be conducted in all immigrants and refugees with eosinophilia or with evidence of IDA. Eosinophilia also occurs commonly in patients with strongyloidiasis,[6] so that disease should also be ruled out by fecal examination and serologic testing.

## Treatment

The benzimidazoles, albendazole (400 mg once) or mebendazole (100 mg b.i.d. × 3 days), are the drugs of choice for hookworm infection (Table 32.2). When used in a single dose, mebendazole is often not effective in removing significant numbers of hookworms.[13] Similarly, *N. americanus* often has low susceptibility to albendazole, and repeat dosing may also be required. Pyrantel pamoate (11 mg/kg [max. 1 g] × 3 d) is also effective as an alternative agent and is available as an over-the-counter medicine (Pin-X; Effcon) for human pinworm infection in the United States.

Albendazole and mebendazole are embryotoxic and teratogenic in pregnant rats at a single oral dose equivalent to the human dose.[14] Therefore, there are potential safety considerations for their use in young children and in pregnancy. The results from a WHO Informal Consultation on the use of benzimidazoles

**Table 32.2 Drugs used in the treatment of hookworm**

| Drug | Dose | Duration | Efficacy | Adverse Events |
|------|------|----------|----------|----------------|
| Albendazole | 400 mg once (200 mg once for children 12–24 months) | Single dose | Albendazole is usually effective in curing hookworm infection. However, for some patients multiple doses are required to effect cure. The median cure rate is 80–90%.[13] However, there is marked heterogeneity in response. | GI discomfort, headache, nausea, dizziness; hypersensitivity reactions uncommon. Praziquantel may increase plasma levels of albendazole active metabolite Albendazole is an approved drug, but considered investigational for the treatment of hookworm infection by the FDA. |
| Mebendazole | 100 mg OR 500 mg | Twice daily for 3 days OR Single dose | Multiple dosing over 3 days improves the cure rate to close to the rates reported for albendazole. The median cure rate for mebendazole is less than 40% when it is used in a single-dose (500 mg) formulation.[13] | Occasional diarrhea, abdominal pain; rare leukopenia, agranulocytosis, hypospermia, hypersensitivity reactions. |
| Pyrantel pamoate | 11 mg/kg (maximum 1 g) | Once daily for 3 days | | Occasional GI disturbance, headache, dizziness, rash, fever. Pyrantel pamoate is an approved drug but it is considered investigational for hookworm infection by the FDA |

in children younger than 24 months have determined that the incidence of side effects in this population is similar to those in older children and that the use of these agents is justified in children as young as 12 months.[14,15] However, it is recommended that healthcare providers read the package inserts for albendazole and mebendazole before treating very young children. A reduction in the albendazole dosage (200 mg single dose) has been recommended for children aged 12–24 months.[11,15]

Both albendazole and mebendazole are contraindicated for pregnant women in their first trimester. When considering their use in the second and third trimester, the risks versus benefits of treatment need to be considered. Christian et al.[12] observed that antenatal anthelmintic chemotherapy for hookworm-infected pregnant women in Nepal resulted in significant improvement in birth weight and infant survival.

Hookworm treatment with anthelmintic drugs followed by normal dietary intake is usually sufficient to restore host nutritional status. However, iron supplementation is recommended for anemia in pregnancy[12] and for other selected patients. In rare cases of profound anemia, blood transfusion is warranted.

## Prevention and Patient Follow-Up

In areas of high transmission, hookworm post-treatment reinfection can occur within a few months. This observation, coupled with the low efficacy of single-dose benzimidazoles and concerns about possible anthelmintic drug resistance[16] provide the rationale for developing a first-generation recombinant hookworm vaccine.[4] In contrast, immigrants to North America and Europe are not typically exposed to larvae in the environment post-treatment and therefore not at risk for reacquiring infection. It has been suggested that *A. duodenale* larvae can arrest their development in the musculature and other tissues, and may enter the gastrointestinal tract where they can develop to adult hookworms several months after treatment. The frequency of this phenomenon among immigrants from *A. duodenale*-endemic regions (e.g. Egypt, Nepal and northern India, China, parts of sub-Saharan Africa, Paraguay, and Northern Argentina) is not known.

An innovative empiric albendazole treatment program has been developed by the US Centers for Disease Control and Prevention (CDC) for refugees prior to their departure from some developing countries.[5] An analysis of such a program among African refugees suggests that overseas pre-departure treatment programs can have a significant impact on hookworm and other parasitic infections.

## Clinical Pearls

- Eosinophilia and anemia are likely to be the most common manifestations of hookworm in immigrants; hookworm pneumonitis would be rare.
- Diagnosis of hookworm infection is by examination of the stool for hookworm eggs.

## Special Considerations for Immigrants

- Hookworm infection is most likely to be found only in those who have lived in poverty in rural areas of sub-Saharan Africa and Southeast Asia.
- Pre-departure treatment of refugees with albendazole has reduced the prevalence of helminth infections in refugees screened on arrival in the US.
- When used as a single-dose formulation, albendazole is considered more effective than mebendazole. For immigrants with hookworm infection, mebendazole should be administered on three consecutive days. In some cases, repeated dosing of albendazole is also required to achieve cures for hookworm infection.

## References

1. De Silva NR, Brooker S, Hotez PJ, et al. Soil-transmitted helminth infections: updating the global picture. Trends Parasitol 2003; 19:547–551.
2. Mabaso MLH, Appleton CC, Hughes JC, et al. The effect of soil type and climate on hookworm (*Necator americanus*) distribution in KwaZulu-Natal, South Africa. Trop Med Int Health 2003; 8:722–727.
3. Hotez PJ, Brooker S, Bethony JM, et al. Hookworm infection. N Engl J Med 2004; 351:799–807.
4. Hotez PJ, Bethony J, Bottazzi ME, et al. Hookworm: 'The great infection of mankind.' PLoS Medicine 2005; 2:e67.
5. Geltman PL, Cochran J, Hedgecock C. Intestinal parasites among African refugees resettled in Massachusetts and the impact of an overseas pre-departure treatment program. Am J Trop Med Hyg 2003; 69:657–662.
6. Nutman TB, Ottesen EA, Ieng S, et al. Eosinophilia in Southeast Asian refugees: evaluation at a referral center. J Infect Dis 1987; 155:309–313.
7. Maxwell C, Hussain R, Nutman TB, et al. The clinical and immunologic responses of normal human volunteers to low-dose hookworm (*Necator americanus*) infection. Am J Trop Med Hyg 1987; 37:126–134.
8. Anyaeze CM. Reducing burden of hookworm disease in the management of upper abdominal pain in the tropics. Trop Doc 2003; 33:174–175.
9. Stoltzfus RJ, Dreyfuss ML, Chwaya HM, et al. Hookworm control as a strategy to prevent iron deficiency. Nutr Rev 1997; 55:223–232.
10. Albonico M, Stoltzfus RJ, Savioli L, et al. Epidemiological evidence for a differential effect of hookworm species, *Ancylostoma duodenale* or *Necator amercanus*, on iron status of children. Int J Epidemiol 1998; 27:530–537.
11. Nkhoma E, van Hensbroek PB, van Lieshout L, et al. Severe anaemia in an 11-month-old girl. Lancet 2005; 365:1202.
12. Christian P, Khatry SK, West KP Jr. Antenatal anthelminthic treatment, birthweight, and infant survival in rural Nepal. Lancet 2004; 364:981–983.
13. Bennett A, Guyatt H. Reducing intestinal nematode infections: efficacy of albendazole and mebendazole. Parasitol Today 2000; 16:71–74.
14. Hotez PJ, Bethony J, Brooker S. Soil-transmitted helminth infections. In: Burg FD, Ingelfinger JR, Polin RA, et al., eds. Current pediatric therapy. 18th edn. Philadelphia: Elsevier; 2005.
15. Montresor A, Awasthi S, Crompton DWT. Use of benzimidazoles in children younger than 24 months for the treatment of soil-transmitted helminthiases. Acta Tropica 2003; 86:223–232.
16. Albonico M, Engels D, Savioli L. Monitoring drug efficacy and early detection of drug resistance in human soil-transmitted nematodes: a pressing public health agenda for helminth control. Int J Parasitol 2004; 34:1205–1210.

# CHAPTER 33

# Leishmaniasis

Gregory Juckett

## Leishmaniasis at a Glance

- *Clinical classification*: cutaneous leishmaniasis (CL), mucocutaneous leishmaniasis (MCL), and visceral leishmaniasis (VL) forms.
- *Other names*: cutaneous forms have many regional names: Baghdad or Delhi boil, oriental sore, *uta* (Peru), Chiclero's ulcer, bay sore, and *saldana* (Afganistan, Iran). MCL in Latin America is usually called *espundia*. VL is called *kala azar*, meaning black fever in Hindi.
- Caused by various species of *Leishmania* protozoa, obligate intracellular parasites of humans and animals.
- Transmitted by female sandflies, genus *Phlebotomus* in the Old World, *Lutzomyia* in the New World.
- Transmission occurs in Central and South America (except Chile and Uruguay), the Mediterranean, North and East Africa, the Middle East, northern India, Bangladesh, Pakistan, Nepal, central Asian republics, and China.
- Clinical manifestation of CL is one or more indolent skin ulcers, whereas MCL produces mucosal ulcerations and deformities of the nose and mouth. VL manifests as fever, splenomegaly, pancytopenia, weight loss, and lymphadenopathy.
- *Diagnosis*: CL and MCL are usually diagnosed by clinical appearance. Punch biopsy from the ulcer margin for pathologic examination and culture confirms diagnosis. VL can be confirmed by microscopy and culture of bone marrow, splenic, hepatic, or lymph node aspirates (Fig. 33.1). Serologic diagnosis can be accomplished with indirect fluorescent antibody testing (IFAT) or ELISA or Western blot. K39 rapid antigen strip testing is utilized in India.
- *Treatment*: Pentavalent antimonials such as sodium stibogluconate (*Pentostam*) are still widely used for VL, MCL, and complicated CL. However, liposomal preparations of amphotericin B may be the most available option for VL in the US (too expensive for most developing countries). Pentamidine is a second-line VL option due to toxicity. Oral miltefosine for VL has replaced pentavalent antimony in India and will eventually be approved elsewhere. Many cutaneous lesions will eventually resolve spontaneously, although some require treatment (Fig. 33.2).

## Epidemiology

Forms of cutaneous leishmaniasis (CL) are widespread with an estimated 1.5 million cases in 88 countries, affecting residents and immigrants from Latin America, the Middle East, the Mediterranean, North and East Africa, Central and South Asia (Figs. 33.3 and 33.4).[1] Unlike many parasitic diseases, leishmaniasis is increasing in prevalence and occurs in urban as well as rural areas. CL is also now appearing in returning US service personnel from Iraq and Afghanistan as well as returning travelers from these areas.[2] Ulcers are usually self-limited (<6–12 months) but often leave conspicuous scars. CL may also occasionally progress over months to years (well after the ulcers have healed), to MCL or *espundia* (literally 'sponge' in Portuguese). MCL is thought to develop through metastasis of the parasite rather

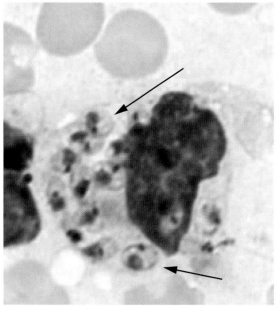

**Fig. 33.1** Leishmaniasis amastigotes in a biopsy specimen.

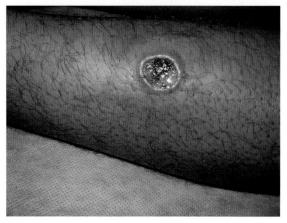

**Fig. 33.3** Cutaneous leishmaniasis of leg in Amazonas, Brazil (photo by author).

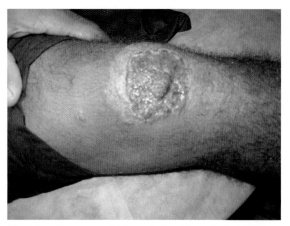

**Fig. 33.4** Cutaneous leishmaniasis of knee in Amazonas, Brazil (photo by author).

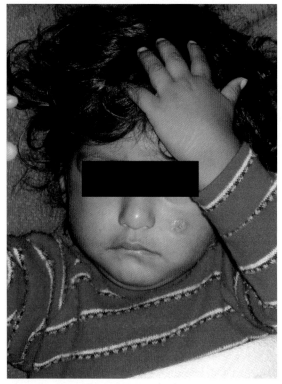

**Fig. 33.2** Resolving cutaneous leishmaniasis on the cheek of a child in Peru (photo by author).

than local spread. Poor nutrition and health, as well as the *Leishmania* species involved (usually subgenus *Viannia* of Latin America), appear to increase the risk of this dreaded complication.

Visceral leishmaniasis (*kala azar*) is thought to be responsible for 80 000 deaths out of 500 000 probable cases per year, most of which occur in South Asia from *L. donovani*.[3] *L. infantum* in southern Europe and North Africa and *L. chagasi* in Latin America also cause visceral disease. Many cases are likely subclinical but malnutrition, poverty, and concomitant diseases intensify symptoms. Coinfection with HIV is an increasing concern, with some VL outbreaks

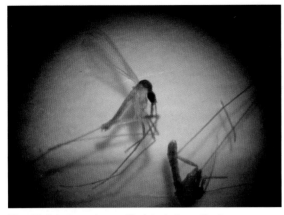

**Fig. 33.5** Lutzomyia sandfly (photo by author).

associated with HIV transmitted via intravenous drug abuse. VL patients with risk factors should be tested for HIV as each disease exacerbates the other. HIV increases the risk of developing VL 100–1000-fold in an endemic area.[4] Even without HIV, the disease is progressive and usually fatal if left untreated.

## Etiology

Leishmania is an obligate intramacrophage parasite (21 species infect humans) transmitted through the bite of sandfly vectors, genus *Phlebotomus* (Old World) or *Lutzomyia* (New World) (Fig. 33.5). Humans are usually incidental victims, with the primary (reservoir) hosts including dogs and rodents, although in the case of *L. donovani* (the cause of *kala azar*) and *L. tropica*, it appears to be an anthroponotic infection (acquired via sandfly vectors from other humans) rather than a zoonotic one.[1] Rarely, VL appears to be congenitally transmitted, and needle sharing, transfusion, and unprotected sex are alternative means of spread.[4]

There are two principal phases in the parasite's lifecycle: the extracellular promastigote stage with flagella, occurring in the gut of the sandfly, and the intracellular 2–4 µg amastigote (without flagella) tissue phase that reproduces in mammalian macrophages (Fig. 33.6). The *Leishmania* species typically resulting in CL grow best at lower temperatures and are considered dermotropic in that they are usually limited to the skin in normal hosts. These include *L. braziliensis*, *L. mexicana*, and *L. amazonensis* in the Americas and *L. tropica*, *L. major*, *L. infantum*,

and *L. aethiopica* in the Old World. Viscerotropic infections are caused by *Leishmania* species adapted to higher temperatures including *L. donovani* (the cause of most *kala azar* in South Asia), *L. infantum* (Mediterranean), and *L. chagasi* (Latin America). Occasionally, skin-adapted species such as *L. tropica* may also result in a mild viscerotropic leishmaniasis.[5]

## Clinical Manifestations

Cutaneous leishmaniasis usually presents as a papule at the site of a sandfly bite, developing into an indolent, often volcano-shaped, ulceration with raised margins. The incubation period between bite and lesion may be several weeks to several months. These ulcers are invariably located on exposed areas of skin (usually face or extremities). Of course, there must also be a history of travel or residence in an endemic area. Men and children are at greater risk, possibly due to increased exposure to sandflies.

'Wet' CL consists of moist ulcers with purulent exudates (e.g. the classic 'oriental sore' of *L. major*), whereas 'dry' forms have a crusted scab (*L. tropica*). Other much less common cutaneous syndromes include diffuse cutaneous leishmaniasis and leishmaniasis recidivans. Diffuse cutaneous disease, caused by *L. mexicana* and *L. aethiopica*, is a nonulcerative progressive condition developing in anergic patients and often resembling lepromatous leprosy. Leishmaniasis recidivans, usually caused by *L. tropica* in the Middle East, is a gradually enlarging facial lesion that may resemble lupus vulgaris or cutaneous tuberculosis (TB).[1]

Mucocutaneous leishmaniasis, better known as *espundia*, attacks the mucus membranes of the nose, mouth, and pharynx to produce facial ulcerations and deformities (Fig. 33.7). Mucosal infections are most common in New World species (sometimes considered as a subgenus *Viannia*) such as *L. (V.) braziliensis*, *L. (V.) guyanensis*, and *L. (V.) panamensis*. Nasal obstruction and bleeding are usually the first symptoms. In the absence of treatment, the infection progresses to destroy nasal cartilage resulting in the so-called 'tapir' nose. Later, the lips and palate may become involved, with secondary infections being a potential cause of death.[5]

Visceral leishmaniasis, or *kala azar*, classically presents with fever, splenomegaly, lymphadenopathy, cachexia, and anemia. Fever may be intermittent or continuous. Other common findings include dark-

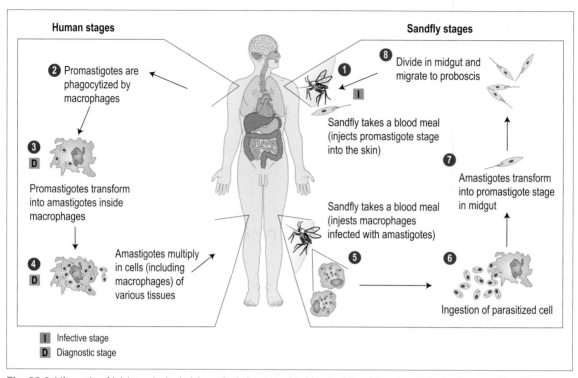

**Fig. 33.6** Life cycle of leishmaniasis. Leishmaniasis is transmitted by the bite of female phlebotomine sandflies. The sandflies inject the infective stage, promastigotes, during blood meals (1). Promastigotes that reach the puncture wound are phagocytized by macrophages (2) and transform into amastigotes (3). Amastigotes multiply in infected cells and affect different tissues, depending in part on the *Leishmania* species (4). This originates in the clinical manifestations of leishmaniasis. Sandflies become infected during blood meals on an infected host when they ingest macrophages infected with amastigotes (5, 6). In the sandfly's midgut, the parasites differentiate into promastigotes (7), which multiply and migrate to the proboscis (8). (From Centers for Disease Control and Prevention DPDx.)

ening of the skin, hemorrhage, diarrhea, and secondary infections. While the onset may be insidious, untreated infections are usually fatal, with death from infection or hemorrhage. Laboratory findings include pancytopenia (normocytic anemia, thrombocytopenia, leukopenia), hypergammaglobulinemia, an elevated sedimentation rate, and elevation of C-reactive protein. Even when successfully treated, 10% of patients may develop post-*kala azar* dermal leishmaniasis (PKDL) 1 year or more after cure. This conspicuous skin condition starts as hypopigmented macules (evolving into papules and nodules that contain many parasites) on the face and upper extremities, later spreading to the entire body. Course is variable, with resolution in 6 months to many years.[5,6]

## Diagnosis

### Who should be tested?

Cutaneous leishmaniasis should be suspected in anyone from an endemic area with one or more chronic skin ulcers on exposed areas. VL is a consideration in patients with weight loss, fever, splenomegaly, adenopathy, and anemia. Most patients with *L. donovani* VL are from South Asia (India, Bangladesh) or East Africa but children under age 5 from the Mediterranean region (southern Europe, North Africa) may be infected with infantile leishmaniasis, *L. infantum*, which has also affected HIV-positive adults in recent years.[1]

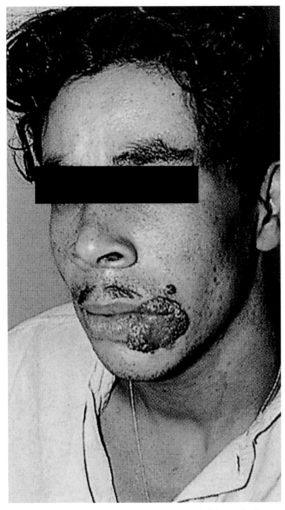

**Fig. 33.7** The lesions of mucocutaneous leishmaniasis due to infection with *L. braziliensis* may first become evident as ulcers involving the mucocutaneous junctions of the mouth and nose. This condition frequently follows a primary cutaneous lesions, which may have healed with or without specific therapy some years earlier. (With permission from Wallace Peters and Geoffrey Pasvol, Atlas of Tropical Medicine and Parasitology, 6th edition, copyright Elsevier Ltd. 2007)

## Differential diagnosis

The differential diagnosis for CL includes infected insect bites, impetigo, myiasis, foreign body reactions, neoplasms (such as basal or squamous cell carcinomas), mycobacterial infections (lupus vulgaris), fungal infections (sporotrichosis, blastomycosis, chromomycosis), yaws, syphilis, sarcoid, and leprosy.

MCL may be confused with many of the same conditions. Nasopharyngeal carcinoma, Wegener's granulomatosis, and lymphoma are also considerations.

VL (characterized by fever and splenomegaly) has an extensive differential diagnosis including malaria, typhoid, TB, systemic lupus erythematosus, brucellosis, histoplasmosis, tropical splenomegaly, and leukemia/lymphoma.[1,5]

## Diagnostic evaluation

Cutaneous leishmaniasis and MCL are usually diagnosed by clinical appearance. Punch biopsy from the ulcer margin for pathologic examination and culture (taking 1–3 weeks) confirms the diagnosis. (A leishmanin skin test [Montenegro test] turns positive in immunocompetent patients but only 2–3 months after the appearance of the ulcer. Skin testing is not available in the US.)

VL can be confirmed by microscopic examination and culture of bone marrow (often most practical), splenic, hepatic, or lymph node aspirates. Identification of the parasite in tissue smears is the standard for diagnosis. Splenic aspirates are the most likely to demonstrate the parasite but are also the most hazardous to obtain.

Increasingly, serologic diagnosis of VL can be accomplished with indirect fluorescent antibody testing (IFAT) or ELISA or Western blot. *Leishmania* rapid strip testing for K39 antigen is utilized in India for moderately sensitive (67–100%) and specific (93–100%) diagnosis. Direct agglutination testing of stained specimens and detection of *Leishmania* antigen in urine by latex agglutination (*Katex*) are methods used in other countries. Species identification, when necessary, may be established through monoclonal antibody testing.[7]

## ICD-9 and ICD-10 Codes

- Leishmaniasis: ICD-9 085; ICD-10 B55
- CL/MCL: ICD-9 085.1-085.5; ICD-10 B55.1, B55.2
- VL: ICD-9 085.0; ICD-10 B55.0

## Treatment

Treatment of cutaneous leishmaniasis is fraught with controversy and there is no ideal therapy (Table 33.1). Fortunately, many of these lesions will resolve spontaneously – albeit with scarring – but some, especially those acquired in the New World, may

**Table 33.1 Drugs used for Leishmaniasis[1,9]**

| Drug | Formulations | Dose | Adverse events | Comments |
|---|---|---|---|---|
| Pentavalent antimony (Sb) i.v. (i.m.) | Sodium stibogluconate (*Pentostam*) or meglumine antimonite (*Glucantime*) – latter is an equivalent drug in Francophone countries and Latin America. Both have availability problems in US. | 20 mg Sb/kg daily i.v. × 20days (CL) or 28 days (VL/MCL); identical regimen for pediatric Rx | Nausea/vomiting, myalgias, fever, rash; 200 mg test dose option; monitor weekly LFTs, ECG, CBC | US first-line drug but available only from CDC (404-639-3670) Ineffective for Indian VL; Pregnancy C D/C if QT >0.50 |
| Amphotericin B deoxycholate (*Fungizone*) i.v. | Parenteral antifungal also serving as an effective but toxic antileishmanial drug | 0.5–1.0 mg/kg i.v. q.d. or q.o.d. × up to 8 weeks (total 20–40 mg/kg) | More toxicity and longer course than liposomal amphotericin B: renal toxicity, hypotension | VL alternative Pregnancy B Not indicated for CL |
| Amphotericin B Lipid formulations i.v. | Liposomal amphotericin B (*AmBisome*) – FDA approved for VL and is available in US. Amphotericin B lipid complex (*Abelcet*) and amphotericin B cholesteryl sulfate (*Amphotec*) are effective but investigational | 3 mg/kg/day i.v. ×5 days and 3 mg/kg/day on day 14 and 21* | Much less toxic than amphotericin B with far shorter course | Alternative agent to pentavalent antimony but perhaps best VL option in US as available and reasonably safe Too costly in developing world |
| Pentamidine isethionate i.m. (i.v.) | *Pentam – 300* | 4 mg/kg i.m. q.d. or q.o.d. for 15–30 doses (VL/MCL) or 3 mg/kg q.o.d. × four doses (CL) | May cause diabetes in 10% | Second-line VL treatment but may be first-line CL option Pregnancy C (rabbit fetal injury) |
| Paromomycin sulfate i.v./i.m. | Aminoglycoside – available in injectable and nonabsorbable oral forms | 15–20 mg/kg/day × 21 days (VL) | Nausea, vomiting nephrotoxic and ototoxic when parenteral | Adjunctive therapy Ineffective against *L. braziliensis* and *L. panamensis* |
| Miltefosine (*Impavido*, *Zentaris*) p.o. | Hexadecylphosphocholine Originally used as an antineoplastic agent but approved for VL in India 2002 – may replace antimonial therapy elsewhere | 100 mg (2.5 mg/kg/day) p.o. q.d. × 28 days no pediatric doses | Nausea, vomiting, diarrhea | Currently very effective treatment of choice for Indian VL (unavailable US) Pregnancy X |
| Ketoconazole (*Nizoral*) p.o. | Antifungal with some antileishmanial effect | 600 mg q.d. × 28 days (adult) | Rash, elevated LFTs | Consider for *L. mexicana* CL |
| Itraconazole (*Sporonox*) p.o. | Antifungal with some antileishmanial effect | 200 mg q.d. × 28 days (adult) | Rash, elevated LFTs | CL: appears less effective than ketoconazole |
| Paromomycin sulfate ointment | *Leshcutan ointment* (paromomycin, methylbenzemonium Cl) (available in Israel) | Apply b.i.d. × 10–20 days (CL only) | May cause skin irritation | Consider for *L. major* and *L. mexicana* – avoid if MCL risk |
| Intralesional pentavalent antimony | Local injection option for CL | Weekly or alternate day injections (CL) | | Infiltrate each side of ulcer until completely blanched |

*The FDA-approved dosage regimen for immunocompromised patients (e.g., HIV infected) is 4 mg/kg/day (days 1–5) and 4 mg/kg/day on days 10, 17, 24, 31 and 38. The relapse rate is high.
b.i.d = twice a day, q.i.d. = 4 times a day, q.o.d = every other day, q.d = once a day

evolve into mucocutaneous disease. If there are numerous, persistent, or conspicuous (e.g. facial) lesions, standard treatment is still intravenous or intramuscular antimony for 20 days. Pentamidine is a second-line option but carries a real risk of provoking diabetes. Ketaconazole and itraconazole are used for *L. mexicana* and *L. panamensis* but are considered less effective for other species. Topical therapies include paromomycin ointment (available in Israel, not the US) and intralesional antimony injections. Imiquimod (*Aldara* cream) was successful (90% cure in a small study) for CL resistant to antimonials in Peru.[7] Excision has also been tried but there is a significant relapse rate. Because CL is dermatropic and temperature sensitive, infrared heat therapy (*L. tropica*) and cryotherapy have been successful in small trials.[7a] Miltefosine oral therapy may also be a future option for CL but this is currently still investigational in the US.[7b]

Visceral leishmaniasis is often treated with pentavalent antimony 20 mg/kg/day i.v. for 28 days outside of India. Availability is problematic in the US where this drug is only obtainable through the CDC. Because of 50–60% resistance to antimonial therapy in India, miltefosine, originally an antitumor drug, is now the best choice for Indian VL. However, this drug also is not currently available in the US. Miltefosine has the advantages of oral administration, mild side effects at usual doses, and satisfactory clinical effectiveness (94% 6-month cure). It may well be effective against other forms of leishmaniasis as well.[8] Liposomal formulations of amphotericin B, given intravenously as a 5-day course, are a very expensive but a relatively convenient and more accessible means of treating VL in the US. Pentamidine, on the other hand, must be obtained from the CDC and is less well tolerated.

Patients who fail conventional therapy with pentavalent antimony are usually treated with amphotericin B (liposomal formulation preferred), pentamidine, or (in India) miltefesone. Coinfection with HIV and *Leishmania*, especially in southern Europe, is a particular problem as each disease accelerates the other. These patients often fail to respond to conventional therapy (>60% failure rate) or relapse repeatedly unless taking antiretroviral therapy.[4,7] Coinfected patients should be started on highly active anti-retroviral therapy (HAART) and treated with 4 weeks of antimonial therapy rather than the usual 21 days.[4]

# Control and Prevention

Avoiding sandfly bites by applying insect repellents is currently the first line of personal defense against leishmaniasis. Proper sanitation and insecticide spraying in cities are also beneficial since these insects breed in moist, dark places such as rodent burrows and rubbish heaps. Unfortunately, sandflies are tiny enough (2–3 mm) to pass through regular house screens or mosquito netting; thus, fine-mesh nets (although they impede air circulation) are necessary for complete protection. Impregnating bed nets with permethrin reduced CL by 65% in Kabul and the current trend is to use regular mosquito nets dipped in insecticide.[5,7] Sandflies are weak fliers that feed after dusk, so limiting evening exposure and sleeping on an upper story is also protective.

Public health measures include community spraying programs with pyrethroid insecticides to minimize sandfly populations. Although these measures can be very effective (60% CL reduction in Kabul) they must be sustainable if control is to be maintained. Zoonotic leishmaniasis, such as *L. infantum* in Italy, may be controlled by the widespread use of deltamethrin-treated dog collars, or by culling infected dogs which serve as reservoir hosts.[7]

A cutaneous leishmaniasis recombinant vaccine is very likely within the next decade, with research already well underway. Leishmaniasis is considered the most amenable of all parasitic infections to control by vaccination. Leishmanization, the ancient practice of inoculating an inconspicuous site to avoid later facial scarring, may also be revived with the development of more standardized, safer, live inoculants. Unfortunately, an effective vaccine for VL appears much further in the future.[7]

---

### Clinical Pearls

- Cutaneous leishmaniasis should be suspected when someone with a travel history to an endemic area presents with a persistent skin ulcer (or ulcerations) with raised margins.
- Visceral leishmaniasis presents with fever, splenomegaly, weight loss, and anemia.
- Pentavalent antimony has been the drug of choice for VL, MCL and complicated CL but this may be changing. Liposomal amphotericin B is more convenient, more available, and better tolerated in the US (albeit expensive) and miltefosine's use may soon expand outside of India.

## Special Considerations for Immigrants

- Many cases of CL will be self-limited in healthy immigrants.
- The type of *Leishmania* parasite and optimal treatment strategy can often be determined by country of origin.
- VL and MCL require immediate parenteral treatment, and infectious disease consultation is recommended.
- Always consider the possibility of HIV coinfection in patients with visceral leishmaniasis.

## References

1. Herwaldt BL. Leishmaniasis. Lancet 1999; 354:1191–1199.
2. Centers for Disease Control and Prevention. Cutaneous leishmaniasis in US military personnel – Southwest/Central Asia, 2002–2003. MMWR 2003; 52(42):1009–1012.
3. Hsia R, Wang NE, Halpern J. Leishmaniasis. eMedicine updated Sep 13, 2005. Available: http://www.emedicine.com/emerg/topic296.htm Accessed 2/7/07.
4. Paredes R, Munoz J, Diaz I, et al. Leishmaniasis in HIV infection. J Postgrad Med 2003; 49(1):39–49.
5. Dedet JP, Pratlong F. Leishmaniasis. In: Cook GC, Zumla A, eds. Manson's tropical diseases. 21st edn. London: Saunders; 2003:1339–1364.
6. Kafetzis DA. An overview of pediatric leishmaniasis. J Postgrad Med 2003; 49:31–38.
7. Davies CR, Kaye P, Croft SL, et al. Leishmaniasis: new approaches to disease control. Br Med J 2003; 326:377–382.
7a. Reithinger R, Mohsen M, Wahid M, et al. Efficacy of thermotherapy to treat cutaneous leishmaniasis caused by L. tropica in Kabul, Afghanistan: A randomized control trial. Clin Infect Dis 2005; 40:1148–1155.
7b. Soto J, Toledo J, Gutierrez P, et al. Treatment of American cutaneous leishmaniasis with Miltefosine, an oral agent. Clin Infect Dis 2001; 33:e57–e61.
8. Sundar S, Jha, TK, Thakur CP, et al. Oral miltefosine for Indian visceral leishmaniasis. N Engl Med J 2002; 347(22):1739–1746.
9. Drugs for parasitic infections. The Med Letter Aug 2004; 46:1–12. Available at: http://www.themedicalletter.com/freedocs/parasitic.pdf. Accessed 2/7/07.

# CHAPTER 34

# Leprosy

M. Patricia Joyce

## Leprosy at a Glance

- Highly curable infectious disease with acute and chronic manifestations that may result in life-long disability.
- Primarily infects skin and peripheral nerves.
- Unique immune complications (reactions) occur separately from infection.
- Typical rash with anesthesia is 70% predictive of diagnosis.
- Reservoir in human population; enzootic in nine-banded armadillo along US Gulf Coast.
- Transmission and infectivity easily interrupted by antibiotics.
- Limited susceptibility in human populations; only 3–5% of people capable of active infection.
- Prolonged incubation is the rule; may require up to 20 years to present clinically.

## Etiology

Leprosy is a curable infectious disease. The causative agent, *Mycobacterium leprae*, primarily infects skin and peripheral nerve, although deep infections (e.g. liver and bone marrow) may be transient occurrences in heavily infected but untreated individuals. The organism is weakly acid-fast, noncultivable, very slow growing (as determined in mouse footpad studies), and in the laboratory appears to be highly susceptible to freezing and probably to drying.

Infection is acquired through close contact with an infected person, but requires prolonged exposure, usually in a household setting. Although the route of transmission has not been clearly determined, both nasal droplet and skin-to-skin contact are considered probable modes. Untreated lepromatous patients have abundant organisms in the nasal mucosa and mucous secretions. *M. leprae* infection is enzootic among nine-banded armadillos in the US Gulf States, and areas of Central and South America, and is a potential, if unusual, source of human infection in these areas.

## Epidemiology

*Mycobacterium leprae*, first identified in Norway by Dr. Gerhard Armauer Hansen in 1873, is a weakly acid-fast, rod-shaped bacterium that has never been grown successfully in artificial media, but can be propagated in the mouse footpad and the nine-banded armadillo. The organism has a long doubling time of 13 days in the mouse footpad, selectively invades peripheral nerves, and grows preferentially at temperatures of 33°–35°C. *M. leprae* does not produce any known toxins, and tissue injury is caused by the host's immune response or by the sheer mass of infecting bacilli. Organisms are identified using a modified acid-fast stain, the Fite-Faraco stain. Under microscopy, viable organisms stain in a uniform, solid manner. Once antimicrobial therapy has been started, most organisms quickly lose their solid staining, appear beaded or fragmented, and are not viable in the mouse footpad. Leprosy is unique in that information available suggests that over 95% of adults are not susceptible to infection even after substantial exposure to large doses of bacilli. In susceptible persons, the infection has a median incubation time of 2–7 years, but may be as long as 20 years.

The US National Hansen's Disease Programs (NHDP) registers approximately 150 new cases per year (Fig. 34.1), the majority of whom are immigrants from endemic countries, although native-born cases are reported from Texas and Louisiana, in particular.[1]

As a result of widespread implementation of multidrug treatment programs and policy changes that remove individuals from the roster of patients to be followed (both promulgated by the World Health Organization [WHO]), the available figures indicate a sharp decline in the prevalence of Hansen's disease (HD) globally over the last two decades. WHO currently identifies nine major endemic countries (Angola, Brazil, Central African Republic, Democratic Republic of the Congo, India, Madagascar, Mozambique, Nepal, and the United Republic of Tanzania) contributing 84% of the new cases detected during 2004, and 74% of registered cases at the beginning of 2005. Globally, the registered prevalence of leprosy was 286 063 cases and the number of new cases detected during 2004 was 407 791, a 21% decrease comparing 2004 to 2003, mainly a result of a reduced number of new cases detected in India, where the detection declined by 29% as compared with 2003. While the majority of world leprosy cases come from India and Brazil, the most endemic areas remain the Federated States of Micronesia, Marshall Islands, and Kiribati, which continue to have the highest new case rate per population (Table 34.1).[2]

WHO pursues a public health goal of leprosy 'elimination' defined as a registered prevalence rate of less than 1 case per 10 000 population. However, a leprosy case is defined as a patient who has yet to receive a minimum therapeutic treatment, followed by his removal from the national case registry. This approach has led to a new cases rate higher than the annual registry prevalence in some countries. While

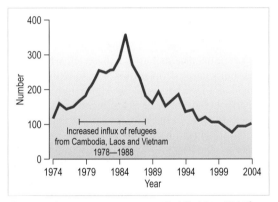

**Fig. 34.1** Leprosy cases reported in US, 1974–2004.[1]

| Table 34.1 World leprosy situation, 2005 | | | |
|---|---|---|---|
| | Registered prevalence at beginning 2005 | Number new cases at beginning 2005 | 2004 new case detection rate per 100 000 population |
| Federal States of Micronesia | 85 | 153 | 139.1 |
| Marshall Islands | 55 | 62 | 103.3 |
| Kiribati (Gilbert Islands) | 29 | 64 | 66.0 |
| Brazil | 30 693 | 49 384 | 26.9 |
| Nepal | 4 699 | 6 958 | 26.2 |
| India | 148 910 | 260 063 | 23.9 |
| Mozambique | 4 692 | 4 266 | 22.0 |
| Democratic Republic of Congo | 10 530 | 11 781 | 21.9 |
| Madagascar | 410 | 3 710 | 20.5 |
| Central African Republic | 438 | 402 | 13.8 |
| Angola | 2 496 | 2 109 | 13.6 |
| United Republic Tanzania | 4 777 | 5 190 | 10.1 |

From: Global leprosy situation, 2005. WHO Weekly epidemiological record 2005; 80(34):289–296.[2]

paucibacillary (tuberculoid) cases may complete treatment by WHO regimens requiring only 6 months of medication, the removal of 'treated' patients from national registries has been highly controversial.[3,4]

## Clinical Manifestations

The clinical features of leprosy are a continuum between the tuberculoid and lepromatous forms of disease. There is substantial overlap in the appearance of the different forms, and careful assessment of clinical and histologic parameters is needed for accurate diagnosis. All clinical forms of leprosy must be correlated with findings on biopsies and skin smears. The disease types may be divided into paucibacillary forms (indeterminate, tuberculoid, and borderline tuberculoid) and multibacillary forms (borderline, borderline lepromatous, and lepromatous). These categories are useful for determining appropriate antibiotic therapy (Table 34.2).

*Tuberculoid leprosy* (TT) is a localized infection in a host with a high degree of cellular immunity. There is usually a single skin lesion or, at most, a few lesions. Lesions are large, flat plaques with well-demarcated, irregular, erythematous, raised borders and an atrophic, scaly center. Hypopigmentation is common, and there is marked anesthesia and anhydrosis of lesions. Plaques are frequently located on the face or extremities. Facial lesions are particularly associated with risk of underlying cranial nerve infiltration and injury, resulting in lifelong disability (Fig. 34.2).

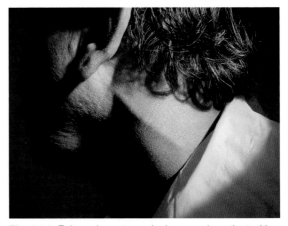

**Fig. 34.3** Enlarged greater auricular nerve in patient with borderline lepromatous disease.

Neural involvement is usually confined to the area of skin lesions, with palpably enlarged peripheral nerves and motor, sensory, and autonomic deficits (Fig. 34.3). Neuropathy may develop without apparent skin lesions in a subset of tuberculoid leprosy termed *pure neuritic*. Testicular and ocular infiltration does not occur, although neuropathy can cause corneal denervation, lagophthalmos, and exposure keratitis. Reactional states do not occur in pure tuberculoid leprosy.

*Borderline tuberculoid leprosy* (BT) patients may closely resemble tuberculoid patients, but have slightly lower host immunity and a higher bacillary load. There are usually several lesions that are smaller and less flat than tuberculoid lesions. Lesions are distributed asymmetrically and are moderately to markedly anesthetic. There may be more than one area of neural involvement. Biopsy shows few bacilli, rather than the rare or absent bacilli characteristic of true tuberculoid cases. Skin smears show few or no bacilli. Reversal (type 1) reactions (movement toward the tuberculoid pole of disease) may occur (Fig. 34.4).

*Borderline*, or *dimorphous*, *leprosy* (BB) is regarded as an unstable form that may move toward either polar form. Patients have moderate numbers of lesions, usually more than 10, of variable morphology. Some lesions resemble the large, irregular, flat plaques of tuberculoid leprosy, while others are smaller and infiltrated or raised. Annular, or ring-shaped, lesions are typical, and lesions are asymmetrically distributed. Neural involvement may occur early or late, involves multiple nerves, and may be severe. Reversal and downgrading reactions

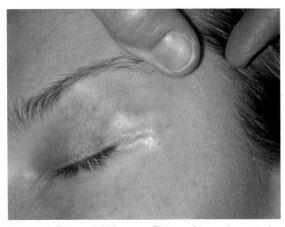

**Fig. 34.2** Tuberculoid leprosy: Picture of hypopigmented anesthetic patch on lateral aspect of eye. (Picture courtesy of Barbara Stryjewska, MD, NHDP, Baton Rouge, LA.)

**Table 34.2 Clinical features of leprosy**

| Feature | Tuberculoid | Borderline tuberculoid | Borderline | Borderline lepromatous | Lepromatous |
|---|---|---|---|---|---|
| Number of lesions | Single or none | Few or single | Usually few or many | Many and generalized | Complete skin involvement |
| Lesion appearance | Large, flat plaque, with irregular border; often scaly and hypopigmented | Large flat plaques, scaly and hypopigmented, erythematous borders | Raised plaques with annular and scaly borders | Highly variable. Lesions may be papules, plaques, or diffuse erythema, often hyperpigmented, with central clearing and scaling | Small, smooth, erythematous or hyperpigmented papules and plaques; diffuse infiltration |
| Distribution | Asymmetric | Asymmetric | Asymmetric | Asymmetric | Symmetric |
| Degree of anesthesia | Marked | Moderate to marked | Variable | Minimal until late | Absent until late |
| Enlarged peripheral nerves | Occurs early; one or two nerves | Occurs early; several nerves | Variable; involves several nerves | Uncommon | Uncommon |
| Stocking–glove neuropathy | Uncommon | Uncommon | Uncommon | Occurs late; several nerves | Occurs late; often diffuse sensory loss |
| Common reactions | None | Reversal | Reversal or downgrading | Reversal or ENL | ENL (50%), rarely Lucio's phenomenon |
| Other features | Corneal denervation or lagophthalmos in 10% | As in tuberculoid | Unstable form of disease; treated similar to lepromatous as may progress over time | As in lepromatous | Ocular, nasal, auricular, and testicular infiltration and thickening; madarosis (eye brow loss) suggestive of chronic disease |
| Skin smears | Bacilli absent or rare | Bacilli rare or few | Moderate bacilli | Many bacilli | Very many bacilli |
| Biopsy results | Frequently non-diagnostic, showing only granulomatous dermatitis | Usually diagnostic | Easily diagnostic | Easily diagnostic | Easily diagnostic |

ENL, Erythema nodosum leprosum.

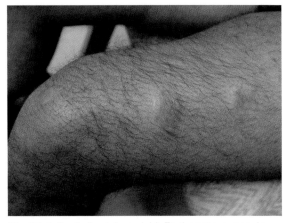
Fig. 34.4 Borderline tuberculoid. Erythematous macular-papular lesions on thigh exhibiting hair loss.

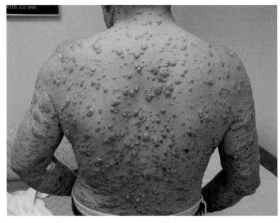
Fig. 34.5 Borderline lepromatous. Multiple scaling nodules generalized over trunk and extremities.

may occur with alterations of cell-mediated immunity to *M. leprae* antigens; they represent changes toward the tuberculoid and lepromatous poles, respectively. The most severe neurologic damage occurs in borderline patients because of the many nerves involved and the tendency for neuritis to occur with reactions. Biopsy and smears show a moderate bacillary load.

*Borderline lepromatous leprosy* (BL) patients resemble lepromatous patients but have fewer bacilli and higher immunity. Skin lesions are usually numerous and may be macules, papules, plaques, or nodules (Figs 34.5, 34.7). Some plaques may appear punched out with a sloping outer margin and a steep inner margin. Nerve involvement occurs late and sensation is often preserved. BL leprosy patients are unique in being susceptible to both type 1 reversal reactions and erythema nodosum leprosum (ENL).

*Lepromatous leprosy* (LL) patients have unrestrained proliferation of bacilli within the skin, peripheral nerves, anterior eye, and testes. Lesions are innumerable, small, erythematous and hyperpigmented macules, papules, and nodules occurring symmetrically. Infiltration is most prominent in cooler areas, such as the ears, upper lip, and forehead (Figs 34.7–34.9). The midline of the back is spared lesions, but all areas of skin, with or without lesions, are heavily loaded with bacilli. Diffuse infiltration of the face may occur, giving the typical leonine facies and loss of the lateral eyebrows (madarosis).

Peripheral nerves are less likely to be infiltrated and enlarged in lepromatous disease, and anesthesia occurs later or may be subtle. When anesthesia occurs, a diffuse pattern is seen, rather than focal

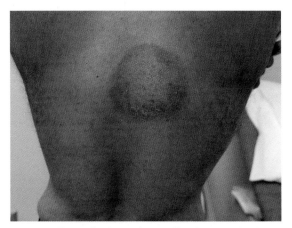
Fig. 34.6 Borderline lepromatous. Flat plaque on back with reactive edges and central clearing with atrophic changes.

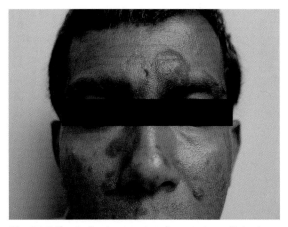
Fig. 34.7 Borderline lepromatous/lepromatous. Raised hyperpigmented plaques on face.

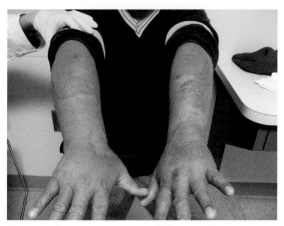

**Fig. 34.8** Lepromatous leprosy. Diffuse erythematous plaques with indistinct edges.

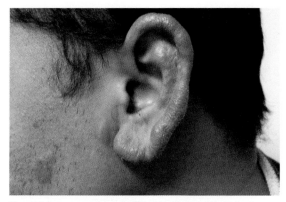

**Fig. 34.9** Lepromatous leprosy. Nodular infiltration of auricular pinna with enlargement of ear lobe.

nerve destruction; it may resemble a stocking–glove pattern. Nasal mucosal involvement causes stuffiness and epistaxis and may lead to septal perforation and collapse. Erythema, nodule formation, and enlargement of the ears may be seen with BL and LL disease (Fig. 34.9). Testicular involvement leads to sterility, impotence, and gynecomastia. Eye involvement includes keratitis, episcleritis, and corneal denervation. ENL, an apparent immune-complex reaction characterized by tender cutaneous nodules and systemic symptoms, occurs in up to 50% of lepromatous patients, usually in the first several years of therapy. ENL may be a chronic complaint on diagnosis of leprosy, or may occur as late phenomena after treatment is completed. Reversal reactions rarely occur in pure lepromatous leprosy.

*Indeterminate leprosy* is the earliest recognizable form of the disease and may be extremely difficult to diagnose. There is typically a single hypopigmented or erythematous macule without abnormal sensation or sweating. Biopsy is non-specific and shows rare or no organisms. The course of indeterminate leprosy is variable. Some lesions heal spontaneously with no further manifestation of disease; others are stable for months or years and some progress into a 'committed' form of persistent leprosy.

*Neural involvement* in leprosy is due to selective proliferation of *M. leprae* in superficial peripheral nerves. Nerve destruction occurs either from inflammation or from infiltration by masses of infecting organisms. Inflammation leads to nerve damage in conditions of high immunity, which are characteristic of tuberculoid or borderline leprosy, and also characteristic of episodes of active neuritis, such as those seen in erythema nodosum leprosum and, particularly, reversal reactions.

Lepromatous and borderline lepromatous patients have massive infiltration of nerves with bacilli, which gradually destroy the nerve. The nerves most affected are those located superficially (hence cooler). They include the ulnar nerve at the elbow; the radial and median nerves at the wrist; the greater auricular nerve; and the olfactory, trigeminal, facial, peroneal, posterior tibial, and sural nerves. Sensory, motor, and autonomic neuropathy may occur together or separately. The first sensory modality lost is hot–cold discrimination, followed by light touch and pain. The central nervous system is never involved.

*Ophthalmic involvement* occurs in all forms of leprosy, but the type of involvement depends on the form of disease. Corneal hypoesthesia and lagophthalmos from denervation are most typical of the tuberculoid end of the spectrum. Bacillary infiltration of the anterior eye occurs in borderline and lepromatous patients, causing nodular keratitis and episcleritis. Erythema nodosum leprosum may cause iridocyclitis and secondary glaucoma. The sensory denervation of the eye results in the absence of symptoms despite progressive ocular injury, thus contributing to vision loss. Patients should be evaluated and followed by an ophthalmologist who is aware of the complications of leprosy. Patients with corneal anesthesia need counseling and measures to prevent exposure injury. Surgery may be useful in lagophthalmos. Inflammatory conditions associated with reactions are managed with steroids.

## Reactional States

Reactional states (also called *lepra reactions*) occur with alterations in host immune response and are important to recognize and treat because they can cause irreversible tissue damage. Several distinct types of reactions occur.

*Reversal reaction* (or type 1 reaction) represents an increase in cellular immune response, with movement toward the tuberculoid pole of disease. This reaction is common in the borderline forms of leprosy and does not occur in the polar forms. Recurrence of skin activity, with erythema, swelling, or worsened anesthesia, at the site of previous lesion is seen in reversal reactions and is treated with corticosteroids. Reversal reactions are said to occur most frequently in the first 6 months after initiation of antimicrobial therapy. An acute flare of sensory loss or motor weakness, particularly involving the face, is considered a true emergency in leprosy and requires immediate immunosuppression to prevent lifelong disability.

*ENL* (or type 2 reaction) is a syndrome of recurrent tender and red nodular skin lesions, occurring in crops over 1–2 weeks, and associated with fever, leukocytosis, myalgias, uveitis, and orchitis. ENL is thought to be an immune-complex disease and associated with elevation in circulating tumor necrosis factor. This type of reaction may occur before the diagnosis of leprosy, and may first present or recur repeatedly even after successful completion of standard multidrug therapy. Thalidomide remains the drug of choice for control of ENL, and treatment may be required for months to years until all ENL activity eventually subsides.

## Diagnosis

### Who should be tested?

The diagnosis of leprosy requires a high index of suspicion when dealing with persons from endemic areas. There is often a delay of 1 or more years after medical attention is sought before the diagnosis is made. The combination of skin lesions and neuropathy should suggest the diagnosis, but neurologic findings may be subtle.

Evaluation of patients should include the following:

- A careful inspection of the skin with diagrams of lesions.
- Areas of anhydrosis should be noted, because this correlates with loss of protective sensation.
- Superficial nerves should be palpated for enlargement and tenderness.
- Detailed sensory testing should be carried out to define deficits. Mapping of sensory deficits is helpful in following the course of neuropathy.
- Motor testing and nerve conduction studies should be performed.
- Examination of insensitive extremities for areas of trauma or pressure injury is important, as is assessment of the adequacy of footwear.
- Ophthalmologic evaluation is indicated in all patients.

### Diagnostic studies

A definitive diagnosis requires demonstration of bacilli in tissue. Biopsy and skin smears should be performed in all patients.

A full-thickness skin biopsy from the active (advancing) margin of the most active lesion, stained with hematoxylin-eosin and Fite-Faraco stains, is the primary laboratory basis for the diagnosis and classification of HD.

*M. leprae* has never been successfully cultured despite many attempts.

If another mycobacterial infection is suspected, a culture should be performed, and growth will exclude leprosy. If fixed in formalin for less than 24 hours, paraffin-embedded tissue may also be satisfactory for polymerase chain reaction (PCR) analysis for *M. leprae* DNA, should that be indicated. PCR has been used experimentally to locate DNA markers for drug resistance as well.

*Slit skin smears*, obtained from tissue fluid and cells from the dermis and stained with Fite-Faraco stain, also aid in diagnosis, in assessment of bacillary load, and in following response to therapy. Skin smears should be performed only by trained, experienced individuals, and are only reliably read at an experienced reference laboratory. A shallow skin incision is made at six standard sites (including ear lobes, elbows and knees), as well as from other selected lesions. A small drop of dermal interstitial fluid is smeared onto a glass slide, and the number of acid-fast bacilli is determined and expressed as a 'bacteriologic index.' Patients with the tuberculoid form of the disease may have negative skin smears even with a skin biopsy diagnostic of leprosy.

*Nerve biopsy* may be useful in tuberculoid leprosy when skin biopsy shows no organisms or when no skin lesions are present. A cutaneous sensory nerve is selected in an area of neuropathy and examined histologically for organisms and typical granulomas.

The *lepromin test* is not commonly used in the United States, but has been used to classify patients already diagnosed with leprosy. Preparations of *M. leprae* antigen from human or armadillo tissue are injected intradermally to assess specific cellular immunity, but the test is too non-selective and non-specific to be useful as a diagnostic test.

*Serologic* assays of antibodies against *M. leprae* cell wall components, such as phenolic glycolipid-1 or lipoarabinomannan, have been useful in epidemiologic studies but are also non-specific or cross-reactive.

*Polymerase chain reaction* testing can be performed by referral laboratories on tissue biopsy samples, but has limited reliability in the setting of tuberculoid disease where few bacteria are seen on standard microscopy.

Once the diagnosis of HD has been confirmed and treatment is being planned, tests for glucose-6-phosphate dehydrogenase deficiency are recommended, as are baseline erythrocyte and leukocyte counts and liver function studies.

Lepromatous patients have a polyclonal increase in antibody production, including antibodies that may produce several false-positive serologic tests, including those for syphilis and HIV.

### Differential diagnosis

The differential diagnosis includes sarcoidosis, syphilis, mycosis fungoides, vitiligo, psoriasis, miliaria profunda, pityriasis alba, tinea corporis, and streptocerciasis, as well as other mycobacterial infections such as those caused by *M. tuberculosis, M. marinum*, and *M. ulcerans*.

### ICD-9 codes

- V74.2 Special Screening examination for leprosy [Hansen's disease]
- 030 Leprosy includes: Hansen's disease, infection by *Mycobacterium leprae*
- 030.0 Lepromatous [type L]: Lepromatous leprosy (macular) (diffuse) (infiltrated) (nodular) (neuritic)
- 030.1 Tuberculoid [type T]: Tuberculoid leprosy (macular) (maculoanesthetic) (major) (minor) (neuritic)
- 030.2 Indeterminate [group I]: Indeterminate [uncharacteristic] leprosy (macular) (neuritic)
- 030.3 Borderline [group B]: Borderline or dimorphous leprosy (infiltrated) (neuritic)
- 030.8 Other specified leprosy
- 030.9 Leprosy, unspecified

## Treatment

Dapsone, rifampin, and clofazimine remain the mainstay drugs of choice (Table 34.3), used in combined multidrug therapy (MDT) regimens depending on the disease classification. Alternative agents can be used in these combinations (see Table 34.3) if there is evidence of drug intolerance or resistance.

Treatment recommendations of the NHDP (http://bphc.hrsa.gov/nhdp) and the WHO are based on the distinction between paucibacillary (PB) and multibacillary disease (Table 34.4), but differ in the length of minimum therapy and the use of monthly witnessed doses of rifampin and clofazimine. The NHDP recommends daily rifampin and only suggests monthly use in the setting of concomitant corticosteroid use for neuritis or control of immune reactions.

Most recently, a single-dose regimen of rifampin, 400 mg, ofloxacin, 400 mg, and minocycline, 100 mg, (ROM therapy) has been recommended by WHO for use in patients with paucibacillary disease limited to a single lesion. The NHDP continues to recommend 12 months of daily therapy for all patients with PB disease, but a third drug (usually clofazimine) may be added if active neuritis develops.[5,6,7]

Mild anti-inflammatory medications may be used for less severe forms of type 1 reactions, but aggressive use of prednisone is indicated to protect nerve function, starting at 60–80 mg per day (1 mg/kg/day). Prolonged low-dose corticosteroids, over 4–6 months, have been shown more effective than very high dosage or very brief courses in the treatment of active neuropathy. Tapering should proceed slowly as the patient's condition permits.

Treatment of ENL may require prolonged use of anti-inflammatory medications as well. These reactions respond only poorly to prednisone even in doses of 60–80 mg daily. Thalidomide (now available in the US only as Thalomid® under the Celgene

**Table 34.3 Antileprosy drugs**

| Agent | Adult Dose | Pediatric Dose | Formulation | Efficacy | Side effects | Pregnancy |
|---|---|---|---|---|---|---|
| Dapsone | 100 mg/day | 1 mg/kg/day, up to adult dosage | 25 mg, 100 mg | Static | Anemia, hemolysis (G6PD), peripheral neuropathy, liver toxicity, methemoglobinemia, sulfone syndrome, agranulocytosis | Category C• |
| Rifampin* | 600 mg/day (given as monthly dose if concurrent steroids used) | 10 mg/kg/day, up to adult dosage | 150 mg, 300 mg | Cidal | Nausea, discolored body fluids, hepatotoxicity, marrow suppression, interstitial nephritis, flu-like syndrome, multiple drug interactions | Category C• |
| Clofazimine | 50 mg/day | 1 mg/kg/day, up to adult dosage | 50 mg | Static | Nausea, skin pigmentation and xerosis, bowel motility/ileus, possible cardiac arrhythmias | IND status+ (previously Category C•) |
| Minocycline* | 100 mg/day | Avoid in children younger than 8 years old | 50 mg, 75 mg, 100 mg | Cidal | Nausea, hyperpigmentation, deposits in bone and teeth, photosensitivity, hypersensitivity, CNS toxicity | Category D: Avoid |
| Ofloxacin* | 400 mg/day | Avoid in children younger than 18 years old | 200 mg, 300 mg, 400 mg | Cidal | Nausea, CNS toxicity, phototoxicity, hypersensitivity, drug interactions | Category C• |
| Levofloxacin* | 500 mg/day | Avoid in children younger than 18 years old | 250 mg, 500 mg | Cidal | Nausea, CNS toxicity, phototoxicity, hypersensitivity, drug interactions | Category C• |
| Ethionamide* | 250 mg/day (Note: for TB, 500–750 mg/day) | 10–20 mg/kg/day as a single dose up to adult dosage | 250 mg | Cidal | Nausea, hepatotoxicity, hypersensitivity, metallic taste, peripheral neuropathy | Category C• |
| Clarithromycin* | 500 mg/dose twice/day | 7.5 mg/kg/day in two divided doses, up to adult dosage | 500 mg | Cidal | Nausea, motility disorder, cardiac arrhythmias, hypersensitivity, drug interactions | Category C• |

* Not FDA approved for this indication.
• Category C: Use approved by the FDA if deemed that potential benefits outweigh potential risks.
+ As of November 2004, clofazimine availability in the USA is limited to use under Investigational New Drug status, and is currently limited to nonpregnant adults despite prior approved use in minors and in pregnancy. Contact NHDP at 1-800-642-2477 for clofazimine IND or for alternative therapy recommendations.

**Table 34.4 Treatment regimens**

| Agent | NHDP regimen | WHO regimen |
|---|---|---|
| **Multibacillary** | | |
| Dapsone | 100 mg/day for 24 mon | 100 mg/day for 12 mon |
| Rifampin | 600 mg/day for 24 mon | 600 mg monthly given under supervision for 12 mon |
| Clofazimine | 50 mg/day for 24 mon (May substitute daily minocycline) | 50 mg/day, plus 300 mg each mon given under supervision for 12 mon |
| **Paucibacillary** | | |
| Dapsone | 100 mg/day for 12 mon | 100 mg/d for 6 mon |
| Rifampin | 600 mg/day for 12 mon | 600 mg monthly under supervision for 6 mon |

NHDP, National Hansen's Disease Programs; WHO, World Health Organization.

STEPS program, at 1-800-4-CELGENE) is indicated for patients with ENL poorly controlled with corticosteroids; 100 mg/day is usually sufficient, although higher doses (up to 400 mg/day, divided in one to three doses) may be used in the initial days of treatment of severe reactions. Thalidomide should be limited to bedtime dosing as soon as possible as it may be severely sedating. Its remarkable anti-inflammatory effect in treating ENL was the major reason that thalidomide was retained in the pharmacopoeia for several decades when it was otherwise generally proscribed due to its teratogenic properties. Clofazimine also has anti-inflammatory effects on type 2 reactions by still unexplained mechanisms and is given in doses of 100–200 mg/day as part of the antibiotic regimen in lepromatous (MB) disease.

## Management of patients who fail initial treatment

Patient compliance with treatment is a major issue because treatment regimens require many months or years of medication. Patient education to encourage compliance when the patient may feel no rapid benefit and to provide support if a reaction complicates the course of the disease is thus a critical part of the overall prevention strategy. Even highly infected patients become noninfectious to others almost immediately upon receiving multidrug therapy; education should emphasize that compliance with treatment is thus also beneficial to family and other close contacts.

If drug intolerance develops, or if resistant bacilli are suspected, the patient should be evaluated by a referral center for alternate combinations of medications. Minocycline or a fluoroquinolone can be substituted in multidrug therapy, but no set guidelines have been established for length of therapy.

## Prevention

Early clinical diagnosis, prompt initiation of multidrug treatment, and vigilant follow-up of contacts are the bedrock of leprosy prevention and control. Although no infectious disease is likely to be eradicated by treatment alone, the evidence clearly indicates that good treatment and follow-up will substantially reduce the number of highly infectious individuals and, in time, this will lead to a decline in transmission and in the number of new patients infected. Evaluation and treatment of infected household contacts remains the mainstay of infection control.

## Infection Control Measures

Because of this long incubation period and gradual, insidious onset, it is often difficult or impossible to identify the source of contact. The long incubation, together with the potential for deformity (greatly exaggerated in the minds of many lay persons), has resulted in an extraordinary stigma and fear of social ostracism that deter many patients from seeking treatment early in the course of the disease. If the disease is not recognized and treated at an early stage, however, some neuropathy and resultant deformity may persist even after antimicrobial treatment has successfully eliminated the pathogen.

### Clinical Pearls

- Skin lesions vary greatly in leprosy, a 'great masquerader' similar to syphilis.
- An asymmetrical skin lesion with anesthesia, even without a visible rash, is highly suggestive of leprosy.
- Prolonged incubation is to be expected.

- With antibiotic therapy, leprosy becomes nontransmissible within days, and is highly curable as an infection but requires prolonged treatment.
- Immune reactions occur during treatment as does neuropathy, but should be considered as separate problems requiring additional therapies to manage.
- Contact tracing should be done of household members, particularly considering children in the household.

### Special Considerations for Immigrants

- Due to prolonged and subclinical incubation, immigrants may present with clinical leprosy long after arriving from endemic areas.
- Immigrants with leprosy may arrive legally in the US after beginning treatment in their home country.
- Cultural stigma against leprosy by immigrants themselves may hamper their being diagnosed and receiving treatment for leprosy, for fear of ostracism in their immigrant communities.

## When to Consider Diagnosis of Leprosy

- Any anesthetic skin patch in immigrant or person residing in southwestern US.

- Unexplained changes in skin pigmentation, particularly if associated with anesthesia.
- Persistent unexplained rash or thickened skin.
- Unexplained peripheral neuropathy in an immigrant.
- Skin nodules or plaques, particularly if generalized, recurrent, or chronic.
- Family history of leprosy or unexplained skin condition or neuropathy.

## References

1. Summary of notifiable diseases – United States, 2004. MMWR 2006; 53(53):1–79.
2. Global leprosy situation 2005. WHO weekly epidemiological record 2005; 80(34):289–296.
3. Lockwood DN. Leprosy elimination – a virtual phenomenon or a reality? Br Med J 2002; 324(7352):1516–1518.
4. Naafs B. Treatment of leprosy: science or politics? Trop Med Int Health 2006; 11(3):268–278.
5. Jacobson RR, Krahenbuhl JL. Leprosy. Lancet 1999; 353(9153):655–660.
6. Joyce MP, Scollard DM. Leprosy. In: Rakel RE, Bope ET, eds. Conn's current therapy 2004. Philadelphia: Saunders/Elsevier Science; 2003:100–105.
7. Moschella SL. An update on the diagnosis and treatment of leprosy. J Am Acad Dermatol 2004; 51(3):417–426.

# CHAPTER 35

# Loiasis

Elizabeth D. Barnett

## Loiasis at a Glance

- Highly endemic in the rainforests of Central Africa and also occurs in western and central Africa.
- Caused by the filarial nematode *Loa loa*.
- Transmitted by the bite of large tabanid (*Chrysops*) flies (known as red flies in Africa).
- Most commonly clinically asymptomatic; characteristic clinical manifestation is Calabar swelling.
- The most distinctive clinical manifestation is caused by the occasional subconjunctival migration of the adult worm, giving rise to the name 'eye worm.'
- Treatment is with diethylcarbamazine (DEC).

## Epidemiology

Loiasis occurs only in Africa, primarily in rainforest areas of Central and West Africa. Isolated cases have been reported in West Africa from Ghana to Guinea, and in Uganda, Malawi, Ethiopia, and Zambia (Fig. 35.1). Chronic infection may occur in 3–13 million residents of these endemic areas. Distribution of disease is affected by the predilection of the vector flies to reside in the forest canopy and lay their eggs in swamps and at river edges. The flies are attracted by movement, dark colors, and wood smoke. Rain forests, with relatively low canopies and scant undergrowth, seem to constitute a particularly desirable habitat for *Chrysops* flies.[1–3] Infection rates are higher in adults than in children, and, in endemic areas, tend to be higher in males.

## Etiology

*Chrysops silacea* and *Chrysops dimidiata* are the most important vector species. Day-biting females inject larvae and pick up microfilariae of *Loa* in their blood meals. Larvae develop into adult worms in 6–12 months; adult worms may live up to two decades (Fig. 35.2). Adult worms migrate through subcutaneous tissue. Microfilariae are released into the bloodstream by adult female worms, but are found most commonly at midday, corresponding to the maximal biting time of the vector flies. Microfilaremia is seen less commonly in travelers or expatriates compared to individuals native to endemic areas.[4]

## Clinical Manifestations

Many of the clinical manifestations of *Loa* infection tend to be more prominent in the recently exposed. Eosinophilia and increased levels of serum IgE are characteristic and are usually more pronounced in symptomatic individuals. Disease manifestations range from asymptomatic infection associated with microfilaremia to severe and life-threatening complications such as encephalitis, cardiomyopathy, and renal failure. Allergic-type symptoms tend to be prominent, especially in those recently exposed. These include pruritus, urticaria, and transient migratory nonpitting edema (Calabar swellings). These swellings are thought to be a hypersensitivity reaction to adult worm antigens and are most common on the extremities. They appear and disappear spontaneously, usually lasting a few days to several weeks.

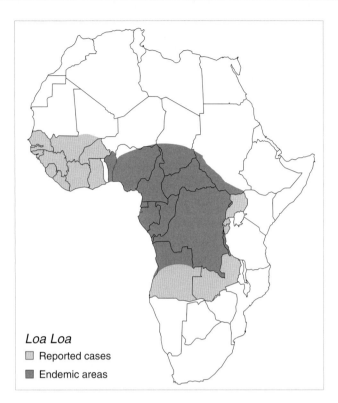

**Fig. 35.1** Distribution of *Loa loa* (Klion AD, Nutman TB. Loiasis and *Mansonella* infections. In: Guerrant RL, Walker DH, Weller PF, eds. Tropical infectious diseases. 2nd edn. Philadelphia: Churchill Livingstone; 2006:1163).

*Loa Loa*
▫ Reported cases
■ Endemic areas

Adult worms may migrate under the conjunctiva, giving rise to the name eye worm for this infection. An intense conjunctivitis may accompany this migration, and most episodes resolve without sequelae. Worms may occasionally be seen migrating under the skin. Unlike the slow progress and intense itching of cutaneous larva migrans (caused by dog or cat hookworm larvae) migration of *Loa loa* is rapid and causes little or no reaction.[2] Complications of infection with *Loa loa* include peripheral neuropathy, encephalopathy, and renal involvement. Peripheral neuropathy tends to occur in association with Calabar swelling and commonly presents as entrapment neuropathy. Encephalopathy occurs most often in the setting of significant microfilaremia and is most often seen following treatment. Microfilariae have been found in the spinal fluid. Encephalitis has also been associated with ivermectin treatment given in mass treatment programs for onchocerciasis.[5] Renal involvement, usually hematuria or proteinuria with a clear sediment, occurs in as many as one-third of those infected. Transient worsening may occur with treatment but is almost always reversible; progression to renal failure is rare.

## Diagnosis

Loiasis may be suspected in anyone who has resided in an endemic area who has transient localized swellings, urticaria, unexplained eosinophilia, or a worm traversing the conjunctiva or skin. Removal of worms can allow definitive diagnosis, as does identifying microfilariae in the blood (best accomplished using concentration or filtration techniques of a midday blood sample).

Immunodiagnosis is of limited utility in individuals from endemic areas because of lack of specificity and inability to distinguish current from past infection. Loa-specific recombinant antigens have been developed, but are not generally available. PCR-based techniques show promise and are highly sensitive, but are not available commercially.

Differential diagnosis includes infection with other filariae, especially those that exist in the same geographic location (*Onchocerca volvulus* and *Wuchereria bancrofti*). Calabar swellings share some characteristics of the angioedema associated with C1 esterase deficiency. Rarely, other nematodes have

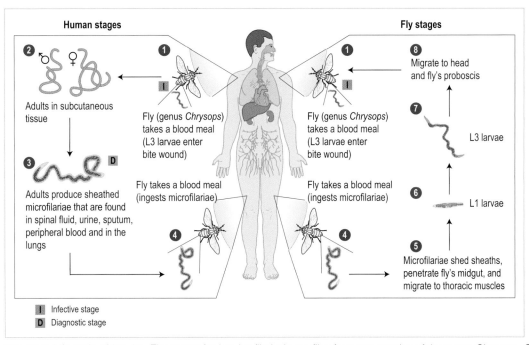

**Fig. 35.2** Life cycle of *Loa loa*. The vector for *Loa loa* filariasis are flies from two species of the genus *Chrysops*, *C. silacea* and *C. dimidiata*. During a blood meal, an infected fly (genus *Chrysops*, day-biting flies) introduces third-stage filarial larvae onto the skin of the human host, where they penetrate into the bite wound (1). The larvae develop into adults that commonly reside in subcutaneous tissue (2). The female worms measure 40–70 mm in length and 0.5 mm in diameter, while the males measure 30–34 mm in length and 0.35–0.43 mm in diameter. Adults produce microfilariae measuring 250–300 μm by 6–8 μm, which are sheathed and have diurnal periodicity. Microfilariae have been recovered from spinal fluid, urine, and sputum. During the day they are found in peripheral blood, but during the noncirculation phase, they are found in the lungs (3). The fly ingests microfilariae during a blood meal (4). After ingestion, the microfilariae lose their sheaths and migrate from the fly's midgut through the hemocoel to the thoracic muscles of the arthropod (5). There the microfilariae develop into first-stage larvae (6) and subsequently into third-stage infective larvae (7). The third-stage infective larvae migrate to the fly's proboscis (8) and can infect another human when the fly takes a blood meal (1). (Adapted from Centers for Disease Control and Prevention DPDx.)

been noted to migrate under the conjunctiva (*Dirofilaria repens* and *Thelazia californiensis*).[1]

Individuals with a compatible exposure, unexplained eosinophilia, migratory angioedema, subcutaneous or subconjuntival worms should be tested for loiasis. Symptoms may continue for years after leaving the endemic area.[6] If the worm can be obtained, diagnosis can be made by identifying the characteristic features of the worm. When this is not possible, examination of the blood for presence of microfilariae is appropriate. Blood samples may be obtained around noon, and a blood smear stained with Wright's or Giemsa stain to allow identification of microfilariae. Of note, individuals with short-term exposure are less likely to have circulating microfilariae. Serologic testing is helpful, especially in amicrofilaremic individuals with short-term exposure.

**Treatment**

The drug of choice for treatment of loiasis is diethylcarbamazine (DEC) (Table 35.1). Examination of blood smears for microfilariae should be done before initiating treatment, as toxicity can be severe in those with significant microfilaremia. In addition, care should be taken to exclude coinfection with *Onchocerca volvulus* as severe adverse events may ensue in patients with onchocerciasis treated with DEC. History of residence in areas where onchocerciasis occurs, as well as signs and symptoms of onchocerciasis, should be sought. If available, serologic testing for onchocerciasis might also be helpful in excluding this disease in selected patients. In patients without microfilaremia, DEC at a dose of 8–10 mg/kg/day, divided into three doses, for 21 days, is considered

**Table 35.1 Drugs used in the treatment of loiasis**

| | Adult dose | Efficacy | Adverse events | Comments |
|---|---|---|---|---|
| DEC | No microfilaremia: 8–10 mg/kd/day for 21 days Microfilaremia: Apheresis and/or gradually escalating doses of DEC up to full dose for total of 21 days | Curative after a single dose in 45–50% | Fever, pruritus, angioedema, arthralgia | Rule out coinfection with onchocerciasis before use Use of steroids and antihistamines may decrease adverse events of DEC |
| Albendazole | 200 mg/dose twice daily for 21 days | Gradual decrease of microfilarial load over months | | |

standard. Some patients may require repeated courses of treatment before all symptoms disappear. Side effects of DEC include fever, angioedema, myalgia, malaise, and pruritus.

When microfilariae are present in the blood, reducing this burden is necessary before beginning DEC to reduce the potential for severe adverse events such as encephalitis. Apheresis (where available) may be used for this purpose. Following reduction of the level of microfilariae in the blood, treatment can begin with small doses of DEC, gradually increasing to standard doses, in combination with steroids.

Ivermectin is effective in reducing levels of microfilariae, but has no effect on the adult worm. Severe adverse reactions to ivermectin have occurred in association with use of ivermectin in mass treatment programs for onchocerciasis, usually in individuals with coinfection with Loa and high-level microfilaremia.[5] Albendazole has been shown to decrease levels of circulating microfilariae in some studies.[7]

## Management of patients who fail initial treatment

Patients who fail initial therapy may respond to one or more additional courses of DEC. Those who are refractory to treatment with DEC may benefit from albendazole at a dose of 200 mg/dose twice daily for 21 days.[8] In addition to reducing the microfilarial load, albendazole may have a direct effect on the adult worm, causing slow death of these worms by inhibition of microtubule formation. Albendazole was superior to placebo in reducing microfilaremia in a small study in Benin.[7]

## Prevention

Vector control measures have not met with much success due to difficulty gaining access to breeding sites of the vector flies. Clearing of forest around dwellings and personal protective measures may have some effect. Chemoprophylaxis with a weekly 300 mg dose of DEC has been shown to be effective in long-term visitors to endemic areas.[9]

### Clinical Pearls

- Unexplained migratory subcutaneous swelling in an individual who has resided in an endemic area suggests *Loa* infection.
- DEC is the treatment of choice.
- Examination of blood for microfilaremia must be done before beginning treatment; if present, reduction of the level of microfilaremia should be done before initiating treatment with DEC.

### Special Considerations for Immigrants

- Symptoms may occur for many years after leaving the endemic area.
- Recrudescence may occur years after treatment.

## References

1. Klion AD, Nutman TB. Loiasis and *Mansonella* infections. In: Guerrant RL, Walker DH, Weller PF, eds. Tropical infectious diseases 2nd ed. Philadelphia: Churchill Livingstone; 2006:1163–1175.

2. Simonsen PE. Filariases. In: Cook GC, Zumla AI, eds. Manson's tropical diseases.21st edn. London: Saunders; 2003:1487–1526.

3. Klion A. Loiasis. In: Strickland GT, ed. Hunter's tropical medicine and emerging infectious diseases. Philadelphia: WB Saunders; 2000:754–756.

4. Klion AD, Massougbodji M, Sadeler B-C, et al. Loiasis in endemic and non-endemic populations: immunologically mediated differences in clinical presentation. J Infect Dis 1991; 163:1318–1325.

5. Gardon J, Gardon-Wendel N, Demanga-Ngangue, et al. Serious reactions after mass treatment of onchocerciasis with ivermectin in an area endemic for *Loa loa* infection. Lancet 1997; 350:18–22.

6. Doan NM, Keiser PB, Bates RA, et al. 33-year-old woman from Nigeria with eosinophilia. Clin Infect Dis 2002; 35:1204,1263–1264.

7. Klion AD, Massougbodji A, Horton J, et al. Albendazole in human loiasis: results of a double-blind, placebo-controlled trial. J Infect Dis 1993; 168:202–206.

8. Klion AD, Horton J, Nutman TB. Albendazole therapy for loiasis refractory to diethylcarbamazine treatment. Clin Infect Dis 1999; 29:680–682.

9. Nutman TB, Miller KD, Mulligan M, et al. Diethylcarbamazine prophylaxis for human loiasis. Results of a double-blind study. N Engl J Med 1988; 319:752–756.

# CHAPTER 36

# Lymphatic Filariasis

Elizabeth D. Barnett

## Lymphatic Filariasis at a Glance

- Lymphatic filariasis (LF) is caused by the filarial nematodes *Wuchereria bancrofti*, *Brugia malayi*, and *Brugia timori*.
- Transmitted by mosquitoes.
- Occurs in tropical Africa, Asia, the Indian subcontinent, many islands of the western and southern Pacific, and some areas of Central and South America.
- Burden of disease is greatest in adults.
- Disease is characterized by chronic and disfiguring lymphedema and hydroceles.

## Epidemiology

About 120 million people worldwide are infected with organisms causing lymphatic filariasis, 90% of them with *W. bancrofti*. *B. timori* occurs only on some small islands in Indonesia, and *B. malayi* is limited to Asia and several Pacific island groups including Indonesia and the Philippines. Infections due to *W. bancrofti* occur in sub-Saharan Africa, the Nile delta in Egypt and Sudan, south Asia, the western Pacific, and Central and South America, including islands in the Caribbean. The largest number of cases occurs in south Asia and tropical sub-Saharan Africa. Large-scale, aggressive control programs recently have decreased the prevalence of disease in many areas. Distribution of disease may be highly focal within affected areas (Fig. 36.1).

Mosquitoes transmit the parasites associated with LF, and several genera are capable of transmitting the infection. In Africa and the Pacific, the *Anopheles* species predominates, whereas in urban areas, including India, *Culex* species are more common.

*Aedes* and *Mansonia* (transmitting only *B. malayi*) species are present in some Pacific islands. The variety of mosquito vectors is a factor in the widespread and patchy distribution of LF. There is no animal reservoir for *Wuchereria bancrofti*, although cats in some parts of Southeast Asia are naturally infected with *Brugia malayi*.

## Etiology

Larvae injected into the skin by the bite of the mosquito migrate to the lymphatics and develop into adult worms. Adult worms reside in the lymphatics and begin to produce microfilariae that are injected into the blood after 8 months in the case of *W. bancrofti* and 3 months in *B. malayi*.[1] Adult worms may produce microfilariae for approximately 5–10 years, and microfilariae may live up to 1 year (Fig. 36.2). Microfilariae show a predominantly nocturnal periodicity, corresponding to the biting habits of the vector mosquitoes, though subperiodic strains are found in some geographical regions. Periodicity may also be influenced by the circadian rhythms of the human host.[2]

The prevalence of disease in a given area depends on a complex interaction of factors including intensity of transmission, genetic susceptibility, immunologic tolerance, prior treatment, and coinfections.[3] Infection rates increase with age, representing the accumulation over a lifetime of adult-stage worms through continued exposure to infected vector mosquitoes. Frequency of disease manifestations also increases with age, though likelihood of developing clinical disease varies geographically. Overall, approximately one-third of those infected have some overt manifestations of disease.[4]

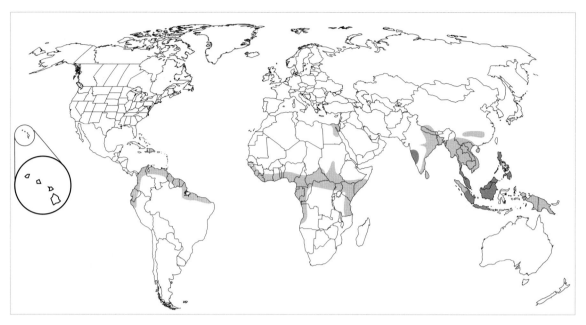

*Lymphatic Filariasis*

☐ *Wuchereria bancrofti*

■ *Wuchereria bancrofti* and *Brugia malayi*

Note: *Brugia timori* is limited to the Timor Island of Indonesia

**Fig. 36.1** Distribution of organisms causing lymphatic filariasis (Courtesy Nutman TB, Kazura JB. Filariasis. In: Guerrant RL, Walker DH, Weller PF, eds. Tropical Infectious Diseases, 2nd edn. Philadelphia: Churchill Livingstone; 2006:1154).

## Clinical Manifestations

Disease manifestations range from clinically asymptomatic infection to severe and disfiguring lymphedema and hydrocele. Each will be discussed in this section.

### Asymptomatic filariasis

This group of infected individuals consists of those who have no overt disease manifestations and who may or may not have microfilaremia. Although disease may not be apparent, this may not be a completely clinically benign condition, as imaging techniques have revealed abnormalities of the structure and function of the lymphatics in affected individuals.[5]

### Acute adenolymphangitis

Acute adenolymphangitis (ADL) covers a variety of clinical entities that present with inflammation. True filarial adenolymphangitis (AFL) presents with inflammation, swelling, and retrograde lymphangitis extending peripherally from the draining node where the parasites presumably reside. Regional lymph nodes are often enlarged, and the entire lymphatic channel can become indurated and inflamed. A second type of acute attack – often labeled bacterial ADL – appears to be caused by bacterial infection through interdigital or other entry lesions. The clinical pattern of bacterial ADL is different from the more classical AFL in that the lymphangitis develops in a reticular rather than in a linear pattern, and the local and systemic symptoms, including edema, pain, fever, and chills are frequently more severe. AFL and bacterial ADL occur in both the upper and the lower extremities with both bancroftian and brugian filariasis, but involvement of the genital lymphatics occurs almost exclusively with *W. bancrofti* infection.

### Hydrocele

Hydrocele is the most common chronic manifestation of lymphatic filariasis due to *W. bancrofti* in many areas, and is uncommon in *Brugia* infection. It

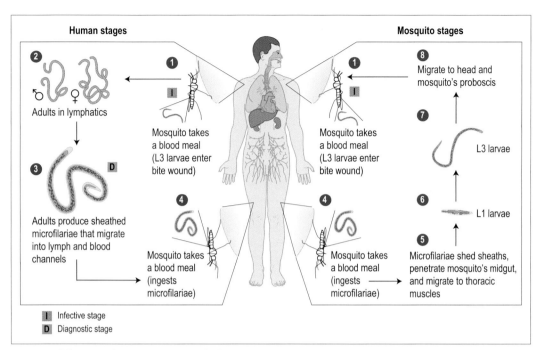

**Human stages**

❷ Adults in lymphatics

❸ Adults produce sheathed microfilariae that migrate into lymph and blood channels

❶ Mosquito takes a blood meal (L3 larvae enter bite wound)

❹ Mosquito takes a blood meal (ingests microfilariae)

**Mosquito stages**

❶ Mosquito takes a blood meal (L3 larvae enter bite wound)

❹ Mosquito takes a blood meal (ingests microfilariae)

❽ Migrate to head and mosquito's proboscis

L3 larvae

❼

❻ L1 larvae

❺ Microfilariae shed sheaths, penetrate mosquito's midgut, and migrate to thoracic muscles

**I** Infective stage
**D** Diagnostic stage

**Fig. 36.2** Life cycle of *Wuchereria bancrofti*. During a blood meal, an infected mosquito introduces third-stage filarial larvae onto the skin of the human host, where they penetrate into the bite wound (1). They develop into adults that commonly reside in the lymphatics (2). The female worms measure 80–100 mm in length and 0.24–0.30 mm in diameter, while the males measure about 40 mm by 0.1 mm. Adults produce microfilariae measuring 244–296 $\mu$m by 7.5–10 $\mu$m, which are sheathed and have nocturnal periodicity, except the South Pacific microfilariae which have the absence of marked periodicity. The microfilariae migrate into lymph and blood channels moving actively through lymph and blood (3). A mosquito ingests the microfilariae during a blood meal (4). After ingestion, the microfilariae lose their sheaths and some of them work their way through the wall of the proventriculus and cardiac portion of the mosquito's midgut and reach the thoracic muscles (5). There the microfilariae develop into first-stage larvae (6) and subsequently into third-stage infective larvae (7). The third-stage infective larvae migrate through the hemocoel to the mosquito's proboscis (8) and can infect another human when the mosquito takes a blood meal (1). (Adapted from Centers for Disease Control and Prevention DPDx.)

may or may not be preceded by episodes of lymphadenitis, epididymitis, or funiculitis. Straw-colored fluid accumulates within the sac surrounding the testicles because of blockage of draining lymphatics. The fluid reaccumulates rapidly if drained. Hydrocele in LF is most often unilateral. Vulvar lesions in females are uncommon.

## Lymphedema

Chronic lymphedema occurs following multiple episodes of swelling of the legs (most common), arms, or breasts. Involvement of the entire leg is typical for bancroftian filariasis, whereas only the lower leg is involved in brugian filariasis. The process usually begins unilaterally, but may proceed to involve both extremities.

A WHO classification scheme grades the progressive phases of lymphedema as follows:

- Grade 1: mostly pitting edema, spontaneously reversible with elevation;
- Grade 2: nonpitting edema that does not resolve with elevation;
- Grade 3: increased swelling compared with grade 2; changes in the skin overlying the swollen extremity (dermatosclerosis and papillomatous lesions).[3]

## Chyluria

Chyluria results from blockage or impairment of the renal lymphatics, leading to passage of lymph into the genitourinary tract. The condition is rare, but loss of protein in the urine may result in significant nutritional deficiencies.

## Tropical pulmonary eosinophilia

Tropical pulmonary eosinophilia (TPE) is a syndrome of peripheral blood eosinophilia (often at very high levels), repeated episodes of coughing and wheezing, usually worse at night, and absence of microfilaremia. It is more common in males. Pulmonary function tests may reveal obstructive as well as restrictive components, and the condition can progress to interstitial fibrosis if untreated. A rapid response to diethylcarbamazine (DEC) is characteristic and can be used to distinguish TPE from other chronic conditions such as asthma.

# Diagnosis

Clinical features of lymphatic filariasis as described in a patient of appropriate age plus residence in an appropriate geographic area should suggest the diagnosis of filarial disease. Diagnosis can be confirmed by identification of microfilariae in the blood, adult worms in biopsy specimens, or by testing for filarial antibodies and antigens. Blood specimens should be obtained at a time corresponding to the periodicity of the organism (usually at night) and examined under a microscope. Concentration and filtration techniques will increase the sensitivity of this technique.[6]

Serologic tests have improved the diagnosis of filarial diseases and have made it possible to diagnose bancroftian filariasis in those who are amicrofilaremic. Testing for filarial IgG alone is limited by lack of specificity due to cross-reaction with nonfilarial nematodes, and because it cannot distinguish between those exposed but not infected, those actively infected, and those successfully treated. IgG4 antibody is more specific and reportedly a good marker for active infection.[7] The most specific serologic tests available are those that identify circulating antigens to *W. bancrofti*.[6,8] Circulating antigen tests are not available for brugian filariasis, for which diagnosis may be aided by IgG4 antibody.[9] PCR techniques have been developed for detection of both *W.* bancrofti and *B. malayi* but require that there be microfilarial DNA in the blood sample tested.[6] Non-specific tests that may aid in the diagnosis include presence of eosinophilia and elevated IgE. Ultrasonography can identify motile adult worms in the lymphatic vessels ('filarial dance sign') in the scrotum of infected males as well as in the breast tissue of females.[10]

## Differential diagnosis

Acute manifestations of filarial disease (AFL) must be distinguished from bacterial infection, trauma, or thrombophlebitis. Leg swelling may be the result of heart failure, kidney disease, blockage of the lymphatics due to other causes, or congenital defects of the lymphatic system (lymphedema praecox, Milroy's disease). Swelling of the scrotum can occur with hernias, malignancies, or infections. Tropical pulmonary eosinophilia must be distinguished from asthma and other helminth infections during the phase of the life cycle involving migration through the lungs. In most cases, a detailed history as well as detailed physical examination, accompanied by antibody or antigen testing, will be diagnostic. Rapid response to DEC distinguishes TPE from other conditions.

# Treatment

The available chemotherapy for LF includes DEC, ivermectin, and albendazole (Table 36.1). DEC (6 mg/kg/day for 12–14 days, or alternatively, 6 mg/kg in a single-day dose) remains the treatment of choice for the individual with active LF (microfilaremia, antigen positivity, or adult worms on ultrasound), although albendazole has also been shown to have some macrofilaricidal efficacy.[11] If the adult parasites survive, microfilaremia along with clinical symptoms can recur within months after conclusion of the therapy. Evidence shows that these drugs used in combination can increase effectiveness.[12]

Most *Wuchereria* and *Brugia* spp. harbor bacterial endosymbionts. These *Wolbachia* are vital for parasite larval development and adult worm fertility and viability. New approaches for treatment use antibiotics (e.g. the tetracyclines) that target the *Wolbachia*, and microfilarial and antigen levels have been seen to reduce with these treatments.[13]

Initially, lymphedema may improve with treatment, but fibrosis of the lymphatics may have produced irreversible changes that do not allow complete resolution. Once lymphedema is established, antifilarial medication is not useful if the patient does not have active infection. Antifilarial medication is also not indicated in management of episodes of bacterial ADL These should be managed with skin care and antibiotics if indicated. Management of lymphedema should concentrate on local skin care with appropriate treatment of entry lesions and on exercise, elevation, and use of fitted stockings where available and pragmatic.[14] Surgical drainage of hydroceles pro-

**Table 36.1 Drugs used for treatment of lymphatic filariasis**

| | Adult dose | Efficacy | Adverse events | Comments |
|---|---|---|---|---|
| DEC | 6 mg/kg/day divided into two or three daily doses, over 12–14 days OR 6 mg/kg in a single day dose Extend length of therapy to 14–21 days for TPE Alternative for mass treatment programs: 6 mg/kg/dose weekly or monthly | 80–90% reduction of microfilaria levels of *W bancrofti* in a few days; slower response with *B. malayi* 74.9% reduction in microfilariae in annual treatment; 90% reduction in biannual treatments with prolonged suppression of microfilaremia Limited activity against adult worms | Fever, malaise, headache, joint and body pains; occasional bronchospasm; local adverse events may include lymphadenitis, abscesses, and lymphedema Reactions most severe with brugian filariasis | Not available commercially in the US Severe reactions may occur in individuals infected with *O. volvulus* or *L. loa*. Ideally limit dose to 3 mg/kg on first day; antipyretics may ameliorate side effects; interruption of treatment rarely necessary; DEC has little effect on adult worms Not recommended for use in pregnancy |
| Ivermectin | 150 mcg/kg/dose | Elimination of microfilaremia; more rapid reappearance of microfilaremia than with DEC | Similar to DEC | Little to no effect on adult worms Microfilariae return more rapidly than with DEC Not recommended for pregnant women or children under age 5 |
| Albendazole | 400 mg in a single dose | Some activity against adult worms | Abdominal pain | Greater efficacy in combination with DEC or ivermectin Treatment of helminths is an added benefit |
| Doxycycline | 200 mg daily for 8 weeks | Activity against both adult worms and microfilariae | GI disturbance; photosensitivity | Not for use in children <8 years, pregnant/nursing women |

duces immediate relief but fluid reaccumulates rapidly. Hydroceles may respond to treatment with DEC, or can be drained repeatedly or managed surgically.[3]

## Control And Prevention

Control measures, including the Global Program to Eliminate Lymphatic Filariasis, are based on the concept of community-based treatment given periodically in order to suppress microfilaremia (thereby interrupting transmission).[1,14] Single agents (DEC or ivermectin) and combination therapy (DEC, ivermectin, and albendazole in multiple combinations) have proven effective in suppressing microfilaremia when used periodically.[11,14,16] Immigrants may have taken part in such programs in their country of origin. Vector control has proven less reliable in providing sustained control, and is used in combination with chemotherapy.

### Clinical Pearls

* Consider LF in individuals with hydrocele or asymmetric limb swelling with history of residence in an endemic area, even if years before immigration.
* Consider LF in the setting of lymphadenopathy or lymphadenitis that does not respond to antibacterial therapy.
* Consider LF when a history of recurrent limb swelling is elicited.
* Consider tropical pulmonary eosinophilia due to filariasis in the setting of coughing and wheezing worse at night accompanied by eosinophilia and increased IgE in an individual from an appropriate endemic area.
* IgG4 and circulating antigen tests are helpful in making a diagnosis and do not require nighttime blood draws.

### Special Considerations for Immigrants

* DEC is not licensed for commercial use in the United States but is available from the CDC under an Investigational New Drug protocol.
* Daily therapy is most appropriate for treatment of immigrants no longer residing in endemic areas.
* Care of affected limbs with hygiene, exercise, and physical therapy is an important component of a treatment regimen of patients with lymphedema.

## References

1. Simonsen PE. Filariases. In: Cook GC, Zumla AI, eds. Manson's tropical diseases. London: Saunders; 2003:1487–1526.
2. Southgate VR, Bray RA. Medical helminthology (Appendix III). In: Cook GC, Zumla AI, eds. Manson's tropical diseases. London: Saunders; 2003:1649–1716.
3. King CL, Freedman DO. Filariasis. In: Strickland GT, ed. Hunter's tropical medicine and emerging infectious diseases. Philadelphia: WB Saunders; 2000:740–754.
4. Nutman TB, Kazura JW. Filariasis. In: Guerrant RL, Walker DH, Weller PF, eds. Tropical infectious diseases 2nd ed. Philadelphia: Churchill Livingstone; 2006:1152–1162.
5. Freedman DO, Filho PF, Besh S, et al. Lymphoscintigraphic analysis of lymphatic abnormalities in symptomatic and asymptomatic human filariasis. J Infect Dis 1994; 170:927–933.
6. Eberhard ML, Lammie PJ. Laboratory diagnosis of filariasis. Clin Lab Med 1991; 11:977–1010.
7. Haarbrink M, Terhell A, Abadi K, et al. IgG4 antibody assay in the detection of filariasis. Lancet 1995; 346:853–854.
8. Weil GJ, Jain DC, Santhanam S, et al. A monoclonal antibody-based enzyme immunoassay for detecting parasite antigenemia in bancroftian filariasis. J Infect Dis 1987; 156:350–355.
9. Rahman N, Anuar AK, Ariff RHT, et al. Use of anitfilarial IgG4-ELISA to detect *Brugia malayi* infection in an endemic area of Malaysia. Trop Med Int Hlth 1998; 3:184–188.
10. Amaral F, Dreyer G, Figueredo-Silva J, et al. Adult worms detected by ultrasonography in human bancroftian filariasis. Am J Trop Med Hyg 1994; 50:753–757.
11. Ismail M, Jayakody R, Weil G, et al. Efficacy of single dose combinations of albendazole, ivermectin and diethylcarbamazine for the treatment of bancroftian filariasis. Trans R Soc Trop Med Hyg 1998; 92:94–97.
12. Fox LM, Furness BW, Haser JK, et al. Tolerance and efficacy of combined diethylcarbamazine and albendazole for treatment of *Wuchereria bancrofti* and intestinal helminth infections in Haitian children. Am J Trop Med Hygiene 2005; 73:115–121.
13. Taylor MJ, Makunde WH, McGarry HF, et al. Macrofilaricidal activity after doxycycline treatment of *Wuchereria bancrofti*: a double-blind, randomized, placebo-controlled trial. Lancet 2005; 365:2116–2121.
14. Shenoy R, Kumaraswami V, Suma T, et al. A double blind, placebo-controlled study of the efficacy of oral penicillin, diethylcarbamazine or local treatment of the affected limb in preventing acute adenolymphangitis in lymphedema caused by brugian filariasis. Ann Trop Med Parasitol 1999; 93:367–377.
15. Melrose WD. Lymphatic filariasis: new insights into an old disease. Int J Parasitol 2002; 32:947–960.
16. Addiss DG, Beach MJ, Streit TG, et al. Randomised placebo-controlled comparison of ivermectin and albendazole alone and in combination for *Wuchereria bancrofti* microfilaraemia in Haitian children. Lancet 1997; 350:480–484.

# CHAPTER 37

# Malaria

William Stauffer

## Malaria at a Glance

- Malaria is common in immigrants and refugees arriving from sub-Saharan Africa.
- Newly arriving immigrants and refugees may have minimal or no symptoms from their malaria.
- Immigrants and refugees who return home to visit friends and family are at high risk of acquiring malaria infection during or following travel.
- The epidemiology of malaria in immigrants and refugees is dependent on migration and travel patterns.

## Introduction

Malaria is a devastating infection that affects over 500 million persons annually, causing more than 2 million deaths.[1,2] Severe morbidity and mortality is predominantly inflicted upon children, particularly those less than 5 years of age in sub-Saharan Africa. It has been estimated that a child dies, on average, every 30 seconds due to this protozoal infection. Despite recent attention malaria continues to plague the developing world and is particularly prominent in areas with limited resources. Immigrants and refugees are increasingly migrating from areas of high malaria endemicity such as sub-Saharan Africa. Unfamiliarity of medical practitioners in nonendemic areas with malaria can lead to delays or errors in diagnosis and appropriate treatment.[3]

## Malaria life cycle

Human malaria is caused by four species of the plasmodia parasite: *Plasmodium falciparum*, *P. vivax*, *P. ovale*, and *P. malariae*. The parasites, in the form of sporozoites, are introduced into the blood through the bite of a female *Anopheles* spp. mosquito. The sporozoites remain in the circulation for approximately 30 minutes before they infect a hepatocyte. For the next 7–10 days the parasites develop in the hepatocytes and are then released into the circulation as merozoites which subsequently invade red blood cells (RBCs). The host does not become clinically ill until the posthepatic phase. Both *P. vivax* and *P. ovale* can become dormant in the hepatocyte, in a form referred to as a hypnozoite. The hypnozoite may emerge months to years after initial infection to cause disease. Signs and symptoms of malaria caused by *P. falciparum*, which does not possess the hypnozoite form, will generally occur within a month of infection (Fig. 37.1).

## Epidemiology

### Global distribution of malaria

Worldwide distribution of malaria is shown in figure 37.2. The four species of malaria vary widely in their intensity and distribution. *Plasmodium falciparum* is prevalent in sub-Saharan Africa (Fig. 37.3) but is also found in South Asia, Southeast Asia and Pacific rim islands, South America and small portions of Central America, as well as in Haiti and the Dominican Republic. *P. vivax* is found predominantly in South Asia, the Middle East, Southeast Asia and Pacific rim islands, and South America, and accounts for a majority of the malaria reported in Central America. *P. vivax* can also be found in Africa, especially in the Horn of Africa and south along the eastern coast. It is interesting to note that it is an unusual infection in a majority of sub-Saharan Africa, in many areas

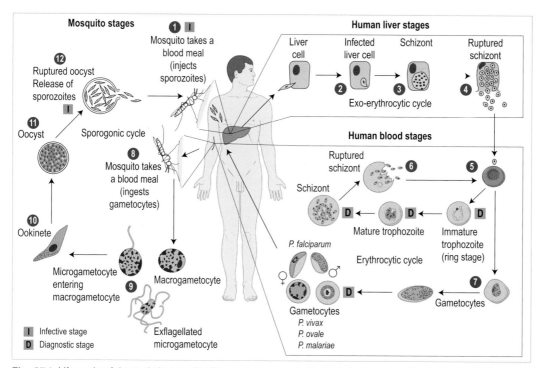

**Fig. 37.1** Life cycle of the malaria parasite. The malaria parasite life cycle involves two hosts. During a blood meal, a malaria-infected female *Anopheles* mosquito inoculates sporozoites into the human host (1). Sporozoites infect liver cells (2) and mature into schizonts (3), which rupture and release merozoites (4). (Of note, in *P. vivax* and *P. ovale* a dormant stage [hypnozoites] can persist in the liver and cause relapses by invading the bloodstream weeks, or even years later.) After this initial replication in the liver (exo-erythrocytic schizogony (A)), the parasites undergo asexual multiplication in the erythrocytes (erythrocytic schizogony (B)). Merozoites infect red blood cells (5). The ring stage trophozoites mature into schizonts, which rupture releasing merozoites (6). Some parasites differentiate into sexual erythrocytic stages (gametocytes) (7). Blood stage parasites are responsible for the clinical manifestations of the disease. The gametocytes, male (microgametocytes) and female (macrogametocytes), are ingested by an *Anopheles* mosquito during a blood meal (8). The parasites' multiplication in the mosquito is known as the sporogonic cycle (C). While in the mosquito's stomach, the microgametes penetrate the macrogametes generating zygotes (9). The zygotes in turn become motile and elongated (ookinetes) (10) which invade the midgut wall of the mosquito where they develop into oocysts (11). The oocysts grow, rupture, and release sporozoites (12), which make their way to the mosquito's salivary glands. Inoculation of the sporozoites into a new human host perpetuates the malaria life cycle (1). (Adapted from Centers for Disease Control and Prevention DPDx.)

accounting for less than 10% of cases. This scarcity of *P. vivax* is thought to reflect evolutionary genetic loss of an antigen on the red blood cell surface termed the Duffy group antigen. The parasite must attach to this antigen to infect a red blood cell and continue its life cycle and, due to its absence in many sub-Saharan African populations, the parasite is unable to cause disease. *P. ovale* is a less common malaria parasite which is restricted to Africa, predominantly West Africa, while *P. malariae* is also found mostly in Africa.

The clinical manifestations of *P. falciparum* malaria depend on many factors including epidemiologic patterns and immune status of the exposed individual. Nonimmune individuals including infants, young children, and persons residing outside of holo- or hyperendemic malarious areas (i.e. travelers) are

at the greatest risk of severe *P. falciparum* malaria. Although several species of malaria infect humans, the burden and consequences of *P. falciparum* predominate. *P. falciparum* may lead to death in a nonimmune host less than 12 hours from onset of symptoms.[4] However, in highly endemic (holoendemic) areas more than 75% of the population may be affected at any given time, with a majority of individuals being asymptomatic due to acquired partial immunity. These variations of clinical disease and asymptomatic infection may, in part, be due to gene expression variation between serotypes of *P. falciparum*.[5] Areas with high malaria endemicity include a majority of West, Central and portions of East Africa. While the less deadly, relapsing forms of malaria (*P. vivax*, *P. ovale*) occur in sub-Saharan Africa, these infections account for a minority of infections.

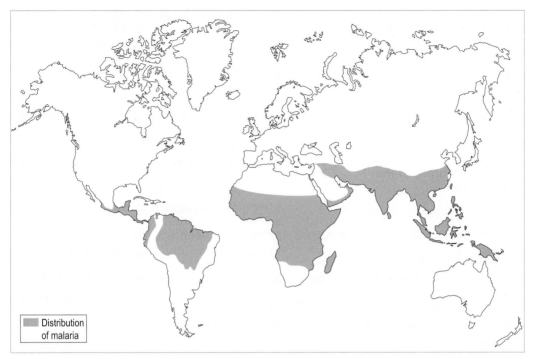

**Fig. 37.2** Worldwide distribution of malaria.

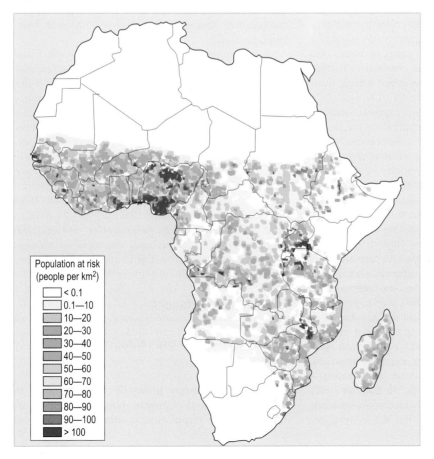

**Fig. 37.3** Sub-Saharan Africa distribution of malaria.

Population at risk
(people per km²)

< 0.1
0.1—10
10—20
20—30
30—40
40—50
50—60
60—70
70—80
80—90
90—100
> 100

Other areas such as Central Asia, South Asia, Southeast Asia, and areas of Latin America and the Caribbean have varying degrees of malaria, although in these areas malaria rarely reaches hyper- or holo-endemic rates. These areas also have varying ratios of deadly *P. falciparum* and nonfalciparum, although most areas outside sub-Saharan Africa have higher percentages of nonfalciparum malaria, particularly *P. vivax*.

## Malaria and the immigrant to the United States

Malaria was endemic in most of the continental United States and Europe into the nineteenth century with sporadic outbreaks as far north as Minnesota. There are several species of *Anopheles* mosquitoes (especially *Anopheles quadramaculus*) endemic to the US capable of transmitting malaria under favorable conditions. There have been a number of recent autochthonous cases and small outbreaks of malaria transmitted in the US including both *P. falciparum* and *P. vivax*.[6,7]

There is concern that resettling immigrants and refugees, especially those from areas of high endemicity, may act as potential reservoirs for malaria. Although sustained malaria transmission would be unlikely, single autochthonous cases or small outbreaks would be possible. This concern is further exacerbated by data recently collected which show that refugees may become clinically ill from *P. falciparum* over 6 months after the last exposure-indicating active infection, and parasitemia for prolonged periods of time after arrival (unpublished data, William Stauffer) suggesting subclinical circulating parasites. As stated, *P. falciparum* may be extremely virulent in nonimmune hosts and autochthonous transmission could lead to severe consequences. Partially due to this concern, in the late 1990s, the Centers for Disease Control and Prevention (CDC) recommended that all refugees departing for the US from sub-Saharan Africa receive presumptive therapy for malaria. These recommendations were implemented in May of 1999 when the International Organization of Migration (IOM) began presumptive treatment of refugees with sulfadoxine-pyrimethamine (SP, Fansidar®). Data collected prior to 1999 (1997–1999) found that >60% of Liberian refugees, arriving from four primary countries of asylum in West Africa, had active infection (parasitemia) 4 weeks after arrival in Minnesota.[8] In another study of refugees arriving in Canada from the less endemic area of Tanzania, it was found that 18% of refugees

three months after arrival had evidence of active infection.[9] Since the implementation of the pre-departure presumptive antimalarial treatment few data are available on malaria imported to the US by newly arriving immigrants or refugees. One study, performed in 2004, compared a rapid antigen test to a single thick and thin blood smear using polymerase chain reaction (PCR) as the gold standard. When 103 newly arrived Liberian refugees were tested 4 weeks after arrival, 8.7% had active *P. falciparum* infection.[10] Therefore, although the implementation of the empiric treatment program seems to be associated with a substantial decrease in the prevalence of active malaria in West African refugees, it does not eradicate the disease from the population. The authors postulate this is due to one, or more, of the following factors: drug-resistant *P. falciparum* with recrudescence of disease (rates of >50% SP resistance have been documented in Freetown, Liberia), failure to receive the medication (although IOM reports 96% treatment rates), and/or reinfection after treatment prior to departure. In 2004, the CDC modified the recommendation for presumptive pre-departure treatment from SP to artemisinin combination therapy due to concern regarding SP resistance. Due to cost concerns and a shortage of artemisinin coagulation therapy, this strategy has not been implemented.

A recent study, at a single county hospital and clinic system in Minnesota, further demonstrates the success of the presumptive therapy program.[11] Prior to 1999, the African refugees arriving in the county experienced rates of 6–9% per year of presentation of clinical malaria, costing this single county hospital ≈$75 000–100 000 per year. Since 1999, the percentage of African refugees who subsequently develop malaria has dropped to 0–2% per year, despite a dramatic increase in the number of African refugees arriving in the county since 1999–2000. In this study it was estimated that for every 15 African refugees treated with presumptive antimalarial therapy prior to departure, one case of clinical malaria is prevented in the United States (number needed to treat = 15).

## Clinical Manifestations

### Common malaria presentations in immigrants

*Plasmodium falciparum* generally presents days to weeks after initial exposure; however, in the partially immune population it may present several months or more after arrival. The classic clinical presentation of *P. falciparum* malaria is high fevers accompanied by chills, rigors, sweats, and headache. Malaria is also commonly associated with generalized weakness, backaches, myalgias, vomiting, pallor, jaundice, and hepatosplenomegaly. However, it is important to note that malaria in partially immune individuals may produce no or minimal clinical symptoms. Children frequently present with a syndrome that includes vomiting and/or diarrhea that may be confused with gastroenteritis. Other common presenting signs and physical symptoms in new immigrants include anorexia and decreased activity in children, isolated splenomegaly with or without a protuberant abdomen, or fever alone. A high clinical suspicion of malaria must be maintained when working with a population from a country where malaria occurs.

*Plasmodium vivax* and *P. ovale* may be detected shortly after arrival but, because they are capable of producing the hepatic hypnozoite stage, they may also present months to years later. *P. vivax* infection commonly presents with paroxysmal fevers, headaches, myalgias, anemia, and hypersplenism. Splenic rupture, a serious complication, may follow trauma, including an overly vigorous splenic examination. *P. malariae* and *P. ovale* generally cause fever but not a toxic appearance. In some individuals *P. malariae* may coexist as a commensal organism causing infection but no clinical disease, though it has been associated with nephrotic syndrome in children.

### Complicated *P. falciparum* malaria

Many factors influence a patient's risk of developing severe *P. falciparum* malaria, particularly the species of malaria and the patient's immune status based on prior exposure to malaria. Severe complications of malaria in newly arrived immigrants are unusual due to preexisting immunity. An exception to this generalization occasionally arises in the young infant or child immigrant with malaria who presents with severe anemia, the main cause of death in children occupying areas of constant, high-intensity malaria.

Severe malaria may occur more commonly, although still infrequently, in the immigrant who returns home to visit family and friends (VFR) (see Ch. 58). The VFR traveler is the highest-risk type of traveler to acquire malaria. Further, preexisting malaria immunity wanes quickly following immigration and the longer the residence outside a malaria-endemic area prior to re-exposure, the higher the risk of severe disease on re-exposure with travel. Children of VFR travelers born in nonendemic areas who may encounter malaria for the first time during their travels are of particular concern. In this population, as with nonimmune travelers, the most common complication is cerebral malaria. This condition is heralded by headache, confusion, and irritability and may lead to precipitous decline from normal sensorium to coma within hours. Seizures are common. Other characteristics of cerebral malaria include decorticate or decerebrate posturing, nystagmus, dysconjugate gaze, papilledema, retinal hemorrhages, and altered respiration. The cerebral spinal fluid (CSF) is generally unremarkable, with less than 20 white blood cells/microliter, a slightly elevated protein level, and a normal glucose level. Imaging studies may reveal nonspecific findings consistent with cerebral edema or ischemia. Even in the face of known malaria parasitemia it is imperative that other causes of neurologic decline be excluded (i.e. bacterial meningitis) since, especially in immigrants, the patient may have incidental malaria that may not be the cause of the neurologic decline. Hypoglycemia and respiratory distress caused by severe metabolic acidosis are other common complications, especially in children. Black water fever (severe hemolysis, hemoglobinuria, and renal failure) and algid malaria (vascular collapse, shock, and hypothermia) are rare presentations in immigrants.

## Diagnosis

In addition to specific tests for malaria, several other laboratory abnormalities are commonly observed which may alert the clinician to the possibility of malaria. These findings include thrombocytopenia, anemia, neutropenia, elevated liver enzymes, hypoalbuminemia, hematuria, albuminuria, elevated C-reactive protein (CRP), and elevated procalcitonin. It is interesting to note that although in acute clinical malaria it is common for patients to have thrombocytopenia, elevated inflammatory markers (i.e. CRP) and a slightly elevated bilirubin, these abnormalities may be absent in a majority of partially immune individuals with asymptomatic infection.

### Specific diagnostic techniques

Diagnostic tests available in the US for malaria include traditional thick and thin blood smears (blood films), PCR, and antibody tests. Rapid antigen testing is expected to be approved by the FDA in the near future. The thick and thin blood smears remain the most widely available and used test, particularly in the United States. Thick blood smears test for the presence or absence of parasites while thin smears allow for speciation and quantification. The sensitivity and specificity of smears range widely and are influenced by many factors such as laboratory skill, timing and quality of smear collection, and level of parasitemia. One negative set of thick and thin blood smears is never sufficient to exclude malaria, even in the most skilled hands. In asymptomatic refugees, it was found that blood films were only 20% sensitive compared to PCR for the diagnosis of malaria.[11]

Many rapid antigen tests are available outside the United States and it is anticipated they will become available in the US in the near future. The test that will be available in the US differentiates *P. falciparum* from nonfalciparum infections. These tests have shown mixed results in multiple trials, but the newer generation of tests seem to compare favorably to blood smears when used by trained personnel under laboratory conditions. The first rapid test is expected to become available for the diagnosis of acute malaria in the US (NOW ICT®). A pivotal clinical trial evaluating the performance of the NOW ICT® (Binax, Inc., Portland, ME, USA) rapid antigen test in over 4000 patients was recently presented at the American Society of Tropical Medicine and Hygiene Annual Conference by the US Army.[12] Overall sensitivity and specificity was 95% and 94% for *P. falciparum* infection and 69% and 99% for *P. vivax*, respectively. For parasite counts >5000 per µL, sensitivity was >99% for *P. falciparum* and 94% for *P. vivax*. The negative predictive value (NPV) also exceeds 99%, making this test ideal for excluding acute symptomatic *P. falciparum* malaria. When compared to PCR for the detection of malaria in asymptomatic immigrants, however, this test, like the blood film, was not sensitive and only detected 20% of the infections.[11] It should also be noted that this test may remain positive for *P. falciparum* for days to weeks after successful treatment due to the persistence of antigen in the blood, which can lead to false positives in recently treated immigrants and refugees.

Polymerase chain reaction tests are felt to be at least as sensitive and specific as the traditional blood smear. The clinical utility of PCR is limited for several reasons: the turn around time for results can be long, it is not currently approved by the FDA for diagnosis of acute malaria, and it has limited availability, located mostly in research and government laboratories. Currently, PCR is utilized mainly for confirming positive blood films and is valuable in identification of malaria species, particularly when smears are not definitive or there is a mixed infection. It is also more sensitive and specific for nonfalciparum species of malaria than blood film or rapid antigen testing.

Antibody tests are of little clinical utility. One exception, where serum immunoglobulin levels may be useful, is in the patient with 'tropical splenomegaly' (hyperactive malarial splenomegaly). Tropical splenomegaly or HMS is a term that has traditionally been used to describe individuals who have a large spleen, are suspected of having chronic malaria, and who have repeated negative malaria smears. In this cohort, the total IgM antibody is markedly elevated. A clinical therapeutic trial of antimalarial treatment will generally decrease IgM levels, and in younger individuals may decrease spleen size (the older the patient, and the more fibrosis, the less likely to observe splenic regression).

## Differential diagnosis

The differential diagnosis of malaria is extensive and is contingent upon presenting symptoms. Fever, a common presenting symptom, has an extensive differential from infection (viral, bacterial, parasitic) to autoimmune disease, among other causes. However, a very high level of suspicion for malaria should be maintained for any immigrant from an endemic area presenting with fever, and the diagnosis of malaria investigated. Thrombocytopenia frequently accompanies fever in the acutely ill patient with malaria.

Hepato- and/or splenomegaly (HSM) is another common presentation for malaria that carries a robust differential diagnosis depending on the person's previous areas of residence and travel. Common causes of HSM in the tropics that must be considered include chronic schistosomiasis, visceral leishmaniasis, and brucellosis, though other common causes must also be investigated (i.e. lymphoma).

Malaria frequently presents with fever, nausea, and vomiting which resembles gastroenteritis, particularly in children. Any child from an endemic area with these symptoms must have malaria considered before receiving the presumptive clinical diagnosis of gastroenteritis.

# Treatment

## Who should be tested/treated?

Although CDC recommendations currently call for all sub-Saharan African refugees to be treated presumptively before departure, this recommendation is fluid and medications may change or not be given due to cost concerns. In addition, immigrants of non-refugee status from similar areas currently receive no pre-departure screening or treatment. Some experts recommend that all newly arriving immigrants and refugees from sub-Saharan Africa receive presumptive therapy upon arrival unless it was given and documented pre-departure. Alternatively, when available and the patient will have follow-up, PCR testing can be considered. Exceptions to this are immigrants who have been living in nonendemic, or less endemic areas such as South Africa and Nairobi proper. The medication of choice for presumptive treatment in the US is atovaquone-proguanil (Table 37.1). Atovaquone-proguanil will be effective against *P. falciparum*, *P. malariae*, and the blood stage of *P. vivax* and *P. ovale* but will not treat the hypnozoite stage of the latter two infections. With the exception of New Guinea, there are few, if any, areas where in refugees *P. vivax* and *P. ovale* have a high enough prevalence to consider presumptive treatment. Therefore, CDC will be issuing new recommendations that all sub-Saharan refugees, with the exception of special groups, receive presumptive pre-departure malaria therapy with artemisinin combination therapy prior to departure to the US.

## Treatment in the acutely ill patient

Treatment of malaria must be based on the *Plasmodium* species, severity of disease, drug sensitivities of the infecting parasites, and by the availability of medications and resources. The severity of illness will influence the drug selected and the route of administration.

## Treatment of *P. falciparum*

*Plasmodium falciparum* treatment should be divided into uncomplicated versus complicated cases. Complicated malaria is less common in migrants as they generally have either partial immunity or, at least, some immunologic memory. Complicated malaria should be suspected when a patient at risk of malaria presents with altered mental status, respiratory distress, signs or symptoms of shock, seizures, gross hematuria or severe laboratory abnormalities including acidemia, profound anemia, signs of disseminated intravascular coagulation, or hyperparasitemia (based on the percentage of red cells which are infected: >2% in non-immune and >10% in partially immune).

## Management of uncomplicated *P. falciparum* malaria

Atovaquone-proguanil (Malarone®) has been shown to be effective, safe, and well tolerated as a single agent. It is approved by the FDA for the treatment of mild to moderate acute *P. falciparum* malaria in adults and children over 5 kg (see Table 37.1). At this time, many experts consider atovaquone-proguanil the drug of choice for uncomplicated *P. falciparum* malaria. When given alone, either drug induces resistance rapidly; it was hoped that the combination would forestall emergence of drug resistance. Unfortunately, within several years of widespread use, several cases of resistance have been reported.[13]

Alternative agents include oral quinine (or quinidine if more readily available) plus clindamycin, or in older children (>7 years), quinidine/quinine plus doxycycline. Oral quinine plus sulfadoxine-pyrimethamine (SP, Fansidar®), once considered the first-line therapy in the US for uncomplicated *P. falciparum*, should not generally be used due to rising SP resistance. Other alternatives include mefloquine, lumefantrine, halofantrine, and the artemisinin compounds; of these drugs, only mefloquine is available in the US at this time. Mefloquine continues to be an effective single agent although it can cause significant gastrointestinal or neurologic adverse effects. Halofantrine demands intensive monitoring because of potentially severe cardiac adverse effects, including prolongation of the QT interval, and should never be used in a patient who has recently received mefloquine as it may precipitate severe arrhythmias. It is helpful to caution travelers who are prescribed mefloquine of this situation and advise them to avoid treatment with halofantrine if offered while traveling. Though not available in many areas, the artemisinin derivatives are extremely effective and inexpensive antimalarials but must be used in combination with a long-acting agent to prevent recrudescence of disease.

Chloroquine-sensitive *P. falciparum* is now encountered rarely. Chloroquine susceptibility may only be assumed and treatment with chloroquine considered if the *P. falciparum* was contracted in Central

**Table 37.1 Guidelines for treatment of malaria in the United States. From Center for Disease Control and Prevention. (Based on drugs currently available for use in the United States)**

| Clinical diagnosis/Plasmodium species | Region infection acquired | Recommended drug and adult dose[1,7] | Recommended drug and pediatric dose[1,7] *Pediatric dose should NEVER exceed adult dose* |
|---|---|---|---|
| Uncomplicated malaria/P. falciparum or species not identified | Chloroquine-sensitive (Central America west of Panama Canal; Haiti; the Dominican Republic; and most of the Middle East) | Chloroquine phosphate (Aralen™ and generics) 600 mg base (=1000 mg salt) p.o. immediately, followed by 300 mg base (=500 mg salt) p.o. at 6, 24, and 48 hours Total dose: 1500 mg base (=2500 mg salt) | Chloroquine phosphate (Aralen™ and generics) 10 mg base/kg p.o. immediately, followed by 5 mg base/kg p.o. at 6, 24, and 48 hours Total dose: 25 mg base/kg |
| If 'species not identified' is subsequently diagnosed as P. vivax or P. ovale: see P. vivax and P. ovale (below) re. treatment with primaquine | Chloroquine-resistant or unknown resistance[1] (All malarious regions except those specified as chloroquine-sensitive listed in the box above. Middle Eastern countries with chloroquine-resistant P. falciparum include Iran, Oman, Saudi Arabia, and Yemen. Of note, infections acquired in the newly independent states of the former Soviet Union and Korea to date have been uniformly caused by P. vivax and should therefore be treated as chloroquine-sensitive infections.) | A. Quinine sulfate[2]: 542 mg base (=650 mg salt) p.o. t.i.d. × 3 to 7 days plus one of the following: doxycycline, tetracycline, or clindamycin Doxycycline: 100 mg p.o. b.i.d. × 7 days Tetracycline: 250 mg p.o. b.i.d. × 7 days Clindamycin: 20 mg kg/day p.o. divided t.i.d. × 7 days B. Atovaquone-proguanil (Malarone™)[4] Adult tablets = 250 mg atovaquone/ 100 mg proguanil 4 adult tablets p.o. q.d. × 3 days C. Mefloquine (Lariam™ and generics)[5] 684 mg base (=750 mg salt) p.o. as initial dose, followed by 456 mg base (=500 mg salt) p.o. given 6-12 hours after initial dose Total dose = 1250 mg salt | A. Quinine sulfate[2]: 8.3 mg base/kg (=10 mg salt/kg) p.o. b.i.d. × 3 to 7 days plus one of the following: doxycycline[3], tetracycline[3] or clindamycin Doxycycline: 4 mg/kg/day p.o. divided b.i.d. × 7 days Tetracycline: 25 mg/kg/day p.o. divided q.o.d. × 7 days Clindamycin: 20 mg/day p.o. divided t.i.d. × 7 days B. Atovaquone-proguanil (Malarone™)[4] Pediatric tablet = 62.5 mg atovaquone/25 mg proguanil 5-8 kg: 2 peds tabs p.o. q.d. × 3 d 9-10 kg: 3 peds tabs p.o. q.d. × 3 d 11-20 kg: 1 adult tab p.o. q.d. × 3 d 21-30 kg: 2 adult tabs p.o. q.d. × 3 d 31-40 kg: 3 adult tabs p.o. q.d. × 3 d >40 kg: 4 adult tabs p.o. q.d. × 3 d C. Mefloquine (Lariam™ and generics)[5] 13.7 mg base/kg (=15 mg salt/kg) p.o. as initial dose, followed by 9.1 mg base/kg (=10 mg salt/kg) p.o. given 6-12 hours after initial dose Total dose = 25 mg salt/kg |

| Clinical diagnosis/Plasmodium species | Region | | |
|---|---|---|---|
| Uncomplicated malaria/ P. malariae | All regions | Chloroquine phosphate: treatment as above | Chloroquine phosphate: treatment as above |
| Uncomplicated malaria/ P. vivax or P. ovale | All regions[7] Note: for suspected chloroquine-resistant P. vivax, see row below | Chloroquine phosphate plus primaquine phosphate[6]; Chloroquine phosphate: treatment as above; Primaquine phosphate: 30 mg base p.o. q.d. ×14 days; G6PD testing must be done and G6PD ruled out before primaquine may be used | Chloroquine phosphate plus primaquine phosphate[6]; Chloroquine phosphate: treatment as above; Primaquine phosphate: 0.5 mg base/kg p.o. q.d. × 14 days; G6PD testing must be done and G6PD ruled out before primaquine may be used |
| Uncomplicated malaria/ P. vivax | Chloroquine-resistant[7] (Papua New Guinea and Indonesia) | A. Quinine sulfate[2] plus either doxycycline or tetracycline plus primaquine phosphate[6]; Quinine sulfate: treatment as above; Doxycycline or tetracycline: treatment as above; Primaquine phosphate: treatment as above; G6PD testing must be done and G6PD ruled out before primaquine may be used; B. Mefloquine plus primaquine phosphate[6]; Mefloquine: treatment as above; Primaquine phosphate: treatment as above; G6PD testing must be done and G6PD ruled out before primaquine may be used | A. Quinine sulfate[2] plus either doxycycline[3] or tetracycline[3] plus primaquine phosphate[6]; Quinine sulfate: treatment as above; Doxycycline or tetracycline: treatment as above; Primaquine phosphate: treatment as above; G6PD testing must be done and G6PD ruled out before primaquine may be used; B. Mefloquine plus primaquine phosphate[6]; Mefloquine: treatment as above; Primaquine phosphate: treatment as above; G6PD testing must be done and G6PD ruled out before primaquine may be used |
| Uncomplicated malaria: alternatives for pregnant women[8,9,10,11] | Chloroquine-sensitive[11] (see uncomplicated malaria sections above for chloroquine-sensitive Plasmodium species by region) | Chloroquine phosphate: treatment as above | Not applicable |
| | Chloroquine resistant P. falciparum[8,9,10] (see uncomplicated malaria sections above for regions with known chloroquine resistant P. falciparum) | Quinine sulfate[2] plus clindamycin; Quinine sulfate: treatment as above; Clindamycin: treatment as above | Not applicable |
| | Chloroquine-resistant P. vivax[8,9,10,11] (see uncomplicated malaria sections above for regions with chloroquine-resistant P. vivax) | Quinine sulfate; Quinine sulfate: 650 mg salt p.o. t.i.d. × 7 days | Not applicable |
| Severe malaria[12,13,14,15] | All regions | Quinidine gluconate[13] plus one of the following: doxycycline, tetracycline, or clindamycin | Quinidine gluconate[13] plus one of the following: doxycycline[3], tetracycline[3], or clindamycin |

**Table 37.1 Guidelines for treatment of malaria in the United States (Based on drugs currently available for use in the United States)—cont'd**

| Clinical diagnosis/ Plasmodium species | Region infection acquired | Recommended drug and adult dose[1,7] | Recommended drug and pediatric dose[1,7] Pediatric dose should NEVER exceed adult dose |
|---|---|---|---|
| | | Quinidine gluconate: 6.25 mg base/kg (=10 mg salt/kg) loading dose i.v. over 1–2 hrs, then 0.0125 mg base/kg/min (=0.02 mg salt/kg/min) continuous infusion for at least 24 hours. An alternative regimen is 15 mg base/kg (=24 mg salt/kg) loading dose i.v. infused over 4 hours, followed by 7.5 mg base/kg (=12 mg salt/kg) infused over 4 hours every 8 hours, starting 8 hours after the loading dose (see package insert). Once parasite density <1% and patient can take oral medication, complete treatment with oral quinine, dose as above. Quinidine/quinine course =7 days in Southeast Asia; =3 days in Africa or South America. Doxycycline: treatment as above. If patient not able to take oral medication, give 100 mg i.v. every 12 hours and then switch to oral doxycycline (as above) as soon as patient can take oral medication. For i.v. use, avoid rapid administration. Treatment course = 7 days. Tetracycline: treatment as above Clindamycin: Treatment as above. If patient not able to take oral medication, give 10 mg base/kg loading dose i.v. followed by 5 mg base/kg i.v. every 8 hours. Switch to oral clindamycin (oral dose as above) as soon as patient can take oral medication. For i.v. use, avoid rapid administration. Treatment course = 7 days. | Quinidine gluconate: same mg/kg dosing and recommendations as for adults. Doxycycline: treatment as above. If patient not able to take oral medication, may give i.v. For children <45 kg, give 4 mg/kg i.v. every 12 hours and then switch to oral doxycycline (dose as above) as soon as patient can take oral medication. For children ≥45 kg, use same dosing as for adults. For i.v. use, avoid rapid administration. Treatment course = 7 days. Tetracycline: treatment as above Clindamycin: treatment as above. If patient not able to take oral medication, give 10 mg base/kg loading dose i.v. followed by 5 mg base/kg i.v. every 8 hours. Switch to oral clindamycin (oral dose as above) as soon as patient can take oral medication. For i.v. use, avoid rapid administration. Treatment course = 7 days. |

[1] NOTE: There are three options (A, B, or C) available for treatment of uncomplicated malaria caused by chloroquine-resistant *P. falciparum*. Options A and B are equally recommended. Because of a higher rate of severe neuropsychiatric reactions seen at treatment doses, we do not recommend option C (mefloquine) unless options A and B cannot be used. For option A, because there are more data on the efficacy of quinine in combination with doxycycline or tetracycline, these treatment combinations are generally preferred to quinine in combination with clindamycin.

[2] For infections acquired in Southeast Asia, quinine treatment should continue for 7 days. For infections acquired in Africa and South America, quinine treatment should continue for 3 days.

[3] Doxycycline and tetracycline are not indicated for use in children less than 8 years old. For children less than 8 years old with chloroquine-resistant *P. falciparum*, quinine (given alone for 7 days or given in combination with clindamycin) and atovaquone-proguanil are recommended treatment options; mefloquine can be considered if no other options are available. For children less than 8 years old with chloroquine-resistant *P. vivax*, quinine (given alone for 7 days) or mefloquine are recommended treatment options. If none of these treatment options is available or is not being tolerated and if the treatment benefits outweigh the risks, doxycycline or tetracycline may be given to children less than 8 years old.

[4] Give atovaquone-proguanil with food. If patient vomits within 30 minutes of taking a dose, the dose should be repeated.

[5] Treatment with mefloquine is not recommended in persons who have acquired infections from the Southeast Asian region of Burma, Thailand, and Cambodia due to resistant strains.

[6] Primaquine is used to eradicate any hypnozoite forms that may remain dormant in the liver, and thus prevent relapses, in *P. vivax* and *P. ovale* infections. Because primaquine can cause hemolytic anemia in persons with G6PD deficiency, patients must be screened for G6PD deficiency prior to starting treatment with primaquine. For persons with borderline G6PD deficiency or as an alternate to the above regimen, primaquine may be given 45 mg orally one time per week for 8 weeks; consultation with an expert in infectious disease and/or tropical medicine is advised if this alternative regimen is considered in G6PD-deficient persons. Primaquine must not be used during pregnancy.

[7] NOTE: There are two options (A or B) available for treatment of uncomplicated malaria caused by chloroquine-resistant *P. vivax*. High treatment failure rates due to chloroquine-resistant *P. vivax* have been well documented in Papua New Guinea and Indonesia. Rare case reports of chloroquine-resistant *P. vivax* have also been documented in Burma (Myanmar), India, and Central and South America. Persons acquiring *P. vivax* infections outside of Papua New Guinea or Indonesia should be started on chloroquine. If the patient does not respond, the treatment should be changed to a chloroquine-resistant *P. vivax* regimen and CDC should be notified. For treatment of chloroquine-resistant *P. vivax* infections, options A and B are equally recommended.

[8] For pregnant women diagnosed with uncomplicated malaria caused by chloroquine-resistant *P. falciparum* or chloroquine-resistant *P. vivax* infection, treatment with doxycycline or tetracycline is generally not indicated. However, doxycycline or tetracycline may be used in combination with quinine (as recommended for nonpregnant adults) if other treatment options are not available or are not being tolerated, and the benefit is judged to outweigh the risks.

[9] Because there are no adequate, well-controlled studies of atovaquone and/or proguanil hydrochloride in pregnant women, atovaquone-proguanil is generally not recommended for use in pregnant women. For pregnant women diagnosed with uncomplicated malaria caused by chloroquine-resistant *P. falciparum* infection, atovaquone-proguanil may be used if other treatment options are not available or are not being tolerated, and if the potential benefit is judged to outweigh the potential risks. There are no data on the efficacy of atovaquone-proguanil in the treatment of chloroquine-resistant *P. vivax* infections.

[10] Because of a possible association with mefloquine treatment during pregnancy and an increase in stillbirths, mefloquine is generally not recommended for treatment in pregnant women. However, mefloquine may be used if it is the only treatment option available and if the potential benefit is judged to outweigh the potential risks.

[11] For *P. vivax* and *P. ovale* infections, primaquine phosphate for radical treatment of hypnozoites should not be given during pregnancy. Pregnant patients with *P. vivax* and *P. ovale* infections should be maintained on chloroquine prophylaxis for the duration of their pregnancy. The chemoprophylactic dose of chloroquine phosphate is 300 mg base (=500 mg salt) orally once per week. After delivery, pregnant patients who do not have G6PD deficiency should be treated with primaquine.

[12] Persons with a positive blood smear or history of recent possible exposure and no other recognized pathology who have one or more of the following clinical criteria (impaired consciousness/coma, severe normocytic anemia, renal failure, pulmonary edema, acute respiratory distress syndrome, circulatory shock, disseminated intravascular coagulation, spontaneous bleeding, acidosis, hemoglobinuria, jaundice, repeated generalized convulsions, and/or parasitemia of > 5%) are considered to have manifestations of more severe disease. Severe malaria is practically always due to P. falciparum.

[13] Patients diagnosed with severe malaria should be treated aggressively with parenteral antimalarial therapy. Treatment with i.v. quinidine should be initiated as soon as possible after the diagnosis has been made. Patients with severe malaria should be given an intravenous loading dose of quinidine unless they have received more than 40 mg/kg of quinine in the preceding 48 hours or if they have received mefloquine within the preceding 12 hours. Consultation with a cardiologist and a physician with experience treating malaria is advised when treating malaria patients with quinidine. During administration of quinidine, blood pressure monitoring (for hypotension) and cardiac monitoring (for widening of the QRS complex and/or lengthening of the QTc interval) should be monitored continuously and blood glucose (for hypoglycemia) should be monitored periodically. Cardiac complications, if severe, may warrant temporary discontinuation of the drug or slowing of the intravenous infusion.

[14] Consider exchange transfusion if the parasite density (i.e. parasitemia) is >10% or if the patient has altered mental status, non-volume overload pulmonary edema, or renal complications. The parasite density can be estimated by examining a monolayer of red blood cells (RBCs) on the thin smear under oil immersion magnification. The slide should be examined where the RBCs are more or less touching (approximately 400 RBCs per field). The parasite density can then be estimated from the percentage of infected RBCs and should be monitored every 12 hours. Exchange transfusion should be continued until the parasite density is <1% (usually requires 8–10 units). I.V. quinidine administration should not be delayed for an exchange transfusion and can be given concurrently throughout the exchange transfusion.

[15] Pregnant women diagnosed with severe malaria should be treated aggressively with parenteral antimalarial therapy.
(From Centers for Disease Control and Prevention.)

America west of the Panama Canal, Argentina, Egypt, Haiti, the Dominican Republic, and selected Middle Eastern countries.

## Managing complicated *P. falciparum* malaria

The patient with complicated malaria demands immediate parenteral antimalarials and aggressive supportive therapy. Quinidine is the only acceptable available parenteral antimalarial in the United States. Quinine and the artemisinin compounds are widely available outside the United States and would be considered the drugs of choice in that setting. Since quinidine is not immediately available on all hospital formularies, temporizing approaches to therapy may need to be implemented immediately until parenteral quinidine becomes available. Parenteral clindamycin may be initiated in this circumstance as well as placement of a nasogastric tube for the delivery of oral quinidine. When parenteral quinidine is unavailable it may be acquired directly from the manufacturer on an emergent basis (Eli Lilly Company 800-821-0538).

The patient should have cardiac monitoring with frequent blood pressure measurements when initiating quinine derivatives. These agents must be given as a gradual intravenous infusion to avoid acute cardiovascular complications, particularly hypotension. Infusion rates should be reduced if the QT interval is prolonged by more than 25% from its baseline value. Oral therapy is initiated as soon as tolerated by the patient. It should be noted that a second agent (i.e. doxycycline) must be used in conjunction with quinine, quinidine, or especially the artemisinin compounds to prevent recrudescence.

Close monitoring and supportive therapy are imperative for good outcome. Initial hypoglycemia should be treated with 25% (infants and small children) or 50% dextrose as a rapid infusion. To prevent and monitor for hyperinsulinemic hypoglycemia patients should be started on a 5% or 10% dextrose solution when initiating quinine derivatives, and blood glucose levels should be monitored frequently. Quinine-induced hypoglycemia may develop several days into treatment. Hypovolemia and lactic acidosis must be managed with intravenous crystalloids or colloids, with vasopressors and bicarbonate occasionally being necessary. Severe anemia may necessitate blood transfusion. Seizures, particularly common in children, may be managed acutely with benzodiazepines and, when repeated or prolonged, other anticonvulsants may be utilized. Renal failure may develop and would necessitate adjustment of drug dosages.

---

**Table 37.2 Poor prognostic criteria for severe *P. falciparum* malaria**

**Clinical features**
  Impaired level of consciousness (LOC)*
  Respiratory distress*
  Jaundice*
  Repeated convulsions
  Shock

**Laboratory features**
  Hypoglycemia* (whole blood glucose <40 mg/dL)
  Elevated bilirubin* (total >2.5 mg/dl)
  Acidosis (plasma bicarbonate <15 mmol/L)
  Lactic acidosis (serum lactate >45 mg/dL)
  Elevated aminotransferase levels (>3 times normal)
  Renal insufficiency (serum creatinine >3 mg/dL)

* Particularly poor prognostic factors in children, particularly if respiratory distress and impaired LOC coexist.

---

Repeated smears with parasite quantification should be followed to monitor therapeutic success. Very high levels of parasitemia or failure to respond to treatment may indicate primary drug failure/resistance and therapy should be adjusted and exchange transfusion considered. Due to lack of objective data, effectiveness and safety of exchange transfusion have been debated, with exact criteria for initiating therapy being unclear. Some authorities have suggested exchange transfusion may be beneficial in any severely ill patient with a parasitemia that exceeds 10% or in any patient with parasitemia in the range of 5–15% with signs of poor prognosis (Table 37.2). When managing a severe case of malaria, an experienced infectious disease or tropical medicine specialist should be consulted and additional support may be obtained through the CDC malaria hotline (770-488-7788).

## Treatment of nonfalciparum malaria

*Plasmodium vivax* and *P. ovale* are usually susceptible to chloroquine. Recent exceptions to this rule have been documented in *P. vivax* from South America and Oceania, particularly New Guinea. In patients with a high likelihood of chloroquine-resistant *P. vivax*, mefloquine or quinine/quinidine plus doxycycline (over age 7 years) may be used. With both *P. vivax* and *P. ovale*, the initial treatment should be followed by treatment with primaquine ('radical cure'). Primaquine is effective against the exoerythrocytic liver phase and is given to prevent relapse, but occasional relapses may still occur despite appropriate therapy. All patients receiving primaquine must have a glucose-6-dehydrozenase (G6PD) level checked prior to drug initiation, as a severe hemolytic anemia may occur in patients with a deficiency of this enzyme. For patients with G6PD deficiency, primaquine should be withheld and each subsequent relapse should be treated with chloroquine or an acceptable alternative.

*Plasmodium malariae* is susceptible to chloroquine, which is the drug of choice. It does not possess the ability to form a hypnozoite in the liver, and therefore radical cure with primaquine is not needed.

## ICD-9 Codes

- 084.8 Blackwater fever
- 084.9 Other pernicious complications of malaria
- 084.5 Mixed malaria
- 084.1 Vivax malaria (benign tertian)
- 084.2 Quartan malaria
- 084.3 Ovale malaria
- 084.6 Malaria, unspecified
- 084.0 Falciparum malaria (malignant tertian)
- 771.2 Other congenital infections
- 573.2 Hepatitis in other infectious diseases classified elsewhere

## Prevention

One of the most high-risk groups of travelers for acquiring malaria is immigrants who return to their home country, frequently referred to as 'visiting friends and relatives' or 'VFR' travelers (see Ch. 58). Insect avoidance and malaria chemoprophylaxis are of paramount importance in persons traveling to malaria-endemic areas. Immigrants, especially those who have experienced malaria, may consider it a minor inconvenience and fail to understand that the more time since their last infection the more likely they are to become significantly ill. Individual and community education regarding the risk of travel should be stressed and pre-travel medical visits encouraged. Although insect avoidance and chemoprophylaxis are beyond the scope of this chapter there are many sources to provide guidance to the provider in assisting travelers to avoid malaria infection and disease (see Chapter 58 and selected reading).

## Infection control measures

Malaria may only be transmitted by a competent mosquito vector after an appropriate incubation period or through direct exposure to a blood product (i.e. transfusion, congenital). Universal precautions are adequate for protection of healthcare providers in the clinical setting.

### Clinical Pearls

- Malaria is currently a common infection in immigrants who migrate from sub-Saharan Africa (with the exception of Nairobi).
- Minimally symptomatic or asymptomatic infection may occur in partially immune populations.
- Immigrants who travel to a country of previous residence (VFR travelers) where malaria is endemic are at particular risk of acquiring infection and disease.

## References

1. World Health Organization. The global malaria situation: current tools for prevention and control. 55th World Health Assembly. Global Fund to Fight AIDS, Tuberculosis and Malaria. WHO document no. A55/INF.DOC./6. Available: http://www.who.int/topics/malaria/en Accessed 2/27/07.
2. Greenwood B, Mutabingwa T. Malaria in 2002. Nature 2002; 415:670–672.
3. Kain KC, MacPherson DW, Kelton T, et al. Imported malaria: prospective analysis of problems in diagnosis and management. Clin Infect Dis 1998; 27:142–149.
4. Warrell DA. Management of severe malaria. Parassitologia 1999; 41:287–294.
5. Kaestli M, Cockburn CA, Cortes A, et al. Virulence of malaria is associated with differential expression of *Plasmodium falciparum* var gene subgroups in a case-control study. J Infect Dis 2006; 193(11):1567–1574.
6. Centers for Disease Control and Prevention. Malaria Surveillance – United States, 1998. MMWR 2001; 50(SS05):1–18.
7. Centers for Disease Control and Prevention. Malaria Surveillance – United States, 2004. MMWR 2006; 55(SS04):23–27.
8. Maroushek SR, Aguilar EF, Stauffer W, Abd-Alla MD. Malaria among refugee children at arrival in the United States. Pediatr Infect Dis J 2005; 24(5):450–452.
9. Ndao M, Bandyayera E, Kokoskin E, et al. Malaria 'epidemic' in Quebec: diagnosis and response to imported malaria. Can Med Assoc J 2005; 172(1):46–50.
10. Stauffer WM, Newberry AM, Cartwright CP, et al. Evaluation of malaria screening in newly arrived refugees to the United States by microscopy and rapid antigen capture enzyme assay. Pediatr Infect Dis J 2006; 25(10):948–950.
11. Collinet-Adler S, Stauffer WM, Boulware DR, et al. Financial implications of refugee malaria: The impact of pre-departure anti-malarial presumptive treatment. Am J Trop Med Hyg. In press.
12. Gasser RA Jr, Magill AJ, Ruebush T, et al. Malaria diagnosis: performance of NOW® ICT malaria in a large scale field trial [Abstract #2338]. 54th Annual Meeting American Society of Tropical Medicine and Hygiene, Washington, DC; Dec 11–15, 2005.

13. Kuhn S, Gill MJ, Kain KC. Emergence of atovaquone-proguanil resistance during treatment of *Plasmodium falciparum* malaria acquired by a non-immune North American traveler to West Africa. Am J Trop Med Hyg 2005; 72(4):407–409.

## Selected Reading

Centers for Disease Control and Prevention. Travelers' health: yellow book. http://www.cdc.gov/travel/yb/

Greenwood B, Mutabingwa T. Malaria in 2002. Nature 2002; 415:670–672.

Greenwood BM, Bojang K, Whitty CJ, et al. Malaria [review] [142 refs]. Lancet 2005; 365(9469):1487–1498.

Honigsbaum M. The fever trail: in search for the cure for malaria. New York: Picador; 2001.

Stauffer WM, Fisher PR. Diagnosis and treatment of malaria in children. Clin Infect Dis. 2003; 37:1340–1348.

Suh KN, Kain KC, Keystone JS. Malaria [see comment] [Review] [52 refs]. Can Med Assoc J 2004; 170(11):1693–1702.

Drugs for Parasitic Infections. The medical letter on Drugs and Therapeutics 2004; 46:e1–e12. Available at: http://www.medletter.com/freedocs/parasitic.pdf

# CHAPTER 38

# Onchocerciasis

Elizabeth D. Barnett

## Onchocerciasis at a Glance

- Also known as river blindness, or enfermedad de Robles.
- Caused by *Onchocerca volvulus*, a filarial nematode for which humans are the only definitive hosts.
- Disease is transmitted by the black fly (*Simulium* spp.).
- Transmission occurs within limited areas of Africa, Central and South America, and the Arabian peninsula.
- Clinical manifestations in those with lifelong exposure include dermatitis, subcutaneous nodules, keratitis, and chorioretinitis.
- Diagnosis is by identifying microfilariae in skin snips, identifying adult worms in tissue, or by serologic tests.
- Treatment is with ivermectin, which acts to kill microfilariae; no specific nontoxic treatment is available to kill adult worms.

## Epidemiology

Almost 18 million people worldwide are infected with *Onchocerca volvulus*; almost 2% of those are blind, and another 3% have severely impaired vision. Almost all cases (99%) of onchocerciasis occur in sub-Saharan Africa, with about half of the cases found in Nigeria and Democratic Republic of Congo (Fig. 38.1). Onchocerciasis is a major public health problem along rivers where black flies breed, and where in some villages close to 100% of individuals may be infected. DNA probes have demonstrated the presence of different strains of the parasite. Blindness occurs more frequently with savanna strains of *O. volvulus*, while forest strains cause blindness less frequently even in heavily infected individuals. Infection is also present in Yemen and Saudi Arabia, though cases in the latter country are likely imported, as no transmission has been documented there. Onchocerciasis control programs have reduced disease burden in the Volta River Basin in West Africa and eliminated the disease from western Kenya.[1]

Isolated foci of onchocerciasis occur in the Americas, the largest of which are in Guatemala, Mexico, and Venezuela. Transmission is about 10-fold less intense in Central and South America than in sub-Saharan Africa, with comparatively lower worm burdens and lower rates of blindness. In contrast to the relative stability of disease distribution in Africa, where vector distribution determines that of the disease, foci in the Americas are enlarging as human habitation expands to rainforest areas where the *Simulium* vector is already present.[1,2]

## Etiology

*Onchocerca* larvae are transmitted by the bite of the *Simulium* fly. The larvae are deposited into the skin where they require at least 6–12 months and a series of molts for development of mature adult worms, with the female worms capable of producing microfilariae. Adult females live inside fibrous nodules located subcutaneously or in deep musculature, while the smaller adult males appear to circulate from nodule to nodule to inseminate the females.[1,2] Adult females may live as long as 14–15 years, producing hundreds of microfilariae each day. Microfilariae, whose lifespan ranges from 6 to 24 months, migrate from the nodules most commonly to the skin and the eye, but may also be found in lymphatic

493

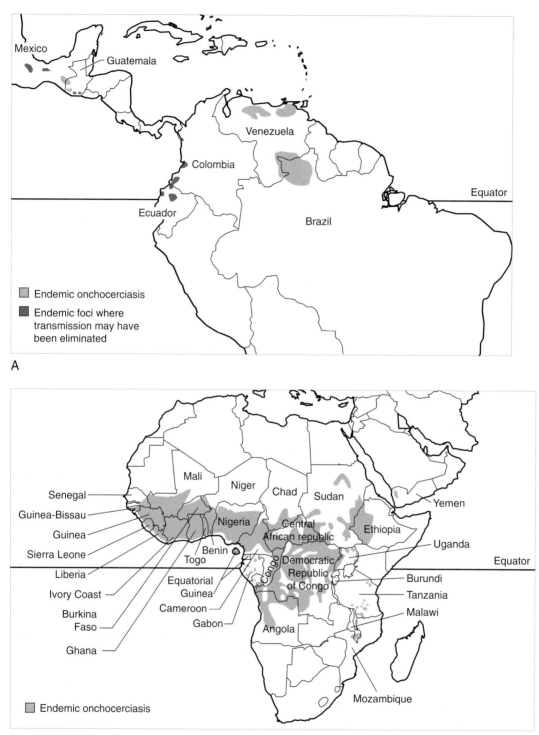

A

B

**Fig. 38.1** Distribution of onchocerciasis. **(A)** Latin America. **(B)** Africa and the Middle East (Freedman D. Onchocerciasis. In: Guerrant RL, Walker DH, Weller PF, eds. Tropical infectious diseases. 2nd edn. Philadelphia: Churchill Livingstone; 2006:1178).

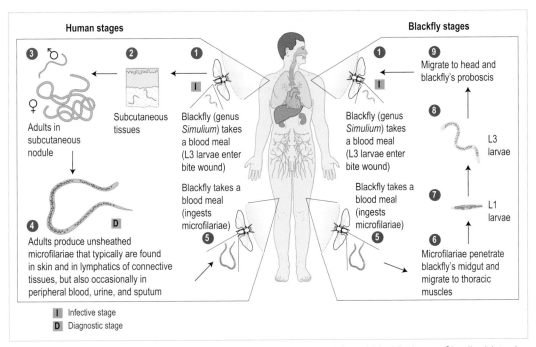

**Human stages**

**Blackfly stages**

❸ ♂
❷ Subcutaneous tissues
❶ Blackfly (genus *Simulium*) takes a blood meal (L3 larvae enter bite wound)

❶ Blackfly (genus *Simulium*) takes a blood meal (L3 larvae enter bite wound)
❾ Migrate to head and blackfly's proboscis

♀
Adults in subcutaneous nodule

❽ L3 larvae

Blackfly takes a blood meal (ingests microfilariae) ❺

Blackfly takes a blood meal (ingests microfilariae) ❺

❼ L1 larvae

❹ D
Adults produce unsheathed microfilariae that typically are found in skin and in lymphatics of connective tissues, but also occasionally in peripheral blood, urine, and sputum

❻ Microfilariae penetrate blackfly's midgut and migrate to thoracic muscles

**I** Infective stage
**D** Diagnostic stage

**Fig. 38.2** Life cycle of *Onchocerca volvulus*. During a blood meal, an infected blackfly (genus *Simulium*) introduces third-stage filarial larvae onto the skin of the human host, where they penetrate into the bite wound (1). In subcutaneous tissues the larvae (2) develop into adult filariae, which commonly reside in nodules in subcutaneous connective tissues (3). Adults can live in the nodules for approximately 15 years. Some nodules may contain numerous male and female worms. Females measure 33–50 cm in length and 270–400 µm in diameter, while males measure 19–42 mm by 130–210 µm. In the subcutaneous nodules, the female worms are capable of producing microfilariae for approximately 9 years. The microfilariae, measuring 220–360 µm by 5–9 µm and unsheathed, have a life span that may reach 2 years. They are occasionally found in peripheral blood, urine, and sputum but are typically found in the skin and in the lymphatics of connective tissues (4). A blackfly ingests the microfilariae during a blood meal (5). After ingestion, the microfilariae migrate from the blackfly's midgut through the hemocoel to the thoracic muscles (6). There the microfilariae develop into first-stage larvae (7) and subsequently into third-stage infective larvae (8). The third-stage infective larvae migrate to the blackfly's proboscis (9) and can infect another human when the fly takes a blood meal (1). (Adapted from Centers for Disease Control and Prevention DPDx.)

vessels and lymph nodes (Fig. 38.2). The *Simulium* fly ingests microfilariae present in the skin when taking a blood meal.

## Clinical Manifestations

The clinical spectrum of disease due to *Onchocerca volvulus* is largely due to inflammatory responses to dying or dead microfilariae. No overt clinical disease is present in many infected individuals. In others, disease may involve the eye, the skin, and the lymph nodes. Short-term exposure rarely results in clinical manifestations of disease; symptoms may not appear until at least 2 years of exposure have occurred and the sole manifestation may be dermatitis.[3] Clinical manifestations in those from endemic areas are a result of the interaction of duration of exposure, parasite burden, and host immune response.

## Dermatitis

Skin lesions are the most common clinical manifestations of onchocerciasis. Itching is the most common complaint, and may be intense and profoundly troublesome. Papular dermatitis may occur along with itching, and may be localized to one part of the body or may be associated with swelling or edema.[4] Recently, development of a classification scheme for dermatitis associated with onchocerciasis has facilitated communication about dermatologic manifestations of the disease.[5] Patients may have manifestations in more than one category. The categories are:

1. *Acute papular dermatitis*: scattered papular lesions that may progress to vesicles and pustules; scratching of lesions can lead to secondary infection and ulceration. May resolve spontaneously without treatment.

2. *Chronic papular dermatitis*: larger papules with more variability in size than acute papular dermatitis; less pruritic. Postinflammatory hyperpigmentation is common.

3. *Lichenified dermatitis (Sowda)*: intensely pruritic eruption usually confined to one extremity (often a leg) consisting of hyperpigmented papules and plaques with edema of the limb and associated regional lymphadenopathy. Bacterial superinfection is common as a result of excoriation. First described in Yemen and most common in Yemen and Sudan.

4. *Atrophy*: loss of elasticity due to degeneration of the structural elements of the skin following chronic infection. Skin appears wrinkled, tissue-paper thin, and may have little subcutaneous tissue.

5. *Depigmentation*: areas of complete or near-complete depigmentation over the anterior shin interspersed with areas of normal skin that are centered around hair follicles ('leopard skin').

Skin manifestations specific to Mexico and Guatemala have been described and include erisipela de la costa (macular rash and swelling of the face) and mal morado (lesions associated with reddish color especially on the trunk and upper limbs).

## Subcutaneous nodules (or onchocercomata)

Subcutaneous nodules develop as a result of tissue reaction to adult worms. They are painless, variable in size, and do not cause medical problems though they may be undesirable cosmetically. The location of the nodules (more commonly on the head in Central America and predominantly in the pelvic girdle in Africa) is thought to reflect the biting pattern of the local vector fly.[6]

## Eye lesions

Microfilariae gain access to the cornea via the skin and conjunctiva. A punctate keratitis develops at sites of inflammation around dying microfilariae and may clear spontaneously as the inflammation resolves. Presence of intraocular microfilariae may be detected by slit lamp examination of the anterior chamber. After years of exposure and infection, irreversible eye changes may occur, including sclerosing dermatitis, optic neuritis or optic nerve atrophy, and chorioretinopathy. Sclerosing keratitis results in gradual opacification of the cornea, beginning at the margins with ingrowth of pigment and vessels. Chorioretinopathy occurs insidiously as a result of inflammation of the retinal pigment epithelium.[7]

## Diagnosis

The diagnosis of onchocerciasis should be considered in individuals who have lived in areas where *O. volvulus* occurs and who have any manifestation of disease, including itching alone. Physical examination may reveal skin or eye manifestations of disease, but these findings are not specific to onchocerciasis and additional diagnostic tests are warranted. Eosinophilia, though associated with onchocerciasis, is present inconsistently and therefore lacks diagnostic specificity.

The most common method of diagnosing onchocerciasis is by demonstration of microfilariae in the skin by examining skin snips taken from the iliac crest (preferred site in Africa) or scapula (preferred site in the Americas). A small piece of bloodless skin is placed on a microscope slide, and normal saline added. It may be examined at least 1 hour later, and if no microfilariae are seen at that time, reexamined periodically over the next 24 hours. Care should be taken to avoid blood in the skin specimen, as blood-borne filariae may be present and be mistaken for *O. volvulus*.

Ultrasound of nodules can distinguish onchocercomata from lymph nodes or other masses. Removal of nodules and identification of adult worms also seals the diagnosis. Microfilariae may be seen in the cornea and anterior chamber of the eye by slit lamp examination. If this is done, the patient should sit with the head bent down and forward for 10–20 minutes to allow microfilariae to move to the anterior chamber.

Serologic tests for *O. volvulus* using specific recombinant antigens are highly sensitive and specific but are not widely available. A rapid card test that detects specific IgG4 antibodies to a recombinant antigen in serum or blood has been shown to be both sensitive and specific.[8] Antibody detection tests are limited by their inability to distinguish between current and past infection, and are therefore most useful for individuals originally from nonendemic areas suspected of being infected. Antigen detection tests currently are not available. Polymerase chain reaction technique is the most sensitive means of detecting parasite DNA, and can distinguish between strains of the parasite, but requires specialized equipment and is not available for general use. Moreover, it must be done on extracted DNA from skin snips.

## Differential Diagnosis

The skin findings, especially early in disease, are nonspecific and must be distinguished from other similar conditions such as atopic or contact dermatitis, scabies, and insect bites. Later changes may resemble findings in leprosy, chronic dermatitis, vitiligo, or yaws. Eye changes may be due to syphilis, toxoplasmosis, or tuberculosis, and optic atrophy may be associated with glaucoma or nutritional deficiencies.[2]

## Treatment

There are no drugs available that kill the adult worms of *O. volvulus*. Therapy is therefore directed against the microfilariae, which serves the dual purpose of preventing the pathologic sequelae of the disease and preventing ongoing transmission if treatment is given to the community at large.[2] Prolonged treatment is required in order to maintain very low levels of microfilariae, thereby preventing pathology.

Ivermectin is the drug of choice for treatment of onchocerciasis (Table 38.1).[9] It reduces rapidly the number of microfilariae, but has little effect on adult worms. Given in a dose of 150 μg/kg, ivermectin results in rapid reduction of microfilariae in the skin and in the eye. The drug suppresses production of microfilariae for about 6 months, and repeated dosing probably is needed for 10 years or more in order to maintain sustained low microfilariae levels. There are some data to suggest that repeated dosing may decrease the lifespan and fertility of female worms.[10] The interval between doses is typically 6–12 months, but may be modified based upon rapidity of return of symptoms.

Ivermectin lacks significant toxicity, but may produce a post-treatment reaction as a response to dead and dying microfilariae. Symptoms occur within the first few days after treatment in 10–15% of those who react after the first dose, and may be severe in 1–5% of those.[1] Pruritus, fever, lymphadenitis, rash, myalgias and, rarely, hypotension, may

**Table 38.1  Drugs used in the treatment of onchocerciasis**

|  | Adult dose | Pediatric dose | Efficacy | Adverse events | Comments |
|---|---|---|---|---|---|
| Ivermectin | 150 mcg/kg/ dose every 6–12 months | Same (no safety data available for children <5 years or <15 kg) | >80% of skin microfilariae eliminated in 48 hrs; slowly increases to 97%; retreatment required every 6–12 months for 10 years or more | Potential severe encephalopathy in patients heavily infected with *Loa loa* Pruritis, rash, fever; rarely hypotension | Active only against microfilariae Probably safe in pregnancy but best to defer until after delivery |
| Doxycycline | 100 mg daily for 6 weeks | 100 mg daily for 6 weeks in children >8 years of age | Sustained reduction of microfilariae 18 months after treatment[12] | GI upset, photodermatitis | Investigational; not approved for this indication Likely most suitable for those who have left endemic areas and are able to adhere to daily regimen Contraindicated in pregnant and nursing women and children <8 years of age |

occur. Reactions tend to be less severe with subsequent doses of ivermectin. There are few safety data available for use in pregnancy or in children under 5 years of age or 15 kg, though the drug is likely safe in these cases.[11]

There is currently no place for use of diethylcarbamazine (DEC), formerly the mainstay of therapy, in treatment of onchocerciasis because of unacceptable toxicity. Severe toxicity also limits the use of suramin, the only available agent that is active against the adult worm. A promising new therapeutic approach targets endosymbiotic bacteria that live with adult worms. When doxycycline was given with ivermectin in Ghana, suppression of microfilariae was prolonged in the doxycycline plus ivermectin compared with the ivermectin only group.[12]

## Control and Prevention

The first efforts to control onchocerciasis were based on elimination of vector flies. The successful Onchocerciasis Control Program in West Africa resulted in dramatic reduction of morbidity from disease in the Volta River Basin. Prolonged (15 years) treatment of rivers with DDT in Kenya and parts of Uganda resulted in elimination of disease.[13] Programs for mass distribution of ivermectin, coordinated by nongovernmental organizations as well as the African Program for Onchocerciasis Control and the Onchocerciasis Elimination Program in the Americas (OEPA), with funding from the World Bank and other UN agencies, now are the mainstay of control and prevention efforts.[14] Sustainability and success of such programs will depend on continued efforts and adequate funding in this era of competing priorities for healthcare resources. Efforts to develop agents effective against the adult worm are ongoing. Investigation of alternatives to current dosing regimens suggests that reducing the interval between doses of ivermectin to 3 months could change the duration of control programs.[15]

### Clinical Pearls

- Itching with or without rash in an individual with prolonged residence in an onchocerciasis-endemic area should suggest onchocerciasis.
- Eye disease is rare in individuals who have not had prolonged exposure.
- Ivermectin is the drug of choice; caution should be used in patients who may have heavy infection with *Loa loa*.

### Special Considerations for Immigrants

- Symptoms may not be present on arrival but may occur weeks to months later, especially in those who were taking part in mass eradication programs in their country of origin.
- Itching, with or without rash or chronic dermatitis, should prompt consideration of onchocerciasis in immigrants from appropriate geographic areas, even as long as 10–15 years after immigration.
- Treatment will need to be prolonged; the interval between doses can be tailored to rapidity of return of symptoms.

## References

1. Cooper PJ, Nutman TB. Onchocerciasis. In: Strickland GT, ed. Hunter's tropical medicine and emerging infectious diseases. Philadelphia: WB Saunders; 2000:756–769.
2. Freedman D. Onchocerciasis. In: Guerrant RL, Walker DH, Weller PF, eds. Tropical infectious diseases 2nd ed. Philadelphia: Churchill Livingstone; 2006:1176–1188.
3. Hoerauf A, Buttner DW, Adjei O, et al. Onchocerciasis. Br Med J 2003; 326:207–210.
4. McCarthy JS, Ottesen EA, Nutman TB. Onchocerciasis in endemic and nonendemic populations: differences in clinical presentation and immunologic findings. J Infect Dis 1994; 170:736–741.
5. Murdoch ME, Hay RJ, Mackenzie CD, et al. A clinical classification and grading system of the cutaneous changes in onchocerciasis. Br J Dermatol 1993; 129:260–269.
6. Simonsen PE. Filariases. In: Cook GC, Zumla AI, eds. Manson's tropical diseases. London: Saunders; 2003:1487–1526.
7. McGavin DDM. Ophthalmology in the tropics and subtropics. In: Cook GC, Zumla AI, eds. Manson's tropical diseases. London: Saunders; 2003:301–361.
8. Weil GJ, Steel C, Liftis F, et al. A rapid-format antibody card test for diagnosis of onchocerciasis. J Infect Dis 2000; 182:1796–1799.
9. Greene BM, Taylor HR, Cupp EV, et al. Comparison of ivermectin and diethylcarbamazine in the treatment of onchocerciasis. N Engl J Med 1985; 313:133–138.
10. Plaisier AP, Alley ES, Boatin BA, et al. Irreversible effects of ivermectin on adult parasites in onchocerciasis patients in the Onchocerciasis Control Programme in West Africa. J Infect Dis 1995; 172:204–210.
11. Pacque M, Munoz B, Poetschke G, et al. Pregnancy outcome after inadvertent ivermectin treatment during community-based distribution. Lancet 1990; 336:1486–1489.
12. Hoerauf A, Mand S, Adjei O, et al. Depletion of *Wolbachia* endobacteria in *Onchocerca volvulus* by doxycycline and microfilaremia after ivermectin treatment. Lancet 2001; 357:1415–1416.
13. Burnham G. Onchocerciasis. Lancet 1998; 351:1341–1346.
14. Abiose A, Jones BR, Cousens SN, et al. Reduction in incidence of optic nerve disease with annual ivermectin to control onchocerciasis. Lancet 1993; 341:130–134.
15. Gardon J, Boussinesq M, Kamgno J, et al. Effects of standard and high doses of ivermectin on adult worms of *Onchocerca volvulus*: a randomized, controlled trial. Lancet 2002; 360:203–210.

# CHAPTER 39

# Schistosomiasis

Drew L. Posey and William Stauffer

## Schistosomiasis at a Glance

- Over 200 million infected worldwide.[1,2]
- Prevalence rates may exceed 50% in highly endemic areas.[3]
- Untreated infections may lead to bladder cancer, obstructive uropathy, or portal hypertension.[1]
- Treatment is with praziquantel.[1]
- Symptoms may be variable and can range from hematuria to failure to thrive.[4]

## Epidemiology

Worldwide, 500–700 million people are at risk for acquiring schistosomiasis, and 200 million people throughout Africa and parts of South America, the Caribbean, the Middle East, and Southeast Asia are infected (Table 39.1).[5–8] The parasite is found in tropical regions in fresh water harboring competent snail vectors.[9] The snail vectors are *Schistosoma* species-specific. For *Schistosoma mansoni*, competent snail vectors are in the genus *Biomphalaria* (Africa, much of the Arabian Peninsula, Brazil, Surinam, Venezuela, and some Caribbean islands); for *S. haematobium*, it is *Bulinus africanus* (sub-Saharan Africa, West Africa), tetrapoloid members of *B. tropicus/truncates* complex (Mediterranean region, Southwest Asia, and West Africa), and *B. forskalii* group (Arabia, Mauritius, and West Africa); for *S. japonicum*, *Oncomelania hupensis* is the vector in China, Indonesia, and the Philippines. *S. mekongi* is transmitted along the Mekong River in Cambodia and Laos by *Neotricula aperta*.[5] Movements of infected human populations and large-scale irrigation projects, which extend the range of competent snail vectors, have expanded endemic areas.[5,10]

Within heavily endemic areas, prevalence rates may exceed 50%. However, high prevalence rates are not confined to native populations, as expatriate communities within endemic areas are also reported to have high prevalence rates.[11]

## Etiology

Schistosomiasis is caused by trematode parasites.[6] Infection occurs after contact with fresh water that contains larval forms, called cercariae (Fig. 39.1).[1] Skin penetration occurs within 3–5 minutes. Approximately 40% of cercariae that penetrate the skin will eventually become viable adult worms. After penetrating the skin, cercariae lose their bifurcated tails and enter capillaries and lymph vessels and travel to the lungs. After several days, the parasites make their way to the portal venous system, mature, and unite. Pairs of worms then migrate to the superior mesenteric veins (*S. mansoni*), the inferior mesenteric and superior hemorrhoidal veins (*S. japonicum*), or vesicle plexus and veins draining the ureters (*S. haematobium*). Approximately 4–6 weeks after infection, male and female worms mate. The worm pairs begin producing eggs and will do so for the life of the worm, producing up to a few thousand eggs per day.[5] The total lifespan of the worm averages 3–10 years, but some may live for more than 30 years.[4] Many eggs may pass from blood vessels into adjacent tissues and then through intestinal or bladder mucosa to be shed in feces (*S. mansoni* and *S. japonicum*) or urine (*S. haematobium*).[1] *S. mansoni* eggs are shed singly, while *S. haematobium* and *S. japonicum* eggs are released in clumps. Approximately 50% of eggs will be viable upon release, but most will desiccate and die if they do not soon come into contact

499

**Table 39.1 Countries endemic for schistosomiasis**

| Region | Region | Region | Region |
|---|---|---|---|
| **Africa** | **Africa, continued** | **Asia** | **Caribbean** |
| Algeria* | Libya[†] | Cambodia[‡] | Antigua[2] |
| Angola[†] | Madagascar[†] | China[§] | Dominican Republic[2] |
| Benin[†] | Malawi[†] | Indonesia[§] | Guadeloupe[2] |
| Botswana[†] | Mali[†] | Laos[‡] | Martinique[2] |
| Burkina Faso[†] | Mauritania[†] | Malaysia[§] | Montserrat[2] |
| Burundi[†] | Mauritius[†] | Philippines[§] | Puerto Rico[2] |
| Cameroon[†] | Morocco* | **Middle East** | Saint Lucia[2] |
| Central African Republic[†] | Mozambique[†] | Iran* | **South America** |
| Chad[†] | Namibia[†] | Iraq* | Brazil[2] |
| Congo[†] | Niger[†] | Jordan* | Surinam[2] |
| Côte d'Ivoire[†] | Nigeria[†] | Lebanon* | Venezuela[2] |
| Democratic Republic of Congo[†] | Rwanda[†] | Oman[†] | |
| Djibouti[†] | Senegal[†] | Saudi Arabia[†] | |
| Egypt[†] | Sierra Leone[†] | Syrian Arab Republic* | |
| Eritrea[†] | Somalia[†] | Turkey* | |
| Equatorial Guinea[†] | South Africa[†] | Yemen[†] | |
| Ethiopia[†] | Sudan[†] | | |
| Gabon[†] | Swaziland[†] | | |
| Gambia[†] | Tanzania[†] | | |
| Ghana[†] | Togo[†] | | |
| Guinea[†] | Tunisia* | | |
| Guinea Bissau[†] | Uganda[†] | | |
| Kenya[†] | Zambia[†] | | |
| Liberia[†] | Zimbabwe[†] | | |

* *Schistosoma haematobium.*
[†] *Schistosoma haematobium* and *S. mansoni.*
[‡] *Schistosoma mekongi.*
[§] *Schistosoma japonicum.*
[2] *Schistosoma mansoni.*

with fresh water.[5] Once in fresh water, the parasite's life cycle is completed when the eggs hatch, releasing miracidia that infect freshwater snails in temperatures between 20° and 30°C.[12] After two generations within the snail, cercariae are then released.[1,5,12,13]

## Clinical Manifestations

Persons with schistosome infection can have a variety of clinical symptoms depending on how recently they were first infected, frequency of re-exposure, and the specific infecting strain of schistosomiasis. In addition, the host susceptibility to disease plays an important role as well as other synergistic comorbidities (such as hepatitis C virus infection). Schistosome infections are frequently asymptomatic for many years while the infection insidiously leads to damage to organs such as the liver or bladder.[4] Only approximately 10% of infected persons will develop severe clinical disease.[5]

## Acute infection

At the time of cercariae skin penetration, individuals may experience mild, transitory reactions or a prickling sensation at the site of entry. Within a few hours to a week after cercariae first enter the skin, a macular rash may appear at the site of entry, which may be followed by papules. The papules may be accompanied by erythema, vesicles, edema, and pruritus and may last 7–10 days.[5]

The adult worms have devised ingenious mechanisms to evade the host immune system and quickly and invisibly migrate to their preordained vessels, where the pair begin to secrete eggs. These eggs are highly antigenic and travel through the blood system until they are deposited. Deposition of eggs produced by the worm pairs, typically 5–7 weeks after infection, causes the symptoms associated with acute schistosomiasis, also known as Katayama fever.[5] These symptoms can include fever, headache, myalgias, abdominal pain (in particular, right upper

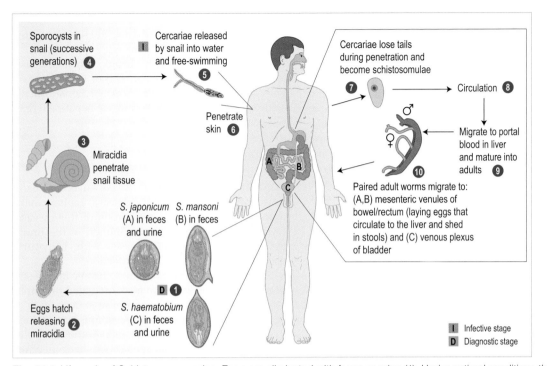

**Fig. 39.1** Life cycle of *Schistosoma* species. Eggs are eliminated with feces or urine (1). Under optimal conditions the eggs hatch and release miracidia (2), which swim and penetrate specific snail intermediate hosts (3). The stages in the snail include 2 generations of sporocysts (4) and the production of cercariae (5). Upon release from the snail, the infective cercariae swim, penetrate the skin of the human host (6), and shed their forked tail, becoming schistosomulae (7). The schistosomulae migrate through several tissues and stages to their residence in the veins (8, 9). Adult worms in humans reside in the mesenteric venules in various locations, which at times seem to be specific for each species (10). For instance, *S. japonicum* is more frequently found in the superior mesenteric veins draining the small intestine (A), and *S. mansoni* occurs more often in the superior mesenteric veins draining the large intestine (B). However, both species can occupy either location, and they are capable of moving between sites, so it is not possible to state unequivocally that one species only occurs in one location. *S. haematobium* most often occurs in the venous plexus of bladder (C), but it can also be found in the rectal venules. The females (size 7 to 20 mm; males slightly smaller) deposit eggs in the small venules of the portal and perivesical systems. The eggs are moved progressively toward the lumen of the intestine (*S. mansoni* and *S. japonicum*) and of the bladder and ureters (*S. haematobium*), and are eliminated with feces or urine, respectively (1). Pathology of *S. mansoni* and *S. japonicum* schistosomiasis includes: Katayama fever, hepatic perisinusoidal egg granulomas, Symmers' pipe stem periportal fibrosis, portal hypertension, and occasional embolic egg granulomas in brain or spinal cord. Pathology of *S. haematobium* schistosomiasis includes: hematuria, scarring, calcification, squamous cell carcinoma, and occasional embolic egg granulomas in brain or spinal cord. Human contact with water is thus necessary for infection by schistosomes. Various animals, such as dogs, cats, rodents, pigs, hourse and goats, serve as reservoirs for *S. japonicum*, and dogs for *S. mekongi*. (Adapted from Centers for Disease Control and Prevention DPDx.)

quadrant), and bloody diarrhea.[4,5] Eosinophilia is usually detected at this stage, but the absence of eosinophilia does not rule out infection.[1] Most persons infected with *S. mansoni* may also experience respiratory symptoms.[14] On physical examination, tender hepatomegaly is a common finding, as is splenomegaly.[1] During this acute illness, many but not all patients may shed eggs, and frequently serologic tests are positive.[1]

Acute manifestations may also include neurologic findings, which may consist of focal or generalized tonic-clonic seizures, especially with infection by

*S. japonicum*.[1] Transverse myelitis is a common neurologic manifestation of *S. mansoni* or *S. haematobium*. Schistosomal myelopathy is due to egg deposition or embolization in the spinal cord or meninges.[4] Neurologic findings have been reported among people with limited exposure to schistosomiasis-infected water, such as soldiers, travelers, and aid workers.[1,15]

A coinfection of schistosomiasis and *Salmonella* may lead to persistent *Salmonella* bacteremia and urinary tract infections. To eradicate the *Salmonella* in this situation, treatment of schistosomiasis is typically required prior to treatment of *Salmonella*.[5]

## Chronic infection

Chronic disease is the most prevalent form of schistosomiasis. Chronic manifestations are due to granulomatous reactions stimulated by the antigens released by schistosome eggs.[5] The duration and intensity of the infections are related to the amount of antigen released and the severity of the fibrotic deposition in host tissues.[12] While granulomas have been detected in tissues throughout the body, including brain, lung, skin, adrenal glands, and skeletal muscle, the species of schistosome and the host susceptibility patterns determine the typical chronic manifestations.[12] For example, children may have some unique characteristics of chronic infection manifested by the development of growth impairment, anemia, and memory deficits.[1,16]

### S. mansoni, S. japonicum, and S. mekongi

Egg deposition from these schistosomes typically occurs in the intestine or liver; thus granulomas are most likely to form in these locations.[5] Most lesions are found in the colon and rectum.[12] Because eggs may be retained in the gut wall, inflammation, hyperplasia, ulceration, microabscesses, and polyposis may be found.[5] Symptoms can include colicky hypogastric pain, melena, diarrhea, or constipation. The frequency of symptoms is associated with the severity of infection.[1,12] Colonic polyposis is common. A protein-losing enteropathy has also been described.[17] Severe colonic or rectal manifestations may result in stenosis.[2]

In the liver, perisinusoidal inflammation and periportal fibrosis may result from the granulomatous response.[5] Hepatomegaly occurs early in the progression of disease.[12] Over time, periportal collagen deposits lead to blood flow obstruction, portal hypertension, varices, variceal bleeding, splenomegaly, and hypersplenism.[1,5] The periportal fibrosis can be detected on ultrasonography, computed tomography, and magnetic resonance imaging.[1] Sustained heavy infection may lead to a condition known as Symmers' pipestem fibrosis in 4–8% of patients with chronic infection.[18] Until the late stages of the disease, hepatocellular function is preserved and lobular architecture is retained.[1] Bleeding esophageal varices is a serious sequalae of fibrotic hepatic schistosomiasis.[12] Pulmonary hypertension may develop as a complication in persons with portal hypertension.[19]

Co-infection with hepatitis B or C virus can lead to accelerated liver damage.[1,6] For example, chronic schistosomiasis caused by S. mansoni and hepatitis B virus (HBV) infection may result in a higher risk of hepatocellular carcinoma than with HBV alone; this effect is not seen in infections with S. japonicum.[20,21] In addition, persons with chronic schistosomiasis may have more severe hepatitis B or C infections.[22] Persons with more severe forms of hepatosplenic schistosomiasis have greater rates of hepatitis B than the general population.[4]

### S. haematobium

While infection with S. haematobium can occasionally cause mild colonic or hepatic disease, genitourinary disease is the classic manifestation of this disease. Dysuria and hematuria are common in the initial manifestations of the disease, with hematuria appearing 10–12 weeks after infection.[1,5]

As with S. mansoni infections, chronic manifestations of S. haematobium are also attributed to granulomatous inflammation in response to deposition of eggs in tissue. Chronic manifestations can include dysuria, hematuria, bladder calcifications, ureter obstruction, proteinuria, renal colic, hydronephrosis, and renal failure. These changes can predispose patients to secondary genitourinary bacterial infections. Areas of roughened bladder mucosa surrounding egg deposits visible on cystocopy are pathognomonic.[1,5]

While there is some controversy regarding the exact role of S. haematobium infections and the development of bladder cancer, squamous cell carcinomas of the bladder are associated with S. haematobium.[5,12]

In females, infection with S. haematobium causes genital manifestations in approximately one-third. Genital manifestations may include hypertrophic, ulcerative, fistulous, or wart-like lesions on the vulva and perineum.[1] While isolated internal disease is less frequent, tubal infertility may be a late complication of chronic infection.[23-25] In males, genital schistosomiasis has also been reported[6] and S. haematobium eggs have been detected in semen specimens and in lesions noted in the prostate and seminal vesicles.[26]

## Diagnosis

### Who should be tested?

Most infected immigrants and refugees are asymptomatic but illness can be detected during a laboratory examination in which a stool or urine sample is examined for eggs.[5] Generally, only newly arriving refugees and international adoptees undergo these examinations, and the presence of schistosomiasis serves to stress the point that all newly arriving immigrants should undergo medical screening (see Ch. 12). Most often, the organism is detected in a screening stool examination for ova and parasites, or when a patient from an endemic area has a persistent eosinophilia, despite repeatedly negative stool examinations. *Schistosoma haematobium* may also be detected when red blood cells are found when urine screening is done on an African immigrant.

The epidemiology of disease plays a crucial role in determining which populations should be tested, or alternatively, empirically treated. For example, because of the high rates of schistosomiasis detected among some refugee groups, CDC has recommended presumptive therapy for schistosomiasis (http://www.cdc.gov/ncidod/dq/refugee_health.htm).[27,28] However, schistosomiasis is very prevalent in many African populations, and it may prove more cost-effective to treat presumptively all, or a majority of, sub-Saharan refugees prior to departure or on arrival to the United States. The World Health Organization has a strategy of presumptive treatment focusing on children based on community levels of prevalence.[3] However, refugees are typically excluded from WHO or in-country control programs and persons may become reinfected.

Although *S. japonicum* is common in some areas of Southeast Asia, especially in areas of China, and *S. mansoni* may be found in the Middle East, as well as Latin America and the Caribbean, clinical experience shows that a vast majority of disease burden in immigrants to the United States occurs in sub-Saharan immigrants and is caused by *S. mansoni* or *S. haematobium*. As mentioned, most immigrants with schistosomiasis are asymptomatic.[4] A majority of patients with schistosomiasis will have an absolute eosinophil count $\geq$450 cells/microliter.[29] All immigrants with absolute eosinophil counts exceeding this number, particularly from sub-Saharan Africa, should be tested for the infection unless another source is identified and the eosinophilia resolves with treatment of an alternative condition.[29]

*S. mansoni* generally causes hepatosplenomegaly and may lead to portal hypertension and its accompanying complications.[1] Clinicians should have a high index of suspicion for *S. mansoni* infection when a patient from sub-Saharan Africa presents with stigmata of liver disease (i.e. variceal bleeding), signs of splenic sequestration (anemia, thrombocytopenia), and enlarged or small liver and/or splenomegaly. Classically, the left lobe of the liver is disproportionately enlarged in early disease. A small cirrhotic liver accompanied by splenomegaly and signs of sequestration indicates late disease, and occasionally surgical intervention is indicated. Ascites heralds end-stage disease, although it can persist for a prolonged period before decompensation. Conversely, splenomegaly only, with a normal liver, may indicate a reactive process in the spleen which may respond to medical therapy alone. Immigrants from endemic areas with any of the above signs or symptoms, especially those from sub-Saharan Africa, should be tested for infection.

Although schistosomiasis may cause acute dysenteric disease, this is uncommon in immigrants because it generally occurs shortly after exposure and infection. However, irritable colonic bowel habits and abdominal pain may indicate infection and should alert the clinician. Also, as immigrants become more integrated into the US healthcare system, it is becoming more common for them to undergo colonoscopy either for symptoms or as a screening test for carcinoma. Colonic polypoid disease (pedunculated or sessile) in this population should be considered schistosomiasis until proven otherwise. This is frequently revealed on histologic examination of a biopsy specimen. Although the polyposis can be severe enough to lead to intestinal obstruction, once outside an endemic area this is rare. Chronic intestinal schistosomiasis, similar to *Entamoeba histolytica*, can closely resemble Crohn's disease, or ulcerative colitis (inflammatory bowel disease (IBD)), leading to profound mismanagement. Any immigrant presenting from endemic areas for schistosomiasis with signs and symptoms consistent with IBD should have schistosomiasis (and amoebiasis) ruled out as a possible diagnosis prior to initiating therapy. Protein-losing enteropathy has been reported with *S. mansoni*.[17]

A patient from sub-Saharan Africa who presents with dysuria, intermittent hematuria (generally terminal), or signs of obstructive uropathy (i.e. abdominal pain, renal failure due to obstruction), recurrent bacteriuria (especially with *Salmonella* spp.), or a diagnosis of squamous cell bladder cancer should be investigated for *S. haematobium*.

Since the pathology of schistosomiasis is based largely on the deposition of highly antigenic eggs (usually in the liver or the bladder), ectopic egg deposition in virtually any organ can lead to disease with accompanying signs and symptoms. This may range from signs of central nervous disease space-occupying lesions or transverse myelitis to appendicitis caused by obstruction of the appendiceal outlet from polyposis. Also, recurrent *Salmonella* bacteremia, cor pulmonale, pneumonitis, genital granulomas, and renal disease (i.e. glomerulonephritis, nephritic syndrome) have all been reported in association with chronic schistosomiasis.[1] Patients who are at risk of schistosomiasis and who have symptoms that are not easily explainable, particularly if they have an absolute eosinophilia, should have the diagnosis of schistosomiasis considered.

In addition, acute disease, while rare in newly arriving immigrants, may be observed in those immigrants who return home to visit friends and relatives (VFRs). An erythematous, itchy, macular contact dermatitis known by various names; swimmers' itch, schistosome dermatitis, clam diggers itch, or sawah itch, may be seen within 24 hours after exposure.[1,4] Schistosome dermatitis can also be acquired in the United States, where it is a zoonotic disease caused by bird specific schistosomes that die in the human epidermis being unable to cause systemic infection or disease.[4]

A distinct illness known as Katayama fever may occur 5–7 weeks after a heavy exposure to human schistosomes. This syndrome is characterized by abrupt onset of fever, chills, abdominal pain, diarrhea, nausea, vomiting, cough, headache, urticaria and may be accompanied by hepatomegaly and lymphadenopathy. This disorder almost invariably is accompanied by a marked eosinophilia.[1,4,5,12]

## Differential diagnosis

The differential diagnosis will depend on the clinical presentation of schistosomiasis. With its myriad of presentations schistosomiasis can, not surprisingly, be confused with many other disorders. The differential diagnosis is extensive for an immigrant from endemic areas with eosinophilia and negative stool examinations.[30,31] Besides schistosomiasis, the most common and important cause of absolute eosinophilia with negative stool examination is *Strongyloides stercoralis*, given its ability to disseminate in the immunosuppressed patient.[30,31] Many other parasitic infections, particularly geohelminths, may also cause this presentation and are variably detected in the stool examination: these infections are, most commonly, hookworm, tapeworm species (i.e. *Hymenolepis nana, Taenia* spp.), hepatic and pulmonary flukes (i.e. opisthorchiasis) among others.[31] Other causes of eosinophilia, less exotic but still common, are ectopic disease (i.e. eczema, asthma) and drug or other allergic reactions. In this population, multiple causes of eosinophilia are the rule rather than the exception, making it necessary to follow the eosinophil count to ensure it returns to normal after treatment of identified pathogens.

A common finding in an otherwise asymptomatic immigrant is hepato- and/or splenomegaly or isolated splenomegaly. The differential diagnosis for this disorder is extensive, but for immigrants and refugees from sub-Saharan Africa, three disorders account for the vast majority of organomegaly: schistosomiasis, malaria, and visceral leishmaniasis. Other etiologies are more common in populations from other endemic areas and include brucellosis, chronic hepatitis (usually hepatitis B or C) and in some populations, alcohol abuse. The remainder of the differential diagnosis, when testing and history have eliminated the aforementioned causes, is quite broad, ranging from malignancy to toxin ingestion.

Intestinal disease must be differentiated from other common disorders such as nonschistosomal polyposis, peptic ulcer disease, IBD, pancreatitis, or other infections such as amoebiasis.

A sub-Saharan immigrant who presents with symptomatic hematuria and/or proteinuria has *S. haematobium* until proven otherwise. This is particularly important because the diagnosis, when considered, is relatively easy to confirm, and invasive studies frequently performed to evaluate nephritic disease, such as biopsy, may be avoided. Also, any patient from an endemic area with obstructive uropathy is also likely to have schistosomiasis. When not apparent from the original presentation, *S. haematobium* must be distinguished from other causes of hemoglobinuria (glomerulonephritis) and proteinuria.

## Diagnostic evaluation

The patient's presentation and suspected species of schistosomiasis will determine the diagnostic evaluation. The three main diagnostic tests used to identify schistosomes are microscopic detection of eggs in urine or stool, biopsy of infected tissue, and serology.[4] Radiologic imaging may be useful in assessing the level of suspicion of infection, as well as assisting in evaluation of the extent of disease.[4] Since the diagnosis can be elusive, under some circumstances, a therapeutic treatment trial may be necessary,

### Laboratory evaluation

Examination of stool and urine for schistosome eggs is the least expensive and most common method of diagnosing schistosomiasis. A stool ova and parasite (O&P) examination is the most widely available method. A wet-prep, performed at some centers, is very insensitive for detecting infection. Most centers in the United States use a 10% formalin, fixed, concentrated, preparation examined microscopically as a wet mount.[1] This technique identifies a variety of geohelminth and protozoal parasites but is not particularly sensitive for schistosomiasis. For a standard technique, three morning stools should be collected, preferably every other day. The Kato-Katz thick-smear stool examination, which requires approximately 40–50 mg of feces, is one of the most widely used techniques outside the United States.[32] The sensitivity of this technique is highly dependent on technical competency. Stool O&P may detect all species that infect humans.

Urine O&P examination is accomplished by one of several simple techniques including microscopic examination of urine after sedimentation (gravity settling or centrifugation) or micropore filter. The excretion of schistosome eggs into the urine is not uniform over time, and samples collected between 10 a.m and 2 p.m. are more likely to be positive.[5]

When stool or urine samples are negative, it is occasionally necessary to perform invasive tests to confirm the diagnosis of schistosomiasis (e.g cystoscopy or biopsy of bladder or rectal mucosa).[4] These tests are particularly helpful when partially treated disease is suspected. These biopsies are usually performed when urine and stool tests are repeatedly negative but the clinical suspicion remains high.

Serologic screening tests for infection with *Schistosoma* spp. are available in US commercial laboratories. Commercial enzyme-linked immunosorbent assays (ELISA) employ *S. mansoni* antigens and should detect most *S. mansoni* infections but may lack sensitivity in the detection of some *S. haematobium* infections and most *S. japonicum* infections.[33,34] Reference testing is available at the Centers for Disease Control and Prevention through the State Public Health Laboratories (PHL). Antigens of all three human species are available for use when appropriate, resulting in increased test specificity. If the results of commercial assays are not compatible with the clinical presentation and infection is still suspected, specimens accompanied by the patient's travel and exposure history and previous lab results may be submitted for testing through the PHL. While serologic tests may be very useful to determine whether the patient has been infected or not, they cannot be used to determine whether the infection is active because antibodies may persist for years after cure.[33,34]

## Radiological and endoscopic evaluation

The most useful radiologic tool for assessment of both hepatic and bladder involvement is sonography (ultrasound). Hepatic ultrasound may demonstrate thickened portal vessel tracts (Symmers' pipestem fibrosis) and increased portal vein diameter, correlating with increased portal pressures.[4,6] Splenomegaly, when missed by physical examination, may also be apparent.[1] In late-stage disease, cirrhosis and ascites may also be seen. Likewise, urologic evaluation also demonstrates findings associated with schistosomiasis.[4]

Other tests may either incidentally identify disease or may be helpful in the diagnostic evaluation. Contrast-enhanced barium enema, barium swallow, and intravenous pyelogram may identify abnormalities, alerting the clinician to possible disease. Advanced methods such as computed tomography (CT) may reveal similar findings to ultrasound but may provide more detail. Esophageal endoscopy may document esophageal varices. Cystoscopy and sigmoidoscopy or colonoscopy may identify granulomatous polyps in either the bladder or the colon. Although liver biopsy may also be diagnostic, this is not a recommended method for confirming diagnosis under normal circumstances.

## Therapeutic trial

An important limitation of serologic testing for *Schistosoma* antibodies is the inability of the tests to distinguish new infections from previous infections. In patients with no prior treatment for schistosomiasis, positive serologic tests are evidence of prior or ongoing infection and treatment is warranted. However, in patients who may have received treatment in the past, a positive antibody test cannot differentiate old from current infection. To help determine if the infection is current, additional tests such as stool and urine examinations and rectal biopsies may be performed. Positive findings on these tests would support the presence of an ongoing infection. Because stool and urine examinations may be insensitive, patients may not want a rectal biopsy, antigen assays are not widely available (and require further study), and praziquantel is safe and effective, presumptive treatment in situations in which the clinical suspicion is high is reasonable. In most cases, patients will have an absolute eosinophilia which, after time, weeks to months, will decrease with successful treatment.

## ICD-9 Codes

- 120 Schistosomiasis
- 120.0 *Schistosoma haematobium*
- 120.1 *Schistosoma mansoni*

**Table 39.2 Table of drug used for schistosomiasis treatment**

| Drug | Adult dose | Pediatric dose* | Formulation | Efficacy | Adverse events | Comments; use in pregnancy |
|------|-----------|-----------------|-------------|----------|----------------|----------------------------|
| Praziquantel | 20 mg/kg/dose orally in two doses†, 6–8 hours apart | 20 mg/kg/dose orally in two doses†, 6–8 hours apart | Tablets | 60–90% | Gastrointestinal | Pregnancy category B |

\* Praziquantel is not recommended for children <4 years of age.
† Three doses 6–8 hours apart for *Schistosoma japonicum* or *S. mekongi* infections.

- 120.2 *Schistosoma japonicum*
- 120.3 Cutaneous schistosomiasis
- 120.8 Other specified schistosomiasis
- 120.9 Schistosomiasis, unspecified
- V75.5 Schistosomiasis special screening examination

## Treatment

Praziquantel is the drug of choice to treat schistosomiasis (Table 39.2).[3] For infections due to *S. mansoni* and *S. haematobium*, the regimen is 20 mg/kg/dose given in each of two oral doses, 6–8 hours apart. For infections due to *S. japonicum* and *S. mekongi*, 20 mg/kg/dose should be given in each of three oral doses, 6–8 hours apart.[1] If the initial regimen is unsuccessful, repeat treatments with praziquantel are warranted.[1]

Praziquantel is effective in treating schistosomiasis and produces cure rates of 60–90%.[1,5,16] Its activity against schistosomiasis is derived from its ability to interfere with the adult worm's ability to elude host immune mechanisms; it also disrupts $Ca^{2+}$ homeostasis.[35] Praziquantel is a very well-tolerated drug and has been used extensively in WHO treatment programs.[3,36] When there are any untoward effects of the medication, complaints such as epigastric or generalized abdominal pain, nausea, diarrhea (which may be bloody), dizziness, fever, headache, and pruritus are the most frequent. Praziquantel is a pregnancy category B drug. In the United States, praziquantel is not approved for use in children less than 4 years of age.[36]

Praziquantel will also kill *Taenia solium* cysticerci, which may provoke seizure activity in patients with neurocysticercosis.[12] Care should be taken to reduce this risk by inquiring about seizure activity in patients and testing for cysticercosis, if necessary.

The only potential alternative to praziquantel available in the United States is oxaminiquine.[1] However, this medication has limited availability and is not as efficacious as praziquantel. In addition, oxaminiquine is only effective against *S. mansoni*.[1,16] If used, a single 15 mg/kg oral dose is recommended.[16] Reported side effects to oxaminiquine include fever, nausea, diarrhea, headaches, and dizziness.[16,35]

Another potential alternative medication for *S. haematobium* is metrifonate. It also has very limited availability and is produced in few countries. If used, 7.5–10 mg/kg/dose, on alternate weeks, for 3 weeks is the recommended regimen.[16] Because this medication is an organophosphate derivative with anticholinesterase activity, side effects include nausea, diarrhea, emesis, bronchospasm, and vertigo.[16,35] This medication is not approved by the Food and Drug Administration for use against schistosomiasis.[16]

Steroids and anti-inflammatory medications may sometimes be given along with antiparasitic therapy. These are most frequently given in the setting of acute infection or when there is central nervous system involvement.[5]

Following treatment for schistosomiasis, it is unnecessary to perform testing to confirm the cure unless the patient demonstrates signs and symptoms suggestive of schistosomiasis. As mentioned, chronic eosinophilia should prompt an evaluation for other potential causes of eosinophilia.

### Management of patients for whom initial treatment is unsuccessful

If the initial regimen with praziquantel is unsuccessful, repeat treatments with praziquantel are warranted.[1,16] The dose and duration may be increased, but discussion with an expert in the field is recommended before altering the recommended treatment protocol.

## Prevention

Schistosomiasis is prevented by avoiding exposure to fresh water contaminated with the cercariae. Travelers to the endemic countries should be instructed to avoid contact with fresh water during their trip. Even limited exposure to heavily contaminated fresh water can result in infection. Prophylactic medication is not recommended.

## Infection Control Measures

Standard hygiene and sanitation precautions, especially hand washing, should be reinforced to infected patients. Because the United States lacks appropriate snail vectors, the parasite cannot be transmitted to others. Persons treated in the United States should be reassured that they cannot transmit the disease to others in the United States.[5] Schistosomiasis may be reportable to local health departments.

### Clinical Pearls

- Infection may be asymptomatic.[12]
- Eosinophilia is a common marker for infection.[1]
- *S. mansoni*, *S. mekongi*, and *S. japonicum* are typically shed in stool.[1]
- *S. haematobium* is typically shed in urine.[5]
- Immigrants from Sub-Saharan Africa have the highest prevalence of infection.[5]
- When the diagnosis is difficult to confirm, a therapeutic trial may be occasionally warranted.

### Special Considerations for Immigrants

- A large proportion of immigrants and refugees settling in the US come from countries endemic for schistosomiasis.
- Most infected immigrants and refugees were likely infected as children and may have asymptomatic infections.[4]
- Infection in the VFR returning traveler is a distinct possibility.[4]

## References

1. Ross AGP, Bartley PB, Sleigh AC, et al. Schistosomiasis. N Engl J Med 2002; 346(16):1212–1220.
2. Chitsulo L, Engels D, Montressor A, Savioli L. The global status of schistosomiasis and its control. Acta Trop 2000; 77:41–51.
3. World Health Organization. WHO Expert Committee on the Control of Schistosomiasis. Prevention and control of schistosomiasis and soil-transmitted helminthiasis: report of a WHO expert committee. 2001: Geneva, Switzerland. Who technical report series: 912.
4. Lucey DR, Maguire JH. Schistosomiasis. Inf Dis Clin N Amer 1993; 7(3):635–653.
5. Strickland GT, Ramirez BL. Schistosomiasis. In: Strickland GT, editor. Hunter's tropical medicine and emerging infectious diseases. 8th ed. Philadelphia: WB Saunders Company; 2000:804–832.
6. Vennervald BJ, Dunne DW. Morbidity in schistosomiasis: an update. Curr Opin Infect Dis 2004; 17:439–447.
7. Centers for Disease Control and Prevention. Health information for international travel 2005–2006. Atlanta: U.S. Department of Health and Human Services, Public Health Service, 2005:266–270.
8. Hopkins DR. Homing in on old helminthes. Am J Trop Med Hyg 1992; 46:626.
9. Centers for Disease Control and Prevention. Schistosomiasis in U.S. Peace Corps volunteers – Malawi, 1992. MMWR 1993; 42:565–570.
10. Oomen JMV, de Wolf J, Jobin WR. Health and irrigatio. ILRI publication 45. Wageningen: ILRI, 1990.
11. Corachan M. Schistosomiasis and international travel. Clin Infect Dis 2002; 35:446–450.
12. Gryseals B, Palman K, Clerinx J, Kestens L. Human Schistosomiasis. Lancet 2006; 368:1106–1118.
13. Jordan P, Webbe G, Sturrock R. Human Schistosomiasis. Wallingford, England: LAB, 1993.
14. Bethlem, EP, Schettino G, Carralho CR. Pulmonary Schistosomiasis. Curr Opin Pulm Med 1997; 3:361–365.
15. Cetron MS, Chitsulo L, Sullivan JJ, et al. Schistosomiasis in Lake Malawi. Lancet 1996; 348:1274–1278.
16. Olds GR, Dasarathy S. Recent advances in schistosomiasis. Curr Infect Dis Rep 2001; 3(1):59–67.
17. Hussein A, Medany S, Abou el Magd AM, et al. Multiple endoscopic polypectomies for schistosomal polyposis of the colon. Lancet 1983; 1:673–674.
18. King CL. Initiation and regulation of disease in schistosomiasis. In: Mahmoud AAF, ed. Schistosomiasis. London: Imperial College Press, 2001:213–264.
19. de Cleva R, Herman P, PUbliese V, et al. Prevalence of pulmonary hypertension in patients with hepatosplenic Mansonic schistosomiasis – prospective study. Hepatogastroenterology 2003; 50:2028–2030.
20. Baldawi AF, Michael MS. Risk factors for hepatocellular carcinoma in Egypt: the role of hepatitis B viral infection and Schistosomiasis. Anticancer Res 1999; 19: 4564–4569.
21. Ye XP, Fu YL, Anderson Rm, Nolkes DJ. Absence of relationship between *schistosoma japonicum* and hepatitis B virus infection in the Dongtong Lake Region, China. Epidemiol Infect 1998; 121:193–195.
22. Kamal SM, Graham CS, He Q, et al. Kinetics of intrahepatic hepatitis C virus (HCV)-specific CD4+ T cell responses in HCV and Schistosoma mansoni coinfection: relation to progression of liver fibrosis. J Infect Dis 2004 2004; 189:1140–1150.
23. King CH. Disease in Schistosomiasis haematobia. In: Mahmoud AAF, ed. Schistosomiasis. London: Imperial College Press, 2001:265–295.
24. Poggensee G, Feldmeier H. Female genital Schistosomiasis: facts and hypotheses. Acta Trop 2001; 79: 193–210.
25. Goldsmith PC, Leslie TA, Sams V, et al. Lesions of Schistosomiasis mimicking warts on the vulva. BMJ 1993; 307:556–557.

26. Vilana R, Grachan M, Gascon J, et al. Schistosomiasis of the male genital tract: transrectal sonographic findings. J Virol 1997; 158:1491–1493.

27. Centers for Disease Control and Prevention. Recommendations for presumptive treatment of schistosomiasis and strongyloidiasis among the Lost Boys and Girls of Sudan. http://www.cdc.gov/ncidod/dq/ lostboysandgirlssudan/updated_presumptive_tx_recc_ 061305.htm. Accessed December 2, 2005.

28. Centers for Disease Control and Prevention. Recommendations for presumptive treatment of schistosomiasis and stronglyoidiasis among the Somali Bantu refugees. http://www.cdc.gov/ncidod/dq/somali_ bantu/presumptive_tx_reccs_061305.htm. Accessed December 2, 2005.

29. Barnett ED. Infectious disease screening for refugees resettled in the United States. CID 2004; 34:833–841.

30. Stauffer WM, Kamat D, Walker PF. Screening of international immigrants, refugees, and adoptees. Prim Care Clin Office Pract 2002; 29:879–905.

31. Walker PF, Jaranson J, Refugee and immigrant health care. Med Clin N Amer 1999; 83(4):1103–1120.

32. Katz N, Chaves A, Pelligrino J. A simple device for quantitative stool thick-smear technique in Schistosomiasis mansoni. Rev Inst Trop Sao Paulo 1972; 14:397–400.

33. Tsang VC, Wilkins PP. Immunodiagnosis of schistosomiasis. Immunol Invest 1997; 26:175–188.

34. Barsoum IS, Kamal KA, Bassily S, et al. Diagnosis of human schistosomiasis by detection of circulating cathodic antigen with a monoclonal antibody. J Infect Dis 1991; 164:1010–1013.

35. Utzinger J, Keiser J. Schistosomiasis and soil-transmitted helminthiasis: common drugs for treatment and control. Expert Opin Pharmacother 2004; 5(2):263–285.

36. Physicians' Desk Reference. Biltricide. In: Murray L, editor. Physicians' Desk Reference. Montvale: Thomson PDR. 839.

# CHAPTER 40

# Strongyloides

David R. Boulware

## Strongyloides stercoralis at a Glance

- Occurs worldwide; exposure is via larvae in contaminated soil penetrating skin.
- Life cycle is autoinfective within the human host requiring no re-exposure or intermediate host. Infection persists for life.
- Screening of immigrants with stool examination for ova and parasites is problematic because of intermittent shedding, with 25–50% of infections missed by three stool ova and parasite (O&P) examinations.
- Unexplained eosinophilia (>450 cells/dL) with negative stool examinations should prompt either:
  1. Strongyloides IgG serology;
  2. Three additional stool O&Ps minimum;
  3. Empiric treatment with re-checking eosinophilia in 3 months.
- Treatment is with ivermectin 200 mcg/kg orally × 1, repeated once.
- Steroid administration can result in hyperinfection with widespread dissemination of Strongyloides larvae, Gram-negative sepsis, and death.

## Epidemiology

*Strongyloides stercoralis* infection is a common cause of morbidity and mortality throughout the world, particularly in developing countries where there are an estimated 100 million cases. Strongyloidiasis is extremely common, particularly in Southeast Asia, but is also endemic to many other tropical and subtropical areas such as Latin America, sub-Saharan Africa, as well as temperate areas such as the Appa-

lachian region of the United States. Death from strongyloidiasis is primarily due to hyperinfection or disseminated disease. Intestinal parasites are very common in immigrants and refugees from developing countries with prevalence rates among untreated Southeast Asian refugees approaching 50%.[1-3] Immigrants from Cambodia, Laos, and northeastern Thailand are at a particularly high risk of *Strongyloides* infection.[4-6] In such immigrants, *Strongyloides* is likely to be the third most common intestinal parasite after *Giardia* and hookworm. Infection in the nonendemic setting is predominately among immigrants or expatriates having previously resided in endemic areas.[7,8]

In developed countries, almost all deaths attributed to helminths occur secondary to *Strongyloides stercoralis* hyperinfection syndrome or dissemination.[8] Hyperinfection occurs in association to immunosuppression, particularly corticosteroids. Although once thought rare, recent evidence suggests that disseminated *Strongyloides* may be relatively common in high-risk populations but may be misdiagnosed as only Gram-negative sepsis.[9] Despite this feared iatrogenic complication of *Strongyloides*, the infection generally presents with diffuse, mild symptoms including gastrointestinal, dermatologic, or respiratory symptoms.[10,11] Most chronic carriers are asymptomatic.[12-14]

## Etiology

Infection occurs via skin contact with contaminated soil containing infective *Strongyloides* larvae. These larvae cause infection by penetrating exposed skin. The larvae burrow until they enter the venous circulation, traveling to the lungs. Once in the lungs, the larvae migrate into the alveoli, ascending the bronchial tree to enter the gastrointestinal system. Within 4 weeks, mature females reside in the small intestine and begin to shed eggs. Eggs may pass into the environment to propagate an external infectious cycle or hatch into rhabditiform larvae in the colon and burrow through the bowel wall repeating an autoinfective cycle. This internal autoinfective cycle is unique to *Strongyloides*,[1] creating the ability for indefinite lifelong carriage among infected hosts and requiring no re-exposure.

With immunosuppression, particularly corticosteroids, increased numbers of larvae can cause hyperinfection, migrating through the bowel wall and frequently causing Gram-negative bacteremia and sepsis. Dissemination can also occur when larvae migrate to end organs not usually involved in the normal cycle of the parasite, including brain and skin.

## Clinical Manifestations

In chronic infection, clinical symptoms are non-specific and generally mild in chronic infection. Abdominal (40%), pulmonary (20–25%), and chronic skin (15%) complaints are very common; however, these complaints are unfortunately very common in immigrants in general. Importantly, up to 10% of patients may present with wheezing or other symptoms mimicking asthma. Previous case-control studies have indicated that asthma does not seem to be caused by strongyloidiasis; however, misdiagnosis with subsequent steroid therapy is problematic. Prior to diagnoses of strongyloidiasis, patients are commonly misdiagnosed with irritable bowel syndrome, somatization disorder, or 'psychogenic pruritus.' Often, frustration may exist for both the patient and the healthcare provider. Among immigrants with eosinophilia, vague diagnoses should prompt exclusion of chronic helminthic infection, such as strongyloidiasis.

## Diagnosis

The traditional diagnostic method is the stool examination for ova and parasites (O&P). Unfortunately, the sensitivity of O&Ps for chronic *Strongyloides* infection is poor. Traditionally, three stool collections yield a detection rate of only 50% for rhabditiform larvae. With experienced technicians and untreated populations, the sensitivity in the largest case series was 50% per stool O&P.[14] However, even

in the same study, 16% of patients had three prior negative stool O&Ps (mean 3.6 ± 2.1; maximum 9) before eventual diagnosis.[14] Institutional variability exists. Interestingly, half of those antecedent specimens negative for *Strongyloides* did harbor other parasites.

In 85% of cases, chronic infection is associated with mild eosinophilia with an absolute count >450 eosinophils/dL.[6,14] Eosinophilia is a non-specific finding but in an immigrant should always prompt an evaluation for intestinal helminths. The positive predictive value of eosinophilia, i.e. the probability of an immigrant with eosinophilia having an intestinal parasite, is >75%.[11] More importantly, this predictive ability of eosinophilia is not just for new immigrants, but anyone with a history of immigration. Among refugees who were initially screened at immigration into Canada and Australia, several studies have shown that 20–25% of immigrants will still harbor intestinal parasites 6–12 years later.[11,15] In the United States, diagnosis is also often delayed, with the average being 4 years after arrival and 25% being identified after 6 years.[14] This delay in diagnosis is typical.

A more sensitive diagnostic technique is the agar plate method ('parasite cultures'), where 3–4 grams of feces are placed on nutrient agar in a Petri dish, sealed, and left at room temperature for 3 days. While the stool flora grows, the rhabitidiform larvae mature and migrate on the plate. The plate is examined daily for the presence of tracks or moving larvae. This is a more sensitive technique than the trichrome O&P. The 'parasite culture' is very simple to perform; however, most microbiology laboratories do not routinely employ the technique. Additionally, larvae are infectious, creating a hazard for laboratory personnel.

The gold standard for the diagnosis of *Strongyloides* is serology.[1,6] *Strongyloides stercoralis* IgG serology is available from commercial reference labs as well as the CDC. The CDC's serologic technique is over 95% sensitive for detecting persons chronically infected.[6] For commercial reference labs, knowledge as to the validity of the test is important. In some cases, 'home brew' assays developed by commercial reference laboratories themselves may lack adequate validation because of a lack of suitable specimens and must be interpreted with caution. In such cases, the clinician should not hesitate to ask for sensitivity, specificity, and validation data from the lab.

If an immigrant presents with unexplained Gram-negative sepsis and is immunosuppressed, one should exclude strongyloidiasis. In cases of hyperinfection, larvae may be found in sputum, stool, or

**Table 40.1 Drugs used to treat strongyloidiasis**

| Drug | Dose | Duration | Efficacy | Adverse events |
|------|------|----------|----------|----------------|
| Ivermectin | 200 µg/kg/day 3 and 6 mg tablets | 1–2 doses | 85%–95% for 1 dose 99% 2 doses | Dizziness, dyspepsia 8% overall. In high burdens of *Loa loa*, encephalitis may be precipitated[a] |
| Albendazole | 400 mg <50 kg: 7.5 mg/kg | 2 × daily for 3–7 days | 62–84% | <2% GI side effects <1% pancytopenia |
| Thiabendazole | 1.5 g <70 kg: 25 mg/kg 500 mg tablets, suspension | 2 × daily for 3 days | 90% | 66% GI side effects Rare, but fatal hypersensitivity reactions resulting in cholestatic hepatitis [18 published cases] |

[a] The incidence of ivermectin-induced encephalitis due to mass *Loa loa* microfilariae death is approximately 1 in 800 000 ivermectin treatments overall in West Africa.[16] However, adverse events are highest in ivermectin naïve populations with high burdens of microfilariae (e.g. >1% adverse reactions in persons with >30 000 mf/mL). Reactions occur 24–36 hours after ivermectin treatment with fever, fatigue, headache, arthralgias, and markedly elevated CRP.[17] Death or disability occurs in 35% with encephalitis.[16]

biopsy specimens that may be diagnostic. Typically at this stage, copious numbers of parasites exist. In persons with respiratory failure, a sputum culture may incidentally reveal the motile larvae. These serendipitous diagnoses usually occur very late and are not 100%, as undoubtedly strongyloidiasis is underrecognized. Eosinophilia may or may not be present, and lack of eosinophilia is associated with a near 100% mortality rate.

# Treatment

The current treatment of choice is ivermectin 200 µg/kg/day orally for 1–2 days for chronic infection (Table 40.1). A one-time oral administration results in eradication rates of 85–95% in infected children. A prudent recommendation is to administer a second dose to insure almost 100% eradication. By tradition, the second dose is often given two weeks after the first; two consecutive days of dosing achieve close to 100% cure rates and likely better compliance.[17a,17b] A suboptimal alternative to ivermectin would be albendazole 400 mg/dose twice daily orally for 3–7 days. In a head-to-head comparison with ivermectin, 3 days of albendazole was 25–30% less effective.[18] Thiabendazole has significant gastrointestinal side effects which make compliance an issue and can decrease efficacy.

There are minimal data on anthelmintic treatment during pregnancy. Both ivermectin and albendazole are teratogenic in animals. If an asymptomatic individual is screened and known to be pregnant, deferring treatment until after completion of the pregnancy is appropriate. Inadvertent administration of ivermectin during the first 2–3 weeks of pregnancy has not resulted in any increased rates of birth defects or developmental abnormalities during the ongoing antifiliariasis campaign in Africa.[19] Ivermectin is not active against hookworm, a common co-pathogen.

## Treatment of hyperinfection/disseminated disease

Persons with hyperinfection typically have a mortality rate of 50%. Treatment ideally should be with ivermectin 200 µg/kg orally for 7 days, although initiating therapy promptly with any agent pending ivermectin availability is recommended. Discontinuation of corticosteroids is imperative. Ivermectin, albendazole, and thiabendazole are all oral agents; thus, in critically ill patients alternative routes of administration are frequently necessary. Daily monitoring for viable rhabditiform larvae should occur during treatment, especially for oral therapy in a critically ill individual, to demonstrate response to therapy. When paralytic ileus precludes oral or nasogastric administration or this therapy fails, rectal administration daily and subcutaneous veterinarian, parenteral formulations every 48 hours for three doses have been used successfully.[18]

## Follow-up

Eosinophilia should resolve with successful therapy within 3–6 months.[6] If eosinophilia persists, failure should be assumed and empiric retreatment given. *Strongyloides* serologic titers should be expected to decrease by >40% by 6 months after therapy.[6]

# Prevention

Any occupation with intimate exposure to soil, classically agricultural workers, is at risk virtually worldwide. Even in developed countries, such as Spain or the southeastern US, agricultural workers may harbor *Strongyloides*. Humans are the only known host for *S. stercoralis*. Larvae are infectious.

## Clinical Pearls

- Strongyloides infection is life long, unlike most helminths.
- Hyperinfection after immunosuppression can occur decades after immigration.[9,20,21]
- Treatment errors occur most frequently when multiple parasites are present.

## Special Considerations for Immigrants

- Infection is lifelong, and may be recognized years to decades after leaving an endemic area.
- Albendazole given previously at emigration may decrease parasite burden but not eradicate all *Strongyloides*. This may increase the difficulty of detection with initial screening O&Ps:
  - *Strongyloides* IgG serology, persistent eosinophilia are helpful diagnostics
- Multiple intestinal helminths may be present in untreated refugees
  - Multiple parasites increase difficulty of treatment options
  - Multiple parasites increase error rate, inadequate strongyloides therapy
  - Non-pathogenic vs. pathogenic parasites may create confusion.

## Refugee camps

Refugees often can be segregated into two groups: those having resided in 'official' camps recognized by international organizations such as the Red Cross, and those in 'unofficial' camps. While the political rationale is extensive, the repercussions are apparent. In the official camps, intestinal parasites are a recognized problem, principally of childhood nutrition. The standard procedure is for refugees to receive intermittent antiparasitic therapy. Since 1999, this typically has been doses of albendazole. Albendazole is a broad-spectrum antiparasitic effective against most helminths. Importantly, a single dose is ineffective against *Strongyloides*. A few doses will decrease the helminth burden but are unlikely to eradicate *Strongyloides* carriage.

The problem with noneradicative therapy for *Strongyloides* is that it makes subsequent detection more difficult. The traditional sensitivity of a series of three standard O&P collections is approximately 50%. Partial therapy will decrease the worm burden, decreasing the likelihood of detection upon subsequent O&P screening. This increases the probability of continued occult carriage of *Strongyloides* in the refugee population.

In unofficial refugees and immigrants, intermittent anthelmintic therapy does not occur. This eliminates the problem with partial therapy and occult *Strongyloides* infection. The opposite problem can be encountered, whereby multiple parasites are present in stool specimens. First, laboratory technicians may miss the rare *Strongyloides* rhabditiform larvae when thousands of *Ascaris* ova are teeming throughout the stool specimen. Secondly, physicians may err with prescribing treatment.

# References

1. Nutman TB, Ottesen EA, Ieng S, et al. Eosinophilia in Southeast Asian refugees: evaluation at a referral center. J Infect Dis 1987; 155:309–313.
2. Hoffman SL, Barrett-Connor E, Norcross W, et al. Intestinal parasites in Indochinese immigrants. Am J Trop Med Hyg 1981; 30:340–343.
3. Lindes C. Intestinal parasites in Laotian refugees. J Fam Pract 1979; 9:819–822.
4. Wiesenthal AM, Nickels MK, Hashimoto KG, et al. Intestinal parasites in Southeast Asian refugees. Prevalence in a community of Laotians. JAMA 1980; 244:2543–2544.
5. Jongsuksuntigul P, Intapan PM, Wongsaroj T, et al. Prevalence of *Strongyloides stercoralis* infection in northeastern Thailand (agar plate culture detection). J Med Assoc Thai 2003; 86:737–741.
6. Loutfy MR, Wilson M, Keystone JS, et al. Serology and eosinophil count in the diagnosis and management of strongyloidiasis in a non-endemic area. Am J Trop Med Hyg 2002; 66:749–752.
7. Hira PR, Al-Ali F, Shweiki HM, et al. Strongyloidiasis: challenges in diagnosis and management in non-endemic Kuwait. Annal Trop Med Parasitol 2004; 98:261–270.
8. Muennig P, Pallin D, Sell RL, et al. The cost-effectiveness of strategies for the treatment of intestinal parasites in immigrants. N Engl J Med 1999; 340:773–779.
9. Lim S, Katz K, Krajden S, et al. Complicated and fatal *Strongyloides* infection in Canadians: risk factors, diagnosis and management. Canadian Med Assoc J 2004; 171:479–484.
10. Siddiqui AA, Berk SL. Diagnosis of *Strongyloides stercoralis* infection. Clin Infect Dis 2001; 33:1040–1047.

11. de Silva S, Saykao P, Kelly H, et al. Chronic *Strongyloides stercoralis* infection in Laotian immigrants and refugees 7–20 years after resettlement in Australia. Epidemiol Infect 2002; 128:439–444.

12. Gyorkos TW, Genta RM, Viens P, et al. Seroepidemiology of *Strongyloides* infection in the South East Asian refugee population in Canada. Am J Epidemiol 1990; 132:257–264.

13. Román-Sánchez P, Pastor-Guzmán A, Moreno-Guillén S, et al. High prevalence of *Strongyloides stercoralis* among farm workers on the Spanish Mediterranean coast. Analysis of the predictive factors of infection in developed countries. Am J Trop Med Hyg 2003; 69:336–340.

14. Boulware DR, Stauffer III WM, Hendel-Patterson BR, et al. Maltreatment of *Strongyloides* infection: Case series and worldwide physicians-in-training survey. Am J Med 2007; In press.

15. Gyorkos TW, MacLean JD, Viens P, et al. Intestinal parasite infection in the Kampuchean refugee population 6 years after resettlement in Canada. J Infect Dis 1992; 166:413–417.

16. Twum-Danso NA. Serious adverse events following treatment with ivermectin for onchocerciasis control: a review of reported cases. Filaria J 2003; 2(Suppl 1):S3.

17. Chippaux JP, Boussinesq M, Gardon J, et al. Severe adverse reaction risks during mass treatment with ivermectin in loiasis-endemic areas. Parasitol Today 1996; 12:448–450.

17a. Igual-Adell R, Oltra-Alcaraz C, Sanchez-Sanchez P, Matogo-Oyana J, Rodriquez-Calabuig D. Efficacy and safety of ivermectin and thiabendazole in the treatment of strongyloidiasis. Expert Opin Pharmacother 2004; 5:2615–2619.

17b. Gann PH, Neva FA, Gam AA. A randomized trial of single- and two dose ivermectin versus thiabendazole for treatment of strongyloidiasis. J Infect Dis 1994; 169:1076–1079.

18. Muenning P, Pallin D, Challah C, Khan K. The cost-effectiveness of invermectin vs. albendazole in the presumptive treatment of strongyloidiasis in immigrants to the United States. Epidemiol Infect 2004; 132:1055–1063.

19. Marty FM, Lowry CM, Rodriguez M, et al. Treatment of human disseminated strongyloidiasis with a parenteral veterinary formulation of ivermectin. Clin Infect Dis 2005; 41:e5–e8.

20. Ferreira MS, Nishioka Sde A, Borges AS, et al. Strongyloidiasis and infection due to human immunodeficiency virus: 25 cases at a Brazilian teaching hospital, including seven cases of hyperinfection syndrome. Clin Infect Dis 1999; 28:154–155.

21. Newberry A, Williams DN, Stauffer WM, Boulware DR, Hendel-Paterson BR, Walker PF. Strongyloides hyperinfection presenting as acute respiratory failure and gram-negative sepsis. Chest 2005; 128:3681–3684.

# CHAPTER 41

# Preventive Healthcare in Children

Rajal Mody

## Introduction

Children in immigrant families are the fastest growing segment of the pediatric population in the United States. From 2002 to 2004, on average, 156 000 children under the age of 16 years legally immigrated to the United States each year and approximately 22 000 foreign-born children were adopted into US families annually.[1] The number of children entering the country illegally is unknown, but has been estimated at 30 000 per year.[2] Over 75% of children in the United States living in immigrant families were born in the United States.[3] These US-born children have similar health disparities to those experienced by foreign-born children. From 1990 to 1997, the number of children in immigrant families grew by 47%, compared to a 7% increase in children of non-immigrant families.[3] In 1997, 14 million, or nearly one in every five children living in the US, were immigrants or had immigrant parents.[3] One in every four children who live in a low-income family has immigrant parents.[4]

Knowledge regarding the unique health needs of immigrant children has lagged behind the staggering growth in their numbers. Understanding of these needs is starting to form as more research accrues. The information available has revealed important health risks. Although it is difficult to translate these findings into a formal comprehensive set of recommendations for preventive healthcare for immigrant children given the enormous ethnic, cultural, and socioeconomic diversity within this group, to a certain extent some common health issues may be shared among children of different backgrounds. The goal of this chapter is to highlight some of these

issues as areas in which to focus efforts to reduce health disparities of immigrant children.

Children in immigrant families face the same health concerns as the general pediatric population. In addition, these children are confronted with multiple factors before, during and after immigration that increase their susceptibility to several health conditions. These factors are complex and interrelated. Categorizing these factors into four broad topics may help form a framework of immigrant children's preventive healthcare needs (Table 41.1). These categories include: (1) preexisting health inequities, (2) acculturation, the process of assimilating into a new culture, (3) unique environmental exposures and injuries, and (4) 'life-course theory,' a developing understanding of how childhood events and growth patterns may influence the development of chronic illnesses later in life.

It is important to remember while examining these topics that children of immigrant families face obstacles in receiving healthcare of any kind, let alone preventive care (Table 41.2). Perhaps the most obvious barrier is lower rates of health insurance. Among foreign-born children with legal citizenship, only 48% were found to have health insurance and only 66% had an identified regular source of healthcare in 1997, compared to 80% and 92%, respectively, among native-born children of the working poor.[5] The disparities are even greater among specific immigrant groups. The largest minority group of children in the United States is Hispanic. Mexican-Americans comprise the largest proportion of this diverse population.[6] In 1995, Mexican-American adolescents were less likely than adolescents of Cuban, Dominican, Puerto Rican, or Central and South American origin to have had a routine physical

**Table 41.1 Key topics in pediatric immigrant preventive health**

1. Preexisting health inequities
2. Effects of acculturation
3. Environmental exposures and injuries
4. Effects of childhood growth patterns and events on the development of chronic illnesses

**Table 41.2 Barriers to preventive healthcare**

1. High rates of uninsured immigrant children
2. Linguistic isolation:
   Decreased awareness of available resources
   Difficulty navigating healthcare systems
   Difficulty understanding recommendations
   Decreased ability of parents to advocate for their child's needs
3. Healthcare providers lack familiarity with different cultures
4. Parental stress related to relocation
5. Fear of apprehension of family members with illegal immigration status
6. Limited caretaking of children and adolescents who have immigrated without their parents

examination, highlighting significant variation in healthcare access within the broad ethnic group of Hispanic-Americans.[7] The low healthcare utilization of Mexican-American adolescents is at least partially explained by poor insurance coverage. Only 36% of first-generation Mexican-American children were found to have medical insurance between 1988 and 1994. Although second- and third-generation Mexican-American children had higher rates of coverage, they were still more likely to be uninsured as compared to non-Hispanic black and white children under 16 years old.[6]

These figures have likely worsened in recent years due to changes in Medicaid coverage. For example, the prevalence of uninsured foreign-born children living with low-educated single mothers has increased by 13.5% in response to the Personal Responsibility and Work Opportunity Reconciliation Act of 1996, without a corresponding increase seen among US-born children.[8] Even in states that have responded with programs to provide insurance to all low-income children, many children in immigrant families have not been insured due to various obstacles experienced by their parents.[9]

In 2000, after adjusting for insurance coverage, Asian, Hispanic, and black children were less likely than white children in the US to have a usual source of care, health professional or doctor visit, and dental visit in the past year.[10] Therefore, other important barriers, in addition to lack of health insurance, are present. One of these obstacles is the significantly lower awareness among immigrant parents of healthcare and other support services available to their families in the US.[11] The same holds true in Canada despite universal healthcare insurance.[12] This decreased awareness of health-related resources may stem from linguistic isolation, defined as the lack of anyone over 14 years of age in a household able to speak English.[11,12] In addition to decreasing awareness, linguistic isolation, present in over a quarter of all immigrant families with school-age children,[13] impairs parents' ability to make medical appointments, understand health recommendations, and advocate for the needs of their children. Outreach efforts are essential to eliminate this isolation.[11]

Additional obstacles to care exist. Over 10% of Hispanic parents may not bring their children in for care if they feel the medical staff is not familiar with their culture.[14] In addition, parental stress associated with resettlement,[15] as well as fear of apprehension of family members with illegal immigration status,[13] may cause parents to avoid healthcare visits. Finally, children who have immigrated unaccompanied by adults, several thousand of whom enter the United States every year, are especially unlikely to access healthcare.[2,15]

## Preexisting Health Inequities

In general, immigration occurs in response to undesirable living conditions in a person's home country. These negative past circumstances may include, among others, any combination of poverty, war, torture, and/or natural disaster. As a consequence, immigrant children often enter their new countries with mental and physical health issues not commonly seen within the native population. Upon arrival, these preexisting health conditions should be screened for so that necessary therapies can be instituted.

As suggested by Jenista, in a thorough review of the topic,[2] the key components of new-arrival screening of immigrant children should include: (1) infectious disease screening, (2) a review and update of immunizations, (3) evaluation of mental health needs, (4) inspection for dental problems, (5) screening for nutritional disorders, (6) assessment of development, (7) screening for possible environmental exposures, (8) vision and hearing screening, (9) consideration of medical conditions common in specific ethnic groups, and (10) a review or request for any pertinent medical records. Most of these topics of new-arrival screening are discussed in other chapters (Table 41.3). It is important to remember that many of these components, such as mental and dental health, nutritional disorders, developmental disorders, and environmental exposures need to be regularly followed well beyond the new-arrival period. In this section, nutritional disorders in new pediatric immigrants are reviewed.

## Chronic malnutrition

Prior to immigration, children, especially those who have come from refugee camps, are at risk for chronic malnutrition (Box 41.1). Chronic malnutrition typically results from a combination of inadequate intake of micro- and macronutrients, recurrent acute infections, chronic infections including intestinal parasitosis, and occasionally a poor mother–child bond.[16] After nutritional reserves are depleted chronic mal-

---

**Box 41.1**

**Case study 1**

An adoptive mother brings her new 7-year-old son from China in for an initial preventive health screening. He arrived 3 weeks earlier and is getting to know his new family. He is a little tentative with trying some new foods, but overall is eating well. His mother is concerned since his height is only at the fifth percentile for his age. She asks if he should be started on a special high-calorie diet.

---

**Table 41.3 Preventative interventions at time of initial healthcare visit(s)**

1. Infectious disease screening (see Ch. 12)
2. Review and update immunizations (see Ch. 13)
3. Screen for mental health needs (see Ch. 48)
4. Evaluate dental health (see Ch. 45)
5. Screen for nutritional disorders
6. Evaluate developmental status and estimate age
7. Consider environmental exposures
8. Vision and hearing screening
9. Consider medical topics common in specific ethnic groups (see Ch. 16)
10. Review or request any past medical records

Adapted with permission from Pediatrics in Review, Vol. 22, Page 424, Copyright © 2001 by the AAP.

---

nutrition leads to impaired height growth, termed 'stunting.' The long-term consequences of stunting include delays in motor and mental development, decreased work capacity, and increased susceptibility to infections.[17]

To screen for malnutrition, it is imperative to check the height and weight of all newly arrived children. Chronic undernutrition can be screened for by plotting a child's height-for-age on growth reference curves. Stunting is technically defined as a height-for-age value less than two standard deviations (–2 Z-scores) below the mean of the reference population. However, since most growth charts used in clinical practice are presented as percentiles, this cutoff is equivalent to the 2.3 percentile, lower than the commonly used fifth percentile threshold used to detect poor growth. (Percentiles can be converted to Z-scores using the dataset available at http://www.cdc.gov/growthcharts) Often, an immigrant child's date of birth is not known, making nutritional assessment difficult. In such circumstances, initially, the reported age on accompanying paperwork should be accepted, unless there is an obvious discrepancy. Determination of true age should be delayed, ideally up to 1 year, to allow time for catch-up growth and development. At that time, age can be estimated by a combination of bone and dental ages, pubertal stages, maturity, and school performance.[2]

Stunting was detected in 143 (8%) of 1767 refugee children arriving in Massachusetts between 1995 and 1998 from locations all around the world. The chronically malnourished children came primarily from Africa, Near Eastern Asia, and East Asia, in which prevalence of stunting was 13%, 19%, and 30%, respectively.[18] Stunting was associated with both infection with intestinal parasites and origination from developing countries. However, when both of these variables were included in a multivariate analysis only origination from a developing country remained a significant predictor of stunting. An earlier study suggested that significant variation in rates of stunting occurs in children from different resource-poor countries. In the early 1980s, high levels of stunting (34% of boys and 33% of girls) were detected in newly arrived children of Southeast Asian ethnicities (Vietnamese, Cambodian, and Laotian). Moderate levels of stunting were seen in children from China and the Philippines. Children of Latin American origin had even lower levels (9% of boys and 8% of girls).[19] This suggested that, in addition to economic conditions in countries of origin, life circumstances, such as time spent in refugee camps, is likely an important determinant of chronic malnutrition.

In the past there have been some requests for the development of separate growth reference curves for people of different ethnicities. However, it has been shown that even among highly stunted Southeast Asian children, significant linear catch-up growth typically occurs after immigration, allowing these children to approach or reach the heights of age-matched native-born children of all ethnicities.[19,20] Close monitoring is needed to ensure that linear catch-up growth occurs. If it does not occur, underlying chronic infections such as tuberculosis, continued food insecurity, and parental or child mental health issues should be considered.

Achieving adequate catch-up growth does not require intake of energy-dense foods in large amounts. In fact, such foods may be detrimental to future health as discussed below in the acculturation and life-course theory sections. Rather, supplementation of a healthy diet with micronutrients has been shown to be effective and sufficient.[16] Interestingly, rapid catch-up growth resulting in hormonal changes has been hypothesized as a possible explanation of precocious puberty occasionally seen in immigrant children soon after arrival. This phenomenon has been documented most frequently among internationally adopted girls.[21]

## Acute malnutrition

Acute undernutrition leads to poor weight gain and is detected by a low weight-for-height, termed 'underweight or wasting.' Wasting, defined as values two standard deviations below the mean, or below the 2.3 percentile, is seen less often than stunting in newly arrived refugee children. Children under the fifth percentile are underweight. Among a group of children from Southeast Asia with a prevalence of stunting >30%, only 3% of boys and no girls showed wasting upon arrival in the 1980s.[19] In Massachusetts, only 23 (2%) of 964 refugee children had wasting. Of these, 83% came from Africa or East Asia. After adjusting for other variables, anemic children were 15 times more likely than nonanemic children to have wasting. Also, older children and those from developing countries were at greater risk of acute malnutrition.[18] Information on treating acute malnutrition in immigrant children is lacking. Clearly, based on studies in developing countries, higher protein diets with at least a moderate proportion of fat are indicated. However, parents should be educated that this type of high-calorie diet is only temporary and that continued overnutrition after

adequate catch-up weight gain is achieved may predispose children to multiple chronic illnesses.

## Anemia

Iron deficiency is the likely cause of anemia in most pediatric immigrant groups. This is supported by the very high rates of iron deficiency and anemia seen among children in refugee camps abroad.[22] Among the diverse groups of refugee children arriving in Massachusetts between 1995 and 1998, 153 (12%) of 1247 children were anemic.[18] The prevalence of anemia varied significantly by region and age. Children from Africa had the highest prevalence (31%), while those from the former Soviet Union had the lowest (10%). Children under 2 years of age from each region had the highest burden of anemia. Fifty percent of African children younger than 2 years of age were anemic. Young adolescents also were relatively more likely to be anemic. If untreated, iron deficiency may lead to cognitive impairments, behavioral problems, and increased susceptibility to lead poisoning.[23] The Centers for Disease Control and Prevention (CDC) has suggested starting all newly arrived refugee children on multivitamins with iron upon arrival.[24] It is important to remember that genetic hemoglobinopathies, thalassemias, and enzyme deficiencies may also account for many cases of anemia, especially among children from Southeast Asia (see Ch. 46).[25]

## Overweight and obesity

It is not uncommon for certain groups of immigrant children and adolescents to arrive with preexisting obesity. This is especially likely among those children originating from more developed countries or those from developing countries experiencing nutritional transitions towards more energy-dense foods as a result of urbanization. Obesity becomes a much greater problem for all immigrant children after arrival and is discussed in the acculturation section.

Obesity, defined as an excess of adipose tissue, is difficult to test for. The costs and availability of the gold-standard methods of quantifying adipose tissue, such as dual energy X-ray absorptiometry and underwater weighing, are prohibitive. The simple body mass index (BMI) [weight(kg)/ height(m)$^2$] is commonly used to screen for obesity. However, this tool is only a surrogate for adiposity and it has several unique limitations for children and adolescents. In the pediatric age groups BMI varies by age, gender, and maturation. The most commonly used BMI classification system in the US is based on the findings from the US National Health and Nutrition Surveys (NHANES) and charts can be found at http://www.cdc.gov/growthcharts.[26] In this system, adopted by the World Health Organization, children are classified by their sex- and age-specific percentile. BMI values greater than or equal to the 85th and less than 95th percentiles denote 'overweight' (or 'at risk for overweight' by the CDC) and values greater than or equal to the 95th percentile indicate 'obese' (or 'overweight' by the CDC).[27] In this chapter, these cutoffs will be referred to as 'overweight' and 'obese' for simplicity.

Children from Eastern Europe may be particularly likely to arrive overweight. In the Massachusetts study of newly arrived refugee children, 15% of 157 and 14% of 374 adolescents from the former Yugoslavia and Soviet Union, respectively, were overweight or obese. Interestingly, a significant positive association between dental caries and BMI values equal to the 85th percentile was noted (OR = 2.6, 95% CI = 1.2–4.4).[18] This may be explained by higher intake of refined sugars in children from more developed areas of the world.[28]

## Acculturation

Despite the preexisting health inequities immigrant children may have at the time of arrival, it is often noted that, on average, new immigrants of all ages have better health status as compared to the native population. This counterintuitive finding has been called the 'healthy migrant effect' and the 'the epidemiologic paradox.'[29] (see Ch. 3). This phenomenon may be associated with the lower rates of low birth weight infants,[30] early postnatal mortality,[31] asthma,[32] and obesity[33] seen in new immigrant children. Reports have also shown that recent adolescent immigrants are less likely to take part in high-risk behaviors.[29] The underpinnings of these findings may be related to the retention of traditional, often healthier, diets and strong support networks within families and immigrant communities.[29] However, part of the 'healthy migrant effect' may also be explained by underreporting bias. For example, although specific illnesses such as ear infections and pneumonia have been reported to occur less often among newly arrived immigrant children, these same children have far fewer healthcare visits while also having the lowest level of perceived health by parents.[6]

Unfortunately, the 'healthy migrant effect' is short lived. As immigrant children and their families assimilate into the culture of their new country, through a process know as acculturation, their health status begins to deteriorate and, in time, will often fall below that of the general population. Acculturation can be defined as the 'process of learning and incorporating the values, beliefs, language, customs and mannerisms of the new country immigrants and their families are living in, including behaviors that affect health such as dietary habits, activity levels and substance use.'[34] Acculturation can be measured in various ways such as language preference, English proficiency, level of ethnic pride and identity, and ethnicity of neighbors and close friends.[29] Several acculturation scales have been validated. For example, the Acculturation, Habits, Interests and Multicultural Scale for Adolescents (AHIMSA) has been designed to quantify the degree of assimilation into the new culture, separation from the old culture, and integration of and marginalization from both cultures.[35]

It is disconcerting that through the act of fleeing negative life circumstance, immigrants are at risk of developing new problems. The aspects of health that are negatively affected by acculturation are often the same as those in which new immigrants fare relatively well. Acculturation has been reported as a potential risk factor for multiple unhealthy behaviors including smoking,[34,36] alcohol[37,38] and other drug use,[39] high-risk sexual activity,[40] violence,[41] suicidal ideation,[42] physical inactivity,[43] and fast-food consumption.[43] Parental acculturation leading to pressures to bottle-feed their toddlers on demand has been suggested as an explanation of high rates of iron deficiency seen in Hmong-Americans.[44] The well-documented effects of acculturation on the development of obesity and high-risk behaviors will be reviewed below (Table 41.4). In addition, possible connections between acculturation and asthma will be discussed briefly.

### Overweight and obesity

Obesity among children has reached epidemic proportions in developed countries throughout the world.[45] The associated health effects of childhood obesity are numerous and include reduced self-esteem, hypertension, dyslipidemia, type 2 diabetes mellitus, sleep apnea, asthma, cholelithiasis, nonalcoholic steatohepatitis, genu varum and slipped capital femoral epiphysis.[27,46] Obese 4-year-old children and adolescents have an estimated 20% and

**Table 41.4 Effects of acculturation on obesity and high-risk behaviors**

| Obesity | High-risk behaviors |
|---|---|
| • Decreased intake of traditional foods | • Decreased ethnic isolation |
| • Increased intake of energy-dense foods | • Impaired parent–child communication |
| • Decreased physical activity | • Acculturative stresses |

80% likelihood, respectively, of remaining obese in adulthood.[46]

In the United States, the prevalence of overweight children and adolescents has doubled from the late 1970s to 1999–2002.[47] The most current data indicate 23% and 31% of children aged 2–5 and 6–19 years-old in the US are either overweight or obese, respectively (BMI for age ≥ 85th percentile).[48] The prevalence varies considerably by ethnicity. Among Mexican-American youths between 6- and 19-years-old, 40% are overweight or obese. This is significantly higher than rates of 35% among non-Hispanic black children and 28% among non-Hispanic white children of the same age group ($p < 0.05$).[48] Socioeconomic factors such as family income and education can only partially explain these differences in over-weight and obesity among both young children and adolescents.[49,50] Acculturation has been identified as an additional factor in overweight and obesity disparities.

Although fewer studies have looked at the influence of acculturation on the development of obesity within pediatric age groups as compared to adult populations, solid data suggest that many children of immigrant families reach or exceed the rates of overweight and obesity of the native populations as they or their families become more acculturated. This has been best studied among Hispanic and Asian adolescents.

In the complex process of acculturation, children and adolescents are likely to adopt attitudes and behaviors considered to be the norm for areas in which they are living. Immigrants to the United States often transition from traditional foods and activities to those that are considered more 'American.'[43] Unfortunately, these 'American' behaviors such as fast-food consumption and physically inactive pastimes, such as television viewing, are known risk factors for obesity. Among adolescents of Mexican, Cuban, and Puerto Rican ethnicity, significant differences in diet have been noted between first- and second-generation immigrants. The less

acculturated first-generation immigrants were more likely to maintain traditional diets containing plentiful rice, beans, fruits, and vegetables, as compared to second-generation adolescents. In addition, second-generation Mexican-American adolescents were more likely to eat fast food as compared with their first-generation counterparts.[51] Immigrants of Asian ethnicity tend to eat less fish, vegetables, and whole grains and more snack foods, fast food, processed meats, and fat after living in the United States.[43] A recent study evaluating the effects of acculturation on the level of physical activity and fast-food consumption among 1385 Hispanic and 619 Asian-American adolescents living in Southern California found that, after controlling for confounding variables, acculturation, measured by the AHIMSA tool, was negatively associated with physical activity ($p = 0.001$) and positively associated with fast-food consumption ($p = 0.001$).[43]

These acculturation-associated effects on diet and physical activity are consistent with findings that second-generation Asian-American and Hispanic-American adolescents are significantly more likely to be obese as compared to foreign-born adolescents of similar ethnicity.[33] This intergenerational difference is most profound for Asian-Americans in whom the percentage of overweight or obese adolescents increased from 12% among first-generation immigrants to 27% among second-generation immigrants, significantly above the overweight and obesity prevalence of 24% seen among the 7726 US non-hispanic white adolescents included in the study.

The association between acculturation and obesity as seen above in Hispanic-American and Asian-American adolescents has not been studied to the same extent among younger immigrant children. The findings that are available suggest the parental acculturation level may be associated with childhood obesity, but the direction of association may vary between different immigrant groups.

There is some evidence that lower acculturation levels among Hispanic-American parents may protect their children from obesity. Although obesity was not specifically assessed in an analysis of 2985 4–16-year-old Hispanic children, investigators did find that children of less-acculturated parents had a lower intake of fat and other macronutrients associated with obesity.[52] Children from the lowest-income households had a significantly increased likelihood of experiencing food insecurity. Food insecurity, which is potentially a common occurrence among many immigrant families, may be associated with obesity by leading families to establish diets with inferior nutritional quality.[53]

However, among the lowest-income families, a lower level of parental acculturation partially negated the effect of food insecurity.[52]

In contrast, among school-aged Chinese-American children three variables have been found to correlate with the likelihood of having a higher BMI: older age, poor communication between children and parents, and less authoritative parenting style. The authors of this study suggested that the more acculturated mothers, who also tended to have a more authoritative parenting style, may be more equipped to utilize healthcare resources and may be more aware of health issues related to being overweight.[54]

To date, very limited data are available on the effects of acculturation on obesity among the more recent immigrant groups from sub-Saharan Africa. The information available indicates that the interaction between acculturation and traditionally held concepts of health may work synergistically among this group of immigrants leading to a high prevalence of obesity.[55] Within many resource-poor countries, including many in sub-Saharan Africa, obesity is not perceived as an adverse health condition. In these countries being heavy is often seen as a marker of success, wealth, and good health.[55] In many parts of Africa, luxury foods, or 'food of white people,' are desired as a means of achieving larger body sizes.[55] These foods, such as meats, soft drinks, butter, sugar, and mayonnaise, are often expensive in resource-poor areas, but are much more affordable after immigrants settle in developed countries. It has been postulated that increased availability and increased exposure to advertising of such foods combined with decreased physical activity in developed countries may explain high rates of obesity among refugee children from sub-Saharan Africa in Australia.[55] Healthier fruits and vegetables are often viewed as food of the poor, a sentiment that may persist after emigration.[55]

Prevention of obesity has become a key aspect of pediatric health maintenance as the childhood and adolescent obesity epidemic continues to worsen. The American Academy of Pediatrics recommends regular BMI monitoring of children at risk for obesity 'by virtue of family history, birth weight or socioeconomic, ethnic, cultural, or environmental factors.'[46] Clearly, acculturating children of immigrant families are exposed to unique cultural factors mandating close monitoring. Even before excessive weight gain is detected in these children their parents should be routinely reminded, in a culturally sensitive manner, of the importance of healthy eating patterns and physical activity. Parents should be

encouraged to offer fruits, vegetables, low-fat dairy products and whole grain foods, to set limits on unhealthy food choices, to model healthy food choices, to limit television viewing and video time to under two hours per day, and to allow for unstructured play time daily.[46] The CDC suggests that children and adolescents incorporate one hour of moderate activity into their daily schedules. Healthcare providers may be able to make an even more significant contribution by advocating for healthy foods in schools and for opportunities and facilities for regular physical activity.

In general, the BMI based on NHANES data has a high specificity for overweight (91.5% for boys and 92.4% for girls) and obesity (96.9% for boys and 97.3% for girls) relative to percent-body-fat measurements.[56] However, the BMI is likely to overestimate (high false positives) obesity in stunted children. Several reports have found a high prevalence of both stunting and overweight or obesity in Hmong children in the United States.[57] The paradoxical finding of simultaneous stunting and obesity has been reported among children undergoing rapid nutrient transitions, in which weight is gained but linear growth is limited.[58] Nevertheless, using the BMI, triceps skin folds, and body fat percentage, the prevalence of overweight or obesity among 72 Hmong-American children aged 4–11 years was 42%, 29%, and 25%, respectively.[57] Therefore, to avoid overestimations of obesity, it has been suggested that among children with short stature those with high BMIs should have additional testing such as triceps skin fold or body fat percentage measurements. A new BMI system, endorsed by the International Obesity Task Force,[59] based on data collected from large surveys from Brazil, Great Britain, Hong Kong, the Netherlands, Singapore, and the United States, has a higher specificity for obesity as compared to the NHANES-derived BMI at the expense of decreased sensitivity.[56]

## Risk-taking behaviors

Most, if not all, adolescents are faced with pressures to try smoking, alcohol, drugs, and sex. Acculturation has been shown to make adolescents of immigrant families more susceptible to these pressures. As is the case for the effects of acculturation on obesity, this has been best studied among Hispanic and Asian-American adolescents.

Unacculturated adolescents may be protected from harmful behaviors by ethnic isolation. These individuals often are members of non-English-speaking families and live among and socialize largely with people of the same ethnicity, thus limiting their exposure to 'American' norms of rebellious behaviors. Also, less-acculturated youths are more likely to be primarily influenced by parents and family rather than peers.[34] As adolescents' English language skills improve they are more likely to form peer groups with more acculturated immigrant and/or native-born youths, people who are more likely to perceive certain risk behaviors as normative.[34] The US-born group into which an immigrant child assimilates frequently is similar to his or her ethnicity and socioeconomic level. Often, these native-born groups have high rates of risk-taking behaviors. For example, both immigrant and native-born Latino adolescents living in Northern California were found to have similar high rates of substance use, unintended pregnancy, and violence, as compared to native non-Hispanic white adolescents.[60]

Not only does acculturation make immigrant children more likely to gain exposure to 'mainstream' behaviors, it may also distance them from their parents. Through immersion in schools and peer groups, immigrant children and adolescents tend to acculturate and learn the new language much more rapidly and thoroughly compared to their parents or caretakers. This dichotomy, or acculturation gap, may lead to poor communication between children and their parents, resulting in less parental insight into their children's needs and concerns and may reduce children's respect for parental authority.

Acculturation gaps can also lead to role reversal in which children become 'cultural brokers' and are relied upon by their parents to help the family navigate many aspects of daily life. Among adolescent girls from Russia, 89% reported performing cultural brokering, with even higher rates among those with mothers who spoke little English.[61] Higher levels of cultural brokering were associated with higher adolescent stress, more reports of problems at home and with friends, and lower feelings of school membership. Cultural brokering, in addition to the stresses of trying to assimilate with peers, and stresses associated with low socioeconomic status as part of an immigrant family, may be considered collectively as acculturative stress.[62] If extreme, acculturative stress may lead to depression and suicidal ideation among adolescents.[42] It may also contribute to maladaptive substance use as discussed below.

The three aspects of acculturation described above: increasing exposure to 'mainstream' behaviors, poor parent–child communication, and acculturative stress, have been shown to affect substance use among adolescents of immigrant families. The effect of increasing exposure to 'mainstream' behaviors is illustrated by a study of Hispanic and Asian-American children aged 8–16 years. Among these youths, the likelihood of ever smoking was found to be strongly associated with the type of language spoken in their homes. Those who spoke only English at home were twice as likely to have tried smoking as compared with those who only spoke other languages (for Asians OR = 1.94, 95% CI 1.19–3.19; for Hispanics OR = 2.07, 95% CI 1.45–2.97).[34] Increases in smoking were noted for each incremental increase of English usage. In addition to smoking, higher levels of English usage were also associated with a higher perceived access to cigarettes, a higher likelihood of having a best friend who smokes, more frequent offers for cigarettes from friends, and a decreased perceived ability to refuse cigarette offers. These additional associations with English usage likely represent some of the ways in which acculturation increases the risk of smoking and other substance use by removing the protections associated with linguistic and ethnic isolation. Others have found similar correlations between language usage at home and the likelihood of using marijuana alone, or in conjunction with cigarettes and alcohol, among Hispanic-American adolescents of primarily Puerto Rican, Dominican, Colombian, and Ecuadoran origins.[39]

The second consequence of acculturation that may lead to substance use is change in the quality of communication between immigrant parents and their children. Among Hispanic migrant adolescents, this was found to be a significant predictor of past alcohol or cigarette use. Adolescents who were satisfied with the quality of communication they had with their parents were 48% less likely to have ever smoked (OR = 0.52, 95% CI 0.31–0.87) and 27% less likely to have ever drunk alcohol (OR = 0.63, 95% CI 0.38–0.98). The authors suggest that acculturation gaps between adolescents and parents may impair communication, thereby impairing the ability of parents to positively influence behaviors.[63]

Similar findings on the effects of communication have been reported for alcohol use by adolescent Asian-Americans. Among those with low parental involvement, highly acculturated youths were 11 times more likely to have used alcohol as compared to the least acculturated youths. However, among adolescents with moderate or high levels of parental involvement, there was no variation in alcohol use by degree of acculturation.[64]

Thirdly, acculturative stress may predispose adolescents to substance use. This is supported by a study of 8th and 10th grade students from Massachusetts. Although US-born adolescents were more likely to use alcohol or marijuana as compared to immigrant adolescents, especially compared to immigrants that had arrived more recently, the recent immigrant group, defined as living in the United States for less than 6 years, was more likely to be affected by factors that may predict future high-risk behaviors. These factors include: greater peer pressure to partake in substance use, sex, and violence; less parental disapproval of these behaviors; and less confidence in the ability to refuse substances that may be offered to them.[65] These stresses may lead to early substance use in some immigrant youths. For example, binge alcohol drinking has been identified as a possible coping mechanism among some recently immigrated Mexican-, Cuban-, and Puerto Rican-American adolescents of Spanish-speaking homes who are confronting new acculturative stresses.[62]

An important window of opportunity exists in which targeted efforts may decrease the risk of future substance use by both foreign-born children and unacculturated native-born children. Foreign-born adolescents who have lived in the US for fewer than 5 years have significantly lower rates of alcohol consumption and use of cigarettes, marijuana, and other illicit drugs as compared to US-born youths.[36] However, by the time foreign-born adolescents have lived in the US for 10 years, their substance use mirrors that of the native-born population.[36] Similar timelines would likely be seen among unacculturated native-born children of immigrant families.

To best help older children and adolescents avoid or at least reduce the consequences of high-risk behaviors, healthcare providers should consider addressing the issues related to acculturation during office visits. Parents and children should be familiarized to the differing rates of acculturation within a family with a goal of improving parent–child communication. Discussing acculturative stress with adolescents may help them understand that such stresses are common. However, even the most skilled clinician will be unable to counterbalance the powerful effects of acculturation on high-risk behaviors in the office. Therefore, it is important to advocate for and help families in accessing community and school-based programs that address these issues. Outreach programs involving both parents and adolescents have shown promising results. For a group of Hispanic migrant adolescents, just eight evening sessions, three of which were also attended by their parents, focusing on the effects of smoking and alcohol and the development of refusal skills and parent–child communication skills, led to improvements in parent–child communication that were estimated to translate into a 10% decrease in susceptibility to future tobacco or alcohol use.[66]

In addition to substance use, acculturation may increase the likelihood of sexual activity among immigrant youths. For example, while Hispanic-American girls in 7th to 12th grade living in Arizona were overall more likely to have had sexual intercourse than age-matched non-Hispanic white girls (OR = 1.4, 95% CI 1.21–1.63), those who spoke primarily Spanish were significantly less likely to have been sexually active compared to non-Hispanic white adolescents (OR = 0.59, 95% CI 0.42–0.82).[67] As with substance use, the effects of acculturation gaps on parent–child communication may be important risk factors for high-risk sexual activity among adolescents. This has been identified as a major barrier to effective communication about sex between Filipino-American teenagers, a population with high pregnancy rates compared with other Asian and Pacific Islander groups, and their parents. The acculturated adolescents felt that open discussions were necessary to learn about their parents' values in regards to sex. However, parents and grandparents felt that these 'values were transmitted best through traditional Filipino respect for parents' and often avoided discussion with their children.[68] The format of community-based family sessions may help to facilitate needed discussions.

## Asthma

It has been well documented that the prevalence of asthma and other atopic illnesses increases over time after immigration to more developed countries. For example, for every year after immigration to Australia the prevalence of wheezing increased by 11% among children originally from Asia, the South Pacific, the Middle East, Africa, and parts of Europe.[69] In addition to duration of time since immigration, birthplace may be an important determinant of atopic illness within immigrant families. Among 4121 Mexican-American children aged 2 months to 16 years, US-born children had twice the prevalence of asthma as compared with those born in Mexico (OR 2.19, 95% CI 1.09–4.40).[70] The US-born children were also more likely to show evidence of sensitization to many indoor and outdoor aeroallergens.

It is known that the prevalence of asthma and atopy have marked global variation. They are generally more common in more affluent countries.[71] This variation may be partly explained by different degrees of infectious illness in different parts of the world.[72] Viral and parasitic infections and exposure to aerosolized bacterial endotoxins from farms have been suggested to alter the immune system in ways that make atopic illness less likely.[71] Therefore, it is conceivable that the increases in asthma prevalence associated with both increasing time since immigration and among second-generation immigrants may result from the loss of these protective events in more sterile environments. The explanation for the observed asthma trends in immigrant groups is likely related to these environmental changes. However, acculturation may be involved in facilitating these changes.

To date, there has been only one study that has specifically looked at the role acculturation may play in the development of atopic illness. The prevalence of atopy and sensitization to common aeroallergens among children of Turkish origin living in Germany was compared to language preferences. Children in families that spoke only Turkish had the lowest rates of wheezing, itchy rashes, and aeroallergen sensitization, while children in immigrant families that spoke German were affected by these conditions at rates similar to that experienced by non-immigrant German children. The ownership of pets increased with increasing German language preference, suggesting one mechanism in which acculturation may promote allergic illnesses.[32] Some have suggested that the effects of acculturation on stress and obesity may be important to the development of asthma in immigrants.[73]

## Unique Environmental Exposures

As a result of a variety of cultural, socioeconomic, and occupational factors, children of immigrant families may be more prone to several environmental hazards (Table 41.5). Such hazards include contact with toxic substances and injuries. Immigrants originating from areas near Chernobyl may have had past radiation exposure.[74] In addition, decreased exposures may have health consequences as well. For example, limited sun-exposure as a result of traditional clothing may result in low vitamin D levels in certain immigrant groups. This section will address some of these unique interactions immigrant children have with their environment with an emphasis on the issue of lead poisoning.

**Table 41.5 Environmental exposures and injuries of importance to immigrant children**

| Exposures | Before arrival | After arrival |
|---|---|---|
| Lead | X | X |
| Pesticides | | X (especially among migrant farm workers) |
| Home toxin poisonings | | X (especially when parents do not read English) |
| Radiation | X | |
| Pedestrian injuries | | X (especially when parents do not read English) |
| Work-related injuries | | X (especially among migrant farm workers) |
| Vitamin D deficiency (insufficient sunlight exposure) | X | X (especially among females who wear veiled clothing) |

**Box 41.2**

**Case study 2**

A 30-month-old asymptomatic Mexican-American boy is brought back to clinic to discuss his elevated blood lead level. He was first found to have a level of 20 µg/dL 6 months ago at his 2-year-old well child visit. A thorough environmental home inspection found no lead sources. His mother has denied administering any folk remedies to him. Today you decide to test the mother's lead level, which comes back elevated.

### Lead poisoning

Immigrant children and children of immigrants comprise a population at high risk for the long-term health effects of lead poisoning (Box 41.2). The threshold of what constitutes a safe blood lead level (BLL) has changed over time. In the 1940s it was widely believed that children with lead poisoning who did not die recovered with no long-term health sequelae. Even as recently as 1970, BLLs as high as 60 µg/dL were considered acceptable since overt clinical symptoms of headaches, abdominal pain, anorexia, constipation, clumsiness, agitation, and lethargy typically are not present below this level.[75] Children with BLLs as low as 70 µg/dL may develop severe neurological complications including seizures, ataxia, mental status changes, coma, and death.[76] Such severe poisonings are now rare. The death of a 2-year-old Sudanese refugee girl with a BLL of 392 µg/dL, the first lead poisoning-related death in the United States in a 10 year period, 5 weeks after arrival to the United States, underscores the importance of this topic.[77]

In 1991, based on data showing negative consequences on intelligence and neurodevelopment at lower levels, the CDC defined lead poisoning as a BLL ≥ 10 µg/dL.[76] Since then, mounting evidence indicates there is likely no safe BLL. An important study revealed that the magnitude of the decrease in intelligence quotient (IQ) for each incremental increase in BLL is greatest among those children with levels below 10 µg/dL. For those children with average BLLs above 10 µg/dL, a 4.6-point reduction in IQ was noted for every increase of 10 µg/dL. However, IQ decreased by 7.4 points as BLL increased from 1 to 10 µg/dL.[78]

Following the phase-out of leaded gasoline from 1975 to 1986 and the ban on lead-based paint in 1977, the prevalence of lead poisoning among children in the US has decreased.[76] The NHANES studies have documented a greater than 70% decline in the prevalence of children aged 1–5 years with BLLs >10 µg/dL from 78% in 1976–1980 to 4.4% in 1991–1994. During the period 1999–2002 the prevalence decreased further to 1.6%.[79] Despite this dramatic reduction, lead-based paints continue to pose the most common environmental source of elevated BLLs among children in the United States.[76] In contrast, foreign-born children, on average, have much higher rates of elevated BLLs at time of arrival due to exposures abroad. In addition, both foreign-born and native-born children of immigrant families are at above average risk for lead poisoning from exposures within the United States.

## Lead exposures before arrival

Among foreign-born children, refugees have been best studied. The overall prevalence of lead poisoning among recent refugee arrivals from diverse locations has ranged from 11% to 22%.[80,81] In refugees from certain locations rates of lead poisoning as high as 40% have been documented.[81] Additionally, other types of pediatric immigrants are likely at increased risk due to similar environmental exposures abroad. In areas of the world from which many immigrants

originate there are several sources of lead exposure including combustion of lead-containing gasoline, industrial emissions, ammunition manufacturing and use, burning of fossil fuels and waste, and lead-containing traditional remedies, foods, ceramic bowls, pots, and utensils.[80,81] Among Cuban immigrant children to the United States, car repair by parents in the home or yard while living in Cuba was also associated with elevated BLL after arrival to the United States.[82] Foreign-born children may also be more susceptible to these exposures due to the high prevalence of concomitant iron deficiency in immigrant children.

Potentially due to increased gastrointestinal absorption, iron-deficient children are more prone to developing lead poisoning.[23,83] This association, which appears to be strongest among young children, may have significant effects on development since iron deficiency and lead poisoning both impair cognitive function.[23] A recent prospective study showed that iron-deficient children in Boston aged 1–4 years were at significantly increased odds of developing lead poisoning (OR = 4.12, 95% CI 1.96–8.65).[83] Iron deficiency does not have to be severe enough to cause anemia for this association with lead poisoning to occur. A low mean corpuscular volume and elevated red cell distribution width, changes that occur at lower levels of iron deficiency, have been associated with increased propensity for children to have higher BLL.[83] There is some evidence that deficiencies in other micronutrients including calcium and zinc may also predispose to lead poisoning.[76] The Centers for Disease Control and Prevention have suggested multivitamins with iron as a possible intervention to decrease lead poisoning among refugee children <59 months old upon arrival to the United States.[24] However, iron supplementation has been shown to delay urinary lead excretion in those with lead poisoning.[23] Therefore, it may be wise to wait to provide iron supplementation until the result of a child's initial BLL is available.

Among the 299 refugee children, from 25 different countries, under the age of 6 years arriving in Minnesota between 2000 and 2002 who had a BLL checked after arrival, 65 (22%) had a BLL of greater than or equal to 10 µg/dl.[80] Among the children with elevated BLLs, 29 (45%) had levels of 10–14.9 µg/dL, 15 (23%) had levels of 15–19.9 µg/dL, and 21 (32%) had levels of 20–44.9 µg/dL. Of those with the highest levels, 19 children were from sub-Saharan Africa and two were from Bosnia and Herzegovina. The 22% prevalence of elevated BLLs in this refugee group was almost 14 times higher than that of US children aged 1–5 years based on the most recent NHANES data.

An earlier study performed in Massachusetts from 1995 to 1999 found a lower prevalence, 11%, of elevated BLLs among newly arrived refugee children under the age of 7 years.[81] However, this was still 2.7 times higher than similarly aged US-born children. The lower prevalence may be explained by differences in the proportion of refugees from the former Soviet Union and former Yugoslavia. The Massachusetts study was comprised predominately of refugee children from these areas of northern Eurasia (78%) while in the Minnesota study only 22% of the participants were from this region. Two-thirds of the children screened in Minnesota were from Africa.

Although children born in northern Eurasian countries who were screened in Massachusetts within 90 days of arrival had a slightly higher prevalence, 6–7%, of elevated BLLs as compared to similarly aged US children, children from other areas had significantly higher rates of lead poisoning: 40% of 15 children from Central America, Cuba, or Haiti, 37% of 43 Asian children (predominantly from Vietnam), 27% of 79 African children, and 25% of 16 children from the Near East (predominantly from Iraq).[83] None of 33 Bosnian children born in Germany had elevated BLL. Therefore, birthplace is a more important determinant than ethnicity.[81]

Other factors, in addition to birthplace, that may be associated with elevated BLLs in newly arrived immigrants include anemia, presence of pathogenic intestinal parasites, lower weight-for-age and lower height-for-age and BLL testing in the warmer months of May through October.[81] The association with lower height-for-age may indicate that children with chronic malnutrition are at increased risk of elevated BLLs, possibly due to associated micronutrient deficiencies including iron deficiency.

## Lead exposures after arrival

Most refugees with elevated BLL detected during new-arrival screening were likely exposed to lead before immigrating. This is supported by the finding that BLLs declined in 73% of 213 children who were retested at least 6 months after arrival.[81] However, it is noteworthy that, among those retested, 5.9% of children with normal BLLs at initial screening were later found to have lead poisoning. This percentage of lead poisoning due to exposures within the US was higher than that of the age-matched general US population.[81]

Within the United States, foreign- and native-born children of immigrant families are at increased risk of lead exposure due to a combination of socio-economic and cultural factors, in addition to less familiarity with lead poisoning among parents. Immigrant families often live in disadvantaged areas within their new country, the same areas with the highest percentage of dwellings with unsafe lead levels.[84] This is likely the single most important factor to account for the higher prevalence of elevated BLLs in children of immigrant families after the new-arrival period.

Cultural factors that pose potential risks of lead exposure include lead-containing foods, therapies, and pottery (Table 41.6). Those who care for immigrant populations must be aware of these additional lead exposures. For example, in 150 of the 1000 reported cases of elevated BLLs in California between May 2001 and January 2002, Mexican candy was a potential source of exposure.[85] Tamarind fruit candies in the form of lollipops, fruit-rolls, and candied jams are especially likely to contain lead, likely due to leaching of lead from wrappers or packaging into the candy (Fig. 41.1).[85,86] Lead may be added to foods to impart a yellow or orange color, as a sweetener, or to add weight to the food. Lozeena, a spice used by Iraqis to color certain rice and meat dishes, has been documented to have caused lead poisoning in an immigrant family.[87] There have also been several reported cases of lead poisoning caused by traditional Mexican remedies named greta[87] and azarcon[87] used for intestinal ailments, or 'empacho,' which encompasses symptoms including constipation, diarrhea, nausea, vomiting, anorexia, and lethargy. Some samples of azarcon and greta have been found to consist of 90% lead.[87,88] An outbreak of lead poisoning of Hmong children in Minnesota was likely linked to the use of 'pay-loo-ah,' a combination of red- and orange-colored powders that is occasionally fed to children for treatment of fever and rashes.[89] At least one reported case of elevated BLL was associated with use of Surma, a black powder applied to the eye of some Asian Indian children to improve vision.[88] Litargirio, a yellow- or peach-colored lead-containing powdery substance commonly used in rural areas of the Dominican Republic as a deodorant and as a remedy for burns and fungal infections of the feet, has been linked to cases of lead poisoning in immigrant children (Fig. 41.2).[90] An ayurvedic medication that may contain lead has been given to Tibetan children to hasten development.[88] Use of lead-glazed terracotta pottery from Latin America is another potential lead source.[91]

**Table 41.6 Examples of culture-specific lead exposures**

| Exposure | Area of origin | Uses | Description |
|---|---|---|---|
| 'Pay-loo-ah' | Southeast Asian | Treatment of fever and rash | Orange-red-colored powder. Administered by itself or mixed in tea. |
| Greta | Mexico | Treatment of digestive problems | Yellow-orange-colored powder. May be administered with oil, milk, sugar or tea. Sometimes it is added to baby bottles and/or tortilla dough for prevention. |
| Azarcon | Mexico | Treatment of digestive problems | Bright orange powder. Administered similarly to greta. |
| Litargirio | Dominican Republic | Deodorant/antiperspirant and treatment of burns and fungal infections of the feet | Yellow or peach-colored powder. |
| Surma | India | Improve eyesight | Black powder administered to inner lower eyelid. |
| Unknown ayurvedic | Tibet | Treatment for slow development | Small gray-brown-colored balls administered several times per day. |
| Lozeena | Iraq | Add color to rice and meat dishes | Bright orange spice. |
| Tamarind candies (multiple brand names) | Mexico | Lollipops Fruit rolls Candied jams | 'Bolirindo' lollipops by Dulmex are soft and are dark brown in color. Candied jams are typically packaged in ceramic jars. |
| Lead-glazed ceramics | Often made in Latin America | Bean pots Water jugs | |

Data from References 86, 87, 88, 89, 90, and 91.

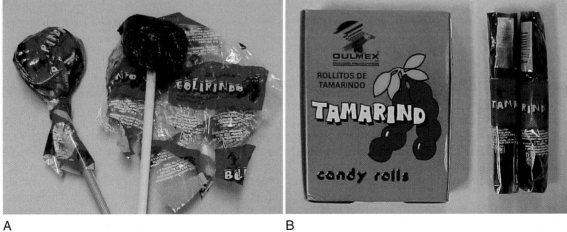

**Fig. 41.1 (A, B)** Examples of lead-containing tamarind fruit candies. Reproduced with permission from the state of Oregon Lead Poisoning Prevention Program.

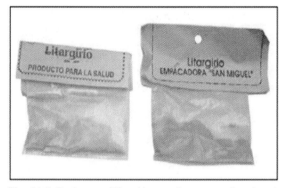

**Fig. 41.2** Packages of litargirio, a yellow or peach-colored powder used as a deodorant, antiperspirant, or remedy in the Dominican Republic. It has been associated with cases of lead poisoning in the United States. (Photo from reference 92.)

Elevated BLLs on screening tests, the presence of continued elevated BLLs in a child after home lead abatements, or findings of anemia, abdominal pain, kidney disease, peripheral neuropathy, or encephalopathy in children of immigrant families should raise suspicion among healthcare providers about possible exposures to culture-specific substances.[87,90] If no lead sources can be identified in children with lead poisoning, clinicians should consider checking BLLs in other family members. If other family members of various ages have elevated levels, a shared source exposure, such as ceramic ware, spices, foods, and remedies, may be present.[86] It is important to ask about these substances using as specific terminology as possible and avoiding terms such as 'traditional or folk remedies.' What a healthcare provider may consider a 'folk remedy' may be perceived as an ordinary product to a parent. This was noted in a case of lead poisoning among two siblings in Rhode Island due to exposure to litargirio. Their mother repeatedly denied exposure to any 'traditional or folk remedies' as she considered litargirio as a common type of deodorant.[90] Other reasons for not disclosing use of such substances may include feeling responsible for the child's lead poisoning, and uncertainty regarding the legality of a particular substance.[88] Therefore, a nonjudgmental approach is indicated. Equally important is to not limit the search for lead sources if parents do report possible exposures to a cultural-specific substance that may contain lead. In such circumstances, environmental inspections of homes often reveal additional sources such as chipping lead paint, and lead-glazed ceramic pots and other large hollow-form ware.[88]

The importance of ongoing lead exposure among immigrant children within the United States has been documented among refugees in New Hampshire.[24] Between October 2003 and September 2004, 242 refugee children resettled in the state. Almost all (98%) of these children were from Africa. Ninety-two (38%) of these children had a BLL checked at their new-arrival screening and then again 2–26 weeks after the first screening. The median age at time of rescreening was 4.9 years. Thirteen (14%) had elevated BLL at both time points. Twenty-seven (29%) initially had levels <10 µg/dL that then increased to >10 µg/dL on repeat testing. Ten (11%) had initially elevated BLL that then decreased to <10 µg/dL. Forty-two (46%) had nonelevated BLLs at both time points. Among the 37 children with an elevated BLL on follow-up testing for which complete information was available, malnutrition was common. Eight children (22%) were wasted and 13 (35%) were stunted (see Malnutrition above for definitions). The median initial BLL was 8.1 µg/dL, increasing to 18.6 µg/dL (range 10–63) on follow-up testing. Three children required chelation therapy for high BLLs detected on their second tests. Of the families who had children with BLLs >15 µg/dL, 89% lived in rental homes built before 1978, 67% noted their children to have one or more behaviors that increase the risk of lead exposure (frequently putting nonfood items into their mouths, picking at loose paint, plaster, or putty, or chewing on painted surfaces). Of eight families who had children with BLLs greater than 20 µg/dL, seven homes were found to have lead hazards in or around the home.

This report indicates that among refugee groups with a high prevalence of malnutrition, nearly 30% of children may develop elevated BLLs after arrival to the US, primarily through exposure to lead paint. Based on these findings, the CDC recommends: (1) checking BLL, hemoglobin, and nutritional assessments of all refugees under the age of 6 years within 90 days of arrival, (2) repeating BLL 3–6 months after residing in a permanent residence, (3) provision of pediatric multivitamins with iron to all refugee children under the age of 59 months immediately upon arrival, (4) consider checking BLL in children 6 years of age if there is any suspicion of possible lead exposures, (5) providing nutritional counseling and referral to the Supplemental Nutrition Program for Women, Infants and Children (WIC), and (6) improving lead-hazard training for refugee and resettlement case workers and healthcare providers.[24] Healthcare providers should consider applying these guidelines to all types of immigrant children who have come from areas of the world where lead hazards are common or who are now living in areas with such hazards.[75]

In addition, at well child visits, providers should spend time educating parents about lead hazards including lead paints in older homes and culture-specific foods, products, or therapies and the potential long-term risks of lead exposures. Meeting the *Healthy People 2010* goal of eliminating BLLs of 10 μg/dl or greater in children aged 1–6 years in the US[76] will require special attention to immigrant children. The important role that new-arrival screening can serve in these efforts is highlighted by the finding that refugee children who underwent new-arrival screening in Minnesota were twice as likely to have their BLLs checked as compared to those children that never had a new-arrival screening appointment. Also, the time from arrival to BLL evaluation was significantly shorter among those children who had new-arrival screens performed.[80]

## Work-related exposures

Migrant or seasonal farm workers comprise a vulnerable population with limited healthcare access (see Ch. 57). There are an estimated 2.5 million seasonal or migrant farm workers in the United States.[92] Over 70% of these individuals are Hispanic, and others are of Haitian, Asian, West Indian, African-American, and Native American backgrounds.[93] Adolescents between the ages of 14 and 17 years account for approximately 7% of this workforce.[92] However, it is notable that children often start working in the fields at the age of 11, and occasionally as early 8 years old.[92] These adolescents and children are prone to injury from tractors, machinery, animals, falls, drowning, heat-related illness, and pesticide-related illness. Annually, an estimated 27 000 adolescents workers under the age of 19 years sustain farm-related injuries and 300 die.[94] Children of migrant workers who live and play on or near these farms are also at risk of injuries and death due to similar hazards, especially when left unattended due to lack of affordable daycare.

The Environmental Protection Agency estimates that up to 300 000 seasonal workers suffer pesticide-related illnesses every year. Both adolescent workers and young children may be particularly susceptible to the harmful effects of pesticides.[93] One-third of adolescent workers interviewed in New York reported pesticide-related illnesses within the previous year. Short-term effects of pesticide exposure may include headaches, nausea, eye irritation, rashes, myalgias, and even death. Long-term consequences

include neurological disorders, liver and kidney disease, cancers, sterility, and birth defects.[94]

Adolescent workers are exposed to pesticides when they eat, drink, or smoke in the farms or by direct exposure[93] to spray. They may decrease exposure risk by regularly washing hands while working. Younger children that do not work in the fields are at risk of exposure due to drift of nearby sprays and by family members who unknowingly bring pesticides home on their clothing, skin, and hair, or in their vehicles.[95] Pesticide levels may be higher inside the homes of migrant farmers than outdoors due to less environmental degradation.[95] Family members can help minimize exposures to children by removing contaminated clothing and shoes before entering their homes.

Healthcare providers can help to decrease pesticide-related illnesses by educating parents and adolescent workers about the relevant health risks and prevention measures. Although employers are required to provide this information, adolescent and adult workers report that if they receive information at all it is often given to them quickly or in English, which they may not understand. Also, even if information is provided, workers often report that decontamination supplies are frequently unavailable, or work-related demands keep them from utilizing them.[92,96]

Given this population's extremely low access to health resources, efforts aimed at decreasing exposures and injury need to be concentrated in the development of outreach programs. For example, to help decrease the risk of childhood poisonings with household toxicants due to illiteracy among parents, the University of California, Davis, has developed the 'Safety Literacy for Migrant Worker Families: Childhood Poison Prevention' project. The project's objectives are to teach parents, in Spanish, how to read safety warnings and emergency first aid instructions as well as to install childproof latches in migrant housing.[97] Advocating for similar programs as well as for increased access to affordable daycare is perhaps the most important way healthcare providers can help prevent injury.

## Pedestrian injuries

Compared to non-Hispanic white children, Hispanic, Asian, African-American, and other minorities have the same overall rates of traumatic head injuries. However, minority children are significantly more likely to sustain injuries as pedestrians or bicyclists struck by vehicles.[98] This has been best studied in Southern California, where Hispanic-American children have been found to have an over three times higher rate of both hospitalization and death due to pedestrian injuries as compared to non-Hispanic white children. After controlling for area of residence, Hispanic children still suffered twice the rate of injury of non-Hispanic children. Therefore, the increased injury risk was only partially related to characteristics of the areas in which the children lived.[99]

A case-control study identified several factors within a Hispanic-American community that may increase the risk of injury. These include: (1) children with parents who could not read English or Spanish, (2) fathers who did not speak English, and (3) a change in a family's residence within the past year.[100] Parental illiteracy or low literacy was the strongest risk factor identified, associated with nearly a four-fold greater risk of injury. The increased risk among those with fathers who do not speak English may be related to lower economic status. Although the children were primarily cared for by their mothers, almost all of the mothers did not speak English, thereby potentially masking associations between maternal English fluency and injury risk. Children who did not speak English were at increased risk of injury, but this is likely explained by the predominance of injuries among pre-school aged children. A change in residence of the family within the past year likely leads to less familiarity with the environment and to less assistance from neighbors with supervision of children.[100]

The study also found that, at the level of the family, poverty, defined by income and household overcrowding, was associated with increased risk of injury.[100] Children living in crowded households may spend more time outdoors, thereby increasing risk of injury. However, the same researchers found that, at the level of the neighborhood, poverty and overcrowding may actually protect Hispanic children from injury.[101] This may be related to the maintenance of traditional childrearing practices characterized by involvement of extended family and community members in the supervision of children within poorer, less acculturated neighborhoods. The link between acculturation and Hispanic-American childhood injuries is further supported by the finding that in neighborhoods in which a large proportion of adults speak some English, as opposed to no English, there is an increased risk of injury.

Since one of the strongest risk factors for injury is parental illiteracy, injury prevention strategies must include nonwritten forms of information that are brought directly to immigrant parents through community health workers or the electronic media.[100] Healthcare providers should also introduce basic safety tips to immigrant parents during office visits since data indicate that minority parents are less likely to be familiar with commonly used safety devices including stair gates and cupboard locks.[102]

## Vitamin D deficiency

Since sunlight is the primary source of vitamin D,[103] vitamin D deficiency in immigrant children is considered briefly in this section on environmental exposure. The ability to synthesize vitamin D is significantly reduced in women and girls who for cultural reasons avoid sunlight or completely cover their skin with clothing.[104] Also, darker skin pigmentation is associated with reduced synthesis of vitamin D when exposed to sunlight.[105] Therefore, female immigrants with dark skin pigmentation from locations, such as Somalia, where women traditionally cover most of their skin with veiled clothing, who have settled in sunlight-deficient northern latitudes, may be at especially high risk for vitamin D deficiency. To date, no studies have been published on the prevalence of vitamin D deficiency among asymptomatic Somali women in northern America. A study from the Netherlands has shown a very high prevalence of severe vitamin D deficiency among asymptomatic veiled Arab immigrant women.[103]

Identifying populations of women with vitamin D deficiency is important to children's health since maternal vitamin D deficiency is an important cause of deficiency in infancy, a period of life in which rickets is likely to manifest. Another risk for vitamin D deficiency in infants is exclusive breast-feeding, since breast milk does not have significant levels of vitamin D.[106] Foreign-born black immigrant mothers are significantly more likely to breast-feed their children compared to US-born white women (OR = 2.6, 95% CI 1.1–6.0).[107] This is clearly a positive finding. However, these women should be familiarized with the importance of supplementing their infants' feed with vitamin D.

Among 17 cases of vitamin D deficiency in toddlers and young children aged 7–33 months seen at a Toronto hospital between 1988 and 1993, all were either of Asian or African origin, darkly pigmented, and had been exclusively breast fed without vitamin D supplementation.[108] Twelve of the children were born to recently arrived immigrant mothers. Every child had characteristic bowing of the extremities and two suffered from hypocalcemic seizures.

Adolescence is another period of life with rapid growth in which rickets or other manifestations of vitamin D deficiency may present. Extraordinarily high rates of vitamin D deficiency were detected among adolescent and adult immigrants in Minnesota from East Africa, Latin America, and Southeast Asia with persistent non-specific musculoskeletal pain.[109] In addition, several cases of limb girdle myopathies caused by vitamin D deficiency have been reported among veiled teenage immigrant girls from Africa living in the Netherlands.[110] Symptoms included pain and weakness in proximal muscles. Diagnosis is made by detecting a low 25-hydroxyvitamin D level and treatment is with ergocalciferol.

Those who care for children should encourage vitamin D supplementation of breast-fed infants. The American Academy of Pediatrics recommends that, starting within the first 2 months of life, 200 international units (IU) of vitamin D be given daily to all exclusively breast-fed infants and nonbreast-fed infants who consume less than 500 milliliters per day of fortified formula.[111] The Academy also recommends that all children and adolescents who do not receive adequate sunlight exposure or do not drink at least 500 mL of fortified milk daily should be supplemented with 200 IU daily.[111] However, there is some evidence that among women without significant sun exposure due to veiled clothing, supplementation of over 600 IU is needed.[103]

## Life-Course Theory

An idea that is receiving increasingly more attention is the possibility that events during critical periods in childhood may affect the likelihood of developing chronic diseases later in life. This concept, known as life-course theory,[112] potentially has important implications for immigrant health. Compelling data from non-immigrant populations suggest an association with low birth weight and accelerated childhood growth rates with hypertension,[113,114] impaired glucose tolerance,[115,116] and coronary events[115] in adulthood.

Researchers in Britain found that the presence of high blood pressure in adults was independently associated with both low birth weight and large weight gain between one and five years of life. Thus, adults with the highest blood pressures had the lowest birth weights and the greatest catch-up weight gain in early childhood.[113] Among a cohort of 13 467 adult women in Shanghai, China, those with the highest risk of early-onset hypertension between the

ages of 20 and 40 years were born with a low birth weight and at age 15 years were more overweight than their peers.[114] A proposed physiological explanation for these observations, based on animal models, is that individuals with low birth weights are born with decreased numbers of glomeruli, and rapid growth in childhood stresses the kidney's capacities, leading to progressive renal damage and hypertension.[114]

Similar growth patterns were seen for coronary events among a cohort of 8760 people born in Helsinki between 1934 and 1944, a period in which malnutrition was relatively common as a result of World War II.[115] The individuals who eventually had coronary events as adults had low mean birth weights. At age 2 years their BMI remained low relative to other children. Subsequently, their BMI rose relative to other children, so that by 11 years of age the BMIs of boys reached the average for the cohort and the BMIs of the girls exceeded the average (Fig. 41.3). Adults with insulin resistance followed this growth pattern as well.[115] The researchers speculate that thin babies are born with reduced amounts of muscle and that, since there is little replication of muscle after birth, rapid weight gain in childhood leads to a disproportionate increase in adipose tissue, increasing the likelihood of insulin resistance.[115]

Any population undergoing rapid transitions in nutritional status may be especially prone to such growth patterns. In many developing countries, urbanization has led to an interesting dichotomy between the nutritional status of young children and adults; underweight children and overweight adults.[117] This may be partially explained by the increased reliance on readily available, cheap, energy-dense, nutrient-poor processed foods among the urban poor. Such foods may place young children, dependent on micronutrients for normal growth, at risk for poor development early in life. With increasing age, the same foods tend to increase adiposity.[117]

This 'nutritional transition' may be involved with the high prevalence of impaired fasting glucose (10.8%) and diabetes (4.4%) among a cohort of 1492 men and women aged 26–32 years in South Delhi, India.[116] Those subjects with the highest rates of impaired fasting glucose and diabetes had the lowest BMIs at age 2 years and the highest BMIs at age 12 years. An increase in BMI by one sex-specific standard deviation from the cohort mean between ages 2 and 12 years was associated with an odds ratio of 1.36 (95% CI, 1.18–1.57, $p < 0.001$) for the development of impaired fasting glucose or diabetes. This association remained significant even after controlling for

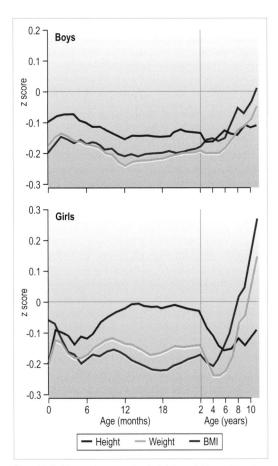

Fig. 41.3 Mean Z-scores for height, weight, and body mass index in the first 11 years after birth among a cohort of Finnish boys and girls who had coronary heart disease as adults. Adapted with permission from reference 115 (Barker, D.J.P. et al. N Engl J Med 2005; 353:1802–1809). Copyright © 2005 Massachusetts Medical Society. All rights reserved.

backgrounds in the US with subsequent growth velocities that exceeded those of US-born Caucasian children.[19,20] Whether rapid growth velocities in immigrant children with initially compromised constitutions place them at risk for future health conditions remains under-studied.

To date, one study has specifically addressed this question. Researchers examined a cohort of 3643 men and 3778 women who had immigrated from the difficult living conditions of southern China to the more economically advantaged environment of Hong Kong at some point in their lives.[112] Those who immigrated before the age of 25 years had an increased risk of developing diabetes as compared with individuals born in Hong Kong after controlling for age, gender, and family history, socio-economic status, comorbidities, smoking, alcohol consumption, and length of stay in Hong Kong. This risk was greatest for those who immigrated as young children. For migration during the life periods of 0–7 years, 8–17 years, and 18–24 years the respective odds ratios were 2.07 (95% CI 1.20–3.57), 1.70 (95% CI 1.16–2.49), and 1.86 (95% CI 1.28–1.96). Furthermore, men who immigrated before 8 years of age were over three times as likely to develop future ischemic heart disease as compared to Hong Kong-born men (OR = 3.25, 95% CI 1.73–6.10). Among women who immigrated before 25 years of age there was a nonstatistically significant increase in ischemic heart disease. Immigration between the ages of 8 to 17 years was associated with increased risk of hypertension and hyperlipidemia. The investigators concluded that 'environmental change through migration in the first two decades of life' was associated with increased risk of several chronic health conditions, indicating 'the importance of specific life-course pathways on the development of the conditions for populations undergoing rapid transition.'

How best to incorporate life-course theory into the preventive care of immigrant children remains unknown. Until more information is available, providers should closely monitor the BMIs of children who started life relatively malnourished with a goal of catching and addressing rapid weight gains early.

adult BMI. A key observation is that, although the children who went on to develop impaired fasting glucose and diabetes as adults had the highest BMIs at age 12 years, only 3.3% of these children were overweight at this age and none was obese.[116] Thus, rapid childhood weight gain, not necessarily excessive childhood weight gain, was a predictor of future illness in this cohort.

Immigrant children, especially those born to malnourished mothers, may be faced with similar life-course pathways resulting in growth patterns that place them at risk for chronic illness. This possibility is supported by studies showing high rates of stunting in newly arrived immigrant children from Southeast Asian, Chinese, Filipino and Hispanic

## Conclusion

- Children of immigrant families are the fastest growing segment of the pediatric population.
- Children of immigrant families face multiple barriers to healthcare, including

insurance coverage, linguistic isolation, and level of providers' cultural competency, leading to health disparities.

- Health disparities among children of immigrant families may stem from preexisting health inequities, acculturation, and environmental exposures. Life-course events, such as the combination of preexisting malnutrition and subsequent acculturation-associated diet and lifestyle changes, may place immigrant children at even greater risk for several chronic health conditions.

- Culturally and linguistically appropriate outreach into immigrant communities is essential to increase awareness of available health resources and to augment preventive health education.

## References

1. Office of Immigration Statistics. Yearbook of Immigration Statistics: 2006. US Department of Homeland Security. http://www.dhs.gov/ximgtn/statistics/publications/Yearbook.shtm Accessed 5/10/07.
2. Jenista JA. The immigrant, refugee, or internationally adopted child. Pediatr Rev 2001; 22:419–428.
3. Hernandez DJ, Charney E. From generation to generation: the health and well-being of children in immigrant families. Washington, DC: National Academy Press; 1998.
4. Reardon-Anderson J, Capps R, Fix M. The health and well-being of children in immigrant families. The Urban Institute. Series B, No. B-52, November 2002.
5. Guendelman S, Schauffler HH, Pearl M. Unfriendly shores: how immigrant children fare in the US health system. Health Affairs 2001; 20:257–266.
6. Burgos AE, Schezina KE, Dixon B, et al. Importance of generational status in examining access to and utilization of healthcare by Mexican American children. Pediatrics 2005; 115:e322–e330.
7. Sarmiento OL, Miller WC, Ford CA, et al. Disparities in routine physical examinations among in-school adolescents of differing Latino origins. J Adoles Health 2004; 35:310–320.
8. Kaushal N, Kaestner R. Welfare reform and health insurance of immigrants. Health Serv Res 2005; 40(3):697–721.
9. Flores G, Abreu M, Brown V, et al. How Medicaid and the State Children's Health Insurance Program can do a better job of insuring uninsured children: the perspectives of parents of uninsured Latino children. Ambul Pediatr 2005; 5(6):332–340.
10. Shi L, Stevens GD. Disparities in access to care and satisfaction among US children: the roles of race/ethnicity and poverty status. Public Health Rep 2005; 120:431–441.
11. Yu SM, Huang ZJ, Schwalberg RH, et al. Parental awareness of health and community resources among immigrant families. Matern Child Health J 2005; 9:27–34.
12. Kobayashi A, Moore E, Rosenberg M. Healthy immigrant children: a demographic and geographic analysis. W-98-20E. Quebec. Canada: Human Resources Development Canada; 1998. Available: http://www.hrsdc.gc.ca/en/cs/sp/sdc/pkrf/publications/research/1998-000133/page00.shtml February 23, 2007
13. American Academy of Pediatrics. Committee on Community Health Services. Healthcare for children of immigrant families. Pediatrics 1997; 100:153–156.
14. Flores G, Abreu M, Olivar MA, et al. Access barriers to healthcare for Latino children. Arch Pediatr Adolesc Med 1998; 152:1119–1125.
15. Davidson N, Skull S, Burgner D, et al. An issue of access: delivering equitable healthcare for newly arrived refugee children in Australia. J Paediatr Child Health 2004; 40:508–509.
16. Lopriore C, Guidoum Y, Briend A. Spread fortified with vitamins and minerals induces catch-up growth and eradicates severe anemia in stunted refugee children aged 3–6 y. Am J Clin Nutr 2004; 80:973–981.
17. Berkman DS, Lescano AG, Gilman RH. Effects of stunting, diarrhoeal, and parasitic infection during infancy on cognition in late-childhood. Lancet 2002; 359:564–571.
18. Geltman PL, Radin M, Zhang Z, et al. Growth status and related medical conditions among refugee children in Massachusetts, 1995–1998. Am J Public Health 2001; 91:1800–1805.
19. Schumacher LB, Pawson G, Kretchmer N. Growth of immigrant children in newcomer schools of San Francisco. Pediatrics 1980; 80(6):861–868.
20. Yip R, Scanlon K, Trowbridge F. Improving growth status of Asian refugee children in the United States. JAMA 1992; 267:937–940.
21. Parent AS, Teilmann G, Juul A. The timing of normal puberty and the age limits of sexual precocity: Variations around the world, secular trends, and changes after migration. Endocrine Rev 2003; 24:668–693.
22. Kemmer TM, Bovill ME, Kongsomboon W, et al. Iron deficiency is unacceptably high in refugee children from Burma. J Nutr 2003; 133:4143–4149.
23. Kwong WT, Friello, Semba RD. Interactions between iron deficiency and lead poisoning: epidemiology and pathogenesis. Sci Total Environ 2004; 330:21–37.
24. CDC. Elevated blood lead levels in refugee children – New Hampshire, 2003–2004. MMWR 2005; 54:42–45.
25. Jeng MR, Vichinsky E. Hematologic problems in immigrants from Southeast Asia. Hematol Oncol Clin North Am 2004; 18:1405–1422.
26. Kuczmarski RJ, Ogden CL, Grummer-Strawn LM, et al. CDC growth charts: United States. Adv Data 2000; 8:1–27.
27. Dietz WH, Robinson TN. Overweight children and adolescents. New Engl J Med. 2005; 352:2100–2109.
28. Cote S, Geltman P, Nunn M. Dental caries of refugee children compared with US children. Pediatrics 2004; 114:733–740.
29. Flores G, Brotanek J. The healthy immigrant effect: a greater understanding might help us improve the health of all children. Arch Pediatr Adolesc Med 2005; 159:295–296.
30. Singh GK, Yu SM. Adverse pregnancy outcomes: differences between US- and foreign-born women in major US racial and ethnic groups. Am J Public Health 1996; 86:837–843.
31. Collins JW, Papacek E, Schulte NF, et al. Differing postnatal mortality rates of Mexican-American infants with United States-born and Mexican-born mothers in Chicago. Ethn Dis 2001; 11:606–613.
32. Gruber C, Illi S, Plieth A, et al. Cultural adaptation is associated with atopy and wheezing among children of Turkish origin living in Germany. Clin Exp Allergy 2002; 32:526–531.
33. Popkin BM, Udry JR. Adolescent obesity increases significantly in the second and third generation US immigrants: the national longitudinal study of adolescent health. J Nutr 1998; 128:701–706.
34. Unger JB, Cruz TB, Rohrbach LA, et al. English language usage as a risk factor for smoking initiation among Latino and Asian-American adolescents: evidence for mediation by tobacco-related beliefs and social norms. Health Psychol 2000; 19:403–410.

35. Ungar JB, Gallaher P, Shakib S, et al. The AHIMSA Acculturation Scale: a new measure of acculturation for adolescents in a multicultural society. J Early Adolesc 2002; 22:225–251.

36. Gfroerer JC, Tan LL. Substance use among foreign-born youths in the United States: does length of residence matter? Am J Public Health 2003; 93:1892–1895.

37. Mokimoto K. Drinking patterns and drinking problems among Asian-Americans and Pacific Islanders. Alc Health Res World 1998; 22:270–275.

38. Guilamo-Ramos V, Jaccard J, Johansson M, et al. Binge drinking among Latino youth: role of acculturation-related variables. Psychol Addict Behav 2004; 18:135–142.

39. Epstein JA, Botvin GJ, Diaz T. Linguistic acculturation associated with higher marijuana and polydrug use among Hispanic adolescents. Subt Use Misuse 2001; 36:477–499.

40. Adam MB, McGuire JK, Walsh M. Acculturation as a predictor of the onset of sexual intercourse among Hispanic and white teens. Arch Pediatr Adolesc Med 2005; 159:261–265.

41. Samaniego RY, Gonzales NA. Multiple mediators of the effects of acculturation status on delinquency for Mexican American adolescents. Am J Community Psychol 1999; 27:189–210.

42. Hovey JD. Acculturative stress, depression, and suicidal ideation among Mexican-American adolescents: implications for the development of suicide prevention programs in schools. Psychol Rep 1998; 83:249–250.

43. Unger JB, Reynolds K, Shakib S, et al. Acculturation, physical activity and fast-food consumption among Asian-American and Hispanic adolescents. J Community Health 2004; 29:467–481.

44. Culhane-Pera KA, Naftali ED, Jacobson C, et al. Cultural feeding practices and child-raising philosophy contribute to iron-deficiency anemia in refugee Hmong children. Ethn Dis 2002; 12:174–176.

45. Janssen I, Katzmarzyk PT, Boyce WF, et al. Comparison of overweight and obesity prevalence in school-aged youth from 34 countries and their relationships with physical activity and dietary patterns. Obes Res 2005; 6:123–132.

46. Committee on Nutrition. American Academy of Pediatrics. Prevention of pediatric overweight and obesity. Pediatrics 2003; 112:424–430.

47. Ogden CL, Flegal KM, Carroll MD, et al. Prevalence and trends in overweight among US children and adolescents, 1999–2000. JAMA 2002; 288:1728–1732.

48. Hedley A, Ogden CL, Johnson CL, et al. Prevalence of overweight and obesity among US children, adolescents, and adults, 1999–2002. JAMA 2004; 291;2847–2850.

49. Baruffi G, Hardy CJ, Waslien CI, et al. Ethnic differences in the prevalence of overweight among young children in Hawaii. J Am Diet Assoc 2004; 104:1701–1707.

50. Gordon-Larson P, Adair LS, Popkin BM. The relationship of ethnicity, socioeconomic factors, and overweight in US adolescents. Obes Res 2003; 11:121–129.

51. Gordon-Larsen P, Mullan Harris K, Ward DS. Acculturation and overweight-related behaviors among Hispanic immigrants to the US: the National Longitudinal Study of Adolescent Health. Social Sci Med 2003; 57:2023–2034.

52. Mazur RE, Marquis GS, Jensen HH. Diet and food insufficiency among Hispanic youths: acculturation and socioeconomic factors in the third National Health and Nutrition Examination Survey. Am J Clin Nutr 2003; 78:1120–1127.

53. Casey PH, Szeto K, Lensing S, et al. Children in food-insufficient, low-income families: prevalence, health, and nutrition status. Arch Pediatr Adolesc Med 2001; 155:508–514.

54. Chen JL, Kennedy C. Factors associated with obesity in Chinese-American children. Pediatr Nurs 2005; 31:110–115.

55. Renzaho AMN. Fat, rich and beautiful: changing socio-cultural paradigms associated with obesity risk, nutritional status and refugee children from sub-Saharan Africa. Health Place 2004; 10:105–113.

56. Zimmermann MB, Gubeli C, Puntener C, et al. Detection of overweight and obesity in a national sample of 6–12-y-old Swiss children: accuracy and validity of reference values for body mass index from the US Centers for Disease Control and Prevention and the International Obesity Task Force. Am J Clin Nutr 2004; 79:838–843.

57. Clarkin P. Methodological issues in the anthropometric assessment of Hmong children in the United States. Am J Hum Biol 2005; 17:787–795.

58. Popkin BM, Richards MK, Montiero CA. Stunting is associated with overweight in children of four nations that are undergoing the nutrition transition. J Nutr 1996; 126:3009–3016.

59. Cole TJ, Bellizzi MC, Flegal KM, et al. Establishing a standard definition of child overweight and obesity worldwide: international survey. Br Med J 2000; 320:1–6.

60. Brindis C, Wolfe AL, McCarter V, et al. The associations between immigrant status and risk-behavior patterns in Latino adolescents. J Adolesc Health 1995; 17:99–105.

61. Jones CJ, Trickett EJ. Immigrant adolescents behaving as culture brokers: a study of families from the former Soviet Union. J Soc Psychol 2005; 145:405–427.

62. Guilamo-Ramos V, Jaccard J, Johansson M, et al. Binge drinking among Latino youth: role of acculturation-related variables. Psychol Addict Behav 2004; 18:135–142.

63. Elder JP, Campbell NR, Litrownik AJ, et al. Predictors of cigarette and alcohol susceptibility and use among Hispanic migrant adolescents. Preventive Med 2000; 31:115–123.

64. Hahm HC, Lahiff M, Guterman NB. Acculturation and parental attachment in Asian-American adolescent alcohol use. J Adolesc Health 2003; 33:119–129.

65. Blake SM, Ledsky R, Goodenow C, et al. Recency of immigration, substance abuse, and sexual behavior among Massachusetts adolescents. Am J Publich Health 2001; 91:794–798.

66. Litrownik AJ, Elder JP, Campbell NR, et al. Evaluation of a tobacco and alcohol use prevention program for Hispanic migrant adolescents: promoting the protective factor of parent-child communication. Preventive Med 2000; 31:124–133.

67. Adam MB, McGuire JK, Walsh M, et al. Acculturation as a predictor of the onset of sexual intercourse among Hispanic and white teens. Arch Pediatr Adolesc Med 2005; 159:295–297.

68. Chung PJ, Borneo H, Kilpatrick SD, et al. Parent–adolescent communication about sex in Filipino American families: a demonstration of community-based participatory research. Ambul Pediatr 2005; 5:50–55.

69. Gibson PG, Henry RL, Shah S. Migration to a Western country increases asthma symptoms but not eosinophilic airway inflammation. Pediatr Pulmonol 2003; 36:209–215.

70. Eldeirawi K, McConnel R, Freela S, et al. Associations of place of birth with asthma and wheezing in Mexican American children. J Allergy Clin Immunol 2005; 116:42–48.

71. Rottem M, Szyper-Kravitz M, Shoenfeld Y. Atopy and asthma in migrants. Int Arch Allergy Immunol 2005; 136:198–204.

72. Cookson WO, Moffatt MF. Asthma: an epidemic in the absence of infection? Science 1997; 275:41–42.

73. Gold DR, Acevedo-Garcia D. Immigration to the United States and acculturation as risk factors for asthma and allergy. J Allergy Clin Immunol 2005; 116:38–41.

74. Weinberg AD, Kripalani S, McCarthy PL, et al. Caring for survivors of the Chernobyl disaster. What the clinician should know. JAMA 1995; 274:408–412.

75. American Academy of Pediatrics Committee on Environmental Health. American Academy of Pediatrics. Lead. In: Etzel RA, ed. Pediatric environmental health. 2nd edn. Elk Grove Village, IL: American Academy of Pediatrics; 2003:249–266.

76. Laraque D, Trasande L. Lead poisoning: Successes and 21st century challenges. Pediatrics Rev 2005; 26:429–436.

77. CDC. Fatal pediatric lead poisoning – New Hampshire, 2000. MMWR 2001; 50:457–459.

78. Canfield RL, Henderson CR, Cory-Slechta DA, et al. Intellectual impairment in children with blood lead concentration below 10 micrograms per deciliter. New Engl J Med 2003; 348:1517–1526.

79. CDC. Blood lead levels – United States, 1999–2002. MMWR 2005; 54:513–516.

80. Minnesota Department of Health. Lead poisoning in Minnesota Refugee Children, 2000–2002. 2004; 32. Anonomous. Lead Poisoining in Minnesota Refugee Children, 2000–2002. Minnesota Department of Health. Available: http://www.health.state.mn.us/divs/idepc/ newsletters/dcn/2004/mar04/lead.html Accessed 2/23/07.

81. Geltman PL, Brown MJ, Cochran J. Lead poisoning among refugee children resettled in Massachusetts, 1995 to 1999. Pediatrics 2001; 108:158–162.

82. Trepka MJ, Pekovic V, Santana JC, et al. Risk factors for lead poisoning among Cuban refugee children. Public Health Rep 2005; 120:179–185.

83. Wright RO, Tsaih SW, Schwartz J. Association between iron deficiency and blood lead level in a longitudinal analysis of children followed in an urban primary care clinic. J Pediatr 2003; 149:9–14.

84. Binns HJ, Kim D, Campbell C. Targeted screening for elevated blood lead levels: Populations at high risk. Pediatrics 2001; 108:1364–1366.

85. CDC. Childhood lead poisoning associated with tamarind candy and folk remedies – California, 1999–2000. MMWR 2002; 51:684–686.

86. CDC. Lead poisoning associated with imported candy and powdered food coloring – California and Michigan. MMWR 1998; 47:1041–1043.

87. CDC. Lead poisoning from lead tetroxide used as a folk remedy – Colorado. MMWR 1982; 30:647–648.

88. CDC. Lead poisoning associated with use of traditional ethnic remedies – California, 1991–1992. MMWR 1993; 42:521–524.

89. CDC. Folk remedy-associated lead poisoning in Hmong children – Minnesota. MMWR 1983; 32:555–556.

90. CDC. Lead poisoning associated with use of litargirio – Rhode Island, 2003. MMWR 2005; 54:227–229.

91. CDC. Epidemiologic notes and reports lead poisoning following ingestion of homemade beverage stored in a ceramic jug – New York. MMWR 1989; 38:379–380.

92. Salazar MK, Napolitano M, Scherer JA, et al. Hispanic adolescent farmworkers' perceptions associated with pesticide exposure. Western J Nursing Res 2004; 26:146–166.

93. Davis S. Child labor in agriculture. ERIC Digest. 1997. Available: http://wdcrobcolp01.ed.gov/CFAPPS/ERIC/ resumes/records.cfm?ericnum=ED405159 February 23, 2007.

94. Wilk VA. Health hazards to children in agriculture. Am J Ind Med 1993; 24:283–290.

95. McCauley LA, Lasarev MR, Higgins G, et al. Work characteristics and pesticide exposures among migrant agricultural families: a community-based research approach. Environ Health Perspect 2001; 109:533–538.

96. Shipp EM, Cooper SP, Burau KD, et al. Pesticide safety training and access to field sanitation among migrant farmworker mothers from Starr County, Texas. J Agric Saf Health 2005; 11:51–60.

97. Thigpen KG. Beyond the bench: keeping migrant families safe. Environ Health Perspect 2004; 112:A618–A619.

98. Howard I, Joseph JG, Natale JE. Pediatric traumatic brain injury: do racial/ethnic disparities exist in brain injury severity, mortality, or medical disposition? Ethn Dis 2005; 15:S5–S51, S56–S61.

99. Agran PF, Winn DG, Anderson CL. Pediatric injury hospitalization in Hispanic and non-Hispanic children in Southern California. Arch Pediatr Adolesc Med 1996; 150:400–406.

100. Agran PF, Winn DG, Anderson CL, et al. Family, social and cultural factors in pedestrian injuries among Hispanic children. Inj Prev 1998; 4:188–193.

101. Anderson CL, Agran PF, Winn DG, et al. Demographic risk factors for injury among Hispanic and non-Hispanic white children: an ecologic analysis. Inj Prev 1998; 4:33–38.

102. Mulvaney C, Kendrick D. Engagement in safety practices to prevent home injuries in preschool children among white and non-white ethnic minority families. Inj Prev 2004; 10:375–378.

103. Glerup H, Mikkelsen K, Poulsen L, et al. Commonly recommended daily intake of vitamin D is not sufficient if sunlight exposure is limited. J Intern Med 2000; 247:260–268.

104. Mishal AA. Effects of different dress styles on vitamin D levels in healthy young Jordanian women. Osteoporosis Internat 2001; 12:931–935.

105. Clemons TL, Henderson SL, Adams JS, et al. Increased skin pigmentation reduces the capacity of skin to synthesize vitamin D3. Lancet 1982; 1(8263):74–76.

106. Wharton B, Bishop N. Rickets. Lancet 2003; 362:1389–1400.

107. Celi AC, Rich-Edwards JW, Richardson MK, et al. Immigration, race/ethnicity, and social and economic factors as predictors of breastfeeding initiation. Arch Pediatr Adolesc Med 2005; 159:255–260.

108. Binet A, Kooh SW. Persistence of vitamin D-deficiency rickets in Toronto in the 1990s. Can J Public Health 1996; 87:227–230.

109. Plotnikoff GA, Quigley JM. Prevalence of severe hypovitaminosis D in patients with persistent, nonspecific musculoskeletal pain. Mayo Clin Proc 2003; 78:1463–1470.

110. van der Heyden JJ, Verrips A, ter Laak HJ, et al. Hypovitaminosis D-related myopathy in immigrant teenagers. Neuropediatrics 2004; 35:290–292.

111. Gartner LM, Greer FR, et al. Prevention of rickets and vitamin D deficiency: New guidelines for vitamin D intake. Pediatrics 2003; 111:908–910.

112. Schooling M, Leung GM, Janus ED, et al. Childhood migration and cardiovascular risk. Internat J Epidemiol 2004; 33:1219–1226.

113. Law CM, Shiell AW, Newsome CA, et al. Fetal, infant and childhood growth and adult blood pressure. Circulation 2002; 105:1088–1092.

114. Zhao M, Shu XO, Jin F, et al. Birthweight, childhood growth and hypertension in adulthood. Internat J Epidemiol 2002; 31:1043–1051.

115. Barker DJP, Osmond C, Forsén TJ, et al. Trajectories of growth among children who have coronary events as adults. New Engl J Med 2005; 353:1802–1809.

116. Bhargava SK, Sachdev HS, Fall CHD, et al. Relation of serial changes in childhood body-mass-index to impaired glucose tolerance in young adulthood. New Engl J Med 2004; 350:865–875.

117. Caballero B. A nutrition paradox – underweight and obesity in developing countries. New Engl J Med 2005; 352:1514–1516.

CHAPTER 42

# Preventive Healthcare and Management of Chronic Diseases in Adults

Patricia F. Walker

## Introduction

Complex interactions between the patient, the healthcare delivery system, and providers all have an impact upon both the ability to, and interest in, participating collaboratively in preventive healthcare and aggressive chronic disease management. This chapter will highlight the dangers of generalization and the need for a disciplined, consistent approach to health promotion and prevention, as well as chronic disease management. Well-documented disparities in preventive healthcare and in chronic disease outcomes exist for immigrants, even after correcting for access to care. Issues of access and language are key determinants of use of preventive health services and chronic disease management, and are discussed elsewhere in detail in this text. However, interesting data on cultural considerations in preventive healthcare and chronic disease management exist, and can assist with the design of culturally competent prevention and treatment programs.

Utilization is also affected by gender, age, race, and ethnicity, as well as by experiences within the healthcare delivery system in an immigrant's country of origin. Prevalence rates for chronic diseases vary by race/ethnicity, country of origin, and time since immigration. It is therefore challenging for clinicians to design preventive health screening programs which are appropriate to patients from many different countries and ethnic and cultural backgrounds. Clinician attitudes and behaviors, skills, and knowledge base also play a role in contributing to health disparities for immigrants.

Other chapters deal with key issues in preventive healthcare and screening including infectious disease screening, women's health, oral health, mental health screening, and screening for injury and violence; this chapter will focus on selected issues of universal concern to adult refugees and immigrants including health promotion and prevention, cancer and osteoporosis screening, as well as management of diabetes and heart disease. Recommended approaches designed to improve preventive health services and chronic disease outcomes will be outlined.

## Preventive Services and Chronic Disease Management: General Considerations

### Access to care

Racial differences in access to care are a primary contributor to health disparities for immigrants, particularly for the undocumented. However, even after correcting for access to care, minority patient outcomes are worse than majority.[1] For example, in one study of primary care office visits utilizing National Ambulatory Medical Care Surveys between 1985 and 2000, neither patient HMO membership nor physician HMO participation was greatly associated with racial disparities in primary care.[2] This study concluded that changes in HMO membership alone are unlikely to affect disparities in receipt of primary care, for better or for worse.

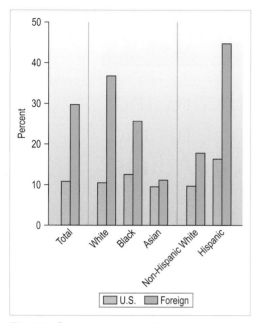

**Fig. 42.1** Persons under age 65 uninsured all year, by race and ethnicity, 2002.[1]

Racial differences in utilization of care are summarized in data from the 2005 National Health Care Disparities report, shown in Table 42.1.

A study of elderly Chinese immigrants in Boston revealed that patients underutilized services for multiple complex reasons including language, transportation, cost, long waits for appointments, and cross-cultural issues including fear and distrust of Western medicine.[6] A prospective study of behavioral risk factors and preventive healthcare practices of immigrants seen in the emergency department at Bellevue Hospital Center, New York, revealed that immigrant women were more likely never to have had a Papanicolaou test (16.1% versus 1.4%) and never to have performed a breast self-examination (20.8% versus 7.5%). Immigrants were more likely not to use condoms (63.4% versus 42.8%) and never to have visited the dentist (21.2% versus 7.8%). These differences were independent of age, gender, marital status, employment, education, income and health insurance status. When analyzing the immigrant group alone, region of origin, length of time in the United States, and English ability were significant independent predictors of higher-risk behavioral profiles and poorer preventive healthcare practices.[7]

Language, job security, and education top the list of concerns for immigrants in successfully adapting to life in a new country. Language is a primary barrier to care, and is related to probability of having a primary care provider (Fig. 42.2).

While the healthy migrant effect has been confirmed in national studies (see Ch. 3), less use of the healthcare delivery system by immigrants is complex and multifactorial, reflecting barriers of access, language, and cultural beliefs which may clash with American healthcare. It is also difficult to separate data specifically for refugees after immigration, as they become subsumed under the foreign-born, or immigrant category.[3]

Health insurance facilitates access to care. The uninsured report more problems getting care, have poorer health status, and are diagnosed at later disease stages (Fig. 42.1).[1]

## Language, transportation, and cross-cultural barriers

Other barriers to care include language, transportation, and cross-cultural issues between providers and patients.[4] Age, gender, country of origin, and length of time in the US all have been shown to impact immigrants' utilization of healthcare services. A recent survey of Latinos in Philadelphia showed income and education determined having health insurance, time in the US and health insurance determined having a regular source of care, and having a source of care and being female determined visits to the doctor in the past year.[5]

## Unequal treatment

In a national survey of physicians in 2002, the majority of doctors tended to say the healthcare system 'rarely' or 'never' treats people unfairly based on various characteristics such as race/ethnicity, language, or country of origin, though significant minorities of physicians, including female physicians and physicians of color, disagreed.[8] African-American physicians, for example, were much more likely than other physicians to be aware of existing disparities in treatment for heart disease and HIV/AIDS based on race. Doctors who said racial and ethnic disparities happened at least 'somewhat often' were most likely to say that a lack of doctors in minority communities and communication difficulties were the primary reasons. Providers are not alone in this belief: in a nationally representative sample of Americans age 18 or over, 68% of Americans were unaware that disparities in the quality of healthcare exist.[9] Forty-four percent of African-

**Table 42.1 Racial and ethnic differences in healthcare utilization[1]**

| Core report measure | Racial difference[a] | | | | | Ethnic difference[b] |
|---|---|---|---|---|---|---|
| | Black | Asian[c] | NHOPI[c] | AI/AN | >1 Race | Hispanic |
| **Dental care** | | | | | | |
| Persons with a dental visit in the past year[d] | ↓ | ↓ | = | ↓ | ↓ | ↓ |
| **Emergency care** | | | | | | |
| Emergency department visits per 100 population[e] | ↑ | ↓ | | | ↑ | |
| **Avoidable admissions** | | | | | | |
| Admissions for perforated appendix per 1000 admissions with appendicitis[f] | ↑ | = | | | | ↑ |
| **Mental healthcare and substance abuse treatment** | | | | | | |
| Adults who received mental health treatment or counseling in the past year[g] | ↓ | ↓ | | ↓ | = | ↓ |
| Persons age 12 and older who received illicit drug or alcohol abuse treatment in the past year[g] | = | | | ↑ | | = |

[a] Compared with whites.
[b] Compared with non-Hispanic whites.
[c] Findings are presented separately for Asians and NHOPI whenever possible. However, some data sources collected data for Asians and Pacific Islanders (APIs) as a single population; in these cases, the Asian and NHOPI cells are merged into a single cell representing APIs.
[d] Source: Medical Expenditure Panel Survey, 2002.
[e] Source: National Hospital Ambulatory Medical Care Survey – Emergency Department, 2001–2002. Missing rates preclude analysis by ethnicity.
[f] Source: HCUP SID disparities analysis file, 2002. This source categorizes race/ethnicity very differently from other sources. Race/ethnicity information is categorized as a single item: non-Hispanic non-white, Hispanic black, Hispanic, Asian or Pacific Islander. These contrasts compare each group with non-Hispanic whites.
[g] Source: Substance Abuse and Mental Health Services Administration, National Survey on Drug Use and Health, 2003.
NHOPI, Native Hawaiian or Other Pacific Islander; AI/AN, American Indian or Alaska Native.
Symbols
= Group and comparison group receive about same amount of healthcare.
↑ Group receives more healthcare than the comparison group.
↓ Group receives less healthcare than the comparison group.
Blank cell: Reliable estimate for group could not be made.

Americans and 56% of Hispanics/Latinos felt they received worse care than whites. Patients' perceptions of bias on the part of providers have been shown in other studies. In a study from the Commonwealth Fund in 2002, African-Americans (15%), Hispanics/Latinos (13%), and Asian-Americans (11%) were more likely than whites (1%) to feel they are treated with disrespect when receiving healthcare, experience barriers to access to care such as lack of insurance or not having a regular doctor, and feel they would receive better care if they were of a different race or ethnicity (Fig. 42.3).[10]

## Pre-emigration healthcare experiences

Generational status, pre-emigration healthcare experiences, and acculturation all play a role in utiliza-

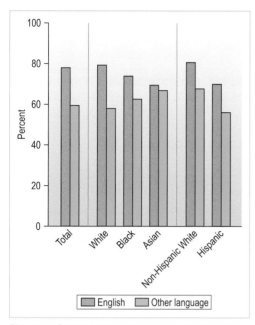

**Fig. 42.2** Persons who have a usual primary care provider, by race and ethnicity, and language spoken at home, 2002.[3]

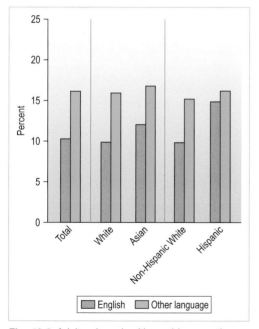

**Fig. 42.3** Adults whose health provider sometimes or never listened carefully, explained things, showed respect, and spent enough time with them, by race and ethnicity, and language spoken at home, 2002.[1]

tion of services. Elderly immigrants from the former Soviet Union extensively utilized health services in one study.[11] Providing support for depression and loneliness, educating immigrants about the role of primary care providers in the US as well as realistic expectations of American medicine, and managing care to decrease the use of unnecessary services were all recommended.

> 'I noticed that Russian patients were more inclined to ask to see a specialist – a request based on the 2 tiered care delivery system of the former Soviet Union, with public insurance being equated with poor care.'
>
> Minnesota physician

One intriguing study of Russian-speaking immigrants across three age groups demonstrated that immigrant women accessed healthcare services based on their patterns of utilization in their countries of origin. Younger and middle aged women tended to utilize the emergency room for episodic care, and older women accessed services at clinics.[12] Lack of connection to a specific primary care provider or clinic, as previously outlined, is a barrier to care for immigrants.

Perceptions of health services attributes were influenced by families' sociocultural referents and pre-emigration experience in one study of immigrants to Montreal. The primary attributes upon which families based their evaluation, selection, and adoption of health services were geographical and temporal accessibility, interpersonal and technical quality of services, and language spoken by health professionals and staff.[13] Many immigrants come from countries where appointments were not utilized, and expectations of the ability to walk in for care without an appointment persist after arrival in the US. Timeliness of care differs by race and ethnicity in the United States, as shown in Table 42.2.

In one study of Bosnian immigrants (more than 300 000 of whom have come to the United States since the 1990s), participants were universally critical of the US system and compared their experience with prewar Bosnian healthcare. They were specifically critical of confusion about health insurance coverage, lack of personalized quality of care, access to primary and specialty care, and a perception of US healthcare as bureaucratic.[14] In 150 Latino immigrant families, even perceived social acceptance, such as being identified as Latino, affected health behavior, emphasizing the complexity of factors which interplay in health behavior.[15]

**Table 42.2 Racial differences in timeliness of care[1]**

| Core report measure | Racial difference[a] | | | | | Ethnic difference[b] |
|---|---|---|---|---|---|---|
| | Black | Asian[c] | NHOPI[c] | AI/AN | >1 Race | Hispanic |
| **Timeliness** | | | | | | |
| Adults who sometimes or never get care for illness or injury as soon as wanted[d] | ↓ | ↓ | | | = | ↓ |
| Emergency department visits in which the patient left without being seen[e] | ↓ | | | | | |

[a] Compared with whites.
[b] Compared with non-Hispanic whites.
[c] Findings are presented separately for Asians and NHOPI whenever possible. However, some data sources collected data for Asians and Pacific Islanders (APIs) as a single population; in these cases, the Asian and NHOPI cells are merged into a single cell representing APIs.
[d] Source: Medical Expenditure Panel Survey, 2002. This source did not collect data for >1 race.
[e] Source: National Hospital Ambulatory Medical Care Survey – Emergency Department, 2001–2002. Missing rates preclude analysis by ethnicity.
NHOPI, Native Hawaiian or Other Pacific Islander; AI/AN, American Indian or Alaska Native.

## Cultural issues affecting use of preventive services

Concepts of prevention vary across cultures, are complex and multifaceted, and relate to beliefs about disease causation. In many immigrant communities, the Western biomedical model of disease causation is alien, and illness may be thought due to bad karma, soul loss, curses such as the evil eye, or punishment for wrong-doing in a previous life (see Chs 7 and 8). Concepts of disease prevention and treatment exist in all cultures, and are based on belief systems of disease causation.

> When Hmong refugees first arrived in Minnesota, mothers would put knives facing outwards in the cribs of their newborn infants, to repel evil spirits. Beautiful Hmong baby hats are designed in part to fool evil spirits into thinking that this is not a child to harm, but a flower to be ignored.

Patients therefore may not be coming to a Western provider with a desire for obtaining a diagnosis (they may already have a belief about what is causing their illness), but specifically for symptom relief. In many cultures, any procedures done in the setting of lack of symptoms, such as mammography and colonoscopy, are considered invasive and unnecessary. A focus group with Iranian women in Sweden revealed that complex relationships and reasoning about health maintenance and disease prevention were related to perceptions of body and self, and to the continual construction of social roles throughout the lifespan. 'Cultural' differences in cancer prevention behavior appear to have been as related to social roles and phases in the life cycle as to ethnicity. Providing information which focused on potential serious diagnoses, such as 'we may find an early cancer,' was viewed as leading to negative outcomes.[16]

Both cross-cultural issues and the state of the care delivery system in an immigrant's home country affect beliefs regarding early diagnosis and intervention. Patients may believe in fate or karma, and may not feel healthcare systems can intervene in destiny. Because of lack of services in their country of origin, they are often not aware of the existence of effective treatments either for cancer or for chronic diseases such as diabetes or heart disease. Other needs including language acquisition, jobs, and childcare issues necessarily take precedence over interaction with the medical care system.

In one study of Russian immigrant women and breast cancer screening in Israel, interviews demonstrated gaps between cognition and behavior. Israeli women aged 50–74 in this study were entitled to a free screening mammography every 2 years. Most respondents were educated women who acknowledged their personal risk, understood the role of screening, but still avoided preventive action.

'I didn't see doctors even when I had high blood pressure, colitis and other problems – since they are all chronic. I know all about the drugs, diet, etc. I have some prescription drugs at home; friends buy them for me in Russia. So you can figure out yourself that I have no time and no right mindset for preventive check ups. I just take it easy – what will be, will be'.

Russian immigrant[57]

Preventive health concerns were low on the personal agenda of female immigrants, burdened by more immediate needs including income, housing, and support of other family members. Other barriers included lack of referral from primary care providers, fear of cancer diagnosis, apprehension regarding irradiation and pain involved in mammography, a fatalistic general attitude toward health and illness, and distrust of current cancer therapies. Older women (60+), whose risks were actually higher, shared a false belief that breast cancer strikes younger women and that they were already past the age of concern. Older informants avoided gynecological clinics because of the male gender of most gynecologists, their poor command of Hebrew, and a belief that gynecological checkups were irrelevant and even shameful at their age. The study concluded that female immigrants, particularly older ones, must be a special target group for preventive health interventions.[17] In another study, intervention with socioculturally tailored breast health articles in Urdu and Hindi in South Asian community newspapers resulted in improved self-reporting of 'ever had' routine physical checkup, clinical breast examination, and knowledge, as well as decreased misperception of low susceptibility to breast cancer, and short survival after diagnosis.[18]

In many non-Western cultures, discussing a diagnosis of cancer or terminal illness is not culturally acceptable, and is thought to cause more symptoms as well as speed up the inevitable dying process. Because of a lack of desire to receive a diagnosis of cancer, patients are less likely to agree to participate in cancer screening. Management of cancer, once diagnosed, becomes problematic, as the therapeutic alliance with the patient and extended family can be broken as informed consent for treatment is provided.

'I received a telephone call from California from an irate middle- aged son of a Russian patient. I had told my patient, aged 83, that he had esophageal cancer. "How dare you tell my father!" expressed his son, "You should have

called me, and I would talk to him and make a plan. You have made him more sick." '

P.F. Walker

In an editorial by Dr. Antonella Surbone, an oncologist from Italy, the observation was made that what is beneficent from a Western biomedical ethics perspective – that patients are given informed consent for diagnosis and treatment of cancer – may actually be maleficent in other cultures.[19]

## End-of-life care/advance directives

Research has identified three basic dimensions in end-of-life treatment that vary culturally: communication of 'bad news'; locus of decision-making (individual versus extended family/community); and attitudes toward advance directives and end-of-life care.[20]

Bosnian immigrants in one study were interviewed about their views of physician–patient communication, advance directives, and locus of decision-making in serious illness.[21] 'It's like playing with your destiny,' one immigrant stated. Many indicated they did not want to be directly informed of a serious illness. There was an expressed preference for physician- or family-based healthcare decisions. Advance directives and formally appointed proxies were typically seen as unnecessary and inconsistent with many respondents' personal values. Findings of this study suggested that the value of individual autonomy and control over healthcare decisions may not be as applicable to cultures with a collectivist orientation. Designing care to be patient-centered is one of six key recommendations from the Institute of Medicine's Quality Chasm report,[22] and yet to do so can create direct conflicts with Western biomedical ethical principles including the principles of autonomy and informed consent. Provision of effective informed consent for patients with limited health literacy has been improved via a 'teach back' method, in which patients are asked to recount information during the informed consent process, in order to demonstrate their level of understanding.[23]

## Unfamiliarity with services

Immigrants may not be as aware of existing community resources, including health promotion resources. In the 1999 National Survey of America's Families, compared to US-born citizens, immigrant

**Table 42.3 Selected factors shown to contribute to differences and disparities in preventive health services for immigrants**

| Patient issues | Care delivery systems issues | Provider issues |
|---|---|---|
| Age | Access/lack of health insurance | Lack of financial alignment to encourage or support providers caring for immigrants |
| Gender | Lack of organizational commitment to disparities reduction | Lack of language concordant providers |
| Language ability | Lack of adequate spoken language resources | Lack of knowledge of immigrant groups' medical issues based on race/ethnicity or country of origin |
| Competing needs: housing, job, education | Lack of adequate data collection on outcomes and satisfaction by population | Lack of knowledge of immigrant groups' cross-cultural issues |
| Transportation | Lack of adequate reimbursement for care and services | The culture of Western biomedicine |
| Cross-cultural beliefs | Lack of adequate resource allocation for safety net populations (social workers/case management/community health workers) | Lack of diverse providers reflecting the cultural perspective of communities served |
| Lack of knowledge of existing resources | Location in areas of need | Time pressures |
| Fear, lack of trust, perceptions of bias, stereotyping and racism | Lack of adequate written language materials | Lack of access to educational resources on a real time basis |
| Previous experiences with health services in country of origin/region of origin | Lack of culturally competent outreach and education programs | Attitudinal issues, including bias, racism and stereotyping |
| Length of time in the US | Lack of connection to communities being served | |

citizens were at highest risk of not being aware of health and community resources for most outcomes.[24] Parental race/ethnicity, education level, employment status, and child age were other significant independent risk factors. This study clearly documented disparate awareness among parents of different immigrant status. Recommendations were made that community and health resources should reach out to immigrant populations, in linguistically and culturally appropriate ways, to alert them to the availability of their services. In one study of the effectiveness of a community-based advocacy and learning intervention for Hmong refugees, participants' increased quality of life could be explained simply by their improved satisfaction with existing resources of which they had been previously unaware (Table 42.3).[25]

## The healthy migrant effect and chronic health conditions

In general, many immigrants arrive in the US healthy (unless they are older immigrants) and their health gradually erodes over time (see Ch. 3). A Canadian study revealed that there is robust evidence that the healthy immigrant effect is present for chronic conditions for both men and women, and results in relatively slow convergence to native-born levels. Region of origin was an important determinant of immigrant health. The healthy immigrant effect was thought to reflect convergence in physical health rather than convergence of screening and detection of existing health problems.[26] The paradoxically low mortality of recent immigrants may be in part due to a temporal advantage. Mortality from treatable, communicable, and maternal conditions, so high in many countries of origin, quickly declines to levels close to those of the host country. Mortality from ischemic heart disease, the most common cause of death in industrialized host countries, takes years to decades to rise to comparable levels. After adopting a Western lifestyle, immigrants face an increasing risk of ischemic heart disease.[27] In one study, Canadian 'new immigrants' (those who immigrated less than 10 years previously) had better health than their longer-term counterparts (those who immigrated 10 or more years previously), whose health status was similar to that of Canadian-born persons. Older (age 65 and over) recent immigrants had poorer overall health compared to Canadian-born persons.[28] A longitudinal analysis of health status and healthcare for immigrants in Canada revealed that health status of immigrants quickly declined after arrival, with a concomitant increase in use of healthcare services.[29] In a US National Health Interview Survey on Asian and Pacific Islander health, the immigrant health advantage consistently decreased with duration of residence.[30] For immigrants whose duration of residence was less than 5 years, 5–10 years, and 10 years or more, the odds ratios for activity limitations were 0.45, 0.65, and 0.73, respectively. Subgroup analysis noted that Pacific Islanders and Vietnamese were found to have less of a healthy immigrant advantage on US arrival.

### Country of origin as a predictor of health

In one intriguing study, the ability to disaggregate health status of black Americans into subgroups (US-born blacks, black immigrants from Africa, the West Indies and Europe) revealed differences in the status of US-born and foreign-born blacks compared to that of US-born whites on three measures of health: US-born and European-born blacks had worse self-rated health, higher amounts of activity limitation, and higher odds of limitation due to hypertension compared to US-born whites.[31] In contrast, African-born blacks had better health than US-born whites on all three measures, while West Indian-born blacks had poorer self-rated health and higher odds of limitation due to hypertension, but lower odds of activity limitation. The study concluded that grouping together foreign-born blacks may result in missing important variations within this population. The black immigrant health advantage varied by region of birth, and by health status measure.

### Self-ratings of health status

Data from the 1992–1995 National Health Interview Surveys revealed significant differences in health characteristics between groups classified by race and nativity.[32] Over 87% of foreign-born black persons assessed their health as excellent to very good, compared with 52% for US-born black persons, and similar to US- and foreign-born white persons (69% for each group). Eleven percent of foreign-born black persons were limited in performing some type of activity, compared with 20% of their US-born counterparts. Among white persons, 14% of foreign-born and 16% of US-born individuals were limited in activity. The study concluded that information about the nativity status of black and white populations may be useful in public health efforts to eliminate health disparities. Most health systems collect data by race and ethnicity, rather than by country of origin, and important population differences may be lost as a result.

## Disease Prevention/Health Promotion

### The danger in generalizing among various immigrant groups

Different immigrant groups have different health behaviors. In one study of newly arrived (less than 90 days) adult refugees in United States, rates of overweight were highest among Bosnians and lowest among Vietnamese.[33] Cubans reported the most physical activity and Kosovars the least. Rates of smoking were highest among Bosnians and lowest among Cubans. Older refugees were more overweight and reported less physical activity and more smoking than younger adults. The study concluded that different groups have different health promotion needs. A 2005 telephone survey of middle-aged and older Asian Indian immigrants to the US showed that average length of residence in the US was over 25 years.[34] Fifty-two percent were of normal weight, 55% incorporated aerobic activity into their daily lifestyle, and only 5% smoked. Younger age, longer length of residence, and a bicultural or more American identity were associated with greater participation in physical activity. Higher income, a bicultural or more American ethnic identity, and depression were associated with higher fat intake. A multitude of factors influenced the practice of healthy behaviors and perceived health of Asian Indian immigrants, and needed to be taken into account when developing culturally appropriate health promotion interventions. One study of refugees' knowledge and perceptions of nutrition, physical activity, and smoking behaviors indicated that they had a realistic perception of their weight (55% felt they were overweight), and none thought obesity was a positive characteristic.[35] For all categories discussed, refugees were in the pre-contemplative stage of change. Health behaviors were expected to change over time after arrival. For Korean immigrant women to the US, needs for and attitudes toward physical activity were influenced by cultural context and immigration, and strongly associated with their daily experiences.[36]

## Obesity in immigrants

Throughout the world, there are now more people who are overweight (1 billion) versus those who are underweight (850 million).[37] The WHO standard classification for obesity in adults, and its relationship to co-morbidities, is as shown in Table 42.4.

As the worldwide move from rural life to urban environments continues, chronic health problems worsen. For thousands of years, Israeli Bedouins lived in the desert, traveled by foot, hauled water from wells, and ate what they could raise.[38] As they moved to cities, the prevalence of high blood pressure, heart disease, and diabetes increased, and 70% of Bedouins in Israel are now overweight or obese.

'The reason is clear. It happened because they changed their lifestyle. Now in the city they live a more sedentary existence. They eat white bread. They don't eat much vegetables and fruit. They eat more meat and that's a problem.'

Dr. Dove Kamir
Israeli Department of Health Promotion[38]

**Table 42.4 WHO standard classification of obesity (1997)**

|  | BMI | Risk of comorbidities |
|---|---|---|
| Normal BMI* | 18.5–24.9 | Average |
| **Overweight** |  |  |
| Pre-obese | 25.0–29.9 | Increased |
| Obesity class I | 30.0–34.9 | Moderate |
| Obesity class II | 35.0–39.9 | Severe |
| Obesity class III | >40 | Very severe |

* Body mass index (BMI) is defined as the individual's body weight divided by the square of their height.

$$BMI = \frac{weight\ (kg)}{height^2\ (m^2)}$$

Obesity is worsening in women and men, and is not limited to industrialized countries. In the past 20 years, the rates of obesity have tripled in developing countries that have been adopting a lifestyle involving decreased physical activity and overconsumption of cheap, energy-dense food.[109] The highest prevalence is in the Pacific Islands, where on the island of Nauru, for example, noted 79% of adults were obese (body mass index [BMI] >30) in 1994.[39] Prentice et al. in this same study noted the lowest rates worldwide are in less-developed Asian countries, with rates elsewhere varying from 3% in Ghana, 10% in Iran, 15% in Canada, 21% in South Africa, 28% in the United States, and 29% in Bahrain (Figs 42.4, 42.5).

Nutrition-related noncommunicable diseases exacerbated by obesity include type 2 diabetes, dyslipidemia, hypertension, coronary artery disease, and selected cancers including endometrial, breast, and colon cancer.[40]

In a cross-sectional national study, prevalence of obesity was 16% among immigrants and 22% among US-born individuals.[41] The age- and sex-adjusted prevalence of obesity was 8% among immigrants living in the United States for less than 1 year, but 19% among those living in the United States for at

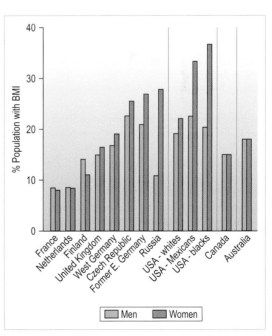

Fig. 42.4 Examples of the prevalence of obesity in adults throughout the world.

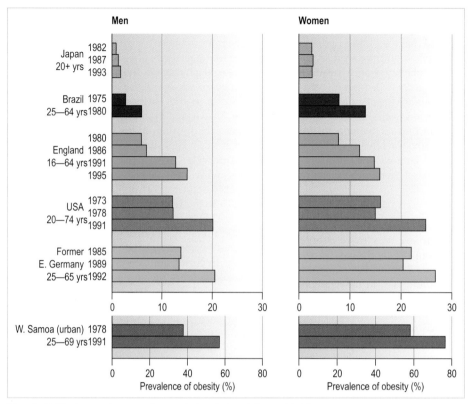

**Fig. 42.5** The increasing prevalence of obesity in adults worldwide.

least 15 years. The prevalence of obesity among immigrants living in the United States for at least 15 years approached that of US-born adults, with the exception of foreign-born blacks. Early intervention with information about diet and physical activity was thought to represent an opportunity to prevent weight gain, obesity, and obesity-related chronic illness. A Seattle, Washington, study on dietary acculturation noted that immigration to the US was usually accompanied by environmental and lifestyle changes that can markedly increase chronic disease risk, particularly adopting dietary patterns that tend to be high in fat and low in fruits and vegetables. Dietary acculturation was found to be multidimensional, dynamic, and complex, and varied considerably based on personal, cultural, and environmental attributes. The authors recommended that practitioners working with immigrants should determine the degree to which dietary counseling should be focused on maintaining traditional eating habits, adopting the healthful aspects of eating in Western countries, or both.[42]

'When I first came, I was overwhelmed by American grocery stores. What is this food? How do I know what is healthy, and how to cook such things?'

> Female participant,
> Russian Heart Health Project, 2001
> Center for International Health,
> St. Paul, Minnesota

A 2005 Canadian study demonstrated that, on average, immigrants are substantially less likely to be obese or overweight upon arrival in Canada.[43] Rates of obesity and overweight converged slowly to native-born levels, but there was marked variation by the ethnicity of the immigrant. The authors found evidence that ethnic group social network effects exerted a quantitatively important influence on the incidence of being overweight and obese for members of most ethnic minorities, tempering the process of adjustment to Canadian lifestyle norms that may be driving excess weight gain with additional years in Canada.

## Perceptions of body image

In many of the world's less-developed countries, being overweight or obese was associated in the past with wealth and better health as outlined in one report from the WHO in Samoa, where obesity is epidemic (Table 42.5).

Hispanics in the United States and sub-Saharan Africans have for centuries considered overweight and obesity to be a sign of success, wealth, and good health.[44] As outlined by Renzaho,[44] the cultural exposure of sub-Saharan Africans to the suffering of HIV, war, natural disasters, and high levels of malnutrition, has been demonstrated to affect cultural perceptions of body image. These cultural preferences for larger body sizes prevalent in people from developing countries were also reported in white people from developed countries at the turn of twentieth century. Unlike the developed world, which has shifted from preferring larger to lean body size, sub-Saharan Africans have maintained their preference for larger body size even after migration to developed countries, regardless of the length of stay in their host country.[45]

However, the dangers of generalizing are again emphasized, as more recent studies indicate that as standards of living improve and obesity worsens, many societies recognize the health dangers of obesity. In a 1996 study, both male and female Polynesians from the Cook Islands preferred to be smaller.[46] For Senegalese women, being overweight was the most desirable body size, however obesity was associated with greediness and the development of diabetes and heart disease.[47] In a study of British Bangladeshis with diabetes, patients saw obesity as unattractive, unhealthy, and linked to diabetes and heart disease.[48] Erroneous stereotypes

regarding patients' perceptions should be abandoned in favor of culturally competent nutritional outreach and education programs.

## Recommended approaches

Recommendations for how to best promote healthy eating in immigrant women were outlined in a Toronto, Canada, literature review, and included the need to consider the social context of immigrant women's experience, address cultural, linguistic, economic, and informational barriers, and consider how these change over time.[49] Another New Zealand study looked at Islamic women's barriers to fitness and exercise, and suggested innovative solutions to facilitate Somali women's access to fitness and exercise opportunities, including exercise classes in a community center used by the Somali community, and trial memberships at a women-only fitness center.[50] Many immigrants become more aware of the need for increased physical activity after adopting sedentary lifestyles after immigration. A study of married Mexican immigrant women revealed that the majority (78%) were not involved in regular physical activity and had, on average, poor cardiovascular fitness (76%).[51] However, 93% had a positive attitude towards exercise, were well informed of the benefits, and perceived physical activity to be a health-promoting behavior. Cultural values and beliefs about physical activity, gender roles, and social and physiologic factors were described as barriers to women's intention to engage in physical activity.

Lastly, the projected trends for obesity prevalence worldwide underscore the importance of concentrated efforts to stem the epidemic (Fig. 42.6).

### Table 42.5 Samoan perceptions of 'big'

| Pacific idea | Western idea |
| --- | --- |
| • Healthy | • Danger to health |
| • Well fed | • Thin is desirable (especially in role models) |
| • Being cared for | |
| • Status of wealth (within the group) | • Low status |
| | • Poor education |
| • Competitiveness within the group | • Gluttony, lack of self-control |
| • The body is a social entity | • The body is an individual entity |

Source: WHO Regional Office for the Western Pacific Report on Workshop on Obesity Prevention and Control Strategies in the Pacific, Apia, Samoa, September 2000.

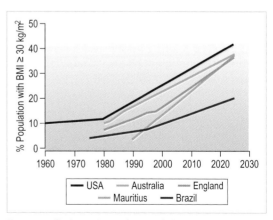

**Fig. 42.6** Projected prevalence of obesity in adults by 2025.[52]

## Tobacco use

Currently, tobacco causes more deaths in developing countries than in developed countries (see Ch. 15). However, immigrants to America have lower rates of tobacco usage compared with native-born Americans. Analysis of a national database using the Tobacco Use of the Current Population Survey revealed that after controlling for many factors, the odds of being a daily smoker were highest among US-born individuals of US-born parents and lowest among foreign-born individuals.[53] Being a second-generation immigrant (i.e. US-born) with two immigrant parents also conferred a protective effect from smoking. Differences in the stage of the tobacco epidemic between immigrants' countries of origin and the US, and anti-smoking socialization in immigrant families were thought to explain the protective effect of being foreign-born and second generation with two immigrant parents.[54] Smokeless tobacco and areca nut usage, such as *paan* and *gutka*, are a major issue in South and Southeast Asian communities.[55] This study from the Center for Immigrant Health in New York City noted that the incidence of oral cancer is higher in new immigrants who use such products, compared with native communities. The authors recommended that prevention programs, as well as research, address the unique sociocultural circumstances of this community. Clinicians should be sure to ask about use of smokeless products including *paan*, *gutka*, *malloo* (a Cambodian betel nut product), and *qat* in the Somali and other African communities.

The 1995–1996 and 1998–1999 Current Population Survey examined smoking prevalence statistics by race/ethnicity and immigrant status.[56] With the exception of male Asian/Pacific Islanders, immigrants exhibited significantly lower smoking prevalence rates than non-immigrants. However, rates varied by country of birth. This research also highlighted the need to disaggregate health statistics by race/ethnicity, immigrant status, and among immigrants, country of birth (Table 42.6).

## Evidence-Based Preventive Services

### General considerations

There is much literature on immigrant health, and providers must learn how to access specific resources for diverse patient populations. A Danish survey of

**Table 42.6 Selected recommendations for health promotion messages and activities in immigrants**

Understand your patient's goals: 'I want to live to see my grandchildren graduate.' Educate patients regarding average lifespan of healthy men and women in developed economies: 'You have the opportunity to live a longer life here.'

Explore cultural attitudes and beliefs regarding weight and exercise, particularly for women: 'Can you exercise as a woman at home or in a community center?'

Emphasize the healthy migrant effect: 'How much did you weigh when you first arrived?'

Emphasize retention of healthy lifestyles where they exist, from their country of origin, focusing on walking, portion size, and food choices: 'Remember how you walked to market back home?'

Refer most patients, even those at their ideal weight, to a dietician with expertise in dietary issues of immigrants. Teach knowledge of nutrition labels, which is often lacking. Discourage Western fast food and 'junk food.'

Emphasize the strength of existing cultural norms which discourage unhealthy behaviors, such as the use of alcohol.

Emphasize the positive effective of anti-smoking socialization which exists in many immigrant communities.

Partner with immigrant organizations to deliver culturally competent health promotion and disease prevention messages in the community.

Utilize bicultural community health workers to teach health promotion, provide home visits for nutrition consultation, and review of food items in the home.

health professionals revealed that doctors, nurses, and assistant nurses obtained their knowledge about immigrants through the media and patient contact, and less through travels, courses, and colleagues.[57] The authors concluded that as preventive health services guidelines are formulated and reviewed, they should routinely address the evidence basis for racial and ethnic considerations, country of origin considerations, as well as cross-cultural issues. As outlined in Chapter 15, the use of race and ethnicity as a proxy for genetic risk for disease, while necessary given current knowledge limitations, is complex and inadequate. In a special communication in the Journal of the American Medical Association, Dr. Mike Bamshad explained that new studies of human genetic variation show that while genetic ancestry is highly correlated with geographic ancestry, its correlation with race is modest.[58]

Particularly in minority populations, Dr. Bamshad hypothesized that geographic ancestry and explicit genetic information are alternatives to race that appear to be more accurate predictors of genetic risk factors that influence health. He concluded by stating that 'operationalizing alternatives to race for clinicians will be an important step toward providing more personalized healthcare.'[58] Healthcare delivery systems can begin by collecting not only race/ethnicity and language data, but demographic data by country of origin, which may be a better proxy for disease risk in new immigrants. Disaggregating health outcomes by country of origin would provide valuable and practical information, and help target interventions to high-risk groups.

## Osteoporosis screening in immigrants

Osteoporosis is underrecognized and undertreated in immigrant communities. Many immigrant communities have multiple risk factors for osteoporosis as shown in Table 42.7. Screening rates for osteoporosis vary by race/ethnicity and income, as outlined in the most recent National Health Disparities Report (Fig. 42.7).[1]

A study of immigrant health in Oslo, Norway, revealed widespread vitamin D deficiency in both men and women born in Turkey, Sri Lanka, Iran, Pakistan, and Vietnam residing in Oslo.[59] Overall prevalence of vitamin D deficiency, defined as 25 (OH) D < 25 nmol/L was 37.2%, ranging from 8.5% in men born in Vietnam to 64.9% in women born in Pakistan. Prevalence was higher in women than in men, higher in those born in Pakistan and lower in those born in Vietnam. Fatty fish intake and cod liver oil supplements were also important determinant factors of vitamin D status. A study in Australia

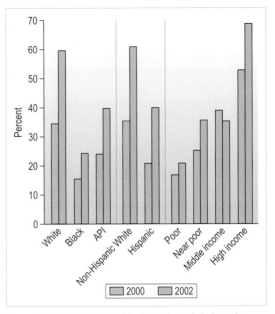

**Fig. 42.7** Elderly female Medicare beneficiaries who reported ever being screened for osteoporosis with a bone mass or bone density measurement by race, ethnicity, and income, 2000 and 2002.[1]
API – Asians/Pacific Islander

of dark-skinned or veiled women attending a prenatal clinic revealed that a remarkable 80% had low levels of vitamin D, and Muslim women presenting with evidence of osteoporosis on bone densitometry were 2.5 times more likely to have severe vitamin D deficiency than women of European descent.[60]

A Danish study of veiled Arab women revealed that 96% had low vitamin D levels, and 57% had vitamin D deficiency osteomalacia with elevated parathyroid hormone (PTH) levels. Major symptoms included difficulty with gait (26%), muscle pain (88%), difficulty rising from a chair or ascending a staircase (32%), paresthesias of the hands and feet (58%), and muscle cramps (72%). Recommendations from the study included supplementing with 1000 units of vitamin D daily for sun-deprived individuals.[61] Ironically, this is not a new issue. In the United Kingdom in the 1970s immigrants from the Indian subcontinent living in the UK began presenting with florid symptoms of osteomalacia including bone pain, myopathy, and pseudofractures.[62] Physicians in the US in northern environments in the early twentieth century were very knowledgeable about the issue, as were mothers, who insisted their children take cod liver oil daily, which has a high concentration of Vitamin D.

---

**Table 42.7 Selected risk factors for osteoporosis in immigrant communities**

White or Asian race
Grand multiparous status
History of prolonged periods of malnutrition/undernutrition
Lactase deficiency and avoidance/lack of access to dairy products
Higher prevalence of tobacco use in some immigrant communites

'My grandfather was a physician at the Peter Bent Brigham Hospital in Boston. I recall my father describing his professorial physician father stopping every day around noon time, going out on the streets of Boston in the 1930s, sitting on the curb in his suit and tie, and rolling up his sleeves and pant legs for 15 minutes. "That's all the vitamin D you need," he would say.'

P.F. Walker

In a Minnesota clinic which serves a large number of immigrants, vitamin D deficiency was highly associated with chronic non-specific musculoskeletal pain, with 140 of 150 patients (93%) reporting chronic pain.[63] Beyond 35° north or south, there is no vitamin D synthesis from November to early March. Clinicians, particularly for patients living in northern environments or caring for veiled women, should have a high index of suspicion for osteomalacia and vitamin D deficiency, and aggressively screen for the same. Treatment of vitamin D deficiency includes options shown below.

Ergocalciferol 50,000 units M, W, F × 4 weeks
OR
Ergocalciferol 50,000 units one po weekly for 8 weeks.
Followed by vitamin D 800 IU daily, chronic supplementation
OR
Ergocalciferol 150,000–300,000 units injected once annually.[110]
Ensure adequate calcium intake necessary to decrease PTH.
Monitor semi-annually with serum calcium and 25 OH vitamin D levels.
Light skin: 5–10 minutes of sunlight on arms, legs and face 3 times weekly
Dark skin: 30–60 minutes of sunlight on arms, legs and face 3 times weekly (sunlight exposure should be between 11 AM–2 PM)

Douglas Pryce, MD
Hennepin Faculty Associates
Personal Communication, July 2006

Providers should have increased awareness of risk factors for osteoporosis in both immigrant women and men, and screen at an earlier age than current US recommendations. Guidelines for first bone densitometry screening based on multiple specific risk factors, such as those experienced by refugees, are not available, but many clinicians experienced with caring for immigrants begin screening patients for vitamin D deficiency with 25 (OH) vitamin D and PTH levels as well as bone densitometry at menopause, or with chronic musculoskeletal complaints.

## Cancer screening in immigrants

### Differences in prevalence by race and country of origin

As outlined in Chapter 15, there were 10.9 million new cases of cancer worldwide, and 6.7 million deaths in 2002, and cancer remains the second most common cause of death in the United States. Cancer prevalence rates may vary by fivefold for men around the world, and fourfold for women. Racial and ethnic differences in prevalence of cancer persist, and cancer patterns change with migration, such as the decreased risk of gastric cancer in Japanese immigrants to the US over time, and increased risk of breast cancer as women migrate to more industrialized countries (Table 42.8).[65]

Cancers which are caused by infections, such as liver, stomach, and cervical cancer, are more common in less developed countries (Table 42.14). In a study of Chinese immigrants in Alberta, Canada, incidence rates for cancers more common in China (gastric, esophageal, and liver) were more similar to those for Canadian-born residents than to rates for Shanghai.[66] For cancers that are traditionally uncommon in China (breast and prostate), disease rates for immigrants were midway between those of the two comparison groups. This study supported observations that the risk of cancer in immigrants tends toward the risk of people in the new host country.

Haiman et al.[67] studied racial and ethnic differences in the incidence of lung cancer. Their study showed African-American males have an increased risk of lung cancer, whereas Latino and Asian males and females have reduced rates compared with whites. When broken down according to smoking history, racial and ethnic differences were attenuated. However, relative rates of lung cancer among smokers differed dramatically by race and ethnicity, and the reasons for these differences remain unexplained (Table 42.9).

**Table 42.8 Increase in breast cancer relative risk with migration to US[64]**

| | |
|---|---|
| New immigrants from urban areas in Asia | 30% |
| Three or four grandparents born in the US | 50% |
| Asian-Americans born in the US | 60% |
| Migrants that have lived in the US >10 years | 80% |

**Table 42.9 Incidence rates\* by site, race, and ethnicity, US, 1999–2003**[68]

| Incidence | White | Black | Asian/Pacific Islander | American Indian/ Alaskan Native | Hispanic/ Latino[†] |
|---|---|---|---|---|---|
| All Sites | | | | | |
| Males | 555.0 | 639.8 | 385.5 | 359.9 | 444.1 |
| Females | 421.1 | 383.8 | 303.3 | 305.0 | 327.2 |
| Breast (female) | 130.8 | 111.5 | 91.2 | 74.4 | 92.6 |
| Colon & rectum | | | | | |
| Males | 63.7 | 70.2 | 52.6 | 52.7 | 52.4 |
| Females | 45.9 | 53.5 | 38.0 | 41.9 | 37.3 |
| Kidney & renal pelvis | | | | | |
| Males | 18.0 | 18.5 | 9.8 | 20.9 | 16.9 |
| Females | 9.3 | 9.5 | 4.9 | 10.0 | 9.4 |
| Lung & bronchus | | | | | |
| Males | 88.8 | 110.6 | 56.6 | 55.5 | 52.7 |
| Females | 56.2 | 50.3 | 28.7 | 33.8 | 26.7 |
| Prostate | 156.0 | 243.0 | 104.2 | 70.7 | 141.1 |
| Stomach | | | | | |
| Males | 9.7 | 17.4 | 20.0 | 21.6 | 16.1 |
| Females | 4.4 | 9.0 | 11.4 | 12.3 | 9.1 |
| Liver & bile duct | | | | | |
| Males | 7.2 | 11.1 | 22.1 | 14.5 | 14.8 |
| Females | 2.7 | 3.6 | 8.3 | 6.5 | 5.8 |
| Uterine cervix | 8.6 | 13.0 | 9.3 | 7.2 | 14.7 |

\* Per 100 000 age-adjusted to the 2000 US standard population.
[†] Persons of Hispanic/Latino origin may be of any race.
Source: Incidence (except American Indian and Alaskan Native): Howe HL, Wu S, Ries LAG et al. Annual report to the nation on the status of cancer 1975–2003, featuring cancer among US Hispanic/Latino populations. *Cancer* 2006; 107:1643–1658. Incidence (American Indian and Alaskan Native 1999–2002): Ries LAG, Harkins D, Krapcho M, et al (eds). SEER Cancer Statistic Review, 1975–2003, National Cancer Institute, Bethesda, MD, http://www.seer.cancer.gov/csr/1975_2003/,2006. Mortality: SEER Program, http://www.seer.cancer.gov SEER* Stat Database: Mortality – All COD, Public-Use with State, Total US (1990–2003), National Cancer Institute, DC CPS, Surveillance Research Program, Cancer Statistic Branch, released April 2006. Underlying mortality data provided by NCHS.
American Cancer Society, Surveillance Research, 2007. American Cancer Society. *Cancer Facts and Figures 2007*. Atlanta: American Cancer Society, Inc. Adapted with permission.

## Disparities in cancer care and outcomes

The Institute of Medicine has outlined cancer disparities in its landmark report 'The Unequal Burden of Cancer.'[69] African-Americans have earlier onset of colon cancer, and yet are offered colonoscopy as a diagnostic tool less frequently.[69] The American College of Gastroenterology has recently recommended that African-Americans receive a first screening colonoscopy at age 45, rather than at age 50.[70] Asian Pacific Islander and Hispanic women are less likely to have received a diagnostic mammogram in the previous 2 years.[1] African-American, Hispanic white, and Native American women with breast cancer present with more advanced disease and have poorer survival rates than non-Hispanic whites. Infrequent or no cervical cancer screening is the most important determinant of invasive cervical

cancer occurrence. Between 1990 and 2002, one study revealed that 50% of Vietnamese-American women have ever had a pap smear, compared with 94.7% of the general American female population.[71] Cervical cancer incidence rates in California were the highest in Vietnamese patients in a 1996 National Cancer Institute Report (Table 42.10).

For Asian Pacific Islander women, outcomes vary by subgroup.[1] As outlined in a study of cancer health disparities among Asian-Americans, Dr. Moon Chen explained that Asians are the only racial/ethnic population in the US to experience cancer as the leading cause of death.[73] This is thought to be due in part to experiencing proportionally more cancers of infectious origin (human papillomavirus-induced cervical cancer, hepatitis B virus-induced liver cancer, and Helicobacter pylori-associated stomach cancer), and also to be experiencing an increasing

**Table 42.10 Cervical cancer incidence rates by country of origin (per 100 000) in California, 1988–1992[72]**

| | |
|---|---|
| Vietnamese | 43.0 |
| Southeast Asians | 35.2 |
| Latinos | 17.1 |
| Koreans | 14.7 |
| Black (non-Latino) | 12.5 |
| Filipinos | 11.8 |
| Chinese | 8.0 |
| White (non-Latino) | 7.5 |
| Japanese | 5.7 |

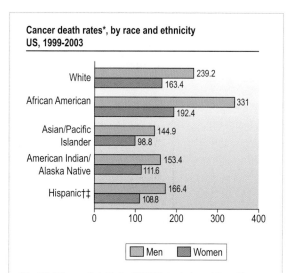

Cancer death rates*, by race and ethnicity
US, 1999-2003

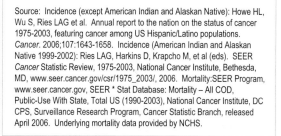

*Per 100,000 age-adjusted to the 2000 US standard population. †Persons of Hispanic/Latino origin may be of any race. ‡Excludes deaths from Minnesota, New Hampshire, and North Dakota due to unreliable data.

Source: Incidence (except American Indian and Alaskan Native): Howe HL, Wu S, Ries LAG et al. Annual report to the nation on the status of cancer 1975-2003, featuring cancer among US Hispanic/Latino populations. *Cancer.* 2006;107:1643-1658. Incidence (American Indian and Alaskan Native 1999-2002): Ries LAG, Harkins D, Krapcho M, et al (eds). SEER *Cancer* Statistic Review, 1975-2003, National Cancer Institute, Bethesda, MD, www.seer.cancer.gov/csr/1975_2003/, 2006. Mortality:SEER Program, www.seer.cancer.gov, SEER * Stat Database: Mortality – All COD, Public-Use With State, Total US (1990-2003), National Cancer Institute, DC CPS, Surveillance Research Program, Cancer Statistic Branch, released April 2006. Underlying mortality data provided by NCHS.

**Fig. 42.8** Cancer death rates by race and ethnicity (American Cancer Society, Surveillance Research, 2007).

number of cancers associated with 'Westernization.'[73] In 1996, the American Cancer Society set a goal of 50% reduction in age-adjusted cancer mortality rates by the year 2015. Focusing on high-risk groups is a key part of many national initiatives at present. As one example, through the ACS Nationwide Asian Americans/Pacific Islander Initiative, numerous ethnically specific recommendations have been developed and initiated. Strategies are available on their website (http://www.cancer.org/apicem).[74]

As is true for other disparities, the causes for cancer disparities remain complex and multifactorial. They include patient-related barriers,[59] clinician-related barriers, and health systems barriers. In one study of Latinas in California, foreign-born Latinas experienced the highest rates of never having been screened for breast and cervical cancer.[75] Lack of health insurance coverage remained the strongest predictor of cancer screening underutilization in this group. Cancer death rates also vary by race and ethnicity (Fig. 42.8).

## Barriers to cancer screening in immigrants

**Foreign birth, gender, and ethnic concordance** In an excellent study from 2003, Goel et al. outline racial and ethnic disparities in cancer screening, emphasizing the importance of foreign birth as a barrier to care.[76] Foreign birth was shown to explain some differences in cancer screening previously attributed to race and ethnicity (Table 42.11).

Hispanic and Asian Pacific Islanders (AAPIs) living in the United States were less likely to report cancer screening.[76] Racial/ethnic subgroups comprised largely of immigrants had lower screening rates for cervical, breast, and colorectal cancer.

Access to care explained some differences in screening by race and ethnicity, but in this study, social factors such as education and income did not play a major role. The observation that disparities in cancer screening were not entirely accounted for by access to care suggested to the authors that there may be additional cultural barriers to care that require addressing. Provider gender and ethnicity have been shown to affect cancer screening rates, as in one study which showed that AAPI women cared for by female or non-AAPI providers have higher rates of breast and cervical cancer screening.[77] In the Goel study,[76] the conclusion was made that general factors such as lack of knowledge about the benefits of cancer screening, the effects of provider gender and race/ethnicity, amount of time spent with patients, frequency with which cancer screening is offered, and cultural differences in patient responses to screening recommendations all should be taken into consideration. In a study from Seattle, Washington,

**Table 42.11 Rates of screening by race/ethnicity and birthplace[76]**

| | Pap smear,[†] % screened | Mammogram,[†] % screened | Fecal occult blood test,[†] % screened | Sigmoidoscopy,[†] % screened |
|---|---|---|---|---|
| Overall | 84 | 72 | 27 | 29 |
| Race/ethnicity | | | | |
| White, non-Hispanic | 86 | 74 | 28 | 30 |
| Black | 88 | 70 | 24 | 26 |
| Hispanic | 77 | 66 | 18 | 20 |
| AAPI | 71 | 62 | 27 | 27 |
| Birthplace | | | | |
| U.S.-born | 86 | 73 | 27 | 30 |
| Foreign-born | 74 | 66 | 21 | 23 |

* All percentages are based on weighted analyses.
[†] $P < .005$ for each type of cancer screening by both race/ethnicity and birthplace.

| | Pap smear, $N = 10\,511$ AOR (95% CI) | Mammogram, $N = 4607$ AOR (95% CI) | Fecal occult blood test, $N = 9835$ AOR (95% CI) | Sigmoidoscopy, $N = 9981$ AOR (95% CI) |
|---|---|---|---|---|
| Race/ethnicity | | | | |
| White | 1.00 | 1.00 | 1.00 | 1.00 |
| Black | 2.34 (1.76 to 3.11)[†] | 1.21 (0.93 to 1.56) | 1.01 (0.83 to 1.22) | 1.11 (0.89 to 1.37) |
| Hispanic | 0.79 (0.67 to 0.94)[†] | 0.97 (0.72 to 1.30) | 0.75 (0.59 to 0.94)[†] | 0.77 (0.62 to 0.96)[†] |
| AAPI | 0.36 (0.26 to 0.49)[†] | 0.50 (0.31 to 0.83)[†] | 0.77 (0.53 to 1.11) | 0.68 (0.47 to 0.99)[†] |

* Analysis adjusted for sociodemographic characteristics (age. marital status, region of residence, education, income) and illness burden (self-reported health status, smoking, concurrent illnesses, body mass index, hospitalizations in past year).
[†] $P \leq .05$.
AOR, adjusted odds ratio; CI, confidence interval.

| | Pap smear, $N = 10\,486$ AOR (95% CI) | Mammogram, $N = 4597$ AOR (95% CI) | Fecal occult blood test, $N = 9823$ AOR (95% CI) | Sigmoidoscopy, $N = 9968$ AOR (95% CI) |
|---|---|---|---|---|
| U.S.-born | | | | |
| White | 1.00 | 1.00 | 1.00 | 1.00 |
| Black | 2.44 (1.81 to 3.28)[†] | 1.18 (0.91 to 1.53) | 1.05 (0.86 to 1.28) | 1.15 (0.92 to 1.43) |
| Hispanic | 0.94 (0.74 to 1.20) | 1.17 (0.76 to 1.80) | 0.77 (0.56 to 1.05) | 0.85 (0.64 to 1.13) |
| AAPI | 1.57 (0.62 to 4.02) | 0.50 (0.17 to 1.47) | 1.36 (0.73 to 2.54) | 0.85 (0.45 to 1.60) |
| Foreign-born | | | | |
| White | 0.58 (0.41 to 0.82)[†] | 0.86 (0.60 to 1.23) | 0.83 (0.64 to 1.07) | 0.98 (0.75 to 1.28) |
| Black | 1.05 (0.49 to 2.24) | 1.62 (0.53 to 4.99) | 0.40 (0.18 to 0.88)[†] | 0.48 (0.21 to 1.09) |
| Hispanic | 0.65 (0.53 to 0.79)[†] | 0.84 (0.58 to 1.22) | 0.72 (0.53 to 0.98)[†] | 0.70 (0.51 to 0.97)[†] |
| AAPI | 0.28 (0.19 to 0.39)[†] | 0.49 (0.28 to 0.86)[†] | 0.61 (0.39 to 0.96)[†] | 0.63 (0.40 to 0.99)[†] |

* Analysis adjusted for sociodemographic characteristics (age. marital status, region of residence, education, income), and illness burden (self-reported health status, smoking, concurrent illnesses, body mass index, hospitalizations in past year).
[†] Unadjusted odds ratios did not differ substantially from the adjusted odds ratios presented in this table.
[‡] $P \leq .05$.
AOR, adjusted odds ratio; CI, confidence interval.

of Asian-American women, a strong association was found between screening mammogram and having had a recommendation made by physicians and nurses.[78]

'I must spend the first 15 minutes of a 20 minute appointment asking, "Who is your family?" for my Somali patients. If I do not do this, patients will think I do not care about them. It is hard to address so many issues in brief appointments.'

Somali American internist, Mohamud Afgarshe, MD Health Partners Center for International Health, St. Paul, Minnesota

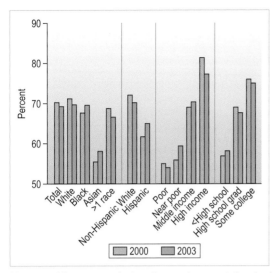

**Fig. 42.9** Women aged 40 and over who report they had a mammogram within the past 2 years, by race, ethnicity, income, and education, 2000 and 2003.[1]

**Access** Access continues to remain a critical determinant affecting immigrants' use of preventive services. Approximately half of recent immigrants to the United States lack health insurance. In a 2004 national telephone survey of foreign-born recent immigrant females, 73% and 78% reported a Pap smear or mammogram, respectively, in the previous 2 years versus 89% and 89% of US-born women.[79] Adjusting for differences in sociodemographics, health attitudes or beliefs, patient or provider communication, and the medical care environment, insurance remained the strongest predictor of screening. The authors recommended increasing awareness of available safety net sources of care to help improve cancer screening among uninsured recent immigrants. A 2005 California study demonstrated US citizen immigrants were significantly more likely to report receiving a Pap smear ever or a mammogram ever as compared to immigrants who were not US citizens.[80] The reasons for differences in cancer screening rates between citizens and non-citizens are not entirely clear, and more research is needed (Fig. 42.9).

### Cross-cultural barriers to screening

**Attitudes and knowledge** Even though there has been a decrease in overall cancer death rates in the US, immigrant minorities continue to experience disproportionately higher cancer incidence and mortality rates. In one detailed New York City study by

Gany et al. of attitudes, knowledge, and health seeking behaviors of five immigrant communities (Haitian, English-speaking Caribbean, Latino, Korean, and Chinese) in the screening and prevention of cancer, health seeking behaviors and the degree to which cultural, linguistic, and systematic barriers impacted behaviors were addressed.[81] The authors concluded that while there were many similarities across immigrant groups, there were also significant variations between groups, and tailored community-based approaches were necessary. Misinformation was observed among all groups, and warranted the development of culturally competent programs for cancer control with immigrant minorities.

Knowledge of risk factors for cancer, as well as knowledge regarding the efficacy of screening tools, is lacking in many immigrant communities. In a 2001 study by Scarinci et al. from Birmingham, Alabama, low-income Latina immigrants displayed significantly less knowledge regarding cervical cancer than non-Latina women.[82] Culturally based knowledge and beliefs regarding cervical cancer and screening were felt to influence obtaining a Pap smear in this population. In a study of immigrant Chinese women in Seattle, despite known high rates of invasive cervical cancer, there were low rates of cervical cancer screening. Twenty-four percent had never had a Pap smear and only 60% had recent screening.[83] In this same study, factors independently associated with cervical cancer screening were marital status, housing type, and age at immigration. A British Columbia study in 2004 revealed the average knowledge level about cervical cancer risks was low in Chinese-Canadian women, especially among those with less education and who received their usual care from a male doctor.[82] Importantly, knowledge of these risk factors was shown to influence Pap screening behavior. Physicians should spend the extra time which may be needed in order to educate immigrant women regarding preventive health services.

> 'As for preventive healthcare, they never went for Pap smears or mammograms because no doctor told them they needed these services.'
>
> Conclusion from a focus group of older Russian immigrant women[12]

Matin and LeBaron conducted focus groups for unmarried Muslim women in San Francisco.[84] Many immigrant Muslim women have low rates of healthcare utilization, especially preventive care such as breast examinations, mammograms, and cervical cancer screening. Religious and cultural values were found to significantly affect healthcare behavior in this study. Themes which emerged included: Muslim values of virginity and bodily privacy are in conflict with standards of American healthcare; family involvement in healthcare is a means to protect against standards of care which threaten Muslim values; and there are unmet needs for access to information.

'The hymen is evidence of your virginity. Virginity is highly expected of women who are not married. Anything that can indicate otherwise is detrimental to your integrity.'

'I want to be assured as much as possible that my hymen wouldn't be broken. That's the underlying fear for a lot of us. I wouldn't really have a fear of going to the gynecologist if I were married and sexually active. After marriage, this won't be much of an issue.'

'I think necessity means different things to different people. Some people might think that preventive care is a necessary reason to go through a pelvic exam and Pap smear. [Some may think] that if there's a medical problem, then it's more permissible for someone to see you there.'

'I actually am concerned that I don't understand and that I don't know how necessary [a pelvic exam] is. I want to know how effective these [tests] are – how necessary they are.'

Comments from a focus group of unmarried
Muslim women, ages 18–25[84]

The authors concluded that, 'despite multiple challenges in obtaining adequate healthcare, Muslim women in this study were enthusiastic and candid in discussing these highly sensitive and taboo topics'.

Patients and physicians may also have different perceptions of the same clinical situation. In a study of Tamil women and physicians providing services to them, the perceived reasons for barriers to screening for breast cancer were different. Women reported a lack of understanding of the role of early detection in medical care, religious beliefs, and fear of social stigmatization. Physicians reported barriers as being women's episodic care, unrelated presenting problems, and women refusing to be screened. Interventions must include an understanding of utilization barriers for both women and their doctors.[85]

In a community-based group education program for Russian patients, we had a one-hour discussion about cancer screening. Twenty of 20 participants at the beginning of the hour did not to want to be told if they had a diagnosis of cancer. After a discussion regarding early detection of cancer, and treatment options available in United States, 18 of 20 participants agreed they would want to be told if they had a diagnosis of cancer.

P.F. Walker
Russian Heart Health Project
Jay & Rose Phillips Family Foundation
Center for International Health
St. Paul, Minnesota

Given the complexity and seriousness of linguistic, structural, and cultural barriers to care, approaches to improve cancer screening must be made from both an individual provider and a care delivery system perspective (Table 42.12).

### Specific recommended approaches for providers

Cancer occurrence varies because of regional, behavioral, and genetic differences, as well as country of birth and socioeconomic status. The complex interactions of genetics, country of origin, and risk factors for specific cancers, such as tobacco use, make it more difficult for clinicians to have screening guidelines which are population and geography specific. Much work remains to be done to improve evidence-based guidelines in this regard.

For clinicians involved in the care of immigrants, providers should keep in mind the global incidence of the most common cancers, as outlined in Chapter 15, and shown again in Table 42.13.

It is also helpful to remember the leading causes of cancer by country of origin, whether that causality is environmental, genetic, or both (Fig. 42.10; Tables 42.14, 42.15):

## Management of Chronic Disease

Management of chronic disease, including diabetes and heart disease, can be very frustrating for both immigrant patient and clinician. For many immigrants with little or no experience with access to regular medical care in their home country, the idea of frequent clinic visits for a problem which is often, at least initially, asymptomatic, is alien. Immigrants more frequently present late with advanced disease, including complications of diabetes, or a late-stage

....................................................................................................................................

**Table 42.12 Selected recommendations for care delivery systems demonstrated to improve cancer screening rates for immigrants**

Address access issues.

Collect demographic data by race/ethnicity and country of origin and monitor treatment equity and outcomes. Disaggregate data as much as possible.

Hire more providers who reflect the communities served.

Help patients have an identified primary care provider and clinic.

Partner with local immigrant self-help agencies to deliver health promotion messages.

Provide point-of-service information in culturally effective ways: videos in native languages, translated health educational materials.

Send personalized form letters with ethnic-specific breast and cervical cancer screening information.[86] Provide financial incentives for low income women to obtain pap smears and mammograms.

Utilize more group education meetings.

Hire more bilingual community health workers, promoters, and social work/case management staff to assist with home visits and logistical support, such as transportation.

Provide active outreach in the community: at soccer tournaments, cultural celebrations, farmers' markets, and health fairs.

Research how immigrant communities receive their news, such as radio or television, and partner with those media resources.

Support providers with point-of-service access to evidence-based recommendations for specific patient populations. Require cultural competence education.

....................................................................................................................................

**Table 42.13 Global incidence of the five most common cancers**

| | Developing | | Developed | |
|---|---|---|---|---|
| | Males | Females | Males | Females |
| 1. | Lung | Breast | Lung | Breast |
| 2. | Stomach | Cervical | Prostate | Colorectal |
| 3. | Liver | Colorectal | Colorectal | Lung |
| 4. | Esophagus | Stomach | Stomach | Stomach |
| 5. | Colorectal | Lung | Bladder | Ovary |

Source: Parkin DM, Pisani P, Ferlay J. Global cancer statistics. CA Cancer J Clin 1999; 49:33–64.

malignancy. Issues of competing priorities including financial pressures, lack of transportation, language, and cultural barriers affect chronic care in much the same way as they impact utilization of preventive services.

## Diabetes in immigrants

### Incidence and prevalence by race/ethnicity

One and a half million new cases of diabetes were diagnosed in individuals age 20 or older in the United States in 2005.[87] US national prevalence data are available for non-Hispanic whites, non-Hispanic blacks, Hispanics/Latinos, and American Indians/Alaskan Natives. National prevalence data are not available for Asian Pacific Islanders or foreign-born Africans (Fig. 42.11).

Minority populations are disproportionately affected by diabetes. Over thirteen million (8.7%) of non-Hispanic whites age 20 or older in the US have diabetes, as do 3.2 million (13.3%) of non-Hispanic blacks. Prevalence rates for diabetes are higher in African-Americans, Hispanics, and Asian Pacific Islanders, as outlined in Chapter 15. From 1980 through 1994, the age-adjusted prevalence of diabetes was highest among black females. Mexican-Americans are 1.7 times more likely to have diabetes than non-Hispanic whites, and in California, Asians were 1.5 times more likely to have diabetes than non-Hispanic whites. From 1980 through 2004, the age-adjusted prevalence of diagnosed diabetes increased for all race/ethnicity and sex groups examined (Fig. 42.12).[87]

Diabetes is more common among many immigrant groups. Among Hispanics, type 2 diabetes is

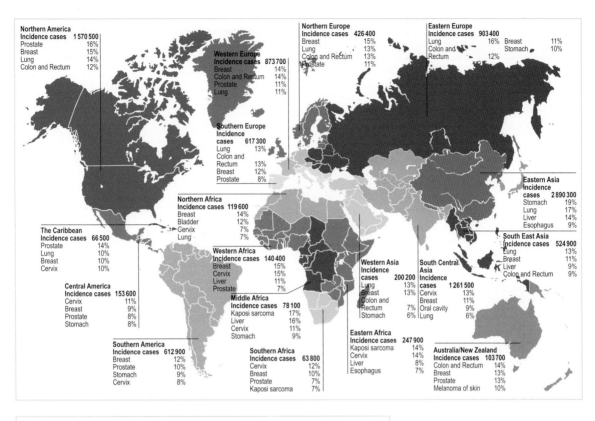

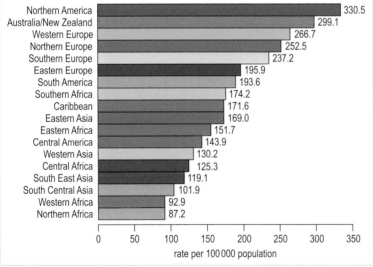

**Fig 42.10** Cancer incidence worldwide.

**Table 42.14  Cancer worldwide: top four cancers, and age-standardized incidence rates (%) by region of origin**

| Country/region | 1 | 2 | 3 | 4 | Remember |
|---|---|---|---|---|---|
| North America | Breast (15%) | Prostate (14%) | Colon (14%) | Lung (13%) | |
| South America | Breast (13%) | Prostate (10%) | Stomach (9%) | Cervix (8%) | |
| Western Europe | Breast (14%) | Colon (14%) | Prostate (11%) | Lung (11%) | |
| Eastern Europe | Lung (16%) | Colon (12%) | Breast (11%) | Stomach (10%) | Thyroid cancer after Chernobyl |
| Southeast Asia | Lung (13%) | Breast (11%) | Liver (9%) | Colon (9%) | Nasopharyngeal cancer in ethnic Chinese, including the diaspora, gallbladder cancer in Northern Thai, Lao, Burmese |
| East Africa | Kaposi's sarcoma (14%) | Cervix (14%) | Lung (8%) | Esophagus (7%) | Burkitt's lymphoma |

Source: http://info.cancerresearchuk.org/cancerstats.
Adapted by PF Walker.

**Table 42.15  Considerations for clinicians to improve cancer screening in immigrants**

Inquire respectfully about cultural beliefs, and address concerns regarding screening. *'Can you teach me about your culture's concerns, if any, with this examination?'*

Taking the time to provide information has been demonstrated to change patient's willingness to agree to have breast examinations, pap smears and colonoscopy.

Demonstrate your understanding of your patient's culture. *'I am aware that many Muslim women are concerned about virginity or physical examinations after circumcision; is that a concern for you?'*

Offer male or female colleagues as resources, to improve gender concordance.

Concepts of time and sense of urgency regarding screening vary by culture; ask about health maintenance at every visit, even in patients who have previously refused screening.

Involve family members as appropriate in discussions. *'Feel free to invite a family member here at your next visit, if that can help with making your decisions.'*

Utilize photographs when possible (Google images and other resources).

Breast cancer is the most common cancer in women around the world; utilize all available resources, outreach, and educational techniques, as described above, to encourage screening.

Lung cancer is the most common cancer in men around the world; ask all male and female patients regarding smoking status, including smokeless tobacco products, and encourage smoking cessation.

Remember the higher incidence of *cancers caused by infections* in developing countries: liver, cervical and gastric.

Screen appropriately as outlined in other chapters in this text.

Specifically target interventions for increasing Pap smear rates for high-risk ethnic communities. Develop an immigrant women's cancer screening clinic, staffed by female providers. Long-term, culturally competent outreach will be necessary.

Colorectal cancer is among the top five cancers for female and male immigrants and current screening levels are inadequate. Utilize all available resources to increase screening rates.

*Remember the more rare cancers* that are more common in immigrants: nasopharyngeal cancer in immigrants of southern Chinese origin (including Hmong from Laos, Vietnamese and Cambodian of ethnic Chinese origin), gallbladder cancer in Hispanics and Southeast Asians, and thyroid cancers among those exposed after the Chernobyl nuclear accident (Ukrainians, Poles, Byelorussia).

PF Walker.

the fifth leading cause of death. Diabetes-related mortality was highest for Mexican-Americans, followed by Puerto Ricans and Cuban-Americans, in one study of Hispanics in the United States.[88] The prevalence of type 2 diabetes is three to six times higher among immigrant South Asians (persons of Pakistani, Indian, or Bangladeshi origin) than whites.[89]

As reported in the study by Mukhopadhyay et al.,[89] one-fifth of the world's population lives in South Asia, and the projected prevalence of type 2 diabetes is set to double in this area over the next 20 years. In 2000, the global burden of patients with diabetes was estimated at 175 million; projections are that this will increase to 353 million, as shown in Figure 42.13.

A study of Russian-speaking immigrants age 40 and older revealed the prevalence of diabetes was 16.9%, obesity (defined by BMI ≥30) was 33.2%, high blood pressure 53.8%, and sedentary lifestyle 69.8%.[90]

After adjusting for age, these rates were significantly higher than rates for non-Hispanic whites in New York State. The authors commented that, 'the literature on Russian immigrants suggests an association between dietary behavior, economic hardship, cultural and linguistic barriers, and less favorable health outcomes.'

### Disparities in diabetes care

Disparities in care and outcomes exist for diabetics by race and ethnicity. Recommended annual ser-

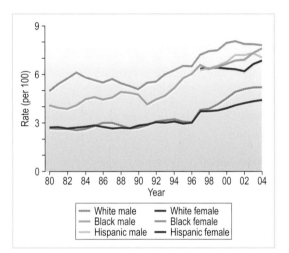

Fig. 42.12 Age-adjusted prevalence of diagnosed diabetes by race/ethnicity and sex, United States, 1980–2004.

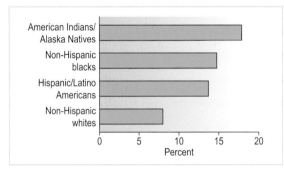

Fig. 42.11 Prevalence of diabetes by race/ethnicity.

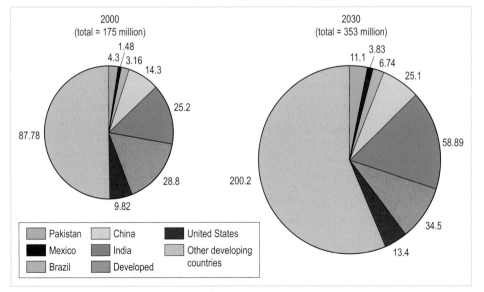

Fig. 42.13 Number of patients with diabetes worldwide, by country of origin.

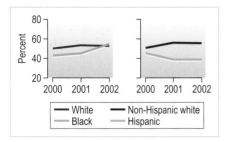

**Fig. 42.14** Adults age 18 and older with diagnosed diabetes who had three recommended services for diabetes in the last year, based on race (left) and ethnicity (right).[92]

vices include measurement of HbA$_1$C and foot and eye examinations (Fig. 42.14).

In 2001 and 2002, the proportion of adults with diagnosed diabetes who had three recommended services was lower among Hispanics compared with non-Hispanic whites. In both years, the proportion of adults with diagnosed diabetes who had all three services was lower among poor compared with high-income adults. The National Healthcare Disparities report notes that only 40% of those diagnosed with diabetes have their HbA$_1$C under optimal control (<7.0%).[1]

Management of blood pressure and high cholesterol is also key to reducing long-term risk for cardiovascular complications of diabetes (Fig. 42.15).

Significant racial/ethnic disparities were not observed in HbA$_1$C control. Fifty percent of diabetics have their total cholesterol under control (<200 mg/dL). Blacks with diabetes were more likely than whites to have their total cholesterol under control. Seventy percent of diabetics have their blood pressure under control, defined as lower than 140/90. Significant racial and ethnic disparities were not observed in this measure.[1]

Clinical inertia in primary care also contributes to poor diabetes control, as seen in one study which compared care of predominantly black patients with type 2 diabetes mellitus receiving treatment at a medical clinic with similar patients being treated at a diabetes clinic. Compared with patients from the diabetes clinic, patients at the medical clinic had worse glycemic control, were less likely to be treated with insulin, and were less likely to have their therapy intensified if glucose levels were elevated, regardless of the type of therapy they received.[91]

### Barriers to care for immigrant diabetics

Many cross-cultural factors affect care for immigrant diabetics. Obstacles to effective diabetes man-

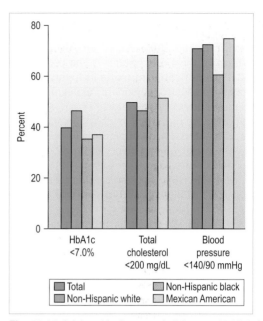

**Fig. 42.15** Adults with diagnosed diabetes with HbA$_1$C, total cholesterol, and blood pressure under control, by race/ethnicity, 1999–2002.[1]

agement have been outlined in a paper from Hawaii (Table 42.16).[93] From the perspective of these authors, issues of access, transportation, affordability of medication co-payments, and understanding of the need for life-long attention to daily management of a chronic illness are primary barriers to improved outcomes. Complicated medication regimens in patients with low health and English literacy are a challenge, and raise major concerns regarding patient safety and adherence to therapy. Comorbidities, including major depression, play a significant role in disparate outcomes, particularly in refugees with a high incidence of major depression, anxiety, and post-traumatic stress disorder.

Health beliefs also influence diabetes self-care. In a first report of immigrant health and illness beliefs of men with diabetes, Swedish researchers revealed dissimilarities in beliefs about health and diabetes which influenced self-care behavior and healthcare seeking.[94] Comparing diabetics born in Sweden, the former Yugoslavia, and Arabic countries, Swedes focused on heredity, lifestyle, and management of diabetes, while non-Swedes claimed the influence of supernatural factors and emotional stress related to the role of being an immigrant and migratory experiences as factors related to development of diabetes and having a negative influence on health. Knowledge about diabetes was limited among men in the study, but Arabs showed active information-seeking

**Table 42.16 Obstacles to effective diabetes management**

| | |
|---|---|
| Transportation | In many immigrant communities, patients rely on public transportation, which may be limited. |
| Culture | Cultural beliefs about health influence behavior. Providers may attempt to impose attitudes or behavioral changes not welcomed by the patient. |
| Family | Health is a family responsibility in many cultures. For example, insulin injections and medically relevant decisions are provided by one or more family members, who are rarely available in the office setting. |
| Economics | Medications, special food, exercise, transportation, diabetic supplies all may be beyond the resources of many patients. |
| Limited access | Chronic disease management requires a team approach, with access to effective medical education and nutrition counseling. This may be lacking in many health care settings. |
| Denial/lack of understanding | Patients may not understand chronic disease pathophysiology, and may choose to underplay long-term consequences, even when understanding is adequate. |
| Social issues | Competing priorities including work and family may affect a persons ability to follow recommendations. |
| Multiple medical problems | Medical therapies and priorities can be confusing for patients with multiple problems, particularly those with limited health and English literacy. Mental health issues can interfere with effective management. |

Adapted with permission pending[94].

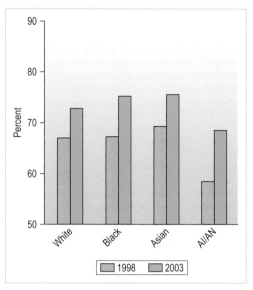

**Fig. 42.16** Adults with blood cholesterol screening in the past 5 years by race, 1998 and 2003.[1]

behavior compared with Swedes and those from former Yugoslavia. The recommendation was made that men's cultural backgrounds and spiritual beliefs need to be considered in diabetes care.

### Strategies to improve outcomes for immigrant diabetics

Numerous pilot programs and interventions designed to improve care for immigrant diabetics have been published, and selected examples which have demonstrated improved outcomes are shown in Table 42.17.

Although it is important for clinicians to serve as champions for culturally competent diabetes intervention programs, such initiatives require intensive team effort, and must be economically feasible to be sustainable in the long term.

### Cardiovascular risk factors

Hypertension and hyperlipidemia are significant risk factors for cardiovascular disease. In the National Health and Nutrition Surveys from 1986–1994 and 1999–2002, the proportion of adults with hypertension whose blood pressure was under control was lower among Mexican-Americans compared with non-Hispanic whites. Between the study periods, the proportion of adults with blood pressure under control increased from 23% to 29%, and improvements were observed among non-Hispanic whites and non-Hispanic blacks.[102,103]

In both 1998 and 2003, the proportion of adults who had their blood cholesterol checked was lower among Hispanics compared with non-Hispanic whites (Fig. 42.16).[87] In 2003, blacks were more likely to receive cholesterol screening compared with whites. From 1998 to 2003, rates of blood cholesterol screening improved from 67% to 73% for all adults. Significant improvements in screening were observed

**Table 42.17 Strategies to improve outcomes for immigrant diabetics**

| Target patient population | Intervention | Outcome | Reference |
|---|---|---|---|
| Chinese in Hawaii with diabetes and hypertension | Survey with Family Behavior Checklist. Education in Chinese by diabetes nurse educator | Increased family support, decreased blood sugar and blood pressure | 95 |
| Low-income Hispanics with diabetes in Boston | 10 group sessions targeting diabetes knowledge, attitudes and self management skills, using culturally specific and literacy sensitive strategies | 6 month statistically significant decrease HbA₁C <0.85, increased physical activity, decreased depression | 96 |
| African-American and Latino adults with diabetes in Detroit | Culturally competent curricula, designed with community input. Five 2-hour group educational meetings | Improved knowledge, and healthy dietary changes. Statistically significant decrease in HbA₁C <7.0. Improved quality of life score | 97 |
| Mexican-Americans along the Texas–Mexico border with type 2 diabetes | 52 hours of culturally competent education over 1 year, provided by bilingual Mexican-American nurses, dieticians and community workers | Statistically significant lowering of HbA₁C, <1.4% below control at 6 months. Higher diabetes knowledge scores | 98 |
| US–Mexico border health strategic initiative for adult diabetics, esp. migrant workers | Cross-border initiative. Community bilingual diabetes classes. Use of promoters for outreach and support. Education linked with clinical care | Statistically significant 0.7 decrease in HbA₁C. Improved self management. Improved self perception of quality of life | 99 |
| Low income ethnic minority populations in California with diabetes | Diabetes case management added to primary care | Statistically significant HbA₁C reduction of 1.88 over 25 month follow-up | 100 |

for all racial, ethnic, income, and education groups except American Indians/Alaskan Natives, for which the change did not reach statistical significance.

Previous research has demonstrated a higher risk of coronary disease in immigrants. In a Swedish study, many immigrant groups showed higher risks of smoking, physical inactivity, and obesity compared with Swedish-born individuals. Certain immigrant groups were found to have preventable increased risk of unhealthy behaviors and risk factors for coronary disease.[53] Immigrants from the former Soviet Union have been the largest group of refugees to come to the US in the last two decades. Lifestyle habits prevalent in Russia, including smoking, alcoholism, (largely in non-Jewish immigrants), and lack of preventive health have prompted studies of Russian-born subjects. In a Denver study, there was a higher prevalence of hyperlipidemia ($p < 0.04$), and hypertension ($p < 0.03$) than in US coun-

terparts.[104] Almost half of participants had two or more cardiac risk factors. In a study of midlife women from the former Soviet Union over a 1-year period after immigration to the United States, leading risk factors for heart disease were obesity, dyslipidemia, and depression.[105] However, interestingly and contrary to findings in other immigrant groups, women from the former Soviet Union were found to decrease their risk for coronary heart disease as they assume a more American lifestyle.

## Conclusion and Recommendations

The compelling reason for continuing both to radically change and improve healthcare in America is that outcomes for all are less than they should be. This is particularly true for minorities and immigrants.

## Choose a framework

For clinicians committed to reducing disparities in satisfaction and outcomes for immigrants, it is critical to have a clear framework for recommended interventions. Chapter 4 offers such an overview and framework for consideration for best practices in refugee and immigrant healthcare. The Institute of Medicine (IOM) 2001 'Crossing the Quality Chasm' report (which states that interventions should be based on six key principles to provide care (i.e. timely, efficient, equitable, effective, and patient centered), and the 2002 IOM 'Unequal Treatment' reports are also excellent references in this regard (http://www.iom.edu). Establishing the urgency of the imperative, including global health equity, as well as the business, legal, and quality case for immigrant healthcare is important to the long-term success of programs. In the context of larger care delivery systems, initiatives for refugees and immigrants should not be isolated, as they may fail long-term as a result. That being said, culturally specific clinics and community clinics have been demonstrated to be very successful nationally (Box 42.1).

Providers should articulate the principle that healthcare quality and satisfaction need to improve for all. They should also be supportive of organizational activities to collect demographic data and analyze satisfaction and quality by race/ethnicity and country of origin.

'When I saw my outcomes were worse for African diabetics in my practice, it made me think about what I could do to improve them.'

## Patient-level recommendations

As outlined above, the Unequal Treatment report acknowledges patient-level variables which contribute to health disparities. For example, if patients choose not to treat a cancer once diagnosed, or not to undergo screening Pap smears for cultural reasons, these may contribute to a difference in health outcomes, but are not considered a disparity in care.

'I am old, and I do not want surgery for this cancer.'

Comment of a 62-year-old Hmong woman, on hearing her diagnosis of colon cancer.

Average life span for a woman in Laos at the time of her diagnosis: age 48.

However, as clinicians, our focus should be on patient education to have an impact on choices regarding preventive health and chronic disease management. Studies have shown that patients' decisions can be affected by education, and providers should spend the time to encourage patients to make informed decisions.

'What appear to be individual or cultural preferences are often substantially shaped by modifiable practices of the healthcare system. True differences in preference that are worthy of respect surely exist between individuals or demographic groups, but some apparent differences in preference may actually reflect problems with the healthcare system that are worthy of remediation.'[106]

Armstrong K, Hughes-Halbert C, Asch DA.

The medical community also must be more diligent about personal cultural competency training. The California Endowment has published principles and recommended standards for cultural competence education of healthcare professionals (http://www.calendow.org). Studies also show that resident physicians do not feel adequately prepared in cross-cultural healthcare,[107] and educational curricula which are widely available nationally should be more extensively utilized. As discussed in Chapter 5, New Jersey and California have mandated cultural competency education for physicians. Providers must also be more aware of diseases seen more commonly in immigrant populations, a key goal of this textbook.

Because many data are not population specific, interventions which are effective and tailored to specific populations are hard to design. Interventions which are effective for Chinese-Americans may not

6. Aroian KJ, Wu B, Tran TV. Healthcare and social service use among Chinese immigrant elders. Res Nurs Health 2005; 28(2):95–105.
7. Jacobs DH, Tovar JM, Hung OL, et al. Behavioral risk factor and preventive healthcare practice survey of immigrants in the emergency department. Acad Emerg Med 2002; 9(6):599–608.
8. The Kaiser Family Foundation. National Survey of Physicians: Part 1 – Doctors on disparities in medical care. 2002. Available: http://www.kff.org
9. Robert Wood Johnson Foundation. Americans' views of disparities in healthcare. Advances e-Newsletter December 2005, Issue 2.
10. Princeton Survey Research Associates. The Commonwealth Fund 2001 Healthcare quality survey. Available: http://www.cmwf.org/surveys
11. Aroin KJ, Khatutsky G, Tran TV, et al. Health and social service utilization among elderly immigrants from the former Soviet Union. J Nurs Scholarsh 2001; 33(3):265–271.
12. Ivanov LL, Buck K. Healthcare utilization patterns of Russian-speaking immigrant women across age groups. J Immigr Health 2002; 4(1):17–27.
13. Leduc N, Proulx M. Patterns of health services utilization by recent immigrants. J Immigr Health 2004; 6(1):15–27.
14. Searight HR. Bosnian immigrants' perceptions of the United States healthcare system: a qualitative interview study. J Immigr Health 2003; 5(2):87–93.
15. Arcia E, Skinner M, Bailey D, et al. Models of acculturation and health behaviors among Latino immigrants to the US. Soc Sci Med 2001; 53(1):41–53.
16. Frisbie WP, Cho Y, Hummer RA. Immigration and Health of Asian and Pacific Islander Adults in the United States, American Journal of Epidemiology 2001; 153(4):372–380.
17. Remennick L. 'I have no time for potential troubles': Russian immigrant women and breast cancer screening in Israel. J Immigr Health 2003; 5(4):153–163.
18. Ahmad F, Cameron JL, Stewart DE. A tailored intervention to promote breast cancer screening among South Asian immigrant women. Soc Sci Med 2005; 60(3):575–586.
19. Surbone A. Letter from Italy: truth telling to the patient. JAMA 1992; 268(13):1661–1662.
20. Searight HR, Gafford J. Cultural diversity at the end of life: issues and guidelines for family physicians. Am Fam Phys 2005; 171(3):429–430.
21. Searight HR, Gafford J. 'It's like playing with your destiny': Bosnian immigrants' view of advance directives and end-of-life decision-making. J Immigr Health 2005; 7(3):195–203.
22. Institute of Medicine. Crossing the Quality Chasm: a New Health System for the 21st Century/Committee on Quality Health Care in America, Institute of Medicine Committee on Quality of Health Care in America. Washington, DC: National Academy Press; 2001.
23. Wu HW, Nishimi RY, Page-Lopez, CM, et al. Improving patient safety through informed consent for patients with limited health literacy. National Quality Forum 2005. Available: http://www.qualityforum.org
24. Yu SM, Huang ZJ, Schwalberg RH, et al. Parental awareness of health and community resources among immigrant families. Matern Child Health J 2005; 9(1):27–34.
25. Goodkind JR. Effectiveness of a community-based advocacy and learning program for Hmong refugees. Am J Community Psychol 2005; 36(3–4):387–408.
26. McDonald JT, Kennedy S. Insights into the 'healthy immigrant effect': health status and health service use of immigrants to Canada. Soc Sci Med 2004; 59(8):1613–1627.
27. Razum O, Twardella D. Time travel with Oliver Twist – towards an explanation for a paradoxically low mortality among recent immigrants. Trop Med Int Health 2002; 7(1):4–10.
28. Gee EM, Kobayashi KM, Prus SG. Examining the healthy immigrant effect in mid- to later life: findings from the Canadian community health survey. Can J Aging 2004; 23(Suppl 1):s61–s69.

Box 42.2

- Examine your own attitudes and beliefs toward immigrant preventive and chronic care.
- Develop a personal self-education plan:

  Culture and belief systems of patients;
  Prevalence of disease by race/ethnicity/country of origin;
  Learn what interventions have been demonstrated to work, and engage teams.

- Develop a standard intervention method:

  Target your interventions towards highest-risk groups;
  Provide cancer screening based on prevalence rates by race/ethnicity or country of origin, not necessarily standard guidelines which may not be as applicable for your patient population;
  Review outcomes by race/ethnicity and assist in the design of interventions to reduce disparities.

PF Walker

be effective for Somali-Americans. However, many studies show that as clinicians, we can influence patient choices regarding preventive health and chronic disease management. In a qualitative study of elderly Chinese-Americans in California, participants revealed a 'genuine adaptability to combining Eastern and Western healthcare modalities.'[108]

## Specific Recommendations for Providers

Emphasizing the strengths and resilience of immigrant communities, and partnering with them to design and implement interventions can be very rewarding. We have much to learn from the healthy migrant (Box 42.2).

## References

1. National Healthcare Disparities Report 2005. Available: http://www.qualitytools.ahrq.gov/disparitiesreport
2. Franks F. Is patient HMO insurance or physician HMO participation related to racial disparities in primary care? Amer J Managed Care 2005; 11(6):397–402.
3. Lipson JG, Weinstein HM, Gladstone EA, et al. Bosnian and Soviet refugees' experiences with healthcare. West J Nurs Res 2003; 25(7):854–871.
4. Walker PF. Preventive healthcare in a multicultural society: Are we culturally competent? [editorial]. Mayo Clin Proc 1996; 71:519–521.
5. Documét Pl, Sharma RK. Latinos' healthcare access: financial and cultural barriers. J Immigr Health 2004; 6(1):5–13.

29. Newbold B. Health status and healthcare of immigrants in Canada: a longitudinal analysis. J Health Serv Res Policy 2005; 10(2):77–83.

30. Frisbie WP, Cho Y, Hummer RA. Immigration and health of Asian and Pacific Islander adults in the United States. Am J Epidemiol 2001; 153(4):372–380.

31. Read JG, Emerson MO, Tarlov A. Implications of black immigrant health for US racial disparities in health. J Immigr Health 2005; 7(3):205–212.

32. Lucas JW, Barr-Anderson DJ, Kington RS. Health status of non-Hispanic US born and foreign-born black and white persons: United States, 1992–95. Vital & Health Statistics – Series 10: Data from the National Health Survey. 2005; 10(226):1–20.

33. Barnes DM, Harrison C, Heneghan R. Health risk and promotion behaviors in refugee populations. J Health Care Poor Underserved 2004; 15(3):347–356.

34. Jonnalagadda SS, Diwan S. Health behaviors, chronic disease prevalence and self-rated health of older Asian Indian immigrants in the US. J Immigr Health 2005; 7(2):75–83.

35. Barnes DM, Almasy N. Refugees' perceptions of healthy behaviors. J Immigr Health 2005; 7(3):185–193.

36. Im EO, Choe MA. Physical activity of Korean immigrant women in the US: needs and attitudes. Int J Nurs Stud 2001; 38(5):567–577.

37. Yach D. Highlights of the 18th international nutrition congress, Durban, South Africa. September 18–23, 2005.

38. Aaron Shackter, BBC reporter broadcast on Public Radio International, The World. June 7, 2006.

39. Prentice AM. The emerging epidemic of obesity in developing countries. Am Int J Epidmigr. 2006; 35:93–99.

40. Popkin BM. The nutrition transition: an overview of world patterns of change. Nutrition Rev 2004; 62(7): S140–S143.

41. Goel MS, McCarthy EP, Phillips RS, et al. Obesity among US immigrant subgroups by duration of residence. JAMA 2004; 292(23):2860–2867.

42. Satia-About AJ, Patterson RE, Neuhouser ML, et al. Dietary acculturation: applications to nutrition research and dietetics. J Am Diet Assoc 2002; 102(8):1105–1118.

43. McDonald JT, Kennedy S. Is migration to Canada associated with unhealthy weight gain? Overweight and obesity among Canada's immigrants. Soc Sci Med 2005; 61(12):2469–2481.

44. Renzaho AM. Fat, rich and beautiful: changing socio-cultural paradigms associated with obesity risk, nutritional status and refugee children from sub-Saharan Africa. Health Place 2004; 10(1):105–113.

45. Powell AD, Kahn AS. Racial differences in women's desires to be thin. Intnl J Eating Disorders, 1995; 17(2):191–195.

46. Craig PL, Swinburn BA, Matenga-Smith T, et al. Do Polynesians still believe that big is beautiful? Comparison of body size perceptions and preferences of Cook Islands, Maori and Australians. NZ Med J 1996; 109(1023):200–203.

47. Holdsworth M, Gartner A, Landais E, et al. Perceptions of healthy and desirable body size in urban Senegalese women. Intl J of Obesity 2004; 28:1561–1568.

48. Greenhalgh T, Chowdhury M, Wood GW. Big is beautiful? A survey of body image perception and its relation to health in British Bangladeshis with diabetes. Psychol Health Med 2005; 10(2):126–138.

49. Hyman I, Guruge S, Makarchuk MJ, et al. Promotion of healthy eating among new immigrant women in Ontario. Can J Diet Pract Res 2002; 63(3):125–129.

50. Guerin PB, Diiriye RO, Corrigan C, et al. Physical activity programs for refugee Somali women: working out in a new country. Women Health 2003; 38(1):83–99.

51. Juarbe TC, Lipson JG, Turok X. Physical activity beliefs, behaviors, and cardiovascular fitness of Mexican immigrant women. J Transcult Nurs 2003; 14(2):108–116.

52. Macdiarmid J. The global challenge of obesity and the international obesity task force. International Union of Nutritional Sciences. Available: http://www.iuns.org

53. Gadd M, Sunquist J, Johansson SE, et al. Do immigrants have an increased prevalence of unhealthy behaviours and risk factors for coronary heart disease? Eur J Cardiovasc Prev Rehabil 2005; 12(6):535–541.

54. Acevedo-Garcia D, Pan J, Jun HJ, et al. The effect of immigrant generation on smoking. Soc Sci Med 2005; 61(6):1223–1242.

55. Changrani J, Gany F. Paan and gutka in the United States: an emerging threat. J Immigr Health 2005; 7(2):103–108.

56. Baluja KF, Park J, Myers D. Inclusion of immigrant status in smoking prevalence statistics. Am J Public Health 2003; 93(4):642–646.

57. Michaelsen J, Krasnik A, Nielsen A, et al. Health professionals' knowledge, attitudes, and experiences in relation to immigrant patients: a questionnaire study at a Danish hospital. Scand J Public Health 2004; 32(4):287–295.

58. Bamshad M. Genetic inferences on health? Does race matter? JAMA 2005; 294:937–946.

59. Holvik K, Meyer HE, Haug E, et al. Prevalence and predictors of vitamin D deficiency in five immigrant groups living in Oslo, Norway: the Oslo Immigrant Health Study. Ur J Clin Nutr 2005; 59(1):57–63.

60. Grover SR, Morley R. Vitamin D deficiency in veiled or dark skinned pregnant women. Med J Aust 2001; 175:251–252.

61. Glerup H, Mikkelsen K, Poulsen L, et al. Commonly recommended daily intake of vitamin D is not sufficient if sunlight exposure is limited. J Int Med 2000; 247:260–268.

62. Preece MA, Mclntosh WB, Tomlinson S, et al. Vitamin D deficiency among Asian immigrants to Britain. Lancet 1973; 1:907–910.

63. Plotnikoff GA, Quigley JM. Prevalence of severe hypovitaminosis D in patients with persistent, nonspecific musculoskeletal pain. Mayo Clin Proc 2003; 78:1463–1470.

64. Ziegler RG, Hoover RN, Pike MC, et al. Migration patterns and breast cancer risk in Asian-American women. J Natl Cancer Inst 1993; 85(22):1819–1827.

65. Hortobagyi GN, de la Garza SJ, Pritchard K, et al. The global breast cancer burden: variations in epidemiology and survival. Clin Breast Cancer 2005; 6(5):391–401.

66. Luo W, Birkett NJ, Ugnat AM, et al. Cancer incidence patterns among Chinese immigrant populations in Alberta. J Immigr Health 2004; 6(1):41–48.

67. Haiman CA, Stram DO, Wilkins LR, et al. Ethnic and racial differences in the smoking related risk of lung cancer. New Engl J Med 2006; 354:333–342.

68. American Cancer Society Report. Cancer prevention and early detection facts and figures 2005. Atlanta: American Cancer Society; 2005.

69. Haynes MH, Smedley BD, eds. The unequal burden of cancer: An assessment of NIH research and programs for ethnic minorities and the medically underserved. Washington, DC: National Academy Press; 1999.

70. Agrawal S, Bhupinderjit A, Bhutani MS, et al. Colorectal cancer in African Americans. Amer J Gastroenterol 2005; 100(3):515–523.

71. Lam TK, McPhee SJ, Mock J, et al. Encouraging Vietnamese-American women to obtain Pap tests through lay health worker outreach and media education. J Gen Int Med 2003; 18:516–524.

72. Miller BA, Kolonel LN, Bernstein L, et al. Racial/ethnic patterns of cancer in the United States 1988–1992. Natl Cancer Inst, NIH Pub No. 96-4104, Bethesda, MD 1996.

73. Chen M. Cancer health disparities among Asian Americans; what we do and what we need to do. Cancer 2005; 104(12Suppl):2895–2902.

74. Vance R. The Asian-American and Pacific Islander population and the American Cancer Society Initiative. Cancer 2005; 104(12Suppl):2905–2908.

75. Rodriguez MA, Ward LM, Perez-Stable EJ. Breast and cervical cancer screening: impact of health insurance status, ethnicity, and nativity of Latinas. Am Fam Med 2005; 3(3):235–241.

76. Goel MS, Wee CC, McCarthy EP, et al. Populations at risk of racial and ethnic disparities in cancer screening:

the importance of foreign birth as a barrier to care. J Gen IM 2003; 18(12):1028–1035 (copyright permission pending).

77. McPhee SJ, Stewart S, Brock KC, et al. Factors associated with breast and cervical cancer screening practices among Vietnamese American women. Cancer Detect Prev 1997; 1:510–521.

78. Tu SP, Yasui Y, Kuniyuki AA, et al. Mammography screening among Chinese-American women. Cancer 2003; 97:1293–1302.

79. Carrasquillo O, Pati S. The role of health insurance on Pap smear and mammography utilization by immigrants living in the United States. Prev Med 2004; 39(5):943–950.

80. De Alba I, Hubbell FA, McMullin JM, et al. Impact of US citizenship status on cancer screening among immigrant women. J Gen IM 2005; 20(3):290–296.

81. Gany FM, Herrera AP, Avallone M, et al. Attitudes, knowledge, and health-seeking behaviors of five immigrant minority communities in the prevention and screening of cancer: a focus group approach. Ethn Health 2006; 11(1):19–39.

82. Scarinci IC, Beech BM, Kovach KW, et al. An examination of sociocultural factors associated with cervical cancer screening among low-income Latina immigrants of reproductive age. J Immigr Health 2003; 5(3):119–128.

83. Do HH, Taylor VM, Yasui Y, et al. Cervical cancer screening among Chinese immigrants in Seattle, Washington. J Immigr Health 2001; 3(1):15–21.

84. Matin M, LeBaron S. Attitudes toward cervical cancer screening among Muslim women: a pilot study. Women Health 2004; 39(3):63–77.

85. Meana M, Bunston T, George U, et al. Older immigrant Tamil women and their doctors: attitudes toward breast cancer screening. J Immigr Health 2001; 3(1):5–13.

86. Jibaja-Weiss ML. Differential effects of messages for breast and cervical cancer screening. J Health Care Poor Underserved 2005; 16(1):42–52.

87. Centers for Disease Control and Prevention. Division of health interview statistics, National Center for Health Statistics. Hyattsville, MD: US Department of Health and Human Services; 2006.

88. Smith CA, Barnet E. Diabetes-related mortality among Mexican Americans, Puerto Ricans, and Cuban Americans in the United States. Pan Am J Pub Health 2005; 18(6):381–387.

89. Mukhopadhyay B, Sattar N, Fisher M. Diabetes and cardiac disease in South Asians. Br J Diabetes Vasc Dis 2005; 5:253–259.

90. Hosler AS, Melnik TA, Spence MM. Diabetes and its related risk factors among Russian-speaking immigrants in New York State. Ethn Dis 2004; 14(3):372–7.

91. Medical Expenditure Panel Survey. 2002. Available: http://www.meps.ahrq.gov

92. Sperl-Hillen J, O'Connor PJ. Factors driving diabetes care improvement in a large medical group: ten years of progress. Am J Managed Care 2005; 11(5)S:S177–S185.

93. Humphrey J, Jameson LM, Beckham S. Overcoming social and cultural barriers to care for patients with diabetes. West J Med 1997; 167(3):138–144.

94. Hjelm KG, Bard K, Nyberg P, et al. Beliefs about health and diabetes in men of different ethnic origin. J Adv Nurs 2005; 50(1):47–59.

95. Wang CY, Abbott LJ. Development of a community-based diabetes and hypertension preventive program. Public Health Nurs 1998; 15(6):406–414.

96. Rosal MC, Olendzki B, Reed GW, et al. Diabetes self-management among low-income Spanish-speaking patients: a pilot study. Ann Behav Med 2005; 29(3):225–235.

97. Two Feathers J, Kieffer EC, Palmisano G, et al. Racial and ethnic approaches to community health (REACH) Detroit partnership: improving diabetes-related outcomes among African American and Latino adults. Am J Public Health 2005; 95(9):1552–1560.

98. Brown SA, Garcia AA, Kouzekanani K, et al. Culturally competent diabetes self-management education for Mexican Americans: the Starr County border health initiative. Diabetes Care 2002; 25(2):259–268.

99. Ingram M, Gallegos G, Elenes J. Diabetes is a community issue: the critical elements of a successful outreach and education model on the US-Mexico border. Prev Chronic Dis 2005; 2(1):A15.

100. The California Medi-Cal Type 2 Diabetes Study Group. Closing the gap: effect of diabetes case management on glycemic control among low-income ethnic minority populations: the California Medi-Cal type 2 diabetes study. Diabetes Care 2004; 27(1):95. Comment in Diabetes Care 2004; 27(4):995.

101. Dietrich AJ, Tobin JN, Cassells A ,et al. Telephone care management to improve cancer screening among low-income women. Ann Intern Med 2006; 144:563–571.

102. Hicks LS, Fairchild DG, Cook EF, et al. Association of region of residence and immigrant status with hypertension, renal failure, cardiovascular disease, and stroke, among African-American participants in the third National Health and Nutrition Examination Survey (NHANES III). Ethn Dis 2003; 13(3):316–123.

103. US Department of Human Services, Centers for Disease Control. National health examination prevention survey, 1999–2006; 1988–1994. available: http://www.cdc.gov/NHANES

104. Mehler PS, Scott JY, Pines I, et al. Russian immigrant cardiovascular risk assessment. J Health Care Poor Underserved 2001; 12(2):224–235.

105. Miller AM, Chandler PJ, Wilbur J, et al. Acculturation and cardiovascular disease risk in midlife immigrant women from the former Soviet Union. Prog Cardiovasc Nurs 2004; 19(2):47–55.

106. Armstrong K, Hughes-Halbert C, Asch DA. Patient preferences can be misleading as explanations for racial disparities in healthcare. Arch Int M 2006; 166(9):950–954.

107. Weissman JS, Betancourt J, Campbell EG, et al. Resident physicians' preparedness to provide cross-cultural care. JAMA 2005; 294:1058–1067.

108. Pang EC, Jordan-Marsh M, Silverstein M, Campbell EG, et al. Health-seeking behaviors of elderly Chinese Americans: shifts in expectations. Gerontologist 2003; 43(6):864–874.

109. Hossain P, Kawar B, Nahas M. Obesity and Diabetes in the Developing World – A Growing Challenge. NEJM 2007; 356(3):213–215.

110. Heikinheimo RJ. Annual injections of vitamin D and fractures of aged bones. Calcified Tissue International 1992; 51(2):105–110.

# CHAPTER 43

# Women's Health Issues

Helen Bruce

## Introduction

The rich patchwork of American immigration history continues into the twenty-first century with a polyglot population unique in its ever changing diversity. This chapter cannot possibly review the cultural, religious, and political nuances of women's immigration journeys as they meet daily with clinicians in hospitals and clinics. Instead, it will ask the reader to become familiar with the particular immigrant group/groups within their catchment community and that they gain knowledge in language, customs, religion, beliefs of wellness, illness, and the role of a woman in that culture from such texts as *Transcultural Aspects of Perinatal Health Care,*[1] *Cultural Diversity in Health and Illness*[2] and, often more interestingly, the clients themselves. A range of issues that are important to women when they meet care providers will be discussed, with the idea of increasing communication and understanding of the woman as an individual within a system of healthcare that should be flexible to her unique needs.

Immigrant mothers represented 21.4% of all births in the US in 2002 (Table 43.1; Fig. 43.1),[3] with the number of births to immigrant mothers increasing dramatically since 1970.[4] An increase continues into 2005, as shown by data from Minnesota (Fig. 43.2), representative of a national trend with women of Hispanic origin having the highest birth rate.

Pregnancy is frequently a woman's initial exposure to the American healthcare system. This first encounter may have a lasting impact on how the women will continue their uptake of the medical and preventive services available to them.

'When I came to America I went to a clinic and hospital because I was told that was the American way when pregnant. Each visit the male doctor looked at and touched me in places that even my husband would not look at or touch. I left the clinic feeling dirty and not good in my body and did not return.'

These words are an explanation given by a small Asian woman looking up at a tall, white-coated OB/GYN resident physician. The physician found it unacceptable that the pregnant woman did not want to be examined by him at a 36-week prenatal visit. In an effort to help the physician understand this woman's need of respect for her modesty and of a female provider, the woman had agreed to explain her wishes via an interpreter. Had the young physician had previous exposure in care of immigrant women, he may have known that touching certain parts of the body is considered disrespectful or insulting to the Hmong and he would have been more aware of the factors which contribute to the response of any immigrant to life in his or her adopted country. This Asian woman, born in the mountains of Laos, was shaped by the belief system of her Hmong childhood. Married as a teenager, she had delivered her first son and daughter at home with assistance from her mother-in-law and husband. She fled from the Pathet Lao soldiers through the jungles of Laos, crossed the Mekong River to a refugee camp and then adapted to resettlement in the US. She had endured the deaths of her son and mother-in-law in the jungle then carried seven other pregnancies, delivering them without complications. Obstetrically, she presented as high risk for grand parity and age. Her strengths, however, were her innate knowledge that she could carry and deliver healthy babies. Motherhood is highly regarded within her family and community, and if she continued the rituals of pregnancy long used by her community, they would keep the pregnancy safe. On the day in mention, she was noted to be wearing new

**Table 43.1 Race/ethnicity and country of origin for immigrant and native mothers, 1970–2002**

|  | 1970 | | 1980 | | 1990 | | 2002 | |
|---|---|---|---|---|---|---|---|---|
|  | Immigrant | Native | Immigrant | Native | Immigrant | Native | Immigrant | Native |
| **Race/ethnicity** | | | | | | | | |
| Non-Hispanic White | 84.5% | 84.3% | 30.1% | 77.0% | 17.8% | 73.1% | 14.5% | 70.1% |
| Non-Hispanic Black | 5.5% | 15.6% | 6.8% | 16.6% | 7.2% | 17.9% | 7.5% | 16.5% |
| Non-Hispanic Asian | 6.6% | 0.9% | 16.8% | 0.3% | 18.8% | 0.4% | 18.9% | 0.9% |
| Non-Hispanic Other | 3.4% | 0.2% | 0.7% | 1.0% | 0.4% | 1.1% | 0.2% | 1.4% |
| Hispanic[2] |  |  | 45.6% | 5.1% | 55.8% | 7.4% | 58.9% | 11.1% |
| **Country** | | | | | | | | |
| Mexico | 23.8% |  | 35.9% |  | 39.5% |  | 44.5% |  |
| Cuba | 3.4% |  | 2.4% |  | 1.5% |  | 0.8% |  |
| Canada | 6.4% |  | 2.6% |  | 1.6% |  | 1.3% |  |
| Balance of world | 66.4% |  | 59.1% |  | 57.4% |  | 53.3% |  |

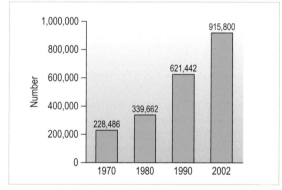

Figure 43.1 Center for Immigration Studies, Analysis of Public Use Natality Files, Provided by the National Center for Health Studies.

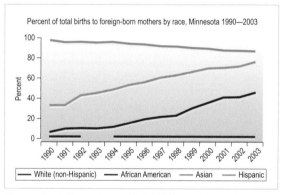

Figure 43.2 Percentage of total births to foreign-born mothers by race, Minnesota, 1990–2003.

white strings and a copper bracelet around her wrists denoting that the traditional shaman ceremony – *Ua neeb* – had taken place in preparation for safety and well-being in labor and birth.

This social history is representative of many refugee new Americans: war, death of family members, years spent in refugee camps, and finally resettlement in the US. Thankfully, missing here was a history of physical violence, rape, starvation, torture, and/or illegal entry into this country. Women who come via voluntary immigration may have no such history of loss. Globalization brings women for education and employment to the US, with the internet encouraging increasing numbers of international marriages. New brides may or may not have language or job skills to enter easily into a new country

or work force. They may or may not join a family of their own ethnic community.

In whatever group, immigration is an overwhelming and stressful experience. The American Refugee Committee in 1990 described stages of adaptation which included euphoria, hostility, recovery, acceptance of, and then integration into a new country. Integration can be rapid in women who are young and come from stability. In older women, or those with a turbulent background, integration can take many years, if it ever happens. When a clinician first meets an immigrant, it is helpful to an ongoing relationship to take time establishing both an immigration and resettlement history. In a first prenatal encounter, many clues to the history await an enquiring examiner. Openness to the first greeting and questions, willingness to undress for the examination, stillness and/or rigidity of expression and/or body in response to touch, acceptance of testing, medication, and repeat appointments will tell of the level of trust and engagement any one client will allow. Declining the same may require bartering by clinicians to meet agreed acceptance with examination and testing deferred until the client can accept with understanding.

Modern obstetrics has benefited from the advances of medical science and research, yet there is a paucity of high-quality population-based studies on refugee women's reproductive health.[3] Immigrant and refugee women are placed together in national data collections with women of the same ethnic background who can be third- or fourth-generation Americans. Indeed, newly arrived African women are placed in the same data base as women whose American roots are centuries old. 'For statistics to be meaningful, we need to take a closer look at each subgroup.' 'Our challenge for the next century is to close the disparities gap without compromising the uniqueness and richness of each culture.'[4] The conclusion of a 2005 study of adverse pregnancy outcomes among Somali immigrants in Washington State echoes Dr. Satcher's words, namely that pregnancy outcomes should be evaluated within ethnically and culturally unique groups. Somali immigrants were found to be a high-risk subgroup.[5]

Many immigrant women are suspicious of aspects of care considered normal to native-born Americans. Venipuncture, pelvic examination, and amniocentesis rank high as techniques that can cause withdrawal of women from a partnership in pregnancy care. All are viewed as invasive as are induction of labor, cesarean birth, and types of contraception which may be considered harmful to the mother and fetus. The aim of prenatal care for all women is to encourage physical, mental, and emotional well-being in the mother and to allow a baby to be nurtured, matured, and prepared for extrauterine life. Visits for prenatal surveillance can allow for melding of standards of care with traditional beliefs. Thus, a partnership develops where mutual respect, dialogue, education, and empowerment can bring acceptance of different types of healing and wellness, and can meet prenatal aims in an immigrant community.

Engagement and partnership in care are essential if the reduction in maternal mortality and morbidity, the Healthy People 2010 goals,[6] are to be achieved. Evident in Table 43.2 are the adverse outcomes well known to clinicians in obstetrics who daily strive to

prevent acute occurrences. Frequently, it is only when the acute occurs that many immigrant mothers will engage in the care that is appropriate. In the interchange between clinician and patient in a clinical setting lie the seeds of change in maternal statistics.

## Physical Examination

The importance of a physical examination is basic to all Western medicine, where the clinician undertakes a full physical examination. Jennifer Potter[7] writes of a lack of knowledge, fear, cultural beliefs, restrictions, taboos, history of sexual abuse, personal violence, or a lack of familiarity or belief in preventive screening as barriers to examinations by women. She gives pointers to performing a sensitive exam which include building rapport, attending to comfort, respect for modesty, and empowering the patient before, during, and after the exam by explanation in simple nonmedical language. Her outline for examination is particularly relevant to women who have a history of rape, violence, or female circumcision.

### Tips for performing a sensitive and comfortable pelvic examination

1. Ask the patient to empty the bladder (also important for accurate pelvic organ palpation).
2. Respect her modesty.
   - a. If the doctor is male, defer exam to a female clinician when requested by the patient.
   - b. Provide the patient with a gown and ask her to change into it in private.
   - c. Pull a curtain around the examining table so that she will not be exposed if someone inadvertently opens the door during the exam.
   - d. Use drapes liberally and appropriately.
3. Demonstrate good hygiene by washing your hands in her presence (even though you will be wearing gloves).
4. Place stirrups in a position that is appropriate for her life stage and in the presence of illness or any disability.
5. Select the smallest possible speculum that will allow adequate visualization of the vagina and cervix.

**Table 43.2 Adverse maternal outcomes of four ethnic groups[a,34]**

| Adverse outcome | White | African-American | Hispanic | Asian |
|---|---|---|---|---|
| **Preterm labor[b]** | 1.00 | 1.71 (1.60, 183) | 0.89 (0.83, 0.97) | 0.89 (0.76, 1.05) |
| **Hypertensive disorders of pregnancy** | | | | |
| Preeclampsia[c] | 1.00 | 1.59 (1.49, 1.69) | 1.00 (0.93, 1.07) | 0.93 (0.81, 1.06) |
| Transient hypertension of pregnancy[c] | 1.00 | 1.13 (1.07, 1.20) | 0.63 (0.59, 0.67) | 0.67 (0.59, 0.76) |
| Pregnancy-induced hypertension[c] | 1.00 1.00 | 1.38 (1.31, 1.46) | 0.79 (0.74, 0.84) | 0.73 (0.62, 0.83) |
| **Gestational diabetes[d]** | 1.00 | 1.26 (1.14, 1.40) | 1.44 (1.32, 1.58) | 2.05 (1.80, 2.32) |
| **Antepartum hemorrhage** | | | | |
| Placenta previa[e] | 1.00 | 1.78 (1.57, 2.02) | 1.20 (1.04, 1.37) | 1.57 (1.27, 1.93) |
| Abruption placenta[c] | 1.00 | 1.52 (1.43, 1.62) | 0.86 (0.80, 0.92) | 0.95 (0.83, 1.08) |
| **Membrane disorders** | | | | |
| Premature rupture of membrane[c] | 1.00 | 1.19 (1.15, 1.23) | 0.87 (0.84, 0.90) | 1.26 (1.19, 1.34) |
| Infection of the amniotic cavity[c] | 1.00 | 1.95 (1.86, 2.05) | 1.15 (1.09, 1.22) | 1.79 (1.64, 1.95) |
| **Mode of delivery – cesarean section[f]** | 1.00 | 1.09 (1.07, 1.11) | 1.06 (1.04, 1.08) | 0.85 (0.82, 0.89) |
| **Other – postpartum hemorrhage[g]** | 1.00 | 0.89 (0.85, 0.94) | 0.87 (0.83, 0.92) | 1.19 (1.09, 1.29) |

[a] n = 1 030 350. Data are expressed as odds ratios and 95% confidence intervals unless otherwise indicated.
[b] Adjusted for maternal age.
[c] Adjusted for maternal age, gestational diabetes, preexisting diabetes, and preexisting hypertension.
[d] Adjusted for maternal age and preexisting hypertension.
[e] Adjusted for maternal age and previous cesarean section.
[f] Risk ratio. Adjusted for [c] plus pregnancy-induced hypertension, preterm labor, placenta previa, abruption placenta, premature rupture of membrane, and infection of the amniotic cavity.
[g] Adjusted for maternal age, coagulation disorders, uterine tumor, and cesarean section.

6. Cover the stirrups with clean and comfortable pads or potholders to cushion her feet.

7. When she is ready, ask her to sit on the exam table and ask her to put her heels into the stirrups. Help guide her feet, if necessary.

8. Ask her to move into position by placing her hand at the end of the exam table and slowly sliding her bottom down until her buttocks are slightly overlapping the edge of the table. Assist her by adjusting the table and pillow, if necessary.

9. Maintain an ongoing dialogue about what you are doing and what she should expect next.

10. Ask frequently how she is doing and make adjustments if she experiences any discomfort.

11. Hand and finger movement should be gentle, slow, and with no quick motions.

12. Reassure her immediately when findings are normal.

13. Replace drapes when the exam is complete, and help her sit up on the table.

14. Explain that it is normal to have some spotting after a pap smear because the brush used to obtain the sample is a little bit abrasive.

15. Show her where tissues, tampons, and sanitary pads are located, ask her to get

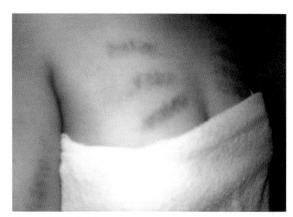

Figure 43.3 Coining.

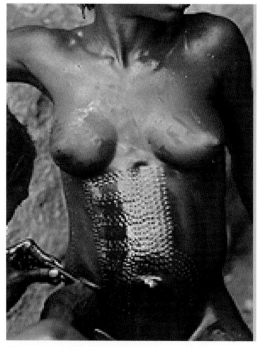

Figure 43.4 Skin decorating.

dressed and let her know you will return in several minutes to finish up.

16. Review findings and explain follow-up procedure.

In many cases, women may not allow a breast or pelvic exam on a first encounter. Gentle, persistent requests will gain access to these examinations, which should be undertaken when there is adequate time to respond to whatever the examination reveals.

## Traditional Practices

Traditional practices such as cupping, coining, and pinching (Figs 43.3, 43.4, 43.5) are frequently seen during examination. Used prior to a clinic visit to give comfort or alleviate symptoms, they show a belief in complimentary healing. Pinching between the eyebrows may relieve headache, coining on the soft tissue between ribs is believed to reduce fever. The resulting dermabrasion, which lasts several days, should not be confused with bruising from domestic violence. Ritual skin decoration and tattooing of face, breasts, and abdomen, performed as rites of passage into womanhood, can be observed in women from Africa.

No other traditional practice, however, has caused as much debate internationally as female circumcision or female genital mutilation. This writer chooses to use 'female circumcision' since it is the term that circumcised women use to describe themselves. It is estimated that 130–140 million women and girls worldwide have undergone some form of circumci-

sion with approximately 190 000 females estimated to be affected or at risk in the US. Despite international efforts to halt this debilitating yet tenacious custom by the World Health Organization since the 1960s, it continues today.

### Female circumcision

Female circumcision (Fig. 43.6) is most commonly performed in Africa, with 98% of all women in Sudan and Somalia being affected,[8] as well as the Middle East and Asia – all areas from which women migrate to the US. Clinicians therefore will be required to observe and treat the long-term effects of circumcision with an understanding that the circumstances under which the 'procedure' was done may not have been conducive to accurate cutting. The end result, then, in any one woman may have features of different types of circumcision, the most common types being:

- Type I: clitoridectomy – excision of all or part of the clitoris;
- Type II: excision – of the prepuce and clitoris with partial or total excision of the labia minora;

571

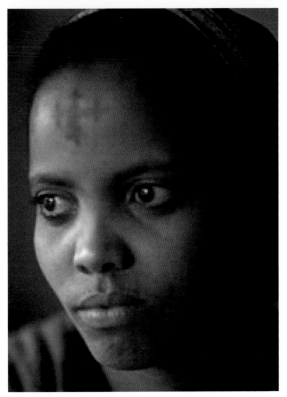

**Figure 43.5** Tattooing.

- Type III: infibulation – excision of part or all of the external genitalia and stitching or narrowing of the vaginal opening;
- Type IV: piercing, cutting, cauterization of the clitoris and surrounding tissue, cutting of the vagina with introduction of substances to tighten or narrow the vaginal introitus.[9]

### Long-term complications of female circumcision[2]

- Recurrent urinary tract infections;
- Generalized tenderness, increased sensitivity of vulva, perineum, and vagina, resulting in vaginismus;
- Cysts – sebaceous, inclusion, or dermoid;
- Neuroma;
- Keloid scarring;
- Vaginal stenosis leading to obstructed labor with resultant fistulae;

- Calculus formation in the vagina;
- Fear of coitus, anxiety, and depression.

### Problems for prenatal care and labor

- Difficult or impossible to obtain either a clean-catch urine or catheter sample to assess for asymptomatic bacteria, urinary tract infection, pylonephritis and preeclampsia in pregnancy.
- Inability to assess gestational age and cervical length by transvaginal ultrasound in pregnancy.
- Difficult or impossible to do pelvic examination in pregnancy and assess labor progress.

Prior to examination, it is important to ask a patient if 'cutting' has taken place, the woman's feelings on the matter, and whether a previous pelvic examination had been undertaken. The patient's knowledge of the type of circumcision may not be accurate and clinical assessment can decide the extent of cutting, and need for defibulation or reduction of circumcision.

Opportunities to discuss and encourage deinfibulation should be taken as they present, which could be pre-marriage and pre-pregnancy, 20–30 weeks' gestation in pregnancy, or at birth. The clinician involved must have an understanding of the highly personal, sensitive, emotive, and individual response to such discussion and allow time for it to unfold. As with many facets of childbirth, in whichever culture, stories abound over what should or should not be done to the vulva and perineum during birth. Circumcised women know by oral tradition of the fistulae that can result from obstructed labor, with resultant incontinence of urine and feces so destructive to women's lives.[9] What they have not yet come to trust is modern obstetrics' ability to recognize and resolve obstructed labor in most cases not caused by circumcision.[10]

### Counseling regarding defibulation

- Explain the problems resulting from circumcision.
- Outline the procedure of deinfibulation.
- Allow time for emotional processing and husband/family consultation.
- Prepare the patient for a new physical state and emotional reactions to same, i.e. the fast stream of urine with resultant sound change.

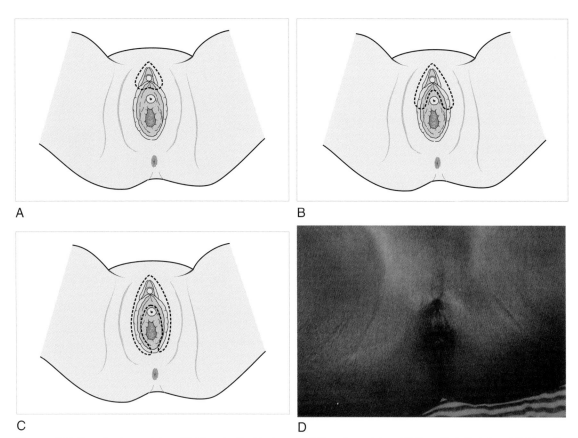

**Figure 43.6** Female circumcision. **(A)** Type I: clitoridectomy. **(B)** Type II: excision. **(C)** Type III: infibulation. **(D)** Type III: healed infibulation.

- Instruct in postoperative care regarding sitz baths and analgesia.

Prenatal visits allow time for discussion and agreement on deinfibulation with complete or partial repair of the incision. Many circumcised women feel their closed appearance is normal and that to be opened would be abnormal. International research has looked at the medical consequences of the physical act; only now is research beginning to look at the psychological and emotional impact of female circumcision and deinfibulation on the woman's body image. K.E. Adams writes that 'until cultural factors that lead to circumcision are understood, the pattern of abuse will continue.'[11] Clinicians must discuss the issue with women who have daughters in the hope that opening the subject to debate will bring pause or cessation to this custom passed from generation to generation. The clinician can also discuss the law

as it stands in the US related to female circumcision by which the practice became a federal crime in March 1997 (Table 43.3).

## Obesity

As female circumcision is of international concern, so obesity is one of the fastest growing national health concerns in the US with one-third of all women considered obese. Obesity has been found to be more prevalent in lower income and minority women, with 49% of African-American women, 38% of Mexican-American women, and 31% of white women found to be obese.[12] Associated disease leads to greater morbidity and when coupled with pregnancy, leads to higher rates of miscarriage, type II diabetes, hypertension, preeclampsia, and macroso-

Table 43.3 **States that have enacted legislation criminalizing female circumcision**

| California [a] | Minnesota | Rhode Island |
|---|---|---|
| Delaware [a] | New Jersey | Tennessee |
| Illinois | New York | Texas |
| Michigan | North Dakota | Wisconsin |

[a] These states have also enacted legislation that criminalizes both the parents and the physician who perform female circumcision.

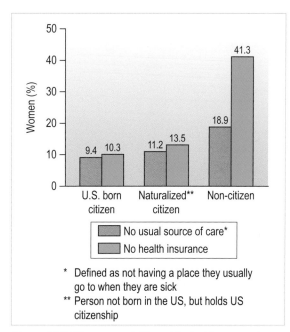

Figure 43.7 Women aged 18 or older lacking a usual source of care and health insurance, by citizenship status, 2001.

mia.[13] Yet in new immigrants, obesity is shown as an 8% prevalence in those with less than 1 year's residence in the US. This rate doubles to 19% with a residency of 15 years and over. Kaplan and colleagues[14] noted a nearly fourfold greater risk of obesity in the Hispanic population between recent immigrants and those of longer term. Being heavy is considered to be a sign of well-being and prosperity in many immigrant communities.

## Cultural concerns

- Being heavy is a sign of prosperity (high number of malnourished people in countries of origin).
- Being heavy is a sign of having somebody care for you.
- Having an appetite should not be restricted; it is a sign of being healthy.
- A child always has to finish the plate.
- Being plump equals being strong.

(Source: MCH Immigrant Health[15])

Acculturation into mainstream American life can lead to unhealthy dietary changes and a more sedentary life style. All immigrant women, when asked, will talk easily of the foods from their country of origin, such as mangos from Asia or camels' milk from North Africa. Preparation of food was a major portion of a woman's work with the often daily walking to market or field, then joint preparation with women from their extended family. This can be lost in the US, where obtaining and preparing food is an entirely different experience. Husbands frequently shop for food and families live as single units with women often experiencing isolation and a sense of loss of their role.

The effects of this isolation frequently cause an increase in symptoms of early pregnancy, particularly nausea and vomiting, commonly affecting up to 70% of pregnant women.[14] Women who in their country of origin coped with this common side effect within an extended family network find their new lifestyle increases the severity of this usually self-limiting problem. Food taste is different, odors disturb more, and a faster pace of life all add to an inability to cope. *Helicobacter pylori*, known to be more prevalent in the immigrant population if present, may aggravate the vomiting.[15] No clear studies of immigrant women in regard to this are available, yet clinical observation suggests that emergency room visits for nausea and vomiting are greater in number in newly arrived immigrants. A 2005 study of hyperemesis gravidarum, where severity in vomiting required a 2.6-day hospital stay to resolve dehydration and electrolyte imbalance, accounted for a major portion of the nondelivery pregnancy-associated hospitalizations in the US in 2000, with resultant expenditure of healthcare dollars.[16]

Lack of medical insurance (Fig. 43.7) and knowledge of the healthcare system available will often lead immigrant women to seek late care, or care in the wrong venue. Assessment, hydration, and medication for hyperemesis with referral to home care hydration, can all be undertaken in a clinic providing prenatal services where continuity of care will be established without emergency room usage.

# Nutrition and Contamination

Dialogue on diet and exercise specific to pregnancy and lactation for a foreign-born mother should also include information on contaminants dangerous to pregnancy. In *Food Safety For Moms-To-Be*[17] the food-borne risk from listeria, toxoplasmosis, and methyl mercury is reviewed with preventions outlined. Cleaning, cooking, chilling, and storing information is also reviewed and is ideal for women who may not have had previous access to the modern equipment of an American kitchen. Many immigrant families supplement their food supply by fishing and it is crucial that the knowledge of dangers to the fetus of methyl mercury and PCBs be made known, preferably in their primary language. More than 300 000 newborns yearly are reported to be exposed to mercury with resultant adverse neurological sequelae.[18] Fish is well recognized as a low-fat source of protein, vitamin E and minerals, all essential in the diet of pregnancy, so should not be forsaken. The recommendations from the Minnesota Department of Health (Table 43.4) are pertinent to the fish found in Minnesota and are in line with national recommendations.[19]

Exposure to pesticides is well documented in migrant workers in rural settings with increased vulnerability in pregnant women and infants.[20,21] Immigrant women in urban settings are also exposed where pesticides are sprayed to reduce rodents, fungi, and insects either in their home, work sites, community, or as residues on food. Many new immigrants live in rented, old homes decorated with lead-based paint and built before 1986 when an amendment to the Safe Drinking Water Act prohibited the use of lead solders and pipes in water systems. Lead is a powerful neurotoxin and it is recommended that women have serum levels tested in pregnancy. Preconceptual assessment would provide a more preventative approach. Elevated serum levels in adults may result in hypertension, in pregnancy increased abortion rate, and in infancy delays of physical and mental development.[22] Persistent organic pollutants (POPs) and polybrominated diphenyl ethers (PBDE) are known contaminates of the food supply with resultant accumulation to the individual body burden. Since women have proportionally more adipose tissue than men, their body composition poses greater risk for uptake and storage of toxins in body fat. Immigrant women's body burden is dependent on contaminants in their country of origin. Studies have shown that American women have a 10–100 times greater level of PBDEs in adipose tissue and breast milk than their European counterparts.[23] The unique make-up of breast

| Table 43.4 Recommendations regarding fish | | | | |
|---|---|---|---|---|
| **For fish caught in Minnesota lakes and rivers** | | | | |
| Amount of each type of fish caught in Minnesota | | | | |
| Pan fish (sunfish & crappie) | | Walleyes *shorter than* 20 in. | | Walleyes *longer than* 20 in |
| Perch | | Northern pike *shorter than* 30 in. | | Northern pike *longer than* 30 in. |
| Bullheads | | All sizes of other species | | Muskellunge |
| 1 meal a week | | 1 meal a month | | **Do Not Eat** |
| **For commercial fish (bought in a store or eaten in a restaurant)** | | | | |
| Amount of each type of fish | | | | |
| Salmon | Catfish | Shrimp | Canned 'white' | Shark |
| Cod | Tilapia | Crab | tuna (6oz) | Swordfish |
| Pollock | Herring | Scallops | Tuna steak | Tile fish |
| Canned 'light' tuna (6 oz) | Sardines | Oysters | Halibut Lobster | King mackerel |
| | 2 meals a week | | 2 meals a month | **Do Not Eat** |

Include all sources of fish you eat when making choices. For example, if you eat one 6 oz can of white (albacore) tuna, then wait 2 weeks before eating another meal of any type of fish. Or, if you eat one meal from an 18-inch walleye, do not eat any other meals of fish for 1 month.

tissue allows for a rapid excretion of stored contaminant in the lipid content of breast milk, as much as 10 times higher than the content in ordinary food.[23] Immigrant mothers have both a higher rate and longer duration of breast-feeding than their native-born sisters. An infant's body burden therefore can begin in utero and increase rapidly when breast-fed. Despite this, the benefits of breast-feeding are still acknowledged to outweigh the disadvantages of contaminants.[24]

It seems, therefore, that advice on consumption of a diet low in fat, meat, and dairy products, safe fish intake, clean water, and adequate selection and preparation of fruit and vegetables would aid women in a slower escalation of body burden, to their own and their infant's benefit. Precautionary principle,[25] if used by clinicians, can begin to raise awareness in women who come from cultures where contaminants such as tobacco, alcohol, and illicit drugs are viewed as negative behavior during reproductive years. Increasing a woman's knowledge in this area can only strengthen her reproductive health.

Use of a folic acid supplement to reduce infant mortality and morbidity in neural tube defects (NTDs) should also be advised by care providers. In the early 1990s, it was recognized that the most important environmental influence on neural tube development was maternal folate levels.[26,27] Genetic, geographic, and ethnic factors also present in the first 28 days of gestation are important, with higher incidence rates found in the British Isles, China, Egypt, and India. Sikhs living in India have more than twice the incidence of NTD than Sikhs living in Canada with a supplemented folate intake.[28] The recommended intake is hard to obtain from food alone despite government regulation to fortify cereal grains.[29] Many immigrant women do not have cereal or bread as part of their daily diet and frequently do not plan their pregnancies. As approximately 50% of all pregnancies in the US are unintended,[30] the American College of Obstetricians and Gynecologists recommends low-risk women in their reproductive years take a daily multivitamin or prenatal multivitamin which contains 400 micrograms of folic acid. Women at high risk with a history of NTD are recommended to take a 400 milligram daily dosage. Multivitamins with a gelatin base from seaweed can be prescribed for women whose religion forbids the ingestion of pork, the base for most gelatins. A 2000 study[31] revealed only 25–40% supplementation uptake in the month prior to conception. Awareness by all clinicians of the importance of prescribing supplementation coupled with public health efforts in languages appropriate to the communities served may assist the Healthy People 2010[6] aim of 75% uptake in prenatal multivitamin supplementation. Prenatal recognition of a fetal anomaly is extremely difficult information to give to any parent. When the information is given to an immigrant family via an interpreter, it is crucial to have visual evidence available and the time needed for such a face-to-face encounter. Some immigrant parents see the fetus with nonlethal anomalies as a special gift given to their family for care.[1] Others know that such a child would frequently die in infancy in their country of origin. The support services available to them in the US should be introduced to the discussion as their initial shock gives way to reality.

## Laboratory Testing

### Recommended laboratory tests for all pregnant women

- Blood type and Rh factor
- Human immunodeficiency virus (HIV)
- Antibody screen
- Rapid plasma reagent (RPR)
- Complete blood count
- Urine analysis
- Rubella titer
- Chlamydia and gonorrhea cultures
- Hepatitis B surface antigen
- Serum lead levels

### Carrier screening offered with informed consent

The following carrier screen applies to people of the indicated ancestries:

- Hemoglobin electrophoresis: African, Southeast Asian, Mediterranean.
- DNA based screen for Tay-Sachs and Canavan disease: Ashkenazi Jew, French Canadian, Cajun.
- Cystic fibrosis screen: Ashkenazi Jew, Caucasians.
- Maternal alpha fetoprotein evaluation: all women.

Foreign-born women may require additional screening in pregnancy if this has not been completed since entering the US. If a woman is hepatitis B nonimmune, vaccination can be initiated and completed during pregnancy. Parasitic infestation can add to anemia, and appropriate screening should be undertaken (see Ch. 11). The placement and reading of a purified protein derivative (PPD) when positive, should lead to a chest X-ray and follow-up care.

An aim of Healthy People 2010[6] is a reduction in preterm births and low birth weight infants. National statistics in 2000[2] found:

- US-born preterm birth rate, 11.9%;
- Foreign-born preterm birth rate, 10.5%;
- US-born low birth weight rate, 7.9%;
- Foreign-born low birth weight rate, 6.4%.

These statistics are reinforced by a 1999 study of immigrant women to France, Belgium, and the US which concludes there are better birth outcomes in immigrant women despite their disadvantaged backgrounds.[32]

## Cultural Behaviors and Beliefs

Thought to be reflective of a healthy migrant effect, those who immigrate may be healthier, with cultural behaviors protective of pregnancy, thus sustaining a more positive pregnancy outcome. As previously stated, the use of tobacco, alcohol, and illicit drugs is viewed as very negative behavior, with other cultural beliefs and behaviors passed from generation to generation believed to safeguard the pregnancy. If Jamaican women fail to satisfy a food craving, there will be a poor pregnancy outcome. Should Hmong women raise their hands above their heads during pregnancy, the baby may not breathe at birth. Mexican women protect their fetus by not crossing their legs in pregnancy, this can cause fetal strangulation. They also will wear safety pins, in the form of a cross, on clothing covering the abdomen to protect the fetus from evil.[33] Common to each cultural group is the importance of food that has specific value in maintaining the balance of physical health at this vulnerable time. Emotional well-being is sustained by ensuring that the pregnant woman is sheltered from unpleasant emotions such as fear, anger, despair, and sadness.[33] Spiritual health is encouraged through prayer, ritual incantation, and the wearing of amulets for protection specific to pregnancy. The fasting from sunrise to sunset during Ramadan ending with the celebration of Idal-Fitr is a time of spiritual renewal and strengthening in the Islamic faith. Exceptions can be made when women are pregnant or ill but pregnant women look forward to this time joyfully.

'Ramadan for me is a phase of time where I reduce my obligations outside and focus inward . . . It's hard to explain to a nonMuslim that fasting is a very kind thing for a Muslim body, spirit, and soul'[34]

Care providers need to be creative during this 1-month period since venipuncture and pelvic assessments are considered to break the fast.

## Recommendations for provider review pre-Ramadan[34]

### Ask pregnant Muslim patients if they plan to fast during Ramadan

- Explore what influences her decision.
- Inquire as to reasons she might decide not to fast.
- Discuss perceived disadvantages of not fasting.
- Assess plan to ensure adequate nutrition and fluids.

### Assess for risk factors that might preclude fasting safely

- Insulin-dependent diabetes.
- Any condition that requires medications during the day.
- History of renal stones, preterm delivery, poor obstetrics outcome.
- Peptic ulcer disease
- Malnutrition.
- Strenuous physical activity.
- Ramadan occurring in summer months.

### Provide information about how to fast safely

- Diet
  1. Stop caffeine and cigarettes gradually in advance.
  2. Get up for *sahoor* (morning meal)
  3. Eat high fiber, whole grains, fruits, vegetables, nuts.
  4. Avoid excess salt, sugar, and caffeine.
  5. Drink water, milk, and juice just before dawn.
  6. Breakfast with water and dates (this is traditional).
  7. Balanced, nutritious evening meal, and plenty of fluids.

8. Bedtime snack including water or juice, protein, and fruit.
- Activity
  1. Avoid strenuous physical activity; get adequate sleep.
  2. Stay cool during day.

Many cultural beliefs have no scientific basis, yet clinicians would be wise to know those that are pertinent to pregnancy and birth, respecting those that are safe and rescinding the unsafe, such as the traditional herbal drink brewed especially for pregnancy and postpartum usage by Cambodian women, which contains high levels of alcohol, or the craving for and eating of clay by West African women, where the clay has high levels of lead.

Just as culture impinges on pregnancy so does it attend labor, birth, and postpartum. Brigette Jordon observes in *Birth in Four Cultures*, 'While the process of childbirth is, in some sense, everywhere the same, it is also everywhere different in that each culture has produced a birthing system strikingly dissimilar from others.' Jordon's belief is that childbirth is grounded in cultural and social settings that channel the biological.[35] No matter how educated in Western medicine an immigrant woman is, she will always rely on family and community for advice.

'The best place to get information is from your doctor. But he is also a human being. So also check with your community, friends, or your parents.'[36]

She often views labor and birth from an entirely different perspective than her biomedically educated provider. Women bring to birthing beliefs from the family.

'You know during my labor, the doctors asked me to 'take a deep breath'. I don't like that. I would rather say the Qur'an [pray] instead of taking a deep breath. Why do I have to waste my time breathing when I can say my prayers?'[36]

A Hmong woman whose labor is prolonged may ask forgiveness from her mother-in-law for a perceived wrongdoing and will labor in silence rather than vocalize, believing the baby will be scared from her cries and will delay being born. Mexican women will be very expressive, with families supportive of their verbalization. Women from the community are birth companions in most developing countries, with husbands and male family members near but not present. Major decisions over care, however, must have the husband or elder male member's approval, and should this person be thousands of miles away, even

with today's high-speed communication, much time can pass before a crucial decision is reached. In American medicine, time is of the essence, while to an immigrant family it may be more elastic. A laboring woman having a protracted latent or active phase of labor may be considered normal by a family yet providers will suggest the use of modern obstetrical aids such as i.v. infusion, Pitocin augmentation, internal fetal and uterine monitoring, amino infusion, and analgesia via intrathecal narcotic or epidural. Modern obstetrical rituals can be considered intrusive by a woman who has birthed normally in her country of origin, and should be discussed with her at prenatal visits or classes to allow time for understanding. Unless time and energy are spent in simple, clear explanation, families can believe that a cesarean birth is the result of these aids rather than the provider's desire to have a healthy mother and baby on completion of the birth. Many misguided stories over cesarean birth also circulate in immigrant communities: 'The doctor makes more money by cesarean birth,' or 'This is the only way the doctor knows how to deliver a baby.'

'[My friends] told me: 'Don't go to that hospital, because they like to do the cesarean section.' And I went to that hospital and I delivered with C-Section.'[36]

The rising cesarean rate (29.1% of all births in the US in 2004[37]) is driven by the fundamental goal of obstetrics to optimize the outcome of pregnancy and is not always appreciated by immigrant families. There is an emotional and spiritual connectedness to the natural birth process which can be lost with surgical delivery. To immigrant women who may have had a life of loss, the inability to birth naturally intensifies a sense of lessening to their womanhood and a loss of standing in their community. Yet these women know only too well the dangers of birth, coming from countries where the maternal mortality rates are always higher than in the US.[38] Eritrean women, for example, face a 1 in 24 chance of death from pregnancy within their lifetime with a mortality rate of 630 per 100 000 live births, compared to their American sisters with a mortality rate of 12.1 in 100 000 live births in 2003.[38,39] Nothing, however, can be as devastating to a woman as a stillborn baby or neonatal death, or to a community the demise of a mother from pregnancy or birth. Immigrant women sustain a higher percentage of maternal deaths than their American-born sisters of like racial grouping.[39] Only in the black population are foreign-born numbers equal and at alarmingly high percent-

**Table 43.5 Pregnancy-related mortality ratios (PRMRs) among five ethnic groups, United States, 1993–1997[a]**

| PRMR | Hispanic | Asian/Pacific Islander | American Indian/Alaska Native | Black | White | Total |
|---|---|---|---|---|---|---|
| US-born women[b] | 8.0 | 6.1[c] | 13.2 | 30.0 | 7.6 | 11.6 |
| Foreign-born women | 11.8 | 12.7 | –[b] | 29.5 | 6.2 | 12.4 |

[a] n = 2334.
[b] The 50 states of District of Columbia.
[c] Fewer than seven pregnancy-related deaths; considered unreliable (relative standard error ≥38%).

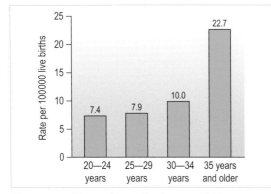

**Figure 43.8** Maternal mortality, by age, 2000.

ages for a developed country with modern medical capabilities (Table 43.5).[2]

Also notable is the higher mortality rate in all women aged 35 years and older with an increase of 3–4% from 2003 to 2004.[40] Unlike their American counterparts who may be having a first or second pregnancy after 35 years, immigrant women are frequently highly gravid, adding to their risk factors (Fig. 43.8).

Loss of hope in the anticipated life of a child or the death of a mother is an excruciating loss in an immigrant community. Grief is expressed in the language and rituals of each culture with wailing and tearing of clothes for some, weeping and beating of self for others, or heart wrenching stoic silence and stillness for others. The American ritual of preserving memory by seeing, holding, or dressing the baby, cutting a lock of hair or obtaining a foot/hand print can be startling to an immigrant family. Many families would consider those rituals as negative to the mother's well-being and they should be gently introduced to a grieving family with giving memories as the foremost aim. Autopsy is seldom performed in an immigrant's home country where death is viewed

as the will of Allah, the intervention of God, or the mandate to any given life, and is frequently refused. Preparation of the body for burial will require input from a community's religious members to give honor to the life lost.

Time is again a dynamic during the postpartum period, which lasts for 28 days for Hmong women, 40 days for African and Hispanic women, and 3 months for Vietnamese and Cambodian women. Since 6 weeks is when most women of lower economic standing return to work in America, this can cause a considerable psychological struggle in a woman who culturally believes she is not yet fully well. Immediately after birth, many foreign-born women are considered vulnerable to an imbalance and weakening of body forces secondary to the birth process. Exposure to various activities such as strenuous housework, room temperature (cold air), weather (wind and rain), or fluids and food (cold food by cultural definition, not temperature) can lead to a further imbalance with longer recovery or, in Chinese women, premature aging of the skin and/or pain in the joints and bones in older age.[1] It is not unusual for Asian women to leave hospital after birth without showering since hospitals set an upper water temperature limit to avoid scalding in showers, so the water is considered 'too cold' by these women. Binding of the abdomen with or without heat application to aid uterine involution and to assist the abdominal muscles in regaining tone is common to many immigrant groups.

## Birth control

Resumption of coitus on completion of the postpartum period is dependent on cessation of bleeding. If present, the woman is not yet fully cleansed and cannot participate in coitus. Discussion regarding contraception and when initiation of a method will begin is made prenatally by most American-born women. This is not so in immigrant women, many of whom will only discuss the topic after the birth is completed. Words are powerful, particularly if heard in a second language with which you are only just becoming fluent. Family planning, family spacing, birth control are all terms used to define a range of options available to prevent pregnancy. To a foreign-born woman and husband the suspicion created by the words 'birth control' can stop a discussion at its very inception. To use or not to use a contraceptive method is commonly not the woman's choice, but resides with the husband or older women (if in an extended family) making the decision. Since pregnancy is often seen as a gift from a higher power, or if a family distrusts Western medicine or the family has seen many of its members die in their country of origin, no interference in the natural process of procreation will be chosen. If a choice is made, clear instruction on any changes in menstrual flow and frequency should be discussed. Many immigrant women believe they must bleed monthly to be healthy and will quickly stop any method that disturbs their menstrual pattern. Fully breast-feeding for up to 2 years prior to coming to the US may have assisted women in spacing their pregnancies. Two factors should be considered when anovulation is used as contraception in the US. Many mothers supplement their breast-feeding with artificial milk (Box 43.1), thus nullifying the anovulatory process. Large numbers of women stop breast-feeding by 6 months (Fig. 43.9) and are therefore no longer safe from pregnancy. Many women have insurance coverage for pregnancy and birth only and can not afford access to contraception when breast-feeding stops. This then perpetuates the cycle of unplanned pregnancies in low income families.

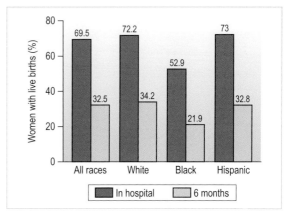

**Figure 43.9** Women breast-feeding in hospital and at 6 months postpartum, by race/ethnicity, 2001.

---

### Box 43.1
#### Breast-feeding: cultural transitions

Perception that infant formula is a sign of economic progress.

Infant formula is thought to be better because American babies are bigger.

Social support for breast-feeding is missing.

Lack of support in the US for breast-feeding.

Bottle-feeding perceived as modern and as a US value.

Bottle feeding gives the mother independence.

(Source: NY Task Force on Immigrant Health[15])

## Preventative gynecological care

Preventative gynecological care in the form of screening for breast, cervical, uterine, and ovarian cancers as well as sexually transmitted disease is also diminished by lack of health insurance and knowledge. To foreign-born women the idea of preventive care is a concept which can be hard to accept. Women seek medical intervention only when symptomatic in the country of origin. Negative experiences give women phrases like 'too probing' for pelvic exams, 'too painful' for mammograms, 'too embarrassing' for pelvic exams and any questions regarding sexually transmitted diseases (STDs). To talk about disease in Asian communities is viewed as bad luck or bad karma. Practitioners need to take time, and use simple, nonthreatening language when discussing screening. It is wise for the clinician to know if a husband/partner is traveling out of the country. The possibility of a second wife or partner, be they male or female, in this or the visited country, can pose an infection risk to the woman who culturally is not allowed to question her husband's behaviors. Cervical cancer is the second most common cancer worldwide with human papillomavirus (HPV) the greatest and most persistent of STDs. HPV is believed to infect 60–80% of all sexually active women at some time. Most infections are transient, therefore benign, and by 24 months after initial infection will have cleared. Molecular testing has aided in identification of the HPV types which gain persistent infection and can result in high-grade cervical cancers or their precursors. Cytological

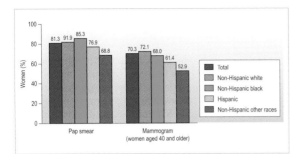

**Figure 43.10** Women's self-reporting of Pap smears and mammograms.

screening has resulted in a major reduction of cervical cancer rates in developed countries. This preventable disease killed 3710 women in the US in 2005, revealing failure in adequate screening and/or follow-up of detected anomalies.[41]

The thought of having a pelvic exam for Pap smear is disturbing to many foreign-born women and is seen as not only invasive but unnecessary. This is reflected in national rates of Pap smear where women of color are noted in smaller numbers (Fig. 43.10), with Asian-American and Pacific Island women at lower Pap smear frequencies than other ethnic groups.

A Healthy People 2010[6] goal is to increase the percentage of women ever receiving Pap tests to 97%. In 2000, the following reported ever receiving a Pap test (age adjusted, aged 18 years and over):

- 95 percent: American Indian or Alaska Native only;
- 95 percent: black or African-American only, not Hispanic/Latino;
- 95 percent: white only, not Hispanic/Latino;
- 87 percent: Hispanic/Latino;
- 77 percent: Asian only.

To reach this goal, grants from the federal government and the Centers for Disease Control are available to communities where disparities in screening and rates of cervical cancer are apparent. This funding is welcome since routine vaccination against the HPV is in its infancy and may take up to 20 years before it is widely utilized as a prevention tool in the general population.

Breast cancer deservedly has gained a higher profile in the national debate and media than cervical cancer. Statistics continue to show that women of color and women from rural areas have less disease but a higher mortality rate than white women.[41] Breast self-examination, clinical breast exam with mammogram, and ultrasound continue to be effective screening tools when used. Both breast and cervical cancer are found in women as they age. For screening to be accepted as part of a healthy life choice, young women need education in school, college and, for immigrant women, in their community newspapers and in their own language. Education also begins when they interface with clinicians for any reason. The following case history is one where the groundwork for such education has begun (Box 43.2).

---

**Box 43.2**

**Case study**

A 19-year-old Ethiopian female, in the country for 3 months, presented with history of dyspareunia for 2 months. Gynecological history was of normal 28-day menstrual cycle beginning at 14 years. Circumcision had been undertaken in a hospital setting at age 12. On clinical examination, type II circumcision with ease of access to introitus was found. Blockage was palpated above lower third of the vagina with inability to perform either digital isolation of the cervix or to obtain a Pap smear. She was referred to a female gynecologist who, after ultrasound and examination, diagnosed a thin transverse septum, with a small central dimple opening. The septum transversed from left upper third to lower-right midsection of the vaginal walls. The gynecologist advised to have the septum

removed and deinfibulation of circumcision prior to pregnancy. The patient declined.

The young woman returned 1 year later for prenatal care to a certified nurse-midwife clinic at 8 weeks' gestation. She complained of inability to swallow prenatal multivitamin capsules, and was therefore given a liquid preparation. Barium swallow, ENT consult and work-up were negative, 6 months prior to her appointment.

At 20 weeks' gestation, she stated swallowing was becoming more difficult and she had not gained weight. Asked why she thought she was unable to swallow, she said, 'Because the jealous girls and their mothers in my home village put a spell on me as I left for marriage in the USA. There is no medicine in

**Box 43.2**

**Case study—cont'd**

America to help me.' When asked what medicine would be given in Ethiopia, she replied, 'My grandmother will make a tea to drink with hair taken from the head of those who were jealous. After I drink it, I will go to the waterfall where we go to bathe and the sickness will go.' The midwife suspected homesickness, and when introducing the idea into the conversation was advised by the patient that she was not crazy.

The patient was referred to an obstetrician for discussion to plan for delivery. Suggestions of cesarean birth, reduction of septum, and circumcision were negated by patient. 'I will have a normal birth; the women from my country do not need surgery for birth.' An interpreter and an aunt of the patient were present for this appointment. On completion of the interview, the interpreter advised the patient to read the Qur'an daily at home.

In the third trimester, swallowing becoming more difficult and the aunt stated that the patient had crying and screaming spells at home when she lay on the floor stating that the curse was getting stronger.

At 32 and 36 weeks' gestation, a shaman ceremony was performed in the clinic with the aunt and

interpreter present. The patient, aunt, and interpreter all agreed the ceremony was very similar to that which would have taken place in the home village in Ethiopia. The patient stated that swallowing was much easier but not yet normal after the 36-week ceremony. Also at 36 weeks' gestation, the obstetrical team, with patient and family, agree to spontaneous labor with epidural for analgesia to allow for incision of septum. The patient was initially unwilling to have the epidural but finally agreed.

At 41 weeks' gestation, spontaneous rupture of membranes occurred. Pitocin augmentation of labor and epidural placement occurred in the first stage of labor. When in second stage, a transvaginal resection of septum and anterior episiotomy of circumcision was performed. A normal birth of an 8 pounds 4 ounce male infant in good condition occurred. On completion of the third stage, inspection and completion of resection was undertaken with suturing of labial lips to prevent circumcision rehealing. Estimated blood loss was 700 mL.

At the second and tenth week postpartum visits, the patient was happy with the birth outcome and could now swallow without difficulty. There was evidence of sound healing in the vagina and vulva with no dyspareunia.

This case history is evidence of skilled obstetrical care combined with respect for a woman's traditional healing beliefs. The outcome was a safe birth of a baby whose mother was healthy in body and mind on completion of her care.

At the beginning of the twentieth century, William Osler[42] taught 'that it is more important to know what sort of a patient has a disease, than what sort of disease a patient has.' Now, one century later, medical science in America has gained amazing knowledge, technology, and skill in giving appropriate care to all of its citizens. It must also gain and sustain the will to increase research specific to the subgroups envisioned by David Satcher[4] if the disparities gap is to be closed and the 2010 initiatives be attained.

Foreign-born women, be they refugee or immigrant, bring an immense wealth in strength, dignity, fortitude, and resourcefulness to their new homeland. There are many opportunities available to a provider to give care that is responsive to each woman's unique individuality. This care will reflect on generations to come: their children are the future of America.

## References

1. Shah MA, Campbell D, Fullerton J. Editors for National Perinatal Association. National Perinatal Association – A Resource Guide. Transcultural Aspects of Perinatal Health Care.
2. Spector RS. Cultural diversity in health and illness. New Jersey: Pearson Prentice Hall; 2004.
3. Births to Foreign Born Mothers – Minnesota Vital Statistics – July 2005 Volume No. 4. Minnesota Center for Health Statistics. http://www.healthstate.mn.us/divs/chs/vitalsigns/index.html
4. Camarota SA. Birth to immigrants in America 1970–2002. Center for Immigration Studies. Hcc/www.cis_org/articles/2005/back805.html
5. Gognon AJ, Tuck J, Barkunba L. A systematic review of questionnaires measuring the health of resettling refugee women. Health Care Women Internat 2004; 25;111–149.
6. Satcher D. American women and health disparities. J Am Med Women's Assoc 2001; 56;131–132.
7. National Institute of Environmental Health Sciences. Health disparities research. Available: http://www.niehs.nih.gov/oc/factsheet/disparity/home.htm
8. Healthy People 2010. Available: http://wonder.cdc.gov/DATA2010
9. Potter J. The pelvic exam. Available: http://www.hmsharvard.edu/coenh/culture
10. Kelly E, Adams Hillar PJ. Female genital mutilation. Curr Opin Obstet Gynecol 2005; 17:490–494.
11. Toubia N. Caring for women with circumcision. A Rainbq Publication; 1999.

12. Miller S, Lester F, Webster M, et al. Obstetrical fistula: a preventable tragedy. J Midwif Women's Health 2005; 50:286–294.

13. Essen B, Sjoberg MO, Gudmundsson S, et al. No association between female circumcision and prolonged labour. Eur J Obstet Gynecol Reprod Biol 2005; 1:121.

14. Adams KE. What's 'normal': female genital mutilation, psychology and body image. J Am Med Women's Assoc 2004; 59:168–170.

15. Hedley AA, Ogden CL, Johnson CL, et al. Prevalence of overweight and obesity among US children, adolescents and adults. JAMA 2004; 291:2847–2850.

16. Goel MS, McCarthy EP, Phillips RS, et al. Obesity among US immigrant subgroups by duration of residence. JAMA 2004; 292:2860–2867.

17. Kaplan MS, Huquet N, Newsom JT, McFarlane BH. The association between length of residence and obesity among Hispanic Immigrants. Am J Prev Medicine Nov 2004; 27(4):323–326.

18. Villanueva H, Norris L. Cross cultural care in Maternal and Child Health Manual. National MCH Immigrant Health Training Project #369303-1. New York University School of Medicine. September 1995 pp. 37–38.

19. Attard CL, Kohli MA, Coleman S, et al. The burden of illness of severe nausea and vomiting of pregnancy in the United States. Am J Obstet Gynecol 2002; 186:S220–S227 (level 11-2).

20. Goodman KJ, O'Rourkek RS, Wang C, et al. Helicobacter pylori infection in pregnant women from a US–Mexico border population. J Immigrant Health 2003; 5:99–107.

21. Gazmararian JA, Petersen R, Jamieson DJ, et al. Hospitalisation during pregnancy among managed care enrollees. Am J Obstet Gynecol 2002; 1000:94–100 (level 11-2).

22. Food safety for moms-to-be. Available: http://www.cfsan.fda.gov/pregnancy.html

23. Environmental Working Group Body Burden. The pollution in newborns. Available: http://www.ewg.org/reports/bodyburden2/ July, 2005.

24. Huffing K. The effects of environmental contaminants in food on women's health. JMidwif Women's Health 1996; 51:26–32.

25. Hanke W, Jurewicz J. The risk and adverse reproductive and developmental disorders due to occupational pesticide exposure. An overview of current epidemiological evidence. Int J Occup Med Environ Health 2004; 17: 223–243.

26. Kirrane EF, Hoppin JA, Umbach DM, et al. Pesticide exposure and women's health. Am J Int Med 2003; 44:584–594.

27. Afzal B. Drinking water and women's health. J Midwif Women's Health 2006; 51:12–16.

28. Nickerson K. Environmental contaminants in breast milk. J Midwif Women's Health 2006; 51:26–32.

29. American Academy of Pediatricians Work Group on Breast Feeding.Breast feeding and the use of human milk. Pediatrics 1997; 100:1035–1039.

30. Kriebel D, Tickner J, Epstein S, et al. The precautionary principle in environmental science. Environment Health Perspect 2001; 109:871–876.

31. Wald NJ, Law MR, Morris JK, Wald DS. Quantifying the effect of folic acid. Lancet 2001; 358:2069–2073.

32. Lumley J, Watson L, Watson M, Bower C. Periconceptional supplementation with folate and/or multivitamins for preventing neural tube defects. (Cochran review) The Cochrane Library, Issue I 2003.l Oxford: Update Software (level I).

33. Nassbaum RL, Mclnnes RR, Willard HF. Genetics of disorders with complex inheritance. In: Thompson and Thompson genetics in medicine. 6th edn. Philadelphia: WB Saunders; 2001:289–310 (level III).

34. Food standards: amendment of standards of identity for enriched grain products to require addition of folic acid. FDA. Final Rule. Fed Regist 1996; 61:8781–8797.

35. Henshaw SK. Unintended pregnancies in United States. Fam Plan Perspect 1998; 30:24–29, 46.

36. Improving maternal healthcare: the next generation of research.
Available: http://www.ahrq.gov/research/maternhlth/

37. Guendelman S, Buekens P, Blondel B, et al. Birth outcomes of immigrant women in the United States, France, and Belium. Maternal Child Health J 1999; 3(4):177–180.

38. Shen JJ, Tymkon C, MacMullen N. Disparities in maternal outcomes among four ethnic populations. Ethnicity Disease 2005; 15:492–497.

39. Robinson Trinka, Raisler J. 'Each a doctor for herself': Ramadan fasting among pregnant Muslim women in the United States. Ethnicity Disease 2005; 15:S99–S103.

40. Jordon B. Birth in four cultures. 4th edn. Prospelt Heights, Illinois: Waveland Press; 1993.

41. Brief Report: 'Somali Women Speak Out'. J Midwif Women's Health 2004; 49(4):345–349. Available: http://www.jmwh.org

42. Hamilton BE, Martin JA, Sutton PD, et al. Birth: preliminary data 2004. Centers for Disease Control and Prevention, National Center for Health Statistics. Natl Vital Stat Rep 2005; 54(8):1–17.

43. State specific trends in US live births to women born outside of the 50 states and District of Columbia – United States, 1990 and 2000. Available: http://www.cdc.gov/mmwr/preview/mmwrhfml/mm5148a3.htm

44. Reproduction, Maternal, Newborn Health. The World Health Report 2003 Statistical Annex 8, p. 215 and 219.

45. Forna F, Jamieson DJ, Sanders D, et al. Pregnancy outcomes in foreign-born and US women. Int J Gynaecol Obstet 2003; 83:257–265.

46. Calligan WM, Berf, CJ. Pregnancy-related mortality among women aged 35 years and older, United States, 1991–1997:1015–1021. Obstetr Gynecol 2003; 102(5 part 1).

47. American Cancer Society. Cancer Facts and Figures 2005. http://www.cod.gov/cancer/nbccedp/nbcam.htm

48. William Osler: A Life in Medicine Toronto: University of Toronto Press; 1999.

49. Johnson EB, Reed SD, Hitt J, et al. Increased risk of adverse pregnancy outcomes among Somali immigrants in Washington State. Amer J Obstet Gynecol 2005; 193:475–482.

50. Chang J, Elamevans LD, Berg CJ, et al. Pregnancy Related Mortality Surveillance United States 1991–1999. MMWR Surveillance Survey 2003. February 2003/vol52/#552.

51. Preventive Care, Women's Health USA 2003, p. 66. Health Resources and Services Administration. US Department of Health and Human Services. http://www.hrsa.gov/womenshealth

52. Kramer EJ, Ivey SL, Ying YW. Immigrants Women's Health. San Francisco: Jossey-Bass; 1999.

# CHAPTER 44

# Women's Reproductive Health

Anita J. Gagnon, Lisa Merry, and Cathlyn Robinson

## Introduction

There are currently fifteen million refugees and asylum seekers worldwide,[1] a percentage of whom will resettle in host countries. The health of resettling refugees is not well known since health data are rarely reported for refugees separate from all immigrants combined. Refugees, individuals forced from their homeland and unable to return for a period of time due to sociopolitical instability (paraphrased from UNHCR[1]), and asylum seekers arriving in resettlement countries, are thought to be at greater risk than the general population for several harmful health outcomes as a result of their migration history. Anecdotal reports from professionals suggest that childbearing and other aspects of reproductive health add an additional burden on female refugees, which places them in a particularly disadvantaged position. These suppositions have not been systematically examined.

Reports would suggest that screening and care provided to resettling refugees is anything but systematic.[2-5] Policy makers and program planners, however, generally see knowledge of health 'events' (including illness episodes and health/social services use) as required for optimal health planning.[6] The extent and nature of health 'events' and their determinants in resettling refugee women and their infants becomes even more relevant when the role of development from birth to 6 months of life on future health outcomes is considered.[7]

## Review of the Literature

### Refugee women's reproductive health prior to resettlement

Refugee women experience several challenges to their health. Published review articles and case studies describe the experience of refugees in transit or in camps. The issues considered can be grouped into five broad categories: (1) fertility regulation, (2) sexually transmitted infections, (3) sex and gender-based violence, (4) pregnancy and childbirth, and (5) health services availability and use.

There are differing opinions of the effects of migration on fertility and family planning.[8] One suggests that forced migration increases fertility as refugees satisfy their desire to repopulate, in order to replace deceased children or soldiers and as migration produces a healthier, more stable environment (for example, in some camp situations) with improved healthcare services and nutrition. The opposing opinion suggests that migration decreases the fertility rate of refugees because of perceived uncertainty of the future, economic instability, and marital separation. Fertility rates have also been found to vary with knowledge and availability of contraception. In sum, there are no known common fertility patterns of refugees.

Refugee women appear to be at greater risk than other women for sexually transmitted infections

(STIs), including human immunodeficiency virus (HIV), for a variety of reasons.[8] Migration often occurs without the accompaniment of spouses, thereby increasing the likelihood of sexual activity outside stable relationships. Military operations have been found to be associated with an increase in STI transmission and many refugees are fleeing war-torn areas or must travel through or encamp in those areas. Economic disruption may require refugee women to be involved in sexual activity to acquire food or other goods for themselves or their children. Psychological stresses, including the need for protection from soldiers or men living in or near the camps, may also lead to the granting of sexual favors. Men entrusted to ensure the travel of refugee women through to a safe haven may demand sexual favors. Migration appears to increase the incidence of sexual and gender-based violence (SGBV; e.g. rape, forced impregnation, and other forms of violence), which in turn promotes the spread of STIs.

The use of SGBV by one group to oppress another has long been in existence in times of war. Incidence is difficult to estimate since it is grossly under-reported. The use of SGBV as a weapon of war has come to light more recently, due to the atrocities in Rwanda and the former Yugoslavia.[9,10] Systematic rape may be used as a weapon for ethnic cleansing. Women younger than 25 years of age, and of a particular ethnic background, are thought to be at greater risk for SGBV, as are women of low socioeconomic status who live in circumstances with poor security. SGBV leads to the spread of HIV and STIs; can lead to genital, anal, and other physical injuries and to unwanted pregnancies; and accounts for a variety of psychosocial difficulties for women.[9]

Domestic violence plagues many women worldwide and this form of violence may begin or escalate during pregnancy, or patterns of abuse may be altered with more injuries to the abdominal area attempted.[11] Physical and psychological torture has been extensively reported to occur to both women and men and takes many forms.[12] All organ systems may be affected and in particular the musculoskeletal and nervous systems. Post-traumatic stress disorder, anxiety, depression, somatization, and other psychological effects are common sequelae. Refugee men may be subject to general physical torture while refugee women are subject to sexual abuse.

Female circumcision affects one hundred million girls and women worldwide and is considered by many to be a form of SGBV. It is performed in 26 African countries and by groups in Oman, South Yemen, the United Arab Emirates, Indonesia, and Malaysia.[13,14] In addition to the chronic health effects of these procedures, including urinary tract infections, painful menstruation, and scarring, difficulties can arise in passing the infant through the birth canal and there is increased risk of uterine rupture.[15]

It is generally assumed that refugee women have poorer pregnancy outcomes than other women, although few data are available to refute or support this claim. It is likely that infant and pregnancy health outcomes such as mortality are poorer in war-affected populations, although perhaps no worse than in refugees' own country of origin once restabilization of the country or population occurs.[8] This may be explained by the relatively greater availability of healthcare services in refugee camps. There is also a dearth of data on other maternal health outcomes such as morbidity and nutritional status. Safe motherhood is thought to be determined by factors shared by settled populations: socioeconomic status, age, education, access to services, and urban versus rural habitation.[8] However, what distinguishes migrating refugee women from settled women is their increased exposure to war, SGBV, abuse and torture, and STIs/HIV.

Several reports have considered the needs of refugee women[16] and the reproductive healthcare services that they are receiving.[17,18] A great deal of effort is now being placed on ensuring that a minimum set of reproductive health services is made available to refugee women in camps.

## Migration and health in resettlement countries

Immigration classifications vary by country, although the concept of the ability to freely return to the country of origin usually distinguishes immigrants, who have that option, from refugees, who do not. The differences in experiences between those in these two broad categories have been reviewed.[19] When examined together, immigrants are multiethnic, their mother tongue and the language used vary, and they have a variety of religious traditions, lifestyles, and political alliances. As opposed to refugees, other immigrants choose to resettle. They are motivated to leave their countries and re-establish themselves in a new country in the hope of a better life. Their departures are planned and they are able to return to their countries of origin if they choose. On the other hand, refugees are forced to leave their countries to ensure their survival. Their arrival in the new country is in many respects involuntary and they are not able to return to their countries of origin.

Their departures from their homelands are often from violent situations in which they have not been able to put closure to important relationships and they may feel guilty for leaving their families or friends. All immigrants will go through phases of adjustment, although the permanent, forced nature of the refugee migration experience makes their integration into society more difficult.[20,21]

There is a paucity of systematically collected data on health statistics as they relate to migration history.[22] Most available reports are of small studies, each with its own objectives, methods, and measurement strategies, dissimilar from the others. One review has summarized some of the apparent trends in health due to migration, specifically migration within the European Union.[22] The quality of individual studies reviewed, in particular sampling strategies, which might suggest that results are representative of the population under investigation, was not addressed. With this limitation in mind, that review suggested that there are trends towards a rise in tuberculosis, HIV/AIDS, cardiovascular diseases, and certain cancers in immigrants. It also suggested that there are a greater number of avoidable accidental injuries at work and at home. Another study suggested that communicable disease prevalence is high in certain immigrant population groups.[23] Also reported are difficulties in communication, problematic interpretations of patient symptoms, lack of healthcare provider understanding of traditional remedies for common ailments, unemployment, depression, and underutilization of services.[24,25]

Psychosocial problems appear to be common and may result from resettlement policies stressing geographical dispersion of migrants to areas where there are few 'like' community members in an effort to quickly integrate them into mainstream society. Separation and divorce are reported to be frequent.[26] Additional family difficulties are said to occur if children are seen to be integrating more quickly than their parents by acquiring the language skills of the new country resulting in a capacity to more easily function in the new society, with a shift in power from the parent to the child.

## Refugee women's health during resettlement

As with studies of migration and health generally, many studies of resettling refugee women's health have also been small, and, for the most part, did not define 'refugee' consistently nor did they rely on representative sampling or make a direct comparison between refugee women and their host-country counterparts. These limitations preclude drawing conclusions with regard to the prevalence of health concerns within the population of resettling refugee women and their relative importance in comparison to host-country women. They do, however, suggest health issues that should be considered with regard to refugee women. These include: conflicts arising in women concerning control of their own sexuality,[27,28] perinatal health,[29] the reintroduction of female circumcision,[14] mental health,[30] health service needs, occupational health risks, and discrimination.

Many immigrant and refugee women are reported to have difficulty controlling their sexuality.[27] There is a great deal of confusion with regards to the maintenance of virginity, with family values and those of the new society often clashing.[28] This can lead to requests for hymenal reconstruction by some women who are expected to be virgins when they marry and must provide evidence of this through blood-stained sheets. Girls may suffer a fear of being put to death if it is determined that they are not virgins.[28] Women from some African countries are not taught or socialized to say 'no' to sexual advances by their husbands.[27] This stands in stark contrast to many refugee-receiving countries in which a woman may refuse her husband's advances and if he forces himself on her, he can be charged with rape. If women suggest the use of condoms to husbands having extramarital affairs, this can lead to violence by the husbands towards the women. These women risk being abused in their attempts to protect themselves against STIs and unwanted pregnancies. Infertility or sub-fertility is also thought to cause a great number of problems, especially in groups in which fertility gives rise to social standing.

Perinatal health outcomes are cited as an area of concern.[29] Infants born to migrants from certain countries have been reported to be of lower birth weight, shorter gestational age, and to experience higher perinatal and postneonatal mortality than infants of nationals. Only limited reference has been made to other areas of reproductive health. Nutrition, including breast-feeding, was cited as another area of concern. Initiation and continuance of breast-feeding is thought to be decreasing in migrants[31] and nutritional problems in their children are reported to be common.

Female circumsicion is being reintroduced into Europe and North America by certain immigrant communities. The Centers for Disease Control in the US, for example, estimates that approximately 168 000 girls and women living in the US in 1990 either had or may have been at risk for female circumcision. An estimated 48 000 of these were under 18, and about 75% of these were born in the US.[31]

Several mental health issues have been cited as important to resettling refugee women. These include anxiety, depression, somatization, social isolation, and domestic violence.[32] A review of childbearing and women's mental health noted studies reporting psychiatric disorders during pregnancy and post-partum.[33] In addition to other psychiatric disorders, post-traumatic stress disorder was reported.

Inadequate health services due to language barriers, or inappropriate sex or culture 'matching' between a woman and her care provider have been reported.[27,28,32] General health services delivery issues relevant to resettling refugee women are reported to include: general attitudes toward disease, attitudes towards receiving care by male healthcare professionals, and religious taboos.[28]

Occupational health issues are another area to consider. Refugee women may be employed in certain types of industry for which they are overqualified and in which the general health risks are important due partially to poor protection by employers.[30] Some of the general health issues include repeated movement injuries, eye, lung, and skin exposure to toxic substances, long hours of factory employment followed by long hours of home care, and accidental injury.[30] Foreign-earned educational credentials, which some refugee women may possess, are an asset to the receiving society in terms of the knowledge base gained.[27] They can, however, lead to psychological problems in women due to the drop in social status when those credentials are not recognized by the receiving society.[30] Unfamiliar environments may pose very real challenges to resettling refugee women. Even household items such as dishwashers and fireplaces and practices such as usual garbage removal may need to be explained to women.[27] Discrimination based on color, physical features, or race is another issue that must be dealt with by many refugee women,[27] not only in the workplace but in every aspect of their lives.[30]

## Summary

Studies reviewed on resettling refugees *suggest* health concerns to consider with regard to women's reproductive health; however, they do not provide insight into *the extent* to which these health concerns prevail across various refugee populations. The studies reviewed were, for the most part, unsystematic and uncritical reviews, published reports, or case reports, which provide insight into the particu-lar situations of certain individuals. Well-conducted population-based studies are required to provide an estimate of the prevalence of reproductive health issues of concern in resettling refugee women and their relative importance when compared to non-refugee host-country counterparts. The literature reviewed thus far suggests that there may be several reproductive health-related factors to consider with regard to resettling refugee women. These are summarized in Figure 44.1.

## Research Question

Are there any differences in reproductive health indicators between refugee or asylum seeking women in countries of resettlement and their non-refugee counterparts?

## Methods

The methods chosen to answer the research question were based not on an interest in the specifics of a particular refugee group, but rather on an interest in the potential similarities of women's health issues across refugees resettling in various countries worldwide and the extent to which issues suggested in the qualitative literature and in nonrepresentative studies were supported in population-based reports. It was thought that identifying common issues across resettling refugee women might enlighten policy makers in various refugee-receiving countries as to the health issues to be considered in defining immigration policies and in planning for resettlement.

### Criteria for considering studies for this review

- *Types of studies*: original research.
- *Types of participants*: refugees and 'unspecified' immigrants (i.e. migration history not specified); sample comprising at least 50% women or data provided separately for women.
- *Types of outcomes*: any quantitative indicator of physical or mental health or health services use.

### Search strategy for identification of studies

Literature was culled from five electronic databases – Medline 1966–2001, CINAHL 1982–2001, Health-Star 1975–2001, PsychInfo 1887–2001, and Sociofile 1963–2001 – after consultation with a university librarian regarding optimal search strategies and

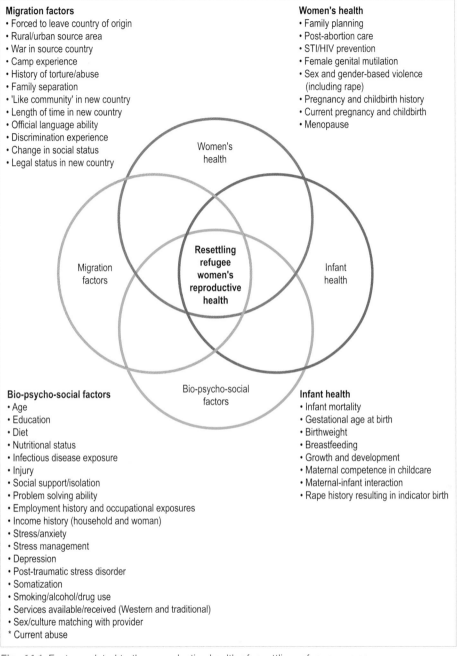

**Migration factors**
- Forced to leave country of origin
- Rural/urban source area
- War in source country
- Camp experience
- History of torture/abuse
- Family separation
- 'Like community' in new country
- Length of time in new country
- Official language ability
- Discrimination experience
- Change in social status
- Legal status in new country

**Women's health**
- Family planning
- Post-abortion care
- STI/HIV prevention
- Female genital mutilation
- Sex and gender-based violence (including rape)
- Pregnancy and childbirth history
- Current pregnancy and childbirth
- Menopause

**Bio-psycho-social factors**
- Age
- Education
- Diet
- Nutritional status
- Infectious disease exposure
- Injury
- Social support/isolation
- Problem solving ability
- Employment history and occupational exposures
- Income history (household and woman)
- Stress/anxiety
- Stress management
- Depression
- Post-traumatic stress disorder
- Somatization
- Smoking/alcohol/drug use
- Services available/received (Western and traditional)
- Sex/culture matching with provider
* Current abuse

**Infant health**
- Infant mortality
- Gestational age at birth
- Birthweight
- Breastfeeding
- Growth and development
- Maternal competence in childcare
- Maternal-infant interaction
- Rape history resulting in indicator birth

**Fig. 44.1** Factors related to the reproductive health of resettling refugee women.

database-specific terminology. Selected terms related to refugees, immigrants, multiculturalism/culture were used, producing 183 361 citations. When these terms were combined with women's health or related terms, 1568 citations were identified. This list of citations was reviewed, and relevant abstracts obtained. Abstracts clearly describing studies not meeting inclusion criteria were excluded from further consideration. All remaining full-text articles (n = 193) were obtained for review. The specific search strategies applied to each database are detailed in Table 44.1. Bibliographies of relevant studies were reviewed

**Table 44.1 Search methodology in electronic databases**

| Variable search terms | Medline 1966–2001 | CINAHL 1982–2001 | HealthStar 1975–2000 | PsychINFO[a] 1887–2001 | SocioFILE[a,b] 1963–2001 |
|---|---|---|---|---|---|
| **Refugee*** | Refugees or asylum.tw. or refugees.tw. | Exp. Refugees | Exp. Refugees or asylum.tw. | Exp. Refugees | Exp. Refugees or Asylum seeker.mp. |
| **Immigrant*** | Emigration & immigration or population dynamics | Exp. Immigrants/or immigrants, illegal.mp. or transient.mp. | Exp. Emigration & Immigration | Exp. Immigrants Exp. Immigration | Exp. Immigrants Exp. Migrants Exp. Emigration |
| **Multicultural*** | Exp. Cultural diversity or exp. Ethnic groups or culture | Exp. Cultural diversity/ or exp ethnic groups/ | Exp. Cross-cultural comparison/ or exp. Cultural diversity/ or ethnic groups.mp. | Multiculturalism[d] Cultural Sensitivity Cross Cultural Diff. Minority Groups | Exp. Culture Exp. Cultural Contrast |
| **Women's Health*** | Exp. women's health[e] | Exp. women's health | Exp. Women's health[f] | Exp. Health and Exp. Human Female | Women's healthcare = 111 Exp. Health/ and exp. Womens' healthcare = 108 Female = 16 106 |
| **Total** | C = 538 = 967[g]; kept = 88 | C = 339; kept 50 | C = 160; kept = 23 | C = 68; kept = 23 | C = 463; kept 9 |

Number of 'combination' articles = 1568.
Number of kept articles = 193.
* And related terms.

Exp, explode term; .tw., text word; C, search term combined with women's health or related term; Kept, the studies that were kept from the search.
[a] No pertinent data from 1887 to 1967.
[b] Difficult search; women and women's health were not relevant search terms; 'female' as a search term was vague; none of the searches produced relevant articles.
[c] Combined all search terms with women's healthcare and with female.
[d] Term is not used before 1984.
[e] Women's health is not a search term from 1966–1974, 1975–1986. Exploded health and exploded women. No relevant articles were found.
[f] Women's health was not a strong search term from 1975–1991. Health/or women's health/ was used as a search term.
[g] Number of hits found when combining health and exp. Cultural diversity, etc. from 1966 to 1986.

and additional articles retrieved. Abstracts from the Conference Proceedings of the Reproductive Health for Refugees Consortium, 2000, were also reviewed. Websites of multilateral and bilateral agencies that address refugees' concerns and academic centers focusing on refugees were searched for relevant literature. A web search was also conducted using the Google search engine, applying the terms 'refugee women and reproductive health.'

## Procedure for consolidating studies identified

The full texts of studies identified from the various sources were reviewed and inclusion criteria were applied to them. Those of refugee women in camps or in transit were removed from further consideration. Remaining studies were subsequently assessed for their methodological quality in terms of providing a population estimate of a health event. Methodological quality was determined through assessment of the likely presence or absence of biases that might have affected the internal validity of the studies' results. These included assessments of (1) the adequacy of the sampling strategy and completeness of follow-up, and (2) appropriateness of the measurement strategy, including the use of reliable and valid questionnaires administered in appropriate language and cultural contexts.

Based on this assessment, studies were graded as 'low quality' in terms of providing a population estimate of a health event if the sampling strategy was not representative of the population of interest *or* if it was not described, *and* if the measurement strategy employed questionnaires or other measurement strategies with no reliability or validity data to support their use in that population *or* was not described. They were graded as being of 'moderate quality' if the sampling strategy was not clearly representative of the population of interest but employed a quasi-representative approach *and* if the measurement strategy included some consideration of cultural/language variations in obtaining needed data *or* if there was representative sampling with weak measurement strategies *or* vice versa. Studies were considered to be of 'high quality' if the sampling strategy was clearly representative *and* if measurement strategies employed were known to be reliable and valid for the population under study. Studies were grouped into low, medium, and high quality for purposes of discussion; no statistical analyses were used to combine the data due to the large variation in health events selected for measure in each of the studies.

As the scoring scheme suggests, those studies not deemed to be of high quality had important limita-

tions, suggesting that health event estimates provided by them might lead to inaccurate conclusions regarding the health status of refugee and other women. Only data from high-quality studies, therefore, were used in attempting to answer the research question.

## Results

The various search strategies employed resulted in a large number of citations potentially eligible for inclusion (n = 1568) and application of initial inclusion criteria resulted in retrieval of a large number of articles (n = 193). Once reviewed, a total of 41 studies met the 'high quality' criteria; 23 met moderate quality criteria; and 25 were found to be of poor quality.

Fourteen of the high-quality studies looked at refugees exclusively, nine of which focused on reproductive health indicators.[34-42] The remaining 27 studies included 'unspecified' immigrants, 19 of which focused on reproductive health indicators and eight of which focused on other health indicators.

Of the 14 'high-quality' studies on resettling refugee women, eight were published in the 1980s,[34-36,38-41,43] five in the 1990s,[37,44-47] and one in 2000.[42] Of the 14, 12 were conducted with Indochinese refugees, including Khmer, Vietnamese, Laotian, Cambodian (Kampuchean), Chinese-Vietnamese, and Thai.[43] Eleven of the 12 were conducted in the United States, and one in Australia.[40] The 12 studies taken together shed some light on the health status of Indochinese refugee women in industrialized resettlement countries. Eight of the studies examined reproductive health and four, mental health. Five of the reproductive health studies made some comparison to the resettlement population.[35,36,39,40,42] These comparisons revealed that Indochinese refugee women have higher fertility rates[36,39] and higher rates of low birth weight infants,[36,40] but lower infant mortality rates[42] when compared with host-country populations. More recent arrivals (e.g. in the resettlement country for less than 3 months) appeared to have the highest levels of fertility[39] and highest rates of low birth weight infants.[36] Other factors found to have affected reproductive health included greater parity, older mothers, shorter interpregnancy intervals, inadequate utilization of prenatal care,[35,36] previous adverse outcomes,[35] and limited education.[36] Moreover, the number of children born prior to arrival in the resettlement country, the number of years married, and the level of economic and cultural adaptation were all shown to be associated with decreased fertility, whereas aspects of migration history (e.g. time spent in refugee camp) were associated with increased fertility.

The three studies of Indochinese refugees that do not make comparisons to the resettlement population suggest that: refugee women from a rural background have higher fertility levels than those of women in urban areas;[41] those in resettlement countries for shorter periods present at greater risk, lacking prenatal care, having more infants of low birth weight and more pregnancy complications;[34,38] and a high number of refugee women are infected with intestinal parasites and other infections.[38,43]

The four studies on Indochinese refugee women focusing on mental health show that a number of these women suffer from somatization,[38] post-traumatic stress disorder,[44,48] depression,[48] and psychological distress.[47] One of these studies compared refugees to immigrants and found that somatization was higher in refugees.[43] Associated with mental illnesses were the following factors: low income,[43,47] low levels of acculturation,[43,49] exposure to violent/traumatic events,[44,47] lengthy time spent in a refugee camp, and older age.[47]

The two studies that do not consider Indochinese refugee women look at Bosnian women[46] and refugee women from Eastern Europe, the former Soviet Union, the Middle East, and Africa,[37] and examine these populations resettling in Sweden and Greece, respectively. Results suggest that Bosnian women have poorer overall health than Swedish women, namely, low quality of life as measured by poor appetite, memory loss, little leisure time, and low levels of mental wellness as evidenced by low energy, patience, sleep, mood swings, and more physical symptoms. Refugee women in Greece, when compared to indigenous Greek women, were found to have similar rates of low birth weight and preterm delivery.

The 19 studies which focus on the reproductive health of 'unspecified' immigrant women defined their population as foreign-born without specifying immigrant status. They are included in this report because of a paucity of evidence specific to refugee women. Two studies indicate that immigrant status was measured, but do not present results based on status differences.[50,51]

Unlike the 14 studies discussed above, these 19 studies were conducted in a wide range of ethnic populations. Eleven included all immigrants in their study (i.e. anyone born outside of the host country)[50–58] and/or described the population by source continent or race.[50–60] The remaining eight studies looked at specific ethnic populations including Mexicans or Puerto Ricans,[61–63] Turks, Filipinos, or Vietnamese,[64–67] and Ethiopians.[68] Study settings also varied, with nine of the studies having taken place in the US, five in Canada, four in Australia, and one in England.

The results of these 19 studies suggest overall that foreign-born women experience the same risk, or better birth outcomes in terms of birth weight and/or incidence of preterm births and/or rate of infant mortality,[51,53–55,58,59,61,62,68] and these positive outcomes progressively worsen as time in the receiving country lengthens and/or they become more acculturated.[51,54] Two studies found foreign-born women to have a significant rate of low birth weight infants,[55,64] while two other studies completely contradicted the above findings, contending that foreign-born women have worse birth outcomes, including higher rates of stillbirths, of peri- and postnatal death,[60] and a higher incidence of low birth weight infants.[65]

As in the refugee-specific studies, fertility rates were found to be high in the 'foreign-born' population and higher for those with shorter periods of time in resettlement countries.[52,56,57,60] Other results included: dissatisfaction with prenatal care;[66,67] reduced prenatal care (fewer than three prenatal visits) associated with a lack of insurance benefits (irrespective of citizenship);[62] infant care behaviors that vary with number of years since immigration;[50] and an increased rate of premarital childbearing amongst immigrant Puerto Rican women when compared to women in their homeland.[63]

The remaining eight high-quality studies which focus on other health indicators do not differentiate refugee women from immigrants and also present results on the 'foreign born' as a whole. Three of these studies looked at psychological illness in immigrants and found them to suffer from somatization[69] and psychological distress.[20,70] Psychological distress is shown to be associated with low sense of coherence, poor sense of control, economic difficulties, trauma and/or violence experienced and/or living,[20] and numerous relocations.[70] Results of these studies also indicate that immigrants are healthier than the host population in terms of chronic illnesses, life expectancy, and disability and dependency, with immigrants in host countries for the shortest time being the healthiest.[71–74]

## Discussion

In this systematic review of refugee women's reproductive health, studies of high quality were identified which provide data on population estimates of a narrow range of health events, and these largely in Indochinese refugee women resettling in the US. Although there is a great deal of literature on refugees, and refugee women's reproductive health is taking on added importance due to massive movements of people across continents, few data are available to inform immigration health policy in this area. Little has been published on the effect of refugee versus nonrefugee migration history on women's health outcomes. In fact, only six studies of high quality comparing reproductive health effects of migration history were identified in this search of five electronic databases and several websites. The current study adds to the existing body of literature on resettling refugee women's health by highlighting the increased risk, over US nationals, for resettling Indochinese refugees to give birth to low birth weight infants and for them to experience somatization. This review also highlights the lack of clarity employed in published literature in defining study populations by immigration status, migration history, and sex. Extremely few high-quality population-based data are available to support the conclusions of smaller reports described in other literature and represented in Figure 44.1. This systematic review suggests that there is extremely little evidence available upon which policy and clinical decisions related to the reproductive health of refugee women can be made given the paucity of high-quality population-based data.

## Limitations

The results of this study are based on the use of electronic databases, which are searched using keywords input by a librarian. It is possible that the keywords used to describe a given article when creating the database and those used for this study could have differed. Further, non-English-language keywords would not have been identified in this search. Extensive consultation with a university librarian and additional searching of citations of literature obtained in the initial search were methods applied to reduce the possibility of missing key studies. Studies that have not been published were not included in this review because no such studies were identified from the non-database searches.

## Clinical/policy implications

The results of this study indicate that health-related indicators identified in non-population-based studies of refugee women are generally not supported in the high-quality population-based studies currently available with the exception of Indochinese refugee women resettling in the US. In that population, care should be taken to ensure adequate assessment for potentially giving birth to low birth weight infants and for the presence of somatization, since both of these health indicators occur more frequently in this population group than in the nonrefugee group.

Other factors identified in non-population-based studies were not confirmed in high-quality population-based studies but likely need to be considered in clinical care until they have been ruled out as having been idiosyncratic to a particular subset of refugee women. A thorough clinical assessment should include bio-psycho-social factors including screening for tuberculosis, intestinal parasites, experience of malaria during pregnancy, and changes in socioeconomic status. Written translations of patient instructions need to be made available to improve comprehension. Risk factors for torture should be assessed including refugee or political asylum seeking status, immigration from a totalitarian regime, civil war in country of origin, residence in refugee camp, prisoner of war, multiple family members deceased due to trauma, history of arrest or detention, and leadership in antigovernment organizations.[74]

Professionals need to affirm that all forms of SGBV are unacceptable in all forums available to them, especially policy forums. Professional bodies need to publicly defend health professionals detained in the performance of their duties and in the maintenance of ethical standards.[75] Legislation to prevent female circumcision needs to be put forward and supported.

## Research implications

The background literature presented suggests that there are several indicators of health to be explored on a population level to determine the extent to which reporting of health problems in a few individual women is, or is not, a widespread problem requiring greater investment in human and financial resources. Several of the issues to be examined are difficult, although not impossible, to address on a population level due to their delicate nature, histories of SGBV and spousal abuse being among them. However, these and others do require confirmation on a larger representative population. Having determined the extent of the problems, implementing and evaluating solutions to them will be required. The weaknesses of several of the studies attempting to provide population estimates must be avoided. These include non-representative sampling strategies and use of culturally inappropriate approaches to obtain needed data. A wide body of literature on translation theory can be tapped for appropriate methodology.

## Conclusion

The results of this systematic review of refugee women's reproductive health suggest there are a woefully inadequate number of studies directly comparing the health events experienced by resettling refugee women to those of their nonrefugee counterparts. This paucity of data prohibits planners and policy makers from making informed decisions regarding the distribution of resources. Results further show that, of a large number of factors suggested by other literature to be important, none has been confirmed in high-quality population-based studies of refugee women from a wide variety of backgrounds. There is an urgent need for more studies examining refugee women specifically. In performing these, better definitions of immigration status should be used, optimal translation procedures and culturally sensitive methodology should be exploited, and sampling of populations should be done in a representative fashion.

## References

1. UNHCR. Who is a refugee? UNHCR web-page: 'Basic Facts'. 2004. Available: http://www.unhcr.ch/cgi-bin/texis/vtx/basics/+DwwBm7ewAbdwwwwnwwwwwwhFqoUfIfRZ2ItFqtxw5oq5zFqtFEIfgIAFqoUfIfRZ2IDzmxwwwwwww1FqtFEIfgI/opendoc.htm Ref Type: Electronic Citation.
2. Thonneau P, Gratton J, Desrosiers G. Health Profile of applicants for refugee status (admitted into Quebec Between August 1985 and April 1986). Can J Pub Health 1990; 81:182–186.
3. Miettinen OS. The need for randomization in the study of intended effects. Statis Med 1983; 2:267–271.
4. Jones J. Asylum seekers in UK receive poor healthcare. Br Med J 2000; 320:1492.
5. Fassil Y. Looking after the health of refugees. Br Med J 2000; 321:59.
6. Neugebauer R. Editorial: The uses of psychosocial epidemiology in promoting refugee health. Am J Pub Health 1997; 87:726–728.
7. National Forum on Health. Canada health action: Building on the legacy. [2]. 1997. Health Canada. Ref Type: Report.
8. McGinn T. Reproductive health of war-affected populations: what do we know? Internat Fam Plan Perspectives 2000; 26:174–180.
9. Center for Reproductive Law and Policy. Reproductive freedom and human rights – rape and forced pregnancy in war and conflict situations. 1996.
10. Palmer CA, Zwi AB. Women, health and humanitarian aid in conflict. Disasters 1998, 22:236–249.
11. Schmuel E, Schenker JG. Violence against women: the physician's role. Eur J Obstetr Gynecol Reproduct Biol 1998; 80:239–245.
12. Weinstein HM, Dansky L, Iacopino V. Torture and war trauma survivors in primary care practice. West J Med 1996; 165:112–118.
13. Jones WK, Smith J, Kieke B Jr, et al. Female genital mutilation. Female circumcision. Who is at risk in the US? Pub Health Rep 1997; 112:368–377.
14. Retzlaff C. Female genital mutilation: not just 'over there'. J Internat Assoc Phys AIDS Care 1999; 5:28–37.
15. Anonymous. A traditional practice that threatens health – female circumcision. WHO Chronicle 1986; 40:31–36.
16. Craig A. Birth spacing and healthcare for refugee women. UNHCR Publications. Refugees Magazine 1994.
17. Courtney H. Spacing children, preventing AIDS. UNHCR Publications. Refugees Magazine 1995.
18. Marshall R. Refugees, feminine plural. UNHCR Publications. Refugees Magazine 1995.
19. Gravel S, Battaglini A. Culture, santé et ethnicité: vers une santé publique pluraliste. Montreal: Régie Régionale de la Santé et des Services Sociaux; 2000.
20. Sundquist J, Bayard-Burfield L, Johansson LM, et al. Impact of ethnicity, violence and acculturation on displaced migrants: psychological distress and psychosomatic complaints among refugees in Sweden. JNerv Mental Dis 2000; 188:357–365.
21. Jones D, Gill PS. Refugees and primary care: tackling the inequalities. Br Med J 1998; 317:1444–1446.
22. Carballo M, Divino JJ, Zeric D. Migration and health in the European Union. Trop Med Internat Health 1998; 3:936–944.
23. Adair R, Nwaneri O. Communicable disease in African immigrants in Minneapolis. Arch Internal Med 1999; 159:83–85.
24. Downs K, Bernstein J, Marchese T. Providing culturally competent primary care for immigrant and refugee women: a Cambodian case study. J Nurs Midw 1997; 42:499–508.
25. Bauer HM, Rodriguez MA, Quiroga SS, et al. Barriers to healthcare for abused Latina and Asian immigrant women. JHealth Care Poor Underserved 2000; 11:33–44.
26. Keely CB. The resettlement of women and children refugees. Migration World 1992; 20:14–18.
27. Simms GP. Aspects of women's health from a minority/diversity perspective. 2000. www.hc-sc.gc.ca/canusa/papers/canada/english/minority.htm Health Canada. Ref Type: Electronic Citation.
28. Huisman WM. Trans-cultural medicine. Curare 1998; 15:21–34.
29. Manderson L, Mathews M. Vietnamese attitudes towards maternal and infant health. Med J Australia 1981; 1:69–72.
30. Gannage CM. The health and safety concerns of immigrant women workers in the Toronto sportswear industry. Internat J Health Serv 1999; 29:409–429.
31. Jirojwong S, Manderson L. Physical health and preventive health behaviors among Thai women in Brisbane, Australia. Health Care Women Intl 2002; 23:197–206.
32. Allotey P. Travelling with 'excess baggage': health problems of refugee women in Western Australia. Women Health 1998; 28:63–81.
33. Zelkowitz P. Childbearing and women's mental health. Transcult Psychiatr Res Rev 1996; 33:391–413.
34. Davis JM, Goldenring J, McChesney M, et al. Pregnancy outcomes of Indochinese refugees, Santa Clara County, California. Am J Pub Health 1982; 72:742–744.
35. Gann P, Nghiem L, Warner S. Pregnancy characteristics and outcomes of Cambodian refugees. Am J Pub Health 1989; 79:1251–1257.
36. Hopkins DD, Clarke NG. Indochinese refugee fertility rates and pregnancy risk factors, Oregon. Am J Pub Health 1983; 73:1307–1309.
37. Malamitsi-Puchner A, Tzala L, Minaretzis D, et al. Preterm delivery and low birthweight among refugees in Greece. Paediatr Peri Epid 1994; 8:384–390.
38. Roberts NS, Copel JA, Bhutani V, et al. Intestinal parasites and other infections during pregnancy in Southeast Asian refugees. JReproduct Med 1985; 30:720–725.
39. Rumbaut RG. Fertility and adaptation: Indochinese refugees in the United States. Internat Migration Rev 1986; 20:428–466.

40. Ward BG, Pridmore BR, Cox LW. Vietnamese refugees in Adelaide: an obstetric analysis. Med J Australia 1981; 1:72–75.

41. Weeks JR, Rumbaut R, Brindis C, et al. High fertility among Indochinese refugees. Pub Health Rep 1989; 104:143–150.

42. Weeks JR. Infant mortality among ethnic immigrant groups. Soc Sci Med 2000; 33:327–334.

43. Lin EHB, Carter WB, Kleinman AM. An exploration of somatization among Asian refugees and immigrants in primary care. Am J Pub Health 1985; 75:1080–1084.

44. Berthold SM. The effects of exposure to community violence on Khmer refugee adolescents. JTraumatic Stress 1999; 12:455–471.

45. Sack WH, Clarke GN, Kinney R, et al. The Khmer Adolescent Project. II: Functional capacities in two generations of Cambodian refugees. J Nerv Mental Dis 1995; 183:177–181.

46. Sundquist J, Behmen-Vincevic A, Johansson SE. Poor quality of life and health in young to middle aged Bosnian female war refugees: a population-based study. Public Health 1998; 112:21–26.

47. Chung RC, Kagawa-Singer M. Predictors of psychological distress among Southeast Asian refugees. Soc Sci Med 1993; 36:631–639.

48. Sack WH, McSharry S, Clarke GN, et al. The Khmer Adolescent Project. I. Epidemiologic findings in two generations of Cambodian refugees. J Nerv Mental Dis 1994; 182:387–395.

49. Hospital stays continue 10-year decline. Am J Pub Health 1992; 82:54.

50. Edwards NC, Boivin JF. Ethnocultural predictors of postpartum infant-care behaviours among immigrants in Canada. Ethnicity Health 1997; 2:163–176.

51. Rumbaut R. Unraveling a public health enigma: Why do immigrants experience superior perinatal health outcomes. Rese Sociol Health Care 1996; 13B:337–391.

52. Ford K. Duration of residence in the United States and the fertility of US immigrants. Internat Migration Rev 1987; 24:34–68.

53. Doucet H, Baumgarten M, Infante Rivard C. Risk of low birthweight and prematurity among foreign-born mothers. Can J Pub Health 1992; 83:192–195.

54. Hyman I. The effect of acculturation low birth weight in immigrant women. Can J Pub Health 1998; 87:158–162.

55. Kleinman JC, Fingerhut LA, Prager K. Differences in infant mortality by race, nativity status, and other maternal characteristics. Am J Dis Child 1991; 145:194–199.

56. Ng E, Nault F. Fertility among recent immigrant women to Canada, 1991: an examination of the disruption hypothesis. Internat Migration Rev 1997; 35:549–579.

57. Ram B, George V. Immigrant fertility patterns in Canada, 1961–1986. 1989:413–425.

58. Singh GK, Yu SM. Adverse pregnancy outcomes: differences between US- and foreign-born women in major US racial and ethnic groups. Am J Pub Health 1996; 86:837–843.

59. Collins JWJ, Shay DK. Prevalence of low birth weight among Hispanic infants with United States-born and foreign-born mothers: the effect of urban poverty. Am J Epid 1994; 139:184–192.

60. Dolton WD. The health and welfare of the immigrant. Roy Soc Health J 1966; 86:22–27.

61. Cervantes A, Keith L, Wyshak G. Adverse birth outcomes among native-born and immigrant women: replicating national evidence regarding Mexicans at the local level. Matern Child Health J 1999; 3:99–109.

62. Kalofonos I, Palinkas LA. Barriers to prenatal care for Mexican and Mexican-American women. J Gender Cult Health 1999; 4:135–152.

63. Landale NS, Hauan SM. Migration and premarital childbearing among Puerto Rican women. Demography 1996; 33:429–442.

64. Mitchell J, Mackerras D. The traditional humoral food habits of pregnant Vietnamese-Australian women and their effect on birth weight. Australian J Public Health 1995; 19:629–633.

65. Henry OA, Guaran RL, Petterson CD, et al. Obstetric and birthweight differences between Vietnam- and Australian-born women. Med J Australia 1992; 156:321–324.

66. Small R, Lumley J, Yelland J, et al. Shared antenatal care fails to rate well with women of non-English-speaking backgrounds. Med J Australia 1998; 168:15–18.

67. Yelland J, Small R, Lumley J, et al. Support, sensitivity, satisfaction: Filipino, Turkish and Vietnamese women's experiences of postnatal hospital stay. Midwifery 1998; 14:144–154.

68. Wasse H, Holt VL, Daling JR. Pregnancy risk factors and birth outcomes in Washington State: a comparison of Ethiopian-born and US-born women. Am J Pub Health 1994; 84:1505–1507.

69. Ritsner M, Ponizovsky A, Kurs R, et al. Somatization in an immigrant population in Israel: a community survey of prevalence, risk factors, and help-seeking behavior. Am J Psychiatry 2000; 157:385–392.

70. Johansson LM, Sundquist J, Johansson SE, et al. Immigration, moving house and psychiatric admissions. Acta Psychiatr Scand 1998; 98:105–111.

71. Chen J, Ng E, Wilkins R. The health of Canada's immigrants in 1994–95. Health Rep 1996; 7:33–45.

72. Sundquist J, Johansson SE. Long-term illness among indigenous and foreign-born people in Sweden. Soc Sci Med 1997; 44:189–198.

73. Chen J, Wilkins R, Ng E. Health expectancy by immigrant status, 1986 and 1991. Health Rep 1996; 8:29–38.

74. Weinstein HM, Sarnoff RH, Gladstone E, et al. Physical and psychological health issues of resettled refugees in the United States. J Refugee Studies 2000; 13:303–327.

75. Geiger HJ, Cook-Deegan RM. The role of physicians in conflicts and humanitarian crises. Case studies from the field missions of Physicians for Human Rights, 1988 to 1993. JAMA 1993; 270:616–620.

# Dental Diseases and Disorders

Susan E. Cote and Harpreet Singh

## Introduction

Dental diseases are the most prevalent chronic diseases worldwide.[1] Despite great improvements in the oral health of populations across the world, problems still persist, particularly among poor and disadvantaged groups in both developed and developing countries. Immigrants and refugees have particularly high rates of dental diseases and unmet dental needs and these groups should be regarded as 'at risk' with regard to oral health. The country of origin, time span of migration and years in transition reflect the accumulated treatment needs. Even people with good oral health under normal situations can experience dramatic decline when under stressful conditions.[2] The high prevalence of dental disease and neglected oral hygiene can also be the result of low priority of oral health compared to the more immediate problems of resettlement.

Although rarely life threatening, dental diseases have a detrimental effect on the quality of life from childhood through old age. Dental diseases affect eating, speaking, nutrition, health, and self-esteem.[3] The interrelationship between oral and general health is well established. Severe periodontal disease is associated with diabetes mellitus, cardiovascular disease, stroke, chronic respiratory disease, and preterm low birth weight babies.[4] Dental diseases can also create excessive financial and social costs on the individual and society. The treatment of dental diseases is extremely expensive, the fourth most costly disease to treat in most industrialized nations.[1] Dental diseases can also affect economic productivity and compromise a person's ability to work at home, at school, or on the job.[5]

An oral health assessment is an important component of a comprehensive physical examination. Since immigrants may be more likely to establish primary medical care before seeking dental care, the medical team is in a unique position to assess the oral health status and facilitate referrals to dental services for the initiation of care. Therefore, it is important for medical and dental practitioners to understand refugee and immigrant oral health needs, as well as their cultural beliefs and practices. This chapter will present the oral health status of immigrants, and manifestations and treatment options of oral conditions that may be present. The chapter will also include examples of the cultural beliefs and practices of some groups of immigrants.

## Oral Health Assessment

A complete assessment of the craniofacial tissues should include observation and palpation for signs of pathology or infection. Assessment should include the head and neck, the dentition and soft tissues of the oral cavity – the mucosa covering the hard and soft palate, lips, tongue, oropharynx, floor of the mouth, and gingiva. Many systemic diseases have oral manifestations that may be the initial signs of clinical disease. A thorough oral examination can detect signs of microbial infections, pathology, oral cancer, manifestations of HIV/AIDS, injury and trauma or torture, as well as nutritional deficiencies.[6] For example, there is evidence that patients who experience signs and symptoms of more advanced oral cancer are more likely to seek initial contact with medical healthcare professionals while patients with asymptomatic early-stage disease are more likely to be detected by oral healthcare providers.[7] The National Institute for Dental Craniofacial Research has a step-by-step guide for health professionals to perform an oral examination, that is available on their website.[8]

## Dental Caries

One of the most common diseases of the oral cavity is dental caries, an infectious disease induced by diet, leading to the destruction of tooth structure. An estimated five billion people worldwide suffer from dental caries.[1] In the United States, dental caries remains the most common chronic disease of children aged 5–17 years (five times more common than asthma)[5] and can progress throughout life. It is no longer accepted that certain races are naturally resistant to dental caries. Differences in the prevalence among different populations can be attributed to behavior, diet, and access to dental care.[9]

The main factors in the etiology of dental caries are cariogenic bacteria, fermentable carbohydrates, a susceptible tooth, and time. A large, carious lesion may progress to the pulp and surrounding bone, resulting in a dental abscess with possible pain and fever. If the pulp of the tooth becomes necrotic, the pain may subside, but the infection is still present (Fig. 45.1). Complications can be the spread of infection causing facial cellulitis, osteomyelitis or, in severe cases, cerebral abscess, endocarditis, or other disorders. In both primary and permanent teeth, an abscess may appear as a fistula on the gingiva and there may be a discharge when the gingiva is pressed. Treatment would be the elimination of infection and restoration of the tooth to function. Immediate referral to a dentist is recommended. Antibiotics may be indicated along with saltwater rinsing to reduce the infection. Over-the-counter pain relievers may be recommended for pain and fever. Aspirin should not be applied directly over the tooth or mucosa as it will increase the irritation and can create mouth ulcers.

Refined sugars are the most important dietary factor in the development of dental caries.[3] The rela-

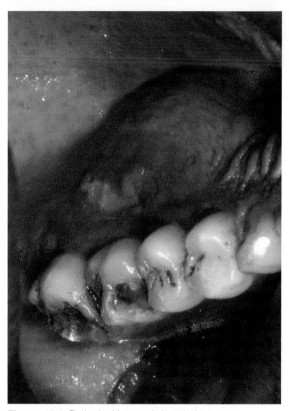

**Figure 45.1** Periapical intraoral dental abscess.

tionship between dental caries and refined sugar consumption has been well documented. An increased prevalence of dental caries has been associated with countries with higher per capita sugar consumption.[10] In some developing countries, as socioeconomic levels rise, so does the amount of sugar in the diet, with corresponding increases in dental caries. In Africa, dental caries is considered a good proxy measure for socioeconomic development.[11] Differences have been noted in caries prevalence between high and low socioeconomic groups. The prevalence and severity of dental caries is generally higher among the privileged residing in urban centers, where sugar is considered a luxury. In contrast, the indigenous rural diet is low in refined sugar and lower levels of caries have been found.[11]

Oral health surveys in a number of countries have found that immigrant children have higher rates of treatment needs, untreated caries, oral pain, and oral pathology than US children.[12-17] Table 45.1 summarizes oral health data collected from different populations of immigrant children and data collected

**Table 45.1 Surveys of oral health needs in child immigrants from several countries**

| Variable | Cote et al.[17] | | | Gomez et al.[28] | Mann et al.[15] | Pollick et al.[12] | Scheer et al.[14] | Watson et al.[13] | US (NHANES III)[17] |
|---|---|---|---|---|---|---|---|---|---|
| Country of origin | African | E. European | Other – primarily South Asia Middle East | Mexican migrants | Ethiopia | Southeast Asia, East Asia, Philippines Central America | Former Soviet Union | Latino immigrant | US |
| Age | 6 mon–17 yr | 6 mon–17 yr | 6 mon–17 yr | 0–6 yr | 0–12 yr | 6–11 yr | 0–3 yr | 3–5 yr | 2–16.9 yr |
| N = | 121 | 60 | 44 | 220 | 345 | 1012 | 514 | 142 | 11 296 |
| **Treatment needed** | | | | | | | | | |
| No obvious problems | 40% | 17% | 34% | | | 23% | | 56% | 78% |
| Treatment needed | 60% | 83% | 66% | | | 77% | | 44% | 22% |
| **Caries experience\*** | | | | | | | | | |
| No caries experience | 62% | 20% | 50% | 44% | | | | 53% | 51% |
| Caries experience | 38% | 80% | 50% | 56% | | | | 47% | 49% |
| **Untreated Caries** | | | | | | | | | |
| No untreated caries | 65% | 24% | 50% | 45% | 74% | | 51% | 54% | 77% |
| Untreated caries | 35% | 76% | 50% | 55% | 26% | | 49% | 46% | 23% |
| **Oral pain present** | | | | | | | | | |
| No pain | 89% | 85% | 92% | | | | | | 99% |
| Pain | 11% | 15% | 7% | | | | | | 1% |
| **Oral pathology** | | | | | | | | | |
| Normal | 82% | 83% | 91% | | | | | | 90% |
| Abnormal | 8% | 17% | 9% | | | | | | 10% |

\* Caries experience determined by the presence of an untreated caries lesion, a restoration (which presumably was once a caries lesion), or missing because it was extracted as a result of dental caries.

from NHANES III of US children. Difference in the distribution of age makes it difficult to compare the data between the groups. Eastern European refugee children presented with particularly high treatment needs, untreated caries, pain, and pathology. African refugees, who originated from more rural areas, had the lowest caries experience and untreated caries. Significant differences were found when comparing the oral health status of refugee children to US children.[17] The African refugee children had only half the dental caries experience of US children. However, when black African refugee children were compared to black US children, they had less of a history of dental caries but similar likelihood of having untreated dental caries, despite the fact that very few African refugee children had previous access to professional dental care.[17]

There are limited published data comparing the oral health status of immigrant adult populations. Adult refugees who had recently arrived in the United States primarily from Africa, the former Soviet Union, and Eastern Europe had an overall prevalence of unmet treatment needs of 87%. Forty-five percent had never been to the dentist and 13% required urgent care within 24 hours. Refugees from Eastern Europe and the former Soviet Union were over eight times more likely to present with a history of dental caries and more than 10 times as likely to have seen a dentist as those from Africa. However, the degree of urgency was greater among the Africans, with 22% who presented to the clinic in pain compared to 11% from Eastern Europe and the former Soviet Union.[18] In a study conducted in New York City, Haitian adult immigrants were found to have low levels of dental caries.[19]

A dental assessment of asylum seekers and refugees receiving care at the Boston Center for Refugee Health and Human Rights documented that 73% of clients had untreated dental caries, with highest rates among Africans.[20] The high rate can be attributed to living conditions prior to coming to the US, their extended time in transition, legal status in the US which makes them fearful to seek care and risk being deported, or lack of access to affordable dental care.

Differing levels of fluoride in the drinking water may also contribute to differences in caries experience between different refugee and immigrant populations. It has been well documented that fluoride at an optimal range of 0.7–1.2 parts per million (ppm) reduces dental caries; however, it does not eliminate risk of the disease.[21] Several countries in Africa and the Eastern Mediterranean have excessively high levels of naturally occurring fluoride in the water supply.[10] Excess fluoride exposure occurring during tooth formation may result in dental fluorosis.[22] While clinically mild cases may appear as white spots and severe cases as discolored teeth or pitted enamel, dental fluorosis should not be misdiagnosed as dental caries.

In some parts of Africa, such as Tanzania, there is a high prevalence of dental fluorosis. One of the contributing factors is the use of fluoride-containing trona (magadi). Magadi is a crude mixture of various salts containing varying amounts of fluoride that is used to reduce cooking time. It is also added to food to add flavor, especially to vegetables and beans. A mixture of beans and bananas cooked with magadi is a traditional food used for weaning babies.[22] There are no reports of this practice continuing in the US.

## Early childhood caries

Early childhood caries (ECC) is a serious form of dental caries that affects the primary dentition of infants and toddlers. Decay of primary teeth can delay children's growth, lead to malocclusion by adversely affecting the correct guidance of the permanent dentition, and cause poor speech articulation and low self-esteem.[16] In many cultures, however, the primary dentition is believed to have no value and parents are not concerned if the child has decay as these teeth will be replaced. For some, the early loss of primary teeth symbolizes a life transition or a brotherhood or sisterhood with other children in that community.[23]

Although ECC affects children from all socioeconomic classes, it is most often found in children of new immigrants, or any US-born individual with lower socioeconomic status.[24] An ongoing study in Boston has shown an overall prevalence of ECC of 8.7% compared to the national average of 4.5%.[25] Differences were seen when the data were stratified by the parents' region of origin (Table 45.2).[25] ECC prevalence of 9% was seen in children whose parents were originally from North America, mainly the United States and Canada. The rate was much lower, at 6%, in children whose parents' region of origin was the Caribbean, primarily from Haiti. The rate was higher, at 11%, in children whose parents' region of origin was Africa, primarily from Nigeria and Cape Verde, and 12% in children whose parents' regions of origin were other countries such as Honduras, Mexico, China, and Vietnam. Latino children have been reported to have very high levels of ECC. Thirty-three percent of Head Start Latinos in

**Table 45.2 Distribution of Boston children's early childhood caries (ECC) by parents' region of origin[25]**

| Parents' region of origin | n | ECC |
|---|---|---|
| Asia | 51 | 13.7% |
| Middle East | 9 | 0.0% |
| Europe | 17 | 17.6% |
| Africa | 142 | 10.6% |
| North America | 301 | 9.0% |
| Central America | 29 | 10.3% |
| Caribbean | 238 | 5.9% |
| South America | 6 | 0.0% |

California presented with ECC compared to 13% of white children.[26] At the California–Mexico border, the prevalence of ECC in Latino children was extremely high at 58% (Ramos-Gomez FJ, et al., unpublished).

Similar to other forms of caries, risk factors for ECC are linked to dietary practices. Feeding practices of infants and also toddlers vary with culture and socioeconomic status and may also be influenced by family, specifically the mother's female relatives. The influence of the extended family is important for some cultures where decisions on health and related issues may be made by older family members. One such situation is the recommendation in the US of discontinuing use of the baby bottle by 12 months of age. This practice is not popular among the Muslim Asians due to fear that the change might cause the infants to stop drinking milk and would not be acceptable in the community or to the older family members. A large milk intake is perceived as desirable since the provision of milk in the Indian subcontinent is associated with wealth.[27] Latino babies have also been found to be bottle-fed for extended periods of time, often until age 2 or 3 years.

Children that are breast-fed at will or bottle-fed at night with milk or formula are at an increased risk of ECC. Studies have shown human milk and baby formula to be more cariogenic than cow's milk.[28] The practice of adding sugar or sugary flavorings to infant's milk further increases the risk. The use of sugary drinks such as juice or soda in bed is also a risk factor. In some cultures, sugar is considered valuable as a source of energy and helpful in treating stomach aches and constipation. Sweetened drinks in bed have been found to be common practice among Latino and Asian populations and are probably a contributing factor to the high prevalence of ECC and untreated dental caries.[26]

## Periodontal Disease

Periodontal disease (periodontitis) is a chronic bacterial infection that affects the gingiva, bone, and other tissues that support the teeth. Infection in these tissues can initiate a series of inflammatory and immunologic changes starting with gingivitis, which presents with swelling and bleeding of the gingival tissues. Periodontitis causes the destruction of connective tissue and bone surrounding the teeth that can result in loss of teeth. Poor oral hygiene or high levels of dental plaque are associated with high prevalence rates and severity of periodontal disease.

During the past 10 years, there has been an increased focus on the link between periodontal disease and systemic health. Research has shown that people with periodontitis are more likely to develop cardiovascular disease. One such study suggests the risk of fatal heart disease doubles for people with severe periodontal disease. Severe periodontal disease in pregnant women may be linked to a sevenfold increase in the risk of delivering preterm low birthweight babies.[6] Diabetics are two to three times more likely to have periodontal disease which progresses rapidly and can worsen glycemic control.[6]

Most adults show some signs of gingivitis or periodontal disease. In the United States, there are disparities in the prevalence of periodontal disease, with rates highest among African-Americans (33%) compared to Mexican-Americans (25%) and Caucasians (20%).[5] Immigrants are particularly at risk due to their interrupted lifestyles, lack of resources, and lack of access to professional dental care. Among newly arrived adult refugees in Boston, 88% had some degree of gingival inflammation, ranging from mild to severe. Nine percent presented with an acute periodontal infection requiring immediate referral to a dentist for treatment [18]

In Africa, gingivitis is widespread and can be severe in children. Acute necrotizing ulcerative gingivitis (ANUG), which is now rarely seen in developed countries, is prevalent among children aged 3 years to puberty in sub-Saharan African countries.[10] ANUG is a progressive, painful gingival infection with ulceration, swelling, and sloughing off of dead tissue that can spread throughout the mouth and throat. Stress, poor oral hygiene, and poor nutrition can induce the onset of ANUG. Symptoms are

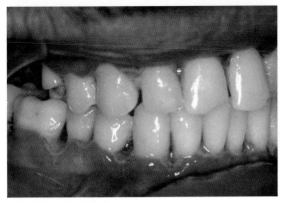

**Figure 45.2** Acute necrotizing ulcerative gingivitis.

painful gingiva, bleeding in response to any pressure or irritation, a swollen, grayish film on the gingiva, crater-like ulcers, foul taste in the mouth, and bad breath. Medical professionals should screen refugee children, particularly from African countries, for ANUG and refer children presenting with these symptoms to a dentist. Treatment usually requires antibiotics, debridement, and, in severe cases, dental surgery (Fig. 45.2).

Noma (cancrum oris), an acute gangrenous infection of the face, may be on the increase in Africa. What begins as ulcers on the gingiva can progress rapidly, becoming necrotic and spreading to the oral mucosa and tissues of the face, causing deterioration, severe disfigurement and, in 90% of the cases, death. Noma is mainly found in children who are malnourished and living in unsanitary conditions. If detected early, it can be treated with antibiotics and proper nutrition, but often it is left untreated. The sub-Saharan area from Senegal to Ethiopia has the highest incidence and is known as 'the Noma belt.' It is estimated that 450 000 children will die each year from Noma.[29] According to the WHO, a few sporadic cases have been reported in the US.[30]

## Edentulism

Edentulism, or complete loss of teeth, is prevalent among older people all over the world and is highly associated with lower socioeconomic status.[4] Severe dental caries and periodontal disease are the major reasons for tooth extractions. Studies show years of smoking is also associated with high numbers of missing teeth.[1] In many countries, access to oral health services is limited and teeth are often extracted because of pain or lack of resources for dental treat-

ment. In many cultures, tooth loss is considered a normal part of the aging process and one should only visit the dentist when in pain to have the tooth extracted.[19,31] In addition, maintaining one's teeth in old age may be viewed negatively. Some Chinese, particularly the elderly, believe that having teeth in old age would eat away their children's fortune, bringing bad luck to the family.

The concept of primary preventive care and restorative treatment for teeth that are asymptomatic is foreign to many and may require extra effort on the part of the health professional to explain that dental diseases are preventable and can be treated with routine dental care.

Edentulous people have difficulty chewing certain foods, which causes changes in the diet. Such changes include reduction in fruits, vegetables, meats, and other foods that are hard to chew and are associated with compromised nutrition and weight loss.[32]

Removable dentures are particularly common among older people from developed countries.[4] A comprehensive examination should include having the patient remove dentures and examining the oral mucosa. Denture stomatitis is a common mucosal lesion where colonization of yeast is observed. Clinically, erythema and edema with possible white plaque are distributed over the mucosa that is covered by the denture. The prevalence of denture stomatitis correlates strongly to denture hygiene and the amount of denture plaque. Wearing dentures at night, neglect of denture soaking at night, and use of defective and unsuitable dentures are also risk factors for denture stomatitis, as are tobacco and alcohol.[4] Due to the disrupted lifestyle of refugees and immigrants and the inability to maintain proper oral hygiene, there is an increased risk of developing denture stomatitis.

## Oral Cancer

Oral cancer is the largest category of those cancers that fall into the head and neck cancer category. Each year in the US, approximately 30 000 people are newly diagnosed with oral cancer and there are over 8000 deaths. Worldwide, the problem is far greater, with new cases annually approaching 300 000. Oral cancer is more common in men and is the eighth most common cancer in the world. The death rate associated with oral cancer is particularly high as it is typically discovered in the later stages.[33] Smoking, using smokeless tobacco, chewing betel, and drinking alcohol are all risk factors for oral cancer and exert a synergistic effect.[1] Oral cancer may appear as

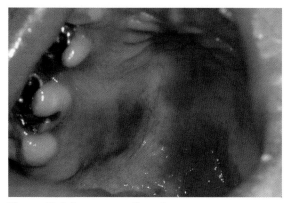

**Figure 45.3** Squamous cell carcinoma.

a persistent sore or lesion in the mouth that does not heal or that bleeds easily; a mass or thickening in the cheek or neck; or a painless white (leukoplakia) or red (erythroplakia) patch on the gingiva, tongue, lips, or lining of the mouth. Anyone with a suspicious oral lesion should be referred to a dentist or doctor for appropriate diagnosis and treatment as early as possible (Fig. 45.3).

In the United States, risk factors primarily include tobacco use, heavy alcohol consumption, poor diet, and sunlight exposure (lip cancer). Higher incidence rates of oral cancer exist within the minority populations in the United States and may be attributed to a higher prevalence of tobacco smoking and heavy consumption of alcohol within minority populations.[7] Acculturation has been shown to be a predictor of poorer health and greater health services use. One study has reported that diet, smoking, and alcohol consumption, as a result of acculturation, were associated with increased cancer risk.[34]

In different parts of the world, risk factors vary and reflect different cultures and practices. The high rates of oral cancer in western and southern Europe and southern Africa reflect the prevalence of the risk factors such as tobacco and alcohol use.[35] In South Central Asia, cancer of the oral cavity ranks among the three most common types of cancer and is related to the chewing of betel quid.[35] It is estimated that 10–20% of the world's population chews betel. In Cambodia, smoking cigarettes is considered to be a male prerogative and chewing betel to be a female habit.[36] In Thailand, the prevalence of smoking is about 60%, betel nut chewing 15%, and alcohol consumption 35%.[1]

Betel quid, also known as 'paan,' is a mixture of areca nut, calcium hydroxide, spices, seeds, and tobacco wrapped in a betel leaf. The areca nut, commonly known as betel nut, grows on an areca palm tree and is both cytotoxic and genotoxic. Betel quid chewing is common through Southeast Asia, India, and New Guinea. 'Gutka' is a powdered or granulated mixture of tobacco, areca nuts, limes, and spices, available in handy foil sachets. Introduced over two decades ago, gutka is immensely popular across all socioeconomic strata of the Indian society with both genders and it is believed to be a harmless 'mouth freshener.' The risk of oral cancer due to paan and gutka use has been clearly demonstrated. In India alone, approximately 30% of the oral cancers are attributed to smokeless tobacco and areca nut use, and an additional 50% to the combined use of smokeless tobacco/areca nut use and smoking.[7]

Smokeless tobacco consumption in South Asia in various forms is an important cultural tradition. Some ethnic groups believe that betel quid chewing is beneficial to health, a 'miracle cure' for most diseases, with an added cosmetic value and aphrodisiac properties. The belief in its ability to relieve pain, reduce fever, and prevent indigestion is also common. Paan also has religious connotations in India and in other parts of Southeast Asia. The distinctive, generalized red staining on teeth may be considered culturally fashionable, a sign of beauty.

Paan and gutka are legal in the United States, and readily available in ethnic enclaves.[32] As South Asian people have emigrated to various countries, they have continued using these products, and clinicians in the United States may see evidence of these practices.[7] As a result, there is evidence of high rates of oral cancer in some immigrant populations, such as those from the Indian subcontinent.

Qat, also referred to as khat, is a leafy narcotic that when chewed produces a feeling of euphoria and stimulation. Qat chewing sessions have become a major cultural phenomenon in the Yemeni and Somali cultures. This tradition originated in Ethiopia and spread to other parts of Africa and the Arabian Peninsula. The social aspect of qat chewing is as important if not more so than the physical high it creates. The leaves are placed in the mouth and held between the molars and the cheeks rather than chewed. This can provoke the development of oral keratic white lesions at the site of placement. In the United States, qat is used among the immigrants from Yemen, Somalia, and Ethiopia. The active ingredient, cathinone, is considered a schedule I drug and is present for only 48 hours after harvesting, and then is quickly converted to cathine, which is a legal substance. It is generally shipped to the US at the end of the week for weekend use.[37]

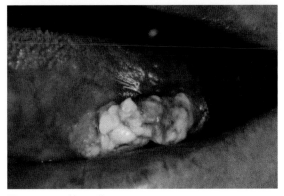

**Figure 45.4** Kaposi's sarcoma.

Regardless of the prevalence of these habits, healthcare professionals may come in contact with patients using these various forms of tobacco and should make a special effort to evaluate and educate regarding the risk factors of oral cancer and screen for oral lesions.

## HIV/AIDS Clinical Manifestations

The HIV/AIDS epidemic is one of the greatest challenges ever to global well-being, and is particularly severe in sub-Saharan Africa and Asia. Oral problems are common among persons with HIV, arising as a result of the weakened immune system. Studies have shown that approximately 40–50% of HIV-positive persons have oral fungal, bacterial, or viral infections, often occurring early in the course of the disease.[38] As a result, oral health providers can contribute effectively to the early diagnosis, prevention, and treatment of this disease.

Kaposi's sarcoma is the most common oral malignancy associated with HIV infection (Fig. 45.4). Some of the other common oral manifestations include oral candidiasis, oral hairy leukoplakia, HIV gingivitis, and periodontitis. Herpes simplex infections occur at a higher frequency in the HIV-positive population and aphthous ulcers are also common, and may be large and painful and may take a long time to heal. Xerostomia, or dry mouth, occurs frequently as a result of reduced salivary flow due to swollen salivary glands and is also induced by the medications used. The reduced salivary flow increases the risk of dental caries and also may lead to difficulty in chewing, swallowing, and tasting food.[38] Regardless of whether the disease has produced oral manifestations, it is important for patients with HIV/AIDS

to visit dental care providers for cleanings and oral health assessments.

## Trauma

Two separate surveys conducted in the United States found that 5–10% of all foreign-born adult patients seen in large urban medical centers suffered some form of torture in their countries of origin.[39,40] Many refugees and asylum seekers report having suffered torture that may be in the form of physical torture, including orofacial trauma, a family history of torture, or sexual trauma. Physical torture may include beatings to the head and face, electric shock and burns to the mouth and lips, intentional fracture or removal of teeth, torture through starvation and thirst, forcible pouring of caustic or non-nutritive products into the victim's mouth, forced oral sexual assault, and the intentional withholding of dental treatment for acute conditions (Lituri K, Garcia R. personal communication) (Box 45.1).

Oral manifestations of physical trauma may include loose, missing, or broken teeth or the inability to chew in comfort. In the mouth, there may be signs of healing or scar tissue from abrasions, lacerations, contusions, fractures, electrical and chemical burns, and puncture wounds. As a result of past trauma experiences, patients may develop oral phobia that may prevent them from seeking dental care. Examination tools and procedures may precipitate memories of the torture implements or methods and cause acute emotional reactions or profound withdrawal anxiety. A health professional who has

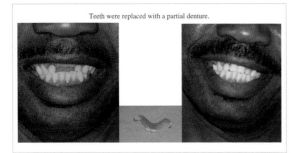

Figure 45.5 Trauma.

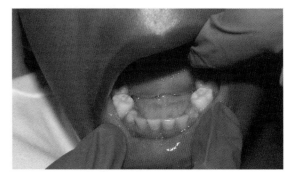

Figure 45.6 Mutilation of primary canines.

established trust and can overcome linguistic and cultural barriers is in an ideal position to initially screen and inquire for signs of trauma to the face and oral cavity (Lituri K, Garcia R. unpublished manuscript) (Fig. 45.5).[41]

## Cultural Beliefs and Oral Health Practices

The countries of origin of refugees and immigrants entering the United States reflect current world conditions. Many are from areas of the world with language, customs, and cultures that are quite different from those residing in the US or immigrating in the past. The changing demographics of refugees and immigrants present healthcare professionals with the challenge of caring for patients with diverse backgrounds, cultural beliefs and practices, and perceptions about health and illness. Understanding of some traditional oral health practices assists healthcare professionals to address the oral health needs of immigrants in a more informed and effective manner.

Traditional oral hygiene practices vary widely in different parts of the world (Table 45.3). Chewing sticks are a common practice in many parts of Africa, the Middle East, and Asia. When properly used, chewing sticks are quite effective in removing plaque.[17] A recent report suggests that 'miswak' chewing sticks may have an inhibitory effect on the levels of oral streptococci, and thus lower the risk of dental caries.[17] Many refugees prefer using chewing sticks as part of their daily oral hygiene regimen rather than adopting the use of a toothbrush.

The Somalis use a stick collected from the branches of a tree called 'roomay' in Somalia, or a stick called 'muswaki' made from the root of another type of tree. Ashes and wood charcoal, derived from tree burning, are also rubbed on the teeth to whiten

them. They may also use a natural medicine derived from a tree called 'havekeddy' on their teeth to ease tooth pain or use cloves, which are kept in most Somali homes and are also used by Somalis in the US.[41] Cloves and clove oil have also been used around the world as an herbal remedy to treat toothaches.

Traditional healing practices are common in many African countries. One such practice in Sudan, Tanzania, and Ethiopia is the extraction of the primary canine tooth buds by a traditional healer. The belief is that swelling in the area of the gums associated with the unerupted primary canines causes diarrhea, vomiting, and fever. In most instances, the lower canines are extracted bilaterally, but extractions of upper canines and lower incisors have also been reported. Instruments used for these procedures include penknives, metal blades made from spoon handles or bike tire spokes, and sharp fingernails. In some cultures, salt or herbs are applied to the area of the gum that is injured following the procedure. The instruments used are often not sterilized, and no anesthesia is used. The age at which the extractions and lancing occurs vary from as early as 1 month to 2–3 years (Fig. 45.6).[42] Uvulectomies (removal of the uvula) are also done on many East African infants, usually at a few weeks of age. Families report that this is done to prevent throat infections and at times to cure a wide range of problems from tonsillar infection to growth retardation. The surgery leaves a variety of anatomic changes in the soft palate.[43]

Another common traditional ritual among the Dinka and Nuer tribes in southern Sudan is the removal of the lower anterior teeth and also sometimes upper anterior canine teeth of male and female children to mark the journey from childhood to adulthood. In the Sudan, the absence of the lower teeth is a tribal identifier, a precursor to marriage and manhood. This is done by the elders in the tribes

**Table 45.3 Cultural practices of immigrants**

| Practice | Region | Description | Manifestation | Treatment |
|---|---|---|---|---|
| Betel nut chewing (paan, gutka) | Southeast Asia, India, New Guinea | Mixture of areca nut, calcium hydroxide, spices, seeds and tobacco wrapped in a betel leaf or in foil sachets | Generalized red extrinsic staining of the teeth | Discourage use Oral cancer screening Refer to dentist for suspicious lesions |
| Qat (Khat) | Africa and Arabian peninsula: Yemen, Ethiopia and Somalia | Leafy narcotic that produces euphoria and stimulation | Leukoplakia | Discourage use Oral cancer screening Refer to dentist for suspicious lesions |
| Chewing sticks (Miswaki, Miswak, Roomay) | Africa, Middle East, Asia | Stick from the branch of a tree to clean teeth | None | Supplement with a toothbrush |
| Havekeddy | Somalia | Natural medicine from tree to alleviate dental pain | None | None |
| Cloves or clove oil | Worldwide | Used to relieve toothache | None | None |
| Missing primary canines | Sudan, Tanzania, Ethiopia | Canine tooth buds of infants or children extracted using penknives, metal blades, bike spokes or sharp fingernails | Missing or mutilated canines | None |
| Uvulectomy | East Africa | Removal of uvula | Missing uvula leads to anatomic changes in the soft palate | None |
| Missing lower anterior teeth and upper canines | South Sudan | Removal of teeth in children at puberty | Missing lower front teeth leading to malocclusion | Refer to dentist for replacement and orthodontic evaluation |
| Trona (magadi) | Eastern Africa | Mixture of salts containing high levels of fluoride to reduce cooking time | Dental fluorosis | None |
| Ashes, wood charcoal | Africa | Rubbed on teeth to whiten | None | None |

without the use of anesthesia by twisting the tip of a spear between the teeth until they fall out. This ritual is thought to have originated in the days when the people of southern Sudan were regularly taken as slaves. Those captives with teeth missing were seen as unhealthy and certainly less valuable and so were often released. The practice continues today but now the lack of front teeth has come to be seen as a sign of beauty. The missing teeth can cause malocclusion with the maxillary anterior teeth, flaring, speech impediments from tongue thrusting, and difficulty biting into foods (Fig. 45.7). When these Sudanese immigrate to the US, one of their top priorities is to have the missing teeth replaced. They are unfamiliar with professional dental treatment as their only dental experience has been by the elders in the tribe with rudimentary instruments and without anesthesia. Dental treatment requires the

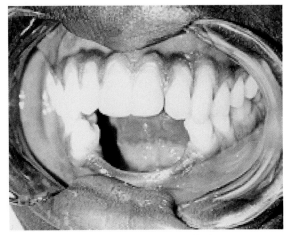

**Figure 45.7** Missing anterior teeth of a Sudanese.

---

**Box 45.2**

**Case study 2**

Before coming to the United States from Sudan, this person had never heard of a dentist or knew about a toothbrush or toothpaste. He cleaned his teeth with chewing sticks and charcoal. The only time he had dental work was when the elders of the tribe pulled the lower anterior teeth. It was an important ritual in the Dinka tribe which was done without anesthesia and only crude instruments were used. He was expected to remain very still and not cry or he would shame his family. When he came to the US, he visited the dentist and had his teeth replaced. He and some of his Sudanese friends named the dentist 'math de lec' ('friend of teeth' in Dinka).

---

time to explain the procedures. Once the teeth are replaced, it is important to recognize there is an adjustment period to adapt to eating and speaking differently (Box 45.2).

The Chinese population is characterized by strong elements of traditional beliefs concerning the prevention and treatment of disease. Problems such as loosening of the teeth are considered to be an imbalance of the kidneys. Remedies would be to take enriching foods (tonics) to strengthen and balance the kidneys. Gingival inflammation and abscesses are believed to be caused by intense heat or flaring fire in the stomach. The traditional Chinese way to cure bleeding or swollen gingiva, bad breath, or an abscess is to take herbal teas to 'cool down the fire.' The concept of foods and herbs having different characteristics such as cold, hot, and poisons extends to all aspects of prevention and the cure for all kinds of health problems.[44] Herbal teas, tiger balm, salt water, Japanese medical plaster, rum, kerosene, white flower oil, melon cream, and other available Chinese medicines are all used for dental problems.[31] There is a trend towards increased use of these remedies with age and among females.

## Management of Dental Needs

Medical practitioners are in a valuable position to assess and prioritize the dental health needs of immigrants and make referrals for necessary treatment. Dental conditions that require immediate care include large dental caries which present with pain, fever, or swelling, dental or periodontal abscesses, and acute necrotizing ulcerative gingivitis (ANUG). These conditions should be treated within 24 hours to alleviate the pain and treat infection. Any suspicious lesions of the lips, cheeks, tongue, or other soft tissue in the oral cavity may be indicative of oral cancer or related to HIV/AIDS infection. These require rapid referral to a dentist for diagnosis and/or treatment. The management of nonurgent dental needs such as dental caries without pain, and preventive dental care can be incorporated into routine health visits and other health promotion activities (Table 45.4).

As immigrants acculturate into the US, changes in lifestyle, diet and behaviors put them at risk for dental diseases as well as other conditions such as cardiovascular diseases, cancer, obesity, and diabetes. As the diet changes, there can be an increase in sugar and processed food consumption, increasing the risk for dental caries. In some immigrant populations, lifestyle changes such as an increase in smoking and alcohol consumption increase the risk for numerous conditions, including oral cancer and periodontal disease. Some immigrants may choose to continue infant feeding practices from their home country which may not be consistent with the recommendations in the US, such as discontinuing use of a baby bottle after 1 year of age. In many cultures, the community and the family have a significant role in decision-making regarding child rearing, health issues, and lifestyles. A community-based approach when combined with individual counseling may be more effective when attempting to promote healthy behaviors.

Immigrants face many barriers when trying to access dental care, such as language and low literacy levels. Many are unfamiliar with the US healthcare

### Table 45.4 Common dental conditions in immigrants

| Dental condition | Region | Description | Treatment |
| --- | --- | --- | --- |
| Dental caries | Worldwide | Dental decay (cavity) | Refer to dentist Immediate referral if pain, swelling or fever present |
| Dental abscess | Worldwide | Infection at the apex of a tooth, gingiva or alveolar bone. | Immediate referral to dentist |
| Early childhood caries | Worldwide (especially in lower socioeconomic status) | Dental caries in infants and toddlers as a result of feeding practices; manifesting as white to brown spots to cavitated lesions | Refer to dentist Diet counseling |
| Fluorosis | Common in Eastern Africa | White spots to pitted discolored enamel | None |
| Periodontal disease | Worldwide | Bacterial infection affecting the gingival and alveolar bone | Refer to dentist |
| ANUG (acute necrotizing ulcerative gingivitis) | Worldwide, especially sub-Saharan Africa | Progressive painful gingival infection caused by stress, poor oral hygiene and poor nutrition | Immediate referral to dentist Antibiotics, debridement, dental surgery |
| Noma | Sub-Saharan Africa (isolated cases in other areas) | Acute gangrenous infection of face found in malnourished children | Immediate referral to dentist Antibiotics, proper nutrition, surgery |
| Oral cancer | Worldwide | Cancer in the mouth, white or red lesions on the oral mucosa, swelling in cheek or neck | Refer to dentist |
| HIV/AIDS | Worldwide | Kaposi's sarcoma, oral candidiasis, leukoplakia, HIV gingivitis and periodontitis | Refer to dentist |
| Trauma | Worldwide | Loose, missing or broken teeth | Refer to dentist |

system and are not able to navigate through the process of receiving dental care. Many immigrants do not have dental insurance, or might have the perception that dental care is costly and beyond their reach. Still others fear that accessing dental public health services will jeopardize their immigration status. Required paperwork may be overwhelming and scheduling appointments in a timely way may be difficult. Some immigrant groups prefer to use traditional remedies as treatment for dental problems, which delays dental visits. Past experiences from painful dental treatments, torture, or tribal rituals may have instilled a fear of dentistry and influenced the immigrant's decision not to receive professional dental care. Furthermore, immigrants could be unfamiliar with the restorative or preventive dental treatment options available to them. Cosmetic dentistry is extremely popular in the US, with a huge demand for whiter teeth. However, some other cultures do not perceive white teeth as desirable. Individuals from Somalia have remarked that the brown staining from dental fluorosis is something to be proud of because it shows that your teeth are strong. Similarly, betel nut staining among some populations is seen as a sign of beauty.

Many commonly prescribed medications have side effects that are manifested in the oral cavity. Pediatric medications including antibiotics may contain sugar to improve palatability, therefore making them potentially cariogenic. Parents and children should be educated regarding the need to brush after each dose, or to take their medications at meal times rather than between meals, and to avoid taking medicines before bed. In addition, there are over 400 prescriptions and over-the-counter medications that have xerostomic effects. Commonly known as dry mouth, xerostomia inhibits salivary flow. Reduction in saliva can place a patient at increased risk for dental caries and infections. Medications for high blood pressure and depression are examples of prescriptions that may cause xerostomia. To reduce the adverse effects, patients could be referred to the dentist for more frequent examinations and fluoride treatments, artificial saliva replacements could be prescribed, or medications could be adjusted.

## Conclusion

Immigrants are confronted with many barriers when attempting to resettle into a new country. Accessing oral healthcare is particularly challenging due to financial constraints and is further compounded with the issues of language, culture, and different care-seeking behaviors. Great diversity exists in the backgrounds and past experiences of refugees and immigrants regarding oral health. Some have never been to a dentist or are unfamiliar with dental procedures in the United States. Medical providers are most likely to be the first introduction to healthcare services for immigrants. Since oral health is a critical component of overall health, an oral health assessment is an essential part of a comprehensive examination. The medical team plays a key role in facilitating the referral for dental services and promoting good oral health habits. When addressing oral health issues, it is important to be culturally sensitive and to be aware that each individual presents with unique backgrounds, experiences and varying degrees of oral health knowledge and literacy. An interdisciplinary, cooperative approach using the skills of both medical and dental practitioners can ensure that the oral health needs of immigrant patients are met.

## References

1. The World Oral Health Report 2003. World Health Organization; 2003.
2. Williams S, Sardo Infirri J. Refugees, immigrants and oral health. Migration World Mag 1996; 24:31.
3. Diet, Nutrition and the Prevention of Chronic Diseases, Report of the Joint WHO/FAO Expert Consultation. Geneva: World Health Organization; 2003.
4. Petersen PE, Yamamoto T. Improving the oral health of older people: the approach of the WHO Global Oral Health Programme. Commun Dent Oral Epidemiol 2005; 33:81–92.
5. Department of Health and Human Services, Oral Health in America: a Report of the Surgeon General, Rockville, MD: US Public Health Services, National Institute of Dental and Craniofacial Research, National Institute of Health; 2000.
6. National Institute for Dental and Craniofacial Research, The Oral-Systemic Health Connection. Available: http://www.nidcr.nih.gov/HealthInformation/DiseasesAndConditions/OralSystemicHealthConnection/OralSystemic.htm Accessed 1/30/07
7. Kerr AR, Changrani JG, Gany FM, et al. An academic dental center grapples with oral cancer disparities: current collaboration and future opportunities. J Dental Educat 2004; 68(5):531–541.
8. National Institute for Dental and Craniofacial Research, Detecting Oral Cancer: A Guide for Health Care Professionals Available: http://www.nidcr.nih.gov/HealthInformation/DiseasesAndConditions/OralCancer/DetectingOralCancer.htm Accessed 1/30/07
9. Burt BA, Eklund SA. Dentistry, dental practice and the community. 5th edn. Philadelphia: WB Saunders; 1999.
10. WHO Oral Health Country/Area Profile Programme, WHO Department of Noncommunicable Diseases Surveillance/Oral Health, Malmo, Sweden, WHO Collaborating Centre, Malmo University.
11. Enwonwu CO, Phillips RS, Ibrahim CD. Nutrition and oral health in Africa. Internat Dental J 2004; 54:344–351.
12. Pollick H, Rice A, Echenberg D. Dental health of recent immigrant children in the newcomers schools, San Francisco. Am J Public Health 1987; 77:731–732.
13. Watson MR, Horowitz AM, Garcia I, et al. Caries conditions among 2–5-year-old immigrant Latino children related to parents' oral health knowledge, opinions and practices. Commun Dental Oral Epidemiol 1999; 27(1):8–15.
14. Scheer M, Phipps K. Oral health disparities among immigrants from the former Soviet Union. Presentation at the APHA Conference, Tuesday, November 18, 2003; San Francisco, CA.
15. Mann J, Cohen HS, Fisher R, et al. Prevalence of dental caries among Ethiopian emigrants. Internat Dental J 1994; 44(5):480–484.
16. Ramos-Gomez FJ, Tomar SL, Ellison J, et al. Assessment of early childhood caries and dietary habits in a population of migrant Hispanic children in Stockton, California. J ASDC Dentistry Childr 1999; 66(6):366, 395–403.
17. Cote S, Geltman P, Nunn M, et al. Dental caries of refugee children compared with US children. Pediatrics 2004; 114(6): e733–e740.
18. Cote S, Geltman P, Lituri K, Barnett E, et al. Program for refugee oral health. Poster presentation at the National Oral Health Conference, April 26–May 1, 2002; Pittsburgh, PA.
19. Cruz GD, Xue X, LeGeros RZ. Dental caries experience, tooth loss and factors associated with unmet needs of Haitian immigrants in New York City. J Public Health Dentistr 2001; 61:203–209.
20. Singh H, Henshaw M, Scott T, et al. Dental health status of asylum seekers at the Boston Center For Refugee Health and Human Rights (BCRHHR). Poster presented at the National Oral Health Conference, May 2–4, 2005; Pittsburg, PA.
21. Centers for Disease Control and Prevention. Recommendations for using fluoride to prevent and control dental caries in the United States. MMWR Recommendations and Reports 2001; 50:1–42.
22. Awadia AK, Bjorvatn K, Birkeland JM, et al. Weaning food and magadi associated with dental fluorosis in northern Tanzania. Acta Odontologica Scand 2000; 58(1):1–7.

23. Casamassimo PS. Dental disease prevalence, prevention and health promotion: the implications on pediatric oral health of a more diverse population. Pediatric Dentistr 2003; 25(1):16–18.

24. DenBesten P, Berkowitz R. Early childhood caries: an overview with reference to our experience in California. J Calif Dental Assoc 2003; 31(2):139–143.

25. Singh H, Kressin N, Nunn M, et al. Early childhood caries (ECC) at two urban medical centers. Oral presentation presented at the FDI World Dental Federation meeting. August 22–27, 2005.

26. Shiboski CH, Gansky SA, Ramos-Gomez F, et al. The association of early childhood caries and race/ethnicity among California preschool children. J Public Health Dentistr 2003; 3(1):38–46.

27. Williams S, Sahota P. An enquiry into the attitudes of Muslim Asian mothers regarding infant feeding practices and dental health. J Human Nutrit Dietet 1990; 3:393–401.

28. Bowen WH, Lawrence RA. Comparison of the cariogenicity of cola, honey, cow milk, human milk, and sucrose. Pediatrics 2005; 116(4):921–926.

29. Noma/Facing Africa. Available: http://www.facingafrica. org Accessed 1/30/07

30. Noma in the World. Available: http://www.who.int/ oral_health/media/en/orh_report-03_en.pdf Accessed 2/6/07

31. Scrimshaw SC. Our multicultural society: implications for pediatric dental practice. Pediatric Dentistr 2003; 25:11–15.

32. Hutton B, Feine J, Morais J. Is there an association between eduntulism and nutritional state. J Cana Dental Assoc 2002; 68(3):182–187.

33. Oral Cancer Foundation. Oral Cancer Facts. Available: http://www.oralcancerfoundation.org July 28, 2005.

34. Stewart DC, Ortega AN, Dausey D. Oral health and use of dental services among Hispanics. J Public Health Dentistr 2002; 62(2):84–91.

35. Parkin DM, Bray F, Ferlay J, et al. Global cancer statistics, 2002. CA Cancer J Clinicians 2005; 55(2):74–108.

36. Pickwell SM, Schimelpfening S, Palinkas LA. 'Betelmania'. Betel quid chewing by Cambodian women in the United States and its potential health effects. West J Med 1994; 160(4):326–330.

37. Qat trade in Africa. Available: http://www.american.edu/ projects/mandala/TED/qat.htm Accessed 2/6/07

38. US Department of Health and Human Services, Health Resources and Services Administration. HRSA Care Action: Providing HIV/AIDS care in a changing environment. Available: http://hab.hrsa.gov/publications/april2002.htm Accessed 2/6/07

39. Randall GR, Lutz EL. Approach to the patient. In: Serving Survivors of Torture. American Association for the Advancement of Science, 1991.

40. Eisenman D. Survivors of torture in the general medical setting: how common and how commonly missed? 8th International Symposium on Torture; A Challenge to Health, Legal, and Other Professionals. New Delhi, India; 22–25 September, 1999.

41. Ethnomed. Somali Oral Health. Available: http://www. ethnomed.org/ehnomed/cultures/somali/som_oral_health. html Accessed 2/6/07

42. Graham EA, Domoto PK, Lynch H, et al. Dental injuries due to African traditional therapies for diarrhea. West J Med 2000; 173(2):135–137.

43. Graham E. Peripartum and infant care issues and practices among refugee groups in Seattle. Harborview Medical Center. August 1996. Available: http://ethnomed.org/ ethnomed/clin_topics/peri.html Accessed 2/15/07

44. Lee KL, Schwarz E, Mak KYK. Improving oral health through understanding the meaning of health and disease in a Chinese culture. Internat Dental J. 1993; 43:2–8.

CHAPTER 46

# Anemia and Red Blood Cell Disorders

Randy Hurley

## Introduction

Anemia is a common manifestation of systemic illness. The World Health Organization (WHO) estimates that the number of anemic people worldwide approaches two billion. Women and children are more commonly affected: the WHO estimates that nearly 50% of women and children from developing nations and perhaps a quarter of men are anemic.[1] Anemia in immigrants can be a result of both acquired and inherited causes (Table 46.1). Unfortunately, comprehensive studies describing the incidence and etiology of anemia in immigrant populations are lacking. However, the worldwide geographic distribution of several genetically based red blood cell (RBC) disorders (thalassemia, hemoglobin C and E, ovalocytosis, and sickle cell disease), the prevalence of iron deficiency, and the geographic prevalence of other diseases affecting the hematologic system (malaria, helminth infection, HIV, TB) are well known.[2,3] Therefore, understanding the prior prevalence and geographic distribution of anemia in the country of origin is helpful when evaluating a new immigrant with a hematologic problem (Box 46.1).

## Geographic Distribution of Red Blood Cell Disorders

Malaria affects the tropical regions of the world and it is postulated that most genetically-based RBC disorders, such as the thalassemias, hemoglobinopa- thies, ovalocytosis, and elliptocytosis provide a selective protective advantage against malaria para- site infection. Indeed, malaria has had one of the most profound evolutionary effects on the human genome: genetic RBC disorders have a high preva- lence in areas of the world where malaria once was or still is a major health concern.[4] It is estimated that 4.83% of the world's population carry globin gene variants, including 1.67% of the population hetero- zygous for α- or β-thalassemia and 1.92% carry sickle hemoglobin.[5] Due to population movement and immigration, these disorders are now seen on all continents of the world. Although accurate epide- miologic data are not available for all parts of the world, it is known that both α- and β-thalassemia are more common in Africa, the Mediterranean, India, and Southeast Asia. Sickle cell disease is seen in 1– 2% of infants born in tropical Africa. However, if the heterozygous state provides a selective protective advantage against malaria, the prevalence in adults may be much higher.[3] Sickle cell disease is also seen to a lesser extent in India and the Middle East. Glucose 6-phosphate dehydrogenase (G6PD) defi- ciency is seen with varying frequency throughout Africa, Asia, and Central and South America. Hemo- globin C is most prevalent in West Africa whereas hemoglobin E is seen most exclusively in Southeast Asia. The red cell membrane defect, ovalocytosis, is more prominent in Southeast Asia whereas hereditary elliptocytosis is more common in West and North Africa. Table 46.2 provides an estimate of the frequency of RBC disorders in the three groups with the highest known prevalence: Southeast Asians, Africans, and people from Eastern

### Table 46.1 Causes of anemia in immigrants

**Common acquired causes**
- Iron deficiency
- Malaria
- HIV
- Anemia of chronic disease

**Genetic RBC disorders**
- α- and β-thalassemia
- Hemoglobin E
- Sickle cell disease and hemoglobin C
- G6PD deficiency
- RBC membrane defects: ovalocytosis, elliptocytosis

Mediterranean countries.[3,6-8] These estimates are a compilation of WHO data and published data from prenatal screening clinics and newborn testing series. It should be emphasized, however, that even within geographic regions, the heterogeneity of ethnic groups leads to a wide variation in the prevalence of these disorders. Indeed, an excellent example in the developed world is from Italy: the prevalence of hemoglobin disorders in Northern Italy is 1–2% but reaches 12% in Sardinia.[6]

## Box 46.1

## Case study 1

**You are asked to see a 33-year-old Laotian woman 1 day postoperative for a drop in hemoglobin. She had been in the United States for 2 weeks visiting relatives when she developed acute cholecystitis and underwent a laparoscopic cholecystectomy without difficulty. The pathology indicated acute cholecystitis with pigmented gall stones. Her preoperative CBC showed:**

WBC 11 900
Hb 10.3 g/dL
RBC 5.10 m/μL (normal 4.0–5.2 m/μL)
MCV 67.6 fl
Plt 240 k

Postoperatively, she feels well but her hemoglobin has decreased to 8.7 g/dL. There is no evidence of abnormal bleeding and her vital signs are normal. She is a para 5005 and has normal monthly menstrual periods. She is not febrile. Her examination is unremarkable. There is no splenomegaly.

### Learning issues
- Given her ethnic background, what are the common hereditary RBC disorders that she could have?
- What is the differential diagnosis of microcytic anemia and how does an RBC number in the upper-normal range help?
- What are this patient's risk factors for iron deficiency?
- What is the significance of pigmented gallstones?
- Describe appropriate evaluation.

### Discussion
Often, anemia is multifactorial and, certainly, in the postoperative setting, could reflect blood loss or a dilutional effect from rehydration. However, Southeast Asians have a high prevalence of globin gene

mutations. Estimates suggest 15–20% of patients may have hemoglobin E, and 25% of patients may carry an α-thalassemia mutation. Glucose-6-phosphate dehydrogenase deficiency can be seen in 10–15% of patients but more commonly produces symptoms in males due to the X-linked recessive inheritance pattern.

The differential diagnosis of microcytic anemia includes iron deficiency, thalassemia/hemoglobin E, severe anemia of chronic disease, as well as less common etiologies such as lead ingestion.

Her multiparity and ongoing menstruation put her at risk for iron deficiency; this could be compounded by poor nutrition and/or intestinal blood loss from helminth infection. The microcytic anemia with a 'normal' RBC number, however, would implicate uniformly small RBCs as is seen in thalassemia/hemoglobin E.

Pigmented gallstones suggest ongoing RBC turnover indicative of thalassemia or G6PD deficiency. Other systemic signs such as persistent fever could suggest other etiologies such as malaria.

### Evaluation
The initial evaluation should begin with a reticulocyte count, peripheral smear evaluation, and a stool specimen for occult blood. Thick and thin smears for malaria were obtained due to her recent arrival from an area endemic for malaria. A total bilirubin and LDH are a quick screen for hemolysis but should be compared to other liver function tests (alkaline phosphatase, AST, ALT) because of the recent gallbladder surgery. A diminished haptoglobin level would help confirm an element of RBC destruction. A ferritin and hemoglobin electrophoresis should be ordered to help distinguish different causes of microcytic anemia. A Heinz body slide, in conjunction with classic peripheral smear findings of spherocytes and 'bite cells' would help

identify G6PD deficiency. A G6PD activity level should not be ordered at this time since it can be misleadingly normal after an acute hemolytic event.

**Additional data**

| | |
|---|---|
| Reticulocyte count: | 2.5% |
| Peripheral smear: | Hypochromic microcytes and 'pencil-shaped cells' No fragmented or 'bite cells' |
| Stool hemoccult: | Negative |
| Malarial smear: | Negative |
| Total bilirubin: | 2.1 mg/dL (normal <1.5) |
| Direct bilirubin: | Normal (elevated indirect bilirubin) |
| LDH: | 275 U/L |
| Alkaline phosphatase: | Normal |
| AST/ALT: | Normal |
| Haptoglobin: | <5 mg/dL |
| Ferritin: | 30 ng/mL (normal 10–150) |
| Hemoglobin electrophoresis: | Normal amounts of HbA1, and HbA2, no Hb F or HbE |
| Heinz body prep: | Negative |

**Discussion**

This patient's anemia is most likely due to a combination of iron deficiency and α-thalassemia: indeed, the peripheral smear suggests iron deficiency. This case is also an example of how laboratory test results, particularly for the reticulocyte count, ferritin, and hemoglobin electrophoresis, need to be put into clinical context to be appropriately interpreted. Isolated iron deficiency is a hypoproliferative anemia typified by a very low reticulocyte count of 1% or less. Depending on the severity of α-thalassemia, the reticulocyte count can be normal to markedly elevated (5% or greater). The reticulocyte count of 2.5% needs to be interpreted in the clinical context: it is a little too high for isolated iron deficiency but suggests an inadequate bone marrow response if the anemia was entirely due to increased RBC destruction (hemolysis). The elevated bilirubin and LDH combined with the absent haptoglobin and pigmented gallstones confirm an element of hemolysis that does not appear to be due to G6PD deficiency (the Heinz body prep is normal). The ferritin is in the 'normal range' albeit the low normal range. As an acute-phase reactant, one would expect the ferritin to be elevated (perhaps above 100 ng/mL) in a patient presenting with inflammation from acute cholecystitis. Therefore, the borderline low ferritin in conjunction with the microcytic indices and peripheral smear morphology would implicate an element of iron deficiency. Lastly, the normal hemoglobin electrophoresis rules out significant β-thalassemia and hemoglobin E; it can be normal, however, in α-thalassemia trait. The normal RBC number in the face of significant microcytosis also lends support for a clinical diagnosis of α-thalassemia as does the evidence of increased RBC turnover (elevated LDH/bilirubin, absent haptoglobin, and pigmented gallstones). A more sophisticated DNA test could be used to confirm a diagnosis of α-thalassemia.

**Table 46.2 Estimates of prevalence of genetic RBC disorders in various regions of the world[3,6,7,8]**

| Disorder | Southeast Asia | Africa | Eastern Mediterranean |
|---|---|---|---|
| α-thalassemia | 8–25% | 5–8% | 1% |
| β-thalassemia | 2–8% | 3–7% | 2–8% |
| Hemoglobin E | 8–45% | <1% | <1% |
| G6PD deficiency | 5–25% | 5–20% | 2–15% |
| Hemoglobin S | <1% | 1–25% | 1% |
| Hemoglobin C | <1% | 1–5% | <1% |
| Ovalocytosis | 1–30% | <1% | <1% |
| Elliptocytosis | 1–30% | 1–4% | <1% |

The wide prevalence range of certain disorders is due to the heterogeneity of ethnic groups and the role of malaria-influencing geographic climates in these regions.

# Common Acquired Causes of Anemia

## Iron deficiency anemia

The WHO estimates that 50% of anemia worldwide can be attributed to iron deficiency; it is the most common nutritional deficiency.[1] Iron balance is a reflection of dietary iron intake, adsorption, and iron (blood) loss. Iron is available in the diet as heme iron from animal protein sources and non-heme iron from vegetable sources. Heme iron is readily absorbed in the diet as is iron in breast milk. In contrast, iron from vegetable sources has low bioavailability. Due to menstruation, lactation, and iron loss during pregnancy, women of reproductive age worldwide have the highest incidence of iron deficiency. This population should be considered for supplementation. Gastrointestinal tract blood loss,

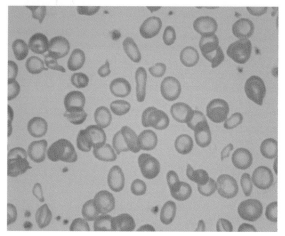

**Figure 46.1** Iron deficiency. The red blood cells are small and poorly hemoglobinized (increased central pallor). Note occasional 'cigar-shaped' or 'pencil cells'.

only is there parasite-mediated RBC destruction and increased splenic removal, malaria infection also suppresses RBC production by the bone marrow.[11] Therefore, the reticulocyte response may not be as vigorous as in a purely hemolytic process. Occasionally, malaria infection is associated with immune-mediated RBC destruction and a positive direct Coombs test due to adsorption of immunoglobulin and complement onto the RBC surface. Severe acute intravascular hemolysis may rarely occur (blackwater fever) leading to hemoglobinemia, hemoglobinuria, and severe hyperbilirubinemia. Recurrent malaria infection can be immunosuppressive and can be complicated by secondary bacterial or viral infection. Fifty percent of patients develop some degree of splenomegaly which contributes to the pancytopenia often seen in chronically infected patients.

## HIV

Human immunodeficiency virus infection and AIDs can cause a plethora of hematologic problems. Early on during HIV infection, immune thrombocytopenia is common as is the development of antiphospholipid antibodies. Anemia is the most common manifestation of HIV infection and is multifactorial due to both direct and indirect effects of the virus.[12] Anemia is most often a hypoproliferative, low reticulocyte anemia due to anemia of chronic disease. Often, there is a blunted erythropoietin response. Coombs-positive autoimmune hemolytic anemia also occurs with increased frequency in HIV infection. Antiretroviral therapy often causes macrocytosis.

the major source of iron loss, has a wide differential diagnosis. This includes peptic ulcer disease and colon cancer as in the general population but also includes helminth infection in immigrant populations. Iron deficiency leads to a microcytic anemia occasionally associated with thrombocytosis. The cells have increased central pallor and occasional elongated 'pencil cells' and target cells (Fig. 46.1). The red cell distribution width (RDW) is elevated and the reticulocyte count is low. Serum ferritin is characteristically low (<15 ng/mL) in uncomplicated iron deficiency and is the single best test for assessing iron stores. Since ferritin is also increased by inflammation, iron deficiency can be identified with greater sensitivity by using a higher cutoff value of ferritin of <30–100 ng/mL.[9] A ratio of soluble transferrin receptor to ferritin level may also be helpful in distinguishing iron deficiency from anemia of chronic disease.

### Malaria

The RBC protozoal infection, malaria, is endemic to most of the equatorial areas of the world. The prevalence of malaria in immigrants, particularly from Africa, has been reported to be as high as 15%.[10] Anemia is the most common manifestation of malaria infection but leukopenia and thrombocytopenia (often from splenomegaly) may also occur. The pathophysiology of anemia is multifactorial: not

### Anemia of chronic disease

Anemia of chronic disease (ACD), perhaps best termed anemia of acute or chronic inflammation, is a hypoproliferative anemia resulting from inflammatory cytokine effects on RBC production.[9] The hallmark is cytokine-induced disturbance of iron homeostasis. Iron, present in the bone marrow, is sequestered in reticuloendothelial cells and is not available for RBC and hemoglobin production. Often, ACD is a normochromic-normocytic anemia but it can progress to a microcytic anemia. The reticulocyte count is low, whereas the ferritin is characteristically >100 ng/mL and is often elevated. The erythropoietin response is blunted. Table 46.3 lists common causes of ACD.

**Table 46.3 Common causes of anemia of chronic disease**

**Infections**
  Viral including HIV
  Bacterial and mycobacterial including TB
  Parasitic
  Fungal

**Cancer**

**Autoimmune**
  Rheumatoid arthritis
  Systemic lupus
  Vasculitis
  Inflammatory bowel disease

**Chronic renal failure**

# Genetic Red Blood Cell Disorders

Red blood cells can simplistically be thought of as 'little bags of hemoglobin.' They are anucleate cells containing virtually only hemoglobin and several RBC enzymes enveloped in an RBC membrane. Therefore, genetic RBC disorders can be characterized as disorders of hemoglobin quantity (thalassemic syndromes) or quality (hemoglobinopathies), disorders of RBC enzyme function (G6PD deficiency), or disorders of the RBC membrane. The increased frequency of genetic RBC disorders is thought to represent a selective evolutionary advantage protecting against malaria infection.

## Thalassemia syndromes

Normal adult hemoglobin (Hb A) is a tetrad consisting of two $\alpha$ globin chains and two $\beta$ globin chains ($\alpha 2 \beta 2$). There are two $\alpha$ globin genes on each chromosome 16 (four per genome) and one $\beta$ globin gene on each chromosome 11 (two per genome). The thalassemic syndromes are a group of autosomal recessively inherited disorders leading to a quantitative decrease in $\beta$ or $\alpha$ hemoglobin chain production. Beta-thalassemia may only manifest several months after birth because of the predominance of $\gamma$ globin chain production in newborns, which gives rise to Hb F, fetal hemoglobin ($\alpha_2 \gamma_2$). In contrast, severe $\alpha$-thalassemia can lead to in utero death (hydrops fetalis). Both $\alpha$- and $\beta$-thalassemia are clinically heterogeneous disorders depending on the severity of decreased globin chain production. Patients may have only mild microcytic anemia (thalassemia trait)

or may have a profound hemolytic anemia with ineffective erythropoiesis, extramedullary hematopoiesis and growth retardation (thalassemia major). Additionally, thalassemia can coexist with other hemoglobin mutations such as sickle cell hemoglobin (Hb S-$\beta$ thal) or hemoglobin E (Hb E-$\beta$ thal) leading to an even more varied clinical course. Beta-thalassemia (due to increased levels of Hb A2 and Hb F) and hemoglobinopathies (due to abnormally migrating Hb bands) are distinguishable by hemoglobin electrophoresis as are severe forms of $\alpha$-thalassemia. The hemoglobin electrophoresis is normal, however, in $\alpha$-thalassemia trait: the diagnosis is often made clinically but can be confirmed with DNA analysis studies.

### Beta-thalassemia

**Beta-thalassemia trait** This condition is due to the deletion of one of the two $\beta$ globin genes.[5] Patients have a mild microcytic anemia but no other major clinical sequelae. They should not be prescribed iron and those of reproductive age should undergo genetic counseling.

**Beta-thalassemia major** Beta-thalassemia major begins to manifest 6 months after birth as $\gamma$ globin chain synthesis declines and is normally replaced by $\beta$ globin chains. The deficiency of $\beta$ globin chain synthesis leads to an excess of unpaired $\alpha$ globin chains that self assemble into $\alpha$-4 tetrads. These tetrads form intracellular inclusions leading to hemolysis in the spleen and ineffective erythropoiesis in the bone marrow. The hemolysis is manifested by microcytic anemia, reticulocytosis, hyperbilirubinemia, and splenomegaly. The ineffective erythropoiesis contributes to anemia and hyperbilirubinemia but also leads to expansion of the marrow space resulting in skeletal abnormalities such as frontal bossing and growth retardation. The peripheral smear shows microcytosis with microspherocytes, polychromasia, target cells, and basophilic stippling of RBCs (Fig. 46.2).

Splenomegaly leads to leukopenia and thrombocytopenia. The chronic extravascular hemolysis and need for RBC transfusions leads to iron overload and hemosiderosis.

### Alpha-thalassemia

**1-chain deletion** Patients with deletion of 1 of the 4 $\alpha$ globin genes are clinically normal without anemia or microcytosis.

**2-chain deletion** Patients with deletion of two $\alpha$ globin genes have $\alpha$-thalassemia trait manifested as

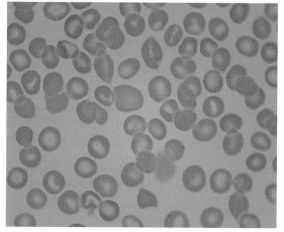

**Figure 46.2** Beta thalassemia. These RBCs are small but, in contrast to iron deficiency, are well hemoglobinized. There is increased basophilic stippling (small blue clumps of ribosomal RNA) in one of the RBCs.

a mild microcytic anemia but a normal hemoglobin electrophoresis. The clinical importance arises when two persons with α-thalassemia trait have offspring. The four α globin genes are situated as two genes on each chromosome 16. Thus, there are two possible deletion patterns: two genes from the same chromosome (αα/–) or a separate gene from each chromosome (α-/α-). Parents each harboring an αα/– deletion are at increased risk for producing an offspring incapable of α chain production (–/–) resulting in hydrops fetalis, leading to death in utero. For antenatal screening purposes in populations where α-thalassemia is prevalent, it is advisable to check the hemoglobin and mean corpuscular volume (MCV) of a pregnant woman's partner as well.[13]

**3-chain deletion** Three-chain deletion (α -/–) leads to α-thalassemia major or hemoglobin H disease. The severe decrease in α chain production leads to accumulation of unpaired gamma chain tetrads in newborns (γ4 or Hb Barts) and unpaired β globin chains (Hb H, β4) in later life. Patients have a significant anemia but the clinical course is not as severe as β-thalassemia major.

**4-chain deletion** Hydrops fetalis: in the past, 4-chain deletion with complete absence of α globin chain production was incompatible with life. Recent in utero techniques have allowed rare live births and attempts at stem cell transplantation.

**Hb constant spring** Hb constant spring (Hb CS) is a nondeletional mutation of the α globin gene leading

to a hemoglobin with separate electrophoretic mobility on Hb electrophoresis. When Hb CS is coinherited with 2-chain deletions, a more severe form of Hb H disease, entitled Hb H-constant spring occurs. This is a more severe thalassemic syndrome than the traditional 3-chain deletion Hb H disease, often with more severe transfusion-dependent anemia and splenomegaly.

## Glucose-6-phosphate dehydrogenase deficiency

Glucose-6-phosphate dehydrogenase (G6PD) is an enzyme in the RBC hexose monophosphate pathway designed to produce reduced glutathione.[14] Glutathione is used to prevent oxidative damage to hemoglobin and other intracellular structures. Thus, in G6PD deficiency, hemoglobin becomes oxidized and precipitates inside RBCs leading to hemolytic anemia; precipitated hemoglobin inside RBCs is identified by light microscopy as 'Heinz Bodies.' G6PD deficiency has a much wider equatorial geographic distribution than the thalassemias, encompassing not only Africa, the Mediterranean, India, and Southeast Asia, but also Central and South America.[3] The G6PD enzyme is located on the X chromosome; therefore, males are typically more symptomatic than heterozygous females. Over 400 variants of G6PD have been identified, leading to a wide clinical spectrum of disease; the WHO has classified these variants into five separate clinical classes ranging from severe chronic hemolysis to varying degrees of intermittent hemolysis to normal or supranormal levels of G6PD.

G6PD deficiency can cause four clinical hemolytic conditions:

1. Neonatal jaundice;
2. Infection-induced hemolysis: increased hemolysis associated with pneumonia, hepatitis B, septicemias, and viremias;
3. Food-induced hemolysis: induced by ingestion of fava beans (favisim);
4. Drug-induced hemolysis: certain oxidant drugs can precipitate hemolysis in G6PD deficient patients (Table 46.4).

Hemolysis is both intravascular and extravascular. The peripheral blood smear may show fragmented cells, microspherocytes, and 'bite cells' (Fig. 46.3). Staining with a supravital dye reveals precipitated hemoglobin as Heinz bodies. In addition to hyperbilirubinemia and reticulocytosis, lab abnormalities may include hemoglobinemia and hemoglobinuria. The diagnosis can be confirmed by measuring G6PD

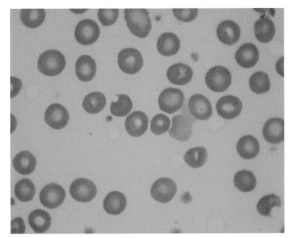

**Figure 46.3** G6PD deficiency. Note several spherocytes: small RBCs with little central pallor as well as two classic 'bite cells.'

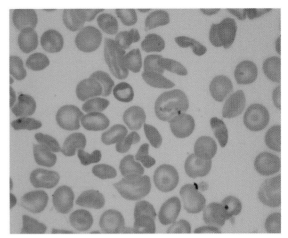

**Figure 46.4** Sickle cell anemia. There are occasional clumped sickle-shaped cells and target cells.

**Table 46.4 Commonly used drugs causing hemolysis in G6PD deficiency\***

| | |
|---|---|
| Antimalarials | Primaquine |
| Sulfonamides | Sulfacetamide, sulfapyridine, sulfamethoxazole |
| Sulfones | Dapsone |
| Antibiotics | Nitrofurantoin, nalidixic acid |
| Others | Phenazopyridine |

\* Avoid use of these drugs in immigrants from areas of high prevalence, or check a G6PD screen prior to use.

levels in RBCs. However, shortly after a hemolytic event, G6PD levels may be falsely elevated since reticulocytes have higher G6PD levels than mature RBCs. Therefore, it may be prudent to delay assaying G6PD levels until several weeks after the hemolytic episode has resolved.

## Hemoglobinopathies

Point mutations in the β globin molecule lead to several distinct clinical syndromes. Often, a diagnosis can be made on clinical grounds and peripheral blood smear morphology then confirmed by hemoglobin electrophoresis

**Sickle cell disease:** Hb S results from the substitution of valine for glutamic acid at position 6 of the β globin chain. The resultant hemoglobin has reduced solubility at low oxygen tensions. Inheritance of one sickle globin gene leads to sickle trait whereas inheritance of two sickle globin genes leads to sickle cell anemia. Sickle trait is characterized by minimal anemia and hyposthenuria but no vaso-occlusive crisis unless severe hypoxia occurs (such as at extreme altitude, etc.). Sickle cell anemia is characterized by a moderate to severe chronic hemolytic anemia with recurrent painful vaso-occlusive crisis. The peripheral smear shows characteristic sickle-shaped cells and increased polychromasia (Fig. 46.4). The sickle cell gene can be coinherited with β-thalassemia (sickle-β-thal).

**Hemoglobin E** Hb E is due to a substitution of lysine for glutamic acid at position 27 of the β globin chain. Hb E is seen primarily in patients from Southeast Asia. Heterozygous and homozygous Hb E produces only a mild microcytic anemia but it is important to identify to prevent unnecessary iron treatment of these patients. Hb E can also be coinherited with β-thalassemia, leading to a moderate thalassemic syndrome (occasionally termed β-thalassemia intermedia).

**Hemoglobin C** Hb C results from a substitution of lysine for glutamic acid at position 6 of the β globin chain. Patients with heterozygous Hb C are clinically normal. Homozygous Hb C produces a mild to moderate normochromic-normocytic anemia with splenomegaly. The peripheral smear shows numerous target cells and, rarely, intracellular hemoglobin crystals (Fig. 46.5).

617

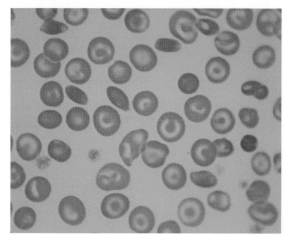

**Figure 46.5** Hemoglobin C. There are numerous 'target cells.'

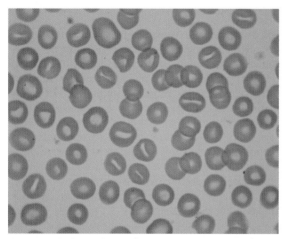

**Figure 46.6** Ovalocytosis. There are numerous stomatocytes: cells with 'slit-like' areas of central pallor.

## Red blood cell membrane defects

Red blood cell membrane defects include hereditary spherocytosis, most common in northern Europeans, hereditary elliptocytosis, seen with increased frequency in northern Africa, and hereditary ovalocytosis, seen in Southeast Asians. Elliptocytosis and ovalocytosis are thought to confer resistance to malaria. Both produce a mild or minimal normochromic-normocytic anemia with characteristic elliptical or oval-shaped erythrocytes on peripheral blood smear (Fig. 46.6). In contrast, hereditary spherocytosis in Northern Europeans can cause a chronic hemolytic anemia.

| Table 46.5 Evaluation of anemia | |
| --- | --- |
| History | |
| Physical examination | |
| Screening tests | CBC, differential, platelet count |
| | MCV |
| | Reticulocyte count |
| | Peripheral smear |
| Tests to evaluate microcytosis | Ferritin |
| | Hemoglobin electrophoresis |
| Tests to evaluate hemolysis | Bilirubin, LDH |
| | Haptoglobin |
| | Direct Coombs test |
| | G6PD tests |
| | Plasma free hemoglobin |
| | Urine hemoglobin |
| | Urine hemosiderin |
| Tests pertinent to recent immigrants | Hemoglobin electrophoresis |
| | Malaria smears |
| | Stools for ova and parasites |
| | HIV serology |
| | G6PD screen |

## The Approach to Anemia

The general approach to anemia includes a history, physical examination, and laboratory investigation to characterize the anemia according to both a morphologic and kinetic classification scheme (Table 46.5).

**History** Severity of symptoms of anemia is related to the rapidity of onset. Anemic patients may have nonspecific symptoms such as fatigue and dyspnea on exertion or may have exacerbation of other chronic underlying diseases such as cardiac, respiratory, or vascular disease. Gastrointestinal symptoms and melena could provide clues to chronic blood loss or malabsorption; pica for ice or clay could suggest iron deficiency; neuropathic or cognitive symptoms could implicate vitamin $B_{12}$ deficiency.

**Physical examination** Pallor, tachycardia, and cardiac flow murmurs are nonspecific signs of anemia. Scleral icterus may suggest hemolysis or underlying liver disease. Splenomegaly or stigmata of chronic liver disease may provide additional clues to the etiology of anemia. Loss of joint position, vibration, and two-point discrimination sense in the lower extremities could suggest vitamin $B_{12}$ deficiency. A sample of stool should be tested for occult blood.

**Table 46.6 Morphologic classification of anemia: what is the MCV?**

*Microcytosis: MCV < 80 fl*
1. Iron deficiency
2. Thalassemia
3. Hemoglobin E
4. Severe anemia of chronic disease
5. Lead poisoning
6. Sideroblastic anemia

*Normochromic-normocytic: MCV 80–100 fl*
1. Anemia of chronic disease
2. Infiltrative disorders
3. Early iron deficiency
4. Sickle cell anemia and hemoglobin C
5. Bone marrow failure (aplastic anemia)

*Macrocytic: MCV > 100 fl*
1. Vitamin $B_{12}$ and folate deficiency
2. Alcohol
3. Liver disease
4. Drug induced (AZT, methotrexate, chemotherapy, anticonvulsants)
5. Myelodysplastic syndromes
6. Hypothyroidism
7. Reticulocytosis

**Laboratory testing** The laboratory diagnosis of anemia focuses on a complete blood count (CBC), platelet count, RBC indices including MCV, reticulocyte count, and review of the peripheral blood smear. This allows the clinician to categorize the anemia based on both the morphologic and kinetic classification of anemia.

## Classification of anemia

### Morphologic classification

This classification scheme uses the MCV to divide anemia into microcytic anemias (MCV < 80 fl), normochromic-normocytic anemia (MCV = 80–100 fl) and macrocytic anemia (MCV > 100 fl). Table 46.6 provides the differential diagnosis of anemia based on these morphologic classifications. The clinician should be reminded that these MCV values are somewhat arbitrary. For example, patients with early iron deficiency may have 'borderline microcytosis' with an MCV of 80–85 fl. Similarly, the differential diagnosis of macrocytosis should be considered in patients with 'borderline macrocytosis' (MCV 95–100 fl). The clinician should recognize that both macrocytic and microcytic causes of anemia can coexist (leading to a dimorphic RBC population on periph-

eral smear). Likewise, multiple causes of microcytosis (example, iron deficiency coexisting with α-thalassemia ) or multiple causes of macrocytosis can occur simultaneously.

**Microcytic anemia (MCV < 80 fl)** The differential diagnosis of microcytosis can be assessed by history, physical examination, and laboratory parameters: a severe 'chronic illness' should be evident in anemia of chronic disease causing microcytosis as should a source of blood loss for microcytic anemia due to iron deficiency. Thalassemia and hemoglobin E have a genetic and familial predisposition. The RBC indices also provide a clue to thalassemia and hemoglobin E: in contrast to iron deficiency where the RBC number is reduced, often the RBC number is normal or slightly elevated in thalassemia and Hb E. Often, the reticulocyte count is elevated in thalassemia and Hb E but may be normal in α-thalassemia trait. In contrast, both anemia of chronic disease and iron deficiency are hypoproliferative anemias characterized by normal to low reticulocyte counts.

Characteristic findings are present on the peripheral blood smear that can help differentiate causes of microcytic anemia. Iron deficiency is characterized by increased poikilocytosis with cigar-shaped cells and occasional target cells. Beta-thalassemia and α-thalassemia major are characterized by increased basophilic stippling of RBCs, increased polychromasia, and target cells.

Additional tests to evaluate microcytic anemias include the serum ferritin and a hemoglobin electrophoresis. Neither a serum iron nor total iron binding capacity is sufficiently sensitive to distinguish iron deficiency from severe anemia of chronic disease. As an acute-phase reactant, serum ferritin is elevated in anemia of chronic disease and is diminished in iron deficiency. The difficulty arises when iron deficiency coexists with anemia of chronic disease, the latter falsely elevating the ferritin from a characteristically low level up into the normal range. Using a cutoff value for ferritin of less than 100 ng/mL will successfully identify 98% of iron deficiency anemias when bone marrow iron stores are used as a gold standard.[9] As previously described, the ratio of soluble transferrin receptor to ferritin concentration may better distinguish isolated ACD from concomitant ACD with iron deficiency anemia.[9] A hemoglobin electrophoresis can identify β-thalassemic syndromes and hemoglobinopathies (Hb C, E, S) but is normal in one- and two-chain deletion variants of α-thalassemia. The hemoglobinopathies and the thalassemic syndrome, Hb constant spring, run as a separate Hb band on gel electrophoresis; beta-

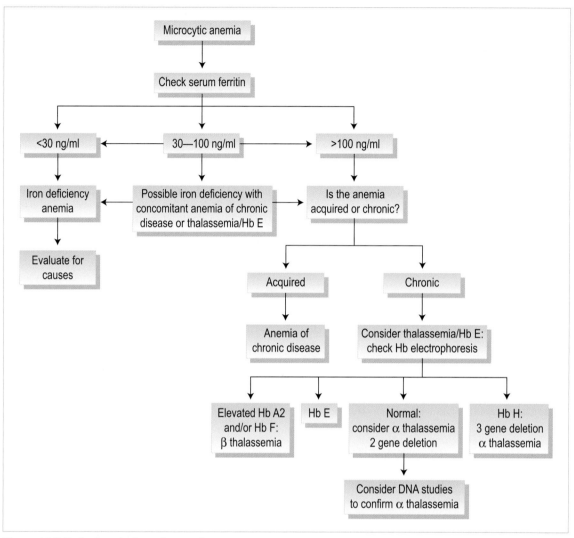

Figure 46.7 Evaluation of microcytic anemia.

thalassemia is detected by increased levels of HbA2 and HbF. Figure 46.7 provides an algorithm for evaluation of microcytic anemia.

**Normochromic-normocytic anemia (MCV 80–100 fl)** This classification is perhaps the most common category of anemia, encompassing acute blood loss and most anemia of chronic disease (it is only severe ACD that truly becomes microcytic). Early on, nutritional deficiencies such as iron, $B_{12}$, and folate deficiency are normochromic-normocytic. Infiltrating disorders of the marrow, bone marrow failure (aplastic anemia), and dimorphic (coexisting microcytosis and macrocytosis) anemias have a

normal MCV. Figure 46.8 provides an algorithm for evaluating normochromic-normocytic anemia.

**Macrocytic anemia (MCV > 100 fl)** After a history and physical examination (reviewing diet, alcohol, medications, assessing for peripheral neuropathy, etc.) a review of the peripheral blood smear is perhaps the first step to evaluating macrocytic anemias. Megaloblastosis from $B_{12}$ or folate deficiency is characterized by oval macrocytes and hypersegmentation of the neutrophils (Fig. 46.9). Vitamin deficiency can be confirmed with vitamin $B_{12}$ and folate levels; however, patients with vitamin $B_{12}$ levels in the normal range can still have 'B$_{12}$-responsive' disease. Elevated levels

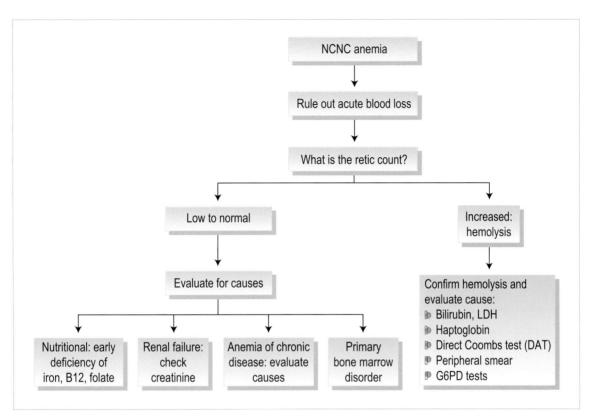

**Figure 46.8** Evaluation of normochromic normocytic (NCNC) anemia.

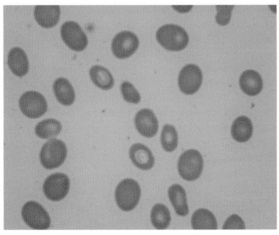

**Figure 46.9** Vitamin B$_{12}$ deficiency. The smear shows large, oval-shaped cells (oval macrocytes).

of methylmalonic acid may be a more sensitive indicator of biochemical B$_{12}$ deficiency. Dysplastic findings in the RBC, WBC, and platelet lines may be a clue to myelodysplasia (MDS) but bone marrow

biopsy and aspiration with cytogenetic analysis is required to confirm the diagnosis. Liver disease is characterized by target cells and occasionally acanthocytes and can be confirmed by history, examination, and evaluation of liver function tests. Patients with ongoing hemolysis and a compensatory reticulocytosis will have an elevated MCV; reticulocytes are larger than normal RBCs, thereby increasing the overall mean cell volume.

## The kinetic classification of anemia

Table 46.7 displays the kinetic classification in which the reticulocyte count is used to characterize anemia based on decreased RBC production, increased RBC destruction (hemolysis), or ineffective erythropoiesis.

**Hypoproliferative anemia** The reticulocyte count is low in hypoproliferative anemias. These are considered low-erythropoietin anemias where the stimulus to RBC production is reduced or where the basic building blocks for RBC production, such as iron, are unavailable.

**Table 46.7** The kinetic classification of anemia decreased production versus increased destruction: what is the reticulocyte count?

| Classification | RBC production Reticulocyte Ct | BM* | Measures of destruction Total bilirubin and LDH | Examples |
|---|---|---|---|---|
| Hypoproliferative (decreased production) | Decreased | decreased | Normal | IDA**, ACD BM failure |
| Hemolysis (increased destruction) | Increased | increased | Elevated | G6PD deficiency Immune Malaria Sickle cell |
| Ineffective erythropoiesis | Normal to increased | increased | Normal to elevated | Thalassemia MDS* $B_{12}$/folate deficiency |

* Bone marrow RBC production.

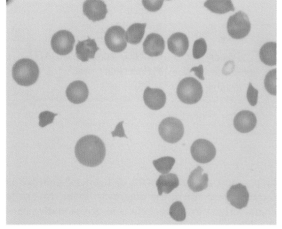

**Figure 46.10** Micro-angiopathic intravascular hemolysis from disseminated intravascular coagulation (DIC). The smear shows numerous RBC fragments and increased polychromasia (large bluish young RBCs).

**Hemolysis** Hemolysis is characterized by a compensatory reticulocytosis. The unconjugated bilirubin is elevated, as is the lactate dehydrogenase (LDH), reflecting RBC breakdown. Decreased levels of haptoglobin, a hemoglobin-binding protein that is rapidly cleared from the circulation, is a more specific indicator of RBC breakdown. There are several classification schemes of hemolysis: immune versus nonimmune, hereditary versus acquired, but perhaps the most practical categorization of hemolysis is the site of destruction: intravascular versus extravascular. Intravascular hemolysis is characterized by breakdown of RBCs in the peripheral circulation: shistocytes and fragmented cells are visible on the peripheral blood smear (Fig. 46.10). There is evidence of free hemoglobin in the serum and free hemoglobin or hemosiderin in the urine (i.e. the 'blackwater fever' of *Plasmodium falciparum* malaria or acute hemolysis in G6PD deficiency). Extravascular hemolysis is characterized by removal of circulating RBCs in the spleen. Microspherocytes are evident on the peripheral smear. RBC membrane defects and sickle cell anemia result in extravascular hemolysis and a portion of the anemia of thalassemia major (although best characterized as ineffective erythropoiesis) is due to extravascular hemolysis.

**Ineffective erythropoiesis** Ineffective erythropoiesis is characterized by intramedullary destruction of RBCs in the bone marrow. The marrow is very hypercellular compared to only a modest elevation of the reticulocyte count. Markers of RBC destruction (unconjugated bilirubin and LDH) may be elevated. The differential diagnosis includes megaloblastosis due to $B_{12}$/folate deficiency, thalassemia, and MDS.

## Pancytopenia

The differential diagnosis of pancytopenia is separated into splenomegaly causing sequestration and underlying bone marrow failure conditions. In immigrants, splenomegaly is the most common cause of pancytopenia. The differential diagnosis of splenomegaly in immigrants from developing nations is varied. It includes prior malarial or leishmaniasis infection, splenomegaly complicating thalassemia major, and portal hypertension from chronic liver disease. A number of bone marrow conditions can cause pancytopenia including $B_{12}$ and folate deficiency, MDS and aplastic anemia, leukemia, complications of HIV, and TB.

## References

1. WHO. Focusing on anemia: towards an integrated approach for effective anemia control. Geneva: World Health Organization; 2004. Available: http://www.who.int/topics/anemia/en/who_unicef-anaemiastatement.pdf November 18, 2005.
2. Jeng MR, Vichinsky E. Hematologic problems in immigrants from Southeast Asia. Hematol Oncol Clin N Am 2004; 18:1405–1422.
3. Fleming AF. Hematologic diseases. In: Strickland GT, ed. Hunter's tropical medicine and emerging infectious disease. 8th edn. Philadelphia: WB Saunders; 2000.
4. Kwiatkowski DP. How malaria has affected the human genome and what human genetics can teach us about malaria. Am J Human Genet 2005; 77:171–229.
5. Rund D, Rachmilewitz E. Beta thalassemia. N Engl J Med 2005; 353:1135–1146.
6. Angastiniotis M, Modell B. Global epidemiology of hemoglobin disorders. Ann NY Acad Sci 1998; 850:251–269.
7. Borna-Pignatti C, Galanello R. Thalassemia and related disorders. In: Greer JP, Foerster J, Lukens JN, et al., eds. Wintrobe's clinical hematology. 11th edn. Philadelphia: Lippincott Williams & Wilkins; 2004.
8. Monzon CM, Fairbanks VF, Burgert EO, et al. Hereditary red cell disorders in Southeast Asian refugees and the effect on the prevalence of thalassemia disorders in the United States. Am J Med Sci 1986; 292:147–151.
9. Weiss G, Goodnough LT. Anemia of chronic disease. N Engl J Med 2005; 352:1011–1023.
10. Lopez-Velez R, Huerga H, Turrientes MC. Infectious disease in immigrants from the perspective of a tropical medicine referral unit. Am J Trop Med Hyg 2003; 69:115–121.
11. Ekvall H. Malaria and Anemia. Curr Opin Hematol 2003; 10:108–114.
12. Claster S. Biology of anemia, differential diagnosis and treatment options in human immunodeficiency virus infection. J Infect Dis 2002; 185(Suppl 2):S105–S109.
13. Leung TN, Lau TK, Chung Tkh. Thalassemia screening in pregnancy. Curr Opin Obstet Gynecol. 2005; 17:129–134.
14. Frank JE. Diagnosis and management of G6PD deficiency. Am Fam Phys 2005; 72:1277–1282.

# Overview of the Mental Health Section

The mental health of immigrants has, as in the field of medicine generally, been relegated to secondary status as the acuity of physical and social needs predominates. It is only later, usually in resettlement, that the immigrants' psychiatric and mental illness needs receive attention. Unfortunately, these needs are often ignored. Partly, this may be due to the chronicity and interrelationship of mental illness and integration or adjustment problems and the concomitant challenges to treatment. It is a testament to the insight of the primary editors of this text that mental health is given considerable priority as a part of immigrant medicine.

This section is intended to be pragmatic and practical but based upon findings in the published literature. The intended audience is primary care practitioners in resettlement countries such as the United States, but the principles should be relevant for social workers, psychiatrists, psychologists, and other mental health professionals, and students in the primary care and mental health professions. In addition, those who work for both governmental and nongovernmental agencies, especially in reception programs, may find this section helpful. Recommended resources for additional information are listed at the end of this overview.

A number of themes and commonalities are noted throughout these chapters, regardless of context, demographics, or time factors. Among them are: (1) the prevalence of major depression and PTSD across gender, age, and ethnic groups; (2) the interrelationship of not only the individual, but also family and community; (3) the interconnection of physical, psychiatric, psychological, and social problems; (4) the central role of culture and problems with equivalence (in concepts, language, metrics, norms) which interfere with the integration of immigrants into their host societies; and (5) the persistent role of trauma and violence history in precipitating long-lasting problems with mental illness and adjustment.

The mental health section includes three chapters which discuss epidemiology and risk factors, screening in primary care settings, and mental illness diagnosis and treatment. Eisenman discusses how to approach the identification of mental health problems and a history of torture in clinical settings where these are often missed. Specific instruments are identified for use in screening. In the chapter by Kinzie et al., the focus is on mental illness in immigrants, in particular major depression and PTSD. Case examples are used extensively to illustrate issues in diagnosis and treatment.

After these overview chapters, three chapters discuss populations selected for particular emphasis. Wenzel et al. discuss survivors of torture. This topic is particularly pertinent with recent debate over the definition of torture and whether its use can ever be morally justified, such as to prevent terrorist attacks. Torture victims have many of the same mental illness and social integration problems as refugees who have been traumatized in other ways, but the very personal nature of torture requires especially sensitive approaches to interviewing and treatment. Most of the authors in the mental health section, not only in this chapter, have worked with both traumatized refugees and specifically with torture survivors, illustrating the importance of this subpopulation. Ekblad et al. discuss interpersonal violence towards women, finding that it leads to more health and mental health problems and poorer integration into host societies. Ellis and Betancourt discuss children and adolescents, who have many of the same mental health problems and integration issues as adults, but require special approaches. Treatment ideally occurs in pediatric clinics or in schools. Another population, which is not discussed in a separate chapter, is the elderly. Although elderly

625

immigrants deserve consideration as a special population, very little has been written about them.[1] Those older than 60 years comprise up to 30% of the refugees in some United Nations camps. They may be unable to meet their basic needs because of physical disability, mental impairment, loss of social support, or malnutrition.[2] Medications for chronic diseases may not be available. Access to health services may be difficult when mobility is limited. Losses after displacement can be more profound, and readjustment challenging, when the elderly have fewer future opportunities for rebuilding their lives. Carlin[3] identifies problem areas for the elderly refugee or immigrant, including: (1) separation from or loss of family members, including disapproval by younger family members who are better able to acculturate, have no time to help, and have greater authority; (2) isolation from friends and problems making new friends; (3) compromised independence because of language difficulties and illness; and (4) loss of job status and productivity with few opportunities left. Interventions should take advantage of the respected position that the elderly have in many societies and cultures, such as in conflict resolution and as heads of extended families. Training for new vocations and skills should not be restricted to the younger members of society: the elderly have much to offer.[39]

Mental health and integration are difficult for immigrants and complicated for their providers. Despite these challenges, caring for immigrants is interesting and rewarding. It is important to adopt an integrated approach to mental healthcare that moves away from just psychiatric care. Even more than for the mainstream population, the responsibility for helping the troubled immigrant falls onto primary care.

## Recommended resources

### Websites

http://www.irct.org International Rehabilitation Council for Torture Victims

http://www.UNHCR.org United Nations High Commissioner for Refugees

### Books and reviews

John P. Wilson and Boris Drozdek, eds. Broken spirits: the treatment of traumatized asylum seekers, refugees, war and torture victims. New York: Brunner-Routledge Press; 2004.

Quiroga J, Jaranson JM. Politically-motivated torture and its survivors: A desk study review of the literature. Torture 2005; 15(2,3):1–111.

Hollifield M, Warner TD, Lian N, et al. Measuring trauma and health status in refugees: a critical review. JAMA 2002; 288:611–621.

Gerrity E, Keane TM, Tuma F, eds. Refugees and asylum-seekers. The Mental Health Consequences of Torture. New York: Kluwer Academic/Plenum Publishers, 2001.

Reyes G, Jacobs GA, eds. Handbook of international disaster psychology. Vol 3. Refugee Mental Health. Westport, CT: Praeger Publishers; 2006.

Jaranson J, Popkin M, eds. Caring for victims of torture. Washington, DC: American Psychiatric Press; 1998.

### Manuals

Iacopino V, Ozkalpipci O, Schlar C. The Istanbul Protocol: Manual on the effective investigation and documentation of torture and other cruel, inhuman or degrading treatment or punishment. Geneva: Office of the United Nations High Commissioner for Human Rights; August 1999. Available: http://www.phrusa.org

Harvard Trauma Questionnaire and Hopkins Symptoms Checklist. Manual from Harvard Program in Refugee Trauma. Available: http://www.hprt-cambridge.org

### Journals

Journal of Nervous and Mental Disease, published by the University of Maryland.

Torture Journal, published by IRCT, Copenhagen.

Transcultural Psychiatry, published by McGill University, Montreal.

World Cultural Psychiatry Research Review.

## References

1. Quiroga J, Jaranson JM. Politically-motivated torture and its survivors: A desk study review of the literature. Torture 2005; 15(2,3):1–111.
2. Burton A. Older refugees in humanitarian emergencies. Lancet 2002; 360:47–48.
3. Carlin JE. Refugee and immigrant populations at special risk: women, children and the elderly. In: Holtzman WH, Bornemann TH, eds. Mental health of immigrants and refugees. Austin, Texas: Hogg Foundation for Mental Health; 1990:224–233.

# CHAPTER 47

# Epidemiology and Risk Factors

James M. Jaranson, Solvig Ekblad, Georgi V. Kroupin, and David P. Eisenman

## Introduction

The immigrant's mental health and integration into a new society are closely intertwined. Patterns of immigration have changed over time, but problems with discrimination and human rights issues often persist and/or have worsened for the immigrant. Traumatic experiences in the home country and in transit, in addition to stressors in final resettlement, are prevalent and increase the chances of developing mental illness and adjusting less successfully to the host society. The influence of these traumatic events may be temporary and manageable with straightforward solutions, or, unfortunately, may be disabling and enduring. It is important to clarify not only the most common psychopathology disorders in the target group, but also the protective and risk factors that differentiate those who are resilient from those who need professional clinical help.[1]

Prevalence and comorbidity of mental illness are discussed. Risk factors reviewed include violence, loss and separation, and socioeconomic status. Issues affecting integration, adjustment, adaptation, and acculturation are cited.

## Changing Immigration Patterns

Study of the mental health effects of immigration is often cited as beginning in the 1930s with the work of Odegaard,[2] who studied the prevalence of schizophrenia among Norwegian immigrants to Minnesota compared with a sample of Norwegians who remained in the home country. He found more schizophrenia among the immigrants, and the finding of greater mental health problems among immigrants has been common in studies of diverse populations ever since.

However, much has changed since Odegaard completed his work. Immigration has changed from predominantly Europeans to those from developing or disadvantaged countries in South America, Africa, the Middle East, Asia, and Eastern or Central Europe. This has meant far greater linguistic, cultural, and religious differences from the mainstream population. Reasons for immigrating have also changed. More are likely to be emigrating because of fear and traumatic experiences than only for economic advantage. Although economic migrants flow across the southern border of the US, many refugees and asylum seekers have left their home countries after experiencing torture or other influential traumatic events. While few in the early part of the twentieth century sought refuge from persecution, many immigrants are now refugees, asylum seekers, or otherwise undocumented immigrants who have been traumatized. The phases of immigration have also become more complicated. Rather than traveling from the home country to the country of final resettlement, many immigrants now have long transitional periods in intermediate countries or refugee camps prior to reaching their final destination. These transitional periods are often filled with stressors, danger, and traumatic experiences in their own right.[3] Intermediate immigration status, e.g. being an undocumented or asylum applicant, may exacerbate mental health problems.[4,5] Final resettlement usually involves poverty, anti-immigrant sentiment, and discrimination based on racial, ethnic, gender, or religious identity. This is further complicated by the increase in terrorism worldwide, and authorities in resettlement countries are becoming more fearful of those who emigrate from countries where terrorists reside.

Consequently, all of these changes in immigration have implications for potentially increased problems with mental health and integration for immigrant populations. Questions which still require answers are how frequent is mental illness in each phase of migration, what are the precipitants, and what can we do to help minimize the occurrence of mental illness for immigrants?

## Prevalence of Selected Psychiatric Disorders

High rates of mental health problems have been well documented in various refugee and immigrant groups. Most studies demonstrate a high prevalence of post-traumatic stress, anxiety, depression, and somatization.[6-9] Wide variations reported in the prevalence of post-traumatic stress disorder (PTSD) (4–86%) and depression (5–31%), for instance, may be ascribed to a number of factors affecting refugees before migration, in the process of flight, and during and after the resettlement, as well as to differences in data collection, analysis, and interpretation. Porter and Haslam[10] used a worldwide study sample in a meta-analysis, compared refugees with nonrefugee comparison groups and concluded that the sociopolitical context of the refugee experience is associated with refugee mental health and humanitarian activities that influence these conditions positively.

### Comorbidity

Many refugees suffer from multiple mental health problems. Patients with PTSD are also frequently diagnosed with major depressive disorder (MDD). Marshall et al.[11] found high comorbidity between these disorders: 71% of subjects in their study who had PTSD also met criteria for MDD, and 86% of

those with major depression met criteria for PTSD. They also reported high comparability in risk factors for depression and PTSD.

While PTSD and comorbid PTSD/depression have similar clinical presentation, results of some studies support the existence of depression as a separate clinical entity.[12] According to these authors, major depression and PTSD are independent sequelae of traumatic events, which have similar prognosis, and interact to increase distress and dysfunction. In one study, patients with comorbid MDD and PTSD were more likely to attempt suicide, and women with both disorders were more likely to attempt suicide than men with the same diagnosis.[13]

High rates of mental health problems are reported both in newly arrived asylum seekers and refugees and in those who resettled many years ago. In a prospective study of mass evacuated Kosovo Albanians, participants with PTSD had significantly lower cortisol levels. Depressive symptoms and aggression followed the same pattern as PTSD, with increasing symptom levels, while sense of coherence scores decreased. Women had worse outcomes regarding both PTSD and depression.[14-16] Aggression among refugees is often neglected in the clinical context. In Western-oriented culture, depression is more acceptable. Thus, aggression in traumatized populations, especially its consequences, needs to be evaluated in more detail. Specifically, Carlson and Rosser-Hogan[17] reported that a high proportion of recently arrived Cambodian refugees suffer from severe psychiatric symptoms (86% PTSD; 96% high dissociation scores; 80% clinical depression), and there is a relationship between the amount of trauma they experienced and the severity of these symptoms.

At the same time, Marshall et al.[11] found that two decades after the end of the Cambodian War and resettlement of refugees in the United States, Cambodians continued to have high rates of psychiatric disorders associated with trauma. In their study, 62% of Cambodian refugees who came to the United States 20 years ago met DSM-IV diagnostic criteria for PTSD in the past year and 51% met diagnostic criteria for MDD.

### Risk Factors

Mental health problems may come just as much from how refugees are approached in the resettlement country as from their past, although in most cases they tend to be attributed to their past experiences. Below, we consider several factors affecting refugees' mental health in all stages of their refugee experience.

## Violence

Of particular concern is political violence. Whether occurring overtly through war and armed conflict, or covertly through the sustained and institutionalized repression of a group of people, political violence includes many violence types such as war-related violence, torture, sexual violence, forced disappearances, and extrajudicial killings. Many, if not most, refugees and asylum seekers have experienced significant pre-migration political violence, including torture, as evidenced by prevalence studies in clinics and community samples.[5,18-21]

In a systematic sample of Latino immigrant adults attending three community-based primary care clinics in Los Angeles, Eisenman and colleagues[22] found that, overall, 54% screened positive for political violence exposure: 8% reported torture, 15% witnessed violence against their family, 27% reported forced disappearance of family members, 26% witnessed mass violence, and 32% reported their life endangered by attacks with bombs or heavy weapons. Five percent reported witnessing torture or an execution and 3% (6 women and 1 man) reported being raped. These results are consistent with earlier estimates from one urban medical clinic in New York City in which 6% of all foreign-born patients had experienced political torture.[23] These estimates are not surprising given that immigrants and refugees widely use public health clinics.[24] These groups experience similarly high rates of intimate partner violence[25] and community violence.[26]

Torture's effect may be additive to other forms of trauma. Jaranson et al.,[9] in their study of Somali and Oromo refugees in Minnesota, reported that in their sample torture survivors were more likely than other refugees to experience physical and psychological problems. Jaranson et al. found torture prevalence ranged from 25% to 69% by ethnicity and gender, higher than usually reported, and torture survivors had more physical and mental health problems.

One of the surprising findings in Jaranson's study was the relationship between gender and torture prevalence. Although it is commonly assumed that men are the primary target of organized violence and experience more psychological problems, some studies of the relationship between gender and trauma yield different results. Specifically, in the above-mentioned study, women were found to be as likely subjected to torture as men. As an example from clinical experience, Vietnamese men who were exposed to the most horrific forms of torture in concentration camps following the Vietnam War usually were the ones who were granted political asylum in the United States through the 'Humanitarian Operation' program. In the meantime, the ordeals their wives had to go through remained to a large degree unnoticed until recently. Gender differences for psychiatric vulnerability among traumatized populations require further investigation for their relationship both to trauma and to psychosocial factors.

## Loss and separation

Often, refugees come from cultures where families and other relatives, not individuals, are the primary social units. The family also has economic responsibility for its members, equivalent to social welfare in some Western societies. In addition, refugees frequently have an economic responsibility for the family members left behind, which may increase the post-migration stress. The topic of loss of roots, and loss of connection to cultural and social traditions, deserves a book, and some have been written. The very fabric of social connection may be broken beyond repair. One author (GVK) had a Russian female patient who said that she now didn't care much how she looked – the opinion of these foreign people in the streets didn't matter much to her.

Loss of family members and close friends, and the commonly prolonged separation from them, has a most profound effect on refugees' health and ability to adapt to a new life by damaging their very roots. Often, patients still have close family members who were left behind and are still exposed to life-threatening risks. As a result, many patients can't even start recovering from trauma because they are still exposed to it.

On an individual level, forced migration results in many, often irreversible, losses. Although few refugees were wealthy people in their own countries, even those who didn't own much often lost their homes, their personal belongings, things that made up everyday life. Some refugees were highly educated and had professional careers only to lose the value of those careers in the process of immigration because degrees, training, and other qualifications gained in other countries were not accepted in the destination country. A direct result of the above changes is a feeling of a profound loss of social status and self-esteem. Many feel that their lives have been useless.

Dealing with issues of trauma, loss (e.g. land, climate, traditions, food, home, family and relatives, social status, material issues, etc.) and separation presents major challenges both for primary care providers and for mental health specialists. The mental health literature presents a wide variety of useful constructive approaches focused on coping skills and adjustment.[27] However, the authors think that therapeutic intervention requires acknowledging and helping refugees deal with the irreversible losses that so many have suffered. Acknowledging that both visible and invisible wounds from these losses may never heal is essential for developing trust in the patient–provider relationship and for successful collaborative work in the future. Culturally sensitive and responsive assessment and treatment models which mix individual and community interventions are essential.[28]

## Socioeconomic factors

Studies of the influence of socioeconomic factors on the severity of mental health problems yield conflicting results. Most studies confirm that lower socioeconomic status (SES), retirement, disability, unemployment, and integration problems make refugees more vulnerable to trauma and its negative effects, including psychiatric symptoms.[29,30] Exposure of immigrants to various traumatic experiences including violence in their new country, in part as a consequence of their lower SES, can be a major contributing factor to their mental health problems. In their study of Cambodians, Marshall et al.[11] found significant rates of exposure to violence in the United States. In their sample, 34% of individuals reported seeing a dead body in their neighborhood, 28% reported having been robbed, and 17% reported having been threatened by a weapon and believing that they might be seriously hurt or killed. However, other authors such as Jaranson et al.[9] did not find a meaningful association between socioeconomic/adjustment factors (high school education, employment and marriage) and the number of psychological problems.

## Integration, acculturation, and adjustment

Among major challenges immigrants and refugees face upon arrival in their new country are language proficiency and other social integration problems,

loss of connection to social traditions, marital problems, and intergenerational conflicts.

Many immigrants, whether highly educated or not, struggle with language and basic communication skills. One can only imagine the damage to self-esteem when an adult person who was competent and confident in his previous life has to get by with a vocabulary of a 3-year-old child and whose intellect is often judged solely by that. The resulting loss of ease of communication and self-sufficiency is hard to overestimate. The single most anxiety provoking moment of the day, e.g. for many educated refugees and immigrants, is a trip to their mailbox. Many times they cannot tell the difference between junk mail and important letters that significantly affect their lives, and they have to wait several days for somebody who knows English to sort through their mail.

Understandably, rates of acculturation are much higher in second-generation refugees.[31] In the most dramatic cases, children as young as 7–9 years old may be the only English-literate family members and consequently are given an immense responsibility to mediate most family interactions with their social environment. The resulting role reversal often leads to parenting crises. In some of the authors' clinical practice, the biggest contributing factor to depression in Hmong women is their powerlessness in parenting their adolescent children.

Although motivation for achievement is high in most immigrant groups, it is mostly younger or/and second-generation refugees who have or can obtain marketable skills and education. Consequently, the physical and emotional gap between the generations increases and family relationships deteriorate. Aging parents who immigrated 'for the sake of children' struggle to 'reinvent' the meaning of their immigration and go through a profound identity crisis.[32]

Immigration presents serious challenges for marital relationships as it brings significant changes in the foundations of marriage. In many traditional cultures, marriages are still more or less arranged, and divorces are rare due to the strong influence of kin and social pressure. Of course, this depends upon how integrated the parents are into their new society. In a new country, the dissolution of many families occurs as forces that kept those families together disappear and they experience major changes in power structure.

Loss of competence, powerlessness, and deterioration of marital and family relationships have a profoundly negative effect on refugee mental health. Among the most important consequences are sharp increases in mental health problems, such as major depression and anxiety, and significant problems in refugees' access to healthcare and utilization of available healthcare services.

While in most cases the emphasis is put on challenges of adapting to a new culture, a number of studies demonstrate that adherence to the original culture can be a resilience factor. Holman et al.[29] found worsening of psychiatric health indices as acculturation into US society increases. Kleinman[33] suggests that lower rates of depression in some immigrant groups compared to their descendants may be seen as evidence that adherence to some aspects of the original culture may serve as protective factors rather than risk factors. In a quantitative review approaching meta-analysis, Ekblad, Belkic and Eriksson[34] found that contact and identification with both the indigenous and host cultures represented the optimal combination for integration and mental well-being. Escobar[35] suggests that strengths such as traditional norms, family structure, and social support may protect individuals against developing psychiatric disorders. Reyes[36] noted that, 'An abundance of intervention programs have been implemented in major American cities to assist refugees with psychosocial concerns, some of which have become particularly influential examples of innovation. Among those is a program in Chicago[37] that employs family therapy and other techniques to apply a framework of intervening with groups composed of multiple families.'

## References

1. Silove D, Ekblad S, Mollica R. Health and human rights. The rights of the severely mentally ill in post-conflict societies. Invited Lancet commentary 2000; 355(9214):1548–1549.
2. Odegaard O. Emigration and insanity. Acta Psychiatry Neurolog Scand 1932; Supplementum 4:1–206.
3. Ward J, Vann B. Gender-based violence in refugee settings. Lancet 2002;. 360(Suppl 1):13–14.
4. Silove D, Steel Z, Watters C. Policies of deterrence and the mental health of asylum seekers. JAMA 2000; 284:604–611.
5. Silove D, Sinnerbrink I, Field A, et al. Anxiety, depression and PTSD in asylum seekers: associations with pre-migration trauma and post-migration stressors. Br J Psychiatry 1997; 170:352–357.
6. Cervantes RC, Salgado de Snyder VN, Padilla AM. Posttraumatic stress in immigrants from Central America and Mexico. Hospit Comm Psychiatr 1989; 40(6):615–619.
7. Mollica RF, Poole C, Son L, et al. Effects of war trauma on Cambodian refugee adolescents' functional health and mental health status. J AM Acad Child Adolesc Psychiatry 1997; 36(8):1098–1106.
8. Holtz TH. Refugee trauma versus torture trauma: a retrospective controlled cohort study of Tibetan refugees. J Nerv Mental Dis 1998; 186(1):24–34.
9. Jaranson JM, Butcher J, Halcon L, et al. Somali and Oromo refugees: correlates of torture and trauma history. Am J Public Health. 2004; 94(4):591–598.
10. Porter M, Haslam N. Predisplacement and postdisplacement factors associated with mental health of refugees and internally displaced persons: a meta-analysis. JAMA 2005: 294(5):602–612.
11. Marshall GN, Schell TL, Elliott MN, et al. Mental health of Cambodian refugees 2 decades after resettlement in the United States. JAMA 2005; 294(5):571–579.
12. O'Donnell M L, Creamer M, Pattison P. Posttraumatic stress disorder and depression following trauma: understanding comorbidity. Am J Psychiatry 2004; 161(8):1390–1396.
13. Oquendo MA, Friend JM, Halberstam B, et al. Association of comorbid posttraumatic stress disorder and major depression with greater risk for suicidal behavior. Am J Psychiatry 2003; 160(3):580–582.
14. Roth G, Ekblad S. A longitudinal perspective on depression and sense of coherence – in a sample of mass-evacuated adults from Kosovo. Brief reports. J Nerv Mental Dis 2006; 194(5):378–381.
15. Roth G, Ekblad S, Prochazka H. A longitudinal study of self-rated aggression in a sample of adult mass-evacuated Kosovars; Submitted.
16. Roth G, Ekblad S, Ågren H. A longitudinal study of PTSD in a sample of mass-evacuated Kosovars, some of whom return to their home country. Eur Psychiatry; in press.
17. Carlson EB, Rosser-Hogan R. Trauma experiences, posttraumatic stress, dissociation, and depression in Cambodian refugees. Am J Psychiatry 1991; 148: 1548–1551.
18. Cunningham M, Cunningham JD. Patterns of symptomatology and patterns of torture and trauma experiences in resettled refugees. Austr NZ J Psychiatry 1997; 31(4):555–565.
19. Mollica RF, McInnes K, Sarajlic N, et al. Disability associated with psychiatric comorbidity and health status in Bosnian refugees living in Croatia. JAMA 1999; 282(5):433–439.
20. Shrestha NM, Sharma B, Van Ommeren M, et al. Impact of torture on refugees displaced within the developing world: symptomatology among Bhutanese refugees in Nepal. JAMA 1998; 280(5):443–448.
21. Allden K, Poole C, Chantavanich S, et al. Burmese political dissidents in Thailand: trauma and survival among young adults in exile. Am J Public Health 1996; 86(11):1561–1569.
22. Eisenman DP, Gelberg L, Liu H, et al. Mental health and health-related quality of life among adult Latino primary care patients living in the United States with previous exposure to political violence. JAMA 2003; 290(5):627–634.
23. Eisenman DP, Keller AS, Kim G. Survivors of torture in a general medical setting: how often have patients been tortured, and how often is it missed? West J Med 2000; 172(5):301–304.
24. Westermeyer J, Williams CL, Nguyen AN. Mental health services for refugees. Vol DHHS: Washington DC: US Government Printing Office; 1991.
25. Bauer HM, Rodriguez MA, Perez-Stable EJ. Prevalence and determinants of intimate partner abuse among public hospital primary care patients. J Gen Intern Med 2000; 15(11):811–817.
26. Shen H, Sorenson SB, Upchurch DM. Violence and injury in marital arguments: risk patterns and gender differences. Am J Public Health 1996; 86(1):35–40.
27. Williams MB, Poijula S. The PTSD workbook: simple, effective techniques for overcoming traumatic stress symptoms. Oakland, CA: New Harbinger Publications; 2002.
28. Silove D. The impact of mass psychosocial trauma on psychosocial adaptation among refugees In: Reyes G, Jacobs GA, eds. Handbook of international disaster psychology. Vol 3. Refugee Mental Health. Westport, CT: Praeger; 2006:1–17.
29. Holman EA, Silver RC, Waitzkin H. Traumatic life events in primary care patients: a study in an ethnically diverse sample. Arch Fam Med 2000; 9(9):802–810.

30. Savin, D, Seymour DJ, Littleford LN, et al. Findings from mental health screening of newly arrived refugees in Colorado. Public Health Reports 2005; 120(3):224–229.

31. Portes A, Rumbaut RG. Immigrant America: A portrait. 2nd edn. Berkley, CA: University of California Press; 1996.

32. Gates R, Esnaola SA, Kroupin G, et al. Diversity of new American families: guidelines for therapists. In: Nichols WC, Pace-Nichols MA, Becvar DS, et al., eds. Handbook of family development and intervention. New York: Wiley; 2000:299–322.

33. Kleinman A. Culture and depression. N England J Med 2004; 351:951–953.

34. Ekblad S, Belkic K, Eriksson N-G. Health and disease among refugees and immigrants. a quantitative review approaching meta-analysis. Implications for clinical practice and perspectives for further research. Part I: Mental health outcomes. National Institute for Psychosocial Medicine, Karolinska Institutet, section for stress research, Stockholm, Stress Research Reports number 267, 1996.

35. Escobar J. Immigration and mental health: why are immigrants better off? Arch Gen Psychiatry 1998; 55:781–782.

36. Reyes G. Overview of the international disaster psychology volumes In: Reyes G, Jacobs GA, eds. Handbook of international disaster psychology. Vol 1. Fundamentals and overview. Westport, CT: Praeger; 2006:xxi–xxxiv.

37. Raina D, Weine S, Kulauzovic Y, et al. A framework for developing and implementing multiple-family groups for refugee families. In: Reyes G, Jacobs GA, eds. Handbook of international disaster psychology. Vol 3. Refugee Mental Health. Westport, CT: Praeger; 2006. 37–64.

# CHAPTER 48

# Screening for Mental Health Problems and History of Torture

David P. Eisenman

## Screening for Mental Health Problems

Primary care clinicians may encounter refugees in a variety of settings delivering primary healthcare services, including community- and hospital-based ambulatory care clinics, public health screening programs, school-based programs, and resettlement agency programs. Evidence for screening – defined here as the early identification of patients with unsuspected and remediable mental health disorders – in any of these service settings is slowly developing. From an evidence-based medicine and public health perspective, screening must be shown to fulfill several criteria. These criteria include: (1) that the screening detects important and treatable disorders; (2) that screening instruments exist that are effective, practical, and acceptable to both patient and provider; and (3) that the screening is effective in routine practice settings, not only in research settings. As discussed elsewhere in this book, the mental health disorders that clinicians might screen for, such as major depression, are prevalent and treatable. However, fulfilling the second and third criteria remains problematic and forms the subject of this chapter.

## Mental Health Instruments

Primary care providers working with immigrants and refugees may select from a wide variety of instruments to assess for mental health problems (Table 48.1).[1-4]

Unfortunately, no instrument has been studied in all the refugee populations that primary care providers will encounter. Choices among instruments include language availability, domains of interest (depression, anxiety, and post-traumatic stress disorder), length, and evidence basis in the target population. For instance, if clinicians are caring for Spanish-language immigrants, modules of the PRIME-MD[7] and the Post-traumatic Stress Checklist–Civilian[8,9] may be useful. Other instruments commonly used in refugee populations include part 4 of the self-report Harvard Trauma Questionnaire (HTQ),[10] the 25-item Hopkins Symptom Checklist (HSCL-25),[11] and the Impact of Events Scale (IES).[12] The HTQ lists 30 symptom items, 16 coming from the *Diagnostic and Statistical Manual of Mental Disorders, Revised Third Edition (DSM-III-R)* criteria for PTSD. However, its sensitivity and specificity in community samples is 16% and 100%, respectively, and it is unknown in primary care populations.[13] The HSCL-25, a self-administered questionnaire originally designed to measure symptom changes in anxiety and depression, has been validated in the general US population and has good reliability and validity in clinical refugee samples. An average-item score greater than 1.75 indicates clinically significant distress. The Impact of Events Scale has been used to screen for PTSD; it has 15 items on 3-point descriptive scales measuring intrusive thoughts and somatic sensations and avoidance behaviors after trauma.

**Table 48.1 Selected instruments for assessing refugee mental health in primary care settings[1-3]**

| Measurement subject | Languages translated | Validity/reliability testing in any refugee groups |
|---|---|---|
| **PTSD** | | |
| Harvard Trauma Questionnaire (HTQ) | Bosnian, Cambodian, English, Dari, Khmer, Laotian, Vietnamese | Yes |
| Impact of Events Scale (IES) | Spanish, Serbo-Croatian, English | Validity, yes; reliability, no |
| Post-traumatic Stress Checklist-Civilian | Spanish, English | Yes |
| Clinician-Administered PTSD Scale (CAPS) | English, Farsi, Pashto | Yes |
| DSM-IIIR PTSD Checklist | Cambodian, English, Laotian, Vietnamese | Validity, no; reliability, yes |
| **Anxiety** | | |
| Hopkins Symptom Checklist (HSCL-25) | Amharic, Bosnian, Cambodian, Dari, English, Khmer, Laotian, Pashto, Tibetan, Vietnamese | Yes |
| Health Opinion Survey | English, Khmer, Laotian, Persian, Spanish, Vietnamese | No |
| PRIME-MD | English, Spanish | No |
| Anxiety disorder module of the Structured Clinical Interview for DSM-IV (SCID) | Spanish, Vietnamese, English | Yes |
| **Depression** | | |
| Hopkins Symptom Checklist, Depression (HSCL-25) | See Anxiety | |
| Zung Depression Scale | Cantonese, English, Hmong, Laotian | Validity, no; reliability, yes |
| Hamilton Depression Rating Scale (HAM-D) | English, German, Russian | No |
| Beck Depression Inventory (BDI) | Dari, English, Hebrew, Pashto, Turkish, Russian | Yes |
| CES-D | Bosnian, Chinese, English, Hebrew, Pashto, Russian, Turkish, Korean, Portuguese, Spanish, Vietnamese | Validity, no; reliability, yes |
| PRIME-MD | See anxiety | |
| Vietnamese Depression Scale (VDS) | Vietnamese, English | Yes |

## Inquiring About a History of Torture

When a mental disorder such as depression or PTSD is diagnosed, primary care providers should inquire about traumatic exposures and human rights violations that may be associated with the disorder. Where such events, such as torture, are reported, it is important to document the events and the resulting mental health problems to support legal claims.[14] This includes asking for details of trauma exposure as well as documenting physical, emotional, and mental health evidence of torture or abuse. Linkages with other health professionals, including professional organizations, local human rights organizations, and international partnerships can be important in addressing this forensic documentation.[15] Organizations such as Physicians for Human Rights (http://www.phrusa.org/) and Doctors without Borders (http://www.doctorswithoutborders.org/) can provide training, resource materials, and even services that assist primary care providers document the effects of torture and abuse. Documentation should only occur if agreed to by the patient.

While often there is an expectation that diagnostic processes may be complicated due to patients' reluctance to speak about their traumatic experiences, in fact patients are usually accepting of physicians' inquiries about violence exposure. Furthermore, research shows that, in the process of screening, refugees are often willing to let health professionals know they are suffering and accept help in the form of mental health intervention.[16,17]

Choosing among trauma detection instruments for use in primary care settings runs into the same gamut of limitations and choices found in choosing among mental health instruments. Trauma detection instruments vary in their length, the completeness of the potential traumas covered, their applicability across cultures, countries, genders, and ages, and their validity and reliability. For example, the Harvard Trauma Questionnaire has been used with multicultural populations as well as specific-country populations (Cambodian, Laotian, Vietnamese, Bosnian) and translated into these and other languages. However, general trauma experiences of women are not well represented, such as traumas to reproductive health, pregnancy, and postpartum outcomes, and the obligation to give sexual favors in return for food, safety, or immigration documents.

Recommendations for torture detection instruments in research settings are that they utilize a 'checklist' approach that includes specific torture and trauma events to determine exposure to torture.[18] This avoids the problem of differing conceptualizations of torture that may exist between cultures. Several traumatic event checklists are available, each developed for a different cultural group with different trauma events. To date, no screening instrument has been tested and validated for its ability to identify persons with a history of torture in primary care settings. Previous studies have used the Harvard Trauma Questionnaire (HTQ) to measure whether or not participants had experienced torture.[10] The HTQ was designed to empirically measure trauma events and PTSD in Indochinese patients referred to a specialty mental heath clinic. It has one item inquiring about a history of torture, embedded within 17 items chosen to be historically accurate for this population's trauma experience. Although the health components of the HTQ have been validated, the torture items have not yet been validated. The HTQ validation study sample, moreover, had a known high prior probability of exposure, and thus the effect of spectrum bias on particular items is uncertain.

Since this study was not conducted in populations that are representative of general clinic populations, we designed and tested a single item inquiring about a history of exposure to torture. Our objective was to validate the use of one question regarding a first-hand experience of torture that is embedded in a context of rapport-building and context-setting questions. We developed the Detection of Torture Survivors Survey (DOTSS) to accurately identify individuals who have been exposed to torture in the heterogeneous populations that attend ambulatory care clinics.[19]

Ambulatory care clinicians interested in detecting survivors of torture among their patients face a dilemma. On the one hand, no single 'event-specific' instrument, such as the HTQ, is appropriate for inquiring about torture in settings with patients from many countries. On the other hand, a checklist of all possible experiences of trauma and torture would be too long if developed for use as a detection tool in a culturally heterogeneous population. Moreover, when individuals visit an ambulatory care clinic where the primary focus of treatment is not torture related, but rather for a medical complaint or emergency, a contextual framework is necessary to provide understanding and a foundation to further query the individual about the experience of torture. The DOTSS offers an alternative by allowing for the common conceptualization of torture that exists between many cultures and embedding the relevant item in contextual statements and questions designed to overcome cultural and torture-related barriers to detection, such as shame and isolation.

Items for the DOTSS were generated by researchers and clinicians from the Bellevue/NYU Program for Survivors of Torture, a program which provides multidisciplinary care to survivors of torture and their families. The DOTSS provides a sequence of questioning that builds a contextual foundation for specific querying about torture. The assessment begins with a statement of why this is of interest to the clinician in order to facilitate the patient's comfort and reduce any fear about the reason for the inquiry. The initial questions are general, asking about any problems that may have occurred in the former country because of religion, political beliefs, or culture, or if any trouble occurred with persons working for the government, military, or police. After this general querying, the individual is asked more specific questions related to torture. This framework builds a foundation for the more specific torture questions to be asked and allows for a natural, conversational flow to the interview.

Data were collected from a convenience sample of foreign-born adult patients (born outside of the United States and US territories) who presented to the emergency department or adult primary care clinic. Patients with altered mental status, or located in the critical care section of the emergency department, were excluded. Interviews were performed in English or Spanish, and interpreters were provided for other languages when necessary.

Inter-rater reliability was determined by having both research assistants score responses to the assessment instruments at the same time. Convergent validity was examined using the Harvard Trauma Questionnaire (HTQ) to determine the presence or absence of a history of torture. This scale was selected as a comparative measure since it currently serves as a screening tool for measuring torture events and trauma. Participants also underwent a blinded in-depth clinical interview to determine criterion validity. The blinded interviewers were all drawn from the clinical staff of the Bellevue/NYU Program for Survivors of Torture and are all trained physicians or psychologists with several years of diagnostic, therapeutic, and research experience with torture. A clinical reference was chosen for criterion validity because a prior study found a clinical interview to have good diagnostic accuracy for defining exposure to torture.[20] The clinical assessment determined whether the participant had been tortured as defined by the World Medical Association, Declaration of Tokyo, which states that torture is: '... the deliberate, systematic or wanton infliction of physical or mental suffering by one or more persons acting alone or on the orders of any authority, to force another person to yield information, to make a confession or for any other reason.'[21] Final clinical assessment of expo-sure to torture was made after discussion with the study investigators. In no cases did the clinical interview or study investigators disagree on exposure status.

The sample consisted of 26 men and 16 women. They were born in 28 countries, represented 7 religious affiliations (including 'no religion'), and were in the United States an average (±SD) of 14.3 ± 10.8 years. The mean age of the entire sample was 44.5 ± 13.5 years, and their average level of education was 11.7 ± 4.4 years. All 42 participated in the study of reliability and convergent validity. Thirty-eight of 42 were included in the analysis of criterion validity, because clinical interviews were not collected on four study participants.

The degree of agreement between the two raters on the DOTSS was determined with Kappa coefficients of inter-rater reliability. The mean Kappa coefficient for the 16 DOTSS items (including DOTSS sub-items) was 0.94 ± 0.09 (range = 0.78–1.00). Results of the blinded, in-depth clinical interview were compared to answers from the 9 DOTSS-base items to evaluate the success of the DOTSS as a screening instrument for a history of torture. 'Were you ever a victim of torture?' was highly predictive of torture/ not tortured status on the basis of the blinded in-depth clinical interview (Table 48.2). In fact, this item correctly classified 37 out of 38 cases (LR+ = 28). The success of the DOTSS as a screening instrument for assessing exposure to torture is demonstrated by its convergent validity with the HTQ. The association between total scores on the DOTSS and HTQ was

**Table 48.2 Sensitivity, specificity, predictive values, and likelihood ratios of the detection of torture survivors survey (DOTSS) items (n = 38)**

Introduction: In this clinic we see many patients who have been forced to leave their countries because of violence or threats to the health and safety of patients and their families. I am going to ask you some questions about this.

| DOTSS item | n | Sensitivity | Specificity | PV+ | PV− | LR+ | LR− |
|---|---|---|---|---|---|---|---|
| 1. In (your former country), did you ever have problems because of religion, political beliefs, culture, or any other reason? | 37 | 0.90 | 0.78 | 0.68 | 0.95 | 4.05 | 0.13 |
| 2. Did you have any problems with persons working for the government, military, police, or any other group? | 37 | 0.89 | 0.82 | 0.62 | 0.96 | 4.98 | 0.14 |
| 3. Were you ever a victim of violence in (your former country)? | 38 | 1.00 | 0.86 | 0.71 | 1.00 | 7.00 | 0.00 |
| 4. Were you ever a victim of torture in (your former country)? | 38 | 1.00 | 0.96 | 0.91 | 1.00 | 28.00 | 0.00 |

PV+, predictive value for positive event; PV−, predictive value for negative event; LR+, likelihood ratio for positive event; LR−, likelihood ratio for negative event; n, number of subjects responding to individual DOTSS item.

examined by calculating a Pearson correlation ($r = 0.94$, $p < .0001$, $n = 39$). This correlation indicates that high total scores on the DOTSS were associated with high total scores on the HTQ.

Results indicate that the DOTSS is a reliable instrument across raters and is valid for distinguishing a history of exposure to torture from the absence of exposure to torture. The DOTSS can be used in order to screen for torture among the heterogeneous nationalities attending primary care clinics. For those clinicians who do not want to routinely use all four items of the DOTSS, the following abbreviated question could be useful if added to routine history taking in the clinical setting: 'In this clinic we see many patients who have been forced to leave their countries because of violence or threats to the health and safety of patients and their families. I am going to ask you a question about this. Were you ever a victim of violence or torture in (your former country)?'

## Feasibility of Mental Health Screening in the Office

The feasibility of mental health screening encounters significant obstacles at the level of the provider, the patient, and the practice setting. From the provider's perspective, the two most common practical barriers to screening for mental health problems in refugees in primary care are lack of time and absence of culturally sensitive and language-specific screening instruments. Overcoming patients' reluctance to be screened for mental health issues is an especially difficult issue in refugee health. Screening by physicians or within a medical office runs the risk of intimidating refugees frightened by the stigmatization and potential implications of the questions. Refugees may be frightened, for instance, that they will be deported or unable to get work if found 'crazy.' At the practice level, it is important that refugees with positive screens are able to obtain treatment. Clinicians who are comfortable with treating these disorders must be available and should have a basic understanding of ethnopsychopharmacology, or, alternatively, refugees with positive screens should have access to mental health services not co-located with primary care. Such mental health services may be more difficult to obtain than co-located services due to structural barriers (lack of transportation, child care, cost) and may not provide services in the appropriate languages or with the requisite knowledge of the refugee's culture, including their traditions, beliefs, and values.

## To Screen or not to Screen?

There is currently insufficient evidence to definitively recommend clinic-wide screening of refugees and immigrants for the prevalent, disabling, and treatable mental health disorders, such as major depression and post-traumatic stress disorder. Still, given the known high incidence of major depression and PTSD in refugee populations, it makes sense to support routine inquiry for these disorders in primary care. Although screening tools generally do not provide much information on functional impact of mental health problems, their simplicity makes it feasible for primary care providers to integrate the quantitative measures into a qualitative clinical interview, thereby enhancing the validity of their overall assessment. Clinicians cannot make accurate diagnoses or treatment plans in other arenas without knowing about the behavior-related problems of their patients; not assessing for the presence of depression in a patient's life is like ignoring the fact that he is homeless and HIV positive. All the information we get from patients, their differentials, and their treatment plans are influenced by psychiatric diseases such as depression. Assessing and treating these disorders early likely decreases clinic visits, reduces somatic complaints and unnecessary work-ups, and generally reduces the clinician's workload.

Since refugees often present with somatic complaints without a physiological basis, completion of the physical work-up may provide a good opportunity to gently inquire about mental health symptoms. Instead of routinely screening all refugee patients as they come into the clinic, it may be better to routinely assess all refugee patients for mental health problems and traumas after completion of the medical evaluation or after a trusting relationship between patient and regular provider has been built. An alternative, if at all possible, is to have the mental health assessment done in the patient's home if home visits are available to the refugee community.

## Conclusion

Routinely assessing for mental health disorders is critical to high-quality primary care practice. A variety of instruments are available for helping clinicians assess patients for mental health problems in selected language groups. Especially if PTSD is diagnosed, understanding the types of traumas experi-

## Box 48.1
### Key messages

- The prevalence of treatable mental health disorders is higher in refugees than in native-born persons.
- Primary care providers should routinely inquire about these mental health disorders.
- Inquiry within the context of routine evaluation is recommended.
- Refugees are often receptive to culturally sensitive screening questions in the context of a trusting primary care relationship.
- Validated screening tools exist for specific disorders in several languages.
- The DOTSS is a valid screening tool for detecting torture survivors in primary care. A single validated question, 'Were you ever a victim of torture?' may be useful in the appropriate clinical setting.

enced is important and a single question from the Detection of Torture Survivors Survey (DOTSS), when delivered in the context of rapport building statements and questions, may be useful for inquiring about a history of torture (Box 48.1).

## References

1. Jaranson J, Quiroga J. Politically motivated torture and its survivors: A desk study review of the literature. Torture 2005; 16:2–3.
2. Gagnon AJ, Tuck J, Barkun L. A systematic review of questionnaires measuring the health of resettling refugee women. Health Care Women Int 2004; 25(2):111–149.
3. Hollifield M, Warner TD, Lian N, et al. Measuring trauma and health status in refugees: a critical review. JAMA 2002; 288(5):611–621.
4. Kroenke K, Spitzer RL, Williams JB. The PHQ-9: validity of a brief depression severity measure. J Gen Intern Med 2001; 16:606–613.
5. Shedler J, Beck A, Bensen S. Practical mental health assessment in primary care: validity and utility of the Quick PsychoDiagnostics Panel. J Fam Pract 2000; 49:614–621.
6. Ware JE, Kosinski M, Keller SD. A 12-item short-form health survey: construction of scales and preliminary tests of reliability and validity. Med Care 1996; 34(3): 220–233.
7. Spitzer R, Kroenke K, Williams J. Validation and utility of a self-report version of PRIME-MD the PHQ Primary Care Study. JAMA 1999; 282:1737–1744.
8. Weathers FW, Litz BT, Herman DS, et al. The PTSD Checklist (PCL): reliability, validity, and diagnostic utility. Paper presented at: 9th Annual Meeting of the International Society for Traumatic Stress Studies: San Antonio, Texas; October 24–27, 1993.
9. Blanchard EB, Jones-Alexander J, Buckley TC, et al. Psychometric properties of the PTSD checklist (PCL). Behav Res Ther 1996; 34:669–673.
10. Mollica RF, Caspi-Yavin Y, Bollini P, et al. The Harvard Trauma Questionnaire. Validating a cross-cultural instrument for measuring torture, trauma, and posttraumatic stress disorder in Indochinese refugees. J Nerv Mental Dis 1992; 180(2):111–116.
11. Mollica RF, Wyshak G, de Marneffe D, et al. Indochinese versions of the Hopkins Symptom Checklist-25: a screening instrument for the psychiatric care of refugees. Am J Psychiatry 1987; 144(4):497–500.
12. Horowitz NJ, Wilmer N, Alvarez N. Impact of Events Scale: a measure of subjective stress. Psychosom Med 1979; 41:209–218.
13. Smith Fawzi MC, Murphy E, Pham T, et al. The validity of screening for post-traumatic stress disorder and major depression among Vietnamese former political prisoners. Acta Psychiatr Scand 1997; 95:87–89.
14. Iacopino V, Ozkalpipci O, Schlar C. The Istanbul Protocol: manual on the effective investigation and documentation of torture and other cruel, inhuman or degrading treatment or punishment. Geneva: Office of the United Nations High Commissioner for Human Rights; August 1999.
15. Iacopino V, Kirschner R, Heisler M. Torture in Turkey and its unwilling accomplices. Boston: Physicians for Human Rights; 1996.
16. Savin, D, Seymour DJ, Littleford LN, et al. Findings from mental health screening of newly arrived refugees in Colorado. Public Health Reports 2005; 120(3):224–229.
17. Barnes DM. Mental health screening in a refugee population: a program report. J Immigr Health 2001; 3(3):141–149.
18. Willis GB, Gonzalez A. Methodological issues in the use of survey questionnaires to assess the health effects of torture. J Nerv Mental Dis 1998; 186(5):283–289.
19. Eisenman DP. Detecting survivors of torture in a primary care setting. 20th Annual Meeting of the Society of General Internal Medicine, Washington, DC, USA, May. 1997; 12(supple 1):131.
20. Montgomery E, Foldspang A. Criterion-related validity of screening for exposure to torture. Danish Medical Bull 1994; 41:588–591.
21. World Medical Association Declaration Guidelines for Medical Doctors Concerning Torture and Other Cruel, Inhuman or Degrading Treatment or Punishment in Relation to Detention and Imprisonment. Adopted by the 29th World Medical Assembly, Tokyo, Japan, October 1975. Available: http://www.wma.net/e/

# CHAPTER 49

# Diagnosis and Treatment of Mental Illness

J. David Kinzie, James M. Jaranson, and Georgi V. Kroupin

## Introduction

The diagnosis and treatment of psychiatric disorders among immigrants is very difficult and challenging. Refugees and immigrants often enter psychiatric treatment reluctantly and fearfully. Many have had severe traumatic experiences and suffer from PTSD and depression, but they may experience disorders along the full range of psychiatric syndromes. Rather than concentrating on stereotypes of behavior in a particular culture, it is better to treat patients as individuals who are interviewed with respect and patience. With patience and sensitivity a mutually agreed treatment plan usually can be formulated and should be spelled out, including the positive effect of medicine, the side effects, and the duration of treatment. Complications often involve the use of interpreters and misunderstanding the role of medications. The doctor–immigrant patient interaction is very complex and may involve somatic preoccupation, hidden psychological trauma, unconscious conversion reaction, physical pathology in addition to psychopathology, and outright deception. It takes time and sensitivity to establish trust in order to understand and treat these patients. A little gentle humor helps both doctor and patient cope (Box 49.1).

## Epidemiological Data

There are enormous numbers of refugees, perhaps 21 million throughout the world.[1] In addition, there are unknown numbers of people internally displaced in their own countries (such as in the United States with the recent hurricanes), and there are a number of people who come to the United States seeking asylum from the chaos and traumas of their own countries. In addition to legal migration there is immigration of undocumented people seeking economic advantages in a new country. The implication of this is that almost every physician will deal with immigrants and refugees of some type. There are now overwhelming data from European studies showing that immigrants, at least those coming from poor countries to the more developed countries of the United Kingdom, the Netherlands, and Denmark, have a much higher rate of developing schizophrenia.[2] Surprisingly, depression seems not to be higher in the first generation but may be higher in the second generation.[3,4]

On the other hand, most refugees who have fled war-torn areas have a very high rate of psychiatric disorders. Prevalence rates have shown that up to 50% of Cambodians have had post-traumatic stress disorder (PTSD) plus depression.[5] A high percentage has also been found among Somali[6] and Bosnian refugees.[7] Perhaps the most vulnerable group has been immigrant school children who have a high exposure to violence. PTSD symptoms in the clinical range of 32% and depression of 16% have been found.[8] These studies indicate high levels of psychiatric disturbances, particularly PTSD and major depressive disorder, among immigrants, especially refugees. Much more psychological distress has been found among asylum seekers whose legal status and ability to stay in the country are often undermined. Living in limbo, they experience additional anxiety.[9] Prevalence rates of post-traumatic stress among traumatized populations are shown in Table 49.1.

**Box 49.1**

**Case history**

'E' is a middle-aged, conservatively dressed Muslim Somali woman who was previously seen in treatment but had dropped out for several months. Her complaint through the Somali counselor was severe headache. She denied any other symptoms and said that all the other treatments had not been helpful. She had received a thorough medical evaluation including an MRI and, for a time, took Tylenol #3 tablets. When asked about other stresses in her life, she denied any and said her only problem was the headache. As we talked more, I asked her if she had seen television images of the situation of the Katrina flooding in New Orleans. At that she became very serious and said that the images, especially of Black (which she emphasized) children separated from their parents, confused and lost, brought back memories of her situation in Somalia during the chaos when families, including her own, were separated. She then went on to describe having nightmares about the situation in Somalia, flashbacks, poor concentration, irritability, and extremely poor sleep. As we discussed her family, she mentioned that a daughter who was married and was living in Saudi Arabia had been deported to Somalia where she was in marked danger and was repeatedly calling 'E,' asking for money. Even to the patient, it became increasingly clear as we talked that the reactivation of her post-traumatic stress and the psychosocial stresses of her daughter had greatly exacerbated her symptoms. In addition, she said that she had stopped taking her psychiatric medicine when she was put on Ibuprofen and Tylenol #3.

## Diagnosis of Post-Traumatic Stress Disorder

Although many reactions to severe stress have been recorded throughout history and more recently in the American Civil War and World War I, PTSD was officially introduced as a diagnostic category into the *Diagnostic and Statistical Manual of Mental Disorders, third edition (DSM-III)*, of the American Psychiatric Association in 1980.[17] Modest modifications have occurred in subsequent revisions of DSM-IV.[18]

Post-traumatic stress disorder requires the existence of a traumatic event to which symptoms can be attributed. In DSM-IV (Criterion A) the person must experience, witness, or be confronted with this event, which involves actual or threatened harm to the person or others. In addition, the person must feel intense fear, helplessness, or horror in response.

ICD-10[19] and DSM-IV differ in their criteria to define PTSD. In DSM-IV, PTSD lasts more than a month and causes 'clinically significant distress or impairment in social, occupational, or other important areas of functioning.'[18] (See p. 429 of cited reference.) PTSD can be specified as acute if symptoms last fewer than 3 months, chronic if duration is 3 months or more, or with delayed onset if symptoms begin after 6 months or longer. Symptoms are grouped into categories or criteria of re-experiencing, avoidance, and hypervigilence and listed in Table 49.2. ICD-10 has two relevant diagnostic categories: (1) 'Post-traumatic stress disorder' (F43.1), which occurs within 6 months of the traumatic event, and (2) 'Enduring personality change after catastrophic experience' (F62.0), which must have been present for at least 2 years. Diagnostic guidelines state that this personality change causes significant interference with daily personal functioning, represents inflexible and maladaptive features, and cannot be attributed to a preexistent personality disorder or to a mental disorder other than PTSD.

The F62.0 category in ICD includes some of the longer-term effects of an unofficial diagnosis often called complex PTSD or disorders of extreme stress not otherwise specified (DESNOS), which had been considered for inclusion in DSM-IV. This is discussed in the chapter on torture survivors by Wenzel, Kastrup, and Eisenman.

From a clinical perspective, the diagnostic category of PTSD is meaningful, and an argument emphasizing the universal aspects of PTSD relates to the many recent research findings on the biological aspects of PTSD.[20] Cross-cultural evidence indicates that PTSD is a useful concept and diagnostic entity that transcends culture. Similar symptoms have been found among Cambodian adolescent refugees,[21] Mexican hurricane survivors,[22] and Kalahari Bushmen.[23] Although some have warned about the dangers of applying Western concepts of trauma to refugees,[24] from both a practical and a heuristic viewpoint, PTSD represents common responses of humans to massive trauma.[25]

PTSD is highly comorbid with depression, occurring together over 80% of the time after trauma (personal data, Intercultural Psychiatric Program). Indeed, depression can occur long after traumatic events. Panic disorder and generalized anxiety disorder are also common comorbid disorders with PTSD. Comorbidity with other anxiety disorders, such as panic disorder, is also common. Table 49.2 compares PTSD, major depression (MDD) and panic disorder, which are among the most frequently diagnosed psychiatric illnesses in immigrants and refu-

**Table 49.1 Traumatized samples with post-traumatic symptoms**

| Primary author | Population sample | Trauma type | Sample size | Country of origin/study | Prevalence total sample (%) | Prevalence non-tortured (%) | Prevalence tortured (%) |
|---|---|---|---|---|---|---|---|
| De Jong[10] | Postconflict | Torture & war | 1200 | Ethiopia/Ethiopia | 16 | Lower | LT Higher ($p < 0.001$) |
| Steel[11] | Resettled refugees | Torture & war | 1161 | Vietnam/Australia | 7–8% with psych dx | | |
| Jaranson[6] | Resettled refugees | Torture & war | 1134 | Somalia & Ethiopia/US | 13 | 4 | 25 |
| Shrestha[12] | Refugees in camp* | Torture & war | 1052 | Bhutan/Nepal | 9 | 4 | 14 |
| Mollica[13] | Refugees in camp | Torture & war | 993 | Cambodia/Thailand | 33 | N/A | N/A |
| Van Ommeren[14] | Refugees in camp* | Torture & war | 810 | Bhutan/Nepal | N/A | 4(C) 15(LT) | 43(C) 74(LT) |
| De Jong[10] | Postconflict | Torture & war | 653 | Algeria/Algeria | 37 | Lower | LT Higher ($p = 0.003$) |
| De Jong[10] | Postconflict | Torture & war | 610 | Cambodia/Cambodia | 28 | Lower | LT Higher ($p < 0.001$) |
| De Jong[10] | Postconflict | Torture & war | 585 | Gaza/Gaza | 18 | Lower | LT Higher ($p < 0.001$) |
| Mollica[7] | Refugees in camp | Torture & war | 534 | Bosnia/Croatia | 26 | N/A | N/A |
| Paker[15] | Prisoners | Torture & prison | 246 | Turkey/Turkey | 33 | 0 | 39 |
| Maercker[16] | Former political prisoners | Torture & prison | 221 | GDR | | | 60(LT) 30(C) |

C, current or within past year; LT, lifetime.
* Case-control study.
Updated from: Modvig J, Jaranson J. A global perspective of torture, political violence and health. In: Wilson JP, Drozdek B, eds. Broken spirits: the treatment of traumatized asylum seekers, refugees, war and torture victims. New York: Brunner-Routledge Press; 2004:38–39.

**Table 49.2 Comparison of DSM IV diagnoses: PTSD, MDD, panic disorder**

| | Post-traumatic stress disorder (PTSD) | Major depressive disorder (MDD) | Panic disorder |
|---|---|---|---|
| Major characteristics | A. Occurs after a traumatic event(s) | Mood disorder: subjective sadness hopelessness, tearfulness | An anxiety disorder: characterized by a discrete period of intense fear |
| Main symptoms B. RE-EXPERIENCING | B1. Distressing recollections<br>B2. Distressing dreams<br>B3. Reliving the experience<br>B4. Distress from cues to the event<br>B5. Physiological reactivity on exposure to reminders | 1. Depressed mood<br>2. Marked decreased interest or pleasure*<br>3. Weight loss or gain<br>4. Insomnia (or hyperarousal)*<br>5. Psychomotor **agitation** or retardation* | 1. Palpitations<br>2. Sweating<br>3. Trembling<br>4. Sensation of shortness of breath<br>5. Feeling of choking |
| C. AVOIDANCE | C1. Avoids thoughts, feelings of event<br>C2. Avoids activities, people, places<br>C3. **Amnesia** for part of the trauma<br>C4. Little interest in activities*<br>C5. Detached or estranged from others<br>C6. Restricted range of affect<br>C7. Sense of foreshortened future | 6. **Fatigue**<br><br>7. Feeling of worthlessness<br>8. **Diminished ability to concentrate**<br>9. Recurrent thoughts of death | 6. Chest pain<br>7. Nausea<br>8. Feeling dizzy<br>9. Feeling of unreality<br>10. Feeling of losing control<br>11. Fear of dying<br>12. Numbness or tingling sensations |
| D. HYPERAROUSAL | D1. Problem falling or staying asleep*<br>D2. **Irritability***<br>D3. **Poor concentration***<br>D4. Hyperviligence<br>D5. Exaggerated startle response | | 13. Chills or hot flashes |
| Criteria for Diagnosis | At least 1in B, 3 in C, and 2 in D | At least five of above symptoms | At least four of above symptoms |

* Symptoms found in both PTSD and MDD.
**In Bold:** Symptoms of PTSD and MDD, which can also be found in brain injury.

gees. The symptoms of PTSD and MDD that are common between the two diagnoses are asterisked in this table.

Unlike American veterans, where alcohol and drug abuse are very common and related to PTSD, alcohol abuse is forbidden in Muslim and Buddhist cultures and may account for its lower prevalence. The prevalence rate is higher among traumatized Hispanic refugees from Central America,[26] where alcohol abuse is a problem.

## Psychosis and organicity

Europeans have found higher rates of schizophrenia in immigrants, rates that have been much higher and cannot be explained by immigrant stress or diagnostic problems related to culture or even racism.[27] We have also found high rates of psychosis among Somalis, which may be related to cultural stress as much as to the use of Khat, an amphetamine-like stimulant known to cause psychotic symptoms. It is sometimes difficult to separate intrusive thought from hallucination, but questioning whether it is a memory or coming from an external source can provide clues. A family member seeing a change in personality provides perhaps the best evidence.

Perhaps it is a disservice to some patients to say that they have a normal reaction to abnormal circumstances, a current approach fashionable in the trauma field. In fact, some patients have a major psychiatric disorder such as schizophrenia or a neurological disorder such as traumatic brain injury (TBI), mild traumatic brain injury (MTBI) (http://www. neuroskills.com/tbi/mtbi.shtml), or organic brain syndrome (OBS). Starvation and chronic malnutrition in refugees and immigrants can also cause significant brain damage, not always irreversible.

Although psychological sequelae might be the most important consequences for the majority of survivors, TBI might be more common than one would expect. Many patients have had multiple head traumas from beatings, shrapnel wounds during war, or falls and accidents during chaotic escapes.[28] Symptoms including poor concentration, loss of recent memory, irritability, and lack of energy can be found in PTSD, depression, and TBI, making the differential complicated. These symptoms are identified in bold type in Table 49.2, indicating how much overlap occurs in the differential with functional disorders such as PTSD and MDD. TBI must be diagnosed to avoid inadequate treatment, but diagnosis can be difficult if there are no neurological soft signs, positive X-ray, MRI or EEG findings. Neuropsychological testing might also be of limited value in refugees and immigrants, but few alternatives exist. We routinely ask about loss of consciousness lasting more than 3 minutes and any symptoms that the patient may relate to this. The patient might also suffer from both PTSD and TBI, limiting the success of treatment.

In addition, many refugees and immigrants have had no education, simply have trouble learning in a new culture, and feel 'dumb' whether or not they have had head trauma. As mentioned, these symptoms may be due to organic factors, to the secondary effects of psychological trauma, or to the confusion of learning a new culture. Many patients also have learning difficulties, which has become an important issue as they apply for citizenship but cannot learn English or history.

## Other diagnostic procedures to rule out concurrent physical disorders

We (JDK and colleagues) have found a very high rate of hypertension among the middle-aged refugees at the ICP at OHSU. Forty to fifty percent have blood pressures in the hypertension range and receive necessary treatment. We also have found an increased rate of diabetes, usually approximately 12–15%, among all refugee groups. This has led us to order a fasting blood sugar or, if not possible, a hemoglobin A1c on all of our patients, in addition to routine blood pressures. Many of our patients have had very poor medical treatment and clearly need an ongoing relationship with a primary care physician.

## Cultural issues in the diagnostic process

There are special issues that are more culturally sensitive to some immigrant groups. Suicide is prohibited in Muslim and Buddhist cultures and, indeed, it is very rare in our experience with them. Nevertheless, ask patients from these religious groups the general question, 'Do you sometimes feel that life is not worth living?' For other groups, particularly Christian or agnostic, suicide may be a real issue and has to be asked more directly. Although drug abuse and alcoholism are rare in Asian and Muslim cultures, these problems are increasing in US immigrant groups, which feel under stress, and should be assessed. Alcoholism seems to be very high among refugees from Latin American and is often associated with domestic violence and subsequent child abuse, direct or indirect. With those groups, we ask about it very directly and make a strong prohibition against the violence. We often have to recommend or initiate alcohol treatment programs for individuals and families from those areas.

## Recommended Knowledge/Required Reading Prior to Seeing the Patient

Physicians should have an overall knowledge of some of the issues involved in the patient populations that they are treating in order to ask sensitive and informed questions about past experiences. For example, clinicians who treat refugees need to know about the Vietnam War, in which hundreds of thousands of Vietnamese left after the fall of Saigon in 1979; the 4 years of the Pol Pot experience in Cambodia, 1975–1979; almost a decade of civil wars in Central America, particularly Guatemala and El Salvador in the 1980s; the Somali wars and the Bosnian wars in 1991–1993; and the Afghani wars under the Taliban ending in 2001. These experiences often include civil unrest, random violence, and forced separation from family members, starvation, witnessing death of friends and family, and refugee status in a second country before finally coming to the United States. In addition, many have suffered torture for reasons including political vengeance or ethnic hostility. Realizing this allows clinicians to consider possible traumas and related diagnoses.

## Interviewing Approaches

Diagnosis of immigrant and refugee psychiatric illness is extremely difficult, with problems on the part of both patients and clinicians. Patients from many cultures are very reluctant to talk about personal issues. Their previous experiences with physicians may lead them to comment only on somatic complaints, such as pain and weakness, and they may expect just a quick diagnosis and a medication prescription. Clinicians, often pressed for time, have much difficulty with the necessity of working through interpreters, often untrained medically and psychiatrically, which will sometimes produce little accurate information. Furthermore, members of some cultures may be reluctant to speak about personal issues with an interpreter who belongs to their own culture and community.

It is not unusual for the patient to present physical complaints as the first symptoms and, as the case in Box 1 demonstrated, to be reluctant to go beyond that. Psychiatric rating scales are usually not very helpful for immigrants,[29] but another argument is offered in the Screening chapter by Eisenman. Most immigrants from severely traumatized areas do not speak English. Many are illiterate in their own languages and have no familiarity with the Likert scales often used as diagnostic tools. Furthermore, if the questions are read to them through a counselor or interpreter, the relationship may affect the answers, e.g. a woman won't tell a male counselor about loss of libido. Indeed, some issues are so sensitive that immigrants may never discuss them even after years of treatment; rape and genital mutilation are two such issues that are very difficult for patients to discuss. In the authors' opinion, the primary diagnosis is made through careful, sensitive, and often lengthy interviewing. Specific cultural approaches (e.g. how to interview Vietnamese, how to treat Somalis) are not as important as the general approach. Refugees often are sensitive to rejection. Impatience, rapid questioning, and expecting quick answers often lead to inaccurate responses and merely increase the level of pressure during the interview. It is very important for the clinician to patiently listen and to encourage the interpreter to do the same. Many times the authors have had to stop an interview and ask the interpreter to be more sensitive or to slow down.

Another primary issue is awareness of the nonverbal communication of the patient. Often, the answer and the nonverbal expression do not match. For example, an interpreter may give a patient's response as, 'I have no problems,' while the patient has a sad look, psychomotor retardation, and long latencies in responding. We have found that it is useful to take the physical symptoms of the patient seriously as a starting point, e.g. 'How long have your headaches lasted, what have you done for them, has anything made them better or worse?' This is a non-threatening approach with which the patient can identify. It is probably not useful to ask about psychosocial stressors immediately, but rather to ask about physical symptoms which may indicate major psychiatric disorders. For PTSD, asking about nightmares, irritability, intrusive thoughts, and avoidance behavior, such as avoiding TV shows of violence or war scenes, can be very useful. These are relatively straightforward and non-threatening questions. For depression, asking about poor sleep, poor appetite, fatigue, and poor concentration rather than the more subjective symptoms of helplessness, hopelessness, negative view of the future, etc. is also less threatening and more universally accepted. When one finds that there are a number of symptoms related to PTSD and/or depression, follow-up can lead to some of the psychosocial events in the patient's life. For example, an affirmative response to nightmares could be followed up by asking whether these nightmares are about real events that happened to the patient in Bosnia (Somali, Cambodia, etc.). Then one can ask, 'Can you tell me more about other things that have happened to you?' Often, the patients will provide additional information but will terminate the process by saying, 'I don't want to talk about it anymore,' or,

'I don't want to be reminded of it.' Avoidance behavior has been a necessary defense mechanism for many refugees. This should be respected and the clinician may simply say, 'I understand that what happened to you in the past is very severe,' and then make an interpretation that most patients have been able to understand, e.g. 'You went through very, very difficult events in the past and now your body and your mind are still reacting to those events, giving you many of the symptoms you have now.' One can list those symptoms such as nightmares, poor sleep, or poor concentration. This connection of psychosocial events with current symptoms has often been helpful for patients. Sometimes, in their chaotic situation of immigrant status and adjustment to a new country, they have not connected the past and the present problems. Additionally, it is useful to ask about ongoing current problems faced by many immigrants. These include language, financial, and housing problems, and concern about the education and socialization of their children, i.e. are they becoming too Americanized?

## Treatment Issues

It is essential to establish a good therapeutic relationship with immigrants or refugees. The drop-out rate for many refugee programs is extremely high, often related to patients' dissatisfaction with the way they were treated, misunderstandings about their treatment, or confusion over what their treatment involves. A kind, gentle, supportive approach, clearly answering the patients' concerns, constitutes by far the best treatment in its own right. We feel that many physicians have under-recognized the importance to the patient of receiving treatment by a highly trained American professional. By giving complete attention and time to the patient during the interview, patients feel respected and listened to.

Next, it is important to negotiate a treatment plan. This usually is uncomplicated, including an agreement about the symptoms that the patient and the physician want to treat. A common approach is as follows: 'I understand that you have nightmares, bad sleep, and are very irritable with your wife. You can't concentrate, your appetite is poor, and you have pain all over your body. Of all these symptoms, which ones are the most important for us to start treating?' Often, patients will say what is most important to them, which may not be what physicians think needs treating first. However, this has started the process of negotiating a treatment plan. It also implies that we can't treat everything at once

and that there will be time later on to approach the other problems.

## Psychopharmacology

Paroxetine, sertraline, fluoxetine, and citralopram are the most commonly used daytime anxiolytic drugs and selective serotonin reuptake inhibitor (SSRI) antidepressants. Depending upon individual drug profiles, side effects such as increased irritability, drowsiness, or vertigo must be considered and explained to the patient. Drugs might not be equally effective against all PTSD symptoms. Recent treatment strategies for PTSD integrate (1) newer antipsychotics, such as olanzapine and risperidone, both of which are sedating, but the latter might reduce flashbacks and mood swings, or (2) antiepileptic/mood stabilizers such as valproic acid that might reduce irritability and flashbacks. As in all contacts with patients from other ethnic groups, ethnopharmacological considerations must be considered, especially cytochrome P450 subtypes and interactions with ethnic medication provided by local healers.[30]

For PTSD, the SSRIs have been considered the gold standard by the guidelines for treatment. They are, in fact, helpful for many but not all symptoms of PTSD. SSRIs also have potential side effects of sexual dysfunction and discontinuation syndromes. Fluoxetine is a good choice, especially since it is long acting and a patient can miss a dose or two without much subjective distress.[31] The tricyclic antidepressants (TCAs) have been underutilized. They have many advantages, including effectiveness for depression, and the more sedating ones are useful for insomnia, anxiety, and panic disorder. Another major advantage is that blood levels are readily available, primarily to ensure medication compliance, which has been a large problem with many groups.[32,33] The adrenergic blocking agents clonidine and prazosin are very helpful in reducing nightmares,[34] which SSRIs do not help. Adrenergic blocking agents also can reduce irritability and daytime flashbacks and help decrease blood pressure; however, the hypotensive effect is counteracted by tricyclics in hypertensive patients. Therefore, TCAs and clonidine probably should not be used together in such patients.

Many patients will complain of the medicines in various ways. A common complaint is, 'I took the pill twice and I didn't get better.' The expectation of immediate relief is based upon an antibiotic model for treatment of infectious disease. Some patients also will complain of side effects, e.g. 'I took the medicine and got constipated,' or, 'I got more nervous.' It is good to anticipate this and tell patients about common side effects, but without excessive detail. If symptoms continue, the patient is told to contact us and we will decide together the best way to help. One should always ask whether they had any problems with the medicine and if, indeed, they took it. Another problem is patients not understanding the need for refills when they run out of medicine. This may be related to the problem of inability to read and not taking the medicine as prescribed, e.g. taking the medicine three times a day instead of taking it all at night as prescribed, then becoming very drowsy during the day (such as with the TCAs or clonidine). It often takes several treatment sessions and considerable education to get patients to take the medicine appropriately. Kinzie and Friedman provide a more complete review of the psycho-pharmacologic treatment of refugees.[35]

Another common problem with medicine has been that patients will be prescribed medicines by other doctors, then stop taking the psychiatric medicine and/or vice-versa. Many refugees do not tell doctors what other medicines they have been prescribed and many clinicians do not ask about this. Patients, in their confusion, will often simply stop taking some or all of their prescribed medication. In addition, many patients take over-the-counter medicines, some of which are compatible while others have difficult interactions with many prescribed drugs. Knowledge of the local herbal medicines for each culture can be very helpful. A specific issue for Muslims has been Ramadan, the month in which most Muslims feel prohibited from eating during the daylight hours. Exceptions can be made for medical treatments. Most Muslim patients, however, will not take a medicine prescribed during the daytime. They can take medicine after supper at sundown and before breakfast at sunrise, usually before 5:00 a.m. One needs to go over the medicines with the patients and try to make the treatment simple and clear during Ramadan.

## Collaborative care

Recent work suggests that collaborative care options can improve adherence to medical treatment, enhance patient satisfaction, and improve treatment outcomes for depressed primary care patients.[36,37] These found co-location of physical and mental health services, experience of clinical staff in com-

municating with culturally diverse populations, communication between providers, and coordination of care to be essential for provision of competent healthcare services for immigrants. Clinics providing best practices in serving immigrants and refugees also include multilingual/multicultural staff and providers, as well as trained medical interpreters on site.

Treatment should be informed by a view of mental health problems as multifaceted issues that can be best understood through the perspectives and contributions of multiple disciplines. Clinics should hold continuing education seminars with local and community experts from health, religion, social sciences (anthropology, history) and other disciplines to learn about how mental health experiences and therapeutic approaches can be shaped by culture, economics, history, gender, religion, historical and social change, and politics. Including traditional healers, in particular, can enhance the development of a culturally appropriate treatment approach.[38]

Families should be understood also in terms of their strengths and the resources they provide to their communities and cultures. For instance, mobilizing support from family members may be an important component of supportive therapy. In most cases, family involvement is likely to enhance recovery and improve adherence to provider recommendations. Exceptions to the goal of family involvement need to be highlighted, such as in cases of incest or domestic violence where the family is part of the trauma exposure. All family involvement requires the patient's permission.

Secondary traumatization in which family members are adversely affected by the trauma directly experienced by someone else in their family may also be associated with mental health problems.

Understanding culture-related resilience and support of patients' cultural identities, together with adaptation efforts, is of paramount importance for providing effective mental health services for refugees and immigrants. In 1999, a US Surgeon General's report[39] concluded that the effects of culture on mental health 'have been historically underestimated – and they do count.' Accessing and utilizing healthcare services in a new country presents many challenges. One of the major challenges is the providers' ability to differentiate barriers to care that are often cultural from the factors that masquerade as such.

In healthcare settings, patients' feelings of isolation, confusion, powerlessness, inability to control or even predict the future result in lack of understanding, and, consequently, lack of trust in the healthcare system. The consequence is two extreme attitudes: isolation and passive non-compliance versus over-utilization of services and conflict.

One of the authors (GVK), a native Russian, was called to a local hospital to mediate a conflict with a Russian immigrant family who was threatening to sue the hospital for what they thought was poor treatment of their mother, a terminally ill patent with liver cancer. The treating physician and the nursing staff were convinced that cultural differences were the major cause of the conflict, as the patient's two sons refused to accept the standards of care in the hospital. Although their mother had been unconscious for several weeks, with days left to live, the patient's sons demanded that she received intensive attention, including taking her vitals three times a day and aggressively treating possible complications (such as pneumonia) if they occurred. Treating physicians and nurses thought that these demands were unreasonable and thought that the sons were trying to take advantage of the situation by threatening to sue the hospital.

The meeting with the family was opened by the treating physician, who, holding his dictaphone to his mouth said: 'Now do we all understand that the patient is dying and there is nothing that could be done to save her?' Everybody agreed. 'Good!' he said with relief. 'No, that's bad!' said one of the sons who sat in grief and despair.

Further discussion revealed differences in how both sides saw the situation. Although certainly being empathic with the patient's suffering, the physician felt that the situation was now clear and easier to manage. He was also relieved to finally come to at least some common ground with the family. Family, on the other hand, was consumed by grief and felt that losing the last bit of hope was unbearable. Further dialogue about specific issues revealed that most of them were easy to resolve. Family members understood that their mother was dying, and they only wanted for her to get enough care to ease her suffering. Taking vitals several times a day, which was certainly medically unnecessary, was the only way for both sons to know when they should rush to the hospital as they wanted to be there when their mother passed away. Besides everything else, a previous treating physician failed to diagnose cancer in this patient and her family came to this new physician angry and mistrustful. In the end, there were not cultural differences, but mostly previous negative experiences, difference in perspectives and lack of dialogue that created the conflict.

## Refugee Patients and Western Physicians: A Complex Interaction

Refugee and immigrant patients bring their own cultural beliefs and expectations to treatment, as do Western physicians. However, the interaction is complicated by the usual medical and psychiatric disorders that a patient has and the expertise and competence that a physician has to manage these disorders. The following case histories illustrate a variety of complex interactions and disorders whose primary purpose is to remind us that treating the patient from another culture involves, first, medical and psychiatric competence and, second, the unique contribution of the cultural expectations of both parties (Boxes 49.2–49.8).

---

**Box 49.2**

**Case study 1**

The patient is a 40-year-old Vietnamese woman who has been seen in clinic for several months. Her unremitting symptoms included backache, headache, poor sleep and multiple pains. It was reported that these symptoms started when her husband was killed serving in the South Vietnamese army. The counselor stated that this was unremitting grief. On one occasion, the counselor was called out of the room. The patient then switched over to fair English, raised her dress, and showed an ugly scar on the leg where her husband had scalded her with boiling water. There was a long history of domestic violence and she actually admitted she was quite relieved when he was killed. Because the expectation was that she would grieve the loss of her husband, she would not share her feelings with the Vietnamese counselor. When the counselor returned to the room, the patient returned to complaining of headache and backache.

ASSESSMENT: Being from a different culture, the psychiatrist could be a neutral sounding board for the patient to vent feelings that she had not been able to tell people from her own culture. This also shows that the interaction between the counselor-interpreter and patient can greatly color the information gathered.

**Box 49.3**

**Case study 2**

The patient is a 55-year-old Bosnian male who experienced considerable torture during the Bosnian war. In the process of psychiatric treatment, it was discovered that he had a tumor on his lung. The surgeon recommended surgery and went through the litany of risks, as was his usual procedure in the American medical/legal setting. The patient was stunned by all the bad things that could happen and refused surgery. The Bosnian counselor who worked with the psychiatrist on the case, herself a Bosnian-trained physician, was appalled. No Bosnian doctor would give such a description of possible negative outcomes but would merely say you have a tumor on your lung, we need to operate, and you are scheduled on Tuesday. A psychiatrist wrote the surgeon, encouraging him to be more authoritarian and to take a more direct approach to ensure the surgery be done. However, neither the surgeon nor the Bosnian patient changed their positions. The surgery was refused and the patient died 18 months later.

ASSESSMENT: This patient illustrates the problems of cultural expectations and information given to patients in other countries versus the complex medical/legal interaction that is standard in the litigious American medical system. Unfortunately, this had the undesirable effect of a patient refusing a possible life-saving surgery.

**Box 49.4**

**Case study 3**

The patient is a mid-50-year-old uneducated Bosnian woman who appeared much older than her stated age. She had multiple medical problems, mostly GI symptoms. Multiple examinations, CAT scans, and endoscopy indicated no pathology. Although it was thought that she was not psychologically sophisticated and was somatizing many of her symptoms, I (DK) tentatively suggested that her symptoms may be related to the loss of her son. About 10 years prior, her 16-year-old son was taken out of their home and village at night by Serbs and never seen again. The patient not only agreed that this was related to her symptoms but agreed it was the entire cause. She said, 'I will never feel good until I know what happened to him.' What followed was a very fruitful discussion of grief and its long-term effects.

ASSESSMENT: This illustrates a tendency of Western physicians to see refugees, especially uneducated immigrants, as psychologically unsophisticated. Therefore, refugees often receive multiple somatic work-ups when, on closer inspection, the symptoms are obviously related to psychological or social events. The patient readily agreed with a psychological interpretation once it was given to her. It also helped greatly in our relationship and in providing education about grief reactions.

**Box 49.5**

**Case study 4**

This patient is a 25-year-old Vietnamese woman who had recently come from Vietnam. She described both trauma and loss and had clear symptoms of depression. She was started on tricyclic antidepressant medicine and, after several months, showed no improvement. At that time, a tricyclic blood level was obtained, showing no evidence of the presence of the medicine, i.e. zero imipramine and desipramine blood levels. When mildly confronted with the fact that she probably wasn't taking any medicine, the patient readily agreed and stated that her uncle in Vietnam had many more symptoms than she did, so she had sent the medicine to him.

ASSESSMENT: Medication non-compliance is a very serious problem, particularly for refugees who have a poor understanding of the need for long-term treatment with medicine. There are many reasons for non-compliance, including saving the medicine for another person.

## Box 49.6
### Case study 5

The patient is a 23-year-old Guatemalan asylee who was first seen in jail on the advice of his lawyer. He was jailed for a recent history of domestic violence. He was a large man but appeared extremely distressed, confused, and cried throughout much of the interview. His hopelessness was clear. After he was released from jail, a further psychiatric evaluation was obtained. He had undergone massive trauma as a child in Guatemala when his village was attacked both by paramilitaries and guerrillas. Many people were killed and he felt his life was in danger. Additional information revealed a strong family history of schizophrenia. On further mental status examination, the patient had auditory hallucinations and paranoid delusions. Specifically, he believed that a witch in Guatemala was putting a hex on him. With antipsychotic medication, the patient's symptoms and behavior greatly improved. He was able to make a compelling case for asylum, which was granted.

ASSESSMENT: It is easy to be overwhelmed by both the legal and the historical aspects of a patient's life, but psychotic symptoms can occur surprisingly frequently in refugees. The response to antipsychotic medicine can be extremely helpful and indeed can profoundly change a patient's life.

## Box 49.7
### Case study 6

The patient, a 55-year-old Cambodian male referred by a family physician, had weakness on his left side, including arm and leg, and a reported visual defect. He also had been confused and disoriented following a stroke. He had a history of severe trauma in Cambodia and other more recent losses. On mental status examination, he did seem very confused and vague about the circumstances of his life. Subsequently, a neurologist's report indicated no neurological findings. A repeat, brief neurological examination on the subsequent visit to the psychiatrist (DK) indicated this was true. No pathological reflexes, no demonstrable weakness, and no deficit in his orientation or recent memory were found when fully tested. The patient was informed that his condition was not permanent and that he should soon improve with medicines including antidepressants and clonidine. He did improve rather rapidly and, in a few months, showed no deficits and no impairment.

ASSESSMENT: The patient represents a rather dramatic form of conversion reaction. Without the documentation of no neurological deficits, he might have been maintained in his presenting state. Antidepressant medicines treated his depression, and encouragement that he was going to improve changed his self-described impairment and his outlook on life completely. He continues to be seen in treatment and is very grateful for his 'cure.'

## Box 49.8
### Case study 7

The patient is a 60-year-old widowed Somali woman who was admitted for severe depression and difficulty functioning. She had a very tramatic past, which included the death of her husband, who was hit in the head with a bullet and died in the patient's arms. In addition to symptoms of post-traumatic stress and depression, the patient gave a long history of burning in the epigastric area, unrelated to any specific event. During treatment, the patient showed much improvement in sleep and nightmares but continued to complain of GI distress. She originally refused to see a general physician for a work-up, fearing that it might be cancer. Eventually, she agreed to a medical evaluation which showed symptoms of ulcer disease, and she was positive for *Helicobacter pylori*. She was started on triple therapy and had much improvement in her GI symptoms.

ASSESSMENT: This indicates the complication of medical and psychiatric disorders. It is important not to overlook ongoing physical disorders, such as ulcer disease, with obvious psychiatric disorders.

## Prognosis

Many of the disorders of refugees are complicated, prolonged, and subject to exacerbations and reoccurrences under stress. Both depression and PTSD tend to be episodic, depending upon the current stressors. Calls from relatives in the home country for money, fighting in their home country, and the television coverage of the tragedies of 9/11 can all lead to complete exacerbation of their symptoms.[40] This means that patients need long-term follow-up and the ability to be seen more frequently during times of stress. Physicians need to maintain an approach similar to the treatment of other chronic diseases such as hypertension and diabetes, in which there will be periodic exacerbations.

Premature termination of treatment can lead to patients feeling abandoned and unprotected. We continue seeing our patients (JDK & colleagues) with brief visits for long periods of time. Patients have become used to regular contact with their doctors, minor changes in medicine, and the ability to make further contact should conditions exacerbate their problems.

## Conclusion

The treatment of immigrants and refugees with psychiatric disorders is challenging and difficult but ultimately very rewarding. In our experience, combined over many years, we have found that our patients are extremely grateful and thankful for being respected and receiving relief from their ongoing subjective distress and discomfort. Of all the misery in the world, one cannot mitigate much of it, but one can help some very distressed individuals feel comfortable and even welcomed in their new country (Box 49.9).

## References

1. Statistics from United Nations High Commissioner for Refugees 2005 Global Refugee Trends. Available: http://www.unhcr.ch/
2. Cooper B. Immigration and schizophrenia: the social causation hypothesis revisited. Br J Psychiatry 2005; 186:361–363.
3. Bhugra D. Migration and depression. Acta Psychiatr Scand 2003; Suppl:67–72.
4. Kinzie JD. Immigrants and refugees, the psychiatric perspective. Transcult Psychiatry 2006; 43(4):577–591.
5. Marshall GN, Schell TL, Elliott MN, et al. Mental health of Cambodian refugees 2 decades after resettlement in the United States. JAMA 2005; 294:571–579.
6. Jaranson JM, Butcher J, Halcon L, et al. Somali and Oromo refugees: correlates of torture and trauma history. Am J Public Health 2004; 94:591–598.
7. Mollica RF, Sarajlic N, Chernoff M, et al. Longitudinal study of psychiatric symptoms, disability, mortality, and emigration among Bosnian refugees. JAMA 2001; 286:546–554.
8. Jaycox LH, Stein BD, Kataoka SH, et al. Violence exposure, posttraumatic stress disorder, and depressive symptoms among recent immigrant schoolchildren. J Am Acad Child Adolesc Psychiatry 2002; 41:1104–1110.
9. Silove D, Steel Z, Watters C. Policies of deterrence and the mental health of asylum seekers. JAMA 2000; 284:604–611.
10. de Jong JTVM., Komproe IH, Van Ommeren M, et al. Lifetime events and posttraumatic stress disorder in 4 postconflict settings. JAMA 2001; 286:555–562.
11. Steel S, Silove D, Bird K, et al. Pathways from war trauma to posttraumatic stress symptoms among Tamil asylum seekers, refugees, and immigrants. J Traumat Stress 1999; 12:421–435.
12. Shrestha NM, Sharma B, van Ommeren M, et al. Impact of torture on refugees displaced within the developing world: symptomatology among Bhutanese refugees in Nepal. JAMA 1998; 280:443–448.
13. Mollica RF, Donelan K, Tor S, et al. The effect of trauma and confinement on functional health and mental health status of Cambodians living in Thailand–Cambodia border camps. JAMA 1993; 270:581–586.
14. van Ommeren M, Jong JT, Sharma B, et al. Psychiatric disorders among tortured Bhutanese refugees in Nepal. Arch Gen Psychiatry 2001; 58:475–482.
15. Paker M, Paker Ö, Yüksel S. Psychological effects of torture: an empirical study of tortured and non-tortured non-political prisoners. In: M. Basoglu, ed. Torture and its consequences: current treatment approaches Cambridge, UK: Cambridge University Press; 1992:73–82.
16. Maercker A, Schutzwohl M. Long-term effects of political imprisonment: a comparison study. Social Psychiatr Psychiatric Epidemiol 1997; 32:435–442.
17. Kinzie JD, Goetz RR. A century of controversy surrounding posttraumatic stress-spectrum syndromes: the impact on DSM-III and DSM-IV. J Traum Stress 1996; 9:159–179.
18. American Psychiatric Association. Diagnostic and statistical manual of mental disorders. 4th edn. Washington, DC: American Psychiatric Association; 2000.

19. World Health Organisation. Tenth revision of the international classification of diseases, chapter V (F): Mental and behavioural disorders. Geneva: WHO; 1991.

20. Friedman M, Jaranson J. The applicability of the posttraumatic concept to refugees. In: Marsella T, Bornemann T, Ekblad S, et al., eds. Amidst peril and pain: the mental health and wellbeing of the world's refugees. Washington, DC: American Psychological Association; 1994:207–227.

21. Sack WH, Seeley JR, Clarke GN. Does PTSD transcend cultural barriers? A study from the Khmer Adolescent Refugee Project. J Am Acad Child Adolesc Psychiatry 1997; 36(1):49–54.

22. Norris FH, Perilla JL, Murphy AD. Postdisaster stress in the United States and Mexico: a cross-cultural test of the multicriterion conceptual model of posttraumatic stress disorder. J Abnorm Psychol 2001; 110(4)L553–L563.

23. McCall GJ, Resick PA. A pilot study of PTSD symptoms among Kalahari Bushmen. J Trauma Stress 2003; 16(5):455–60.

24. Eisenbruch M. Toward a culturally sensitive DSM: cultural bereavement in Cambodian refugees and the traditional healer as taxonomist. J Nerv Ment Dis 1992; 180(1):8–10.

25. Boehnlein JK, Kinzie JD. Commentary. DSM diagnosis of posttraumatic stress disorder and cultural sensitivity: a response. J Nerv Mental Dis 1992; 180:597–599.

26. Farias PJ. Emotional distress and its socio-political correlates in Salvadoran refuges: analysis of a clinical sample. Culture Med Psychiatry 1991; 15:167–192.

27. Eaton W, Harrison G. Ethnic disadvantage and schizophrenia. Acta Psychiatr Scand 2000; Suppl: 38–43.

28. Mollica RF, Henderson DC, Tor S. Psychiatric effects of traumatic brain injury events in Cambodian survivors of mass violence. Br J Psychiatry 2002; 181:339–347.

29. Kinzie JD, Manson SM. The use of self-rating scales in cross-cultural psychiatry. Hosp Commun Psychiatry 1987; 38:190–196.

30. Lin K-M, Poland RE, Nakaski G. Psychopharmacology and psychobiology of ethnicity. Washington, DC: American Psychiatric Press; 1993.

31. Van der Kolk BA, Dryluss D, Michaels M, et al. Fluoxetine in post-traumatic stress disorder. Clin Psychiatry 1994; 55:517–522.

32. Kroll J, Habenicht M, Mackenzie T, et al. Depression and posttraumatic stress disorder in Southeast Asian refugees. Am J Psychiatry 1989; 146:1592–1597.

33. Kinzie JD. Antidepressant blood levels in Southeast Asians: clinical and cultural implications. J Nerv Mental Dis 1987; 175:480–485.

34. Boehnlein JK, Kinzie JD. Pharmacologic reduction of CNS noradrenergic activity in PTSD: the case for clonidine and prazosin. Under editorial review.

35. Kinzie JD, Friedman MJ. Psychopharmacology for refugee and asylum-seeking patients. In: Wilson J, Drozdek B, eds. Broken spirits: the treatment of traumatized asylum seekers, refugees, war and torture victims. New York: Brunner-Routledge Press; 2004:579–600.

36. Holman EA, Silver RC, Waitzkin H. Traumatic life events in primary care patients: a study in an ethnically diverse sample. Arch Fam Med 2000; 9(9):802–810.

37. Savin, D, Seymour DJ, Littleford LN, et al. Findings from mental health screening of newly arrived refugees in Colorado. Public Health Reports 2005; 120(3):224–229.

38. Fairbank JA, Friedman MJ, de Jong JTVM, et al. Intervention options for society, communities, families, and individuals. In: Green B, Friedman M, De Jong JTVM, et al., eds. Trauma interventions in war and peace: prevention, practice, and policy. New York, Boston, Dordrecht, London, and Moscow: Kluwer Academic/Plenum Publishers; 2003:57–72.

39. Mental Health: A Report of the Surgeon General. 1999. Available: http://www.mentalhealth.samhsa.gov/publications/cite.asp

40. Kinzie JD, Boehnlein JK, Riley C, et al. The effects of September 11 on traumatized refugees: reactivation of posttraumatic stress disorder. J Nerv Ment Dis 2002; 190:437–441.

# CHAPTER 50

# Survivors of Torture: A Hidden Population

Thomas Wenzel, Marianne C. Kastrup, and David P. Eisenman

## Introduction

Working with migrants and refugees clearly demonstrates that extreme life experiences clustered around war and different forms of persecution are frequently found in many of the groups encountered. Torture, an act forbidden by numerous international declarations and conventions, such as the United Nations Convention against Torture,[1,2] remains a frequent and destructive form of persecution despite ratification of the Convention by a large number of countries. It has been documented that even children are submitted to torture in many countries.[3] Although common, torture cannot be seen as a simple phenomenon, and the sequelae represent a complex challenge for treatment.

## Definitions of Torture and Ethics Guidelines for Physicians

Conceptions of torture vary among cultures, legal systems, and organizations. Nevertheless, the essential elements of torture include the following: it is purposeful and systematic; it occurs in captivity, usually face-to-face; and it intends to destroy the victim's personality through the infliction of psychological or physical suffering.

The UN Convention Against Torture defines in Article 1: 'For the purposes of this Convention, torture means any act by which severe pain or suffering, whether physical or mental, is intentionally inflicted on a person for such purposes as obtaining from him or a third person information or a confession, punishing him for an act he or a third person has committed or is suspected of having committed,

or intimidating or coercing him or a third person, or for any reason based on discrimination of any kind, when such pain or suffering is inflicted by or at the instigation of or with the consent or acquiescence of a public official or other person acting in an official capacity.'[1] The World Medical Association (WMA) in its declaration of Tokyo offers a similar definition: 'For the purpose of this Declaration, torture is defined as the deliberate, systematic or wanton infliction of physical or mental suffering by one or more persons acting alone or on the orders of any authority, to force another person to yield information, to make a confession, or for any other reason. The declaration of Tokyo as well as a later WMA declaration underline the duty of physicians not to participate in any such act, but to take an active stance in the fight against torture.'[4]

The importance of an active and responsible role of physicians against torture – prohibited without any exceptions – has been underlined in a recent WMA document.[5] The same document, referring also to regional documents such as the American Convention on Human Rights in paragraph 19, specifically recommends that 'National Medical Associations support the adoption in their country of ethical rules and legislative provisions:

19.1 aimed at affirming the ethical obligation of physicians to report or denounce acts of torture or cruel, inhuman or degrading treatment of which they are aware;

19.2 establishing, to that effect, an ethical and legislative exception to professional confidentiality that allows the physician to report abuses, where possible with the subject's consent, but in certain circumstances where the victim is unable to express him/herself freely, without explicit consent.

19.3 cautioning physicians to avoid putting individuals in danger by reporting on a named basis a victim who is deprived of freedom, subjected to constraint or threat or in a compromised psychological situation.

20. Disseminate to physicians the Istanbul Protocol.

21. Promote their training on the identification of different modes of torture and their sequelae.

22. Place at their disposal all useful information on reporting procedures, particularly to the national authorities, nongovernmental organisations and the International Criminal Court.'[5]

These ethics guidelines support the increasing criticism about attempts of some governments, and physicians in those countries, to justify exceptions. The guidelines also refer to the Istanbul Protocol as the recommended UN standard for documentation of torture: 'In some cases, two ethical obligations are in conflict. International codes and ethical principles require the reporting of information concerning torture or maltreatment to a responsible body. In some jurisdictions, this is also a legal requirement. In some cases, however, patients may refuse to give consent to being examined for such purposes or to having the information gained from examination disclosed to others. They may be fearful of the risks of reprisals for themselves or their families. In such situations, health professionals have dual responsibilities: to the patient and to society at large, which has an interest in ensuring that justice is done and perpetrators of abuse are brought to justice. The fundamental principle of avoiding harm must feature prominently in consideration of such dilemmas. Health professionals should seek solutions that promote justice without breaking the individual's right to confidentiality. Advice should be sought from reliable agencies; in some cases this may be the national medical association or non-governmental agencies. Alternatively, with supportive encouragement, some reluctant patients may agree to disclosure within agreed parameters (Istanbul Protocol, paragraph 68).[6]

While the political discussion might at times lead to a blurring of standards,[7] clear definitions of torture are a key precondition to prevention and legal guidelines, and partly overlapping concepts such as that of organized violence[7,8] can be applied in situations such as the development of treatment programs.

Freedom from torture in this context should be seen as a major factor in healthcare and at the same time as a contribution to a civil society.

It might be noted that trends in perpetrator research – an issue of importance for, among other reasons, prevention – indicate that, especially in mass violence or systematic torture, many torturers are literally the neighbor next door. They may have been mistreated, tortured themselves, or exposed to psychological manipulation, convincing them of the need to torture to protect society or as a moral obligation.[9]

## Aims of Torture

Reasons for the use of torture vary. There may be individual motives such as greed, personal cruelty, or monetary gain. In cases of more systematic torture, political aims take precedence, including creating terror, stigmatizing, and damaging the assertiveness of opponents or non-consenting minorities. Sometimes the victims are mistaken for someone else. Situations where torture occurs are not restricted to premises where one is deprived of liberty, such as prisons, police stations, and prison camps, but also to the public sphere, the streets, or even the homes of victims. Especially in these latter situations, friends or family members might witness torture and suffer psychological stress or traumatization without having been directly tortured themselves. Being forced to witness the torture of family members was a common method of indirect torture in the war-torn countries of Central America during the 1980s.

## Prevalence of Torture

Every year, Amnesty International lists countries that practice torture and usually the list exceeds 120 countries. Table 50.1 displays selected studies documenting the prevalence of torture survivors among community samples of refugees. Estimates vary due to methodological issues and differences in the use of torture in those countries. In the 1990s, there were approximately 14 million refugees living in Western Europe and North America, of whom 5% to 35% (700 000 to 4.9 million) were believed to have been tortured.[10] If this 5–35% figure is applied to more recent calculations of 23 million refugees, then up to 8 million tortured refugees exist worldwide. At the primary care practice level, a study of three urban medical clinics in Los Angeles, California, found that 7% of all foreign-born Latino patients had experienced political torture.[11] None of the patients recalled their primary care provider ever inquiring about their exposure to political violence or torture. It seems safe to say, therefore, that primary care

**Table 50.1  Empirical studies including torture prevalence estimates in selected population samples**

| Primary author | Setting and sampling method | Sample size | Country of origin/study | Torture prevalence |
|---|---|---|---|---|
| Thonneau et al., 1990[13] | Western refugee setting: all applicants for refugee status in Quebec, Canada, referred to obligatory medical examination | 1994 | Composite/Canada | 18% |
| Montgomery & Foldspang, 1994[14] | Western refugee setting: consecutive sampling of asylum seekers arriving in refugee reception center | 74 | Middle East/Denmark | 28% |
| Kjersem, 1996[15] | Western refugee setting: all asylum-seekers arriving in Denmark 1.1.86–30.6.88 | 9579 | Composite/Denmark | 10.1% |
| Shresta et al., 1998[16] | Near-area refugee setting: identification of all physically tortured refugees in UNHCR camps in Southern Nepal | 85078 | Bhutan/Nepal | 3% |
| Hondius et al., 2000[17] | Western refugee setting: refugees recruited to treatment center by flyers | 156, dominated by non-help-seeking refugees | Turkey, Iran/Holland | 76% |
| de Jong et al., 2001[18] | National sample: random selection from community populations in four countries | 653<br>610<br>1200<br>585 | Algeria<br>Cambodia<br>Ethiopia<br>Gaza | 8%<br>9%<br>26%<br>15% |
| Modvig, 2001[19] | National sample: random population sample | 1033 household representatives | East Timor | 30% |
| Iacopino et al., 2001[15] | Near-area refugee setting: random sample of households in Macedonian and Albanian refugee camps for Kosovars | 1180 household representatives | Kosovo/Macedonia and Albania | 4% |
| Tang & Fox, 2001[16] | Near-area refugee setting: Random sample of Senegalese refugees in two camps in Gambia (n = 242) | 80 | Senegal/Gambia | 16% |
| Ekblad et al., 2002[38] | Western refugee setting: random selection from airline lists of pre- accepted refugees arriving in Sweden (n = 2930) | 402 sampled, 218 participated<br>98 participated in phase 2 follow-up | Kosovo/Sweden | 51% |
| Lie, 2002[39] | Western refugee setting: all settled refugees in 20 municipalities of Norway, May 1994–December 1995 | 791 invited, 462 contributed data | Composite/Norway | 6% (14% witnessed torture) |
| Jaranson et al., 2004[37] | Western refugee setting: representative community sample | 1134 | Ethiopia & Somalia/US | 44% |

Updated from Modvig J, Jaranson J. A global perspective of torture, political violence and health. In: Wilson JP, Drozdek B, editors. Broken spirits: the treatment of traumatized asylum seekers, refugees, war and torture victims. New York: Brunner-Routledge Press; 2004:42–43.

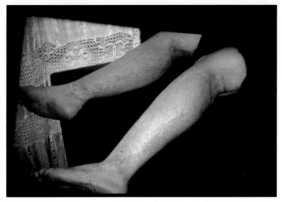

**Figure 50.1** A victim of 'falanga.' (We are grateful for Dr. Maria Piniou-Kalli of MRCT in Athens for supplying this photograph.)

physicians may be treating persons who survived political torture without knowing this and consequently may not fully meet their patients' needs. Studies in primary care populations from a mixture of countries find similar estimates of prevalence in primary care.[12]

## Methods of Torture

While beatings are the most common form of torture, more specific techniques can be observed in many countries. Examples are shown in Table 50.2 but a listing of torture methods can never be complete because torturers are constantly inventing and varying methods.

Regional variation occurs in the specific forms of torture – often characterized by special names – such as 'telefono' (beatings to both ears with subsequent injuries to the outer and inner ear) and 'falanga' (beatings to the soles of the feet, leading to swelling, extreme and often chronic pain) (Fig. 50.1). Mutilating injuries consisting of, for example, amputation of limbs or other body parts are common in some regions, such as Rwanda or Iraq, and are, as is usually the case with torture, intended to punish or to create impairment and stigma.

In the realm of psychological torture methods, regional variations occur with cultural and social differences in what is considered shameful, unhealthy, or dangerous, or as a function of cultural and religious taboos. For instance, one of the authors (DE) interviewed and examined Tibetan nuns tortured by Chinese authorities. They reported that their torture included discarding their supplies used during menstruation in manners inconsistent with

their Tibetan Buddhist beliefs about discarding such bodily fluids. This led to imbalances in their spirit that were believed to cause their chronic symptoms similar to fatigue and depression. Hindu authorities in India cut the hair of Sikh men, another example of psychological torture that is regionally specific.

Though the physical aspects of torture might be more obvious, psychological techniques and psychological aspects of physical torture are nearly always present and strongly interact with the physical symptoms. Because psychological torture is so easy to hide and deny, it is often used instead of physical torture. As evidenced by recent debates in the United States and Europe, there is little agreement on what constitutes psychological torture, making it easier for it to be denied and called other things. Still, torture survivors have often told us that it was the psychological methods, such as mock execution or being forced to witness the torture of a friend, that caused them the most lasting harm.

## Overall Health Effects

Torture may have both immediate and long-lasting physical and psychological consequences. As clinicians in countries receiving refugees, we rarely encounter the most immediate phases, and those coming for treatment may have undergone torture years prior to accessing care. The survivor may have been fleeing, lack money to pay for treatment, suffer stigma, or experience a refusal for treatment by the healthcare system. Injuries encountered, therefore, might be complicated by lack of timely treatment.

For many survivors, a visit to the primary healthcare clinic may be their only contact with healthcare services.[20] Help-seeking[21] and the pattern of reporting of symptoms might be determined by interrelated factors such as gender, culture, and trauma-related factors such as shame or avoidance.[21,22] Impairment can be caused by combinations of both physical and psychological factors.

### Physical health effects

Certain types of torture may give rise to specific symptoms and signs and will usually be related to the severity of the applied method. 'Telefono' torture, for example, has been linked to tinnitus.[23] Violent shaking, a common torture technique in some countries, might lead to cerebral edema and subdural and retinal hemorrhage.[24] Some techniques may 'only' cause scars, but the more specific forms, such

**Table 50.2 Overview of torture methods**

| Physical methods | Psychological methods |
|---|---|
| Blunt trauma<br>  Unsystematic (beatings all over)<br>  Systematic (e.g. under the soles of the feet, i.e. 'falanga;' on both ears, i.e. 'telefono') | Humiliation<br>  Verbal humiliations, e.g. sexual humiliations and mocking<br>  Forced humiliating actions (e.g. breaking taboos, renouncing ideological, political or religious foundation)<br>  Depersonalization/dehumanization (e.g. being called by number instead of name, blindfolded for weeks or months)<br>  Interrogation in the nude |
| Penetrating trauma<br>  Stinging (e.g. under nails)<br>  Cuttings (mutilation)<br>  Amputations<br>  Shots | |
| Crushing trauma<br>  Mutilation of, e.g. extremities by trampling | Threats<br>  Against the victim (e.g. death threats, threats of rape, torture)<br>  Against the victim's family |
| Positional torture<br>  Fixation/restriction of movement by use of ropes, chains, straps<br>  Fixation in forced unphysiological positions, e.g. in small boxes, rooms or cages (the tortoise)<br>  Suspension with arms tied behind the back (Palestinian hanging), on a stick in the hollows of the knees, locked with tied wrists (the parrot stick), in feet or hair | Mock executions<br><br>Deprivation<br>  Of light and sound<br>  Of food and drink<br>  Of access to toilet facilities<br>  Of sleep<br>  Of company<br>  Of access to medicine and medical assistance |
| Shaking<br>  Shaking of the head for a long time | Experiencing the torture of others |
| Asphyxiation<br>  Near-drowning, e.g. in polluted water (submarino)<br>  Near-suffocation, e.g. by use of ropes or plastic bags (dry submarino) | |
| Chemical and physical torture<br>  Chemical tissue damage (e.g. skin, mucous membranes, underlying tissue) by use of acids, bases, inhalation of chili, kerosene, etc.<br>  Physical tissue damage by use of electricity, cold, heat, or fire (burns) | |
| Pharmacological and microbiological torture<br>  Forced intake of toxic doses of, e.g. neuroleptics<br>  Inoculation of pathogenic bacteria or viruses (e.g. HIV)<br>  Deprivation of access to necessary medicine (e.g. insulin) | |
| Sexual Torture<br>  Rape, possibly forced between two victims<br>  Instrumentation of genitals | |
| Animal torture<br>  Enticing animals (dogs, rats, insects etc) to assault or attack a fixated victim | |

From: Modvig J, Jaranson J. A global perspective of torture, political violence and health. In: John P, Wilson and Boris Drozdek, editors. Broken spirits: the treatment of traumatized asylum seekers, refugees, war and torture victims. New York: Brunner-Routledge Press, 2004:38–39.

as 'falanga' and hanging by a limb, may lead to lasting impairment and chronic pain.

Among the most frequently encountered complaints are chronic pains in the head and back. The chronic pain and tension may be accompanied by fibrositis and myofascial pain.[25-28] In those who have been exposed to 'falanga,'[25] we observe damage to connective tissue and damaged heels, thereby rendering walking painful and difficult, even years after the torture. Genital torture can be followed not only by psychological sequelae and sexual dysfunction, but also by chronic pain syndromes.[29] Especially in the identification of factors leading to chronic pain, an interdisciplinary and transcultural approach must be followed, as the expression of distress, emotions such as shame, and physical changes in tissue and neuroanatomical structures must be taken into consideration. For example, rhabdomyolisis after beatings has been observed to be linked to life-threatening renal failure.[30-32]

To document specific physical sequelae, detailed or digital imagery of superficial injuries and skin lesions can be augmented by specific radioimaging and other diagnostic techniques. Magnetic resonance imaging has been proven effective in many forms of injuries such as 'falanga' and blunt brain injuries.[33] Bone scintigraphy has been demonstrated to be effective in the documentation of injuries not detected by regular X-rays.[34,35]

## Psychiatric and psychosocial health effects

The psychological consequences following torture are frequently the most important sequelae as they are long-lasting and disabling. However, many torture survivors initially present with physical complaints and describe in detail various physical symptoms, while it is later that the psychological problems may be revealed.[20] Thus, Salvadoran refugees who suffered from war-related traumas may express their emotional distress with somatic complaints, though without connecting these complaints to their traumatic experiences. Still, persons who survive torture may suffer from functional disability simply due to their psychiatric symptoms, independent of both physical effects of the torture and of medical health status. Commonly, survivors exhibit a collection of psychological symptoms that do not fit a single psychiatric disorder or do not fulfill DSM-IV criteria[36] for a disorder, such as somatic symptoms with no obvious cause, depressed mood, insomnia, nightmares,

anxiety, difficulty concentrating, and avoidance of trauma reminders.

Torture destroys trust so that survivors may not trust others in their community or social networks, thus greatly reducing their resources for social support, employment, friendship, and adjustment to a new society. They may feel estranged from members of their own culture. This may be due to feelings of shame or to fear – often based on fact – that there are members of rival political groups in the country of exile who could threaten their family's safety back in their home country. Progressing through the asylum application process may be adversely affected if the survivor is afraid of government officials and persons in uniforms or if their post-traumatic stress disorder symptoms are provoked when encountering these reminders. These unique consequences of torture are often manifested in ways that are misinterpreted by non-health service providers. For example, our clients have encountered lawyers who do not fully appreciate how trauma impairs memory, social workers who may not understand why a torture survivor refuses to use an interpreter provided by the consulate of the survivor's country, and job placement services that erroneously ascribe a survivor's reluctance to wear a security guard uniform to an unwillingness to work.

## Post-traumatic stress disorder

Diagnostic issues for refugees and immigrants are discussed elsewhere (see Ch. 49). However, there are aspects of diagnosis that need special emphasis when assessing torture survivors.

Post-traumatic stress disorder (PTSD) has been shown to be the most important but not the only diagnostic category in survivors of torture (for example, see references 16, 18, 20–22, 24, 26, 27). Estimates of PTSD prevalence among samples of torture survivors vary greatly due to differences between populations (see Table 49.1). The differences include the forms of torture and trauma exposure, the time that has passed since torture, the frequency and severity of exposure, and several other factors occurring before and after torture.[17,18,22,37] Refugee status and exile must be seen as especially important factors, contributing to mental health symptoms[17,37-39] and may influence mental health through their effects on social support or continued danger because of the risk of forced return. Symptoms might fluctuate, depending on coping strategies, social support, and stressors. News reports from the home country, war pictures, court situations, or asylum procedures can trigger intrusive phases, while distraction through activity and work can lead to avoidant phases.

The development of PTSD might also be related to other protective and risk factors in survivors of torture. Basoglu et al. showed an increase in diagnoses of PTSD among tortured nonrefugees compared to matched controls (18% versus 4%, $p = 0.04$).[40,41] In a nonrefugee group of Turkish political activists and nonactivists, Paker et al. found significant differences between those who had been tortured and those who had not been tortured in current PTSD (20% versus 4% in activists, 30% versus 0% in nonactivists) and current major depression (8% versus 0% for activists, and 23% versus 0% for nonactivists).[42] Despite significant differences in mental health outcomes in the tortured and nontortured groups of Basoglu's and Paker's studies, the most striking finding was that the severity level of psychopathology was lower than expected, especially in the context of very severe and prolonged torture experiences. One explanation for this finding is that higher levels of political activism are associated with less severe levels of psychological symptoms. A matched-control study of tortured Tibetan nuns compared to nontortured Tibetan nuns found a differential effect of torture on forms of distress, with statistically nonsignificant differences in the rates of depression.[43] Protective factors such as strong belief systems (monastic Buddhism) and life in an environment that supported and nurtured their beliefs and culture (a monastery in Dharamsala, India) may have mitigated the occurrence of psychiatric symptoms. Dedication to Buddhist religion was recently shown to be a protective factor for both anxiety and depression in a study of tortured and nontortured Bhutanese refugees.[16]

Post-traumatic stress disorder does not adequately encompass the entire symptomatology of torture survivors.[44-46] The category of 'complex' PTSD or DESNOS (disorder of extreme stress not otherwise specified) has been proposed to cover the complexity of torture and similar forms of extreme trauma.[47,48] In spite of this extension of concepts, many important sequelae observed can best described on a descriptive level. PTSD – especially after sexual violence – is often accompanied by 'associated symptoms' including shame and guilt feelings.[48] The last are of major importance as they appear to be responsible for much of the chronicity observed and interfere with social functioning, leading to treatment avoidance, low treatment compliance, and other forms of self-punishing behavior. Such symptoms are also at least partly included in the complex PTSD list of symptoms. In addition, dissociative symptoms that are frequent in trauma and torture survivors are also not completely covered by the DSM-IV PTSD concept and might require attention. Complex changes in behavior and personality, partly overlapping with some of the symptoms mentioned before, are covered by the new WHO ICD-10 category of 'Enduring personality change after catastrophic experiences' (F 62.0).[49]

Comorbidity, especially with depression (MDD), with possible suicidality, is high and should not be neglected by a singular focus on PTSD.[45,50] Brain trauma can create symptoms similar to PTSD and depression, especially impaired concentration, irritability, and a feeling of lack of energy, and must be diagnosed to avoid inadequate treatment.[51,52]

Substance abuse, especially of alcohol or benzodiazepines, can be common in some populations, frequently as an effort of 'self-treatment' of symptoms of PTSD or depression. Suicidal ideation might be high, especially if there is no perspective of a future life.

## Assessment of Torture Survivors

It is important to begin the assessment of torture with a caveat. To focus attention on torture above and beyond the other stressors and traumas commonly experienced by refugees may not always be to the patient's advantage. Torture may be just one of many traumatic stresses experienced by patients who have frequently endured years of persecution, war, exile, death of loved ones, immigration to a foreign culture with the attendant insecurities and threats to health and well-being, not to mention loss of property, position, and existential place in the world. In this context of years of stress and trauma, torture can be just one factor contributing to their current health status (Box 50.1).

General considerations discussed below should be kept in mind when offering treatment. Standard physical treatment approaches might be very effective if they include psychological help and assistance with legal and social needs. First, primary care clinicians must suspect that a patient was tortured. Given the high prevalence in refugee samples from both the community and primary care settings, one's suspicion should be raised often when evaluating refugees. Patients are unlikely to offer this information so clinicians should inquire (see Ch. 48). Some survivors may assert that they have 'put their experiences behind' them and don't want to be reminded about the pain. They don't believe that

---

**Box 50.1**

**Case study 1**

A Bosnian woman had been repeatedly raped and tortured by soldiers for the express purpose of genocide. Some weeks before, neighbors had advised her to flee, but she did not want to leave the village she loved. Shortly after the rape, she lost contact with her husband, who had been taken away by soldiers, imprisoned, and then 'disappeared.' She decided to abort a child she had conceived during rape, since she could not deal with this. She escaped to a neighboring country, found work, but felt 'strange' and 'unreal.' She could not speak about these events, especially about the rape, and, since she could not get any news about her husband, she could not start to mourn or remarry. She had frequently consulted physicians for chronic lower back pain, but physical therapy and analgesic medication provided only limited reduction of symptoms. A gastroscopy recommended for gastric pain and a suspected abuse of analgesics was first avoided, and then refused shortly before the examination, because the patient experienced extreme fear, trembling, and sweating. In a consultation with a female psychiatrist, previously undiagnosed symptoms of severe PTSD, shame, and guilt feelings were identified. The 'normality' of such a reaction was discussed as part of a focused intervention, treatment with a selective serotonin reuptake inhibitor was recommended, and she was referred to a psychotherapist. At a later stage, family therapy was added, since the older of the patient's two daughters reported increasing problems at school. After 2 years, the patient was free of pain, had secured a better job, and had started a new relationship with a Croatian neighbor.

---

torture is still influencing their physical and mental health. Clinicians should not compel patients to discuss details but, instead, allow them to disclose events as they become comfortable, possibly over months or years.

Countries with widespread persecution create a climate of general distrust among their citizens. This may even compromise the trust in physicians, who, in their home countries, refused to treat torture survivors for fear or ideological reasons. Physicians were even suspected of giving confidential information to agents of the state or to other persecutors. Physicians may have been directly involved in their torture or have been present during the torture (to help torturers determine when their pain infliction

is approaching death). As a first step, trust has to be restored. It is especially important to affirm the safety and confidentiality of the doctor–patient relationship in primary care practice. Increasingly, torturers use methods that leave no scars or grossly visible evidence that torture has occurred. Consequently, survivors may feel that clinicians will not believe them if they tell the horrible truth.

It is also important to consider who is present in the treatment setting. Shame, fear of overburdening family members, or fear of stigma in the case of sexual torture or psychological symptoms might require a setting with only 'safe' members of the family. This must be balanced with the need for reassurance and cultural patterns regulating visits to the physician. Both mental health problems and known sexual violation might in some cases even lead to a threat to the victim's life and endanger the social standing or marriage prospects of other family members. Persistent reporting of somatoform or dissociative symptoms that do not respond to direct treatment again might be an indicator of such undisclosed sexual trauma and require a very sensitive approach. Specific to severe trauma, apparently harmless situations such as an ECG, a gastroscopy, or a general examination can lead to reactivation of unprocessed memories of torture.

Torture survivors often need a wide variety of service providers, including healthcare workers, social workers, immigration lawyers, job placement specialists, and English as a Second Language (ESL) teachers. This is beyond the resources of most primary care clinics and often the survivors themselves to coordinate these services toward the common goal of achieving healing. Communication between these health services, legal services, and social services is often difficult. Therefore, referral to specialized torture treatment programs and centers might be advisable.

The case management services offered by torture treatment centers help create a more seamless delivery of services and ensure that clients receive referrals in a timely manner. Often these centers provide an integrated team of physicians, mental health specialists, social workers, and a network of immigration lawyers who provide multidisciplinary care for survivors. For instance, social workers may assist them with job training and obtaining citizenship, and lawyers may help solve legal problems. These centers are often eager to receive referrals from primary care clinicians and often provide training about torture survivors for the primary care staff. Our clinical experience is that a high proportion of survivors who are able to attend these centers improve significantly in a year or two. This may reflect selection biases (persons who can attend these centers on a regular basis may be intrinsically different from those who can not), or the value of integrated and multidisciplinary services beyond medicine and psychology. Empirical evidence is lacking that specialized centers achieve improved treatment outcomes over standard care. Centers can be found in most major cities in the US, although access to these may be difficult for many survivors due to limited hours or transportation obstacles. Websites include the National Consortium of Torture Treatment Programs (NCTTP) http://ncttp, Doctors of the World http://www.doctorsoftheworld.org/, and Physicians for Human Rights http://www.phrusa.org. In other countries, IRCT and IRCT-affiliated centers can offer advice or treatment (http://www.irct.org). When referring, care should be taken to avoid a feeling of inadequacy or stigma in the patients. Benefits should be carefully explained.

Irritation, disbelief, avoidance, or aggression by the therapist or treating physician can indicate counter-transference feelings, which strongly influence the interaction with the patient. Calming down, discussion with colleagues, or supervision can help to maintain a therapeutic attitude and keep treatment effective. Especially if working with severely traumatized clients on the longer term, therapists or physicians risk vicarious traumatization or secondary traumatic stress (STS), the psychological, spiritual, and social effects of working with trauma victims and of exposure to the traumatic stories they tell. Burn-out prevention strategies, and possibly special training, are required. According to Charles Figley,[53] STS is the constellation of emotional and behavioral responses that can result from *knowledge about* a traumatizing event experience[d] by a significant other. It is the stress resulting form *helping or wanting to help* a traumatized or suffering person.' Also termed 'compassion fatigue' and 'co-victimization,' it is *secondary* trauma because the trauma is experienced vicariously, through a person being a witness or a recorder to another's story. The manifestations of STS can mirror the psychological symptoms experienced by the victim. For instance, STS may include feelings of depression, irritability, intrusive recollections ('I can't get it out of my head'), sleep disturbances, nightmares, emotional numbing, or intolerance of others' experiences, especially the stresses of daily life. It might be noted that culture shock can work both ways and create an additional element of stress in both the patient and the therapist.

## Treatment of Mental Health Sequelae of Torture

Besides the special care necessary to form a positive general environment and interaction, disturbed sleep patterns, as part of PTSD, MDD, or more specific reactions to imprisonment, might be the first target symptoms. The fear of memories and nightmares related to the torture experience and exhaustion due to sleep deprivation can impair any self-healing and coping strategies. Trazadone and similar antidepressants can help to re-establish normal sleeping patterns and avoid dependency problems.[54] Other pharmacological treatment strategies are discussed in Chapter 49.

An integrated treatment package would necessarily include counseling and/or culturally adequate forms of psychotherapy, which even might be first-line interventions in many cases.

Support should be given to the survivor in finding a therapist experienced in trauma or torture treatment. Specific therapeutic strategies might consist of modifications of standard therapeutic modalities such as cognitive behavior therapy (CBT) and could be augmented by newly developed techniques such as eye movement desensitization and reprocessing (EMDR)[55] and testimony therapy,[56] the last a specific approach for the treatment of survivors of torture.

The stigmatization common in many cultures to mental health remains an important issue that requires careful handling and providing adequate information to the patient. Again, brain trauma must be considered in patients with a history of beatings or falling, especially if symptoms such as irritability and concentration difficulties persist in spite of otherwise adequate treatment and recovery.

## Forensic Evaluations

Forensic issues, although not common in everyday practice, might be important in several situations. Particularly, two situations might still require a precise and complete reporting outside of general documentation and treatment needs: asylum procedures and documentation for courts.

Many survivors of torture seek asylum or other forms of protection in host countries. During asylum procedures, documenting sequelae can be a key factor in offering help. In many asylum cases, victims are denied or financially unable to access an independent expert, and documentation can be seen as the next best alternative. The special trust developed with an independent expert can help with a forensic strategy that avoids retraumatization.

Compensation for physical and psychological injuries encountered might require forensic documentation as an important form of evidence and can provide support for the victim.

The international standard recommended in the forensic documentation is the Istanbul Protocol (IP) that can be downloaded from the UNHCR website.[5] The IP gives detailed explanations about different sequelae, diagnostic and documentation strategies, and can also be a helpful tool in the general medical work with torture survivors.[6]

Lawyers and judges in this context frequently question statements by victims of torture, not understanding the importance of typical sequelae. Post-traumatic disorders and brain injury can interfere with a complete or uncontradictory reporting of the experiences encountered by the survivor through physical or psychological mechanisms. Negative findings might also reflect a discrepancy between memories and physical sequelae. Factors influencing incomplete recall, especially of physical violence, include shame or guilt feelings, the natural course of healing, and efforts to hide torture techniques. Opinions must be formulated with care to avoid discrediting survivor. Information about the general medical and psychological status of torture survivors might be helpful for lawyers and judges, who commonly model their approach to decision-making and fact finding on assumptions that do not apply to torture survivors.

## Conclusion

Torture affects the physical, mental, and social well-being of survivors. Primary care clinicians, when sensitized to the unique needs of torture survivors, can help the survivor overcome physical, psychological, and psychosocial dysfunction and disability.

## References

1. Convention Against Torture and Other Cruel, Inhuman or Degrading Treatment or Punishment, adopted by the General Assembly on 9 December 1975 (resolution 3452) Available: http://www.hrweb.org/legal/cat.html
2. United Nations, Universal Declaration of Human Rights, Adopted and proclaimed by General Assembly resolution 217 A (III) of 10 December 1948. Available: http://www.un.org/Overview/rights.html
3. Blaauw M. Sexual torture of children – an ignored and concealed crime. Torture 2002; 12:37–45.
4. The World Medical Association Declaration of Tokyo. Guidelines for Physicians Concerning Torture and other Cruel, Inhuman or Degrading Treatment or Punishment in Relation to Detention and Imprisonment, Adopted by the 29th World Medical Assembly, Tokyo, Japan, October 1975, and editorially revised at the 170th Council Session, Divonne-les-Bains, France, May 2005, Available: http://www.wma.net/e/policy/c18.htm
5. The World Medical Association. The world medical association resolution on the responsibility of physicians in the denunciation of acts of torture or cruel or inhuman or degrading treatment of which they are aware. Helsinki, 2003. Available: http://www.wma.net/e/policy/t1.htm
6. United Nations, Manual on the Effective Investigation and Documentation of Torture and Other Cruel, Inhuman or Degrading Treatment or Punishment. Availaable: http://www.ohchr.org/english/about/publications/docs/8rev1.pdf
7. Quiroga J, Jaranson JM. Politically-motivated torture and its survivors: A desk study review of the literature. Torture 2005; 15(2,3):1–111.
8. Jaranson J, Kastrup M. Psychological consequences of torture and persecution. In: Christodoulou GN, ed. Advances in psychiatry. New York: World Psychiatric Association; 2005:(2):155–161.
9. Haritas Fatouros M. The official torture: a learning model for obedience to the authority of violence. J Appl Psychol 1988; 18:1107–1120.
10. Baker R. Psychosocial consequences for tortured refugees seeking asylum and refugee status in Europe. In: Torture and its consequences: current treatment approaches. Basoglu M, ed. New York, NY: Cambridge University Press; 1992.
11. Eisenman DP, Gelberg L, Liu H, et al. Mental health and health-related quality of life among adult Latino primary care patients living in the United States with previous exposure to political violence. JAMA 2003; 290:627–634.
12. Eisenman DP, Keller AS, Kim G. Survivors of torture in a general medical setting: how often have patients been tortured, and how often is it missed? West J Med 2000; 172:301.
13. Thonneau P, Gratton J, Desrosiers G. Health profile of applicants for refugee status (admitted into Quebec between August 1985 and April 1986). Can J Pub Health 1990; 81:182–186.
14. Montgomery E, Foldspang A. Criterion-related validity of screening for exposure to torture. Dan Med Bull 1994; 41:588–591.
15. Kjersem HJ. Migrationsmedicin i Danmark: Vurdering af nogle migrations- medicinske problemstillinger blandt asylsøgere og flygtninge [Migration medicine in Denmark: evaluation of a number of migration medicine problems among asylum seekers and refugees]. Copenhagen, Denmark: Danish Red Cross; 1996.
16. Shrestha NM, Sharma B, van Ommeren M, et al. Impact of torture on refugees displaced within the developing world: symptomatology among Bhutanese refugees in Nepal. JAMA 1998; 280:443–448.
17. Hondius AJK, Willigen LHM, Kleijn WC, et al. Health problems among Latin-American and Middle-Eastern refugees in the Netherlands: relations with violence exposure and ongoing sociopsychological strain. J Traum Stress 2000; 1:619–634.
18. de Jong JTVM, Komproe IH, Van Ommeren M, et al. Lifetime events and posttraumatic stress disorder in 4 post conflict settings. JAMA 2001; 286:555–562.
19. Modvig J, Pagaduan-Lopez J, Rodenburg J, et al. Torture and trauma in post-conflict East-Timor. Lancet 2000; 356:1763.
20. Gavagan T, Martinez A. Presentation of recent torture survivors to a family practice center. J Fam Pract 1997; 44(2):209–212.
21. Priebe S, Esmaili S. Long-term mental sequelae of torture in Iran – who seeks treatment? J Nerv Ment Dis 1997;185: 74–77.

22. Van Ommeren M, de Jong JT, Sharma B, et al. Psychiatric disorders among tortured Bhutanese refugees in Nepal. Arch Gen Psychiatry 2001; 58:475–482.

23. Sinding R. The late ear, nose, and throat region sequelae of torture. Torture 2000; 9:20–22.

24. Moreno A, Grodin MA. Torture and its neurological sequelae. Spinal Cord 2002; 40:213–223.

25. Amris K. Physiotherapy for torture victims: chronic pain in torture victims, possible mechanisms of pain. Torture 2000; 10:73–76.

26. Thomsen AB, Eriksen J, Smidt-Nielsen K. Chronic pain in torture survivors. Forensic Sci Int 2000; 108:155–163.

27. Leth PM, Banner J. Forensic medical examination of refugees who claim to have been tortured. Am J Forensic Med Pathol 2005; 26:125–130.

28. Roche P. Survivors of torture and trauma: a special group of patient with chronic pain. Austr Physiother 1992; 38:156–157.

29. Norredam M, Crosby S, Munarriz R, et al. Urologic complications of sexual trauma among male survivors of torture. Urology 2005; 65:28–32.

30. Malik GH, Reshi AR, Najar MS, et al. Further observation on acute renal failure following physical torture. Nephrol Dial Transplant 1995; 10:198–202.

31. Malik GH, Sirwal IA, Reshi AR, et al. Acute renal failure following physical torture. Nephron 1993; 63:434–437.

32. Bloom AI, Zamir G, Muggia M, et al. Torture rhabdomyorhexis: a pseudo crush syndrome. J Trauma 1995; 38:252–254.

33. Savnik A, Amris K, Rogind H, et al. MRI of the plantar structures of the foot after falanga torture. Eur Radiol 2000; 10:1655–1659.

34. Lok V, Tunca M, Kumanlioglu K, et al. Bone scintigraphy as clue to previous torture. Lancet 1991; 337:846–847.

35. Mirzaei S, Knoll P, Lipp RW, et al. Bone scintigraphy in screening of torture survivors. Lancet 1998; 352:949–951

36. American Psychiatric Association. Diagnostic and statistical manual of mental disorders. 4th edn. Washington, DC: American Psychiatric Association; 2000.

37. Jaranson JM, Butcher L, Halcon DR, et al. Somali and Oromo refugees: Correlates of torture and trauma. Am J Pub Health 2004; 94(4):591–598.

38. Ekblad S, Prochazka H, Roth G. Psychological impact of torture: A 3-month follow-up of mass-evacuated Kosovan adults in Sweden. Lessons learned for prevention. Acta Psychiatr Scand 2002; 106(Suppl. 412):30–36.

39. Lie B. A 3-year follow-up study of psychosocial functioning and general symptoms in settled refugees. Acta Psychiatr Scand 2002; 106:415–425.

40. Basoglu M, Mineka S, Paker M, et al. Psychological preparedness for trauma as a protective factor in survivors of torture. Psychol Med 1997; 27:1421–1433.

41. Basoglu M, Ozmen E, Sahin D, et al. Appraisal of self, social environment, and state authority as a possible mediator of posttraumatic stress disorder in tortured political activists. J Abnorm Psychol 1996; 105:232–236.

42. Paker M, Paker O, Yuksel S. Psychological effects of torture: an empirical study of tortured and non-tortured non-political prisoners. In: Basoglu M, ed. Torture and its consequences: current treatment approaches. Introduction. Cambridge, UK: Cambridge University Press; 1992:72–81.

43. Holtz TH. Refugee trauma versus torture trauma: a retrospective controlled cohort study of Tibetan refugees. J Nerv Ment Dis 1998; 186:24–34.

44. Summerfield DA. Coping with the aftermath of trauma: NICE guidelines on post-traumatic stress disorder have fundamental flaw. Br Med J 2005; 331:50.

45. Wenzel T, Griengl H, Stompe T, et al. Psychological disorders in survivors of torture: exhaustion, impairment and depression. Psychopathology 2000; 33:292–296.

46. Silove D, Steel Z, McGorry P, et al. Trauma exposure, postmigration stressors, and symptoms of anxiety, depression and post-traumatic stress in Tamil asylum-seekers: comparison with refugees and immigrants. Acta Psychiatr Scand 1998; 97:175–181.

47. Jongedijk RA, Carlier IVE, Schreuder BJN, et al. Complex posttraumatic stress disorder: an exploratory investigation of PTSD and DESNOS among Dutch war veterans. J Traum Stress 1996; 9:577–586.

48. Ide N, Paez A. Complex PTSD: a review of current issues. Int J Em Men Health 2000; 2:43–49.

49. World Health Organisation. Tenth revision of the international classification of diseases, chapter V (F): mental and behavioural disorders. Geneva: WHO; 1991.

50. Ferrada-Noli MF, Asberg M. Suicidal behaviour after severe trauma part 2: the association between methods of torture and of suicidal ideation in posttraumatic stress disorder. J Traum Stress 1998; 11:113–124.

51. Moreno A, Peel M. Posttraumatic seizures in survivors of torture: manifestations, diagnosis, and treatment. J Immigr Health 2004; 6:179–186.

52. Weinstein CS, Fucetola R, Mollica R. Neuropsychological issues in the assessment of refugees and victims of mass violence. Neuropsychol Rev 2001; 11:131–141.

53. Figley CR, ed. Compassion fatigue: coping with secondary traumatic stress disorder in those who treat the traumatized. New York, NY: Brunner/Mazel, Inc.; 1995.

54. Saletu-Zyhlarz GM, Anderer P, Arnold O, et al. Confirmation of the neurophysiologically predicted therapeutic effects of trazodone on its target symptoms depression, anxiety and insomnia by postmarketing clinical studies with a controlled-release formulation in depressed outpatients. Neuropsychobiology 2003; 48:194–208.

55. Korn DL, Leeds AM. Preliminary evidence of efficacy for EMDR resource development and installation in the stabilization phase of treatment of complex posttraumatic stress disorder. J Clin Psychol 2002; 58:1465–1487.

56. van Dijk JA, Schoutrop MJ, Spinhoven P. Testimony therapy: treatment method for traumatized victims of organized violence. Am J Psychother 2003; 57:361–373.

# CHAPTER 51

# Interpersonal Violence Towards Women

Solvig Ekblad, Marianne C. Kastrup, David P. Eisenman,
and Libby Tata Arcel

## Introduction

Violence pervades the lives of many around the world. A review of domestic violence suggests that it happens to women of all socioeconomic and educational backgrounds, in all types of communities, including egalitarian societies and among different groups and countries. However, there is little research about this issue among different ethnic groups and among economically disadvantaged communities.[1] In this chapter we will concentrate on violence, which is one of the most frequent traumatic stressors for displaced, immigrant, and refugee women. Violence is many things, including a social issue, exemplified by statements from the World Bank and United Nations (UN). In November 2004, World Bank[2] President James Wolfensohn concluded in a workshop to mark the International Day for the Elimination of Violence Against Women: 'The workshop made it clear that violence against women exacts enormous cost to economies, to women's health and to women's rights, and that we need to join forces to combat this pressing development concern . . . women should no longer have to live in fear, their children should no longer witness daily acts of violence, and men should enjoy the dignity and freedom from want that enables them to use peaceful means to resolve conflicts.' The former UN Secretary General Kofi Annan[3] has called violence against women the most pervasive, yet least recognized, human rights abuse in the world. To stay out of harm's way some may be able to lock their doors; others have no possibility of escape. The threat is

behind the closed doors (Brundtland foreword WHO World Report on Violence,[4] Beijing Declaration; see Box 51.1). Frequently hidden from the public eye, interpersonal violence is permeating the lives of a large proportion of women. Rape and sexual assault of women are also used as weapons of war and interpersonal violence. Such violence is a social issue and adversely influences general health, mental health, ability, and successful adaptation and integration. The violent abuses exacerbate discrimination against women, e.g., by intensifying women's exclusion from the public sphere and rendering access to social and health services more difficult.[6]

## Setting the Scene

### Types of violence against women

According to the UN Declaration on the Elimination of Violence Against Women, violence is defined as: '. . . any act of gender-based violence that results in, or is likely to result in, physical, sexual or psychological harm or suffering to women.'[7]

It is important to bear in mind that women are exposed to different kinds of violence and that violence may be rooted in gender inequality. The fact that women are frequently economically or emotionally dependent upon their perpetrators has implications for the dynamics of the abuse and ways to deal with it.[4] This report discusses two kinds of interpersonal violence: family violence and community violence, i.e., violence outside the home. The first

### Box 51.1

'. . . Violence against women both violates and impairs or nullifies the enjoyment by women of their human rights and fundamental freedoms . . . In all societies, to a greater or lesser degree, women and girls are subjected to physical, sexual and psychological abuse that cuts across lines of income, class and culture.' Beijing Declaration and Platform for Action, Paragraph 112.[5]

kind relates particularly to women, but, in areas of war and conflict, women are also more likely to face threats of community violence outside the home. There is increasing recognition and understanding of the particular risks that displaced and refugee women are facing in zones of conflict, in refugee camps, and in asylum centers[8] as they are disproportionately affected by violence. Women who seek shelter from the hardships of armed conflicts and strife may end up experiencing further harassment in what, from an outside perspective, should be a safe environment. According to findings by Basoglu et al.,[9] fear of threat to safety and loss of control over life appear to be the most significant mediating factors for PTSD and depression. Therefore, these findings highlight the importance of the combination of political action against impunity and attention to mental health consequences. Both from a public health as well as a judicial point of view these are issues requiring further attention.

### Prevalence of violence

Violent acts against women and girls are reported worldwide. Numerous surveys have consistently demonstrated a high prevalence of physical assaults by intimate partners. Prevalence figures typically rely on self-reports and it is well known that in some cultures violence is frequently kept hidden from outsiders. This may be related to traditional views of a man's right to punish his wife, with victimization often being considered part and parcel of the daily burden of women. As a consequence, the violated women may be reluctant to identify themselves, as it may bring shame on the family and more victimization.[4]

According to Amnesty International,[10] 'domestic violence is the major cause of death and disability for European women aged 16–44 and accounts for more death and ill-health than cancer or traffic accidents. In South Africa more women are shot at home in acts of domestic violence than are shot by strangers on the streets or by intruders.' In other words, 'the prevalence of such violence suggests that globally, millions of women are experiencing violence or living with its consequences.'[11]

Unfortunately, many health professionals are not trained to discover consequences of violence. Thus, despite women's visits to health facilities, many incidents may go unnoticed.

Immigrant and refugee women, as well as those displaced within their own countries, are not beyond experiencing this kind of violence. But they are subjected to further atrocities as the nature of war and violent conflicts has changed, and an increasing proportion of reported casualties are no longer soldiers but civilians. Thus, such women may experience violent acts as seen in recent conflicts, including the ongoing one in the Darfur region of Sudan, as well as in the former Yugoslavia, the Democratic Republic of Congo, Rwanda, Sierra Leone, Liberia, northern Uganda, Chechnya, and the Russian Federation.[12] A global view starts to be evident among different UN organizations and non-governmental organizations (NGOs): in areas of conflict, 'because of the sensitivity of the subject, violence is almost universally under-reported.'[11] Conducting research on these sensitive matters (i.e., sexual violence) is an extraordinary challenge even in relatively stable settings. During conflict and related crises, when there is a lack of stability and disruption of family and community support, such research may be impossible.[13]

### Types of violence

Violence has many faces, and Watts and Zimmerman[11] have reviewed the magnitude of some of the most common and severe kinds of violent acts against women: intimate partner violence; sexual abuse by non-intimate partners; harmful traditional practices; trafficking; forced prostitution; exploitation of labor; debt bondage of women; physical and sexual violence against prostitutes; forced marriage; sex-selective abortions and dowry murders; and rape during war. Characteristically, women living in abusive relationships may be the targets of multiple acts of violence over time. The violence typically involves physical, psychological, and social aspects and frequently involves sexual abuse.[4]

In refugee women, experiences of sexual violence during armed conflicts are commonplace. The aggressor may use sexual assault to show superiority, to humiliate, to force abortions or to force pregnancy upon women as a strategy of war towards another ethnic group.[14] Women may also feel forced to render sexual services to survive, in return for assistance or to protect their children. Traditionally, abusing the conquered women has been seen as part of the realities of war, and it was not until recently that rape in times of war was recognized as a war crime. Many women may face the threat of ostracism by their own families if sexual assault is revealed, leaving the women in question vulnerable and fragile. Women in armed conflicts are at extreme risk of sexual violence[8] and, therefore, impunity for rape and sexual violence must end.

## Influence of culture and sociopolitical context on interpersonal violence

Culture influences the interaction of risk factors with social support and protective psychological factors that contribute to symptoms. While some studies suggest that acculturation decreases the likelihood of interpersonal violence,[15] recent studies find that acculturation actually increases this likelihood.[16] Increased opportunities for the woman may make the man increase his control in order to keep power in the patriarchal family model. This is a method of exerting control over and disempowering women.

Culture can confound diagnosis and management of care by influencing definition of diseases and delineation of abuse or symptoms. Culture also influences help-seeking patterns, perspectives on and expectations of the role of healthcare providers, and patient–practitioner communication. A recently arrived refugee woman may, for instance, expect a hierarchical relationship with a health professional and experience a sense of stigma and shame when confronted with the more egalitarian, consumer-oriented clinical model in Western society. The health staff must, in this context, evaluate the culturally relevant aspects of stress and encourage the protective factors in the present life of the abused woman.

Women of immigrant and refugee background are heterogeneous groups and do not share a common background or similar problems. What they may share are common influences of interpersonal violence within a sociopolitical and structural context.

Usually, migrant women carry a triple burden because of their gender, class, and ethnic background, and they often experience different kinds of psychosocial challenges due to prejudice and discrimination.[17] Women in minority communities may experience sexism from within their communities based on cultural values, beliefs, practices, etc. In addition, as members of minority communities, women may be affected by institutional racism from the dominant culture, 'as expressed through institutional policies, culture norms and prejudicial treatment.'[18] According to Sorenson,[19] institutional racism and sexism are not mutually exclusive; rather, the intersectionality of their multiple identities complicates immigrant and refugee women's experiences of violence.

## Health Consequences of Interpersonal Violence

Violence may have a profound impact on health and functioning. Women who have survived interpersonal violence may display elevated rates of fear, depression, anxiety, post-traumatic stress disorder, substance abuse, tobacco and drug use, hormonal irregularities (e.g., bleeding), and suicide attempts. Perceptions of poor health and worsened health status are also common. The prevailing psychological symptoms include lack of energy, fear, anxiety, depression, feelings of hopelessness, apathy, cognitive dysfunction, insomnia, and somatization.

Physical manifestations may be related to the sexual abuse and include various complaints of the reproductive organs such as chronic pelvic pain, sexual dysfunction, and other types of pain. Musculoskeletal symptoms are also frequent, and some may further suffer a distorted body image.

Refugee women are often heads of households or single providers and are at particular risk of encountering psychological problems when their capacity to cope is overwhelmed or when they have no time to consider their own needs while protecting their immediate families.[14] Refugee women may be particularly vulnerable to stressors related to gender role conflicts and adverse life events and have an increased risk of affective disorders.[20] In a cross-sectional study, Johansson-Blight, et al.,[21] used postal survey questionnaires distributed to a community sample (n = 650, 63.5% response rate) of participants who came to Sweden in 1993–1994 from Bosnia-Herzegovina. They showed that, while job occupancy might be important to the mental health of men in the study, job occupancy and living in an urban region appear to be associated with poor mental health for the women.

Having a job for women may be another stressor because of the traditional family model in which they live. On the other hand, not all who have suffered trauma become victimized and need professional help. Among the protective coping mechanisms are reality orientation, motivation for survival, and the existence of an inner locus of control.[22]

## Therapeutic Aspects

### Barriers to help-seeking

Barriers to help-seeking are related to the cultural context and may include social isolation, language fluency, beliefs about the woman's role in the family, loyalty to the husband and other male relatives, shame related to the abuse, lack of resources and lack of access to them, concerns about separation from extended family, and cultural stigma (Box 51.2). There is often a general distrust of governmental agencies due to previous experiences and the fear of deportation. Women may assume that legal proceedings will be decided in favor of the man. Female victims often believe that reporting their abuser to the police will increase the perpetrator's anger and escalate his violence or that the police may disbelieve the woman's story, resulting in further humiliation. For similar reasons, women may be unwilling to disclose their experiences to health professionals, fearing loss of confidentiality. Some immigrant women believe they have no right to legal protection and feel trapped in their abusive relationships; thus, much interpersonal violence remains unreported.[23]

Furthermore, granting permission to stay in a country may be linked to the male head of the household, thereby endangering the legal status of the woman if she decides to leave her violent husband.

### Clinical implications

#### Communication with patients

One of the main public mental health issues today is to identify displaced, immigrant, and refugee women as well as hidden and/or illegal foreign women who have been abused by interpersonal violence. Refugee women in mental health settings often share common denominators that are a challenge to health professionals.[14] As clinicians, we recommend the following approach for routine abuse screening (Box 51.3) in primary care settings (revised from[24]).

- Introduce yourself, your professional role, what your clinic can offer, your neutrality, and your respect for confidentiality. The

---

> **Box 51.2**
>
> **Barriers for disclosure to healthcare providers**
>
> - Fear of bringing shame to their families, other relatives, and communities.
> - Fear of reinforcing stereotypes.
> - Discourse between linear/individual and relational/collectivist contexts.
> - Loss of socioeconomic status, poverty, and powerlessness may challenge the link between domestic violence and culture.
> - Assumption by the woman of the role of primary family breadwinner, motivating her partner into using interpersonal violence to keep his dominant role in the traditional family.
> - Lack of access to social care and healthcare.
> - Loss of the social support previously received before migration and feeling marginalized from the mainstream culture may result in the woman increasing reliance on her partner.
> - Reluctance to contact police or other legal authorities due to fear of these authorities from previous experiences of abuse, including torture, rape, and other forms of discrimination in her country of origin.
> - Not speaking the mainstream language runs the risk that the abuser is the translator, which negates the woman's chance to reveal the abuse.
> - Risk of deportation and fear of losing custody of their children discourages undocumented women from revealing their abuse because their partners may use threats of deportation to maintain control.
> - Value conflicts between the mainstream culture and the culture of origin may increase levels of stress for more acculturated immigrant women due to loss of social control, alienation from traditional culture, and discrimination by the dominant culture.
> - Abuse in the mainstream country by racial and ethnic discrimination and social class bias.

---

concept of clinician–patient confidentiality may be alien to immigrant and refugee women if this is not the case in their home countries; therefore, it is important to discuss this concept and promise confidentiality in specific terms.
- Establish trust by listening to the woman's trauma story but always keep current stressors in the foreground.
- Assess the safety of the victim immediately and completely, as with any situation of ongoing violence.

## Box 51.3

### Women abuse screening tool

Note: Numeric scores ranging from 3 to 1 can be assigned to the answers below. The women can also complete numeric comfort ratings on each question, ranging from very uncomfortable (1) to very comfortable (4).

1. In general, how would you describe your relationship?
   A lot of tension    Some tension    No tension
2. Do you and your partner work out arguments with:
   Great difficulty    Some difficulty   No difficulty
3. Do arguments ever result in you feeling down or bad about yourself?
   Often          Sometimes      Never
4. Do arguments ever result in hitting, kicking, or pushing?
   Often          Sometimes      Never
5. Do you ever feel frightened by what your partner says or does?
   Often          Sometimes      Never
6. Has your partner ever abused you physically?
   Often          Sometimes      Never
7. Has your partner ever abused you emotionally?
   Often          Sometimes      Never
8. Has your partner ever abused you sexually?
   Often          Sometimes      Never

From Reference 1, page 103, also in Spanish.

- Try to get a view of the woman's expectations and hopes of this meeting (she may have unrealistic beliefs of a swift recovery or 'quick fix').
- Be sensitive to the possibility that the woman may feel forced to tell her story and mitigate this perception or experience.
- Pay attention to the woman's suicidal thoughts, somatization, and silence.
- Act in a humane and professional way, avoiding the waste of precious time resources due to communication difficulties. The woman may simultaneously visit other doctors, i.e., 'doctor shopping,' as long as she feels she is not getting the help she needs.
- Ensure that there is access to competent interpreters if the woman is not fluent in your language and explain the role of the interpreter, including that of confidentiality.

- Have a focus on normalization and empowerment and try to get a view of the woman's capabilities and economic resources (e.g., for transportation and medication) needed to complete treatment.
- Never end a meeting before the woman has the chance to communicate her perception of present and future (i.e., what does she plan to do next, after the meeting).
- End the diagnostic assessment phase by describing the options for intervention and by which local collaborative organizations.
- Pay attention in the assessment of key concepts such as attachment, security, identity/roles, human rights, and existential meaning systems, which have been more or less threatened on different intervention levels.[25]
- Give time to listen and reflect.
- Develop competence working with interpreters for immigrant and refugee patients.
- Do not work alone or full-time with severe traumatic patients, as this risks burn-out or vicarious traumatization.
- Recognize that many women may be polytraumatized, suffering from several traumatic experiences acting simultaneously.
- Be aware that refugee women may live under familial social control that may increase in the host country.
- Respect the cultural and social distances between clinician and client.

Interpersonal violence is described in this chapter, as mentioned earlier, as a traumatic event. Harvey's ecological model for psychosocial trauma postulates that reactions and recovery to trauma are related to person, event, and environment. In concrete, 'the efficiency of trauma-focused interventions depends upon the degree to which they enhance the person–community relationship and achieve "ecological fit" within individually varied recovery contexts.'[26] This is in line with Bracken, who emphasizes that responding to trauma need not be a pathological sign but may also be a reflection of learning, growth, and resilience.[27] According to Moos, 'we need a fundamental paradigm shift in how to construe and examine the aftermath of life crises.'[28] Ekblad and Jaranson[17] interpret this as meaning 'that theories of posttraumatic development and maturation differ from theories of learned helplessness and posttraumatic stress disorder.[17]

## Services

The coordination of victim services between general health, mental health, social services (for example, victim assistance) and the justice system is critical to ensure quality of care. For instance, a lack of financial resources affects women's ability to respond to abuse. Financial independence and employment facilitate escape from an abusive relationship. Linking women to victim services may provide assistance in obtaining crime victim compensation for their healthcare bills. An immigration lawyer can assist immigrant women whose petitions for residency may depend on the abuser's petition. The abused women may be invited to contact cultural, professional, and neutral interpreters, indigenous healers, women's organizations, culture brokers, and other local cultural resources to facilitate short-term and long-term interventions. Healthcare providers and care delivery systems should be aware of and have relationships with culturally competent resources in the community specific to patients' cultural groups and countries of origin.

## Recommendations

We recommend that identification and management of potential risk factors during pre- and post-migration experiences, such as interpersonal violence including rape, be addressed by acceptable and available health systems. Institutionalizing this approach will help alert clinicians and other professionals dealing with immigrant women to possible treatment options. Care providers should also be aware that cultural context may exacerbate the consequences of violence and may limit preventive measures. Cultural traditions may also be protective.[4] Care providers should focus on the most vulnerable groups and recognize the role of poverty and inequality in rendering women more vulnerable.[4]

An important research step will be to agree on the collection of data on violence. The development of an inventory for measuring war-related events, including domestic discord and violence as well as sexual trauma or other abuse in refugees, may be useful but needs further testing.[29] The conventional use of current instruments fails to grasp cultural variations in question content, scale formats, and norms, and can lead to false-positive and false-negative cases of abuse.

Resolving the extensive public health problems of interpersonal and sexual violence in refugee women requires the collaboration of many agencies. The commitment of civil society and governments must focus on changing community and societal norms and on raising the status of women.[4] With migration in an interconnected world, new directions for action are needed.[30]

## References

1. Fogarty CT, Belle Brown J. Screening for abuse in Spanish-speaking women. J Am Board Fam Pract 2002; 15:101–111.
2. The World Bank Examines the Development Implications of Gender-Based Violence, 2 pages. http://web.worldbank.org
3. Annan K. Review of the implementation of the Beijing Platform for Action and Women 2000: Gender, Equality, Development and Peace for the 21st Century. E/CN.6/2005/2, p.22, December 2004.
4. WHO World Report on Violence and Health. Geneva: WHO; 2002.
5. Beijing Declaration and Platform for Action, 2000, § 112.
6. Arcel LT, Kastrup C. War, women and health. NORA 2004; 12(1):37–40.
7. United Nations. Declaration on the Elimination of Violence against Women. New York: United Nations General Assembly, 1993, 5 pages. Available: http://www.un.org
8. UNHCR. Global consultations 25.04.2002. Available: http://www.unhcr.org
9. Basoglu M, Livanou M, Crnobaric C, et al. Psychiatric and cognitive effects of war in former Yugoslavia. Association of lack of redress for trauma and posttraumatic stress reactions. JAMA 2005; 294(5):580–590.
10. Amnesty International. Available: http://web.amnesty.org
11. Watts C, Zimmerman C. Violence against women: global scope and magnitude. Lancet 2002; 359:1232–1237.
12. WHO Information Bulletin Series. Sexual violence in conflict settings and the risk of HIV. Number 2, November, 2004.
13. Reis C, Vann B. Sexual violence against women and children in the context of armed conflict. In: Reyes G, Jacobs GA, eds. Handbook of international disaster psychology. Vol 4. Interventions with special needs populations. Westport, Connecticut: Praeger; 2006:19–44.
14. Kastrup M, Arcel L. Gender specific treatment. In: Wilson JP, Drozdek B, eds. Broken spirits. The treatment of traumatized asylum seekers, refugees, war and torture victims. New York: Brunner Routledge; 2004:547–571.
15. Kantor GK, Jasinski JL, Aldarondo E. Sociocultural status and incidence of marital violence in Hispanic families. Violence Vict 1994; 9(3):207–222.
16. Lown EA, Vega WA. Intimate partner violence and health: self-assessed health, chronic health, and somatic symptoms among Mexican American women. Psychosom Med 2001; 63(3):352–360.
17. Ekblad S, Jaranson J. Psychosocial rehabilitation. In: Wilson JP, Drozdek B, eds. Broken spirits. The treatment of traumatized asylum seekers, refugees, war and torture victims. New York: Brenner-Routledge; 2004:609–636.
18. Kasturirangan A, Krishnan S, Riger S. The impact of culture and minority status on women's experience of domestic violence. Trauma Violence Abuse 2004; 5(4):318–332.
19. Sorenson SB. Violence against women: examining ethnic differences and commonalities. Evaluation Rev 1996; 20(2):123–145.
20. Matthey S, Silove DM, Barnett B, et al. Correlates of depression and PTSD in Cambodian women with young children: a pilot study. Stress Med 1999; 15:103–107.

21. Johansson-Blight K, Ekblad S, Persson J-O, et al. Mental health, employment and gender. Cross-sectional evidence in a sample of refugees from Bosnia-Herzegovina living in two Swedish regions. Social Sci Med 2006; 62(7):1697–1709.

22. Arcel LT, Folnegovic-Smalc V, Tocilj-Simunkovic G, et al. Ethnic cleansing and posttraumatic coping. In: Arcel LT, ed. War violence, trauma and the coping process. Copenhagen: IRCT; 1998:45–78.

23. Bauer HM, Rodriguez MA, Quiroga SS, et al. Barriers to healthcare for abused Latina and Asian immigrant women. J Health Care Poor Underserved 2000; 11(1):33–44.

24. Ekblad S, Roth G. Transkulturell psykiatri/transcultural psychiatry och/and flyktingpsykiatri/refugee psychiatry. In: Psykiatri/Psychiatry. Herlofson J, Åsberg M, Ekselius L, et al. eds. Lund: Studentlitteratur (accepted).

25. Silove D. The psychosocial effects of torture, mass human rights violations and refugee trauma – toward an integrated conceptual framework. J Nerv Mental Dis 1999; 187(4):200–207.

26. Harvey MR. An ecological view of psychological trauma and trauma recovery. J Traumatic Stress 1996; 9:3–23.

27. Bracken P. Hidden agendas: deconstructing PTSD. In: Bracken P, Petty C, eds. Rethinking the trauma of war. London: Free Association Books; 1998:38–59.

28. Moos RH. The mystery of human context and coping. An unravelling of clues. Am J Commun Psychol 2002; 30(1):67–88.

29. Hollifield M, Eckert V, Warner TD, et al. Development of an inventory for measuring war-related events in refugees. Comprehensive Psychiatry 2005; 46:67–80.

30. Global Commission on International Migration. Migration in an interconnected world: new directions for action. Report of the Global Commission on International Migration. Geneva, 5 October 2005. Available: http://www.gcim.org

# CHAPTER 52

# Children and Adolescents

B. Heidi Ellis and Theresa Stichick Betancourt

## Introduction

As increasing numbers of immigrants and refugees become a part of the fabric of the United States, pediatric and adolescent mental health services have needed to adapt and respond to the demand for culturally appropriate services. Mental health services must also respond to the specific social stressors and mental health needs encountered by immigrant youth; in addition to a base rate of psychopathology, the specific circumstances of migration and resettlement may contribute to some immigrant and refugee children being at higher risk for certain disorders. Some immigrants and refugees have experienced or witnessed violence or atrocities in their home country or faced significant danger and adversity during the migration process. All immigrant youth must face the challenges of adjusting to a new culture and navigating the sometimes profound cultural divide between their family's culture and the culture of their new home. Stressors both prior to leaving the home country and after resettlement can contribute to an increased risk for a variety of disorders, in particular post-traumatic stress disorder and depressive disorders. This chapter will briefly review the prevalence of mental health problems in child and adolescent immigrants and refugees and then present current treatment modalities and special treatment considerations in working with this population.

## Mental Health of Child and Adolescent Immigrants and Refugees

Studies of refugee youth suggest that they are at heightened risk for developing mental health problems.[1] In a recent study of 300 children ages 5–18 attending schools in the UK, 100 of whom were refugees, more than 25% of refugee children reported experiencing significant psychological disturbance – more than three times the national average and significantly greater than non-refugee students surveyed.[2] Studies of refugee youth resettled in the United States show rates of post-traumatic stress disorder (PTSD) ranging from 25% to 50%.[3,4] What little longitudinal work has been done suggests that PTSD, in particular, remains relatively persistent in refugee youth over time.[4,5] Sack and colleagues[4] assessed Cambodian adolescents four times over a period of 12 years, with the first assessment occurring a few years after resettlement; they found that at initial assessment and 3 years later around half of the youth met criteria for PTSD (50% and 48%, respectively), and 12 years later this remained as high as 35%. Depression has also been found to be of significance in refugee and immigrant child and adolescent populations, though somewhat less frequently than post-traumatic stress disorder.[3,4]

Studies of immigrant children, in contrast, have shown mixed findings. Several studies report no difference in rates of psychopathology in immigrants compared to non-immigrants.[6,7] Exposure to particular risk factors, such as trauma, increases the likelihood that an immigrant child will experience mental health problems following resettlement.[8] A recent study by Jaycox and colleagues found that immigrant children and adolescents were at risk for both violence exposure and the development of PTSD, with 32% of 1004 immigrant schoolchildren surveyed reporting symptoms in the clinical range.[9]

In light of the extremely high rates of trauma that have been identified within many refugee and immigrant communities, the fact that many of these children do not develop mental health problems points to a great resilience among some children and families. Indeed, within the child refugee field, scholars have pointed out the need to avoid overpathologizing refugees and the importance of not assuming that the experience of trauma necessarily leads to disturbances in mental health.[10] For the subset of children who do present with symptoms of mental health problems, however, the provision of culturally consonant, trauma-informed mental healthcare is critical.

## Mental Health Interventions for Immigrant and Refugee Youth

Before embarking on a discussion of models of intervention for immigrant youth, the following questions must be addressed: who is receiving the intervention, what is the problem to be targeted, and within what service system will the intervention be delivered?

### For whom is the intervention?

This question, while seemingly basic, addresses several fundamental variables that must be considered in choosing an intervention approach. On one level, the interventionist must decide whether the intervention is for the individual child, the family, or even more broadly for a whole community. Appropriate conceptualization of mental health, illness, and healing among diverse cultural groups is important for ensuring the relevance and effectiveness of interventions.[11] For example, in many of the regions from which today's immigrants and refugees originate, more emphasis is placed on the community and collective relationships rather than on the indivi-

dual, which is common in Western cultures.[12,13] In this light, cultural views of mental health, trauma, and healing may be quite different from those in Western host countries, which place a great deal of emphasis on the self as a focal point for treatment. Sensitivity to how a given culture thinks about individuality versus collectivity can also be applied to improve the structure and delivery of mental health services for different immigrant groups. For example, individual therapy approaches may not be the most comfortable starting point for some groups, whereas interventions that integrate psychoeducation into existing community-based activities may be more palatable and can provide a pathway for those needing a higher level of care to be screened and introduced to other forms of services. Interventions that overlook such fundamental cultural differences may be counterproductive for treating multicultural immigrant and refugee populations and fail to tap existing resources to promote mental health and healing.

Once the level of intervention has been decided, additional cultural or historical factors may influence the intervention approach. Culture can greatly influence a family's willingness to engage in treatment, perceptions of mental health services, and explanatory models regarding the child's problems and path to healing.[14] Within some cultures, such as Central Americans, a family therapy model has been identified as particularly consonant with cultural values and practices.[15] Other factors that may influence the treatment approach relate to the historical experience of a child. Recently immigrated families may best benefit from a treatment that focuses on initial adjustment, orientation, and an establishment of safety and security.[16] Indeed, given the many pressing logistical challenges for new arrivals, families may prefer not to engage in treatment soon after arrival despite identified mental health problems.[17] Mental health service providers may find that providing initial case management and linking families to other needed services may present important opportunities for building a treatment alliance. Thus, before identifying an appropriate treatment approach, these factors must be assessed.

### What is the problem to be targeted?

Refugee and immigrant children may present to treatment with any of a variety of mental health or adjustment problems. As detailed above, experiences of loss and trauma have been linked to an increased rate of depressive disorders and post-traumatic stress disorder. However, one must be cautious not to assume the presence of these problems in immigrant children without a diagnostic assessment. A careful assessment of the child's social and developmental history, trauma exposure, and current mental health presentation is essential in order to determine the primary problem in need of treatment. Challenges in acculturation can sometimes confuse the assessment, as in the example of a recently arrived young refugee boy who frequently gets into fights. This behavioral problem could be a manifestation of a mental health problem such as PTSD, in which the child becomes easily emotionally dysregulated and hyperaroused, or could be the result of a learned survival skill within a resource-poor setting such as a refugee camp. Assessing the timeline of the course of the problem, the child's functioning within multiple contexts, the specific antecedents to a behavior, cultural understandings of the problem, as well as behavioral observations can all contribute to a more accurate diagnosis. In particular, mental health providers must avoid equating forced migration experience, particularly that of refugees, with trauma. At times, issues related to grief, loss, and subsequent adjustment issues may be the most appropriate framework for capturing a client's experience. Without question, many immigrants and refugees can and do encounter physical and emotional hardship and exposure to violence that may lead to traumatic reactions during all phases of migration. However, a focus on trauma as an issue in treatment must be established following careful and sensitive assessment, rather than assumed.

A careful approach to trauma-focused treatment is particularly indicated in light of research demonstrating that interventions which encourage the ventilation or retelling of traumatic events at the urging of a therapist, such as critical-incident debriefing may do more harm than good.[18] Furthermore, anthropological evidence has indicated that in some cultures the discussion of past traumatic events may be imbued with very different cultural meanings. Research among war-affected populations in Southern Mozambique found that many people viewed discussion of past traumas as inviting evil spirits to be enlivened.[12] Even if clinical judgment indicates that processing of past traumatic events is indicated for treatment to be successful, the timing, pace, and mechanism by which these memories are engaged must be given careful consideration and planning when working within any cultural group.

## Within what service system will the intervention be delivered?

Many refugee and immigrant families do not seek specialized mental healthcare services for their children.[7,19] This may be the result of the stigma associated with mental illness in many cultures, unfamiliarity with mental health services within the US, or problems identifying a given presenting problem as related to mental health.

Mental health service providers have addressed this challenge in a variety of ways. Some mental health programs have expanded their services such that mental healthcare becomes part of a broader service package. Partnering with existing service systems that have pre-established relationships with refugee children is another means of facilitating the provision of mental health services. Two service systems that have been identified in the literature as key areas for mental health intervention delivery for immigrant and refugee youth are schools and pediatric primary care settings. Collaboration with resettlement agencies and local mutual assistance organizations also presents a possibility for expanding opportunity to bring refugee children into care.

Given the numerous considerations regarding who and what the treatment is for, as well as where the treatment is delivered, there is no single model to be followed in providing mental healthcare for immigrant children and adolescents. In addition, despite the demonstrated need for effective mental health interventions with immigrant and refugee youth, relatively few empirical studies have been conducted that elucidate the best treatment modalities for this population.[20] Despite these challenges, the field has begun to provide some models for consideration in treating immigrant and refugee children. These models, along with the specific populations and treatment targets for which they have been used, are described here.

## Models of Interventions

### Trauma-focused interventions

Within the child trauma literature, there is evidence that trauma-focused cognitive behavioral therapy (TF-CBT) is an effective treatment for traumatized children and adolescents.[21-23] TF-CBT is designed for children and adolescents 3–18 years of age, and has been adapted for use with children who have experienced a variety of different types of trauma such as traumatic loss, community violence, and terrorist attacks. Basic components of the TF-CBT model include skills training, psychoeducation, and stress management, followed by exposure-based exercises and relapse prevention.[24-26] A recent large-scale evaluation of TF-CBT with sexually abused children showed greater improvements in children's PTSD symptomatology, as well as depression, behavioral problems, shame, and abuse-related attributions compared to child-centered supportive therapy.

While this model is very promising for traumatized children generally, there are several limitations that must be considered in its application to refugee and immigrant children. First, the treatment has yet to be specifically evaluated for refugees and immigrants who have experienced trauma associated with war or migration. A series of case studies using imaginal flooding with children exposed to war in Lebanon provides preliminary support for the application of CBT methods to war-traumatized children, showing reduction in PTSD and other related trauma symptoms.[23,25] However, differences in culture, in types of trauma experienced, in stigma associated with seeking treatment, or in complicating life circumstances associated with resettlement may affect the success of implementing this model across different groups of immigrant and refugee children. Furthermore, this model is specific to children experiencing distress related to a traumatic event and does not include addressing other social or emotional issues that may be central to a refugee or immigrant child's experience, such as acculturative stress or cultural bereavement.

Another model of treatment that specifically seeks to address the political nature of trauma experienced by many refugees is testimonial psychotherapy. Originally developed with adult survivors of political atrocities, where the model has been more widely implemented and evaluated, it has been adapted for and used with adolescents. To date, this form of psychotherapy has been pilot tested with Sudanese adolescents, suggesting that it is safe and feasible for this age group.[27] The intervention is premised on the idea that refugees experience healing through giving a testimony of the persecution they experienced. The testimony can then be used for the purposes of education and advocacy. Reduced depression and PTSD over time were seen in adult Bosnian refugees who participated in testimonial therapy.[28] There is no empirical evidence of the effectiveness of this model with adolescents.

## Interventions that promote stability in the family and social environment

Even if an immigrant or refugee child has experienced traumatic events, trauma and related sequelae are not always the presenting problem. Rather, families may identify social issues such as economic stability, a child's school placement, or the threat of deportation as the primary problems in need of assistance. There is some evidence that environmental factors such as unemployment or day-to-day stressors may precipitate or contribute to PTSD or depressive symptomatology.[29,30] Until these basic needs are attended to, psychotherapy may not be sought by refugee and immigrant families.[16,31,32] Clinical consensus in the refugee mental health field asserts that interventions must assess and address the broader socioecological needs of families.[20,27,32,33]

Where war or immigration has affected the functioning of a whole family, family therapy may be the therapeutic modality of choice. Nieves-Grafals suggested that typically a whole family system is affected by distress. As the family system is one of the most central elements of a child's social ecology, directly addressing stress within the family can greatly benefit children.[34] Barenbaum and colleagues identified reducing family distress and promoting parental well-being as important avenues to promoting the well-being of children who have been affected by war.[35] Interventions that attend to the needs of the whole family are particularly compelling in situations where distress in children may be exacerbated by indirect exposures to violence such as the torture of family members and subsequent mental health problems in caregivers.[36] Boothby suggested that particularly when children are faced with ongoing instability in the environment, as might be seen with refugee families facing significant resettlement stressors, interventions that provide direct assistance to parents may be of great benefit to children.[37]

In an empirical study by Dybdahl examining a preventive intervention implemented in war-time Bosnia, the intervention aimed to help young children through addressing their mothers.[38] The intervention targeted 5-year-olds and their mothers who had been internally displaced by war. Parent–child dyads were randomly assigned to one of two conditions: a 5-month psychosocial intervention group along with basic medical care or a control group receiving medical care only. The intervention consisted of psychoeducation about topics such as child development, followed by an opportunity for mothers to discuss each topic. Evaluations of children's functioning showed significant improvement on measures of mental health, physical health, and psychosocial functioning as compared to controls. Maternal mental health improved as well. While this intervention was used within a war-time setting overseas, and has not been implemented following resettlement, it nonetheless suggests the potential value in directly addressing maternal knowledge and well-being as a means of improving child mental health. Particularly in contexts where whole cultural groups may similarly be experiencing dislocation and immigration, approaches that bring together parents and provide psychoeducation and preventative assistance may be particularly cost-effective. More studies are needed to discern whether or not treatment models focusing on mothers might have the similar effects for older children and adolescents compared to the younger children.

A variety of other family therapy approaches with immigrant and refugee families have been described in the literature. Variations in families within and between cultures, cultural views of family and healing, and differences in levels of acculturation require flexibility in applying family therapy models cross-culturally.[16,39] Family roles, as well as what constitutes a family, may differ greatly from one culture to another.

Trauma systems therapy is a treatment approach developed to directly address the social ecology and the ways in which instabilities in the social environment contribute to a traumatized child's emotional difficulties.[40] This treatment model has been adapted for refugees, with a particular emphasis on how to integrate different service systems in promoting a stable, supportive environment for refugee children. While a preliminary study shows support for this treatment model for use with a general population of traumatized children,[41] the adaptation of this model for refugees has not been empirically evaluated.

## Interventions within the service system: schools and primary care

One of the primary challenges in providing mental health services to refugee and immigrant youth is treatment engagement. Research examining service utilization shows that despite high rates of symptomatology, refugee youth greatly underutilize specialized mental health services.[7,17,19] Given this,

interventions developed solely within the context of specialized mental health services are unlikely to address the needs of the majority of refugee youth.[20] Some research suggests that refugees and immigrants may be more likely to seek help for mental health problems through service systems such as schools or pediatric primary care settings.[20,42] Hodes has proposed a tiered system of care in which service systems such as primary care settings and schools serve as the primary site for treatment of less acute emotional and behavioral needs, with more specialized services managing more acutely symptomatic youth.[42] While the model of integrating primary care and mental health has received some attention in the general child mental health literature[43] and the adult refugee literature,[44] at present there are no published studies of models of providing immigrant and refugee child mental health services in pediatric primary care settings.

Research suggests that schools may be a setting in which mental health services can effectively reach immigrant and refugee youth. Problems in treatment engagement associated with the stigma of mental healthcare, as well as practical barriers such as transportation, are minimized or eliminated through the provision of school-based services.[40] Kataoka and colleagues[45] describe a school-based mental health service designed for Latino immigrant children with mental health problems associated with trauma (depression or PTSD). Students were in the third through eighth grades, and received either eight sessions of CBT delivered by Spanish bilingual and bicultural counselors, or were part of a waiting list comparison group. Psychoeducation was also made available to parents and teachers. Students who received the intervention showed significant improvement in symptoms of PTSD and depression compared with those on the waiting list.

O'Shea and colleagues describe a pilot study of a school-based mental health program implemented in the UK with immigrant and refugee children.[46] The program served students aged 7–11 years old who were identified for services by teachers or if they were noted as having special needs. A range of treatment modalities were available, such as family therapy or cognitive processing of loss. All treatment began with meeting parents. Fourteen refugee children with significant exposure to war and violence were enrolled in the program. Length of treatment was not specified. The program was evaluated using a Strengths and Difficulties Questionnaire (SDQ) pre- and post-intervention. For the seven children for whom pre- and post-assessments were available, scores showed improvement. There are a number of methodological problems that limit the generalizability of this study, including the very small sample size, the use of a brief outcome measure that does not specifically capture psychopathology, and heterogeneity of intervention design. Nonetheless, this study suggests that school-based services may be an important means of circumventing logistical barriers to treatment engagement for refugee and immigrant children.

## Psychopharmacology

For many children, psychopharmacology either alone or in conjunction with therapy can provide symptom relief. Particularly for families who are more comfortable seeking mental healthcare within a primary care setting, psychopharmacology may be a viable option for treating some problems. Symptoms with biological underpinnings, such as depressed mood, can respond well to medication. Cultural views of medication may vary widely. Medication may be more familiar and accepted than therapy in some cultures, or in other cultures seen as a sign of serious illness and highly stigmatized. Little empirical research guides the use of psychopharmaceuticals in children and adolescents, particularly cross-culturally. Some clinical observations suggest that people of different ethnic backgrounds respond differently to medications and may be sensitive to side effects.[47] Cultural beliefs that may affect compliance to a prescribed regimen, such as expectations that medication need not be taken once symptoms remit or fasting during Ramadan, are also important considerations.

## Culture and language barriers in providing mental health services

Regardless of the modality of treatment chosen, language and culture must be considered. For recently arrived refugee and immigrant families, English may not be spoken by anyone in the family. Sometimes, the presenting child speaks English fluently, but a parent does not. Each of these scenarios presents problems and challenges to providing mental health services. A number of approaches to overcoming language and cultural barriers in treatment have been described. Two of the key approaches are to use interpreters or bicultural counselors.

For agencies that see clients from a diversity of cultures, using interpreters may be the most con-

venient way to accommodate the many languages represented. Working with interpreters can pose challenges to confidentiality in very small communities. Being able to offer a family a choice of an anonymous phone interpreter may be helpful if a face-to-face interpreter is well known to a family. Clan affiliation, class status, or the religion of an interpreter may be very meaningful to clients and present barriers to their speaking openly and comfortably. It is also important to consider the effect of including an interpreter in a therapeutic dyad. A qualitative study of the use of interpreters with refugee clients found that therapists often view an interpreter as an integral part of the therapy relationship. The client's experience of therapy is sometimes mediated by the interpreter, such that trust or distrust in the therapy relationship may depend on the nature of the client's relationship to the interpreter.[48]

Some agencies have adopted a model of bicultural counselors, where a trained clinician is paired with a layperson or paraprofessional from the community being served. In addition to interpretation, a bicultural counselor may provide case management, consultation to the provider regarding cultural issues, and community-based care. As they become seasoned and develop skills in counseling under the guidance of a trained clinician, bicultural counselors may be able to deliver culturally-sensitive interventions enriched by the fact that they are in the native tongue of the population served. The use of trained, local paraprofessionals also presents a cost-effective option for use in low-resource environments. In a recent study, Bolton and colleagues[49] demonstrated that local lay counselors could be successfully trained and supervised to deliver interpersonal therapy (IPT) for the treatment of depression among adults in Uganda. Randomized clinical trials demonstrated that participants in the IPT groups led by local paraprofessionals showed a significant decrease in symptoms of depression following 16 weeks of IPT group treatment compared to waiting list controls. A current study is underway to examine how such treatment effects might be replicable in adolescents. Many of the same challenges of using interpreters, such as possible loss of confidentiality, remain challenges with this model. However, with careful training and close guidance, bicultural counselors hold a great deal of promise for improving care among diverse immigrant and refugee populations while also building resources within the community rather than relying on outside professionals.

## Future Directions

• • • • • • • • • • • • • • • • • • • • • • • • • • • • • • • • •

Although the empirical base for selecting treatments is limited, clinical experience and a growing body of literature describing mental health interventions have begun to form a repertoire of approaches that can be utilized in treating refugee and immigrant children. As the diversity of the American population continues to increase, and with the sad reality of continuing war and violence globally, the provision of thoughtful, culturally-informed interventions for refugee and immigrant youth will be essential. Immigrant and refugee populations bring with them a host of complex challenges which remain underserved by the current system of mental healthcare. Future directions for the field include the need for services-relevant research to examine the essential components of interventions that are effective among diverse cultural groups and service settings that can best provide these services. The complex challenges of working within such populations presents a window of opportunity for children's mental healthcare to be more culturally competent by investing in the training and involvement of people from the community and moving treatment opportunities out of the office to home, health clinic, school, and community settings.

## References

1. Lustig S, et al. Review of child and adolescent refugee mental health. J Am Acad Child Adolesc Psychiatry 2004; 43(1):24–36.
2. Fazel M, Stein A. Mental health of refugee children: comparative study. Br Med J 2003; 327:134.
3. Weine SM, et al. Adolescent survivors of 'ethnic cleansing:' observations on the first year in America. J Am Acad Child Adolesc Psychiatry 1995; 34(9):1153–1159.
4. Sack WH, Him C, Dickason D. Twelve-year follow-up study of Khmer youths who suffered massive war trauma as children. J Am Acad Child Adolesc Psychiatry 1999; 38(9):1173–1179.
5. Almqvist K, Broberg AG. Mental health and social adjustment in young refugee children 3 1/2 years after their arrival in Sweden. J Am Acad Child Adolesc Psychiatry 1999; 38(6):723–730.
6. Anagnostopoulos D, et al. Psychopathology and mental health service utilization by immigrants' children and their families. Transcult Psychiatry 2004; 41(4):465–486.
7. Munroe-Blum H, et al. Immigrant children: psychiatric disorder, school performance, and service utilization. Am J Orthopsychiatry 1989; 59(4):510–519.
8. Hicks R, Lalonde R, Pepler D. Psychosocial considerations in the mental health of immigrant and refugee children. Can J Comm Mental Health 1993; 12(2):71–87.
9. Jaycox LH, et al. Violence exposure, posttraumatic stress disorder, and depressive symptoms among recent immigrant schoolchildren. J Am Acad Child Adolesc Psychiatry 2002; 41(9):1104–1110.
10. Summerfield D. A critique of seven assumptions behind psychological trauma programmes in war-affected areas. Social Sci Med 1999; 48:1449–1462.
11. Kirmayer L. The cultural diversity of healing: meaning, metaphor and mechanism. Br Med Bull 2004; 69:33–48.
12. Honwana A. Discussion guide 4: non-Western concepts of mental health. In: Refugee children: guidelines on protection and care. Geneva: United Nations High Commissioner for Refugees; 1998.
13. Markus HR, Kitayama S. Culture and the self: implications for cognition, emotion, and motivation. Psycholog Rev 1991; 98(2):224–253.
14. Morris P, Silove D. Cultural influences in psychotherapy with refugee survivors of torture and trauma. Hospit Comm Psychiatry 1992; 43(8):820–824.
15. Arrendondo P, Orjuela E, Moore LJ. Family therapy with Central American war refugee families. J Strategic Systemic Ther 1989; 8(2):28–35.
16. Bemak F. Cross-cultural family therapy with Southeast Asian refugees. J Strategic and Systemic Ther 1989; 8(1):22–27.
17. Geltman PL, et al. War trauma experience and behavioral screening of Bosnian refugee children resettled in Massachusetts. Development Behavior Pediatr 2000; 21(4):255–261.
18. Raphael B, Meldrum L, McFarlane AC. Does debriefing after psychological trauma work? Br Med J 1995; 310(6993):1479–1480.
19. Coard SI, Holden W. The effect of racial and ethnic diversity on the delivery of mental health services in pediatric primary care. J Clin Psychol Medical Settings 1998; 5(3):275–294.
20. Birman D, et al. Mental health interventions for refugee children in resettlement: White Paper II. National Child Traumatic Stress Network: Los Angeles, CA, 2005.
21. Cohen J. Practice parameters for the assessment and treatment of children and adolescents with posttraumatic stress disorder. J Am Acad Child Adolesc Psychiatry 1998; 37(10):4S–26S.
22. Deblinger E, McLeer SV, Henry D. Cognitive behavioral treatment for sexually abused children suffering post-traumatic stress: preliminary findings. J Am Acad Child Adolesc Psychiatry 1990; 29(5):747–752.
23. Saigh PA, Yasik AE, Oberfield RA. Behavioral treatment of child–adolescent posttraumatic stress disorder. In: Bremner JD, ed. Posttraumatic stress disorder: a comprehensive text. Needham Heights, MA: Allyn & Bacon; 1999:354–375.
24. Cohen JA, Mannarino AP. A treatment model for sexually abused preschoolers. J Interpersonal Violence 1993; 8(1):115–131.
25. Saigh A, Yule W, Inamdar SC. Imaginal flooding of traumatized children and adolescents. J School Psychol 1996; 34(2):163–183.
26. Cohen JA, et al. Trauma-focused cognitive behavioral therapy for children and adolescents: an empirical update. Cognitive Behavioral Therapy 2000; 15(11):1202–1223.
27. Lustig S, et al. Testimonial psychotherapy for adolescent refugees: a case series. Transcult Psychiatry 2004; 41(1):31–45.
28. Weine SM, et al. Testimony psychotherapy in Bosnian refugees: a pilot study. Am J Psychiatry 1998; 155(12):1720–1725.
29. Westermeyer JJ. Mental health for refugees and other migrants: social and preventive approaches. Springfield, IL: Charles C Thomas; 1989.
30. Sack WH, Clarke GN, Seeley A. Multiple forms of stress in Cambodian adolescent refugees. Child Develop 1996; 67:107–116.
31. Sveaass N, Reichelt S. Refugee families in therapy: From referrals to therapeutic conversations. J Fam Ther 2001; 23:119–135.
32. Watters C. Emerging paradigms in the mental healthcare of refugees. Social Sci Med 2001; 52:1709–1718.

33. Kinzie JD, et al. A three-year follow-up of Cambodian young people traumatized as children. J Am Acad Child Adolesc Psychiatry 1989; 28(4):501–504.

34. Nieves-Grafals S. Brief therapy of civil war-related trauma: a case study. Cultural Diversity Ethnic Minority Psychol 2001; 7(4):387–398.

35. Barenbaum J, Ruchkin V, Schwab-Stone M. The psychosocial aspects of children exposed to war: practice and policy initiatives. J Child Psychol Psychiatry 2004; 45(1):41–62.

36. Quiroga J, Jaranson JM. Politically-motivated torture and its survivors: a desk study review of the literature. Torture 2005; 15(2,3):1–111.

37. Boothby N. Trauma and violence among refugee children. In: Marsella AJ, Bornemann T, Eklad S, Orley J, eds. Amidst peril and pain: the mental health and well-being of the world's refugees, Washington, DC: American Psychological Association; 1994:239–259.

38. Dybdahl R. Children and mothers in war: an outcome study of a psychosocial intervention program. Child Develop 2001; 72(4):1214–1230.

39. Arredondo P, Orjuela E, Moore LJ. Family therapy with Central American war refugee families. J Strategic Systemic Ther 1989; 8(2):28–35.

40. Saxe GN, Ellis BH, Kaplow J. Collaborative treatment of traumatized children and teens: a trauma systems therapy approach. New York: Guilford Press; 2006.

41. Saxe GN, et al. Comprehensive care for traumatized children: an open trial examines trauma systems therapy. Psychiatr Ann 2005; 35(5):443–447.

42. Hodes M. Three key issues for young refugees' mental health. Transcult Psychiatry 2002; 39:196–213.

43. Garralda ME. The interface between physical and mental health problems and medical help seeking in children and adolescents: a research perspective. Child Adolesc Mental Health 2004; 9(4):146.

44. Murphy D, Ndegwa D, Kanani A. Mental health of refugees in inner-London. Psychiatr Bull 2002; 26(6):222–224.

45. Kataoka SJ, Stein BD, Jaycox LH. A school-based mental health program for traumatized Latino immigrant children. J AM Acad Child Adolesc Psychiatry 2003; 42(3):311–318.

46. O'Shea B, et al. A school-based mental health service for refugee children. Clin Child Psychol Psychiatry 2000; 5(2):189–201.

47. Lin K-M, Anderson D, Poland R. Ethnicity and psychopharmacology: bridging the gap. Psychiatr Clin North Am 1995; 18(3):635–647.

48. Miller KE, et al. The role of interpreters in psychotherapy with refugees: an exploratory study. Am J Orthopsychiatr 2005; 75(1):27–39.

49. Bolton P, Bass J, Neugebauer R, et al. Group interpersonal psychotherapy for depression in rural Uganda: a randomized controlled trial. JAMA 2003; 289(23): 3117–3124.

# CHAPTER 53

# Religion and Spirituality in the Lives of Immigrants in the United States

Linda L. Barnes

## Introduction

In the history of the United States, religion has frequently played a key role in decisions to emigrate, whether to be able to practice in a particular way, or to avoid ways of life imposed by other religious groups. As Jasso et al. observe, 'The religious composition of the US population thus reflects the evolving history of infringements on religious liberty around the world and the steadfast American freedoms.'[1] (It bears adding that, in some cases, immigration is driven not simply by the appeal of such freedoms, but by US interventions in overseas labor markets and/or by the deadly effects of regimes trained or supported by the US.)

Physicians whose patients include immigrants and refugees rarely need to be told that developing effective cross-cultural knowledge and related skills is imperative to providing effective care. For some, it may seem self-evident that such knowledge and skills must include patients' religious and spiritual worldviews. For others, accustomed to a longstanding separation of religion and medicine in Europe and the United States, such worldviews may seem clinically irrelevant, unless related to patients' reluctance to adhere to a particular medical intervention. Medical literature in recent years has also included summaries of issues to take into account when treating patients who have identified themselves with a particular religious tradition.

This chapter will draw from recent scholarship in the field of religious studies to look at broader issues faced by different immigrant and refugee communities in relation to their religious and spiritual traditions. After reviewing the term 'religion,' the chapter will discuss key characteristics of immigrant/refugee religious experience in the United States, concluding with some reflections on related implications for clinicians.

## Defining Terms

In the history of Europe and the United States, 'religion' has often been conceptualized, on the one hand, in terms of its meaning for the individual, as a largely private matter. It is frequently equated with a person's 'belief system' in general and his or her belief in God in particular. On the other hand, descriptions of different traditions may try to identify a core set of tenets, a sacred book or books, religious authorities similar to ministers or priests, and the conducting of group worship services. The underlying assumption here is that 'religion' consists of a universal set of variables. When religion is defined in this way, it is often contrasted with 'spirituality' as a personalized, more universal phenomenon.

Such definitions have crossed over into medical literature in a variety of ways. In some instances, 'religion' and 'spirituality' go undefined and undifferentiated,[2] or are treated as functionally synonymous.[3] Authors sometimes acknowledge a 'lack of conceptual clarity in the research literature,' but bypass the issue by suggesting that individuals have 'little difficulty rating themselves on their own level of spirituality.[4] Citing the Multidimensional Measurement of Religiousness/Spirituality for Use in Health Research,[5] Kilpatrick et al. suggest that 'religiousness has specific behavioral, social, doctrinal, and denominational characteristics that are shared by a group. By contrast, spirituality is concerned with the transcendent, addressing ultimate questions about life's meaning, with the assumption that there is more to life than what we see or understand.'[6] Koenig, too, differentiates between the social and the individual: 'Spirituality is more individualistic and self-determined, whereas religion typically involves connections to a community with shared beliefs and rituals.' He goes on to recommend the term 'spirituality,' in conversations with patients, construing it as the broader and more inclusive of the two terms.[7] Peterman acknowledges, though, that such meanings have changed over recent decades.[8]

Up until the 1960s and 1970s, religion was seen as a broad construct, encompassing individual and institutional elements as well as spirituality. More recently, religion has become more narrowly defined, and spirituality has become distinguished from religiousness, or the practice of religious behavior. Recent definitions of spirituality include dimensions such as a personal search for meaning and purpose in life, connections with a transcendent dimension of existence, and the experiences and feelings associated with that search and that connection. Religion is seen, in contrast, as participation in the institutionally sanctioned beliefs and activities of a particular faith group.[8]

It is less common for medical authors to address the challenges posed by the growing religious pluralism of the United States, and to link such challenges with the broader issues of cross-cultural practice, although some do point to the problems of positing universal, normative definitions.[9,10]

The work of religion scholars, however, points in a number of different directions. First, it is difficult if not impossible to come up with a definition – or even a group of variables – that fits all traditions for either 'religion' or 'spirituality.' We might better say that religions may grow out of relationships with nature, or with God or gods. Religions reflect the deepest or highest human concerns, as responses to something sacred. Religions both express and shape people's sense of meaning, their understanding of what life is about. Religions can bring about profound experience, and find expression in rich systems of symbols. Religions may hold communities together, and influence surrounding societies. In some cases, they serve to justify power disparities; in others, they motivate groups to challenge those very disparities.[11] People kill in the name of religions; they also heal.

Second, 'religion' comes from the Latin religare – to bind fast, as in a bond between humans and the gods – and from religio – referring both to ritual observance and a spirit of reverence. By the thirteenth century, the term was used to characterize Christian faith and practice governed by monastic vows. But many traditions did not grow out of that particular history. Consequently, some languages do not have a word that corresponds directly to the term 'religion.' Indeed, immigrants and refugees may come to define their worldview and lifeways as a religion only when they arrive in the United States, or if they have previously come into contact with Christian missionaries or religious communities.

In Chinese, for example, the different traditions were historically referred to as jiao, or teachings; daojiao, the teaching of the Dao (Daoism); Fojiao, the teaching of the Buddha (Buddhism); and rujiao, the teaching of the scholars (Confucianism). The life of a Chinese individual may be profoundly shaped by what he or she thinks of as a moral code, which is not identified as a religion, but rather is rooted in one of these traditions as a 'Way,' or path, to becoming a profound person. Practicing taijichuan early in the morning may be associated with health; it may also have to do with keeping oneself in balance, a desired spiritual state. Such a person may not think of himself or herself as religious in the sense often meant in the United States, but in this broader sense may be deeply so.

Third, religions are constantly changing in relation to local factors and influences encountered when groups migrate. There is no single, static 'Christianity,' 'Islam,' 'Judaism,' or 'Buddhism.' Religious life in the countries of origin may often be characterized by considerable pluralism, involving not only diverse religions, but also different branches within a single tradition. Sephardic and Ashkenazic Jews, Catholic, Eastern Orthodox, and Protestant Christians, Sunni and Shi'ite Muslims are all instances of such internal pluralism. Nor are any of these branches or groups any more static than are their representatives in the US.

For that matter, people may pick and choose from within a given tradition, customizing their worldview and practice in response to new influences and needs. They may also borrow from other traditions – an increasingly common phenomenon in American communities where different cultural groups live in proximity to one another. Or, people may shore up and tighten the boundaries of their religious group in new ways, in order to assert their identity in a new place. Immigrants and refugees may take great pains to relocate their religious communities and practices, while also modifying them in the process. Where temples proliferated in the country of origin, a group in the US may have to adjust to using a private home, or a collectively purchased suburban ranch house, as its religious center. Home-based practice may take on increased importance. For some people, 'religion' may come to serve as the operative term for what they do, and for what matters to them; for others, 'spirituality' captures key features; and for still others, both are meaningful. Religions, spiritualities, and how people employ both terms are routinely in a state of flux. For clinicians, therefore, it becomes particularly important not to assume that generic definitions capture the lived experience of patients.

## Religious Globalization

Developments abroad may have a profound impact on immigrant and refugee groups, especially in a transnational world, where people cross and re-cross borders, and where internet connectivity and media outlets alert one almost instantly to events around the globe. This transnational reality has several key characteristics. For example, immigrants are better able to sustain strong ties with their homelands than ever before.[12] In many cases, therefore, their social, political, economic, and cultural frames of reference include not only their place of residence in the US, but also other sites where relatives and compatriots have settled, as well as the home culture abroad. Thus, transnationalism entails networks throughout the US and overseas.

In this connection, people may maintain active connections with the religious communities back home. As McAlister observes of Haitian immigrants in New York, for example, religious festivals such as the Fèt Vièj Mirak (the Feast of the Miraculous Virgin) on East 115th Street do not simply replace the corresponding celebration in Haiti. Rather, the Fèt both increases the options for where one can commemorate the event, and expands Haitian sacred space into a new territory – an American city.[12] Such festivals allow people 'to create the proper setting to honor the saint, to renew life, to reaffirm identity even in exile, and to create greater unity among the saint's people.'[13] As they do so, they transform the American religious arena as well.

Moreover, when they return to Haiti, people do so with a redefined, internationalized understand-

ing of their religious world, and visits may be planned accordingly. For those involved in the tradition of Vodou, for example, certain kinds of spiritual work can be undertaken in the US, such as healings, or personal crises involving work or love. However, events such as initiations, funeral rituals, becoming an *oungan* (priest) or *manbo* (priestess), or dealing with a problem that interventions in the US have not resolved, all require travel to Haiti.[14] Members of different religious communities may increasingly participate in what Marquandt refers to as 'transnational religious circuits.'[15]

Within such circuits, the new religious sites provide the opportunity to recreate a part of the home country – a potential refuge into which one can step. There, one can imagine oneself relocated back into a familiar space, where one is recognized and welcomed. Altars, religious iconography of other kinds, and ritual space come together to transplant a setting in which a person's identity can be asserted. In some cases, where numerous family members and friends from a given location have resettled in American cities, as is the case with migrants moving from Michoacán in Mexico to the Metro-Atlanta area, the result is an internationalized 'village.'[15] Similarly, Fuzhounese immigrants recreate Protestant and Catholic church communities, as well as Buddhist, Daoist, and popular-religion temples in New York City and in other urban centers around the US.[16] Transplanted religious communities provide a common ground where people can come together, generate support networks, and tap into often publicly invisible channels for immigration, resettlement, work, and support for engaging governmental and civic institutions.

The gods and saints accompany their devotees, migrating to American soil. The Vièj Mirak is now known to reside in New York City and to extend her blessings from there, as well as from Haiti. The Vodou *lwa* (guardian spirit) Ezilie Dantò (also represented as Our Lady of Lourdes) once spoke through an *oungan* to say that she was spending 3 days every week in Miami, to watch out for migrants there.[17] The saints' festivals organized by Mayan exiles in California and the Southwest are grassroots activities that not only assert ethnic pride, but also honor the holy patrons who have made the journey with the immigrants and the refugees.[13]

Spirit mediums from the Fuzhou area of mainland China have resettled in such disparate places as New York and Indiana. There, they accept questions – either in the form of handwritten notes or through telephone calls – which they then direct to the god He Xian Jun through trance possession. Petitioners may ask the god's opinion 'about everything from business ventures to children's names to the potential success of petitions for political asylum. They come to pray for the health of sick relatives and to give thanks for safe passage across the ocean with snakeheads from China.'[18] On the birthday of Guan Yin, Bodhisattva of compassion and mercy, immigrants from Fuzhou come together at the temple of He Xian Jun to celebrate. The establishment of such religious sites in the US in turn may elevate the standing of related groups in the home country. That a large Chinese Buddhist temple now flourishes in Houston, attracting Westerners as well as Chinese immigrants and, on occasion, being covered by American media, serves as a sign to Taiwanese Buddhists that Buddhism is seen as both legitimate and important in the US.[19]

Communication between adherents both in the country of origin and in the US is enhanced by the use of cassette and video recorders. Not only do tape recordings take the place of written letters, for immigrants who are illiterate, but they may also record religious and healing ceremonies for those who cannot be present, but who 'attend' vicariously. Not infrequently, the person making the recording will provide voice-over commentary for the viewer. In traditions involving spirit possession, as in Vodou, the spirits may speak to the tape or video recorder, conveying messages and advice to those who are absent. Chinese Buddhists involved with the *Hsi-nan* temples record talks and ceremonies, and videotape special events, storing the tapes in a growing library and, not infrequently, copying them and sending them to Taiwan and, sometimes, to mainland China.[19] Practitioners, spirits, and gods thus speak to one another across a transnational space.

Moreover, those who avail themselves of these different kinds of religious resources do not necessarily do so instead of seeking biomedical care. For some, biomedicine was available in their country of origin, albeit in a culturally inflected form. Insofar as biomedicine itself is a cultural system,[20,21] immigrants enter the US, in many cases, with preexisting ideas about physicians, clinics, and biomedical interventions, and their relationship to religious systems of healing. The customized combinations designed by patients reflect their understandings of a given health problem, and the different things they believe need to be done for it, within the constraints of social and economic barriers to care. The nature of these customized solutions may remain invisible to biomedical care providers, insofar as patients selectively disclose only what they assume providers need to know or will be open to hearing about. Cul-

tural assumptions about the role and nature of physicians may further influence patients' decisions about how much to tell doctors about the role of religious involvement in their lives. Generally speaking, however, patients are often delighted to discover that physicians have even a basic awareness of some of the different ways in which religious communities have entered US culture, and of their place in immigrant life.

## Institutional Adaptations

Many of the non-Western religious traditions prioritize home-based or small-group religious observance, as is often the case, for example, for Muslims, Hindus, and Buddhists. Such practices may be among those that transplant the most readily and easily to the US. For groups who remain migrants in the US, as with seasonal farm workers from Mexico, collective religious expression may involve lay specialists 'from *curanderas* (healers) to *rezadoras* (prayer specialists) and *espiritualistas*, who work in the large gaps left by religious institutions.'[22] Some groups, in contrast, have well-established congregational systems and experiences that provide models for religious association in the US. This is the case with the Presbyterian Church in Korea as the result of US missionary influence, and with Latin American Catholic congregations influenced by the participatory models of liberation theology. As Vásquez observes, the latter group may challenge church hierarchies more familiar to Irish- and Italian-American Catholics.[22]

But it also happens that the dominant model of Protestant Christianity in the US filters into the awareness of new religious groups, clad in the mantle of culturally and sometimes politically sanctioned authority. As these groups acclimate to their new surroundings, as they observe and interact with other religious bodies, they may adopt practices previously unknown to them. They may, for example, borrow the organizational form of the congregation. They may move toward professionalizing their religious authorities, even hiring the equivalent of Christian clergy. They may develop a more formal membership system, take steps to attain 501(c)3 status as a nonprofit organization, and schedule events for Sundays. Such reorganizations may represent substantial departures from practices in a home country.

A commonly cited example is Islam, which in Muslim countries does not generally have professional ministers for mosques. Imams are unpaid individuals recognized for their knowledge of the Qur'an and the sayings of the Prophet (*hadith*).[23] By professionalizing the role, and by congregationalizing mosque communities, American Muslims locate themselves within religious frameworks more familiar to the surrounding culture and, by extension, assert their legitimacy. Similarly, Hindu immigrants from India may rework their religious lives to accommodate to the new environment. Raymond Brady Williams characterizes the resulting practices as 'made in the USA ... assembled ... by relatively unskilled labor (at least unskilled by traditional standards) and adapted to fit new designs to reach a new and growing market.'[24] In India, for example, religious practice generally occurs at home, or through individual or family visits to a temple. Large gatherings are more often reserved for temple festivals, as opposed to weekly gatherings.

The Rev. Tai-Xu (1889–1947), a reformer within *Hsi-nan* Buddhism, adopted various organizational and social service practices from Christianity, such as founding seminaries and religiously sponsored hospitals, proselytizing in prisons, and officiating at wedding ceremonies (instead of primarily at funeral rituals).[19] Conversely, as Yang[25] notes, some Christian groups in their countries of origin adopt traditional cultural practices from other religious groups, because these practices are so widespread. Such is the case, for example, among Chinese Christians, who may have observed *Qingming*, a spring commemoration for the dead and for one's ancestors, rooted in the Confucian and Buddhist traditions. In the US, however, such practices are not part of the surrounding culture, allowing Chinese Christians to abandon them without feeling out of step.

## The Flow of Political, Economic, and Social Capital

For some groups, meaningful international connections exist primarily at the level of local groups abroad. Such ties can be characterized as horizontal. For others, equal or more significant connections may be more vertically organized, as is the relationship between local Catholic churches and Rome. Stepick illustrates the point by comparing a local church in Los Angeles that sends money to a sister church in El Salvador with the Catholic Church as a whole raising money for hurricane relief in Nicaragua.[26]

Still other international ties intersect with political movements – in some cases, terrorist; in others,

nationalist. The Federation of Hindu Associations, for example, was organized in Southern California in the mid-1990s, and primarily involved 'wealthy, middle-aged, upper caste, north Indian businessmen,'[24] whose goal was to support the political aims of Hindus. In 1998, the group split, with the FHA advocating for a Hindu state in India.

The religious pluralism that characterizes home countries regularly migrates to the US, although not necessarily in proportional numbers. If, that is, a group suffers persecution for religious reasons, its members may emigrate in larger numbers than do members of the persecuting group. Nevertheless, religiously based tensions, along with political antagonisms between groups, make their way into the US.[27]

Religious groups may play key roles in facilitating the settling, and promoting the economic success, of their own members. Protestant Haitian immigrants may assist fellow congregants with food, money, work, childcare, and other forms of networking. Where Catholic charities are active, parishes may become the base for social service agencies that provide language and citizenship classes, adult education, job-seeking skills, health-related services, and childcare. In contrast, Chinese immigrants may more readily turn either to family and friends, or to Chinese civic groups, which have a long history of assisting immigrants. They may, therefore, be less likely to turn to Buddhist temples for such help. Here is where the *Hsi-nan* incorporation of Christian approaches to the provision of social services represents a new model. In turn, Chinese churches are likely to provide training in how to accommodate to life in the US, as well as 'how to maintain a happy marriage, educate children, better communicate with your boss and co-workers, make investments, take care of your health, etc.'[25]

The flow of monetary remittances from immigrants to communities in the countries of origin has been a longstanding and well-studied phenomenon. Undocumented Mayan workers in Los Angeles, for example, organized themselves into multiple committees, many of them with specific responsibilities related to collecting and sending money to Guatemala. Their efforts enabled their home parish to rebuild the church and staff a clinic.[13] The Temple of Heavenly Thanksgiving, part of a Fuzhounese religious network, supports larger projects in the home village, including not only the expansion of the home temple, but also a charitable foundation, and the provision of services for those back home. All of these measures enhance the standing of those abroad, who are often otherwise marginalized by the host society.[16]

Vietnamese-Americans are estimated to send some US$700 million a year to relatives – and, gradually, to others seen as being in need – building what have been called 'transnational kinship groups' that have helped those in Vietnam set up businesses and rebuild the economy.[28] Religious institutions have been seen as more trustworthy than other agencies for the distribution of monetary remittances. As the relationship between the governments of the two countries changed, and American banks were allowed to set up branches in Vietnam, religious groups could establish international accounts, further simplifying and securing the transaction of funds. Although churches and temples had not historically functioned as social service centers, they have assumed this role in response to the immigrant community in the US, thereby modifying their function, identity, and influence in Vietnam.[28]

Physicians who work with immigrant and refugee groups may be well aware of social service agencies operating within local communities, and in some cases may have well-developed networks of referral. It may be less obvious, however, that religious communities sometimes provide extensive parallel social networks and resources. An awareness of how different local religious groups function can add to the resources that care providers can recommend to their patients.

## Identity Matters

### Religion and nationality

Religious engagement is rarely a static phenomenon, and religious identity may reflect individual and group efforts to navigate their relationship with relocation and different options for assimilation. Stepick suggests that recent research points to 'flexible identities,' with 'individuals emphasizing some aspects of their cultural heritage in one context, but different aspects in another.'[26] Accordingly, he adds, the issue is not so much whether or not immigrants are religious, but rather, in what contexts they are more or less likely to emphasize that aspect of their identity, and in what ways.

Immigrants and refugees who come from a relatively undifferentiated religious environment, and who find themselves in a setting where there is greater religious difference, may feel compelled to define their identities particularly in relation to religion. Indeed, religious identity can take on levels of meaning it may not have had in the country of origin.

For some, it may come to serve as a primary identity, trumping cultural, racial, and even national identities, as is the case for some Afghani Muslims[29] and some Pentacostal Christians.[26] For others, it can become equated with national identity, as happens for some Indian-Americans. Despite the complexity of religious pluralism in India, Hindu immigrant organizations in the US tend to define Indian-American identity *as* Hindu, and particularly as 'upper-caste, upper-middle-class Brahmans,'[22] and to characterize Indian Muslims and Christians as 'resident aliens' whose traditions originated outside of India.[24] Consequently, American Hindu organizations are also prone to promoting a Hindu nationalism in relation to India.

### Religion, race, and ethnicity

Nineteenth-century immigrants to the US from Ireland, Italy, and Eastern-European Jewish communities were frequently categorized as belonging to separate racial groups, distinct from 'white Americans.' In Tallulah, Louisiana, for example, five Sicilian men were lynched for 'having violated the protocols of racial interaction.'[30] Puerto Ricans would later encounter the imposition of a binary racial typology quite different from classification along a color continuum that characterized racial concepts in the former French, Spanish, and Portuguese colonies. Those whose phenotype permitted were therefore likely to take steps toward being perceived as more similar to normative 'whiteness.' Those unable to do so, then and since, have found themselves thrust into racial identities that have little meaning for them, and that may carry the burdens of both stigma and degrees of exclusion. In particular, African and African-descended immigrants discover that they become 'black' or 'African-American' in the US, positioning them to be the targets of racial bias in new ways.

At the same time, the exponential increase in the number of immigrants and their descendents since 1965 has also increased resistance to such classifications, resulting in a greater perception of the US as multiracial, multiethnic, and multicultural. Immigrants may strategically emphasize different dimensions of their identity in order to distance themselves from the impact of a black–white form of racialization.[31] The children of interracial, interethnic, and intercultural marriages are also more vocal in insisting on recognition of the different facets of their identities, challenging the binary of black–white. Where does religion enter this picture?

On the one hand, some religious communities may serve specific racial–ethnic groups, as is the case for some of the Chinese-American churches within larger Christian denominations. Such groups may emphasize their national or regional origins, rather than accepting an 'Asian' identity. Some Hindu Americans emphasize religious identity as a way of rejecting a nonwhite racial classification. Some may also identify as 'Aryan,' pointing to the Central European nomadic people who invaded both Greece and northern India in around 1500 BCE. In this way, they claim a historical connection with the peoples (and racial groups) of Europe.[24]

In still other cases, a group may use religious events to differentiate itself from African-American racial identity, particularly as immigrants with some African descent become aware of the historic and current impact of racism on African-Americans. For example, Haitian immigrants who participate in some of the Italian saints' festivals in New York City may emphasize their Haitian Catholic identity, and are welcomed as devout visitors by the Italians who organize the feast, in contrast with hostility expressed by the same Italian community toward Puerto Ricans, when the latter took up residence in East Harlem in large numbers.[12] If nothing else, the immigrants' or refugees' religious community may provide a refuge from the impact of being racialized and/or marginalized by the surrounding culture. Insofar as 'religious values and rituals are inseparably tied to their ethnic values, customs, holidays, food, dress, and even music and dance,'[32] the community may play an important part in helping a group preserve its ethnic identity.

This is by no means to say that a particular ethnic group will invariably choose only one way of using religion to preserve ethnic identity, as is illustrated by tensions between Chinese Protestants and Chinese Buddhists in Houston.[19] For that matter, even within a particular Chinese Protestant church, there may be considerable heterogeneity, reflecting the corresponding complexity of the Chinese diaspora, which includes 'Chinese and their descendents who left different regions of their homeland for indentured servitude in North America and Southeast Asia a century ago, for refuge in Taiwan and Hong Kong after the 1949 revolution, and to the United States for high-tech jobs today,' and who have, since 1980, also come from the People's Republic of China.[33,34] Such internal differences may contribute to tensions within the particular religious community in relation to worship style, practice, and community objectives.

Clinicians may want to explore immigrant experience of racialization, in order to learn not only about the impact of this added stress, but also about how individuals, families, or groups may strategically be repositioning themselves through their religious identities.

## Religion and gender

Because clinicians rarely enter their practice with training in world religions, they may be as susceptible as the ordinary citizen to stereotypes conveyed through popular media. This is particularly true not only of religious traditions that have suffered general stigmatizing, as happens, for example, with Vodou; it occurs as well in relation to the reporting of gender relations as defined and influenced by different religious traditions. Another influence has been feminism as it has emerged in the United States and Europe, according to which women's rights are largely defined from a Eurocentric point of view. Consequently, some traditions more than others are assumed to be oppressive in relation to women. Practices such as veiling are taken to reflect the subjugation of women, to the degree that some feminist conferences have rejected participation by Muslim feminists who choose to wear the head scarf (*hijab*).

It is certainly the case that religious communities can play a critical part in defining gender roles and relations. In some cases, they may favor the consolidation of more traditional arrangements while, in others, they may actually raise women's status in new immigrant settings. Traditional cultures in South Asia, for example, may be more likely to socialize a woman to identify herself in terms of her relationships as a 'mother, daughter, niece, sister, and so on,' and to encourage her to cultivate herself within these roles, in exchange for respect and support. Women who step outside of these roles may face censure. Some South Asian immigrant parents may send overly independent teenage daughters back to the country of origin, and may set up an arranged marriage.[35] Religiously defined gender norms may be called upon to reinforce these views and actions. Similarly, religious rationales may be used to persuade women who experience domestic violence to suffer in silence. Some of the more conservative church groups oppose women taking on leadership roles or speaking when men are present.[25]

At the same time, immigrant women's standing may actually rise in new ways within their religious world. For example, in Houston's *Hsi-nan* temple, there are women lay leaders, trustees and executive trustees, and administrators. Members of the temple explain that restrictions on women's roles were due to historical circumstances that contradicted Buddhism's core promotion of the equality of all living beings – among them, women.[19] In the Islamic Center of Connecticut, many of the teachers are women, and some serve on the board of directors, growing out of a more widely held view that women are 'important custodians of traditions.'[23] Indeed, religion may afford some women the opportunity to expand their role beyond their families, particularly when these women also have careers and incomes independent from those of their husbands. Chen, for example, describes 'Tina' who volunteers 1 day a week at Dharma Light Temple, where 'her identity revolves around her Buddha nature rather than her kinship obligations.'[36]

## The Second Generations

First-generation immigrants are especially likely to worry about the impact of American culture, as they understand it, on their children. In particular, such worries encompass perceived sexual permissiveness, indifference to education, disrespect for authority, the absence of more traditional values, a high tolerance for (if not also the sanctioning of) violence, and drug and alcohol abuse. In the face of such threats, immigrant parents may become all the more concerned with passing on the culture and values of the home society. Religious communities often function as settings within which worldviews, values, and practices are transmitted.

In turn, the children of immigrants – whether born in the US, or coming from what George calls 'the 1.5 generation' (those born abroad, but who have grown up in the US[37]) – may find themselves caught between 'family dissolution, cultural alienation, racism, a sense of dislocation and disempowerment, loss of familiarity, isolation, and acculturation stress,'[38] on the one hand and, on the other, the desire to assimilate and to turn away from what seem to be the more restrictive practices of their parents. Indeed, what feels reassuring and familiar to the first generation may, to the second generation, feel overly confining and not fully 'American.' The very emphasis on ethnic identity may be precisely what alienates this generation.[39] Conversely, the feeling of ethnic marginality in relation to the larger culture can also lead them to adopt more extreme versions of the religion, as a sharply defined form of identity.[24]

Language usage may become a focal point in these intergenerational challenges. Generally speaking, in contrast with religion, and other cultural practices, the language from the country of origin is more likely to be abandoned by later generations. The second generation of many groups assimilates linguistically, while third-generation members often retain little more than a small number of words and phrases.[39] Some groups attempt to sponsor language schools, and their children may, in turn, go on to study that language in college, but it nevertheless usually functions as a second language in relation to English.

Accordingly, second-generation members of religious groups are more likely to prefer bilingual religious leaders who are also more familiar with the surrounding culture. In some of the church settings, the English-language services adopt practices more common in mainstream congregations, whether or not these have played a part in churches in the home country. Religious communities then face the challenge of whether to try to integrate bilingualism into the primary gatherings, along with such practices, or to hold separate language-based services or rituals. Over time, as members become increasingly involved in other civic and social organizations, the importance of an ethnically based religious group may diminish. The group may then wither, or it may become home to other groups, resulting in a multiethnic community.

Clinicians treating children routinely inquire into how a child or adolescent is doing in school, as an indicator of whether or not the patient is operating successfully within a common social sphere. Problems between parents and children may emerge in some of these discussions. Rarely, however, do intergenerational tensions in relation to religious communities enter the discussion, even though such tensions may reside at the heart of some parents' concerns about their children's orientation to their cultures of origin.

## Civic Engagement and the Larger Culture

Some immigrant religious communities seek institutionalization and legal recognition as a means of securing greater legitimacy and standing for their members. Although there remain branches within US Christian groups who continue to disparage non-Christian faith traditions, the country has nevertheless become what Diana Eck characterizes as 'the world's most religiously diverse nation,'[40] and it is no longer publicly acceptable to challenge the right of those traditions to the full protections of religious freedom.

Religious communities may provide different routes to engagement in the larger surrounding culture. Marquandt,[15] for example, provides contrasting cases of two churches in the Southwest, both in the same town, both of whose members were primarily recently arrived, undocumented Catholic Mexican immigrants who sustained strong, ongoing ties with their home towns. One, the *Misión Católica*, provided a refuge from the negative identities often imposed by that surrounding culture – where, instead of experiencing themselves as unwanted and excluded, they could come together as valued and loved. The church provided them with practical organizational tools with which to protest second-class status, and engaged them in planning protests, coordinating the distribution of resources throughout their community, and taking English classes. The church thereby helped them to challenge political and economic inequities, as one way of engaging in American culture.

In contrast, the Lutheran church, *Sagrada Familia*, promoted engagement by teaching its members 'the rules of engagement with the broader public, with the expectation of someday being invited to participate.'[15] The pastor used his sermons to teach congregants about the Constitution, the Bill of Rights, and their own rights – even as undocumented persons – so that they might participate more fully and with greater confidence.

For the undocumented Fuzhounese immigrants described by Guest, transnational religious organizations provide alternatives to full incorporation into US culture. Networks of Fuzhounese already established in cities such as New York assist newcomers in securing jobs in different regions of the country, often keeping them well below the legal radar. At the same time, by sending remittances home, and assisting their religious communities, they achieve a status otherwise denied them.[16]

The *Hsi-nan* Temple of Houston, on the other hand, not only retains strong ties with official representatives of the Taiwanese government, but also seeks connections with local and state governments. At the temple's dedication ceremony, Houston's mayor proclaimed 'Houston Buddhist Day' and, on behalf of the US government, bestowed 'honorary citizen and goodwill ambassador certificates to the Abbot, a monk, and a founding lay member, in recognition of their contributions to the Houston community,' while a local senator conveyed the governor's proclamation of 'Texas Buddhist Day.' Houston's largest daily dedicated the full Religion Section page

to the ceremony.[19] Altogether, these events secured public standing for the temple and, by extension, for its members.

For Muslim communities, civic engagement has proved challenging, particularly since September 11, 2001. Many have felt the burden of having to provide repeated public statements rejecting terrorism, while still suffering the experience of being perceived as a threat. As Stepick notes, however, it is not the first time that immigrant religious groups have had to fend off discrimination, as was the case for 'Irish papists' during the nineteenth century and 'Jewish anarchists' during the twentieth,[26] and to find ways to redefine themselves in public opinion.

To the extent that Muslim immigrants must also contend with now being a religious minority – a new experience for many of them – there have emerged new needs to define their religious identity and to reflect on the options for engagement in civic processes. Such decisions often cannot be made outside of religious frameworks. As Mattson tellingly observes:

> In order to understand their role in America, Muslims need to define not only Islam but also America. Muslims need to place America in its proper theological and legal category so they can determine what kind of relationship is possible and desirable for them to have with this country. Whether or not integration initially seems like a desirable goal, this process will be affected by the immigrant's race, ethnicity, financial means, linguistic ability, and, most important for our study, what religious paradigms are available to them to interpret their particular experience with America.[41]

That some religious groups within the US denounce American popular culture in its more decadent forms can lend support, for some, to a preference for staying at a remove from that larger culture. The process may be further complicated for those who have experienced the direct effects of American military power either in their own lives, or in those of friends and family. Mattson adds that the impact of US foreign policy resonates in complex ways for different American Muslim groups.[41] Although much the same could be said for other immigrant groups, a key difference for Muslims lies in the explicit connection between policy decisions and the role played by religious differences in Muslim groups abroad.

For some, there can be no full allegiance to American law, insofar as it conflicts with Islamic law. Others cite the Prophet Mohammed as having emigrated himself, and having dispatched followers to live in a non-Muslim country and to obey its Christian ruler in Ethiopia, a story that provides a paradigm for Muslim–Christian cooperation. Still others affirm parallels between American democratic principles and the ideal Islamic state.[41] In each case, the challenge involves determining the degree of civic engagement, and the religious foundation upon which to make the decision to do so.

Such intra- and intergroup negotiations are often not apparent to the surrounding mainstream population, unless a particular group has come to public attention because of political tensions, as has happened for Muslims since September 11, 2001. Conflicts between groups abroad have sometimes led branches of those groups in America to engage in interfaith dialogues in ways that may be reported on in the media. Accordingly, clinician perceptions may be influenced by media accounts of specific religious groups in a general way, and clinicians themselves may know about specific interfaith initiatives in their own towns, while remaining unaware of broader civic roles played not only by these groups, but also by other religious communities among immigrant and refugee populations.

## Hybrid Outcomes

Each of these examples involves complex negotiations and the balancing of different facets of identity, whether *within* a specific religious community, or *between* religious groups serving the same immigrant community as a whole, or between such groups and the surrounding racial/ethnic and religious cultures of the US. Both the erecting of new boundaries, as well as borrowing, imitating, and mixing, result at every step of the way. As noted in the introduction, there are no pure or absolute forms, but rather constantly changing configurations, in relation to local factors and influences. Hybridity, rather than being the exception, is far more often the norm. Paradoxically, such hybrid outcomes may be precisely the means chosen by a community to preserve what it views as core to its identity.

For other groups, it is a matter of course to move back and forth between different religious worlds, as do some Haitians who navigate between Catholicism and Vodou – what McAlister characterizes as being 'bireligious,' or able to speak in multiple religious 'languages.' In such instances, the traditions are not viewed as being in conflict, so much as complementing each other, each with its own linguistic

and behavioral 'codes.' Members, therefore, engage in 'code-switching' as a matter of course.[12]

Some Chinese immigrants also code-switch between Confucian rituals, Buddhist ceremonies, and Christian services, viewing their participation in each as something like what one of this author's interviewees once referred to as 'covering all their bases – sort of like taking out insurance.' Such movement has long characterized Chinese religious life, where the different traditions each offered different resources for different life challenges. Yet even when groups define themselves in inflexible, bounded terms – as is the case in some Protestant evangelical Chinese churches that may fully reject other Chinese religious traditions – exceptions may still be made when a congregant has a family member belonging to another tradition. Yang, for example, cites the case of a woman who undertook Buddhist rituals for her mother, because her brother was actively Buddhist, while the brother, in turn, requested a Christian service followed by Buddhist chanting. Both siblings attended both ceremonies.[25] In such instances, boundaries can prove to be contingent and circumstantial.

We all have different forms of code-switching, many of which we employ relatively seamlessly, in moving from one domain to another in our lives. In clinical settings, immigrants and refugees bring with them these kinds of code-switching skills. They have learned that the more they can employ such skills in different settings, the better their chances of finding the supports they need to adapt to living in the US.[42] For that very reason, rarely are they likely to introduce these topics into discussions with a clinician, despite the centrality that religious communities and practices may play in their lives in the different ways described above.

## Conclusion

Religious engagement has frequently been identified as a factor that can contribute both to individual and group resilience, and to the capacity to cope better in the face of challenging circumstances. Similarly, discussions of specific religious groups have sometimes focused on their opposition to particular medical interventions. Some of the cultural competence literature highlights issues that may arise with adherents of certain traditions. Each of these facets is important. Indeed, one could well go farther and suggest that throughout the entire lifespan of a person, religious dimensions may intersect almost inseparably with cultural ones, shaping many health-related choices.[43,44] Likewise, the many variables so ably detailed by Culhane-Pera in this volume (see Ch. 7) frequently also involve a patient's and family's religious worldviews.

What this chapter has attempted to address are some of the other ways in which religion and spirituality enter into the lived worlds of immigrants and refugees. The first of these ways involves the transnational networks of communities, practitioners, and sacred entities – often much more significant in the lives of their patients than clinicians may realize. The flow of political, economic, and social capital reach public attention primarily in relation to groups targeted by law enforcement and the media, but as we have seen, religious groups may play a central role in helping their members settle and find a foothold in the US. That religious tensions may also migrate can surface in a clinical setting if medical interpreters from one group are brought in to interpret for members of another. Clinicians may be aware of the political dimensions of such conflicts; the significance of the religious dimensions may be less well understood.

Religious identity may serve as a primary identity, overriding cultural, racial, and even national identities. At very least, it may deeply influence how these other aspects of identity are construed and acted upon.[45] Religion may define gender roles either in constraining ways, or in providing immigrant and refugee women with new, expanded social roles or with ways of stepping outside of other social constraints. For members of a second generation, religion may lie at the core of their own struggle with and for an identity *as* Americans.

What one can assume is that each of these variables will undergo ongoing change. A patient from a particular religious community may, in certain ways, be like many other members of that community. At the same time, he or she can also be expected to differ from other members of that community in key ways. To the extent that religion and/or spirituality may constitute both conscious and unconscious components at the foundation of a patient's identity, the clinician would do well to hypothesize that each choice a patient or family makes may grow out of religious worldviews and convictions. To explore whether this is the case – and, if it is, to ask what is at stake – can potentially make all the difference in negotiating the choices related to care.

## References

1. Jasso G, Massey DS, Rosenzweig MR, et al. Exploring the religious preferences of recent immigrants to the United States: evidence from the new immigrant survey pilot. In: Haddad YY, Smith JI, Esposito JL, eds. Religion and immigration: Christian, Jewish, and Muslim experiences in the United States. Walnut Creek: AltaMira; 2003:217–253.

2. Ellis MR, Campbell JD. Concordant spiritual orientations as a factor in physician–patient spiritual discussions: a qualitative study. J Relig Health 2005; 44:39–53.

3. Thoresen CE, Harris AHS. Spirituality and health: what's the evidence and what's needed? Ann Behav Med. 2002; 24:3–13.

4. Lawrence RJ. The witches' brew of spirituality and medicine. Ann Behav Med 2002; 24:74–76.

5. John E. Fetzer Institute. Multidimensional measurement of religiousness/spirituality for use in health research. Kalamazoo, MI: John E. Fetzer Institute; 1999.

6. Kilpatrick SD, Weaver AJ, McCullough ME, et al. A review of spiritual and religious measures in nursing research journals: 1995–1999. J Relig Health 2005; 44:55–66.

7. Koenig HG. Religion, spirituality, and medicine: research findings and implications for clinical practice. South Med J 2004; 97:1194–1200.

8. Peterman AH, Fitchett G, Brady MJ, et al. Measuring spiritual well-being in people with cancer: the functional assessment of chronic illness therapy–spiritual well-being scale (FACIT-Sp). Ann Behav Med 2002; 24:49–58.

9. Hodge DR. Developing a spiritual assessment toolbox: a discussion of the strengths and limitations of five different assessment methods. Health Soc Work 2005; 30:314–323.

10. Mills PJ. Spirituality, religiousness, and health: from research to clinical practice. Ann Behav Med 2002; 24:1–2.

11. American Academy of Religion. What is Religion? Available: http://www.studyreligion.org/what/index.html December 13, 2005.

12. McAlister E. The Madonna of 115th street revisited: Vodou and Haitian Catholicism in the age of transnationalism. In: Warner RS, Wittner JG, eds. Gatherings in diaspora: religious communities and the new immigration. Philadelphia: Temple University; 1998:123–160.

13. Wellmeier NJ. Santa Eulalia's people in exile: Maya religion, culture, and identity in Los Angeles. In: Warner RS, Wittner JG, eds. Gatherings in diaspora: religious communities and the new immigration. Philadelphia: Temple University; 1998:97–122.

14. Brown KM. Mama Lola: A Vodou priestess in Brooklyn. Berkeley: University of California; 2001.

15. Marquandt MF. Structural and cultural hybrids: religious congregational life and public participation of Mexicans in the new south. In: Leonard KI, Stepick A, Vásquez MA, et al., eds. Immigrant faiths: transforming religious life in America. Walnut Creek: AltaMira; 2005:189–218.

16. Guest KJ. Religion and transnational migration in the new Chinatown. In: Leonard KI, Stepick A, Vásquez MA, et al., eds. Immigrant faiths: transforming religious life in America. Walnut Creek: AltaMira; 2005:145–163.

17. Richman K. The Protestant ethic and the dis-spirit of Vodou. In: Leonard KI, Stepick A, Vásquez MA, et al., eds. Immigrant faiths: transforming religious life in America. Walnut Creek: AltaMira; 2005:165–187.

18. Guest KJ. Transnational religious networks among New York's Fuzhou immigrants. In: Ebaugh HR, Chafetz JS, eds. Religion across borders: transnational immigrant networks. Walnut Creek: AltaMira; 2002:149–163.

19. Yang F. The Hsi-nan Chinese Buddhist temple: seeking to Americanize. In: Ebaugh HR, Chafetz JS, eds. Religion and the new immigrants. Walnut Creek: AltaMira; 2000:67–87.

20. Rhodes LA. Studying biomedicine as a cultural system. In: Johnson TM, Sargent CF, eds. Medical anthropology: a handbook of theory and method. New York: Greenwood Press; 1990:165–180.

21. Ali IF. Constructing pious identities through biomedicine: a case study of the Ismailis of Hunza, Pakistan. Doctoral dissertation. New Orleans: Tulane University; 2004.

22. Vásquez MA. Historicizing and materializing the study of religion: the contribution of migration studies. In: Leonard

KI, Stepick A, Vásquez MA, et al., eds. Immigrant faiths: transforming religious life in America. Walnut Creek: AltaMira; 2005:219–242.

23. Abusharaf RM. Structural adaptations in an immigrant Muslim congregation in New York. In: Warner RS, Wittner JG, eds. Gatherings in diaspora: religious communities and the new immigration. Philadelphia: Temple University; 1998:234–261.

24. Kurien P. 'We are better Hindus here': religion and ethnicity among Indian Americans. In: Min PG, Kim JH, eds. Religions in Asian America: building faith communities. Walnut Creek: AltaMira; 2002:99–120.

25. Yang F. Chinese gospel churches: the sinicization of Christianity. In: Ebuagh HR, Chafetz JS, eds. Religion and the new immigrants. Walnut Creek: AltaMira; 2000:89–107.

26. Stepick A. God is apparently not dead: the obvious, the emergent, and the still unknown in immigration and religion. In: Leonard KI, Stepick A, Vásquez MA, et al., eds. Immigrant faiths: transforming religious life in America. Walnut Creek: AltaMira; 2005:11–37.

27. Janzen JM, Ngudiankama A, Filippi-Franz M. Religious healing among war-traumatized African immigrants. In: Barnes LL, Sered SS, eds. Religion and healing in America. New York: Oxford University; 2005:159–172.

28. Ha T. The evolution of remittances from family to faith: the Vietnamese case. In: Ebaugh HR, Chafetz JS, eds. Religion across borders: transnational immigrant networks. Walnut Creek: AltaMira; 2002:111–127.

29. Morioka-Douglas N, Sacks T, Yeo G. Issues in caring for Afghan American elders: insights from literature and a focus group. J Cross-Cult Gerontol 2004; 19:27–40.

30. Orsi RA. The religious boundaries of an inbetween people: street feste and the problem of the dark-skinned. Am Q 1992; 44:313–347.

31. Torres V, Howard-Hamilton MF, Cooper DL. Identity development of diverse populations. San Francisco: Jossey-Bass; 2003.

32. Min PG. A literature review with a focus on major themes. In: Min PG, Kim JH, eds. Religions in Asian America: building faith communities. Walnut Creek: AltaMira; 2002:15–36.

33. Warner RS. Immigration and religious communities in the United States. In: Warner RS, Wittner JG, eds. Gatherings in diaspora: religious communities and the new immigration. Philadelphia: Temple University; 1998:3–34.

34. Yang F. Tenacious unity in a contentious community: cultural and religious dynamics in a Chinese Christian church. In: Warner RS, Wittner JG, eds. Gatherings in diaspora: religious communities and the new immigration. Philadelphia: Temple University; 1998:333–361.

35. Ayyub R. Domestic violence in the South Asian Muslim immigrant population in the United States. J Soc Distress Homeless 2000; 9:237–248.

36. Chen C. A self of one's own: Taiwanese immigrant women and religious conversion. Gend Soc 2005; 19:336–357.

37. George S. Caroling with the Keralites: the negotiation of gendered space in an Indian immigrant church. In: Warner RS, Wittner JG, eds. Gatherings in diaspora: religious communities and the new immigration. Philadelphia: Temple University; 1998:234–261.

38. Thompson NE, Gurney AG. 'He is everything': religion's role in the lives of immigrant youth. New Dir Youth Dev 2003; 10:75–90.

39. Ebaugh HR, Chafetz JS. Dilemmas of language in immigrant congregations: the tie that binds or the tower of Babel? Rev Relig Res 2000; 41:432–452.

40. Eck DL. A new religious America: how a 'Christian country' has now become the world's most religiously diverse nation. San Francisco: HarperSanFrancisco; 2002.

41. Mattson I. How Muslims use Islamic paradigms to define America. In: Haddad YY, Smith JI, Esposito JL, eds. Religion and immigration: Christian, Jewish, and Muslim experiences in the United States. Walnut Creek: AltaMira; 2003:199–215.

42. Zou Y. Multiple identities of a Chinese immigrant: a story of adaptation and empowerment. Qual Stud Educ 2002; 15:251–268.

43. Barnes LL, Plotnikoff GA, Fox K, et al. Religious traditions, spirituality and pediatrics: intersecting worlds of healing: a review. J Ambul Ped Assoc 2000; 106:899–908.

44. Barnes LL. Spirituality and religion in healthcare. In: Bigby J, ed. Cross-cultural medicine. Philadelphia: American College of Physicians-American Society of Internal Medicine; 2003:237–267.

45. Espiritu YL. The intersection of race, ethnicity, and class: the multiple identities of second-generation Filipinos. Identities 1994; 1:249–273.

# CHAPTER 54

# School Readiness and Bilingual Education

Marilyn Augustyn

## Introduction

Schools are typically the first setting of sustained contact with the new culture for immigrant children. Their success and performance are often shaped by these very early first experiences. School performance is perhaps more important in the era of 'No Child Left Behind' (NCLB) than ever before, and there may be no group for whom this is *more* important than the children of immigrants. Completing and going beyond high school is critically important to job success today[1] and yet some of the highest drop out rates occur among immigrant children. Foreign-born students had a dropout rate of 26% in 2003, compared with 17% for children born in the US to foreign-born parents, both of which are higher than the national average (10.3% in 2004).[2] While foreign-born students make up 12% of the total population of high school students, they make up 30% of the dropout population. These numbers may be suspect since many immigrant children never 'drop in' to US schools; that is, children who immigrate later in life begin working immediately and never officially enter the US school system.[3] Among Latino youth who are educated in US schools, there is no statistically different dropout rate for the immigrants versus the US born; in fact, immigrant children drop out at a rate of 14% versus 18% for US-born Latino youth.[4] This is potentially linked to a shifting in family and individual values as adolescents lose the hope for 'obtaining the American dream' as the reality of poverty and inequality sink in.

NCLB attempts to address these very issues among immigrant children.[5] It attempts to provide for both immigrant children and limited English proficient (LEP) youth. Under NCLB, LEP youth are one of the key groups that must be tested. The law mandates that LEP testing scores must improve over time and that schools be held accountable for their performance. Schools that don't 'make this grade' must offer families other options including transfer to other schools immediately, after-school tutoring, and other supplemental programs. In theory, NCLB will effect change on bilingual and English as a second language (ESL) (sometimes called sheltered English) programs as students in these programs will be held to the same standard as English learners. In addition, teachers in these programs must be highly qualified to teach in their subject. Many believe that in order to succeed in these goals, NCLB must place more emphasis on school readiness among immigrant children, including pre-kindergarten and the early grades, as well as parental involvement.

## Who are These Youth?

The more than two million immigrant youth who enrolled in US public schools over the past decade represent significant challenges for local school systems. Like earlier waves of immigrant students, most are concentrated in a few large cities; they are typically poor; many have suffered the traumas of war, civil strife, or economic deprivation; and all must learn the language and customs of a new country. Recent newcomers hail from a more diverse range of cultures than earlier groups, which were primarily European, and many refer to these as the 'new immigration' which intensified in the 1990s. To clarify, when the term 'immigrant children' is used, it refers to foreign-born children who have migrated either as immigrants or refugees. 'Children of immigrants' on the other hand, refers to both US-born and foreign-born children who share a common denominator: immigrant parents. Among children of immigrants, 25% are foreign-born and 75% are born in the USA. These two groups currently make up 20% of all youth in the US and 25% of all low-income children (family incomes under 200% of the poverty level).[6] It is estimated that by 2015 they will make up 30% of the nation's school population.

Seventy-eight percent of all immigrant students who have been in the United States for 3 years or less attend school in just five states, with 45% enrolled in California.[7] As of 1990, 11% of all youth living in California were born outside the United States; the proportions for New York, Florida, Texas, and Illinois range between 6% and 3%. Together, these five states are home to over 1.5 million immigrant youth. In the large city school districts of Los Angeles and Miami, immigrant students represent 20% of the total enrollment.

These children face unique challenges to their educational success compared with those from American-born families. For example, children from immigrant families must attempt to negotiate American schools without benefit of parents raised in this society. They face additional challenges such as limited parental English proficiency, lower educational attainment by their parents, and questions of legal status.

## The Issue of Bilingualism

The overarching challenge for all children of immigrants is the issue of language. The definition of 'limited English proficient' (LEP) includes all children who speak a language other than English at home and speak English less than 'very well.' The LEP share is highest in kindergarten with 10% of kindergarteners classified as LEP. The proportion of LEP children falls to 6% in the lower grades and 4% in the upper grades.[5] In addition, 8 out of 10 LEP children in kindergarten and 6 out of 7 in grades 1–5 are also linguistically isolated – members of families in which all those over 14 are LEP. This challenge is further exacerbated by the fact that over half (53% according to the 1999–2000 Schools and Staffing Survey) of LEP students attend schools where over 30% of their fellow students are LEP.

This brings us to the issue of bilingualism. Few areas in education are as hotly debated and passionately pursued as this. In reality, very few people are considered 'balanced bilinguals'; most speakers are in fact dominant in one language. For many, language use is divided according to very specific domains: family and emotional matters in one, with conversations about work and school in another. It is important to recognize, too, that language skills atrophy quickly if they are not exercised; thus, a child may quickly become 'monolingual' if the parent language is de-emphasized or devalued.

In learning a second language, most experts agree that the best predictor of success is skill and attained milestones in the first language. A common myth is that native language use at home interferes with the acquisition of a second language at school. In a comprehensive review of bilingualism by the National Research Council, they conclude that 'the use of the child's native language does not impede the acquisition of English.'[8] Furthermore, they add that the use of a child's native language in school does not impede the acquisition of English but 'the key issue is not finding a program that works for all children and all localities but rather finding a set of program components that works for the children in the community of interest.'

There are several types of bilingual and immersion educational models[9] including:

- EARLY-EXIT TRANSITIONAL: first-language literacy first then rapid switch to English; 2–3-year program.
- LATE-EXIT TRANSITIONAL (also known as developmental or maintenance program): first-language literacy first then gradual switch to English; 4–6-year program.
- BILINGUAL IMMERSION: (two-way bilingual): minority language first for each group; that is, instruction will begin in the native language of the child with a rapid switch to the 'new' immersion language in all subject areas.
- ENGLISH AS A SECOND LANGUAGE (ESL): specified period in English for development of English language skills.
- SHELTERED ENGLISH INSTRUCTION (in California, often called 'specially designed academic instruction in English' or SDAIE): teaching of grade-level subject matter in English in ways that are comprehensible and engage students academically, while also promoting English-language development.

# Effective Bilingual Schools

In spite of sometimes heated political debate, school systems continue to struggle with how best to educate bilingual children – or oftentimes more specifically, how best to educate English language learners (ELLs), as many school systems refer to children who are LEP students – shifting from a deficit to an asset model. Most research has shown that it takes 4–9 years for ELLs to achieve full proficiency in English.[10] As above, schools have utilized a variety of instructional approaches to assist these students to achieve their full potential. There is considerable local variation and interpretation of the above approaches. Hornberger more broadly classifies bilingual education into three types: transitional, maintenance, and enrichment.[11] The overriding goal of transitional bilingual education is learner achievement in English as quickly as possible, and thus they are often called 'early-exit' bilingual programs. Early-exit programs advocate using the non-English language as a medium of instruction only until the learners are able to function exclusively in English-medium classrooms. The most common medium for delivery of early-exit classrooms is a self-contained classroom taught by a bilingual teacher. In some schools, however, native language instruction is provided by bilingual assistants or resource teachers who remove children from the classroom to instruct them in their native language. Most early-exit programs strive to transition learners out of bilingual education in 3 years or less. The decision of when a child is ready to exit is often based on performance on a standardized test which ranks children's language abilities in English and the native language as well. Children usually need to reach some minimal level in English before they are transitioned out. Usually, though, this minimal language level is based on understanding and speaking English, and this may not adequately reflect the child's ability to read and write in English, which often lags behind oral skills and is critical to academic success.

In contrast, maintenance bilingual education has as a major goal the development of proficiency in both languages and the utilization of both languages in the learning of significant content. This model is also called 'late-exit' because languages other than English are valued and linguistic pluralism is encouraged. In the elementary setting of this type, children begin their literacy and content learning in the native language and then expand on it in English.

The third type of program, an enrichment program, is bilingual immersion or 'two-way immersion.' This is designed for both ELLs and native English-speaking children. The basic goals of this type of program are to develop a high degree of proficiency in both the native and the second languages, achieve academically in both languages, and come to appreciate both cultures. These programs tend to adopt one of two models: the fifty–fifty model where instruction is in each language 50% of the time, or the ninety–ten model where 90% of the instruction is in the minority language in the primary grades with time distribution moving to about equal by fourth grade.

The final two types of programs listed above, ESL and sheltered English, are often referred to as 'non-bilingual settings' since children are being schooled almost exclusively in English with some additional support in their native language. In ESL pullout or resource, second-language learners are assigned to mainstream English-medium classes. In addition, they receive regularly scheduled ESL instruction where they are 'pulled out' of the classroom. Sometimes, the ESL teacher may come to the student and be 'pushed in' to the regular curriculum, providing translation for the ESL students. In sheltered English classrooms, also called self-contained ESL classrooms, the ESL teacher is the classroom teacher and as such assumes responsibility for all curriculum, attempting to address the individual needs of learners at many levels of English and academic proficiency.

These five types of programs are similarly implemented at both the primary and secondary school levels. What may change is the proficiency level in the native language for older children. That is, a child who enters an English-speaking system in high school may be literate in the native language in most subject areas. A significant challenge exists when children and adolescents arrive illiterate in *both* their native language and English, making placement and transition a difficult operation – often resulting in the high dropout rate referred to above. School systems dealing with significant numbers of students in this category have devised specific classrooms to address these needs, but in smaller locales where the number of students in this group is lower, students often languish and quickly give up. In general, research has found that it takes 5–7 years for second-language learners who have received at least 2–3 years of schooling in their native language to compete with native speakers.[12] Unfortunately most programs do not allow this time.

## Supporting Immigrant Children

It is commonly accepted that children's skills in kindergarten and their achievement at the end of third grade are important predictors of their school success. Thus, if policymakers hope to improve the school success of immigrant children, it will be important to intervene early and on many levels. Takanishi, president of the Foundation for Child Development, wrote: 'the three-legged stool of child well-being by age 8 is thus: family economic security, access to healthcare, and access to sound early education. Unfortunately, immigrant children tend to be disadvantaged in all three areas.'[13]

Immigrant children have many strengths, though. Estimates from the Urban Institute's 1999 National Survey of America's Families (NSAF) indicate that children of immigrants are significantly more likely to have two parents in the home versus children of natives (80 versus 70%).[14] Children of immigrants fare as well or better than natives on measures of school engagement including doing homework, caring about school, and frequency of suspension or expulsion from school. However, the NSAF also reports that, compared with children in native-born families, children in immigrant families are generally poorer, in worse health, and more likely to experience food insecurity and crowded housing. Younger children are more likely to live in families that entered after 1996 when welfare legislation barred immigrants from receiving many public health benefits.

Unfortunately, many studies have shown that the use of early education and after-school programs varies by immigrant group and by generational status, but that in general these programs are less well utilized by immigrants. For example, the participation of immigrant children in the Head Start program is lower than their percentage in the eligible population with 36% of Latino children living in official poverty and only 26% attending Head Start.[16]

An additional challenge facing clinicians when screening LEP children is determining a language delay. It is estimated that communication disorders (including speech, language, and hearing disorders) affect 1 of every 10 people in the United States, yet the detection of these disorders is often tragically delayed. Detection is compounded in the non-English speaker who may be cared for in a medical system that does not have the capacity to screen in the native language. It is critically important that clinicians use the same benchmarks for referral in LEP children as they would in English speakers; that is, attributing a child's delay to bilingualism often only results in delayed referral for a subsequently identified disability. Bilingual children learn language at the same rate as monolingual speakers – they may 'code switch' (a phenomenon of switching from one language to another in the same discourse) – but their combined level should be commensurate with their age.

The final challenge of this puzzle lies in the fact that some families may not be as concerned about their child's development because of differing expectations. In one study, Puerto Rican mothers expected their children to name colors at a significantly later age than white mothers, but white mothers expected their children to achieve toilet training at a significantly later age than Puerto Rican and African-American mothers, with mean differences in maternal expectations of these milestones of 6 months or more.[16] These differences can compound a clinician's ability to detect delays since the family may not consider it an issue worthy of discussion (Boxes 54.1; 54.2).

## Conclusion and Next Steps

Policymakers and researchers have identified several areas that must be addressed if we are to improve the educational outcome of the children of immigrants. These include:

- Establishing two-generational early educational and family literacy programs that include the parents in literacy efforts, both for their own literacy and to help them support their child's advancement.
- Screen children for communication delays early and often.
- Provide early education for all children.
- Improve teacher education to work with diverse immigrant children.
- Encourage parental engagement in schools. Often, this may involve a 'culture shift' for families who feel school and family, like church and state, need to be separate. It is important to advocate for families, but most important to help them understand they must be their child's best advocate through the system.

If we care about the success of immigrant children, the future cannot wait.

## Box 54.1

### A tale of two travelers

#### Case study 1

This young boy is a wonderful and funny 8-year-old who came to the US 18 months before from Costa Rica. His parents divorced when he was 6 and his mother and he came to the US alone. He is an only child and the mother has very limited support in the US. She is literate in both English and Spanish and has a professional job which enabled her to find employment in the US. On arriving here, he was placed in the March of the school year into an age-appropriate classroom of first grade. He did not speak any English in a school district with very few LEP students. He received 'push in' support from an ESL teacher who came into the classroom during instruction to 'translate' for him. By the end of second grade, he was reading in English and functioning above grade level in mathematics. Socially, he had significant challenges. Though he tried very hard to interact, he had no friends and ate alone every day. By second grade, he became aggressive when other children teased him and became singled out as a 'trouble maker.' He also was very fidgety in class, unable to sit still and always out of his seat, jumping to raise his hand with an answer. In third grade, his grades began to drop. He was not completing assignments and his aggression towards peers was increasing. The school suggested an alternative placement for 'behavior problems.' When asked, he stated that 'nobody in my school speaks Spanish and here, they don't like Spanish kids.' His mother requested a special education evaluation which showed above average intelligence and achievement but also revealed hyperactivity and marked difficulties maintaining attention. In addition, it showed significant difficulty reading social skills and interacting socially. He began a social skills group outside of school, joined the Cub Scouts at a Latino community center in an neighboring town, and began medication for ADHD. His grades improved remarkably and he feels more confident.

#### Case study 2

This 32-month-old boy presented to a new pediatrician for well child care. He was born in the US and his immunizations were up to date but the majority of his care prior to this examination had been delivered in public health settings for immunizations. His family was well educated in China and had been in the US for about 6 years. The parents had no developmental concerns. The pediatrician was immediately struck by the child's lack of language and eye contact. On further questioning of the family they stated that he did not point and usually 'pulled them' to an object using their hands to get what he wanted. His father stated that 'we do not make eye contact so I think it is something I taught him.' They stated he was fairly easy going, liked to watch TV for 8–10 hours a day, and also enjoyed lining up his cars and trucks but 'never really played with them.' When he was excited he would bang his head on the floor. On a Denver Developmental Screening test he showed marked delays in language and self-help skills. He had no words and was unable to pull off his clothes or assist in dressing. His parents fed him from a spoon and he did not eat finger foods. He was not toilet trained and showed no interest in such. He slept with his mother and cried excessively whenever he was separated from her so that was very rare. The child was referred immediately to Early Intervention where he received speech and language therapy, occupational therapy, and entered a play group. They also helped transition him to the public school system at 3 years of age. Prior to his third birthday his family took him to China for 'acupuncture therapy' for his delays. He received a diagnosis of autistic disorder at 3 years of age and has benefited from significant educational and emotional support.

## Box 54.2

### Tips for supporting immigrant children

#### Clinicians

- Screen children using culturally appropriate measures and standardized tools.
- Do not attribute delays to 'bilingualism' but dig deeper.
- Encourage families to consider early out-of-home education programs.
- Counsel families to limit television time as a 'teacher of English.'
- Encourage families to know their options concerning schooling and to know their child's school and become involved.

#### Teachers

- Advocate at a school level for curriculum that is sensitive to the pace at which LEP children learn English.
- Help families maintain their native culture and language by encouraging diversity of experience in the classroom.

#### Allied health professionals

- Encourage families to consider early out-of-home education programs such as Head Start.
- Support parental efforts to become literate in English.

#### Parents

- Encourage the value of literacy and school performance by being an example for your children.
- Become and remain involved in your child's school, contributing information about your native culture to enhance the education of all children and help your child maintain his/her own cultural identity.

## References

1. Kaufman P, Alt MN, Chapman CD. US Department of Education, National Center for Education Statistics, 2001. Dropout rates in the United States: 2000, NCES 2002–114. Washington, DC: Available: http://nces.ed.gov/pubs2002/droppub_2001/
2. Available: http://www.childtrendsdatabank.org/indicators/1HighSchoolDropout.cfm January 19, 2007.
3. Pew Hispanic Center Fact Sheet. Available: http://pewhispanic.org/reports/report.php?ReportID=55 Accessed January 19, 2007.
4. US Department of Education, National Center for Education Statistics. Generational studies and education outcomes among Asian and Hispanic 1988 Eighth Graders. NCES 199–020, Washington DC: 1998.
5. Capps R, Fix M, Murray J, et al. Promise or peril. Foundation for Child Development, The Urban Institute-Washington, DC; 2004. Available: http://www.fcd-us.org/PDFs/NCLBandImmigrants.pdf January 19, 2007.
6. Suarez-Orozco C, Suarez-Orozco M. Children of immigrants. Boston: Harvard University Press; 2001.
7. McDonnell LM, Hill PT. Newcomers in American Schools. Rand Corporation; 1993. Available: http://www.rand.org/publications/MR/MR103/ January 19, 2007.
8. August D, Hakuta K. Improving schooling for language minority children: a research agenda. Washington, DC: National Academy Press; 1997.
9. Faltis CJ, Hudelson SJ. Bilingual education in elementary and secondary school communities. Boston: Allyn and Bacon; 1998.
10. Collier V. A synthesis of studies examining long-term-language-minority-student data on academic achievement. Bilingual Res J 1992; 16:187–212.
11. Hornberger J. Extending enrichment bilingual education: revisiting typologies and redirecting policy. In: Garcia O, ed. Bilingual education: focusschrift in honor of Joshua A. Fishman on the occasion of his 65th birthday. Amsterdam/Philadelphia: John Benjamins Publishing; 1991:215–234.
12. Thomas W, Colier V. Language minority student achievement and program effectiveness. Washington, DC: National Clearinghouse for Bilingual Education; 1995.
13. Takanishi R. Leveling the playing field: supporting immigrant children from birth to eight. In: Children of immigrant families. Vol. 14. The Foundation for Children; Summer 2004.
14. Reardon-Anderson J, Capps R, Fix M. The Health and well-being of children in immigrant families. Washington, DC: Urban Institute; 2002.
15. Flores G, Fuentes-Afflick E, Barbot O, et al. The health of Latino children. JAMA 2002; 288(1):82–89.
16. Pachter LM, Dworkin PH. Maternal expectations about normal child development in four cultural groups. Arch Pediatr Adolesc Med 1997; 151:1144–1150.

# CHAPTER 55

# Vocational Considerations

Linda A. Piwowarczyk, George Clark, and Nerissa Caballes

## Introduction

Immigrants make up an increasing proportion of the US workforce. Approximately 25% of the US population is either born outside of the United States or a child of someone born outside of the United States. Over one-half of the foreign-born come from Latin America (53%), one-quarter from Asia, 13% from Europe, and 8% from Africa, Oceania, and elsewhere. As the native work population is aging, the contributions of the foreign-born labor force are becoming more significant. Moreover, immigrants contribute to the tax base of the economy[1] as well as to the American Social Security System.[2] Immigrants tend to live at both ends of the social spectrum. In 2004, four-tenths of all scientists were foreign-born (38%), as were three-tenths of those with a Master's degree.[3] At the same time, according to 2004 estimates, foreign-born workers gravitated toward farming, fishing, and forestry (41%), building, grounds cleaning, and maintenance (33%), food preparation and serving (22%), computer and mathematical occupations (19%), and life, physical, and science occupations (17%).[4] Although some immigrants may not find the transition to the US difficult, for others the differences between the society they left behind and the society they have entered can present significant obstacles to successful employment.

Across generations and across cultures, families strive to provide a better life for their children and the families they left behind in their own countries. For example, in 2003, gross flows to developing countries amounted to US$142 billion, compared to US$18.4 billion in 1980. The annual average figure increased from US$7.8 million in 1975–1979 to a recorded total of US$98 billion in 1998–2003. According to World Bank projections, international remittances received by developing countries were expected to reach US$167 billion in 2005 – a more than ninefold increase over the past 25 years.[5] Between 2000 and 2003, new immigrants accounted for more than half of the job growth in the nation's labor force.[6] Despite their high rate of participation in the job market, in many cases their wages and job benefits are low.[7] In practical terms, this often translates into working long hours and two or three jobs in an effort to provide.

This chapter will address barriers faced by immigrants in seeking employment and remaining employed, components of vocational rehabilitation programs, and some of the special considerations needed in vocational counseling for trauma and torture survivors.

## Employment Barriers

Barriers to employment of immigrants include language barriers, inability to transfer qualifications in the country of origin to the US, differences in culturally-shaped work ethic, influence of the family on career selection, lack of sufficient job skills, mismatch between qualifications and expectations, and misperceptions about the process of applying for a job, interviewing, and keeping a job.[8–13] Poor health may also be a barrier to employment, and some of the types of employment found by immigrants may pose health hazards (see Ch. 57). Underemployed workers report lower levels of health and well-being,[14] and the effect on health seems to be greater for immigrant women than for immigrant men.[15] Immigrants who have experienced trauma may face additional challenges including lack of trust of authority figures, difficult living situations, lack of family or group support, and mental health issues that interfere with successful functioning on the job.

Language skills are particularly central as described in a paper highlighting challenges faced by Bosnian refugees resettling in Sweden.[16] For Southeast Asians in Canada, even 10 years after resettlement, language fluency was a significant predictor of depression and lack of employment, particularly among refugee women and among people who did not become engaged in the labor market during their earliest years of resettlement.[17] In the same population, job loss was also shown to lead to an increased risk of depression, leading to more difficulty staying employed.[18] Among Iraqi asylum seekers in Sweden, lack of work, family issues, and the asylum process itself were positively associated with psychopathology.[19]

Different barriers to the work force exist across ethnic groups. Immigrants may arrive with differences in educational attainment, family composition, work experience, vocational training, English language fluency, and ability to drive.[20–22] Previous life experiences can also serve as barriers. Attitudes in the host culture and in the workplace environment can affect how newcomers adapt. Immigrants may face stereotyping.[23] New experiences such as competition, territoriality, and interaction fatigue can make adjustment to the workplace especially challenging.[24] Many newcomers have expectations of what the United States would be like, and these may not match the reality they must face.[24]

Many of the stresses associated with resettlement in a new country affect the process of employment. Stress is created by acculturative tasks such as learning a new language, seeking employment, rebuilding social supports, and defining roles.[21] Culture shock and loss of status have been shown to affect general adjustment of immigrants and refugees.[25] The migrant process also raises issues related to security and comfort, self-worth and self-acceptance, competence, identity and belonging, and the meaning of life.[26] Some immigrants miss the emotional support of loved ones left behind and the former cultural way of life[27] as they are simultaneously challenged by employment. Changes in family dynamics can occur in a new country when men formerly with high status struggle with establishing themselves, and their wives become breadwinners.[28] Others remain isolated until improving their English skills and upgrading their employment status, which later enhances integration.[29]

In an effort to cope with barriers, immigrants may use both family and ethnic groups as resources to search for employment. Those who enlist the aid of families and trusted groups often obtain higher-quality employment than those who rely on themselves. Though these networks are helpful in employment adjustment, they are not always able to compensate for downward occupational mobility and societal restrictions related to credentialing.[30] In fact, some investigators have found that social networks, workplace ethnic composition, and informal and formal assistance have minimal impact on economic adaptation.[31] The prevailing job market has an important effect on employment of immigrants, as differences in employment rate probabilities between recent immigrants and non-immigrants heightened in recession years.[32,33]

## Trauma and Work

As a result of war and human rights violations, some newcomers may come to the United States with significant histories of trauma experienced in their countries of origin and during flight. Although many exhibit extraordinary resilience, a trauma history can be predictive of post-traumatic stress disorder (PTSD), which may negatively influence quality of life and self-sufficiency.[34] In asylum seekers, PTSD has been associated with premigration trauma, delay in processing refugee applications, obstacles to employment, racial discrimination, loneliness, and boredom.[35] A significant relationship has been shown between trauma variables and employment status. For example, among Cambodians, those who continued to have disturbing thoughts about their trauma and spent more time in refugee camps were more likely to be unemployed. The number of years in the refugee camp did not predict income or health.[36] Trauma can affect one's ability to make social connections. Social supports have been shown to affect economic adaptation differently than psychological adaptation.[37]

## The Potential Role for Vocational Rehabilitation for Immigrants

Modern vocational rehabilitation now concentrates on several main components: community-based integrated work, individual choice and decision-making, meaningful work and full participation, flexible customized supports, and career-oriented employment. Goals include the ability for immigrants to choose the career paths they desire and receive the supports necessary to accomplish their goals. Current vocational rehabilitation programs emphasize supported education and employment.

Integrating supported education and employment into one program allows people to explore their career options, obtain the required education and employment skills, and finally seek and maintain employment in their chosen field. It allows each aspect to serve as a counterpart to the other, to link one goal to another, and to offer an extensive continuum of choices and services.[38] Programs following the supported education and training model centralize both short- and long-term educational and vocational goals, maximizing choice, increasing competency, and offering unconditional support. Achieving empowerment and normalization – making individual decisions and reaching goals, fully participating in the process of attaining those goals, achieving those goals in mainstream society, and determining for oneself how much support and assistance is needed to maintain those successes – is the core theory behind vocational rehabilitation services.

## Preparation for Work

Receiving work authorization opens the door to seeking employment in the United States. At this point, the tasks of identifying marketable skills, finding jobs matching the language skills and educational level of the immigrant, and providing job training become important. Optimizing opportunities for immigrants to become self-sustaining can help to prevent dependence on others or on the welfare system and can reduce disillusionment, anger, anxiety, and depression. The following sections will describe specific interventions that can be made to assist immigrants in finding employment.

### Addressing language barriers

Most immigrants are motivated to learn English and there are programs available in many communities to teach adult learners of English. An initial step in the employment process may be to help immigrants identify such programs in their neighborhoods. Speaking English does not necessarily mean a fluent understanding of the language. For example, if an interviewer has explained the tasks of a potential job and then asks the client, 'How do you feel about the responsibilities of this position?,' it can leave the applicant at a loss for an answer. The term 'how do you feel' can be interpreted as a question of health, or physical sensation, as well as a measure of accept-

ability. English terms should be clarified and practiced, with English classes as necessary. For example, what is 'work *ethic*?' What does '*conditional* employment' or '*moderate* physical strength required,' mean? What exactly are 'position *guidelines*?' Does 'employer's/supervisor's *discretion*' mean that the job is dependent upon the whim of another individual? What is a '*team player*?' Many phrases taken for granted by fluent speakers of English may be challenging to our nation's newcomers.

### Assessing work history and expectations about employment

Information about an immigrant's work history, keeping in mind that the jobs that were done in the country of origin may not even exist in the United Status, will be helpful in directing the job search. It is important to address any differences between expectations of the kinds of work an individual would like to do and the reality of what work is available. Although some newcomers may be aware of the need for retraining, recredentialing, accreditation, and reschooling, others may be surprised and disappointed to realize what a barrier this can be. Although some immigrants may eventually be able to work in their former professions, for many a process of vocational transition is more likely. If this issue is not addressed early, immigrants may waste time, effort, and in some cases money, in misdirected pursuit of an expectation.

Some immigrants come to the United States with a preconceived notion that everyone has a good job, and that employment is plentiful. It may be helpful to clarify an individual's understanding of the work situation in the US, of how jobs are obtained, and what their expectations are of the job search process. Often, the competitive process of obtaining a job is unfamiliar. Clarifying these issues as early as possible while at the same time not undermining hope may result in more realistic views as the process of job hunting is navigated.

Information about the home environment may be helpful when assisting immigrants with the employment process. The home environment affects the ability as well as the willingness of the individual to seek and keep a job. Immigrants may be living in borrowed space and relying on the host and others for food, money for transportation, and other items such as winter clothing. Whether there is access to enough food and a comfortable place to rest and sleep can affect alertness and physical stamina. In addition, pressures may be placed on immigrants by their hosts to find work that may not be appropriate, simply to produce an immediate income to pay to the host.

## Assessing the motivation

The reason that an individual seeks certain kinds of employment may not be straightforward. In many instances the individual will identify a particular kind of employment for which they would like to look and limit their willingness to search beyond that area. For example, an individual may insist on looking for a job as a Certified Nursing Assistant and nothing else, based on the fact that he or she has a certificate in that field. Quite often it may become apparent that it was upon the insistence of the host or someone from their country that a particular field was chosen. Broadening the job search to include all areas for which an individual is qualified hastens the ability to reach the ultimate short-term goal of producing an income. Producing an income from any employment source can reduce the burden of the feeling of dependence on others and allow the dignity of making one's own choices.

## Finding a job

Vocational counseling includes helping new arrivals in developing a short-term goal for employment, as well as a long-term goal for vocation. Immediate needs serve as the motivator for short-term employment. Information about the client's abilities, limitations, and language skills can help to direct the job search. For example, religion may prevent ability to work on Sundays, a traumatized back could limit ability to lift, lack of access to transportation could limit the geographic area of the search, and minimal English skills lead toward jobs which require more manual than verbal skills.

The purpose of the job application and employment interview should be made clear. Divulging so much personal information can be confusing and frightening to someone who comes from a society that does not require such a process or who has been interrogated in the past. Explaining why the information is needed and how it is processed takes the individual away from the idea that it is just the immigrant who is being scrutinized.

It is important to explain the process of multiple application submissions in order to get one invitation for an interview and the normalcy of this process. Practice completing several different types of generic applications will increase familiarity with the types of applications that may be encountered.

## The interview

Preparing the new arrival for the interview is an extremely important part of the process. Facing a stranger and talking about themselves may be a new, unfamiliar, and frightening experience for immigrants. Preparing a list of standard interview questions (30 to 50), reviewing a few initially, and giving the individual a few to take home to practice is a method of building skills in this area. Role-playing is another method for learning interview techniques and can be used over time to develop a full interview, depending on the progress of the individual. Allow the client to have some fun with it by letting him or her become the interviewer, with oneself as the applicant. Explaining the dress code that is expected in an interview, that the interview will likely take place as a dialogue, and the role of body language are important parts of interview preparation.

Body language is variable across cultures. The message that some body language relays can be detrimental or positive, dependent on the cultures of the people who are interacting. For example, in some cultures displaying the sole of the shoe (as when seated and legs are crossed) during a conversation is considered rude or disrespectful. Eye contact is considered a challenge of authority or disrespectful of an individual's status in many cultures. In some US cultures, however, lack of eye contact may be viewed as a lack of interest, dishonesty, or as inattention and can be a barrier to a successful interview. Immigrants vary in their ability to pick up these nonverbal cues in their new country, and these are topics to address in detail in job counseling.

Immigrants and the native born both carry their cultural teachings and habits with them to the job site but may be unaware that in some settings the message conveyed may be different from the intended message. Many immigrants, as well as people native to the US, are not aware that they are speaking by way of body motion and positioning. Sitting slouched over or leaning into the side of a chair may mean a lack of concern with appearance or a lack of interest in what the interviewer is saying. Looking away from the interviewer or looking at the floor while speaking could make an interviewer think the applicant is avoiding something or not being truthful. Excessive hand and arm motioning may mean anxiety and can be distracting. Holding tightly to the armrests of the chair may suggest nervousness. Crossing the arms over the chest while the interviewer is speaking may imply lack of belief or interest in what the interviewer is saying. A stern, fixed facial expression or a frown could imply a difficult attitude or give the impression of a lack of cooperation. A very smiley, flighty expression could indicate a lack of seriousness or an effort to try too hard to make a positive impression. Potential cultural conflicts between individuals can relate not only to body language but also to personal space.[39] Interpretations of cues are often so automatic and neurologically imbedded in one's own culture that specific attention has to be paid toward addressing awareness to the cultural context in which these responses occur in order not to misunderstand their meaning.[40]

Specific information that can be given to immigrants about interviewing for jobs in most US employment situations can include:

1. In an interview it is best to sit straight but relaxed while the interviewer is speaking and while you are speaking. This implies that you are paying attention to what is being said and that you are interested.

2. Eye-to-eye contact with the individual without appearing to stare would indicate that you are speaking directly to that person, that the person has your full attention, and that you are responding to the best of your ability.

3. Avoid constant motion with hands and arms by simply clasping your hands together in a relaxed fashion across your waist, which implies confidence and calmness, or by holding a pen and pad to take notes, which means that you want to remember all the information that you are given and gives your hands something to do that is not distracting.

4. Be aware of your facial expression. A relaxed and pleasant or thoughtful expression makes the interviewer comfortable and implies that you are not difficult to talk to. Facial expressions can be practiced at home while looking in a mirror.

5. Explaining to a potential employer polite nonverbal cues from one's own culture can also be empowering for the immigrant being interviewed, as well as to the potential employer, who may appreciate learning this information (Box 55.1).

Role-playing may be helpful in addressing the challenges presented by differences in body languages in different cultures. Once individuals understand the concept of differences in body lan-

---

**Box 55.1**

**Case study 1**

While working with a young Sudanese man, we came to the interview phase and addressed facial expressions. I asked him if he was aware that he had a constant sternness, almost a frown when he spoke to others and he said that he was aware of it. It was explained how expressions can leave a positive or negative impression. When asked if there was a reason that he maintained that facial expression, he said that his Bible training has taught him 'it is wrong to bear a false smile.' Religion was a very strong force in the lives of young Sudanese men, and many understood every written word to be literal, so there was little room for interpretation. In his opinion a frown is neutral, that is to say that it's not a frown, as we know it, but an absence of a false smile. It was explained that in his new society such an expression means that the person may be angry, displeased, or worried. He said he did not realize that it could have so many meanings. He was asked if going to a job interview would make him happy, or pleased. With his response that it would make him pleased, we further asked if he thought that such a positive experience would be worthy of practicing a more welcoming expression on his own, to which he agreed. In this case we did not want to encroach on his religious beliefs, but at the same time wanted to introduce a Western standard. The personal and religious beliefs of an individual should be respected, and never trivialized.

---

guage, they are able to observe ways in which it is displayed and begin to attach meaning to it. Body language should never be presented as a fault, but rather another way in which people communicate either consciously or unconsciously. The interview should not be viewed as an interrogation, but as an opportunity for the employer, as well as the applicant, to get to know each other. The applicant should know that at this time the employer is starting to formulate an opinion, but at the same time, this is the applicant's opportunity to form his or her own opinion about the potential employer.

## Clarify rejection

Seeking employment in the US is a daunting task for the native-born population, and anxiety and depression may accompany making application after application, only to face rejection after rejection. An immigrant who is a torture survivor, for example, has already been devalued as a person by people who are adept and skilled at reducing an individual's self-worth and self-esteem. With each promise from employers of phone calls within a few days, which rarely come, clients may wonder more and more if there is something wrong with them. For the person whose self-esteem has already been reduced, rejection can be the catalyst to stopping the application process. It is critical to explain that application rejection is simply a part of the competitive process in which they are now involved. It may be helpful to use concrete examples, such as: if 20 people have applied for one job, then 19 will be rejected and one will be accepted; this does not mean that 19 were unqualified, but simply that there was only one position to fill. It is important to reiterate this as many times as needed, to reinforce the idea that the job search is about availability and not a personalized search for flaws in the individual. The fact that almost everyone who has a job has gone through this same process needs to be stated in order to take away the individuality of rejection and add normalcy to this part of the search.

## Special Considerations for Survivors of Trauma and Torture

Survivors of trauma and torture have additional and specific challenges in finding employment. The Boston Center for Refugee Health and Human Rights is a multidisciplinary program working with survivors of torture and trauma. It has evolved in response to the needs of its patient population from over 60 countries. The incorporation of vocational rehabilitation evolved out of the observation that the provision of employment services through resettlement did not fully address the varied needs of this population. It remains a work in progress as we have come to understand the immediate needs and long-term goals that uprooted individuals have as they come to another country. The next section will address some of the specific challenges faced by this population and some of the techniques that may be used to facilitate vocational rehabilitation.

For those who have been tortured, recovery involves safety, reconstruction, and reconnection.[41] The experiences faced by trauma and torture survivors present specific challenges. For example, avoidant behavior may be present in those who have PTSD. A safe environment during the vocational rehabilitation process will be particularly critical. Feelings of helplessness, impulsivity, and a sense of

foreshortened future may make an individual look accident prone, passive, or dependent.[42] Irritability can lead to difficulty with supervisors or coworkers. Individuals can be triggered by elements of their physical environment, as well as work relationships. The positive elements of work justify the effort of providing intensive vocational rehabilitation services to these new immigrants. Work can help someone enter a new culture. It can strengthen one's family. It can help one control one's anxiety and can help one to deal with the trauma and control one's emotions. It helps one to communicate with others and to gain meaning.[43]

The supported education and supported employment models, mentioned earlier, may be especially applicable to the population of trauma and torture survivors. The supported education model follows the psychosocial rehabilitation structure and is designed to provide the necessary assistance, preparation, and supports in pursuing higher educational goals. It offers individuals the opportunity to adopt a more positive self-definition and the role of a student as opposed to a consumer of mental health services.[44] It has been defined as 'the provision of postsecondary education in integrated educational settings for people with psychiatric disabilities whose education has been interrupted, intermittent, or has not yet occurred because of a severe psychiatric disability, and who, because of this psychiatric impairment, need ongoing support services in order to be successful in the education environment.'[45]

One of the cornerstones of success for the supported education model lies within the mobile support model where students attend regular classes while receiving support from staff members of mental health agencies. This allows for immersion into normalizing social and interpersonal environments; enhancement of basic educational competencies; exploration and development of individual vocational interests; access to leisure, recreational, and cultural resources; and ongoing support from staff and peers. By engaging in advanced education and training, immigrants also develop increased self-esteem and improved long-term vocational outcomes, with the potential to obtain skilled jobs that may offer more longevity, stability, and financial security.[44]

Supported employment programs also focus on providing ongoing supports and integration into a normalizing, competitive arena. Federal legislation identified the core components to be 'competitive work, integrated work setting, and ongoing support.'[46] The widely used model of supported employment follows individual and/or group placement

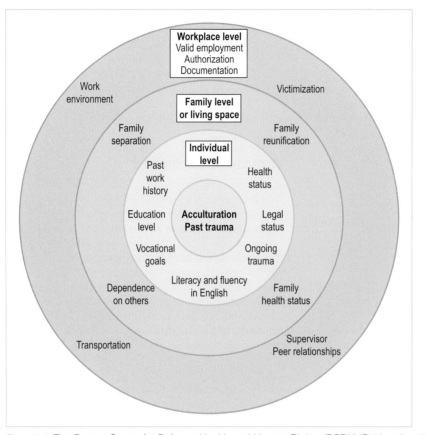

**Fig. 55.1** The Boston Center for Refugee Health and Human Rights (BCRHHR) Vocational Wheel.

approaches, which entail employment-training specialists working with clients on the job site. The advantages of this model include: socialization opportunities, opportunities to work in normative business settings, greater diversity of employment options, improved equal access to the employment market, enhanced learning and transfer of critical job skills, job placement outcomes, productivity, and economic self-sufficiency.[47] A key element of supported employment comes from the implementation of matching jobs to individuals' specific interests and skills, and this model carries the flexibility and structure to meet the needs of the client to ensure success on the job.

## Addressing Occupational Issues with Trauma and Torture Survivors: Lessons Learned

Vocational rehabilitation for the survivor population requires the provider to obtain a clear understand-

ing of the level of impact that the trauma has had on the individual's ability to interact in the social/work setting. Vocational rehabilitation for foreign-born clients seen through the Boston Center for Refugee Health and Human Rights is a multistep process involving the interaction of the immigrant, provider, employer, and all available support resources. There are many components to the workforce experience; it cannot simply be seen as helping an individual to get a job. These components are depicted in Figure 55.1. Vocational rehabilitation differs from rehabilitation for the general population in that refugees, immigrants, and asylum seekers have a different support network and skill set than that of the native-born population. Some of the specific challenges seen by immigrants in the program are described below:

1. The newcomer may have been alone at the worst possible times, particularly if a survivor of refugee trauma or torture. They may be very isolated in the absence of

family members, in a new country, with no means to support themselves. The rehabilitation specialist becomes a resource of sorts, to give advice, support, guidance, and assistance in stepping out into a new community and re-starting a productive lifestyle. It is important that the client does not feel alone in this process, but part of a team. When working with immigrants seeking employment, clarifying that successful entry into the workforce does not terminate your availability is also important.

2. Legal status can greatly influence what options may be available for an individual. For example, if a decision has not been made, asylum seekers must wait 150 days before applying for a work authorization.

3. Newcomers may live in environments that are unsafe. They may be at risk for re-victimization through discrimination or coercion related to immigration status.

4. Separation from family and recent re-unification can be major stressors. It is important to understand why families may be separated. Newcomers desire to support family members left behind or ones who have arrived to join them, but it adds additional stress to do so.

5. Untreated illness may be a cause of absenteeism; although in some settings absenteeism may be lower for immigrants, especially in settings lacking a system for paid sick time. Help finding affordable medical care and reviewing insurance-related issues for immigrants and their families can improve readiness for employment.

6. When not working, individuals may be dependent on others so as to avoid becoming homeless. This may set up situations in which victimization can occur. Over time, pressures can mount, whereby just eating the food in the home can be frowned upon unless one is contributing. Tensions can arise between the host and the guest. It is important to clarify relationships in the household.

7. New immigrants may follow suggestions about employment made by members of their household and community that may result in uninformed decisions and ill-suited vocational goals.

8. Immigrants with a history of trauma may be especially sensitive to environmental triggers and workplace dynamics that could affect relationships with supervisors or peers. Not knowing the job culture also can result in misunderstanding and sometimes being taken advantage of by coworkers or employers.

## Appropriate Employment

For immigrants, as well as refugees and torture survivors, not all employment is good employment. Although newcomers are encouraged to make their job search as broad as possible, some attention should be given to the client's past trauma history. Some environments may act as triggers to re-traumatization. For example, an individual who was tortured by uniformed police or soldiers may be in the wrong environment in an establishment that has a high uniformed presence (corrections, security, etc). Individuals sensitive to loud noises such as those found in a machine shop, or to crowded or confining areas such as busy retail stores and office space cubicles, should attempt to seek positions in other settings. This is particularly important in the primary employment phase, when an adverse placement could distance newcomers from continuous employment (Box 55.2).

## Additional Issues for Torture and Trauma Survivors

Vocational counseling sessions provide the opportunity to address some of the specific workplace challenges for survivors of trauma. A handshake, a commonplace gesture in the US, may not have the same meaning for all. For example, a woman who has been sexually traumatized may be reserved about extending her hand to men who offer a handshake as a greeting. For her, this physical contact with a stranger is unwelcome and stressful. In this instance, a sensitive employer might turn the offer of a handshake into a simple gesture to have a seat, but others might interpret the reluctance to shake hands as unfriendliness or rudeness. In many traditional Islamic cultures, men should not shake the hand of a women unless she is their family member, and in Buddhist societies, monks are forbidden to touch women. Strategies to address anxiety about this important greeting in the US culture may need

**Box 55.2**

**Case study 2**

A woman with whom we worked was unwilling to apply for a cashier's position that was available because she was afraid of making mistakes with customers, which might cause her to be reprimanded by her supervisors. She said that, with every new customer encounter, there was a new opportunity to make a mistake. Even though she was willing and ready to work, this match was not an optimal one for her first job. Recognizing and respecting the clients' fears allows the provider to guide them towards appropriate, nonstressful employment while working to develop workforce skills and understanding.

**Box 55.3**

**Case study 3**

Ideally, vocational rehabilitation programs would offer choice of provider gender to traumatized people. A team of male and female providers would initially interview together, both facing the client frontally. Responses of the clients can be revealing, even in situations where clients do not declare a preference. Sometimes, when a question was posed to a female client from the male provider, she would look directly at the female provider and provide the information, never looking at the male. In other instances, answers as well as focus from a male client to questions posed by the female provider would be directed to the male provider only. This body language indicates a choice as to the gender of the provider with whom the client was most comfortable.

to be developed. Employers who hire a multicultural work force should also inquire as to cultural norms in other countries.

Observing body language and reactions to various topics of discussion during the counseling sessions can yield information about the cultures in which the newcomer was raised or adapted to, or about trauma they may have experienced. The establishment of rapport, confidence, and interest may be seen in the distance that a client keeps, extends, or lessens from the interviewer in the initial and subsequent meetings. For example, a client who initially sits back in the chair and remains pressed back in it, and then starts to lean forwards towards the interviewer, may be developing a certain ease with the provider. It may also indicate a desire to hear more or a developing of confidence in the dialogue. Listening to the level of aggressiveness or subdued passiveness in the voice helps to reveal the ability or inability to speak freely and confidently, but may also reflect cultural norms about appropriate social behavior. A meeting in which the client is fidgeting, his eyes focused on different objects in the room, suggests uneasiness in this environment or with the interviewer, or both. Giving short answers to interview questions such as yes, no, fine, okay, may indicate further that one is not sure about what the depth of dialogue should be or whether it is all right to describe one's thoughts. In many traditional Asian cultures, keeping a low, calm voice is a sign of respect for the other person, and raising one's voice or acting excited can be interpreted negatively.

In an instance like this, we would invite the client to become a participant as opposed to simply a respondent in the following manner. *'How has the job search been for you? Fairly easy, or more difficult than you expected?'* (Wait for response) *'It's important that you remember that my purpose is to help you to make this an easier, successful process, so that you can earn your own money and support yourself. If it has been difficult for you, what do you think would help it be easier?'* At this time, the client has been openly invited to speak in his own terms, and to think about himself rather than the environment, or the interviewer, and to relax. At the same time, you will be able to determine important assessment information. The client's responses will provide level of English competency, level of understanding of the system, perception of barriers, as well as expectations (Box 55.3).

## After Finding Work

Vocational counseling extends beyond the period of the job search. Immigrants need to know that you will be working together after they get a job. Problems that arise at work are sometimes overpowering to immigrants and they may have difficulty considering options for addressing issues at work. For example, if a supervisor displays dissatisfaction with the work of the individual and states this, what should one do? In this situation the client may quit, become frightened of being fired, or aggressively challenge the supervisor, simply by not knowing how to deal with feedback, particularly negative feedback, in a new society. Some societies advance workers based on age and seniority, and immigrants may be unaccustomed to the concepts of new job probationary periods or annual job performance reviews. Other immigrants may face discrimination in the workplace. A young African man who had recently gained employment in a hotel kitchen came to us one day to say that he was too tired every day to continue with his new job. We asked if the eight hours was tiring to him or the labor itself. He explained that when he completed his shift his coworkers would not allow him to leave until he completed *their* assigned tasks as well. He subsequently was working more than 12 hours on some days. This issue was resolved by reviewing peer relationships with him, in addition to involvement of the supervisor. Unfortunately for the immigrant population, unfamiliarity and vulnerability can allow for exploitation. The workplace is not always the safe haven that we want and expect for our clients. People can be coerced into doing the work of their peers, sexually harassed, verbally abused, underpaid (cheated out of overtime, etc.), threatened, and otherwise ill-treated. Advise your clients that if 'something is wrong' to not hesitate to bring it to your attention. If the service provider is in a position to develop an employer/business that can serve your population as a routine referral source, then the relationship between the provider and the employer serves to protect the new arrival from exploitation.

## Conclusion

Immigrants face barriers to employment that differ from those faced by US job applicants. Newcomers may benefit from vocational counseling focusing on introduction to the culture of work in the US, addressing language and other barriers to employment, and identifying optimal job options. Immigrants who are survivors of trauma or torture may have additional needs and may benefit from coordinated vocational rehabilitation programs that draw upon resources in the community, workplace, resettlement agencies, healthcare facilities, schools, and recreational and therapeutic facilities. Close collaboration of healthcare providers with a network of referral resources that extends beyond the clinical setting can help immigrants gain optimal employment. Focusing on the strengths of immigrants, particularly work ethic and eagerness to learn, can help ease the adaptation to work in a new country.

## Acknowledgement

We would like to acknowledge the Office of Refugee Resettlement for its support of our work and Sara Itkin for her contributions during the early development of our program.

## References

1. Ewing, WA. The economics of necessity: economic report of the president underscores the importance of immigration. Immigration Policy Brief. Immigration Policy Center; 2005. Available: http://www.ailf.org/ipc/economicsofneccessity.asp 5/25/2005.
2. Anderson S. The contribution of legal immigration to the social security system. Arlington, VA: National Foundation for American Policy (revised March 2005); 2005.
3. National Science Board. Science and engineering indicators, 2004. Arlington, VA: National Science Foundation; 2004.
4. 'Labor Force Characteristics of Foreign-Born Workers in 2003.' Table 4. Employed foreign-born and native-born persons 16 years old and over by occupation and sex. 2003 annual average. Bureau of Labor Statistics. US Department of Labor News Release. December 1, 2004.
5. Migrant Remittances and Development: Myths, Rhetoric and Realities. International Organization for Migration (IOM); 2006.
6. Sum A, Khatiwada I, Harrington P, et al. New immigrants in the labor force and the number of employed new immigrants in the US from 2000 through 2003: continued growth amist declining employment among the native-born population. Center for Labor Market Studies. Northeastern University; 2003.
7. Facts About Immigrant Workers. National Immigration Law Center; April 2004.
8. Atkins C, Kent R. Attitudes and perceptions in the hiring process. J Employ Counsel 1989; 26:63–70.
9. Vinokurov A, Birman D, Trickett E. Psychological and acculturation correlates of work status among Soviet Jewish refugees in the U.S. Internat Migration Rev 2000; 34(2):538–559.
10. Cobas JA. Ethnic enclaves and middleman minorities: alternative strategies of immigrant adaptation? Sociological Perspectives 1987; 30(2):143–161.
11. Chow J, Bester N, Shinn A. Asian works: a TANF program for Southeast Asians Americans in Oakland, California. J Comm Pract 2001; 9(3):111–124.
12. Stepick A, Portes A. Flight into despair: a profile of recent Haitian refugees in south Florida. Internat Migration Rev 1986; 20(2):329–350.
13. Westwood M, Ishiyama FI. Challenges in counseling immigrant clients: understanding intercultural barriers to career adjustment. J Employ Counsel 1991; 28(4):130–143.
14. Friedland DS, Price RH. Underemployment: consequence for the health and well-being of workers. American Journal of Am J Comm Psychol 2003; 32(1–2):33–45.
15. Akhavan S, Bildt CO, Franzen E, et al. Health in relation to unemployment and sick leave among immigrants in Sweden from a gender perspective. J Immigr Health. 2004; 6(3):103–118.
16. Kivling-Boden G, Sundbom E. Life situation and posttraumatic symptoms: a follow-up study of refugees from the former Yugoslavia living in Sweden. Nordic J Psychiatry 2001; 55(6):401–408.
17. Beiser M, Hou F. Language acquisition, unemployment, and depressive disorder among Southeast Asian refugees: a 10-year study. Social Sci Med 2001; 53(10):1321–1334.

18. Beiser M, Johnson PJ, Turner RJ. Unemployment, underemployment, and depressive affect among Southeast Asian refugees. Psychological Med 1993; 23(3):731–743.

19. Laban CJ, et al. Postmigration living problems and common psychiatric disorders in Iraqi asylum seekers in the Netherlands. J Nerv Mental Dis 2005; 193(12):825–832.

20. Emeka N, McAdoo H. Acculturative stress among Amerasian refugees: gender and racial difficulties. Adolescence 1996; 31(122):477–487.

21. Nicholson BL. The influence of pre-emigration and post-emigration stressors on mental health: a study of Southeast Asian refugees. Social Work Res 1997; 21(1):19–31.

22. Garcia JA, Harris RD. Barriers to employment for welfare recipients. The role of race/ethnicity. J Ethnic Cultural Diversity Social Work 2001; 10(4):21–41.

23. Sue D, Sue D. Counseling the culturally different: theory and practice. New York: Wiley; 1990.

24. Boekestijn C. Intercultural migration and the development of personal identity. The dilemma between identity maintenance and cultural adaptation. Internat J Internat Rel 1988; 12(2):83–105.

25. Yost AD, Lucas MS. Adjustment issues affecting employment for immigrants from the former Soviet Union. J Employment Counsel 2000; 39(4):153–170.

26. Ishiyama F, Westwood M. Enhancing foreign adolescents' difficulties in cross-cultural adjustment. A self-validation model. Can J Psychol 1992; 5:41–56.

27. Matsuoka JK, Ryujini DH. Vietnamese refugees: an analysis of contemporary adjustment issues. J Appl Social Sci 1989–90; 14(1):23–45.

28. Dolo E, Gilgun JF. Gender-linked status changes among Liberian refugees in the United States. J Social Work Res Evaluat 2002; 3(2):203–213.

29. Nontapattamadul K. The integration of Laotian refugees in Calgary. Dissertation Abstracts International, Section A: The Humanities and Social Sciences. 2000; 61(5):2040A.

30. Lamba NK. The employment experiences of Canadian refugees: measuring the impact of human and social capital on the quality of employment. Can Rev Sociolog Anthropol 2003; 40:1.

31. Pootocky-Tripodi M. The role of social capital in immigrant refugee economic adaptation. J Social Service Res 2004; 31(1):59–91.

32. Samuel TJ. Economic adaptation of refugees in Canada: experience of a quarter century. Internat Migration 1984; 22(1):45–55.

33. McDonald JT, Worswick C. Unemployment incidence of immigrant men in Canada. Canadian Public Policy/Analyse de Politiques. 1997; 23(4):353–373.

34. Cusack KJ. Refugee experiences of trauma and PTSD: effect on psychological, physical, and financial well-being. Dissertation Abstracts International, Section B: The Sciences and Engineering. 2002; 62(10):4778B.

35. Silove D, Sinnerbrink I, Field A, et al. Anxiety, depression, and PTSD in asylum seekers: associations with pre-migration trauma and post-migration stressors. Br J Psychiatry 1997; 170(4):351–357.

36. Uba L, Chung RC. The relationship between trauma and financial and physical well-being among Cambodians in the United States. J Gen Psychol 1991; 118(3):215–225.

37. Takeda J. Psychological and economic adaptation of Iraqi male refugees: implications for social work practice. J Social Service Res 2000; 26(3):1–21.

38. Egnew R. Supported education and employment: an integrated approach. Psychosocial Rehabil J 1993; 17(1):121–127.

39. Juckett G. Cross-cultural medicine. Am Fam Phys 2005; 72(11):2267–2274.

40. de Gelder B. Towards the neurobiology of emotional body language. Nature Rev Neurosci 2006; 73(3):242–247.

41. Gorman W. Refugee survivors of torture: trauma and treatment. Professional Psychol Res Pract 2001; 32:443–451.

42. Ressler TJ. Post-traumatic stress disorder: vocational considerations. J Appl Rehabil Counsel 1995; 26(1):9–12.

43. Piwowarczyk L, Keane T. Vocational rehabilitation of torture survivors. Monograph: Boston Center for Refugee Health and Human Rights. (ORR grant # 90ZT008). 2004. Available: http://www.bcrhhr.org

44. Collins M, Bybee D, Mowbray C. Effectiveness of supported education for individuals with psychiatric disabilities: results from an experimental study. Commun Mental Health J 1999; 34(6):595–613.

45. Sullivan A, Nicolellis D, Danley K, et al. Choose-get-keep: a psychiatric rehabilitation approach to supported education. Psychosocial Rehabil J 1993; 17(1):55–68.

46. Marrone J. Creating positive vocational outcomes for people with severe mental illness. Psychosocial Rehabil J 1993; 17(2):43–62.

47. Hursh N. Course lecture: RC 604 Career Development. Boston University. Sergeant College of Health and Rehabilitation Sciences. 1999.

# CHAPTER 56

# Health Literacy

Kevin Larsen

## Introduction

Health literacy has been defined as 'the degree to which individuals have the capacity to obtain, process, and understand basic health information and services needed to make appropriate health decisions.'[1] The American Medical Association (AMA) defines it as 'a constellation of skills including basic reading and numerical tasks required to function in the healthcare environment.'[2] These definitions are carefully worded to articulate that health literacy is more than just the ability to read. As our healthcare system gets more complex and as a larger share of responsibility for self-management is moving into patients' hands, the ability to understand and process complex information is becoming increasingly important. 'Like a driver trying to reach a destination, a patient must learn how to navigate his or her way to health.'[3] A patient must be able to get to appointments on time by reading appointment slips and finding the way to a clinic. He or she must be able to read and fill out clinic forms, communicate with staff, and understand insurance and billing information. The patient also needs to follow directions which are often given in written form, i.e. medication instructions, home care instructions, and follow-up instructions. He or she may be asked to check blood sugars then calculate an insulin dose based on the result. All of this and more is health literacy (Box 56.1).

Health literacy has only recently been the focus of study. A landmark article by Williams et al. in 1995 tested English and Spanish health literacy in patients at public hospitals in Los Angeles and Atlanta. They interviewed patients seeking acute care and excluded anyone whose first language was something other than English or Spanish. In Atlanta they interviewed

only English speakers and found that nearly half (47.4%) of them had inadequate (34.7%) or marginal (12.7%) health literacy. The questions on their survey required patients to read things such as appointment slips and prescription instructions and accurately convey what 'take twice a day,' meant. In Los Angeles, they found that nearly three quarters (71.7%) of the Spanish-speaking patients, when tested in Spanish, had limited (41.9%) or marginal (19.8%) health literacy.[4]

There is now strong evidence that low health literacy correlates with poorer health and worse outcomes. The consequences of inadequate health literacy include less health knowledge, poorer health status, higher rates of health services utilization, and higher healthcare costs.[5] People with low health literacy are more likely to be hospitalized,[6] are less knowledgeable about hypertension goals,[7] symptoms of hypoglycemia, and less able to use an inhaler,[8] and more likely to report poor health.[9] They are also likely to have larger medical bills, largely due to increased hospitalization.[5]

This mounting evidence has brought health literacy to the attention of government, and providers and organized medicine. In its *Unequal Treatment: Confronting Racial and Ethnic Disparities in Health Care* the Institute of Medicine highlights health literacy as one of the factors leading to disparities.[10] They later developed an entire report on the issue of health literacy.[11] The AMA has undertaken a large initiative to develop tools and resources to provide care for patients with low health literacy. They have also produced a book, *Understanding Health Literacy, Implications for Medicine and Public Health*.[12]

Immigrants face many barriers to effective healthcare including logistical, cultural, and linguistic.[13-16] Although the data are not nearly as robust for immi-

---

**Box 56.1**

**Case study 1**

A 60-year-old immigrant from Ecuador has been in primary care for several years. He has few medical problems, and is quite compliant. His primary doctor refers him for a screening colonoscopy to look for asymptomatic colon cancer, as is recommended for people his age. The doctor's clinic hands him instructions for the medicine he will take to clean out his colon so that they can see during the colonoscopy. The Ecuadorian arrives at the appointed day, completely unprepped. They are unable to perform the colonoscopy. When asked why he didn't take his medicines as the directions described, he sheepishly admits, 'I can't read.'

---

**Box 56.2**

**Case study 2**

A 55-year-old Somali immigrant with diabetes was receiving care in our Somali clinic. She came regularly, took her medication faithfully, and all of her visits were with a trained Somali interpreter. She had been instructed how to use her glucometer and its use had been demonstrated reliably during her diabetes education. She was also shown how to adjust her insulin, based on her glucometer readings. She repeatedly came back to clinic with poor glycemic control and had never self-adjusted her insulin. Finally she admitted that she could not read numbers nor do the arithmetic required to adjust her insulin doses.

---

grant groups, there is every reason to believe that immigrants have higher rates of low health literacy than do US-born people. The impact on immigrants is likely greater as they often have fewer ways to access health information. Low health literacy, compounded by issues of culture, language, and education, means that communication with immigrants is complex. Written materials add more complexity rather than less.

## Term Definitions

Health literacy was defined above, but it is important to remember that in this context it implies more than just the ability to read; it also includes the ability to appropriately understand and act on information. A related term is numeracy, also called quantitative literacy. This is the ability to read and understand numbers and perform simple arithmetic. Examples of this include balancing a checkbook, reading a peak flow meter, or using an ATM machine (Box 56.2).

Literacy is also subdivided into components: prose literacy, the ability to locate information in a section of text; and document literacy, the ability to locate information on a form or in a graphic (e.g. a map). Health literacy at times is described as 'functional health literacy' which is simply a way to emphasize that literacy is more than just answering questions on a reading test; it is crucial to comprehending and navigating the modern world.

To function in the complex and multidimensional healthcare environment, one must possess a combination of individual-level attributes including abilities in prose, document, and quantitative literacy; ability to engage in two-way communication; skill in media literacy and computer literacy; motivation to receive health information and freedom from impairments and/or communicative assistance from others (surrogate reader).[12]

The Test of Functional Health Literacy in Adults (TOFHLA)[17] is a frequently used test of health literacy and numeracy. It categorizes patients into inadequate, marginal, or adequate health literacy. People who score in the inadequate range often misread dosing instructions on medicine bottles, appointment slips, and phone numbers. Those who score in the marginal range can do the above tasks, but struggle with other information on medicine bottles (i.e. take 2 hours after eating) and legal documents such as a Medicaid rights and responsibilities handout. Those in the highest category, adequate health literacy, may still have trouble with more complex documents such as informed consent and financial eligibility.[17]

Not only are the health literacy terms confusing, so too are the words that describe immigrants. Here the author will use the terms immigrants and foreign-born interchangeably. Limited English proficiency (LEP) typically refers to someone whose primary language is not English, and struggles some in English. ESL means English as a second language. ELL refers to English language learners. It is important to remember that there are many ESL and ELL people in the US who are not immigrants nor foreign born. Interestingly, according to the National Assessment of Literacy, if one is born in the US, but English is your second language, your literacy is likely to be the same as that of a US-born English speaker. This is also true of immigrants who arrive before age 12. This seems to be an effect of the US education system.[18] It is also important to remember that some immigrants come from English-speaking countries (Jamaica, India, Liberia) and are therefore not ESL or LEP. They still may struggle with health literacy, however.

Interpretation and translation are two more key terms for immigrants, but will largely be covered elsewhere in this book. Interpretation is the act of *verbally* conveying the meaning of words spoken in one language into another. Translation is doing the same with *written* text. These skills have much overlap, but also many differences, Interpretation must be done quickly, in real time, and often tries to convey both verbal and nonverbal communication (tone, body language, etc.). Translation can be edited and checked for accuracy in ways that interpretation cannot, such as translation and back translation.

## Health Literacy in Immigrants

There has been a rapid increase in the number of non-native English speakers in the US. In the 2000 census, nearly 18% of the US population reported speaking a language other than English at home, up from 14% in the 1990 census. Twenty-three percent of this group said they speak English not well or not at all. Over two-thirds of these non-native English speakers speak Spanish and the other 30% have an amazing variety of more than 300 languages. The census also reports that there are 31 million foreign-born in the US and that 47 million citizens and non-citizens speak a language other than English at home (Figs 56.1, 56.2, 56.3).[19]

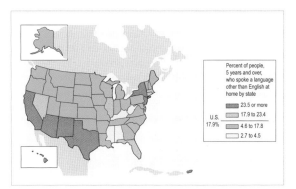

**Figure 56.1** Percentage of people 5 years and over who spoke a language other than English at home by state.

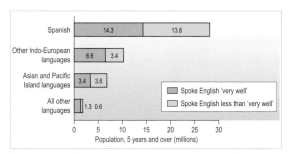

**Figure 56.2** Speakers of languages other than English at home and English ability by language group, 2000.

One question to raise with the Ecuadorian colonoscopy patient (see Box 56.1, above) is, 'Did they give him his instruction in English or Spanish?' This begs the question, when studying health literacy in immigrants, if we should look at their English health literacy, or literacy in their native tongue? The answer may depend on the context of care. If a healthcare environment is entirely in English with all English signs, all English forms, and all English prescription bottles, then English literacy must be what we care about. If, however, the healthcare environment is providing information in another language then we must address the immigrant's literacy in the native tongue.

Unfortunately, the answers to both of these questions are not as well studied as they could be. There is as of yet no validated health literacy questionnaire in any language other than English or Spanish. Also, in nearly all of the health literacy studies in the US, ESL patients have been excluded. This is due to an idiosyncrasy of the test. The REALM (Rapid Assessment of Adult Literacy in Medicine) is a valuable and widely used test. However, its scoring is based on how well someone can pronounce a list of words. Therefore, it has only been validated in native English speakers. It also cannot work in Spanish as Spanish is nearly entirely phonetic. The TOFHLA has a validated Spanish version with a number of studies of Spanish-speaking patients, but as yet none in other LEP populations.

Therefore, for the one in five US residents who don't speak English in their home, we have only partial data. The National Assessment of Adult Literacy (NALS) from 1993 is the best source of information for the foreign-born. In this US-wide survey of general literacy in immigrants and US-borns, questions were asked about education level, immigration history, language spoken at home, and self-reported literacy in English and a native tongue. Literacy in English and Spanish was measured, but

713

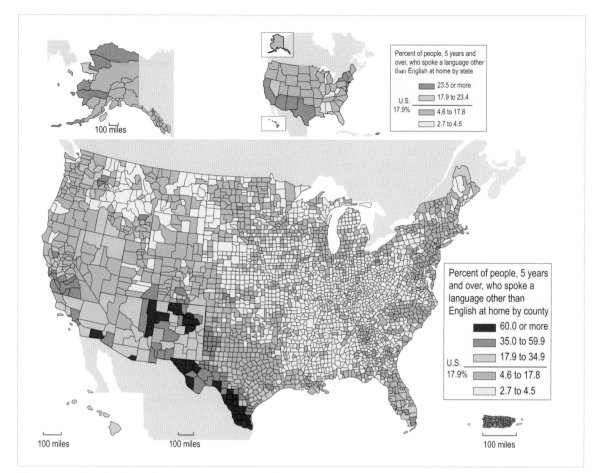

Figure 56.3 People who spoke a language other than English at home, 2000.

not literacy in other languages.[18] The survey was re-done in 2003 and renamed NAAL, National Assessment of Adult Literacy. To date there is only some analysis of ESL people in the updated survey. There were marginal improvements in most of the groups, but a slight decline in literacy in Spanish speakers. Their English-language literacy is shown in Figure 56.4.

From this point on the author will refer only to the 1993 NALS data, as there is much more analysis than for the later 2003 data. Overall, in NALS few people described themselves as illiterate; however, of those that did, most appeared to be ESL. 'When we defined literacy using people's self-assessment of their reading and writing skills, at least 95% of the non-literate population of the United States spoke a language other than English before starting school.'[18]

NALS has limited demographic breakdown for respondents, but these data showed that 6% of Hispanics report they are illiterate compared with 2% Asian/Pacific Islanders and 0% of whites or blacks. However, 16% of Asian/Pacific Islanders reported literacy only in their native tongue. In fact, 0% of the US-born respondents said that they are illiterate. The national estimates of illiteracy are much higher than this. It is unclear whether immigrants are more or less likely to accurately report illiteracy, but like the US-born, the foreign-born are likely to have much higher illiteracy rates than they self-report (Fig. 56.5).

Within the Hispanic group, there was variation by country of origin. Seven percent of Mexicans, 6% of Puerto Ricans and South and Central Americans, and 4% of Cubans reported they were illiterate in any language. Twenty-seven percent of Hispanics

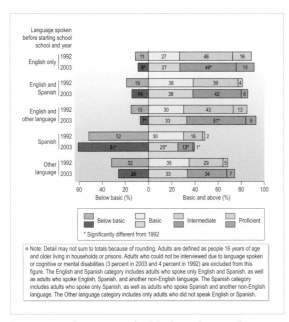

Figure 56.4 Percentage of adults in each prose literacy level, by language spoken before starting school, 1992 and 2003.

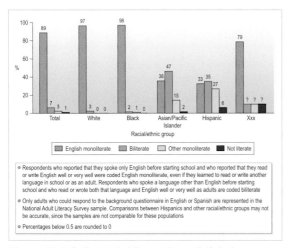

Figure 56.5 Self-reported literacy by racial/ethnic group.

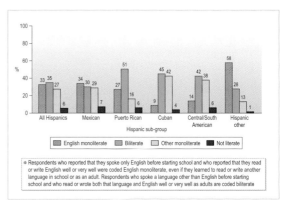

Figure 56.6 Self-reported literacy by Hispanic subgroup.

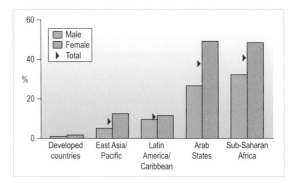

Figure 56.7 Adult literacy rate by gender, 2000.

reported they were literate only in Spanish and 42% of Cubans reported Spanish-only literacy (Fig. 56.6).

Overall, the strongest predictor of low literacy in immigrants is level of education attained. In fact, when adjusted for maximum education level, nearly all of the difference between US-born respondents and immigrants disappears. Around 70% of immigrants with less than 9 years of education scored in the lowest level of prose literacy when tested. Also, immigrants with a postsecondary education scored at equivalent literacy levels as non-immigrants and on some measures scored higher than US-borns. This is not a surprise, considering that many immigrants with post secondary training moved here for their training or started their education as young children in the US.

There are wide variations in educational attainment and literacy across the world. There are also likely differences between immigrant groups who choose to move and refugees whose lives and education have been disrupted. The UN reports literacy rates across countries. Figure 56.7 shows a sample of that information. Worldwide, men have higher literacy rates than women. There are wide differences between literacy rates, with a low of 10% to a high of nearly 100%. Therefore, it is difficult to make generalizations about immigrants.[20] However, Figure 56.8 points out some clear trends by region of the world. In many developing countries the average

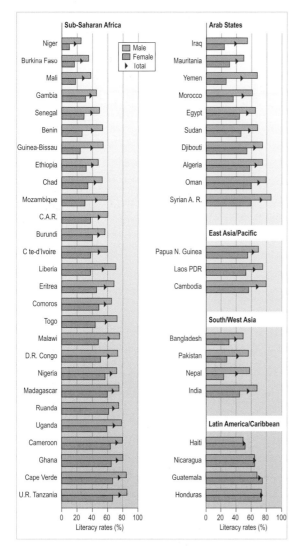

**Figure 56.8** World literacy rates by region and gender, 2000–2004.

The education effect also explains differences between immigrant groups. For example, Hispanics were less likely to speak, read, and write English, in part because Hispanic immigrants have, on average, less education than immigrants from non-Spanish-language countries.[18]

Education prior to arrival in the US is also strongly correlated with literacy attained here. The majority of immigrants who reported fluency and literacy only in their non-English native tongue completed less than 9 years of education prior to arrival in the US. Also, having little or no pre-immigration education is strongly associated with not being able to read or write in any language.[18]

Immigrants not only start with less education, but are also less likely to complete education in the US. US-born adults have higher levels of education attainment, are more likely to have completed high school, and are more likely to have attended some college.[18]

However, on average, immigrants and refugees have higher levels of education than those that stay at home. This is true for all countries that immigrants come from except Puerto Rico, where those that move to the mainland US tend to have lower rates of education. There is variation, however; immigrants from Asia tend to have much higher education rates than Asians that stay at home, while the difference is much less pronounced in Latin American and Caribbean immigrants.[21]

NALS also helps understand the interplay between language spoken at home and English literacy. English is not the primary language spoken in the homes of 41% of Hispanics, 34% of Koreans, 29% of Vietnamese, and 20% of Chinese.[18] Not surprisingly, there is a strong correlation with speaking some English while growing up at home and being literate in English as an adult. Regardless of the language at home, Spanish, Asian, or European, if the non-English language was the only one spoken in the house while a child, that child will have lower English literacy than those who grew up in a bilingual home.[18] However, not all bilingual backgrounds were the same. Those growing up in a bilingual home with English and an Asian or a European language had on average comparable English literacy skills to the English-speaking native-born. Those from bilingual Spanish and English homes tend to have lower English literacy than native English speakers.[18]

Being bilingual did not equate to being biliterate. The average score of self-reported biliterate immigrants placed them in level 2 literacy proficiency. English monoliterates averaged level 3 literacy pro-

female literacy rate is about 50% compared with rates in developed countries in the 90% range.

This education effect explains many of the differences found in the literacy testing. For example, if people immigrate to the US before the age of 12, they are likely to have a much higher level of literacy. In fact, there is no measurable difference in measured literacy between US-born adults and immigrants who arrived prior to age 12. This effect is likely due to greater exposure to the US education system and increased English fluency. These young arrivals are also more likely to complete high school than those who come to the US between the ages of 12 and 18.

ficiency.[18] This was true across all racial and ethnic designations, with black and Hispanic biliterates scoring the lowest.

There were also other striking differences between immigrant groups, most notably Hispanic versus non-Hispanic:

Hispanics were less likely than those from other ethnic groups to claim proficiency in spoken and written English. Hispanics were more likely to retain exclusive use of Spanish than were native speakers of other non-English languages. Hispanics were less likely to speak, read, and write English because Hispanic immigrants were less educated than immigrants from non-Spanish-language countries.[18]

The key findings from NALS that are important to immigrant health literacy are:

- Immigrants are much more likely to report being illiterate in any language than are US-born adults.
- Immigrants who came to the US after age 12 are likely have equal literacy to US-born adults.
- Immigrants who came to the US before age 12 are likely to have lower literacy in any language than US-born adults and be less likely to complete school (including high school, college, and ESL classes) while here.
- Immigrants who report less than 9 years of education are likely to have low levels of English literacy and also likely to report low literacy in their native language.
- Spanish-speaking immigrants from Latin America (Hispanics) are likely to have lower levels of English proficiency and literacy than other immigrants, are more likely to stay monolingual, and on average have less pre-immigration education than other immigrants.
- Children raised in a bilingual home will have higher levels of English literacy than those raised in a home where only the native language is spoken.

## Health Literacy and Medical Literature

In ESL patients whose primary language is other than Spanish, there is little direct study of health literacy. Lindau looked at English health literacy in non-native English speakers. Of 54 women 48% had below adequate health literacy at an urban Chicago site (compared with 38% in native English speakers).[22] As predicted by the NALS, 50% of women who had 9–12 years of education had inadequate literacy.

As there are only validated health literacy tests in English and Spanish, not speaking one of these languages fluently has been an exclusion criteria for nearly all of the health literacy research to date. To study English health literacy in ESL patients requires using the longer, more involved TOHFLA test rather than the shorter, more popular REALM, which relies on correct pronunciation to determine literacy levels. Therefore, this author will summarize the Spanish health literacy research, with the context from the NALS, that Hispanics are likely have lower literacy than other immigrant groups in part due to lower pre-immigration education. However, the mechanisms by which ESL Spanish patients struggle with getting health information are likely applicable to many other ESL populations.

In a 1995 landmark article by Mark Williams et al.[4] on health literacy, researchers interviewed 1892 English speaking and 767 Spanish-speaking patients at Grady Memorial Hospital in Atlanta and Harbor-UCLA Medical Center in Torrance, California, where 30% of the population is Latino. All of the Spanish-speaking patients were interviewed at the California site using the Spanish-TOFHLA. Questions included reading and comprehending a section of a Medicaid application, understanding prescription instructions, clinic appointment slips, and blood glucose test results. Overall, about 40% of the Spanish-speaking patients had the lowest level of health literacy (inadequate) with another 20% scoring marginal. Less than 40% of the Latinos had adequate health literacy in Spanish, compared with nearly 80% of the native English speakers studied in Los Angeles. (The native English speakers in Atlanta had only 50% adequate health literacy.) There was strong correlation with education level, but 20% of high school graduates had inadequate or marginal health literacy. Also, the differences between the English speakers and Spanish speakers disappeared when corrected for years of education. Older age also predicted worse health literacy. Seventy-one percent of Spanish-speaking patients over age 60 had inadequate literacy, as did 51% of the 18–30-year-olds. Interestingly there was minimal difference by socioeconomic status.

In the same study, screening questions were tested for validity, none of which performed very well. Asking if they could read a newspaper was 16% sensitive and 99% specific for inadequate health literacy.

Ability to read forms and written materials from the hospital was 20% sensitive and 99% specific. Responding that they have a surrogate reader was 51% sensitive and 88% specific. A sample of questions is enlightening. Thirty-one percent of Spanish-speaking patients could not describe when a follow-up appointment was scheduled after reading an appointment slip.

This study also helped put in context the case of the Ecuadorian patient scheduled for a colonoscopy from the beginning of this chapter. In this study, 33% of the Spanish speakers could not read well enough to understand an upper GI endoscopy prep. As a colonoscopy preparation is even more difficult, it is no wonder that some people come unprepped when only given written instructions. In one Minnesota hospital, the high fail rate and inadequate preparation for colonoscopy is dealt with by requiring a specific appointment for education with GI nursing staff prior to the actual procedure (Walker PF, personal communication).

Another study at San Francisco General on health literacy and diabetes control found similar results, with 70% of Spanish-speaking patients having marginal or inadequate health literacy. Overall, the study showed that patients with poor health literacy had worse glycemic control of their type 2 diabetes.[23]

Literacy level predicted how Hispanic women would respond to an abnormal Pap smear. Thirty percent of women with inadequate health literacy stated they would not seek medical attention for an abnormal result, compared with 19% of women with adequate literacy.[22] Not surprisingly, Hispanic women with low English proficiency are also less likely to get a Pap smear than those with high English proficiency.[24]

A few studies have included Spanish speakers in their overall analysis, but do not break down the rates of low literacy in Spanish speakers, or differentiate the associations by language or ethnicity. For example, one study of diabetic and hypertensive patients' knowledge of their disease showed less knowledge in patients with low health literacy about both chronic diseases.[7] Another showed more depressive symptoms in Medicare enrollees with low literacy.[25] Yet another looked to see if patients with low health literacy used more healthcare. It did not find such a correlation, but those with low health literacy did report poorer health. The Spanish-speaking patients at all literacy levels were less likely to be admitted to the hospital than were English-speaking patients.[26]

Work in California with Latino patients with HIV showed a strong relationship between level of education and ability to distinguish fact from myth in HIV and its treatment. Understanding prescriptions was associated with age and level of education.[27] This study also showed that high-quality provider communication (noting that all providers in these clinics were bilingual) was related to understanding of HIV terms but time on therapy and time since diagnosis were related to understanding of directions on prescription bottles.[27] This study tried to identify predictors of low health literacy in these patients. Interestingly, education outside of the US, level of acculturation, and Spanish language spoken at home did not predict lower levels of literacy regarding HIV knowledge in their study.

Patients went on to try a program to improve the specific health literacy in these patients (Es Por La Vida). The program consisted of 5 weeks of instruction in Spanish by a bilingual treatment advocate and nurse practitioner, followed by 6 months of nurse case-management. The instruction was to improve knowledge and skills, to build confidence in ability to follow a treatment regimen, and teach assertive communication skills to enhance interaction with physicians and nurses. The study found increased HIV knowledge (especially recognition and understanding of HIV terms) and decreased misperceptions. However, there was no difference in understanding prescription terms, adherence mastery, or adherence behaviors.[28]

## Factors Other than Literacy that May Affect Health or Healthcare of Immigrants

**Acculturation** This is the cultural learning that takes place when people come in contact with a new group, nation or culture. Level of acculturation has been shown to predict utilization of healthcare in the new country and likely affects an immigrant's ability to learn and comply with medical care.[29]

**Ethnicity** In one study at UCLA, Hispanics were twice as likely as non-Hispanic whites not to receive enough pain medicine for the same type of broken bones. Interestingly, Hispanic ethnicity was the only factor that statistically predicted this. The effect size of ethnicity was also much stronger than primary language or insurance status.[30]

**English language proficiency** Latinos with fair and poor English proficiency reported 22% fewer physician visits than non-Latino native-English speakers. This effect was as large as the one seen for having no health insurance or no usual source of care.[31] They are also less likely to get Pap smears or seek care for abnormal Pap smear results,[24] and less likely to have medication side effects explained.[32]

**Provider–patient language concordance** Spanish-speaking LEP patients who saw a bilingual physician had much higher recall of information from the encounter than did patients who saw an English-only-speaking doctor. Patients also asked more questions of the former doctor.[33] Latino patients with language-concordant providers reported better functioning on three overall health scales than did those seen by a provider who did not speak their language.[34]

## Translation and Literacy

The National Standards for Culturally and Linguistically Appropriate Services (CLAS), established by the US Department of Health and Human Services, states that 'healthcare organizations must make available easily understood patient-related materials . . . in the languages of commonly encountered groups . . .'[11] They further mandate that these materials must be culturally responsive and at appropriate literacy levels.

Translation and health literacy are separate but inextricably linked concepts. Translating written materials from English to another language is a more complex task than it appears at first glance. Many languages do not have the large number of words that English possesses. Norway, a country of around four million people, has a much smaller lexicon of words than we do in English, a language spoken by hundreds of millions of people. Norwegians call this 'ord fattig,' literally translated as 'word poor.' By extension, many English words simply do not have an equivalent in other languages. This can make translation out of English difficult and the resulting text often longer than the original English, as a paragraph may be needed in the other language where a word will do in English.

A related problem is one of false fluency. Anyone who has read English instructions for electronic equipment written in Asia can relate to the difference between a native speaker's writing style and that of a non-native speaker. The turn of phrase or the unintended secondary meaning can be funny at times, but at other times confusing or downright incorrect. Therefore, most experts advocate that materials translated into another language be at least edited if not translated by a native speaker of the language into which they are being translated.

The converse is also true; ESL patients assume they understand something because it looks familiar, when in fact it does not mean what they think it does. For example, a Spanish-speaking patients reads on a bottle 'take once daily' and interprets this to mean take eleven pills daily, as *once* is eleven in Spanish.

> Culture gives meaning to health communication. Health literacy must be understood and addressed in the context of culture and language.[11]

In health literacy, especially of immigrants, it is important to understand the interplay between culture and language. Cultures differ in styles of communication, in understanding of health and disease, and even in the meaning of words. Culture, or the shared ideas, meanings, and values of a group, is the context through which we all ascribe meaning to words. For example, the word 'cancer' conjures up in most of us a whole range of feelings, associations, and prior knowledge. We may think about death, chemotherapy, or uncontrolled cell replication. The Hmong language has no word for cancer. Traditional Hmong may not have a concept of the disease, let alone the same shared ideas we have in the US. Imagine translating a document advocating breast cancer screening into Hmong. How can all of the associated ideas and feelings about cancer be translated when the concept doesn't exist? How can the sense of importance of screening be conveyed?

Other examples are less dramatic, but show just how difficult this connection of language and culture can be. For example, to appropriately give their child 'one teaspoon' of medicine, immigrants must have experience with a teaspoon. Does their language have a word for teaspoon? Have they ever seen a teaspoon? Is it the same size as the US standard? Even if their language has a word for teaspoon, does it imply specific measurement as the word does to a native English speaker? An example from the author's experience is the Somali word for fever. The English-speaking healthcare providers give fever a specific meaning of high temperature. Our Somali colleagues tell us that fever has a more general meaning of 'not feeling well' in Somali. This has led to innumerable medical work-ups in Somali patients for infections that we may not have been suspicious of in native English speakers.

Providers are also constantly struggling with how to discuss mental health with Somali-speaking patients. There is only one mental health word commonly used in Somali, roughly translated as 'crazy.' This has a similarly negative cultural connotation as it does in English, making discussion of depression, anxiety, and post-traumatic stress disorder very difficult.

This is one area of health literacy in which native speakers of English from other countries may face the same issues as non-English-speaking immigrants. Medical information and instructions in English often assume a cultural context or knowledge of our system that an immigrant doesn't have. For example, many immigrants' prior experiences with healthcare have largely revolved around treatment for acute illnesses. When the provider suggests taking a medicine for high blood pressure, the patient, not having prior knowledge of hypertension, nor the cultural understanding that treatment is life-long medication, may take the medicine for a week or a month and assume the problem is solved.

## What Can be Done to Improve the Health and Healthcare of People with Low Literacy?

There are a number of studies of community-based interventions aimed at improving health literacy including a few in Spanish-speaking patients. One of these was a literacy training program for low-income Hispanic families in Chicago. Families were randomized to a 12-week dietary education intervention versus a standard nutrition pamphlet. Unfortunately, the study did not show a difference between families in the two groups.[35] Another study showed plays in Spanish with educational messages about health and safety to Hispanic farm workers. Not only did they like the plays, they also tested better on the health and safety knowledge than controls who did not see them.[36] The mixed results are not surprising, considering the number of complex issues of not just literacy, but culture, education and prior experience at play.

An appealing strategy is to make or translate material into easily readable patient handouts. Most English-language patient education material is supposed to be aimed at a sixth grade reading level, but is often written at a much higher level. The same appears to be true for translated documents or those written in other languages. Most studies that have looked at readability and comprehension of patient education materials written for specific ethnic groups have found these materials aimed at inappropriate reading levels.[37-42] Translated materials may also

inadequately address cultural issues and the subtleties of language differences.

To address these challenges, a group in Minnesota, the International Health Education Alliance (IHEA), has partnered with immigrant communities to jointly develop materials. Its mission is 'to assist underserved populations, especially immigrants and refugees; to identify and define, in culturally appropriate ways, their community's health needs in regard to chronic conditions; and to establish new education programs to address these needs.' This group works with many healthcare provider organizations and many cultural groups. It has become a developer and clearinghouse of patient education material and strategies in many languages. It has also worked to translate materials into many languages. Beyond just translation, it then went on to partner with leaders of immigrant communities and modified the education materials 'to fit the "culture" of each target group – culture here encompassing everything from a group's religious sanctions to esthetical preferences to even its conception of body and wellness' (visit: http://ihea.info/). A similar program by the Asian Health Services in Northern California has materials in first language as well as group education and health information (visit: http://www.ahschc.org).

Another Minnesota initiative is the Multilingual Health Resources Exchange, a collaborative of healthcare organizations, community groups, individuals and government agencies. The exchange maintains an index of health materials in many languages as a shared resource. Their website contains free guides to developing material in other languages and for other cultures. For members, or for a membership fee, users can have access to a large library of materials in many languages (visit: http://www.health-exchange.net).

There is federal money to help states with such programs. The federal government provides matching funds through the State Children's Health Insurance Program (SCHIP) and Medicaid for interpretation and translation. Nine states have so far obtained funds for these services: Hawaii, Idaho, Maine, Massachusetts, Minnesota, Montana, New Hampshire, Utah, and Washington.[43] These programs focus on translating material in a culturally appropriate way. None of them specifically deals with issues of literacy in languages other than English.

The AMA, as part of its health literacy materials, has some guidelines for making patient education materials appropriate for patients with limited literacy; although meant as English materials they likely apply to any language (Box 56.3). The AMA recommends four basic rules:[44]

## Formatting checklist for easy-to-read written materials

### General content

- Limit content to one or two key objectives. Don't provide too much information or try to cover everything at once.
- Limit content to what patients really need to know. Avoid information overload.
- Use only words that are well known to individuals without medical training.
- Make certain content is appropriate for age and culture of the target audience.

### Text construction

- Write at or below the 6th grade level.
- Use one- or two-syllable words.
- Use short paragraphs.
- Use active voice.
- Avoid all but the most simple tables and graphs. Clear explanations (legends) should be placed adjacent to each table or graph and also in the text.

### Fonts and typestyle

- Use large font (minimum 12 point) with serifs. (Serif text has the little horizontal lines that you see at the bottom and top of letters, as with this text.)
- Don't use more than two or three font styles on a page. Consistency in appearance is important.
- Use uppercase and lowercase text. ALL UPPERCASE TEXT IS HARD TO READ.

### Layout

- Ensure a good amount of empty space on the page. Don't clutter the page with text or pictures.
- Use headings and subheadings to separate blocks of text.
- Bulleted lists are preferable to blocks of text in paragraphs.
- Illustrations are useful if they depict common, easy-to-recognize objects.
- Images of people, places, and things should be age appropriate and culturally appropriate to the target audience. Avoid complex anatomical diagrams.

- Limit the depth and detail of the content.
- Minimize the complexity of the text itself.
- Use simple, easy- to-read formats.
- Test on the target reader audience (user testing.).

## What Can be Done at the Clinic or Provider Level?

Most importantly, providers need to be aware that limited health literacy can be a problem for patients. Physicians unfortunately are not good at estimating a patient's literacy. In one study in immigrants, physicians routinely overestimated patients' reading levels, and only correctly identified 26% of the inadequate readers.[22] Therefore, it is critical that clinics and hospitals develop a plan to address health literacy. Most experts don't recommend assessing each patient's literacy level and attempting to tailor a plan to that level. Rather, the 'universal design' strategy is best. This is a concept that makes the environment work best for all. Each clinic and hospital should have a plan in place for assessing patient education material and formatting it appropriately. It should also avoid forms, especially complex ones, as much as possible. Thirdly, there should be a policy of helping everyone with written materials. Again, the AMA has a list of suggestions (Box 56.4).[44]

Interventions aimed at those with limited health literacy are a fairly recent area of clinical research; therefore, there are not yet many data about which are effective. A recent review by Pignone, in the Institute of Medicine Report, examined the studies looking at approaches to health literacy.[11] In general, material that is written at a lower reading level with simplified illustrations has a modest effect on understanding. However, this effect is most dramatic and consistent in people at the highest reading levels. People at the lowest reading levels often don't improve their comprehension with simplified materials.[45,46]

Pictograms, pictures like those showing to take medicine with food on pharmacy bottles, do not fare much better. Patients with limited health literacy often have particular difficulty understanding pictograms.[47] People of all reading levels do fairly well with pictograms of simple concepts such as 'poison,' but everyone fares much worse with more complex concepts such as 'take on an empty stomach, 2 hours after or 1 hour before eating.'

Another strategy has been video or CD-ROM versions of educational materials. These too have produced mixed results. Simply transferring text versions of educational pamphlets into CD-ROM does not improve understanding among patients with limited health literacy.[48] Others have shown increased knowledge, but this increase occurred for all participants, regardless of level of health literacy.[49,50]

**Box 56.4**[51]

**Checklist for patient-friendly office procedures**

**Exhibit a general attitude of helpfulness**

**When scheduling appointments**
- Have a person, not a machine, answer the phone.
- Collect only necessary information.
- Give directions to the office.
- Help patients prepare for the visit. Ask them to bring in all their medications and a list of any questions they may have.

**Use clear and easy-to-follow signage**

**Ask staff to welcome patients with a general attitude of helpfulness**

**During office check-in procedures**
- Provide assistance with completing forms.
- Collect only essential information.
- Provide forms in patients' languages.
- Provide forms in an easy-to-read format.

**When referring patients for tests, procedures, or consultations**
- Review the instructions.
- Provide directions to the site of referral.
- Provide assistance with insurance issues.

**When providing patients with information**
- Routinely review important instructions.
- Provide handouts in an easy-to-read format.
- Use nonwritten modalities.

The simplest and most straightforward method for improving outcomes in patients with limited health literacy is an 'interactional' patient education strategy.[50,51] After introducing a new concept, recommendation, or change in therapy, the provider asks questions of the patient to test the patient's understanding. For example, if a provider says, 'I want you to increase your blood pressure medication to two pills a day,' the provider would then ask the patient, 'How many blood pressure pills should you take now?' or 'Show me how much of this medicine you will take.' It is not unusual for a patient to incorrectly recall or demonstrate what he or she is supposed to do. When this happens, the provider should clarify or repeat the information and again ask the patient to explain or demonstrate the teaching. Through such clarification, patients will be more likely to understand what is expected. When patients can recall and comprehend instructions, adherence improves.[51]

Another key resource is the AMA Foundations *Health Literacy Toolkit* available at http://www.ama-assn.org/ama/pub/category/9913.html This includes a video education tool for providers, as well as a free manual for clinicians. This manual is primarily focused on techniques to improve the care of patients with limited health literacy. Suggestions include to:

- Ask about health literacy in the social history portion of a patient assessment.
- Review medications, noting whether the patient remembers the medications by name or by color and shape.
- Routinely offer all patients help in filling out forms.
- Collect information in a patient's preferred language.
- Assure that written information is clear, simple, and reviewed verbally by the clinic staff.

They also suggest six steps to improve interpersonal communication:

- Slow down.
- Use plain, nonmedical language.
- Show or draw pictures.
- Limit the amount of information provided, and repeat it.
- Use the teach-back or show-me method.
- Create a shame-free environment.

## Conclusion

The goal is of healthcare is healthy patients. In the US, the model of care is patient self-management and lifestyle change to avoid disease and disability. This model presupposes that patients have the same understanding of disease and prevention that providers have. It also assumes that patients are not only consumers of healthcare, but also of healthcare information. Immigrants, especially those who speak a language other than English, may not have the same understanding or beliefs about health and disease. They may also have steep challenges as consumers of US health information. Health literacy is a model for understanding these challenges. By being conscious of our immigrant patients' health literacy issues, we can provide better, more patient-involved healthcare.

# References

1. Ratzan SC. Health literacy: communication for the public good. Health Promot Int 2001; 16(2):207–214.
2. Gazmararian JA, et al. Health literacy among Medicare enrollees in a managed care organization. JAMA 1999; 281(6):545–551.
3. Brownfield ED, et al. Direct-to-consumer drug advertisements on network television: an exploration of quantity, frequency, and placement. J Health Commun 2004; 9(6):491–497.
4. Williams MV, et al. Inadequate functional health literacy among patients at two public hospitals. JAMA 1995; 274(21):1677–1682.
5. Weiss BD, Palmer R. Relationship between healthcare costs and very low literacy skills in a medically needy and indigent Medicaid population. J Am Board Fam Pract 2004; 17(1):44–47.
6. Baker DW, et al. Functional health literacy and the risk of hospital admission among Medicare managed care enrollees. Am J Public Health 2002; 92(8):1278–1283.
7. Williams MV, et al. Relationship of functional health literacy to patients' knowledge of their chronic disease. A study of patients with hypertension and diabetes. Arch Intern Med 1998; 158(2):166–172.
8. Williams MV, et al. Inadequate literacy is a barrier to asthma knowledge and self-care. Chest 1998; 114(4):1008–1015.
9. Baker DW, et al. The relationship of patient reading ability to self-reported health and use of health services. Am J Public Health 1997; 87(6):1027–1030.
10. Smedley BD, Stith AY, Nelson AR. Unequal treatment: confronting racial and ethnic disparities in healthcare. The National Academies Press. Ref Type: Serial (Book,Monograph); 2003.
11. Institute of Medicine. Health Literacy. A prescription to end confusion. Nielsen-Bohlman L, Panzer MA, Kindig DA, eds. New York: National Academies Press; 2004.
12. Schwartzberg JG. Understanding health literacy: implications for medicine. VanGeest JB, Wang CC, eds. Am Med Assoc; 2003.
13. Garrett CR, Treichel CJ, Ohmans P. Barriers to healthcare for immigrants and non-immigrants: a comparative study. Minn Med 1998; 81(4):52–55.
14. Ngo-Metzger Q, et al. Linguistic and cultural barriers to care. J Gen Intern Med 2003; 18(1):44–52.
15. Flores G, et al. The importance of cultural and linguistic issues in the emergency care of children. Pediatr Emerg Care 2002; 18(4):271–284.
16. Kandula NR, Kersey M, Lurie N. Assuring the health of immigrants: what the leading health indicators tell us. Annu Rev Public Health 2004; 25:357–376.
17. Parker RM, et al. The test of functional health literacy in adults: a new instrument for measuring patients' literacy skills. J Gen Intern Med 1995; 10(10):537–541.
18. Greenberg E, Macias R, Rhodes D, et al. English literacy and language minorities in the United States, results from the National Adult Literacy Survey (NALS). US Department of Education, Office of Education Research and Improvement. Ref Type: Report; 2001.
19. Shin H, Bruno R. Language use and English-speaking ability: 2000. Census 2000 Brief. US Census Bureau. Ref Type: Report; 2003.
20. Unesco Global Literacy Statistics. UNESCO Institute for Statistics. Ref Type: Report; 2006.
21. Feliciano C. Educational selectivity in US immigration: how do immigrants compare to those left behind? Demography 2005; 42(1):131–152.
22. Lindau ST, et al. The association of health literacy with cervical cancer prevention knowledge and health behaviors in a multiethnic cohort of women. Am J Obstet Gynecol 2002; 186(5):938–943.
23. Schillinger D, et al. Closing the loop: physician communication with diabetic patients who have low health literacy. Arch Intern Med 2003; 163(1):83–90.
24. De Alba I, et al. Impact of English language proficiency on receipt of Pap smears among Hispanics. J Gen Intern Med 2004; 19(9):967–970.
25. Gazmararian J, et al. A multivariate analysis of factors associated with depression: evaluating the role of health literacy as a potential contributor. Arch Intern Med 2000; 160(21):3307–3314.
26. Baker DW, et al. Health literacy and the risk of hospital admission. J Gen Intern Med 1998; 13(12):791–798.
27. van Servellen G, et al. Health literacy in low-income Latino men and women receiving antiretroviral therapy in community-based treatment centers. AIDS Patient Care STDS 2003; 17(6):283–298.
28. van Servellen G, et al. Program to enhance health literacy and treatment adherence in low-income HIV-infected Latino men and women. AIDS Patient Care STDS 2003; 17(11):581–594.
29. Pachter LM, Weller SC. Acculturation and compliance with medical therapy. J Dev Behav Pediatr 1993; 14(3):163–168.
30. Todd KH, Samaroo N, Hoffman JR. Ethnicity as a risk factor for inadequate emergency department analgesia. JAMA 1993; 269(12):1537–1539.
31. Derose KP, Baker DW. Limited English proficiency and Latinos' use of physician services. Med Care Res Rev 2000; 57(1):76–91.
32. David RA, Rhee M. The impact of language as a barrier to effective healthcare in an underserved urban Hispanic community. Mt Sinai J Med 1998; 65(5–6):393–397.
33. Seijo R. Language as a communication barrier in medical care for Hispanic patients. In: Padilla A, ed. Hispanic psychology: critical issues in theory and research. Thousand Oaks,CA: Sage Publications; 1995.
34. Perez-Stable EJ, Napoles-Springer A, Miramontes JM. The effects of ethnicity and language on medical outcomes of patients with hypertension or diabetes. Med Care 1997; 35(12):1212–1219.
35. Fitzgibbon ML, et al. Involving parents in cancer risk reduction: a program for Hispanic American families. Health Psychol 1996; 15(6):413–422.
36. Elkind PD, Pitts K, Ybarra SL. Theater as a mechanism for increasing farm health and safety knowledge. Am J Ind Med 2002; Suppl 2:28–35.
37. Delp C, Jones J. Communicating information to patients: the use of cartoon illustrations to improve comprehension of instructions. Acad Emerg Med 1996; 3(3):264–270.
38. Jolly BT, et al. Functional illiteracy among emergency department patients: a preliminary study. Ann Emerg Med 1993; 22(3):573–578.
39. Jolly BT, Scott JL, Sanford SM. Simplification of emergency department discharge instructions improves patient comprehension. Ann Emerg Med 1995; 26(4):443–446.
40. Logan PD, et al. Patient understanding of emergency department discharge instructions. South Med J 1996; 89(8):770–774.
41. Powers RD. Emergency department patient literacy and the readability of patient-directed materials. Ann Emerg Med 1988; 17(2):124–126.
42. Spandorfer JM, et al. Comprehension of discharge instructions by patients in an urban emergency department. Ann Emerg Med 1995; 25(1):71–74.
43. Morse A. Language access: helping non-English speakers navigate health and human services. National Conference of State Legislature's Children's Policy Initiative. Ref Type: Report; 2003.
44. Weiss BD. Schwartzberg JG, et al., eds. Health literacy, a manual for clinicians. 2003: American Medical Association.
45. Davis TC, et al. Informed consent for clinical trials: a comparative study of standard versus simplified forms. J Natl Cancer Inst 1998; 90(9):668–674.
46. Eaton ML, Holloway RL. Patient comprehension of written drug information. Am J Hosp Pharm 1980; 37(2):240–243.

47. Price S, Raynor DK, Knapp P. Developing effective medicine pictograms for the UK. Health Serv Res Pharm Pract Ref Type: Abstract; 2003.

48. Kim SP, et al. Health literacy and shared decision making for prostate cancer patients with low socioeconomic status. Cancer Invest 2001; 19(7):684–691.

49. Wydra EW. The effectiveness of a self-care management interactive multimedia module. Oncol Nurs Forum 2001; 28(9):1399–1407.

50. Schillinger D, et al. Association of health literacy with diabetes outcomes. JAMA 2002; 288(4):475–482.

51. Ley P. Communicating with patients: improving communication, satisfaction, and compliance. New York: Croom Helm; 1988.

# CHAPTER 57

# Healthcare for Migrant Workers

Nancy Piper Jenks , Anne Kauffman Nolon,
and Allison Dubois

## Introduction

The delivery of healthcare to migrant workers in the USA presents a unique challenge to those caring for the population. This chapter will address a number of those challenges and give examples of best practices that have been shown to improve outcomes for migrants. The populations we are addressing are largely from Central and South America and have migrated to the USA to work, in order to support local family members as well as those that have remained in their native countries. The migrant workers described in this chapter include migrant and seasonal farmworkers and day laborers. The vulnerability of this population stems in part from the nature of their work, their method of arrival into the country, and their documentation status.

## Demographics and Trends

### Migratory patterns

The nation's immigrant population reached a new high of more than 35 million in 2005, accounting for 12.1% of the total population, the highest percentage in eight decades. If current trends continue, within a decade it will surpass the high of 14.7% reached in 1910.[1] The data also indicate that the first half of this decade has been the highest 5-year period of immigration in American history.[1]

Disparities in health, health insurance, and income for immigrants present barriers to both immigrants and healthcare professionals to obtaining and providing healthcare services. One-third of immigrants lack health insurance – two-and-one-half times the rate for natives. Immigrants and their US-born children account for almost three-fourths of the increase in the uninsured population since 1989. Reflecting low levels of coverage, workers and their families use very little healthcare compared to other low-income people. Immigrants may make significant economic progress the longer they live in the United States, but even immigrants who have lived in the United States for 15 years still have dramatically higher rates of poverty, lack of health insurance, and welfare use than natives.[1]

Immigrants are not evenly represented across the United States, with only a few states having the majority of the foreign-born population. More specifically, there are nearly 10 million immigrants in California, accounting for 28% of the nation's total immigrant population, followed by New York, Texas, Florida, and New Jersey. These five states account for 63% of the nation's total foreign-born population, but only 35% of the native-born population. States with the largest increase in immigrants are California, Texas, Georgia, New Jersey, Maryland, North Carolina, Pennsylvania, Washington, Virginia, Arizona, Tennessee, Minnesota, Nevada, New Mexico, South Carolina, and Mississippi.[1]

### Mexico–US migration and health

Mexican migration to the US has been part of the relationship between the two countries for more than a century. The US demand for workers and Mexico's inability to absorb workers into the workforce due to its own economy converge to create a rapid increase in the migratory flow and in the Mexican population residing in the US. Increased border security and pressure suggest an increasing undocumented population with even higher risks and costs associated with border crossings and integration into society. Unfortunately, this situation contributes significantly to limiting access to medical services and to increasing the health risks of migrants.[2]

Most workers who enter the country end up in jobs that require manual labor. The National Population Council of Mexico reports that even though the rate of employment for Mexican migrants is higher than US-born whites (71% versus 67%), these migrants are employed in lower paid manual jobs such as agriculture, landscaping, construction, office cleaning, food preparation, maintenance and repair, and production jobs that tend to have lower wages and no health insurance.[2]

Historically, the US has valued caring for the health needs of foreign-born workers during times of labor shortages such as World War II. This led to the recruitment of farm workers from Mexico, and later, from Puerto Rico and the British West Indies. During this era, the health needs of migrant farm workers were recognized, and met with clinics, housing, and sanitation, first by the Farm Security Administration and then by the War and Food Administration. At the end of the war, funding for these programs evaporated. The nation's attention turned to the peacetime priority of re-employing returning veterans. Although the health status of migrant farm workers received occasional attention from various agencies and committees through the years, no new broad national programs were initiated to replace the system of healthcare lost after World War II. Conditions deteriorated rapidly in the migrant streams following the discontinuation of the federal programs. Today, farm work remains one of the highest risk occupations with farm workers, and their suburban/urban counterpart, the day laborer, having little healthcare coverage and no Federal promise of support as in the past.

Good health is essential for a healthy workforce. In the twenty-first century, the flow of Mexican and other Latin American immigrants into the US requires that attention be given to the health and welfare of the migrant and the public health impact of the influx and assimilation of poorer, more mobile immigrants into US communities and into the workforce. Providing appropriate care for immigrants reflects the commitments and values to the immigrant workforce that were evident during World War II.

## Description of the Population

The higher incidence of poverty among immigrants as a group has significantly increased the overall size of the population living in poverty. Immigrants account for about one in six persons living in poverty. The data by country indicate that there is enormous variation in poverty rates among immigrants from different countries. For example, the 26% poverty rate for Mexicans is more than five times that of persons from Canada or the Philippines.[1] Perhaps the fastest growing segments of the new immigrant population in rural and suburban/urban areas are in two special populations. In rural communities, migrant and seasonal farm workers are immigrants and their families working in agriculture, migrating from Mexico and other Latin American countries to the US, and then state-to-state, at times staying in the area over a season (called 'seasoning over'). Entering more or less in the same manner from the same places, but moving to more suburban and urban areas, are day laborers. For the practitioner treating these special populations of immigrants, understanding of health practices in the migrants' home communities and barriers to healthcare they experience from living in the US, such as poverty, lack of health insurance coverage, and language and cultural differences, can help in guiding treatment planning, provider expectations of setting patient self-management goals, and follow-through and referral practices.

### Migrant and seasonal farm workers

Almost all migrant and seasonal farm workers are foreign born, with only 6% reporting being born in the United States. The majority (70%) remain in the United States and do not return to their country of origin. Although concentrated in certain areas of the country, migrant and seasonal farm workers reside in all states. They travel frequently between states for their employment. As a group, migrant and seasonal farm workers face significant language barriers. Approximately 90% say they read and speak little or no English. They are predominantly male (88%), over half are married, and over 40% have children. Even though migrant and seasonal farm workers report working 5–6 days a week, they are extremely poor. In 2000, the median income for migrant and seasonal farm workers was US$6250, compared to US$42 000 for US workers overall.[3] Migrant and seasonal farm workers and their families are overwhelmingly uninsured. In 2000, 85% of migrant and seasonal farm workers were uninsured, compared to 37% of low-income adults nationally. Further, nine in ten children in farm worker families were uninsured compared to less than a quarter (22%) of low-income children nationally.[3]

## Day laborers

There is a national system of day labor in the United States, encompassing men and women looking for employment in open-air markets by the side of the road, at busy intersections, in front of home improvement stores and in other public spaces. A recent report from the Center for the Study of Urban Poverty at the University of California at Los Angeles, analyzing data from the National Day Labor Survey, provides a portrait of day labor in the United States based on a national survey of 2660 day laborers. The study found that on any given day approximately 117 600 workers are either looking for day-labor jobs or working as day laborers. Seventy-five percent of the day laborer workforce are undocumented migrants. The dimensions of the day labor market are fluid; on a daily basis new workers enter this market while others leave it. Similarly, hiring sites diminish in size or disappear, while new ones emerge. The largest concentration of day laborers is in the West (42%), followed by the East, Southwest, South, and Midwest. Day laborers search for work in different types of hiring sites. Seventy-nine percent of hiring sites are informal, as described above, and are located near residential neighborhoods. One in five day laborers search for work at day labor worker centers. Nearly half of all day laborers are employed by homeowners/renters and 43% by construction contractors. Their top five occupations include construction laborer, gardener and landscaper, painter, roofer, and drywall installer.[4]

The vast majority of day laborers (83%) rely on day labor work as their sole source of income, with 70% searching for work five or more days a week. Three-quarters of day laborers have worked in this market for less than 3 years, suggesting that many make the transition into jobs in other sectors of the economy. Day labor pays poorly, with the median hourly wage approximately US$10. Even so, employment is unstable and insecure, resulting in annual earnings less than US$15 000, usually below the federal poverty threshold. Many day laborers support themselves and families through this work, with a significant number of day laborers married (36%) or living with a partner (7%); almost two-thirds (63%) have children. Twenty-eight percent of the children of day laborers are US citizens. The need for day laborers to earn an income, in most cases, is made all the more urgent by the responsibility to support their families.[4]

Day laborers regularly suffer abuse related to their employment. Almost half of all day laborers experienced at least one instance of wage theft in the 2 months prior to being surveyed. In addition, 44% were denied food/water or breaks while on the job. Workplace injuries are common, with one in five day laborers having suffered a work-related injury, and more than half of those who were injured in the past year did not receive medical care. More than two-thirds of injured day laborers have lost time from work.[4]

## Access to Health Care

### Cultural, language, and legal barriers

Cultural, linguistic, and legal characteristics of new immigrant populations present a multitude of barriers limiting the ease with which immigrants can enter and stay in the healthcare system; providers must engage the new immigrant in a linguistic and culturally sensitivity manner and be cognizant of the legal status of the individual to the extent that this status affects continuity of care, acceptance into referred health services, and insurance coverage.

Successful models must produce positive short-term outcomes while ultimately assimilating patients into a larger public healthcare system.[5] A 'culturally sensitive model' often demands language assistance or translations. As a result, patients require linguistic flexibility (often in the form of Spanish–English bilingualism), either with a bilingual healthcare provider or translation available through the medical team. In addition, many cases require an understanding of the cultural norms and the economic and political environment from which immigrant populations come.[6] This requires research and understanding of the identity of the individual being served. For example, reactions to conventional medical treatment may reflect the cultural taboos and practices of religious groups. An understanding of these beliefs and practices facilitates medical treatments in terms of scheduling appointments and phrasing explanations of treatments. On a more clinical level, certain pharmaceutical treatments may be less effective among certain Latin populations due to genetic and sociocultural factors.[7] This can be seen in the arena of mental health, where it is often difficult for this population to address clinical depression through psychotherapeutic and pharmaceutical interventions. In addition, one recent study in pharmacogenetics and asthma demonstrated different responses to asthma medications in Latinos with certain genetic backgrounds.[8]

Although Mexican immigrants may travel home frequently, many individuals from more distant countries, such as Ecuador and Guatemala, have neither resources nor the will to repeat the long journey from their respective countries. 'Andando por la pampa' (walking the plains) means years of separation from family and home and expresses the sense of vast distance and isolation of the migrant who does not have the ability to travel back and forth on a yearly basis.[9] This also takes a toll on medical outcomes. Because of these disparities of outlook and culture, providers must assist the Latin community one by one, as individuals, taking into consideration the uniqueness of each particular situation.

## Lack of insurance

Table 57.1 reports the percentage of immigrants and natives who were uninsured for all of 2004. The table shows that lack of health insurance is a significant problem for immigrants from many different countries. Overall, 33.7% of the foreign-born population lack insurance compared to 13.3% of natives. Immigrants now account for 26% of the uninsured. The lower portion of the table reports the percentage and number of immigrants and the US-born children (under 18) of immigrant mothers who are uninsured. In 2005, 29.3% of immigrants and their minor children were uninsured. In total, the 13.6 million uninsured immigrants and their children account for 30% of the uninsured, nearly double their 15.9% of the overall population.[1]

Because of the limited value of their labor in an economy that increasingly demands educated workers, many immigrants hold jobs that do not offer health insurance, and their low incomes make it very difficult for them to purchase insurance on their own. The 2005 Center for Immigration Studies reports that nearly 47% of immigrants and their

**Table 57.1 Immigrants without health insurance**

| Country | Number uninsured (in thousands) | Percentage uninsured |
|---|---|---|
| Guatemala | 316 | 58.0 % |
| México | 5812 | 53.8 % |
| Honduras | 191 | 50.4 % |
| El Salvador | 507 | 45.2 % |
| Ecuador | 151 | 44.5 % |
| Haití | 243 | 42.6 % |
| Brazil | 139 | 39.2 % |
| Peru | 122 | 37.0 % |
| Colombia | 149 | 31.1 % |
| Dominican Republic | 212 | 30.5 % |
| Cuba | 243 | 25.6 % |
| Jamaica | 154 | 25.4 % |
| Poland | 126 | 24.2 % |
| Vietnam | 240 | 24.1 % |
| Korea | 149 | 22.1 % |
| China | 397 | 21.7 % |
| Iran | 56 | 16.9 % |
| India | 232 | 16.4 % |
| Russia | 89 | 14.3% |
| Philippines | 211 | 13.8 % |
| Italy | 42 | 10.7 % |
| Great Britain | 55 | 9.3 % |
| Japan | 32 | 9.1 % |
| Canada | 55 | 8.2 % |
| Germany | 25 | 4.8 % |
| All Immigrants | 11 858 | 33.7 % |
| All Natives | 33 191 | 13.3 % |
| Children (under 18) of immigrant mothers[1] | 2849 | 19.6 % |
| Children (under 18) of native mothers[2] | 5420 | 9.1 % |
| Immigrants and their US-born children[1] | 13 629 | 29.3 % |
| Natives and their children[2] | 32 191 | 13.2 % |
| Immigrants and their US-born children uninsured or on Medicaid[1] | 21 639 | 46.7 % |
| Natives and their children uninsured or on Medicaid[2] | 61 639 | 25.2 % |

Source: Center for Immigration Studies analysis of March 2005 Current Population Survey.
[1] Includes all children of immigrant mothers under age 18, including those born in the US.
[2] Including the children of native mothers under 18. The US- born children of immigrant mothers are not included.

children either have no insurance or have it provided to them through Medicaid.[3]

# Health Issues of the Migrant

In 2000, only 20% of migrant and seasonal farm workers reported using any healthcare services in the preceding 2 years. Further, one study found that only 42% of women in farm worker families reported seeking early prenatal care compared to over three-quarters (76%) nationally. Data show a nearly one in four incidence of undesirable birth outcomes and elevated rates of low birth weights and preterm births among this population.[10-12]

The low utilization patterns among farm workers and migrants are not a reflection of limited healthcare needs. Many migrants are often in poor health and they are at elevated risk for an enormous range of injuries and illnesses due to the nature of their jobs. The two most significant reported barriers to care among migrants are cost and language.

## Health issues among new arrivals

Undocumented migrants who come into the country overland often experience arduous and traumatic journeys. Travel from their countries of origin to their destination cities in the USA can take many weeks. Individuals may endure such things as heat exhaustion, lack of adequate and safe food and water, vehicular accidents due to unsafe modes of transportation, effects of overcrowded and inadequate lodging, rape, and other exposure to violence. When migrants reach their points of destination there can be both physical and psychological health outcomes associated with their difficult journey that are often not adequately addressed due to lack of access to professional healthcare. When migrants are able to access care shortly after arrival, musculoskeletal problems such as broken bones, joint problems, and muscle sprains are not uncommon. Gastrointestinal infections from the journey often include acute and chronic diarrhea from, for example, helminth infections, amoebiasis, and enteric bacteria. Sexually transmitted diseases in women who have been victims of rape have been diagnosed, as well as unplanned pregnancies. Migrants may also suffer from skin infections such as fungal infections, scabies, and contact dermatitis contracted during their trip. General fatigue and weight loss are also problems among those who have been traveling for weeks or months to get to their destination.

# Health concerns of agricultural workers

There is much research to substantiate the fact that workers in the agriculture industry are at high risk of death and injury.[10-12] The National Institute for Occupational Safety and Health ranks agriculture among the most hazardous industries. Farm workers are at high risk for fatal and nonfatal injuries, work-related lung disease, noise-induced hearing loss, skin diseases, and certain cancers associated with chemical use and prolonged sun exposure.[10-12]

Production agriculture, a segment of the agriculture industry, is the sector which commonly represents farming. Production agriculture has been shown to have higher rates of fatalities than the agriculture industry as a whole.[13,14] Studies have shown young workers in agriculture to incur more serious injuries and a greater proportion of injury than the general young worker population.[15-18] Reasons for the higher rates have been suggested as being inexperienced in the job/work method, a more hazardous work environment, and risk-taking behavior due to a feeling of invincibility by young workers.[19,20]

Although agricultural crop and livestock production constitutes only 2% of the workforce, from 1994 to 1999 it represented 13% of all occupational deaths.[21] It is among the most dangerous occupations in the nation.[22] In 2001, for every 100 000 agricultural workers in the US there were 22.8 deaths for a total of 228 occupational deaths in agriculture. This compares to a rate of 4.3 deaths for every 100 000 workers in the total US workforce during this same period.[23] Injuries are not limited to adults. Child labor laws differ from state to state and many children work in the fields, sometimes alone, other times accompanied by parents. In Agricultural Safety Information published by NIOSH in 2001, it was reported that an average of 103 children are killed annually working on farms (1990–1996).[24] Every day, about 500 agricultural workers suffer lost-worktime injuries, and about 5% of these result in permanent impairment.[24] In a study of 287 migrant workers, 25 had reported an injury in the previous 3 years. Of these, 17 considered medical attention necessary. Forty-one percent of the injured workers did not receive medical attention within 24 hours, and 24% received no attention at all.[25] Another study found sprains and strains to be the most common occupational injury, constituting 43% of agricultural injuries. Fieldwork was the activity most commonly associated (39%) with injury.[22]

## Musculoskeletal

Musculoskeletal injuries are inherent to agricultural labor. Harvesting requires heavy and repetitive lifting and quick wrist and hand movements, and the piece-rate wage system encourages a rapid work pace. Such ergonomic conditions lend themselves to back and muscle pain. 'In 1996, 34% of lost-time injuries were sprains and strains and 24% were back injuries.'[22]

## Respiratory illness

Agricultural work exposes laborers to pesticides, dust, plant pollen, molds, and other respiratory irritants. Prolonged exposure can lead to chronic respiratory illness.[21] Obstructive lung disease has been linked to livestock and grain work, and asthma, hypersensitivity pneumonitis, and other respiratory problems have been linked to organic dusts.[22]

## Skin disorders

Skin disorders are common in agricultural workers, who have the highest incidence of skin disorders of all industrial classifications. In 1996, the incidence rate for all agricultural production workers was 27.6 per 10 000 workers, climbing to 28.1 per 10 000 workers for crop production. Comparatively, the rate was 6.9 per 10 000 workers for all private industry.[22] A 1991 study published by the Migrant Clinicians Network concluded that dermatitis was the primary cause for clinic visits for males ages 20–29. Dermatitis was 150% more likely in the migrant group than in the general population.[26]

## Eye injury

Farm workers are exposed to potential eye irritants, including dust, pollen, and chemicals, as they work. Untreated chronic eye problems can lead to serious damage; tree branches and accidents with agricultural tools can cause abrasions.[21] Eye problems caused by exposure to chemicals, pesticides, dusts, and plant materials are common in agricultural workers.[27] In 1996, eye injury rates in agricultural employees were 14.2 per 10 000 workers, representing 4.8% of all lost-workday injuries.[22]

## Pesticide exposure

Pesticide exposure is the cause of a variety of occupational illnesses, including eye injuries, cancer, respiratory illnesses, and dermatitis. Between 1982 and 1993, California averaged 1500 reports of pesticide exposure each year. Forty-one percent of these exposures occurred in agricultural workers.[22] Despite improvements in the enforcement of the Worker Protection Standard, many workers have not received training in pesticide application.[21] Between 1992 and 1996, nearly one-fifth of all hired crop workers had mixed or applied pesticides. Only 50% of these received training, and only 79% were able to read English well.[22] 'The result is that agricultural workers are often ill prepared to protect themselves from the potentially hazardous chemicals found around them.'[22] High air temperatures and humidity put agricultural workers at special risk of heat stress. Pesticide workers and early-entry workers are at particularly great risk. The special clothing and equipment worn for protection from exposure to pesticides can restrict the evaporation of sweat, block the body's natural way of cooling itself, and result in increased body temperature. Exposure to certain pesticides can also produce sweating, and there can be combined effects with exposure to heat. In addition, pesticides are absorbed through hot, sweaty skin more quickly than through cool skin.[21] Although high cancer incidence rates indicate a link between cancer and agricultural labor, the migrant lifestyle has made conclusive studies difficult.[21] Finally, exposure to pesticides is a common cause of eye injuries. 'About 25% of Californian reports of pesticide effects involve the eye.'[21]

## Infectious diseases

Infectious diseases have been found to be associated with agricultural employment. Such diseases are often due to poor sanitation at work and home sites, including inadequate washing and drinking water.[21] In the 2000 National Agricultural Workers Survey (NAWS) 15% of farm workers reported having no access to water for washing, while 16% had no access to toilets in the fields.[28] In an examination of 27 North Carolina labor camp water supplies, 44% tested positive for coliform contamination. A study in Utah 'found that workers on farms without sanitation facilities had a clinic utilization rate for diarrhea 20 times higher than that of the urban poor.'[22] Urinary tract infections are common among migrant farm workers due to the lack of toilet facilities; they are particularly prevalent among women because their shorter urethra allows bacteria easy access to the bladder. These infections during pregnancy may contribute to miscarriages, fetal or neonatal deaths, and premature delivery.[22] In one study, 28% of migrants surveyed had some form of parasitic infection. It is estimated that this rate is anywhere from 11 to 59 times higher than the rate of parasitic infection in the general population of the United States.[22] In one study, 28% of a California farm worker community lived in 'back houses' – sheds, garages, and shacks. Such poor, crowded living conditions are conducive to the spread of infectious diseases, particularly tuberculosis. A Centers for Disease Control and Prevention (CDC) study suggests that farm workers are six times more likely to become infected with tuberculosis than the general population.[22]

**Tuberculosis among migrants** There were a total of 14 093 tuberculosis (TB) cases reported in the United States for 2005. Although this is the lowest TB rate since national reporting began in 1953, the decline has slowed. In 2005, foreign-born persons in the USA had a TB rate that was 8.7 times that of a US-born person. Twenty states in the US had more cases in 2005 than 2004, including California, Florida, New York, and Texas. The proportion of cases contributed by foreign-born persons has increased each year since 1993. For the second consecutive year, more TB cases were reported among Hispanics than any other racial/ethnic population.

The CDC has recommended, among several strategies, the testing of recent arrivals from high-incidence countries for latent TB infection and treating them to completion.[29]

In adult immigrants, the first 5 years after immigration carry the highest risk for developing active TB.[30] Identifying active TB in this population can be difficult. Many migrants from high-risk countries do not migrate with symptomatic TB. They may, however, come to the US with latent TB infection (LTBI). Active TB may develop at a later date, with an increased risk among those who develop other chronic diseases. The population with LTBI may serve as an ongoing reservoir for active TB cases. Neither the CDC nor other public health departments maintains a national registry of reported cases of LTBI.

Undocumented migrants who enter the US are not screened for TB. Among 1255 undocumented migrants who attended a weekly evening clinic (Casa de Salud) at Hudson River HealthCare, a community health center in Westchester, NY, from 2001 to 2005, 1.5% were diagnosed with active TB, both pulmonary and extrapulmonary. Twenty-eight percent of those with active TB had arrived in the USA within 6 months of their diagnosis.[31] These cases of active TB cases were reported to the local health department, who organized treatment and screened contacts.

Migrants with symptomatic TB may delay seeking treatment due to lack of access to outpatient care; or, if TB is suspected, they may fear deportation if they are aware of the local health department's involvement with active cases. Delay in treatment has obvious public health consequences, particularly in communities where large numbers of new immigrants are living in crowded housing conditions.

Undocumented migrants who present to Hudson River HealthCare are not routinely screened for TB. Those who are screened with tuberculin skin tests (TSTs) and who test positive are often unable to follow up with the recommended chest X-ray and treatment regime due to issues such as cost barriers, misunderstanding of infection and treatment, and lack of follow-up. Effective TB control and prevention will require sufficient resources and collaborative measures to reduce the burden of disease among this population.

**Infectious disease risk in their new environment: the case of Lyme disease** The migrant population does not have the benefit of pre-trip counseling regarding infectious disease risks they face in their new environment. Lyme disease is the most common vector-borne disease in the United States. A recent study examined the awareness of this infection among migrant workers from Central and South America who had recently moved to an area of New York State where Lyme disease is endemic. The study demonstrated that 80 migrants who had come into the country within the past 4 years were neither familiar with signs and symptoms of Lyme disease nor were aware of how this infection is transmitted. Moreover, the majority of those individuals polled in this study worked as landscapers or in construction, placing them at an even higher risk for Lyme disease than others in the community.[32] This study demonstrated that a short educational intervention was effective in teaching the recognition of Lyme disease as well as strategies to avoid infection.

## Health screening and prevention

The utilization of health services for various health screening tests is lower among immigrants. A number of barriers to, for example, cancer screening, has been demonstrated, including low income or educational level and lack of health insurance.[33] Other barriers related to culture, knowledge, and attitudes as well as low English proficiency have also been shown to play a role.[34,35] Health literacy (defined as the degree to which individuals have the capability to process and understand basic health information and services needed to make appropriate decisions) has been shown to affect rates of cancer screening.[36] In addition, immigrants may find it difficult to navigate healthcare systems. Undocumented immigrants may be disproportionately affected by these barriers in comparison to those immigrants who have become US citizens.[33] A recent study found that not being a US citizen is a barrier to receiving cervical and breast cancer screening among immigrants in California. When the data were adjusted for sociodemographics, access to care, proficiency in language, undocumented immigrants were less likely to receive cervical or breast cancer screening as compared to immigrants who were US citizens.[33]

In addition to screening for breast and cervical cancers, according to data from the National Health Interview Survey (NHIS) recent immigrants have the lowest rates of screening for colorectal and prostate cancers.[37]

Another area of prevention which is often overlooked is routine vaccination. Without health screening prior to a migrant's arrival in the US, immunity to diseases such as measles, mumps, rubella, and varicella is not routinely assessed. Immunizations are not given prior to arrival into this country and it is likely that similar barriers to receiving vaccines as seen with cancer screening exist among this population. Susceptibility to some vaccine-preventable infections has been shown to be higher among immigrants.[38] One study looking at vaccine rates during an outbreak of rubella at a meat-packing factory found that all 83 cases were in the unvaccinated, 83% of whom were born in Latin American countries.[39]

Preventive services are not generally accessed among the migrants and screening for health problems such as high cholesterol, diabetes and depression are not routinely performed. This lack of prevention among the population undoubtedly impacts on overall morbidity and mortality.

## Primary care: the Hudson River HealthCare Experience

Reasons for migrants to seek medical care in an outpatient setting may be due to symptomatic acute or chronic health problems. A study of 1255 undocumented migrants presenting to Hudson River HealthCare's weekly session for migrants between 2001 and 2005 demonstrated that most migrants

**Table 57.2 The most frequent diagnoses of recent arrivals presenting for care**

| Condition | Percentage (%) |
|---|---|
| Positive PPD | 12 |
| Acute respiratory infection | 5 |
| Depression | 5 |
| Back pain | 5 |
| Skin conditions | 4 |
| Gastritis (+ *Helicobacter pylori*) | 4 |
| Hypertension | 3 |
| Diabetes | 3 |
| Fractures/sprains/lacerations | 3 |
| Sexually transmitted infections | 3 |
| Acute gastritis | 2 |
| Fungal dermatitis | 2 |
| Pyodermas | 2 |
| Headache | 2 |
| Pregnancy | 2 |
| Anemia | 2 |
| Active TB | 1.5 |
| Violence exposure | 1 |
| Heart disease | 1 |
| Urinary tract infection | 1 |
| Thyroid disease | 1 |
| Cancer | 1 |

sought care when symptoms were interfering with their daily lives. Table 57.2 lists the most frequent diagnoses of recent arrivals presenting for care.[31]

As mentioned above, undocumented migrants are not routinely screened for tuberculosis. Those who are screened include contacts of individuals with active TB, women who enroll in prenatal care, workers who are required to be tested for pre-employment and students enrolling in school.

The prevalence of depression in this population is significant. In the data shown here, depression was among the second most commonly diagnosed problems. There is clearly an under-recognition of this problem, perhaps related to cultural and language barriers, health literacy barriers, and somatic presentations. New arrivals commonly suffer from a post-traumatic stress disorder as a result of their arduous overland journey. Undocumented status can add to the difficulty of cultural adaptation, as do language barriers. Migrants may come into the US owing large sums of money to individuals who helped them over the border. This additional stress of financial obligations adds to their initial anxiety and depression. The psychological impact of separation from family members left behind in their countries of origin has been documented.[40] Women frequently leave their children behind with family members. These women can experience significant depression as a result of separation from their children.[41]

When depression has been diagnosed, treatment options are often limited. Although migrants may well benefit from counseling and/or pharmacotherapy, treatment adherence is often met with financial barriers and inability to set aside nonworking hours to therapy sessions.

Those with chronic problems such as diabetes and hypertension often present at a time when symptoms are interfering with their daily lives. In the case of diabetes, it is not uncommon to see migrants coming in with blood glucose well above normal. At Hudson River HealthCare, glycosylated hemoglobins (A1c) are measured and tracked on all diabetic patients and among the undocumented migrant population average A1cs are significantly higher than in other diabetics. For type 2 diabetics, oral medication is the mainstay of treatment and regimes need to be adhered to in order to control glucose levels. These medications are expensive and are often taken until symptoms are relieved or until the medication runs out. Diabetics may then wait to return for care when symptoms are again intolerable.

Blood pressure is routinely screened at all visits and hypertension is among the top ten diagnoses. Often asymptomatic, patients may not understand the importance of treatment and do not adhere to medication recommendations. Other cardiovascular risks include hyperlipidemia, which is not routinely screened for. For those diagnosed with high cholesterol, there is again difficulty in maintaining adherence to medical regimes due to costs and understanding the importance of lowering lipids.

## Models That Work

### Community/migrant health centers

Federally Qualified Health Centers are nonprofit, consumer-directed healthcare corporations that provide comprehensive primary and preventive healthcare services and either (1) receive grants under the US Public Health Service Act or (2) do not receive federal PHSA grants, but meet the standards for funding. To receive federal funding, a community health center must:

- Be located in a federally designated medically underserved area (MUA) or serve a federally designated medically underserved population (MUP).
- Have nonprofit, public, or tax exempt status.
- Provide comprehensive primary healthcare services, referrals, and other services needed to facilitate access to care, such as case management, translation, and transportation.
- Have a governing board, the majority of whose members are patients of the health center.
- Provide services to all in the service area regardless of ability to pay and offer a sliding fee schedule that adjusts according to family income.

Unique to community and migrant health centers (C/MHCs) is the federal mandate that over 50% of the Board of Directors must be consumers of the service. For this reason, patients are engaged in guiding the community/migrant health center in its mission of improving the health status of farm workers and in increasing access to healthcare services. Community/migrant health centers have learned to overcome the barriers that separate recent immigrants from healthcare by using creative programs. Health centers often take services to their patients rather than waiting for the patients to come to them. Outreach programs in the community and labor camps provide education and disease screening. Clinic visits may be facilitated by clinic vans for those who have no means of transportation. Bilingual staff care for non-English-speaking patients. In order to bridge the cultural gap, new immigrants and farm workers are recruited to work as health aides in the migrant labor camps.

### Comite Latino and Casa de Salud outreach programs: a community health center approach to culturally competent care

Many patients require not only the primary and preventative healthcare provided on-site by a community/migrant health center but also other medical services in the region. This often includes referrals, billing management, and transportation. As a community/migrant health center committed to serving its new immigrant populations, Hudson River HealthCare created the Comite Latino and the Casa de Salud programs.

Although Hudson River HealthCare is a community health center focusing on provision of primary healthcare, many new immigrant patients require additional social services. In order to address their medical issues adequately, the health center must make the effort to treat the 'total' person. Many psychological stressors (i.e. occupational, legal, housing, economic, etc.) lead to mental health conditions such as anxiety, depression, and alcohol abuse. Addressing social needs, therefore, not only treats specific problems but also serves as a form of early intervention and preventive healthcare. The Comite Latino is the mechanism by which the health center provides a number of social services.

The Comite Latino is the community service arm of the health center created to assist patients with the negotiation of the healthcare arena, including accessing community health centers, assistance with hospital bills, making appointments, and other medical case management needs. Comite Latino community health workers also help in completing medical insurance forms (for example, Medicaid and Child Health Insurance Programs that new immigrants are eligible to receive) and, in some cases emergency Medicaid, as it is needed.

The Casa de Salud program is a completely bilingual clinic within the community health center. All services and staff are bilingual and additional services that support new immigrant access to healthcare services are provided on site. The Comite Latino is closely integrated with the Casa de Salud program and community health workers can make appointments for Casa de Salud and assist patients with the completion of clinical history forms. Some patients (and also healthcare workers) require translation assistance during patient appointments, and the community health workers from the Comite Latino provide these services.

In addition to the on-site services, outreach and blood pressure screenings are performed at 'La Parada' (the site where day laborers congregate to look for work). These community-based services facilitate the integration of new immigrants into the healthcare system. Finally, in an effort to forestall serious yet preventable conditions, Comite Latino provides educational seminars on themes significant to the Latin populations, such as sexual health, Lyme disease, and workplace safety in community-based settings at the community health center.

The Comite Latino has identified key elements in the Hispanic culture that should be recognized in order to maximize healthcare:

- *La familia*: Family involvement is often critical in healthcare, and when ill or injured, many Hispanics frequently consult with other family members and ask them to come along to medical visits. Including family members in the consultation is often critical to the care of the patient.
- *Respeto*: As a mutual and reciprocal sense of respect is important, healthcare personnel and officials are often afforded great respect. However, many patients may avoid disagreeing with or expressing doubts to a healthcare provider or be reluctant to ask questions or reveal confusion about medical care.
- *Personalismo*: Interpersonal relationships are important, and are the basis for the community-based initiatives and centers for primary care. Health providers are expected to be warm and personal. It may be hard to establish a personalized relationship in managed care, and if a health professional that a patient has come to trust is suddenly unavailable they may stop treatment all together.
- *Confianza*: Time spent with healthcare providers is often highly valued, and great trust is instilled in those who help with treatment.
- *Espiritu*: Hispanic culture tends to view health from a synergistic point of view, incorporating body, mind, and spirit. Within the Hispanic community there is an extensive system of traditional medicine. Many Hispanics will combine traditional medicine with other approaches, and it is important to consider use of these products and discuss them in a nonjudgmental way.[42]

## Patient care partner program

The Hudson River HealthCare network of community health centers also utilizes a patient care partner (PCP) program to provide a bridge from the community-based outreach encounter to the medical provider and to help maintain ongoing care management for patients. Once recruited and hired, the PCP undergoes an extensive orientation process, and receives any necessary additional training, such as cultural competency, medical interpretation, and data management. The PCP acts as the patient's navigator through the healthcare system, and:

- ensures that the patient understands provider recommendations and prescription instructions;
- provides health education and nutrition counseling, as well as language-appropriate health and wellness information and materials;
- works with patient and provider to develop a self-management plan for chronic conditions, and track and monitor the patient's progress towards goals, taking into consideration migratory patterns;
- facilitates access to discount prescription medication programs, helping patients to access free or low-cost medications;
- monitors and manages the information generated from the patient's electronic medical record (EMR, Cliniflow®) and from other clinical information systems;
- conducts patient screening to assess risk for depression;
- ensures availability of appropriate health and wellness materials and health education and information on topics relevant to the populations served; and
- conducts other activities to ensure patients are active participants in their health maintenance.

The patient care partner program at Hudson River HealthCare (HRHCare) has resulted in improvements to care coordination and management, and it is anticipated that these improvements will result in improved health outcomes. Outcomes to date include:

- Ninety percent of patients that work with the care partner access prescription medications through manufacturer and federal discount programs.
- All patients in the target community have been screened for depression and linked to mental health services.
- All patients have documentation of smoking status in their medical record and referrals to smoking cessation programs.
- Significant increases in the number of patients with diabetes that have had two HbA1cs in the past 12 months.

## Hospital-based community care partner

The patient care partner program has been further expanded to local emergency rooms to identify patients without a medical home. Local hospital emergency rooms are often utilized as a source of medical care for many new immigrants who are not familiar with outpatient services at, for example, community health centers. The patient care partner acts as a liaison for the community health center and helps links the emergency room patient to primary care. If migrants with nonemergency problems present to the emergency room, the PCP can introduce them to outpatient services, which are less costly and more comprehensive. The care partner is able to set up follow-up appointments for these migrants for primary care services. When ER patients were able to meet with a patient care partner, 85% had a medical appointment in a primary care setting within 3 months of the ER visit. Patients who did not meet with patient care partners had primary care visits scheduled only about 40% of the time. The healthcare partners are able to facilitate the establishment of a medical home for migrants, which can reduce inappropriate ER utilization and may result in better health outcomes for patients.

## Promotora model

*Promotores* and *Promotoras* are community members who promote health in their own communities. In English, most call themselves Community Health Workers. They provide leadership, peer education, and resources to support community empowerment, or *capacitación*. As members of minority and underserved populations, they are in a unique position to build on strengths and to address unmet health needs in their communities. *Promotores(as)* integrate information about health and the healthcare system into the community's culture, language, and value system, thus reducing many of the barriers to health services. They provide peer education, support, and links to services. They also help make healthcare systems more responsive. With the appropriate resources, training, and support, *Promotores(as)* improve the health of their communities by linking their neighbors to healthcare and social services, by educating their peers about disease and injury prevention, by working to make available services more accessible and by mobilizing their communities to create positive change.

The nature of the training, roles, responsibilities, and duties of *Promotores(as)* varies considerably by community and organization. Paid and volunteer *Promotores(as)* may work part or full time with clinics, nonprofit organizations, public health departments, or other organizations. *Promotores(as)* conduct outreach in clients' homes, community centers, clinics, hospitals, schools, worksites, shelters, and farm worker labor camps. Many *Promotor(a)* programs focus on serving the needs of specific ethnic or racial groups, while others focus on vulnerable segments of the population or prominent health problems. Although *Promotores(as)* engage in a broad range of activities, they share a number of common roles. *Promotores(as)* provide: a link between communities and health and human service agencies; informal counseling and support; culturally competent health education; advocacy; and capacity-building on individual and community levels.

## Collaboratives

The Health and Resource Services Administration (HRSA) Bureau of Primary Health Care has developed the Health Disparities Collaboratives (HDCs) program in an effort to eliminate racial and ethnic health disparities. Under this effort to improve the quality of care and reduce disparities, community health centers participate in the HDCs and implement the chronic care model for patients with certain health conditions, e.g. diabetes. The model works to ensure that patients receive evidence-based care for their condition and to empower patients to participate in their own care.

Successful implementation of the model is dependent on six inter-related elements. One is patient self-management, whereby patients learn about their disease and how to prevent problems. Patients set goals for themselves and the clinical team supports them in attaining these goals. The second element is decision support such as evidence-based practice guidelines and protocols that are provided to clinicians so that they can apply the most current knowledge to help their patients. The third component is clinical information systems. Health centers create a registry that is used by the care team to guide treatment, anticipate problems, and track progress for the entire population with the chronic condition. Fourth, the delivery system must be designed to support improved chronic care. Visits are planned in advance, based on patients' needs and self-management goals. Group visits allow patients to see their clinicians and meet with others with similar health problems. Organization of care is a critical element. Health centers, including their leaders and clinical champi-

ons, commit to improving clinical outcomes and making organizational goals for chronic illness part of their business strategy. Last, health centers form partnerships with state programs, local agencies, schools, faith-based organizations, business, and social groups.

*Outcomes*: While specific data on outcomes for migrants are not available, outcome studies of other populations demonstrate significant improvements in health indicators. From 1999 to 2001, the Washington State Diabetes Collaboratives helped reduce blood glucose for patients in participating health centers by 10% on average. The estimated annual cost savings from this improvement are roughly US$419 000 a year. Other studies have demonstrated that reducing HbA1c levels by 10% in people with diabetes can result in savings of more than US$1200 per patient. The savings can be as much as US$4000 in patients with a combination of diabetes, heart disease, and hypertension, which are common comorbidities of diabetes.[43]

CareSouth, a health center system that had participated in the Diabetes Collaborative, had annual health costs of US$343.00 per patient, while patients of other providers had a cost of US$1600 and specialists had a cost of US$1900. The health center had produced those results by reducing the average blood sugar level of their diabetic patients from 11 to 8 – a 3 point drop (a 1 point decrease translates into a 17% decrease in mortality, an 18% decrease in heart attacks, and a 15% decrease in strokes).[44]

## Conclusion

It is likely that migration to the United States will continue at an aggressive rate during the next decade and beyond. The healthcare system and the practitioners within it hold answers to making healthcare services accessible, affordable, and of the highest quality. The challenges for the provider are many and range from communicating with the patient in a linguistically and culturally competent manner, locating financial and health-related resources such as discounted prescription drugs and specialty care so that the continuity of care will not be compromised, to identifying uncommon illnesses and disease and developing a treatment plan. This calls upon the practitioner to be more than an office doctor; it calls the practitioner to see *medicine as social service*.[45] The poverty, legal status, insurance coverage, and other administrative barriers that may keep a patient away from a health provider could seem overwhelming at first, but the knowledgeable, well-connected community practitioner can create a healthcare home for the immigrant using innovative outreach and care strategies. Creating a medical home for the immigrant and family with a support system that enables usage of the system in a cost-effective and rational way makes an inestimable contribution to society and the hard working people who have become a vital part of it. Well-trained practitioners who are sensitive to the complexity of immigrant life, and who can access, navigate, and fully utilize services and resources on behalf of the patient, will shape the healthy future of our nation.

## References

1. Camarota Steven. Immigrants at mid-decade: a snapshot of American's foreign-born population in 2005. Center for Immigration Studies. 2005.
2. Zuniga Elena, et al. Mexico–United States migration: health issues. UCLA Center for Health Policy Research. October, 2005
3. Rosenbaum JD, Shin P. Migrant and seasonal farm workers: health insurance coverage and access to care. Kaiser Commission on Medicaid and the Uninsured. Center for Health Services Research and Policy, George Washington University. 2005.
4. Valenzuela A Jr,Theodore N, Melendez E, et al. On the corner: day labor in the United States. University of California at Los Angeles, Center for the Study of Urban Policy. 2006.
5. Kim MJ, Cho HI, Cheon-Klessig YS, et al. Primary healthcare for Korean immigrants: sustaining a culturally sensitive model. Public Health Nursing 2002; 19(3):191–200.
6. Kyle D, Zai L. Migrant merchants: human smuggling from Ecuador and China. San Diego: The Center for Comparative Immigration Studies; 2001.
7. Reyes C, Van de Putte L, Falcon AP, et al. Genes, culture and medicines: bridging gaps in treatment for Hispanic Americans. Washington, DC: National Alliance for Hispanic Health; 2004.
8. Hall IP. Pharmacogenetics and ethnicity. Am J Resp Crit Care Med 2005; 171:535–536.
9. Miles A. From Cuenca to Queens: an anthropological story of transnational migration. Austin: University of Texas Press; 2004.
10. National Institute for Occupational Safety and Health (NIOSH). Summary of traumatic occupational fatalities in the United States, 1980–1989: a decade of surveillance. DHHS, NIOSH publication number 93–108S, Cincinnati, OH. 1993.
11. Runyan JL. Review of farm accident data sources and research (BLA-125). Washington, DC: US Department of Agriculture; 1993.
12. National Safety Council. Accident facts 1997 edition. Itasca, IL: National Safety Council; 1997.
13. Myers JR, Hard DL. Work-related fatalities in the agricultural production and services sectors, 1980–1989. Am J Ind Med 1995; 27:51–63.
14. US Department of Labor. Fatal workplace injuries in 1994: a collection of data and analysis. Report No. 908. Washington, DC: Bureau of Labor Statistics; 1996.
15. Hoskin AF, Miller TA, Hanford WD, et al. Occupational injuries in agriculture: a 35 state summary. Report prepared by the National Safety Council under NIOSH contract #DSR-87-0942. Itasca, IL: National Safety Council; 1988.
16. Heyer NJ, Franklin G, Rivara FP, et al. Occupational injuries among minors doing farm work in Washington State: 1986 to 1989. Am J Public Health 1992; 82:557–560.
17. Belville R, Pollack SH, Godbold JH, et al. Occupational injuries among working adolescents in New York State. JAMA 1993; 269:2754–2759.
18. Castillo DN, Landen DD, Layne, LA. Occupational injury deaths of 16- and 17-year-olds in the United States. Am J Public Health 1994; 84:646–649.
19. Pollock S, Landrigan PJ. Child labor in 1990: prevalence and health hazards. Ann Rev Public Health 1990; 11:359–375.
20. Murphy DJ. Safety and health for production agriculture. ASAE Textbook No. 5, St. Joseph, MI: American Society of Agricultural Engineers; 1992.
21. Larson A. Environmental/occupational safety and health. Migrant Health Issues. Monograph Series 2002; 2:8–13.
22. Villarejo D, Baron SL. The occupational health status of hired farm workers. Occupational Medicine: State of the Art Reviews, 1999; 14:613–635.
23. Centers for Disease Control and Prevention. Occupational injury deaths and rates by industry, sex, age, race, and Hispanic origin: United States, 1992–2001. National Center for Health Statistics, 2003.
24. Agricultural Safety Information, National Institute for Occupational Safety and Health, 2001. Available: http://www.cdc.gov/niosh/injury/traumaagric.html Accessed 2/8/07.
25. Ciesielski S, Hall SP, Sweeney M. Occupational injuries among North Carolina migrant farm workers. Am J Public Health 1991; 81:926–927.
26. Dever GE. Migrant health status: profile of a population with complex health problems. Migrant Clinicians Network, 1991.
27. Wilk VA. The occupational health of migrant and seasonal farm workers in the United States: progress report. Farm Worker Justice Fund, Washington, DC; 1988.
28. Mehta K, Gabbard SM, Barrat V, et al. Findings from the National Agricultural Workers Survey (NAWS) 1997–1998: a demographic and employment profile of United States farm workers. US Department of Labor, Washington, DC; 2000.
29. Trends in Tuberculosis – United States 2005 Centers for Disease Control and Prevention. MMWR Morb Wkly Rep 2006; 55(11):305–308.
30. Talbot EA, Moore M, McCray E, et al. Tuberculosis among foreign-born persons in the United States, 1993–1998. JAMA 2000; 284:2894–2900.
31. Data from GeoSentinel Surveillance Network, the Global Surveillance Network of the International Society of Travel Medicine. January 2006.
32. Jenks NP, Trapasso J. Lyme risk for immigrants to the United States: the role of an educational tool. J Travel Med 2005; 12:157–160.
33. DeAlba I, Hubbell FA, McMullin JM, et al. Impact of US citizenship status on cancer screening among immigrant women. J Gen Inter Med 2005; 20(3):290–304.
34. Gany FM, Herrera AP, Avallone M, et al. Attitudes, knowledge, and health-seeking behaviors of five immigrant minority communities in the prevention and screening of cancer: a focus group approach. Ethn Health. 2006; 11(1):19–39.
35. Luquis RR, Villanueva Cruz IJ. Knowledge, attitudes, and perceptions about breast cancer and breast cancer screening among Hispanic women residing in south central Pennsylvania.. J Community Health 2006; 31(1):25–42.
36. Garbers S, Chiasson MA. Inadequate functional health literacy in Spanish as a barrier to cancer screening among immigrant Latinas in New York. Prev Chronic Dis 2004; 1(4):A07.
37. Swan J, Breen N, Coates RJ, et al. Progress in cancer screening practices in the United States: results from the 2000 National Health Interview Survey. Cancer 2003; 97:1528–1540.
38. Danovaro-Holiday MC, Gordon ER, Jumaan AO, et al. High rate of varicella complications among Mexican-born adults in Alabama. Clin Infec Dis 2004; 39(11):1640–1641.

39. Danovaro-Holliday VC, LeBaron CW, Allensworth C, et al. A large rubella outbreak with spread from the workplace to the community. JAMA 2000; 284(21):2733–2739.

40. Sullivan MM, Relum R. Mental health of undocumented immigrants: a review of the literature. Adv Nurs Sci 2005; 28(3):240–251.

41. Miranda J, Siddiqu J, Der-Martirosian C, et al. Depression among Latina immigrant mothers separated from their children. Psychiatr Serv 2005; 56(6):717–20.

42. Management Sciences for Health. Getting to know Hispanic/Latino culture. The providers guide to quality and culture. 2003. http://Erc.msh.org.

43. Matthews T. Diabetes: A Case for Quality Health Care. Improving the quality of care for patients can prevent complications and reduce costs. The Council of State Governments. May 2004. http://www.csg.org/pubs/Documents/sn040SDiabetes.pdf Accessed 2/13/07.

44. Agency for Healthcare Research and Quality (AHRQ), Economic and Health Costs of Diabetes, Health Resources and Services Administration, 2003. http://www.ahrq.gov/data/hcup/highlight1/high1.htm

45. Mullan F. Immigration pediatrics. Health Affairs 2005; 24(6):1619–1623.

# CHAPTER 58

# Visiting Friends and Relatives

Jay S. Keystone

## Introduction

Patterns of migration to developed countries have shifted dramatically over the past half century. Since 1980, the number of international migrants more than doubled, mostly from developing to developed countries, rising from 100 million in 1980, just 25 years ago, to 200 million in 2005.[1]

Migration patterns to the US have reflected the changes in global migration patterns. In 1960, 4.5% of the US population was foreign-born (9.7 million) of whom 9.3% came from Latin America, 5% from Southeast Asia, 9.8% from Canada, and the vast majority, 74.5%, from Europe. By 2004, the US foreign-born population numbered 34.2 million, accounting for 12% of the total US population.[2] Currently, in the United States, 20% of the population are either foreign-born, or the children of the foreign-born.[3] Within the foreign-born population, 53% were born in Latin America, 25% in Asia, 14% in Europe, and the remaining 8% in other regions of the world, such as Africa and Oceania (Australia, New Zealand, and the island nations in the Pacific). In addition, second-generation Americans, natives with one or both parents born in a foreign country, numbered 30.4 million, or 11% of the total US population.

In this chapter we will define and describe the characteristics of those visiting friends and relatives (VFRs) in their countries of origin, outline the reasons why they are at greater risk for infection than other travelers, describe the barriers that keep them from obtaining pre-travel advice, identify ways in which health advice might be provided in a more effective way, and provide specific pre-travel health recom-

mendations tailored to this important category of travelers.

Many immigrants will at some point return to their country of birth to visit family and friends. This population of international travelers returning to their country of origin has been given a specific designation as VFRs (visiting friends and relatives). By definition, a VFR is an immigrant, ethnically and racially distinct from those in the country of residence, who returns to his/her homeland to visit friends and/or relatives. This definition excludes immigrants returning to their homeland purely for the purpose of tourism, conducting business, as well as for educational or missionary work. Although strictly speaking, European immigrants might be considered VFRs, for the purpose of discussion in this chapter, VFRs are those who have immigrated to a developed country from a developing country. In spite of making up approximately 10% of the US population, in 2002 VFRs made up 44% of all US international air travelers.[4] Similarly, in the United Kingdom, VFRs made 13% of 59 million visits for the same purpose, reflecting an annual growth rate of 4.3% annually from 1998 to 2002.[5]

VFR populations will vary according to immigration patterns. For example, in the United States, more than half of foreign-born residents are from Latin America and one-quarter are from Asia.[6] In 2002, the top five sources of documented immigrants were Mexico, India, China, the Philippines, and Vietnam.[7] In the UK, in 2003 30% of the immigrants were from Africa, and 24% from the Indian subcontinent.[8]

It is somewhat controversial as to whether first- or second-generation members of an immigrant family born in the receiving country are considered to be VFRs. Although VFRs are often immune or partially immune to infections in their country of birth, they also have greater health risks because they usually travel to remote areas of the developing world and live in conditions that put them at risk of local infections. On the other hand, children of VFRs born in a developed country are like the native-born population because they are not immune to most overseas infections. However, they are also similar to the immigrant population because their living conditions overseas will often approximate those of nationals in the developing world.

## Barriers to Pre-Travel Healthcare

What makes VFR travelers so different from other travelers that they have their own unique category? VFRs are often at greater risk than native-born travelers partly because of their perceptions of risk, health beliefs, and socioeconomic status (the traveler) and partly because of their specific destination risks (the travel). VFR travelers may mistakenly believe that they are immune to many of the infectious diseases endemic to their country of origin, and may be unaware of the true health risks when they return to their homeland. A large Canadian travel survey found that VFRs estimated their risk to be the same as that for intermediate and low-risk travelers.[9] These are two of the major reasons why they will not seek pre-travel health advice or adhere to recommendations made by healthcare providers, especially if those practitioners have little or no knowledge of the conditions in their homeland.

For example, multiple past malaria infections ('like flu to an African') may deter VFRs from seeking pre-travel health advice and taking malaria prophylaxis; however, they often bring their children, but not themselves, for pre-travel health advice.[10-12]

Surprisingly, even when VFRs visit healthcare providers from their birthplace they may receive incorrect advice since the healthcare provider also may have the same mistaken beliefs as the patient.[13] A survey of 2000 travelers in Amsterdam found that almost one-third were VFRs traveling back to their country of origin, particularly Morocco and Turkey, and that 70% had not sought pre-travel advice.[14] Even when pre-travel advice is sought, adherence to travel recommendations, suboptimal in many travelers,[15-17] may be worse in VFRs.[14,15] A study of 307 Canadians of Asian origin traveling to India showed that only 31% intended to use malaria chemoprophylaxis and fewer than 10% mosquito bite prevention. For those

who did seek pre-travel advice, the majority sought this advice from family practitioners rather than from travel medicine providers; this might explain why 76% of the time the malaria chemoprophylaxis prescribed was inappropriate.[9]

Financial considerations are one of the most important factors in limiting the use of pre-travel health services among VFRs, particularly when they travel with family members and the cumulative cost of immunizations and antimalarials is considerable.[18,19] Language barriers, lack of knowledge or access to healthcare, health beliefs, and fear of immigration authorities may influence pre-travel health-seeking behavior as well.

Healthcare systems and providers may also be responsible for barriers to care. Many immigrants have not received an adequate health screening upon arrival in an industrialized country, have not completed primary vaccinations series, or lack immunization records.[19,20] Inadequate use of medically trained interpreters limits a healthcare provider's ability to impart information, and patients may be illiterate even in their own language. Primary healthcare providers are often not knowledgeable about travel medicine, or the geography and disease epidemiology of the destination country.[21] Although many clinicians have access to the CDC or other websites that provide broad country-based disease prevention recommendations, they may not have the expertise to interpret this information in the context of type of travel, local itinerary, living conditions, and other factors.[22] Most do not have access to regularly updated pre-travel health databases that give detailed information on regional disease distribution, seasonal factors, and epidemics within a country (Table 58.1). However, in spite of these barriers to adequate pre-travel health advice, there are a number of practical approaches that may be utilized by primary care and public health practitioners that will enable the VFR to obtain and adhere to pre-travel health advice (Table 58.2).[23]

## Health Risks for Those Visiting Family and Relatives

Those visiting family and relatives may assume more risk than traditional travelers, and have higher levels of morbidity and mortality related to travel. They often choose to travel despite multiple medical problems, during pregnancy, and with small infants and children. VFRs frequently return to visit spouses, parents or children left behind, to introduce 'new

**Table 58.1 Pre-travel health advice resources for healthcare providers**

| | |
|---|---|
| ***Interactive web-based*** | |
| CDC travel Info | http://www.cdc.gov/travel |
| WHO international travel | http://www.who.int/ith |
| Health Canada Travel | http://www.TravelHealth.gc.ca |
| National Travel Health (UK) | http://www.nathnac.org/healthprofessionals/index.html |
| Malaria maps | listserv@wehi.edu.au |
| Travax UK (fee) | http://www.travax.scot.nhs.uk |
| SOS Travelcare (fee) | http://www.travelcare.com |
| Travax US (fee) | http://www.shoreland.com |
| GIDEON (fee) | http://www.gideononline.com |
| EXODUS (fee) | http://www.exodus.ie |
| | |
| ***Surveillance/outbreak information*** | |
| MMWR (CDC) | http://www.cdc.gov/mmwr |
| Weekly Epidemiological Review | http://www.who.int/wer |
| EuroSurveillance Weekly | http://www.eurosurv.org/update |
| Canada CDR | http://www.hc-sc.gc.ca/hpb/lcdc/publicat/ccdr |
| ProMedmail | majordomo@promedmail.org |
| | |
| ***Listserv discussion groups for travel med*** | |
| TravelMed (ISTM) | listserv/@yorku.ca |
| TropMed (ASTMH) | listserv/@yorku.ca |
| ProMedmail | majordomo@promedmail.org |
| | |
| ***Medical assistance /physicians for travellers*** | |
| International Soc Travel Med (ISTMH) | http://www.istm.org |
| Am Society of Tropical Medicine and Hygiene (ASTMH) | http://www.astmh.org |
| SOS Travel Care (fee) | http://www.internationalsos.com |
| IAMAT (donation requested) | http://www.iamat.org |
| State Department (Washington, DC) | http://www.travel.state.gov/medical.html |
| | |
| ***Book references*** | |
| CDC Health Information for International Travelers | http://www.cdc.gov/travel/yb/toc.htm |
| Travel & Routine Immunizations | Thompson R. Milwaukee, WI: Shorland; 2002 |
| Red Book (Am Acad of Pediatrics) | Pickering L, ed. 27th edn. Grove Village, IL: AAP; 2006 |
| Travel Medicine | Keystone JS, et al. Philadelphia: Mosby; 2004 |
| A World Guide to Infections | Wilson M. New York: Oxford University Press; 1991 |
| Travel Medicine Health | DuPont HL, Steffen R. 2nd edn. London: Decker; 2001 |
| Tropical Infectious Diseases | Guerrant RL, et al. Philadelphia: Churchill Livingstone;1999 |
| Manson's Tropical Diseases | Cook GC, et al. Edinburgh: Elsevier Science Ltd; 2003 |
| Hunters' Tropical Medicine | Strickland TG, et al. Philadelphia: Saunders; 2000 |

additions' to their family or to attend weddings and other life cycle events. Last minute travel to visit a sick relative or to attend a funeral is common, allowing little time for pre-travel health advice. Furthermore, many VFRs stay with family members in rural or remote settings where they frequently encounter suboptimal sanitary conditions and are at increased risk of malaria and other infections. Windows may not be screened and bed nets may be in disrepair. Food may be prepared by persons with poor personal hygiene or who are carriers of hepatitis A or other infections, and travelers may be reluctant to eat differently from their hosts. Close contact with the local population puts VFRs at higher risk for respiratory infections such as tuberculosis and meningococcal meningitis.[24,25] Also, VFRs tend to have prolonged stays, thereby increasing the risk for morbidity and mortality.[26,27]

In addition to the greater risk of infectious diseases, injuries among VFRs may also be a problem. Motor vehicle accidents are a frequent cause of injury among travelers and are the single most important

| |
| --- |
| **Table 58.2  Decreasing barriers to pre-travel advice and care** |
| ***For patients*** |
| Community education |
| Patients returning to their communities ('word of mouth') |
| Community/ethnic newspapers, radio programs, postings |
| Reassurance that the provider/clinic has the person's best interest in mind and will not inquire about legal status but will provide services regardless of documentation of legal status |
| ***For primary clinicians*** |
| Access to interactive pre-travel, updated websites and resources |
| Train specific provider in travel medicine or develop close relationship with travel clinic |
| Increase education of providers |
| Providing pre-travel care (generalists) |
| Cross-cultural health issues |
| Immigrant and refugee health issues |
| ***Structural and service changes*** |
| Financial |
| Assist in prioritizing preventive health strategies |
| Sliding fee scales |
| Refer for less costly services (i.e. to public health departments for vaccines) |
| Physical |
| Provide welcoming environment to populations served (e.g. artwork, pictures) |
| Locate travel medical clinics or trained providers in communities of need |
| Locate clinics close to public transportation |
| Address language and cultural barriers |
| Employing multilingual, bicultural staff |
| Medically trained interpreters |
| Prescriptions and handouts in patient's language as well as English |

cause of death of travelers in developing countries.[28-31] The risk of injury may be higher for VFRs because they often utilize high-risk, public transportation and travel in rural areas on poor roads without proper lighting. Also, there is an additional risk due to lack of safety devices within motor vehicles that all too often are poorly maintained.[32] Furthermore, medical care following an injury or severe illness, especially in remote areas, is frequently inadequate.[33-35]

Many refugees who become VFRs have experienced upheaval, armed conflict, and torture prior to emigration, and may have residual post-traumatic stress disorder (PTSD).[36,37] Stress-related health problems may be exacerbated by travel, or by seeing impoverished family members; as a result, some may experience recurrence of pre-existing psychiatric symptoms.

## Health Issues and Recommendations for Those Visiting Family and Relatives

The major challenge is convincing VFR travelers that they would benefit from pre-travel counseling. This is difficult especially if there is a cost involved. Information about the benefits of travel medicine services might be disseminated in appropriate languages through leaflets, posters in places of worship or stores selling ethnic foods, and popular ethnic radio programs or newspapers. The paradigm of separating travel advice as a 'specialty service' from primary care practice is likely to be least effective for VFRs. Ideally, travel medical services should be offered in primary care clinics frequented by immigrants, preferably by physicians caring for those individuals on a regular basis.[38] Familiarity, ease of access, and an established doctor–patient relationship are most likely to encourage use. Essentially, an immigrant should be viewed as a future traveler. Since the majority of VFRs return to their country of birth on one or more occasions, the primary care provider is in the ideal position to screen for their immunization needs well before travel abroad, making travel vaccines an integral part of routine childhood and adult immunization programs. In some primary care clinics, particularly those associated with public health departments, the cost of the travel clinic consultation (coded as health counseling) and many of the vaccines may be covered as part of the clinic service. Finally, since VFRs often seek pre-departure advice for their children and not for themselves, child counseling provides an excellent opportunity to encourage risk management strategies for the parents as well as their children.

When available, it is best to use medically trained, cross-cultural interpreters or multilingual healthcare providers. Family members should be used to translate only when absolutely necessary. Pre-travel advice, medication instructions, prescription bottles, as well as health information about the destination abroad should be written in appropriate languages.[39] For VFRs on limited budgets, providers may help prioritize which vaccines they should receive, choose affordable malaria prophylaxis, or refer them to public health clinics where available.

Although the risk assessment of a VFR is similar to that of a national, there are some minor differences. Additional reasons for travel should be explored. For example, is the traveler planning to undergo medical procedures that are costly in their country of residence, such as dental work, elective surgery, or therapeutic interventions (e.g. angioplasty or tattooing of eyebrows)? Also, it is important to determine whether the VFR is staying in a local home or an upscale hotel, since the risk factors for infection vary considerably.

The following abbreviated discussion of travel health risks is focused on issues that are particularly relevant to the VFR traveler. For more comprehensive and general travel health information, the enthusiastic reader is encouraged to consult official government travel medicine web sites such as those of the US Centers for Disease Control and Prevention (CDC) (http://www.cdc.gov), the Public Health Agency of Canada (http://www.travelhealth.gc.ca), or the UK National Travel Health Network and Centre (NaTHNaC) (http://www.nathnac.org).

## Food and water-borne illnesses

Travelers' diarrhea (TD) is the most frequent illness among travelers to the developing world, affecting 30–60% of all travelers.[40,41] Although the problem may be less of an issue to recent immigrants because of their acquired immunity, it has been shown that when repeated exposure to enteric pathogens ceases, the risk of TD increases.[42] Travelers' diarrhea is a much greater risk for nonimmune children born in a developed country. The greatest risk for VFR travelers is likely to occur when they eat in local homes where the hygiene practices or the health status of the 'cook,' often a poor relative or housekeeper, may be substandard. The typical advice often quoted by healthcare providers, 'boil it, cook it, peel it, or forget it,' is often impractical in a household setting, especially when one is a guest. It is interesting to note that a critical review of the literature on TD prevention concluded that there are few or no data to show that increased food precautions and fewer mistakes actually decrease the frequency of TD.[43] A recent study of long-stay travelers to India supported this concept that TD was not correlated with the degree of attention to food precautions.[44] However, it would be sensible for VFR travelers to try to ensure that food is served hot and that water for home use has been boiled and filtered in their place of residence abroad. It may be more practical to stress the effectiveness of frequent hand washing. or

the use of alcohol and nonalcohol-based hand-sanitizing solutions.[45,46] Avoiding food sold by street vendors would certainly be prudent.[47] Equally important as prevention would be information about management of diarrhea, especially for young children.

Given the paucity of data showing that travelers' diarrhea can be prevented by food and water precautions, it is even more important to ensure that VFR travelers are provided with information on the management of illness during travel, particularly concerning their children. For cost-containment purposes, it is advisable to recommend to adults the use of loperamide and a single dose of levofloxacin 500 mg or another fluoroquinolone for self-treatment of TD. Several studies have shown that a single dose of antibiotic with loperamide is as effective as a standard 3-day course of therapy. Azithromycin 1000 mg in one dose or 500 mg daily for 3 days is recommended for Thailand[48–50] where more than 80% of *Campylobacter* species are now resistant to quinolones.[51,52]

Until recently, fluoroquinolone antibiotics were considered to be contraindicated in children. However, recent reviews suggest that these drugs are safe even with long-term use in children.[53,54] For this reason, many travel medicine practitioners and pediatric infectious disease consultants increasingly are comfortable recommending off label, 1–3-day quinolone regimens in appropriate doses for children. For children who require a liquid preparation, azithromycin (one daily dose of 10 mg/kg per day) is recommended. By using single dose therapy, VFR travelers with limited communication skills are more likely to utilize treatment regimens correctly. For VFRs with small children, it is important to stress the importance of oral rehydration solutions (ORSs). Many VFR parents may be much more familiar with ORS than are their counterparts born in developed countries.

Specific cultural food practices may put the traveler at risk of specific infectious diseases. For example, one might advise Latin Americans to avoid white cheese (queso fresca) to prevent brucellosis and listeriosis,[55,56] and uncooked pork to prevent cysticercosis. Cerviche and other preparations of raw, freshwater fish (sushi, koi pla), common cultural delicacies in many parts of the world, can transmit vibriosis, gnathostomiasis, liver flukes, and other organisms.[57,58] Raw or poorly cooked shellfish may contain hepatitis A or *Salmonella typhi*, posing additional risks for VFRs.[59,60] Although ciguatera poisoning is a common problem among those who eat large, carnivorous reef fish found in subtropical and tropical waters,[61,62] it is rarely seen in VFRs and is more likely to affect tourists.

## Insect-borne diseases

### Malaria

Returned VFR travelers now make up the largest proportion of malaria cases reported in developed countries. In 2003, they accounted for 53.9% of civilian cases in the United States and 35% of 1140 travelers reported to the Geosentinel Surveillance Network of the International Society of Travel Medicine.[63,64] VFR travelers from the UK visiting West Africa had a tenfold greater attack rate than tourists[65] and made up 82% of cases in children.[66] In a review of malaria cases imported into Brescia, Italy, between 1990 and 1998, 71% were in migrants compared to 12% among nonimmune Italians.[67] Pooling of malaria cases in European centers found that 43% occurred in non-nationals, frequently immigrant VFRs.[68] The Geosentinel Surveillance Network showed an eightfold relative risk of acquiring malaria in VFRs compared to tourists.[69]

Although the high proportion of malaria cases among VFR travelers can be partly explained by their travel patterns to endemic areas, their rates of prophylaxis use are lower than nonimmunes from developed countries. Low rates of chemoprophylaxis use among VFRs have been the consistent in several studies, i.e. Canada (31%), Italy (8%), and the UK (46–48%).[17,64,69]

The reasons for inadequate use of chemoprophylaxis are multifactorial: cost,[10,18] lower perception of risk by the traveler[9] and the healthcare provider,[13] and inappropriate medication.[9,12]

Studies show that severe and fatal malaria is uncommon in VFR travelers, who frequently possess partial immunity to malaria prior to emigration. Although this immunity may be maintained for many years, even in the absence of re-infection, protection is clearly incomplete as evidenced by the high rates of clinical malaria in this group. Due to immunological priming, VFRs appear to have far lower mortality rates from malaria than do nonimmune nationals from developed countries.[68,70]

However, increasingly, severe malaria and deaths are being reported among VFRs who have either lost their immunity or have been inoculated with a high load of parasites, or both. The Canadian Malaria Network reported that between 2001 and 2005, 49.2% of 31 severe malaria cases occurred in foreign-born individuals from malarious areas (Anne McCarthy, personal communication, 2005). Of the 185 deaths

from malaria reported in the US from 1963 to 2001, only 13.8% were VFRs However, between 1989 and 2001, 21.3% of fatal cases were VFRs who made up the largest group of travelers to die from malaria.[71] It is important to understand that in few areas of the world is malaria hyperendemic to the point that locals acquire a clinically significant degree of immunity to the infection. The most important of these areas is sub-Saharan Africa and parts of Oceania (e.g. Papua New Guinea and Irian Jaya). Those living in malarious areas in the rest of the world are for the most part nonimmune with respect to malaria and are as likely to die from *Plasmodium falciparum* malaria as are those born in nonendemic areas. Since, as noted above, malaria immunity wanes in the absence of re-infection, even those VFRs returning to sub-Saharan Africa require chemoprophylaxis. The question that has yet to be answered is how long does it take to completely lose one's immunity to malaria. From a clinical perspective, the question has little relevance, since exposure to a heavily infected mosquito is likely to lead to clinical disease, an outcome that is preventable with appropriate medication.

As a way of encouraging VFRs to use prophylaxis, perceptions of immunity should be explored as well as the changing patterns of drug resistance and malaria species. For example, VFRs returning to India need to know that over the past decade the life-threatening form of malaria, *P. falciparum*, has replaced *P. vivax* as the predominant species.[72] As far as VFRs are concerned, the risks and benefits of antimalarials appear to be similar for those born in developed countries. Mefloquine is relatively inexpensive and convenient, but due to neuropsychiatric side effects cannot be used in individuals with depression, anxiety, and PTSD, which are common in VFRs.[73-75] An effective strategy, if time permits, is to start prophylaxis with mefloquine 3–4 weeks prior to departure to allow time to switch to another drug if side effects develop. However, one interesting anecdotal observation among travel medicine practitioners is that neuropsychiatric adverse events from mefloquine appear to be distinctly uncommon in those of African descent.

Doxycycline is generally well tolerated, and is the least expensive of the antimalarials, but has the disadvantage of daily dosing, GI upset, and vaginal candidiasis in women. Atovaquone/proguanil (Malarone®) is prohibitively expensive for most VFRs, especially with prolonged stays, and is not covered on many formularies. Chloroquine remains an affordable choice for travel but is effective in only a few areas of the world. The use of primaquine,

30 mg/day, for malaria prophylaxis in adults is a welcome new option, especially in VFRs who are unable to afford atovaquone-proguanil or tolerate mefloquine.[76] A glucose-6-phosphate dehydrogenase (G6PD) level *must* be determined prior to use of primaquine. It is a second-line agent due to concerns about toxicity in G6PD deficient patients and the fact that it is about 5–10% less effective than other agents. For some long-term visitors, stand-by, self-administered malaria treatment will be the only affordable option, although several studies have shown it is often used incorrectly.[77–79]

It is important to advise VFRs to continue malaria prophylaxis even if diagnosed with malaria while abroad because of the likelihood of an incorrect diagnosis due to a false-positive smear. Several recent studies have shown that the false-positive rate of blood films done by local laboratories in developing countries may be as high as 75%.[80,81] This is a particular problem for those traveling to sub-Saharan Africa.[82] The most important practical advice that one can give VFR travelers concerning this situation is to advise them that even if they were to be diagnosed with malaria during travel, they should continue their antimalarial drug as directed and not assume that it had failed to protect them. Finally, VFRs should be advised to avoid buying their antimalarials overseas, even though they might be cheaper, because of the high risk of obtaining counterfeit or low-quality drugs.[83] A recent survey of counterfeit drugs in Asia showed that 53% of antimalarials sold commercially were counterfeit or contained a substandard amount of the active drug.[84]

Barrier precautions and insect repellents not only protect travelers from malaria, but also from many other infections, some of which are more common in and dangerous to VFRs. Because some VFRs will find it challenging to locate outdoor recreational stores, it may be helpful to sell the insect repellent DEET, and the clothing insecticide permethrin at low cost in the clinic setting. Insecticide-treated bed nets (ITNs) are inexpensive and readily available in endemic countries. Currently, the WHO estimates that fewer than 10% of African children and women at risk use ITNs; unfortunately, it is likely that VFRs would follow the example of their hosts and not use ITNs.[85] Those who don't stay in major cities or air-conditioned hotels are at particular risk of insect-borne diseases such as malaria.

## Dengue

Dengue fever and dengue hemorrhagic fever (DHF) are increasingly recognized as major public health problems in over 100 countries in the tropics and subtropics. Approximately 50 million people are infected annually, with 25 000 deaths.[86,87] The dengue virus has four different serotypes, dengue 1, 2, 3, and 4. Exposure to one dengue virus confers immunity to that serotype but not to the others. One or more serotypes may circulate in an endemic area simultaneously. Second infections of dengue with a different serotype from the first have been associated with DHF and shock syndrome (DSS); blocking antibodies produced during the first infection interfere with the immune response to the second, leading to enhanced viral replication accompanied by increased morbidity and mortality.[88,89] Therefore, since VFRs from a dengue endemic area are more likely to have been exposed to the virus prior to emigration, one might expect them to be at greater risk for DHF and DSS on return to their homeland, especially when a new dengue serotype is present. Furthermore, since the majority of those who acquire dengue have few or no symptoms, most VFRs will not be aware of their prior immune status.[90] Data from The European Network on Imported Infectious Disease Surveillance (TropNetEurop) and several case reports support this theory by suggesting that non-Caucasian travelers have a higher risk of developing DHF than Caucasian travelers.[91,92]

Dengue, often found in urban areas, may be prevented by the use of insect precautions, particularly the use of DEET-containing repellents during daylight hours, especially at dusk and dawn. The CDC website has an excellent downloadable handout on dengue and other diseases that may be provided to travelers (visit http://www.cdc.gov/ncidod/dvbid/dengue/).

## Tuberculosis

One-third of the world's population is infected with tuberculosis (TB), most of whom have a latent infection.[93] In recent years, immigrants to developed countries from high-incidence areas have become the highest risk group for active disease, developing symptoms most frequently within the first 5 years of immigration.[94,95] The contribution of this infection in developed countries from VFR travelers has not yet been determined. Theoretically, their close contact with infected, local populations, long-term travel, and stay in overcrowded, poorly ventilated homes should put them at higher risk. A study of Asian immigrant tuberculosis in the UK in 1984 showed that the onset of tuberculosis among VFRs was strongly associated temporally with their return to the Indian subcontinent.[96] Another review in the UK of more than 1000 cases of active TB without a known contact showed that 60% of UK-born ethnic (South Asian) travelers had visited the Indian subcontinent within 3 years of illness.[97,98] An excellent review of illness in VFRs by the GeoSentinel Surveillance Network showed that they were at greater risk of active tuberculosis compared with non-VFR travelers.[99]

## Blood and body fluid-transmissible disease

Lifestyle activities and illness during travel may increase the risk of contacting body fluid-transmissible diseases (HIV, hepatitis B and C, etc.) from tattoos, sexual encounters, especially with commercial sex workers, improperly sterilized medical equipment (including acupuncture treatments) and personal care such as manicures and shaves; the latter are more likely to occur among VFRs.[100-103] Also, VFRs are more likely to have sexual encounters with locals (in whom infection rates may be higher) than with other non-VFR travelers and use condoms bought in developing countries that may be of poor quality.[104] In addition, VFR children may be at greater risk for hepatitis B due to shared secretions with hepatitis B-infected children in their extended family.[105]

## Other travel precautions and recommendations

A frequent and serious problem in the developing world is the sale of counterfeit and substandard drugs.[106,107] A recent Southeast Asian study showed that samples of the antimalarial drug, artesunate, purchased from shops in five Southeast Asian countries did not contain artesunate 38% of the time, even though packaged in standard blisterpacks.[108] In an urban area in Nigeria, 48% of 581 pharmaceuticals were found to be substandard.[109] It has been estimated that 10–20% of drugs manufactured in China and India are counterfeit, but rates may exceed 40–50% in some areas.[110] Since it is common practice for VFRs to purchase medications and traditional remedies while abroad, they may be at increased risk of drug failure and adverse effects.

Due to the high risk of motor vehicle accidents, VFRs should be advised to avoid overcrowded public vehicles if possible, riding on motorcycles, and travel by road in rural areas after dark.[28] Travel health advisors frequently include advice to reduce motor vehicle accident injuries by encouraging the use of seat belts, car seats for children, and helmets when riding motorcycles during travel. However, it is important to point out that such standard equipment in developed countries is often not available or a luxury in developing countries.

Asthma and allergies may be exacerbated by environmental smoke and pollutants, and burns may occur from indoor open cooking stoves.[111] VFR travelers with asthma need to be prepared for asthma exacerbations, including the use of standby steroids.

Overseas care is likely to be better at large, well-recognized medical facilities. However, in many developing countries, government hospitals provide substandard care because of poor facilities and inadequate resources. Private clinics, some mission hospitals, and physicians serving the expatriate and embassy personnel often are able to provide the best care. Where injections are required, it is advisable to ensure that both the needles and syringes have not been reused and are taken from a sealed package. Although travel/evacuation insurance is ideal, and often provides access to physicians abroad, the fees may be too high for many VFRs. Finally, it is important to remind parents to stress to overseas healthcare providers that their children are not immune to locally acquired infections such as malaria

# Immunizations

## Routine childhood vaccine-preventable diseases

Until recently, immigration services in the US did not require immigrants to have completed their primary immunizations before entry. However, in 1996 an amendment to the Immigrant and Naturalization Act required some categories of new immigrants, but not refugees, to show proof of having received vaccines before immigration. It has been shown that some immigrant children destined to become VFR travelers have incomplete immunization schedules, and some internationally adopted children lack protective antibodies despite vaccination records documenting vaccination.[112-115] In the United States, foreign-born and subsequent American-born generations rank among those with the lowest rates of routine immunization.[20,116] Most experts recommend that, with few exceptions, documented incomplete vaccination courses be completed rather than checking titers or repeating the series. These issues are described in detail in chapter 13.

Under some circumstances it may be cost-effective to measure antibody titers, such as when the vaccination series is suspect, when immunity to infection may be present (e.g. varicella or hepatitis A and B), or when the vaccine is costly. Often, in the case of travelers, there is little time to check titers and still provide adequate immunization before departure.[117,1118] 'Accelerated' vaccination schedules are available in cases of imminent VFR travel.[103]

Routine vaccinations that should be up to date in all VFR travelers include diphtheria, tetanus, polio, measles-mumps-rubella, and hepatitis B as well as pneumococcal, *Haemophilus influenza* type B, and pertussis in their children.

## Varicella

Lack of varicella immunity is a particular issue for VFR travelers. In some rural tropical areas, infection is less common and the age of onset is delayed.[119] In the UK and North America almost 95% of children will be immune by the age of 10, compared with only 50% in parts of the developing world, notably South and East Asia and Latin America.[120] Barnett et al. found that of 668 newly arrived refugees aged 1–20 years, 82% had antibodies to measles, and 64% had antibodies to varicella.[121]

It is noteworthy that adults have a 25-fold greater risk of death compared with young children due primarily to complications such as pneumonia, encephalitis, and hemorrhage. A review of varicella mortality rates in the United States between 1980 and 1989 showed that foreign-born individuals over the age of 45 had a fivefold greater mortality than those born in United States.[122]

## Hepatitis A

Hepatitis A (HAV) is one of the most frequent vaccine-preventable illness in travelers.[123,124] Behrens and colleagues showed that the risk of hepatitis A in UK travelers to India between 1990 and 1992 was tenfold higher among VFRs under 15 years of age than among native-born tourists of the same age.[125] Previously, immigrants from hepatitis A endemic countries were assumed to be immune in childhood.[126-128] A recent small study of 129 VFRs found that 95% were already immune to hepatitis A.[124] However, as the standard of living in developing countries improves, the prevalence of infection is declining, even in some rural areas.[129] A study in Bangkok showed that the prevalence of HAV antibodies in medical students decreased from 77% in 1981 to 7% in 2001.[130] Another recent multicenter study in six countries in Latin America found that

20–70% of pre-adolescents were not immune to hepatitis A.[131]

VFR risk of hepatitis A is based on duration and location of residence in the country of origin, age, year of immigration, and a previous history of jaundice. Serological testing for hepatitis A IgG antibodies or vaccination is indicated in VFR travelers less than 20 years old. In older VFRs, it is cost-effective to test for antibodies if time permits.[132,133] A single dose of vaccine for the last-minute traveler will provide excellent protection for at least 5 years and is not harmful even if the patient is already immune.

## Hepatitis B

Hepatitis B infects more than 350 million people worldwide, with infection rates as high as 80% and carrier rates for the virus of more than 15% in some developing countries.[134] These data suggest that many VFRs will be immune to hepatitis B (HBV) prior to travel. However, for those not immune, hepatitis B is a significant risk during travel for those who engage in high-risk activities, such as unprotected casual sex, or receive tattoos or piercings.[103] Less well known is the high risk of acquiring infection during medical care abroad from unsterile medical equipment. A recent WHO study showed that up to 75% of equipment used for medical injections in developing countries was unsterile.[102] These latter data alone would suggest that all VFRs should be tested for HBV immunity, and immunized for hepatitis B when the traveler is not immune.

## Cholera

Although cholera is a rare occurrence among travelers, a review of cases imported into the United States from 1992 to 1994 showed that, of the 160 cases reported, 78% occurred in VFRs returning from endemic areas.[135] However, given the rarity of the infection, the vaccine (available in Europe and Canada as Dukoral™) is not recommended for VFRs except those planning to work in refugee camps or healthcare in cholera-endemic areas.[136]

## Typhoid fever

Typhoid fever is a considerable problem for VFRs, especially with travel to South Asia. In a recent review of cases of typhoid fever imported into the United States between 1994 and 1999, 77% of the cases were shown to occur among VFRs.[137] Almost half of the cases were acquired in less than 4 weeks of travel and 25% occurred in children under 10 years.

Since the majority of imported cases of typhoid fever in industrialized countries are in VFRs, the vaccine should be recommended in almost all instances. Duration of travel should not be a major consideration in determining the need for vaccination since 1% and 27% of travelers acquired their infection in the first 2 and 3 weeks of travel, respectively.[137,138] Both the injectable polysaccharide and multidose live oral vaccines provide only about 70% protection for at least 2 and 5 years, respectively. For many patients, it is often simpler and more effective to use the single-dose injectable vaccine because adherence to a multidose schedule may be problematic.[139]

## Rabies

Reliable data on rabies are scarce in many areas of the world. According to a recent WHO study in 2004, the annual number of deaths worldwide caused by rabies is estimated to be 55 000, mostly in rural areas of Africa and Asia. Each year an estimated 10 million people receive postexposure therapy after being exposed to possibly rabid animals.

Asia had the greatest number of cases (with an estimated 31 000 deaths), although the estimate for Africa (24 000 deaths) was much greater than initially believed.[140] There is consistent evidence that 30–60% of the victims of dog bites in rabies-endemic areas are children under 15 years of age. Since 1977, there have been 19 cases of imported rabies in France; the most recent cases were in French VFRs returning from their country of origin.[141]

Pre-exposure rabies vaccination should be a serious consideration for VFR children traveling to rabies-endemic areas in the developing world, particularly those traveling for prolonged periods. Children are more likely to approach animals, less likely to report a bite or scratch, and more likely, because of their size, to be bitten on the head or neck. Vaccination is less important for adults who are better able to avoid animal bites. Unfortunately, the cost of the vaccine has become prohibitive for most, although some centers use intradermal immunization (off label) which is one-tenth the cost of the intramuscular route.[142] Therefore, it is very important to stress other aspects of rabies prevention. Children should be kept away from dogs, monkeys, and other animals. The wound, even a lick or scrape, should be cleaned with soap and water for at least 10 minutes. In many developing countries, human or purified equine rabies immune globulin (RIG) is not available and therefore an animal bite may become a trip-ending experience, as the bitten traveler may have to return

home or to a nearby country to receive appropriate therapy. The advantage of pre-exposure immunization is that immune globulin is not necessary for postexposure prophylaxis; in most developing countries rabies vaccine is available, albeit perhaps not the human tissue culture preparation. In the case of an animal bite, whether provoked or unprovoked, VFR travelers should consider the need for rabies immunization. If the animal is a domestic dog or cat (with a history of adequate rabies immunization) that can be observed for 10 days, immunization may be delayed. Otherwise, postexposure treatment, including RIG, should be sought as soon as possible. Because a discussion of the need for rabies immune globulin may be complicated and difficult to understand for those with language problems, some clinicians simplify the discussion by recommending that any animal bite is an indication to return home for postexposure rabies management. In addition to this advice, it would be prudent to recommend that the VFR traveler obtain airline cancellation insurance.

## Meningococcal meningitis

Meningococcal meningitis, usually due to serogroups A, C and W-135, occurs worldwide, but most of the morbidity and mortality occurs in 15 countries included in Africa's sub-Saharan meningitis belt.[143] Large epidemics occur periodically throughout the region, predominately during the dry season.

Vaccination is recommended for travelers to Saudi Arabia for the Hajj and to the meningitis belt during the dry season, and during epidemics.[144] Some experts recommend that the quadrivalent vaccine (ACYW-135) be given year-round (not only in the dry season) to VFRs traveling to sub-Saharan Africa because of increased risk due to their close contact with the local population.

## Conclusion

Those visiting friends and relatives account for a high proportion of international travelers, many of whom have significantly increased travel health risks. For VFRs in particular, financial considerations, accessibility to culturally sensitive healthcare, language, and health beliefs appear to play an important role in determining pre-travel health-seeking behavior and adherence to preventive measures. New strategies are needed to address the health issues of VFR travelers. Medical and public health organizations should use the media to increase public awareness, and to disseminate information not only to VFRs but also to healthcare providers.

It would be ideal for travel medicine services to be housed in clinics providing primary care to VFRs. Alternatively, a primary care practice might wish to designate a healthcare provider (physician, nurse, or physician's assistant) to become knowledgeable in travel medicine, utilizing expert back-up as needed. Medical schools should expand their curriculum to include knowledge about diseases and disease prevention among immigrant populations and VFRs.

More research is needed into how to overcome the barriers that keep VFRs from seeking and adhering to pre-travel health advice. It would be helpful if public health services would assist by providing low-cost travel immunizations and malaria chemoprophylaxis. Until these issues are satisfactorily addressed and ultimately resolved, VFRs will continue to be at high risk for travel-related illness, with potentially serious personal and public health implications.

## References

1. UN Global Commission on International Migration Report, 2005; New York.
2. US Census Bureau data. February 22, 2005.
3. US Census Bureau. Profile of the foreign-born population, 2000. Available: http://www.census.gov/prod/2002pubs/p23–206.pdf. Accessed 5/8/07.
4. Profile of US resident travelers, survey of international air travelers. Office of travel and tourism industries, US Department of Commerce. Available: http://tinet.ita.doc.gov/cat/f-2002-101-001.html Accessed 2/9/07.
5. World Travel Market 2005 UK and European Travel Report. http://www.etc-corporate.org//DWL/WTM2005_Report.pdf Accessed 2/12/07
6. Schmidely AD. Current population reports P23–206 profile of foreign-born population in the United States: 2000. US Consensus Bureau. Washington, DC: US Government Printing Office; 2001.
7. US Department of Homeland Security. Yearbook of Immigration Statistics, 2002. Washington, DC: US Government Printing Office; 2004.
8. National Statistics. Persons granted British Citizenship, United Kingdom, 2003. Available: http://www.homeoffice.gov.uk/rds/pdfs04/hosb0704.pdf. Accessed 2/9/07.
9. Dos Santos CC, Anvar A, Keystone JS, et al. Survey of malaria prevention measures by Canadians visiting India. Can Med Assoc J 1999; 160(2):195–200.
10. Backer H, Mackell S. Potential cost savings and quality improvement in travel advice for children and families from a centralized travel medicine clinic in a large group-model health maintenance organization. J Travel Med 2001; 8(5):247–253.
11. Leonard L, VanLandingham M. Adherence to travel health guidelines: the experience of Nigerian immigrants in Houston, Texas. J Immigrant Health 2001; 3:31–45.
12. Farquharson L, Noble LM, Barker C, et al. Health beliefs and communication in the travel clinic consultation as predictors of adherence to malaria chemoprophylaxis. Br J Health Psychol 2004; 9(Pt 2):201–217.
13. Campbell H. Imported malaria in the UK: advice given by general practitioners to British residents travelling to malaria endemic areas. J Roy Coll Gen Practitioners 1987; 37:70–72.
14. Dijkshoorn H, Schilthuis HJ, van den Hoek JA, et al. Travel advice on the prevention of infectious diseases insufficiently obtained by indigenous and non-native inhabitants of Amsterdam, the Netherlands. Nederlands Tijdschrift voor Geneeskunde 2003; 147(14):658–662.
15. Duval B, De Serre G, Shadmani R, et al. A population-based comparison between travelers who consulted travel clinics and those who did not. J Travel Med 2003; 10(1):4–10.
16. Hughes NJ, Carlisle R. How important a priority is travel medicine for a typical British family practice? J Travel Med 2000; 7(3):138–141.
17. Laver SM, Wetzels J, Behrens RH. Knowledge of malaria, risk perception, and compliance with prophylaxis and personal and environmental preventive measures in travelers exiting Zimbabwe from Harare and Victoria Falls International airport. J Travel Med 2001; 8(6):298–303.
18. Badrinath P, Ejidokun OO, Barnes N. Change in NHS regulations may have caused increase in malaria. Br Med J 1998; 316(7146):1746–1747.
19. Stauffer WM, Kamat D, Walker PF. Screening of international immigrants, refugees, and adoptees. Prim Care Clinics in Office Practice 2002; 29(4):879–905.
20. Strine TW, Barker LE, Mokdad AH, et al. Vaccination coverage of foreign-born children 19 to 35 months of age: findings from the National Immunization Survey, 1999–2000. Pediatrics 2002; 110(2 Pt 1):e15.
21. Keystone JS, Dismukes R, Sawyer L, et al. Inadequacies in health recommendations provided for international travelers by North American travel health advisors. J Travel Med 1994; 1(2):72–78.
22. Health Information for International Travel 2005–2006. US Department of Health Human Services CDC, NCID, Atlanta, Georgia.
23. Horvath LL, Murray CK, Dooley DP. Utility of services provided by a free travel medicine clinic. Abstract #521. Philadelphia: American Society of Tropical Medicine and Hygiene; 2003.
24. Cobelens FG, van Deutekom H, Draayer-Jansen JW, et al. Risk of infection with *Mycobacterium tuberculosis* in travelers to areas of high tuberculosis endemicity. Lancet 2000; 356(9228):461–465.
25. Robbins JB, Schneerson R, Gotschlich EC, et al. Meningococcal meningitis in sub-Saharan Africa: the case for mass and routine vaccination with available polysaccharide vaccines. Bull World Health Org 2003; 81(10):745–749.
26. Valerio L, Guerrero L, Martinez O. Travelling immigrants. Aten Primaria 2003; 32(6):330–336.
27. Bouchaud O, Cot M, Kony S, et al. Do African immigrants living in France have long-term malarial immunity? Am J Trop Med Hyg 2005; 72(1):21–25.
28. Hargarten SW, Baker TD, Guptill K. Overseas fatalities of United States citizen travelers: an analysis of deaths related to international travel. Ann Emerg Med 1991; 20(6):622–626.
29. McIness RJ, Williamson LM, Morrison A. Unintentional injury during foreign travel. J Travel Med 2002; 9(6):297–306.
30. Odero W, Garner P, Zwi A. Road traffic accidents in developing countries: a comprehensive review of epidemiological studies. Trop Med Int Health. 1997; 2(5):445–460.
31. Steffen R, Lobel HO. Epidemiologic basis for the practice of travel medicine. J Wilderness Med 1994; 5:556–566.
32. Andrews CN, Kobusingye OC, Lett R. Road traffic accident injuries in Kampala. East Afr Med J 1999; 76(4):189–194.
33. Kolars JC. Rules of the road: a consumer's guide for travelers seeking healthcare abroad. J Travel Med 2002; 9(4):198–202.
34. McFarlane S, Racelis M, Muli-Muslime F. Public health in developing countries. Lancet 2000; 356:841–846.

35. Razzak JA, Kellermann AL. Emergency medical care in developing countries: is it worthwhile? Bull World Health Org 2002; 80(11):900–905.

36. Walker PF, Jaranson J. Refugee and immigrant healthcare. Med Clin NA 1999; 83(4):1103–1119.

37. Eiseman DP, Gelberg L, Lui H, et al. Mental health and health related quality of life among adult Latino primary care patients living in the United States with previous exposure to violence. JAMA 2003; 290(5):627–634.

38. Christenson JC, Fischer PR, Hale DC, et al. Pediatric travel consultation in an integrated clinic. J Travel Med 2001; 8(1):1–5.

39. McFarlane S, Racelis M, Muli-Muslime F. Public health in developing countries. Lancet. 2000; 356:841–846.

40. Steffen R, deBernardis C, Banos A. Travel epidemiology – a global perspective. Int J Antimicrob Agents 2003; 21(2):89–95.

41. Steffen R. Epidemiology of traveler's diarrhea. Clin Infect Dis 2005; 41(Suppl 8):S536–S540.

42. Ericsson CD, DuPont HL, Mathewson III JJ. Epidemiologic observations on diarrhea developing in US and Mexican students living in Guadalajara, Mexico. J Travel Med 1995; 2(1):6–10.

43. Shlim DR. Looking for evidence that personal hygiene precautions prevent traveler's diarrhea. Clin Infect Dis 2005; 41(Suppl 8):S531–S535.

44. Hillel O, Potasman I. Correlation between adherence to precautions issued by the WHO and diarrhea among long-term travelers to India. J Travel Med 2005; 12(5):243–247.

45. Hammond B, Ali Y, Fendler E, et al. Effect of hand sanitizer use on elementary school absenteeism. Am J Infect Control 2000; 28(5):340–346.

46. White CG, Shinder FS, Shinder AL, et al. Reduction of illness absenteeism in elementary schools using an alcohol-free hand sanitizer. J School Nursing 2001; 17(5):258–265.

47. Mensah P, Yeboah-Manu D, Owusu-Darko K, et al. Street foods in Accra, Ghana: how safe are they? Bull World Health Org 2002; 80(7):546–553.

48. Adachi JA, Ericsson CD, Jiang ZD, et al. Azithromycin found to be comparable to levofloxacin for the treatment of US travelers with acute diarrhea acquired in Mexico. Clin Infect Dis 2003; 37:1165–1171.

49. Bennish ML, Salam MA, Khan WA, et al. Treatment of shigellosis: III. Comparison of one- or two-dose ciprofloxacin with standard 5-day therapy. A randomized, blinded trial. Ann Intern Med 1992; 117(9):727–734.

50. Bhattacharya SK, Bhattacharya MK, Dutta D, et al. Single-dose ciprofloxacin for shigellosis in adults. J Infect 1992; 25(1):117–119.

51. Bodhidatta L, Vithayasai N, Eimpokalarp B, et al. Bacterial enteric pathogens in children with acute dysentery in Thailand: increasing importance of quinolone-resistant *Campylobacter*. Southeast Asian J Trop Med Public Health 2002; 33(4):752–757.

52. Sanders JW, Isenbarger DW, Walz SE, et al. An observational clinic-based study of diarrheal illness in deployed United States military personnel in Thailand: presentation and outcome of *Campylobacter* infection. Am J Trop Med Hyg 2002; 67(5):533–538.

53. Sabharwal V, Marchant CD. Fluoroquinolone use in children. Pediatr Infect Dis J 2006; 25(3):257–258.

54. Leibovitz E. The use of fluoroquinolones in children. Curr Opin Pediatr 2006; 18(1):64–70.

55. Young EJ. Brucella species (Brucellosis). In: Long S, Pickering LK, Prober CG, eds. Principles and practice of pediatric infectious diseases. 2nd edn. New York: Elsevier; 2003:877–878.

56. MacDonald PD, Whitwam RE, Boggs JD, et al. Outbreak of listeriosis among Mexican immigrants as a result of consumption of illicitly produced Mexican-style cheese. Clin Infect Dis 2005; 40(5):677–682.

57. Ansdell V. Food-borne illnesses. In: Keystone JS, Kozasky PE, Freedman DO, et al., eds. Travel medicine. London: Elsevier; 2004:443–446.

58. Morris JG. Cholera and other types of vibriosis: a story of human pandemics and oysters on the half shell. Clin Infect Dis 2003; 37:272–280.

59. Koopmans M, Duizer E. Foodborne viruses: an emerging problem. Int J Food Manage 2004; 90(1):23–41.

60. Eastaugh J, Shepherd S. Infectious and toxic syndromes from fish and shellfish consumption. A review. Arch Intern Med 1989; 149(8):1735–1740.

61. Pottier I, Vernoux JP, Lewis RJ. Ciguatera fish poisoning in the Caribbean islands and Western Atlantic. Rev Environ Contam Toxicol 2001; 168:99–141.

62. de Haro L, Pommier P, Valli M. Emergence of imported ciguatera in Europe: report of 18 cases at the Poison Control Centre of Marseille. J Toxicol Clin Toxicol 2003; 41(7):927–930.

63. Centers for Disease Control and Prevention. Malaria surveillance – United States, 2003. 2005; 54:25–39.

64. Leder K, Black J, O'Brien D, et al. Malaria in travelers: a review of the GeoSentinel surveillance network. Clin Infect Dis 2004; 39(8):1104–1112.

65. Phillips-Howard PA, Radalowicz A, Mitchell J, et al. Risk of malaria in British residents returning from malarious areas. Br Med J 1990; 300(6723):499–503.

66. Ladhani S, El Bashir H, Patel VS, et al. Childhood malaria in East London. Pediatr Infect Dis J 2003; 22(9):814–819.

67. Castelli F, Matteelli A, Caligaris S. et al. Malaria in migrants. Parasitologia 1999; 41(1–3):261–265.

68. Schlagenhauf P, Steffen R, Loutan L. Migrants as a major risk group for imported malaria. J Travel Med 2003; 10:106–107.

69. Jelinek T, Schulte C, Behrens R, et al. Imported *falciparum* malaria in Europe: sentinel surveillance data from the European network on surveillance of imported infectious diseases. Clin Infect Dis 2002; 34(5):572–576.

70. White NJ. Malaria. In: Cook GC, Zumla A, eds. Manson's tropical diseases. 21st edn. Philadelphia: WB Saunders; 2003:1205–1296.

71. Newman RD, Parise ME, Barber AM, et al. Malaria-related deaths among US travelers, 1963–2001. Ann Intern Med 2004; 141(7):547–555.

72. Singh N, Nagpal AC, Saxena A, et al. Changing scenario of malaria in central India, the replacement of *Plasmodium vivax* by *Plasmodium falciparum* (1986–2000). Trop Med Int Health 2004; 9(3):364–371.

73. Schlagenhauf P, Tschopp A, Johnson R, et al. Tolerability of malaria chemoprophylaxis in non-immune travellers to sub-Saharan Africa: multicentre, randomised, double blind, four arm study. Br Med J 2003; 327:1078–1083.

74. Overbosch D, Schilthuis H, Bienzle U, et al. Atovaquone-proguanil versus mefloquine for malaria prophylaxis in nonimmune travelers: results from a randomized, double-blind study. Clin Infect Dis 2001; 33(7):1015–1021.

75. Petersen E, Ronne T, Ronn A, et al. Reported side effects to chloroquine, chloroquine plus proguanil, and mefloquine as chemoprophylaxis against malaria in Danish travelers. J Travel Med 2000; 7(2):79–84.

76. Baird JK, Fryauff DJ, Hoffman SL. Primaquine for prevention of malaria in travelers. Clin Infect Dis 2003; 37(12):1659–1667.

77. Schlagenhauf P, Steffen R. Stand-by treatment of malaria in travellers: a review. J Trop Med Hyg 1994; 97(3):151–160.

78. Schlagenhauf P, Steffen R, Tschopp A, et al. Behavioural aspects of travellers in their use of malaria presumptive treatment. Bull World Health Organ. 1995; 73(2):215–221.

79. Jelinek T, Amsler L, Grobusch MP, et al. Self-use of rapid tests for malaria diagnosis by tourists. Lancet 1999; 354:1609.

80. Keystone JS. The sound of hoof beats does not always mean that it is a zebra. Clin Infect Dis 2004; 39(11):1589–1590.

81. Causer LM, Filler S, Wilson M, et al. Evaluation of reported malaria chemoprophylactic failure among travelers in a US university exchange program, 2002. Clin Infect Dis 2004; 39(11):1583–1588.

82. Reyburn H, Mbatia R, Drakeley C, et al. Overdiagnosis of malaria in patients with severe febrile illness in Tanzania: a prospective study. Br Med J 2004; 329(7476):1212.

83. Aldhous P. Counterfeit pharmaceuticals: murder by medicine. Nature 2005; 434(7030):132–136.

84. Dondorp AM, Newton PN, Mayxay M, et al. Fake antimalarials in Southeast Asia are a major impediment to malaria control: multinational cross-sectional survey on the prevalence of fake antimalarials. Trop Med Int Health 2004; 9(12):1241–1246.

85. Simon JL, Larson BA, Zusman A, et al. How will the reduction of tariffs and taxes on insecticide-treated bednets affect household purchase? Bull World Health Org 2002; 80(11):892–899.

86. Alejandria M. Dengue fever. Clin Evid 2004; (12):1062–1071.

87. Ligon BL. Dengue fever and dengue hemorrhagic fever: a review of the history, transmission, treatment, and prevention. Semin Pediatr Infect Dis 2005; 16(1):60–65.

88. Stephenson JR. Understanding dengue pathogenesis: implications for vaccine design. Bull World Health Org 2005; 83(4):308–314.

89. Halstead SB. Neutralization and antibody-dependent enhancement of dengue viruses. Adv Virus Res 2003; 60:421–467

90. Jelinek T, Muhlberger N, Harms G, et al. for European Network on Imported Infectious Disease Surveillance. Epidemiology and clinical features of imported dengue fever in Europe: sentinel surveillance data from TropNetEurop. Clin Infect Dis 2002; 35(9):1047–1052.

91. Stephenson I, Roper J, Fraser M, et al. Dengue fever in febrile returned travelers to UK regional infectious diseases unit. Trav Med Infect Dis 2003; 1:89–93.

92. Wichmann O, Jelinek T. Dengue in travelers: a review. J Travel Med 2004; 11(3):161–170.

93. Maher D, Raviglione M. Global epidemiology of tuberculosis. Clin Chest Med 2005; 26(2):167–182.

94. Long R, Njoo H, Hershfield E. Tuberculosis: 3. Epidemiology of the disease in Canada. Can Med Assoc J 1999; 160(8):1185–1190.

95. Centers for Disease Control and Prevention. Division of Tuberculosis Elimination Surveillance report 2002. Available: http://www.cdc.gov/nchstp/tb/surv/surv.htm Accessed 2/7/07.

96. McCarthy OR. Asian immigrant tuberculosis – the effect of visiting Asia. British J Dis Chest 1984; 78:248–253.

97. Ormerod LP, Green RM, Gray S. Are there still effects on Indian subcontinent ethnic tuberculosis of return visits?: a longitudinal study 1978–97. J Infect 2001; 43(2):132–134.

98. Singh H, Joshi M, Ormerod LP. A case control study in the Indian subcontinent ethnic population on the effect of return visits and the subsequent development of tuberculosis. J Infect 2005.

99. Leder K, Tong S, Weld L, et al. Illness in travelers visiting friends & relatives. A review of the GeoSentinel Surveillance Network. Clin Infect Dis 2006; 43:1185–1193.

100. Thompson MM, Hajera R. Travel and the introduction of human immunodeficiency virus type I non-B subtype genetic forms into Western countries. Clin Infect Dis 2001; 32:1732–1737.

101. Correia JD, Shafer RT, Patel V, et al. Blood and body fluid exposure as a health risk for international travelers. J Travel Med 2001; 8(5):263–268.

102. Hutin YJF, Hauri AM, Armstrong JL. Use of injections in healthcare settings worldwide, 2000: literature review and regional estimates. Br Med J 2003; 327:1075–1078.

103. Keystone JS. Travel-related hepatitis B: risk factors and prevention using an accelerated vaccination schedule. Am J Med 2005; 118(Suppl 10A):63S–68S.

104. High condom quality essential to reduce HIV spread. Network 1988; 10(2):6–7.

105. Franks AL, Berg CJ, Kane MA, et al. Hepatitis B virus infection among children born in the United States to Southeast Asian refugees. N Engl J Med 1989; 321(19):1301–1305.

106. Newton PN, White NJ, Rozendaal JA, et al. Murder by fake drugs: Time for international action. Br Med J 2002; 324(7341):800–801.

107. Shakoor O, Taylor RB, Behrens RH. Assessment of the use of substandard drugs in developing countries. Trop Med Int Health 1997; 2(9):839–845.

108. Newton P, Proux S, Green M, et al. Fake artesunate in Southeast Asia. Lancet 2001; 357:1948–1950.

109. Taylor RB, Shakoor O, Behrens RH, et al. Phamacopoeial quality of drugs supplied by Nigerian pharmacies. Lancet 2001; 357(9272):1933–1936.

110. Shakoor O, Taylor RB, Behrens RH. Assessment of the use of substandard drugs in developing countries. Trop Med Int Health 1997; 2(9):839–845.

111. Chen BH, Hong CJ, Pandey MR, et al. Indoor air pollution in developing countries. World Health Stat Q 1990; 43(3):127–138.

112. Albers LH, Johnson DE, Hostetter MK, et al. Health of children adopted from the former Soviet Union and Eastern Europe. Comparison with preadoptive medical records. JAMA 1997; 278(11):922–924.

113. Schulpen TW, van Seventer AH, Rumke HC, et al. Immunisation status of children adopted from China. Lancet 2001; 358(9299):2131–2132.

114. Miller LC. International adoption: infectious diseases issues. Clin Infect Dis 2005; 40(2):286–293.

115. Chen LH, Barnett ED, Wilson ME. Preventing infectious diseases during and after international adoption. Ann Intern Med 2003; 139(5 Pt 1):371–378.

116. Centers for Disease Control and Prevention. Racial/ethnic disparities in influenza and pneumococcal vaccination levels among persons aged ≥ 65 years – United States 1989–2001. MMWR 2003; 52:958–962.

117. Hamer D. Connor BA. Travel health knowledge, attitudes and practices among United States travelers. J Trav Med 2004; 11:23–28.

118. Van Herck K, Castelli F, Zuckerman J, et al. Knowledge, attitudes and practices in travel-related infectious diseases. Eur Airport Survey J Travel Med 2004; 11:3–11.

119. Mandal BK, Mukherjee PP, Murphy C, et al. Adult susceptibility to varicella in the tropics is a rural phenomenon due to the lack of previous exposure. J Infect Dis 1998; 178(Suppl 1):S52–S54.

120. Lee BW. Review of varicella zoster seroepidemiology in India and Southeast Asia. Trop Med Int Health 1998; 3(11):886–890.

121. Barnett ED, Christiansen D, Figueira M. Seroprevalence of measles, rubella, and varicella in refugees. Clin Infect Dis 2002; 35(4):403–408.

122. Meyer PA, Seward JF, Jumaan AO, et al. Varicella mortality: trends before vaccine licensure in the United States, 1970–1994. J Infect Dis 2000; 182:383–390.

123. Ryan ET, Kain KC. Health advice and immunizations for travelers. N Engl J Med 2000; 342(23):1716–1725.

124. Barnett ED, Holmes AH, Geltman P, et al. Immunity to hepatitis A in people born and raised in endemic areas. J Travel Med 2003; 10(1)11–15.

125. Behrens RH, Collins M, Botto B. Risk for British travelers of acquiring hepatitis A [letter]. Br Med J 1995; 311:193.

126. Sawayama Y, Hayashi J, Ariyama I, et al. A ten year serological survey of hepatitis A, B, and C viruses infections in Nepal. J Epidemiology 1999; 9(5):350–354.

127. Batra Y, Bhatkal B, Ojha B, et al. Vaccination against hepatitis A virus may not be required for school children in northern India: results of a seroepidemiological survey. Bull World Health Org 2002; 80(9):728–731.

128. Kosuwan P, Sutra S, Koralaraksa P, et al. Seroepidemiology of hepatitis A virus antibody in primary school children in Khon Kaen Province, northeastern Thailand. Southeast Asian J Trop Med Public Health 1996; 27(4):650–653.

129. Poovorwan Y, Theamboonlers A, Sinlaparatsamee S, et al. Increasing susceptibility to HAV among member of the younger generation in Thailand. Asian Pacific J Allergy Immunol 2000; 18(4):249–253.

130. Chatchatee P, Chongsrisawat V, Theamboonlers A, et al. Declining hepatitis A seroprevalence among medical students in Bangkok, Thailand, 1981–2001. Asian Pacific J Allergy Immunol 2002; 20(1):53–56.

131. Ruttimann RW, Clemens RL. Argentine and Latin American hepatitis A. J Travel Med 2002; 9(4):220–224.

132. Lee KK, Beyer-Blodget J. Screening travelers for Hepatitis A antibody. West J Med 2000; 173:325–329.

133. Jacobs RJ, Saab S, Meyerhoff AS, et al. An economic assessment of pre-vaccination screening for hepatitis A and B. Public Health Rep 2003; 118(6):550–558.

134. Custer B, Sullivan SD, Hazlet TK, et al. Global epidemiology of hepatitis B virus. J Clin Gastroenterol 2004; 38(10 Suppl): S158–S168.

135. Mahon BE, Mintz ED, Greene KD, et al. Reported cholera in the United States, 1992–1994: a reflection of global changes in cholera epidemiology. JAMA 1996; 276:307–312.

136. Statement on new oral cholera and travelers' vaccination. Committee to advise on tropical medicine and travel. Can Commun Dis Rep 2005; 31:1–11.

137. Steinberg EB, Bishop R, Haber P, et al. Typhoid fever in travelers: who should be targeted for prevention? Clin Infect Dis 2004; 39(2):186–191.

138. Keystone JS. VFR travelers. In: Health information for international travel 2005–2006. CDC; 2005.

139. Stubi CL, Landry PR, Petignat C, et al. Compliance to live oral Ty21a typhoid vaccine, and its effect on viability. J Travel Med 2000; 7(3):133–137.

140. WHO rabies fact sheet No 99. Available: http://www.who.int/mediacentre/factsheets/fs099/en/ Accessed 2/7/07.

141. Ministère de la santé, de la famille et des personnes handicapées, Direction Générale de la Santé. Un cas de rage dans le Rhône. Press release, October 23, 2003.

142. Meslin FX. Rabies as a traveler's risk, especially in high-endemicity areas. J Travel Med 2005; 12(Suppl 1): S30–S40.

143. Pollard AJ, Shlim DR. Epidemic meningococcal disease and travel. J Travel Med 2002; 9(1):29–33.

144. Wilder-Smith A. Meningococcal disease in international travel: vaccine strategies. J Travel Med 2005; 12(Suppl 1): S22–S29.

# Index